Rosenblum +
Film

Rosenblum +
Film

TEXTBOOK OF

Ophthalmology

Section Editors:

Edward G. Buckley

George A. Cioffi

Eugene de Juan, Jr.

Bradley N. Lemke

Thomas J. Liesegang

Narsing A. Rao

Donald N. Schwartz

David T. Tse

E. Michael Van Buskirk

Kenneth W. Wright

Consultants:

Kenneth C. Chern

Marshall Wareham

Geoffrey Brent

Dean Fiergang

Malcolm R. Ing

Illustrator:

Timothy C. Hengst, CMI, FAMI

TEXTBOOK OF

Ophthalmology

Kenneth W. Wright, MD
Head, Pediatric Ophthalmology and
Strabismus Department
Division of Ophthalmology
The Cleveland Clinic Foundation
Cleveland, Ohio

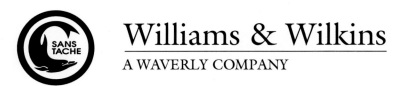

Williams & Wilkins

A WAVERLY COMPANY

BALTIMORE • PHILADELPHIA • LONDON • PARIS • BANGKOK
BUENOS AIRES • HONG KONG • MUNICH • SYDNEY • TOKYO • WROCLAW
1997

Editor: Darlene Barela Cooke
Managing Editor: Frances M. Klass
Production Coordinator: Danielle Santucci
Book Project Editor: Robert D. Magee
Designer: Suan Blaker
Cover Designer: Tom Scheuerman
Typesetter: Maryland Composition, Inc.
Printer: RR Donnelley
Binder: RR Donnelley

Copyright © 1997 Williams & Wilkins

351 West Camden Street
Baltimore, Maryland 21201-2436 USA

Rose Tree Corporate Center
1400 North Providence Road
Building II, Suite 5025
Media, Pennsylvania 19063-2043 USA

Accurate indications, adverse reactions, and dosage schedules for drugs are provided in this book, but it is possible that they may change. The reader is urged to review the package information data of the manufacturers of the medications mentioned.

Printed in the United States of America

First Edition,

Library of Congress Cataloging-in-Publication Data

Textbook of ophthalmology / [edited by] Kenneth W. Wright.
      p.   cm.
    Includes bibliographical references and index.
    ISBN (invalid) 0-06-839292-8
    1. Ophthalmology.   I. Wright, Kenneth W. (Kenneth Weston), 1950–.
    [DNLM: 1. Eye Diseases.   WW 140 t355 1997]
    RE46.T27   1997
    617.7—dc20
    DNLM/DLC
    for Library of Congress   96–24216
                                      CIP

The publishers have made every effort to trace the copyright holders for borrowed material. If they have inadvertently overlooked any, they will be pleased to make the necessary arrangements at the first opportunity

To purchase additional copies of this book, call our customer service department at **(800) 638–0672** or fax orders to **(800) 447–8438**. For other book services, including chapter reprints and large quantity sales, ask for the Special Sales department.

Canadian customers should call **(800) 268–4178**, or fax **(905) 470–6780**. For all other calls originating outside of the United States, please call **(410) 528–4223** or fax us at **(410) 528–8550**.

Visit Williiams & Wilkins on the Internet: **http://www.wwilkins.com** or contact our customer service department at **custserv@wwilkins.com**. Williams & Wilkins customer service representatives are available from 8:30 am to 6:00 pm, EST, Monday through Friday, for telephone access.

          97 98 99
    1 2 3 4 5 6 7 8 9 10

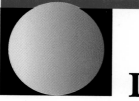

Dedication

To my beautiful wife, Donna, whose love, honesty, and friendship I deeply cherish.
And,
To my wonderful children, Jamie, Matthew, Lisa, Michael and Andrew, for their unselfish support.

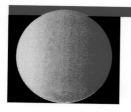

Preface

Ophthalmology is a fascinating and dynamic specialty. Mastering this field requires an understanding of a broad range of diverse topics. Knowledge of embryology, gross anatomy, microbiology, and even the physics of optics are required building blocks for understanding ocular disease. The *Textbook of Ophthalmology* is designed to provide a concise, yet detailed and comprehensive single-volume textbook to teach ophthalmology. The book begins with the basics: chapters on Anatomy, Embryology, and Optics and Refraction. Important clinical correlations are provided, so these sometimes "dry" subjects become more interesting and clinically relevant. Next, the book is divided into the subspecialties of ophthalmology: Neuro-ophthalmology, Strabismus-Pediatric Ophthalmology, Oculoplastics, Ocular Inflammation-Uveitis, Glaucoma, Anterior Segment-External Disease, Retina-Vitreous, and Ocular Trauma. A major goal throughout the book is to present the material clearly. Complex issues are broken down into smaller, digestible steps. Special emphasis is placed on an understanding of the pathogenesis of the disease. Glaucoma is presented as an optic neuropathy, not just as a disease of increased ocular pressure. Emphasis on a mechanistic approach to disease is present throughout the text.

Another unique aspect of this book is that in addition to the standard index, there is a section of clinical problem-oriented tables. The clinical charts are indexed according to clinical presenting sign or symptom. For each presenting sign or symptom listed, the chart provides a differential diagnosis, key differentiating features, and treatment. The reader can use the problem-oriented chart to identify the differential diagnosis and treat the patient without turning the page. In addition, the chart references page numbers in the text for further reading.

A variety of readers will find this single-volume text useful. Ophthalmology residents can use it as their core textbook, for it is manageable in length, yet detailed and comprehensive enough to thoroughly cover each subject. Practicing ophthalmologists will also find this text an invaluable resource, providing a quick update on a specific clinical topic or as a general review of the latest developments in ophthalmology. The book was specifically designed as a single volume so it can be easily transported and used in the clinic or private office setting. As virtually all important topics in ophthalmology are covered, this book provides a great review for Boards or recertification.

As editor, I would like to personally thank the outstanding contributions from the section editors and chapter authors. A good teacher must both have a profound and fundamental understanding of the material, a passion for work, and an ability to simplify and explain. We are extremely fortunate to have such teachers as authors for our book. Special thanks to Dr. Kenneth Chern, chief resident at the Cleveland Clinic Foundation, and Dr. Marshall C. Wareham, clinical ophthalmologist, Dayton, Ohio, whose insight and critical detailed reviews enhanced each chapter. Thanks also to Dr. Dean Fiergang, pediatric ophthalmology fellow, Dr. Geoffrey Brent, ophthalmology resident Cleveland Clinic Foundation, and my administrative assistant, Kelly McNeil from the Cleveland Clinic Foundation for their help. It is my sincere hope that the reader will find this textbook complete, informative, clear, and enjoyable.

Kenneth W. Wright, MD

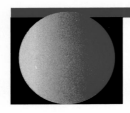

Contributors

Steven Awner, MD
Clinical Assistant Professor
Departments of Ophthalmology and Pediatrics
University of Buffalo
Children's Hospital of Buffalo
Buffalo, New York

Edward G. Buckley, MD
Professor of Ophthalmology
Associate Professor of Pediatrics
Pediatric Ophthalmology and Strabismus, Neuro-
    Ophthalmology
Duke University Eye Center
Durham, North Carolina

Delyse R. Buus, MD
Eye Care Center
Kaiser Permanente
Oakland, California

Kenneth C. Chern, MD
Chief Resident, Division of Ophthalmology
The Cleveland Clinic Foundation
Cleveland, Ohio

George A. Cioffi, MD
Director, Ocular Microcirculation Unit
Devers Eye Institute
Legacy Portland Hospital
Associate Scientist
R. S. Dow Neurological Sciences Institute
Portland, Oregon

Eugene de Juan, Jr., MD
Professor of Ophthalmology
Johns Hopkins University School of Medicine
Co-Director, Vitreoretinal Service
Wilmer Eye Institute/Johns Hopkins Hospital
Baltimore, Maryland

Thomas A. Deutsch, MD
Professor of Ophthalmology
Rush Medical College
Program Director, Department of Ophthalmology
Rush-Presbyterian-St. Luke's Medical Center
Chicago, Illinois

John M. DeVaro, MD
Associate in Pediatric and Neuro-Ophthalmology
Nevyas Eye Associates
Philadelphia, Pennsylvania

Steve Gilberg, MD
Ocular Plastic Surgeon
Ottawa General Hospital Eye Institute
Ottawa, Canada

Saunders L. Hupp, MD
Professor of Ophthalmology and Neurology
Department of Ophthalmology
University of South Alabama
Mobile, Alabama

Thomas E. Johnson, MD
Assistant Professor of Ophthalmology
Bascom Palmer Eye Institute
University of Miami
Miami, Florida

Marilyn C. Kincaid, MD
Clinical Professor of Ophthalmology & Pathology
St. Louis University School of Medicine
Department of Ophthalmology
St. Louis, Missouri

Bradley N. Lemke, MD
Clinical Professor
Department of Ophthalmology and Visual Sciences
University of Wisconsin - Madison
Davis Duehr Dean Clinic
Madison, Wisconsin

Thomas J. Liesegang, MD
Professor and Chairman
Department of Ophthalmology
Mayo Clinic, Jacksonville
Jacksonville, Florida

Timothy J. Martin, MD
Assistant Professor of Surgery/Ophthalmology
Neuro-Ophthalmology
Department of Ophthalmology
Wake Forest University Eye Center
Winston-Salem, North Carolina

Melissa L. Meldrum, MD
Fellow, Ophthalmic Plastic and Reconstructive Surgery
Bascom Palmer Eye Institute
University of Miami
Miami, Florida

Ramana S. Moorthy, MD
Midwest Eye Institute
Indianapolis, Indiana

Stuart Noorily, MD
Retina Associates of New Jersey
Teaneck, New Jersey

Than-Lan T. Quan, MD
Clinical Instructor
University of California at Irvine
Irvine, California

Jyoti Raina, MD
Fellow, Pediatric Ophthalmology and Strabismus
The Cleveland Clinic Foundation
Cleveland, Ohio

Narsing Rao, MD
Professor of Ophthalmology and Pathology
University of Southern California School of Medicine
Director of Ophthalmic Pathology Labs, Doheny Eye
  Institute
Los Angeles, California

Donald N. Schwartz, MD, OD, M.OPT
Associate Clinical Professor
University of California at Irvine
Irvine, California
Clinical Instructor, Doheny Eye Institute
University of Southern California
Los Angeles, California
Chairman, Department of Ophthalmology
Memorial Medical Center
Long Beach, California

Angela Scott, MD
Assistant Professor of Ophthalmology
Duke University Eye Center
Durham, North Carolina

Kevin R. Scott, MD
Assistant Clinical Professor of Ophthalmology
Georgetown University Medical Center, Center for
  Sight
Washington, DC
Attending Surgeon, Fairfax Hospital
Fairfax, Virginia

Bryan S. Sires, MD, Ph. D
Clinical Instructor
University of Washington
Deputy Chief of Ophthalmology
Harborview Hospital
Seattle, Washington

William Townsend-Pico, MD
Vitreoretinal Fellow, Kresge Eye Institute
Department of Ophthalmology
Detroit, Michigan

David T. Tse, MD
Professor of Ophthalmology
Bascom Palmer Eye Institute
Miami, Florida

E. Michael Van Buskirk, MD
Chief, Department of Ophthalmology
Legacy Portland Hospitals
Director, Devers Eye Institute
Clinical Professor of Ophthalmology
Oregon Health Sciences University
Portland, Oregon

Kenneth W. Wright, MD
Head, Pediatric Ophthalmology and Strabismus
  Department
Division of Ophthalmology
The Cleveland Clinic Foundation
Cleveland, Ohio

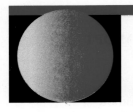

Contents

XI
OCULAR TRAUMA

PROBLEM ORIENTED CLINICAL TABLE

ANTERIOR SEGMENT AND EXTERNAL DISEASES

Differential Diagnosis	Historical Features	Key Findings	Treatment	Chapter Number
FILAMENTARY KERATITIS				
Keratoconjunctivitis sicca (common)	Associated with xerostomia and arthritis (Sjögren's syndrome)	Decreased tear production (Schirmer's test), interpalpebral staining with fluorescein or rose bengal	Punctal occlusion, artificial lubricants	49
Prolonged occlusion	Patching or ptosis	Filaments scattered in areas of occlusion	Removal of patch, topical lubricants	51
Superior limbic keratoconjunctivitis	May have associated thyroid dysfunction	Injection and thickening of superior bulbar conjunctiva, filaments on superior limbus and cornea	Dilute silver nitrate solution, mechanical scraping of the bulbar conjunctiva, surgical resection of affected conjunctiva	50, 51
Neurotrophic keratopathy	CN VII palsy or post-herpes zoster infection	Trophic ulcers in interpalpebral fissure	Bandage contact lens, lateral tarsorraphy	51
Herpes simplex keratitis	Skin lesions (vesicles)	Precede formation of dendritic lesions, decreased corneal sensation	Antiviral therapy	51
Recurrent erosions or rupture of bullae		Located in areas of erosions	Hypertonic saline	51

BULLOUS KERATOPATHY

Differential Diagnosis	Historical Features	Key Findings	Treatment	Chapter Number
Fuchs' endothelial dystrophy	Elderly patients, progressive decrease in vision	Bilateral central endothelial guttae (may be asymmetric), polymegathism	Hypertonic saline, corneal transplantation	51
Epithelial downgrowth	Intraocular surgery	Retrocorneal membrane, edema in areas of membrane, membrane on iris and angle, glaucoma	Very difficult to eradicate membrane, often requiring extensive surgery	45, 52
Chronic uveitis	Uveitis	Intraocular inflammation	Transplantation	31
Vitreous touch	Intraocular surgery with vitreous in anterior chamber	Vitreous to wound or touching cornea	Anterior vitrectomy, lysis of vitreal bands	52
Congenital corneal dystrophy	Present at birth or progressive	Lack of endothelial cells	Penetrating keratoplasty	51
Silicone oil in anterior chamber	Vitrectomy with injection of silicone oil	Silicone oil in anterior chamber	Vitrectomy with removal of silicone oil	63

Differential Diagnosis	Historical Features	Key Findings	Treatment	Chapter Number
FOLLICULAR CONJUNCTIVITIS				
Adenovirus (EKC, PCF)	Acute onset, may follow cold or flu-like illness	Pre-auricular node, watery discharge, bilateral	Highly contagious, resolves spontaneously in 2–3 weeks	50
Toxic follicular conjunctivitis	Use of antiviral, miotic, adrenergics, or atropine drops	Stenotic punctum, scarring of conjunctiva	Discontinuation of drops	50
Herpes simplex	May be accompanied by skin lesions	Multinucleated giant cells on scrapings	Supportive, or antivirals	50
Chlamydia/Trachoma	May be acute or chronic	Follicles on upper and lower tarsal conjunctiva and limbus	Oral tetracycline or erythromycin	50
Newcastle's disease (uncommon)	Exposure to poultry	chemosis, follicles	Supportive	50
Acute hemorrhagic conjunctivitis (uncommon)	Explosive onset	Subconjunctival hemorrhages	Highly contagious, symptomatic treatment	50
CORNEAL DENDRITE				
Herpes simplex virus	Skin lesions	Branching ulcerated epithelial dendrite, terminal bulbs	Antivirals	51
Herpes zoster virus	Dermatomal distribution of skin lesions	Coarse, less branching epithelial plaques	Antivirals	51
Corneal erosions	Corneal trauma, recurrent erosions	Irregular and loose epithelium	Patching, lubricants	51
Acanthamoeba keratitis	Soft contact lens use, use of contaminated or tap water	Disproportionate amount of pain, epithelial cysts and lines early	Epithelial debridement, multidrug medical therapy	51

Differential Diagnosis	Historical Features	Key Findings	Treatment	Chapter Number
RED TEARY EYE, IN THE NEWBORN (Neonatal Conjunctivitis)				
BACTERIAL				
Gonococcal	Onset 3–5 days of age, purulent discharge	Culture and Gram stain	I.M. ceftriaxone or I.V. penicillin	50
Chlamydia	Onset 5 days to 2 weeks of age, clear discharge	Giemsa stain for intracytoplasmic inclusion bodies. Direct immunofluorescent antibody stain	P.O. erythromycin + topical erythromycin Treat parents even if asymptomatic	50
E. Coli Staphylococcal		Gram stain culture	Antibiotics	50
VIRAL				
Herpes Simplex type II	Onset 6 to 14 days of age, clear discharge, usually unilateral	Superficial keratitis with dendritic or geographic epithelial defect. Viral cultures	Systemic acyclovir Topical Viroptic®	50
CHEMICAL				
Silver nitrate prophylaxis	Onset birth to 2 days. Clear tears.	Punctate corneal staining	None	50
CONGENITAL GLAUCOMA	Onset, birth to several months of age. Clear tears and photophobia	Enlarged cornea, > 12.5 mm. Cloudy cornea. IOP > 22 mm Hg C/D ratio > .4	Stabilize with topical beta blockers (Betopic®) and carbonic anhydrase inhibitors, then surgery.	45
DACRYOCYSTITIS (AMNIOTOCELE)	Onset, birth as a bluish nasal bulge. May become infected turning red and inflamed by 3 to 6 days.	Nasal bulge in the area of the nasolacrimal sac, with warmth and erythema.	Trial of massage, but if infected, or if the bulge persists, then: I.V. antibiotics and immediate NLD probing.	24

GLAUCOMA

Differential Diagnosis	Historical Features	Key Findings	Treatment	Chapter Number
MONOCULAR GLAUCOMA				
ICE syndrome	Blurred vision, female > male, 20–40 years old	Corneal edema, iris atrophy, corectopia, PAS	Medical therapy, often need filtration surgery	45, 51
PXF syndrome	Scandinavian ancestry	Pseudoexfoliation material on anterior lens capsule (usually bilateral but asymmetric), Sampaolesis' line, peripupillary iris atrophy	Conventional POAG therapy, ALT works well, cataract extraction may be complicated by vitreous loss	45
Neovascular glaucoma	Diabetes mellitus, trauma or intraocular inflammation	Rubeosis irides, retinal vascular disease (especially CRVO and PDR)	Suppress inflammation, PRP, frequently require filtration with antimetabolites or Seton	45, 60
Uveitic glaucoma	Recurrent uveitis	PAS, intraocular inflammation,	Suppress inflammation, medical therapy, ALT not recommended	45, 31
Traumatic glaucoma	Blunt ocular trauma	Chamber angle deformities or recession	Medical therapy, ALT not recommended	45, 64
Fuchs' heterochromic iridocyclitis	Blurred vision, 20–30 years old	Heterochromia, mild uveitis, No PAS, stellate keratic precipitates, early cataracts	Early cataract extraction, steroid-resistant uveitis	32, 45
Glaucomato-cyclitic crisis (Posner-Schlossman syndrome)	20–50 years old, intermittent ocular pain and blurred vision, halos	Mild uveitis (very few cells in anterior chamber)	Acute self-limited attacks, short-term medical therapy	45
Elevated episcleral venous pressure (Sturge-Weber syndrome)	Trauma, audible bruit, family history (seizures)	Marked dilated episcleral veins, orbital bruit, blood in Schlemm's canal (port wine stain involving lid)	Medical therapy rarely effective, filtration surgery with prophylactic sclerotomies	45, 23
Steroid-induced glaucoma	Steroid use (especially topical)	May precede primary open angle glaucoma	Discontinue steroids and medical therapy	45
Angle closure glaucoma	Episodes of pain, blurring, halos	Shallow anterior chamber, closed angle, iris bombé	Laser iridotomy	45
Intraocular tumor and glaucoma (mainly choroidal melanoma)	Previous diagnosis of cancer	Posterior segment ultrasonography	Radiation vs. enucleation	45, 62

ICE—Iridocorneal Endothealial Syndrome, PXF—Pseudoexfoliative Glaucoma, PDR—Proliferative Diabetic Retinopathy, POAG—Primary Open Angle Glaucoma, PRP—Panretinal Photocoagulation, ALT—Argon Laser Trabeculoplasty, CRVO—Central Retinal Vein Occlusion

Differential Diagnosis	Historical Features	Key Findings	Treatment	Chapter Number
OCULAR HYPOTONY				
Postoperative over-filtration	Previous filtration surgery (especially antimetabolites)	Diffuse or thin-walled filtration bleb	Spontaneous resolution common, shell or pressure tamponade, surgical revision	46, 47
Inadvertent filtration Bleb	Recent cataract extraction	Conjunctival filtration bleb with microcystic changes	Spontaneous resolution common	46, 47
Cyclodialysis cleft	Ocular trauma or surgery	Gonioscopy: cyclodialysis cleft	Cycloplegia, laser closure, surgical closure	45, 46, 64
Uveitis	Pain, photophobia, blurred vision	Significant intraocular inflammation	Suppress inflammation	31, 46
Ciliary body detachment (serous or hemorrhagic choroidals)	Pain, blurred vision	Fundoscopic visualization or ultrasonography	Spontaneous resolution common, surgical drainage	46
Myotonic dystrophy	Normal vision, systemic stigmata of M.D.	Polychromatic cataracts	No treatment	46
Retinal detachment	Photopsia, metamorphopsia blurred vision	Fundoscopic visualization or ultrasonography	Surgical repair	46, 61
Wound/bleb leak	Previous ocular surgery, "watery" eye	Positive Seidel test	Topical antibiotics and aqueous suppressants (possible surgical closure)	46
COMMON SECONDARY OPEN ANGLE GLAUCOMAS				
Pseudoexfoliation glaucoma	Scandinavian ancestry	Pseudoexfoliation material on anterior lens capsule (usually bilateral but asymmetric), Sampaolesi's line, peripupillary iris atrophy	Conventional POAG therapy, ALT works well, cataract extraction may be complicated by vitreous loss	45
Pigmentary dispersion glaucoma	20–40 years old, males > females, myopia, blurred vision with exercise	Pigment granules throughout anterior segment, Krukenberg's spindle, very deep anterior chamber, concave iris	Conventional POAG therapy, ALT works well	45

Differential Diagnosis	Historical Features	Key Findings	Treatment	Chapter Number
Inflammatory glaucoma	Pain, photophobia, tearing and blurred vision	Anterior segment inflammation, synechiae, inflammatory cell precipitates	Intensive cortico-steroid therapy and medical antihypertensives	45
Steroid-induced glaucoma	Steroid use (esp. topical)	—	Discontinue steroids and medical therapy	45
Glaucoma associated with intraocular hemorrhage	Ocular trauma or diabetes mellitus	Hyphema, RBCs or ghost cells in anterior chamber	Consider aminocarproic acid, sickle prep, anterior chamber washout for large nonclearing hyphemas	45, 60, 61
Elevated episcleral venous pressure (Sturge-Weber syndrome)	Trauma, audible bruit, family history (seizures)	Marked dilated episcleral veins, orbital bruit, blood in Schlemm's canal (port wine stain involving lid)	Medical therapy rarely effective, filtration surgery with prophylactic sclerotomies	23, 45
LOW INTRAOCULAR PRESSURE (EXCESS AQUEOUS RUNOFF)				
Wound or bleb leak	Antimetabolite therapy used	Low IOP, positive Seidel test, deflated bleb	Spontaneous closure infrequent, surgical closure with atraumatic vascular needle	47
Overfiltration of glaucoma filtering procedure	Antimetabolite therapy used	Low IOP, large diffuse bleb or thin-walled bleb	Spontaneous resolution common, contact lens or shell tamponade, pressure patching, surgical revision	47
NORMAL OR ELEVATED INTRAOCULAR PRESSURE (INCREASED POSTERIOR PRESSURE)				
Choroidal detachment (hemorrhagic or serous)	Sudden pain and decreased vision, visual field defect, pain with eye movement	Normal or high IOP, poor red reflex, choroidals seen by fundoscopic examination or ultrasonography	Spontaneous resolution frequent, maximal cycloplegia and steroids, drainage for persistent or "kissing" choroidals	47
Angle closure glaucoma with pupillary block	Preoperative narrow anterior chamber angle, hyperopia	Normal or high IOP, occluded peripheral iridectomy	Laser or surgical iridotomy	45
Malignant glaucoma	Filtration surgery for angle closure glaucoma	Normal or high IOP, flat AC despite patent iridectomy, occurs with cessation of postop cycloplegia	Maximal cycloplegia laser vitrotomy in pseudo- or aphakia, vitrectomy frequently required	47

Differential Diagnosis	Historical Features	Key Findings	Treatment	Chapter Number
CONGENITAL/INFANTILE GLAUCOMA (DIFFERENTIAL DIAGNOSIS)				
Congenital/infantile glaucoma	Classic Triad—epiphora, photophobia and blepharospasm	Elevated IOP, corneal edema, Haab's striae, increased corneal diameter, enlarged cup, anterior chamber angle anomalies	Therapy almost always surgical (trabeculotomy or goniotomy)	45
Nasal lacrimal duct obstruction	Excessive tearing, frequently photophobia and blepharospasm	Lacrimal sac fullness and purulent drainage, normal IOP and cornea	Tonometry, nasal lacrimal duct intubation and irrigation	24
Birth trauma and corneal edema	Difficult birth or forceps delivery	Normal IOP, normal corneal diameter, mild corneal edema, tears in Descemet's oriented vertically or oblique	No therapy, spontaneous resolution common	51
Corneal opacification (corneal dystrophies, developmental anomalies, inborn errors in metabolism, intrauterine infection)	Family history of dystrophies or metabolic disorders, maternal history of infection	Usually normal corneal diameter, normal or elevated IOP (if secondary glaucoma present)	Metabolic and infectious evaluation, may require keratoplasty and cataract extraction	23, 51
Enlarged cornea (megalocornea)	Epiphora, photophobia and blepharospasm uncommon	Normal IOP, increased corneal diameter but cornea is clear	No therapy	51

NEURO-OPHTHALMOLOGY

ACUTE UNILATERAL VISUAL LOSS
(Normal Anterior Segment)

ADULT

Differential Diagnosis	Historical Features	Key Findings	Treatment	Chapter Number
Optic neuritis	Pain on eye movement Color vision cat scratch Tick bite Age: 18–45	± Disk edema MG Pupil Visual field defects, color vision defects MRI—paraventricular white matter lesions Positive serology	Observe or steroids if MRI pos. Antibiotic if serology +	7
Anterior ischemic optic neuropathy	Altitudinal visual loss Hypertension Diabetes Age: 50–70	Disk edema with hemorrhage VF defect MG Pupil	Observe	7
	Temporal arteritis Age: >70	Sed rate + Temporal artery biopsy +	Steroids	
Lebers optic neuropathy	Young adult Family history Painless Males > females	Telangiectatic microangiopathy VF defect MG pupil	Observe	7
Papillophlebitis	Painless Post viral	Disk edema Vitreous cells MG pupil visual field defect Positive ANA, sed rate	Steroids	7
Retinal Detachment	Curtain or veil, flashing lights Trauma	Detached retina	Retinal surgery	61
Uveitis	Post viral Collagen/vascular disease Cat/dog exposure Tick bite Sexual contacts	Vitreous cells Retinal lesions disk swelling Serology (syphilis) ELISA (Toxo, toxocara)	Steroids Antibiotics	29–40
Central serous retinopathy	Stress, illness Micropsia Metamorphopsia	Macular fluid FA—hyperfluorescence smoke-stack	Observe ± laser	59
Vitreous Hemorrhage	Diabetic Sickle cell Trauma	Vitreous blood Iris neovas.	Observe	60, 64, 61
Retina artery occlusion	Sudden Painless May wax and wane	Cherry red spot Vessel narrowing Macular edema	Lower IOP Massage	60

Differential Diagnosis	Historical Features	Key Findings	Treatment	Chapter Number
ACUTE UNILATERAL VISUAL LOSS (Normal Anterior Segment)				
CHILD				
Optic neuritis	Pain on eye movement Post viral	± Disk edema MRI—paraventricular white matter lesions MG pupil	Observe Steroids	7
Leber's neuroretinitis	Post viral Headache	Disk edema Macular star MG pupil	Steroids	7
Retinitis	Cat/dog exposure	Vitreous cells Retinal lesions Positive parasite titers, eosinophilia	Steroids Antibiotics	34
Retinoblastoma	Strabismus Leukocoria	White retinal mass, Calcium CT Scan—calcified mass	Radiation or enucleation	22
Retinal detachment	Curtain or veil, flashing lights Trauma	Detached retina	Retinal surgery	61
ADULT PROPTOSIS (see Oculoplatic section for proptosis in children)				
Thyroid Orbitopathy	Females 4:1 Slow progression Diplopia Painless Hyperthyroid	Lid retraction Strabismus + forced duction Chemosis Lid edema Superior limbic keratoconjunc. CT—enlarged EOM (medial, inferior)	Observation Steroids, radiation orbital surgery for optic nerve compromise	9, 25
Pseudotumor/Myositis	Rapid Painful Diplopia Photophobia	Strabismus + forced ductions Episcleral injection, chemosis CT—enlarged EOM or diffuse retrobulbar enhancement	Steroids Radiation if unresponsive	25
Lymphoma	Subacute Painless Diplopia + ptosis Age: 50–60	Firm, rubbery mass Salmon-colored Conj. mass CT/MRI—homogeneous infiltrate, enhances	Biopsy Radiation ChemTx	25
Orbital cellulitis	Rapid (days) Painful Fever Sinusitis Diplopia Trauma	Marked lid edema, erythema chemosis, epiphora Decreased Vision Strabismus Elevated WBC CT—sinusitis, orbital abscess	Drainage Antibiotics	25

Differential Diagnosis	Historical Features	Key Findings	Treatment	Chapter Number
Dural sinus fistula	Subacute Painless Females Age: 40–60 Diplopia Trauma	Lid swelling Chemosis, conjunctival arterialization Sixth nerve palsy Elevated IOP CT/MRI—enlarged superior ophthalmic vein	Observe or embolization	25
Carotid-cavernous sinus	Rapid (hours) Painful Diplopia Trauma	Marked chemosis Ophthalmoplegia MRI—Enlarged cavernous sinus with dilated orbital blood vessels and enlarged EOM Elevated IOP	Embolization	25
Varix	Slow (years) Intermittent Hemorrhage Painless	Prominent conj. vessels, lower lid Pulsation Increased proptosis with valsalva CT—enhancing serpinginous mass	Observe	25
Meningioma	Slow growth Diplopia Blurred vision Painless	Decreased vision VF defects MG pupil Optic atrophy Temporal fossa fullness CT/MRI—enlarged optic nerve Optociliary shunt vessels	Observe if vision good, excision if poor vision	8, 25
Hemangioma (cavernous)	Slow growth Blurred vision Painless	Visual loss Choridal straie Ultrasound—high internal reflectivity CT—intraconal non- enhancing mass	Excision	25
Lacrimal gland tumor—benign	Slow growth Blurred vision Painless Diplopia	Visual loss Supratemporal mass—firm smooth Strabismus CT—lacrimal fossa	Excision	25
Malignant	Subacute Painful	Mass, bone erosion	Biopsy Radiation, ChemTx	25
Metastatic	Acute/subacute Diplopia Painful	Lid retraction (Breast) Hemorrhage CT—poorly circumscribed mass	Treat Primary	25

Differential Diagnosis	Historical Features	Key Findings	Treatment	Chapter Number
Mucocele	Slow growth Eyelid edema Painful Diplopia Sinus history Allergies	Hard mass Strabismus Lid edema CT—sinusitis, orbital cyst	Drainage Antibiotics	25
Neurofibroma Schwannoma	Slow growth Mild pain Ptosis Diplopia Age: 20–60	"Bag of worms" mass CT—well- circumscribed, roundish lesion, usually extraconal	Excision	25

ACQUIRED ABDUCTION DEFICIT

CHILD

Differential Diagnosis	Historical Features	Key Findings	Treatment	Chapter Number
Sixth nerve palsy	Post viral Headache Ear ache Trauma	Facial weakness Otitis media Disk edema Stiff Neck	MRI Observe	9, 20
Duane's syndrome	Head position Asymptomatic	Palpebral fissure narrowing on adduction	Observe	20
Accommodative esotropia	Variable esotropia	Hyperopia	Glasses	17
Orbital myositis	Pain Chemosis	Proptosis Orbital fullness CT scan—Enlarged medial rectus muscle	Steroids	25
Blowout fracture	Trauma Orbital hemorrhage	Enophthalmos Positive forced ductions CT Scan—orbital wall fracture	Observe Strabismus surgery if stable	26

Differential Diagnosis	Historical Features	Key Findings	Treatment	Chapter Number
ACQUIRED ABDUCTION DEFICIT				
ADULT				
Sixth nerve palsy	Pain Headache Acute onset History of diabetes, hypertension	Negative forced duction Positive neuro exam Disk edema	Sed rate Blood count MRI Scan if not isolated or persists	9, 20
Thyroid myopathy	Hyperthyroidism Gradual onset Variable diplopia	Proptosis Lid retraction Positive forced duction CT Scan—enlarged muscles (medial, inferior)	Observe Strabismus surgery if stable	9, 25
Blowout fracture	Acute onset Trauma	Enophthalmos Positive forced duction CT Scan—Medial Orbital wall fracture	Observe Strabismus surgery if stable	26
Accommodative spasm	Variable symptoms Stress	Variable deviation Unable to sustain	Observe Cycloplegia	9
Orbital myositis	Pain Acute onset	Proptosis Chemosis CT Scan—enlarged muscle	Steroids	25
Myasthenia	Variable onset Fatigability	Ptosis Variable motility Exam Positive tensilon test	Mestinon Steroids Thymectomy	9

Differential Diagnosis	Historical Features	Key Findings	Treatment	Chapter Number
PROPTOSIS				
CHILD				
Pseudotumor/Myositis	Acute Painful Diplopia Photophobia Visual loss	Chemosis Strabismus Episcleral injection CT scan—diffuse post. involvement or enlarged muscle	Steroids	25
Orbital cellulitis	Acute Painful Fever History of sinusitis, dental work, trauma Diplopia	Marked lid edema, erythema Chemosis CT scan—sinusitis orbital abscess Strabismus Decreased vision	Antibiotics (H. Flu, strep staph)	25
Histiocytosis X Eosinophilic granuloma (Hand-Schüller-Christian)	Palpable mass Tender Rash Runny nose Fever Subacute	Firm mass CT—lytic bone lesion Diabetes insipidous Palpable lymph nodes	Excision Radiation ChemTx	25
Hemangioma/lymphangioma	Purplish mass Enlarges with crying Rapid growth Non-ophthalmic strawberry marks Age: <6 months	Lid mass Soft, nontender CT—Enhancing diffuse mass Anisometropia	Steroids interlesional or systemic	25
Optic glioma	Slow growth Non-painful Visual loss Headaches	Firm to retro pulse Decreased vision Pulsatile MG pupil Optic atrophy	Observe Radiation	8

Differential Diagnosis	Historical Features	Key Findings	Treatment	Chapter Number
Rhabdomyosarcoma	Rapid growth Painful Age 5–10 Ptosis (33%)	Firm Lid edema CT—mass retro bulbar space Biopsy—striated muscle	Radiation ChemTX	25
Dermoid cyst	Slow growth Diplopia May have acute inflammation	Rubbery mass Proptosis with mastication (if temporal wall involved) CT—cyst with bone scalloping	Excision	25
Leukemia (chloroma)	Rapid growth Fever Irritable	Axial proptosis Firm Blood count—elevated WBCs CT—diffuse orbital mass	ChemTx	25
Neuroblastoma	Jerky eyes Rapid growth Abdominal mass Spontaneous lid ecchymosis Lid swelling	Opsoclonus Horner's CT—diffuse orbital mass with bone destruction lid edema	ChemTx Excision primary lesion	25

OCULAR INFLAMMATION

ANTERIOR UVEITIS

Differential Diagnosis	Historical Features	Key Findings	Treatment	Chapter Number
HLA-B27–associated	Severe pain, photophobia, recurrent episodes, arthritis, GI disease	Severe conjunctival injection, hypopyon +HLA-B27, ±Sacroiliac x-rays	Corticosteroids—topical, periocular, systemic, mydriatics	32
JRA-associated	White, quiet, young girls, pauciarticular	Insidious, relentless, mild, chronic anterior segment cells and flare, +ANA, ±HLAB27	Corticosteroids, mydriatics complications may be severe	32
Herpetic	Moderate pain, photophobia, past labial lesion	Dendrite, disciform scar, iris atrophy, diffuse KPs, + HSV cultures on Hanks medium	Topical trifluorothymidine, ± topical steroids if disciform, mydriatics	32
Syphilitic	Moderate pain, photophobia	+VDRL if recent infection, +FTA	Penicillin, topical steroids, mydriatics	32
Tuberculous	Moderate pain, photophobia. chronic	+ Chest X-Ray, +PPD	Triple or quadruple anti-tuberculous therapy, topical steroids, mydriatics	32
IOL-related (UGH)	Moderate pain, photophobia to no pain, blurry vision, ACIOL	hyphema, iris chafing, glaucoma	Removal/exchange of IOL	32
Posner-Schlossman	Moderate to severe pain, photophobia, recurrent episodes, self-limited	Very mild ant. uveitis, increased IOP	Lower IOP, mild topical steroids, mydriatics	32
Traumatic	Mild to moderate pain, photophobia, history of blunt trauma	Mild anterior uveitis, self limited	Mild topical steroids and mydriatics	32
Fuchs' heterochromic iridocyclitis	White, quiet eye, blurry vision, chronic	Stellate, diffuse KPs, heterochromia (more blue eye, less brown eye), glaucoma, cataract	Avoid corticosteroids—may make glaucoma and cataract worse	32
Idiopathic	Mild to moderate pain, photophobia		Topical corticosteroids, mydriatics	32

INTERMEDIATE UVEITIS

Pars planitis	White, quiet eye to mild pain, floaters, variable loss of vision	Rule out sarcoidosis, lyme, tuberculosis, MS	Topical, periocular, systemic steroids, ±mydriatics	33

Differential Diagnosis	Historical Features	Key Findings	Treatment	Chapter Number
POSTERIOR UVEITIS				
Toxoplasmosis	Floaters, loss of vision, any age	Focal Retinochoroditis, old scar, vitritis, "headlight in fog", +ELISA (IgM, IgG)	Pyrimethamine, sulfadiazine, clindamycin, ± prednisone esp. if optic nerve or macula involved	34
Toxocariasis	Floaters, vision loss, Age <15 (often <10), amblyopia, strabismus	Focal retinitis, vitritis, elevated granuloma, endophthalmitis, tractional RD	Topical, systemic steroids	34
OHS (Histoplasmosis)	Metamorphopsia, loss of vision	chorioretinal scars (histo spots), peripapillary atrophy, CNVM on Fl. angiography	MPS—focal laser to CNVM, submacular surgery, corticosteroids	34
ARN	Loss of vision, acute, rapidly progressive, Age 20–50, can be bilateral	Multifocal retinitis, perivasculitis	IV acyclovir	34
Retinal Vasculitis	Loss of vision, any age, associated rheumatologic disorders (Wegner's, relapsing polychondritis, PAN)	Retinal venous or arteriolar sheathing, rule out Behçet's (aphthous ulcers, genital ulcers, +HLAB5)	Corticosteroids, immunosuppressives	34
Serpiginous choroiditis	Loss of vision, progressive, acute flares,	Geographic, peripapillary, snake-like retiochoroidal scars and active lesion edge, CNVM	Systemic, periocular corticosteroids, immunosuppressive, laser for CNVM	34
Large cell Lymphoma (Masquerade Syndrome)	Chronic floaters, vision loss, Age >65, Neurologic deficit	Vitritis, may be progressive, retinal pigment epithelial level lesions, +MRI, +LP, +Vit. Biopsy	Combination chemotherapy and radiation therapy	34
PANUVEITIS				
Sarcoidosis	Acute or chronic, mild to severe pain, photophobia, gradual vision loss if chronic, Shortness of breath, Blacks	Anterior—66%, posterior—33%, mutton-fat KPs, conj. biopsy, +ACE, +CXR, +gallium scan, ±neuro	Corticosteroids (topical, periocular, systemic), mydriatics, rarely immunosuppressives	36
Behçet's	Acute episodes with quiet periods, aphthous ulcers, genital ulcers, skin lesions, patients from "old silk route"	Hypopyon, retinal vasculitis (esp. vein occlusions), +HLAB5	corticosteroids, immunosuppressives (cyclosporine), colchicine	36

Differential Diagnosis	Historical Features	Key Findings	Treatment	Chapter Number
Lens-induced uveitis, phacoanaphylactic phacolytic, phacotoxic	Acute to chronic onset of pain, photophobia, long-standing morgagnian cataract, retained lens material after trauma or surgery	Phacoanaphylactic-hypopyon, granulomatous inflammation, after cataract surgery,	Cortisteroids, removal of retained lens material, mydriatics	36
Lyme disease	Acute to chronic, deer tick bite, erythema chronicum migrans, systemic illness (any system)	Anterior uveitis, intermediate uveitis, or pan uveitis, +Lyme serology	Penicillin, doxycycline, topical corticosteroids, mydriatics	36
Sympathetic ophthalmia	Chronic relentless, with acute flare-ups of pain, photophobia, vision loss, history of penetrating trauma	Bilateral, granulomatous panuveitis, rarely has cutaneous findings of VKH, but + trauma	Corticosteroids, immunosuppressive, mydriatics	36
Vogt-Koyanagi-Harada syndrome	Prodromal stage—CNS symptoms, acute, convalescent, and chronic phases, subacute to rapid bilateral visual loss, Age—20–50	Acute—bilateral serous RD's, tinnitus, meningismus, Chronic—granulomatous inflammation, Cutaneous—vitiligo, poliosis, alopecia Labs—normal	Corticosteroids, occasionally immunosuppressive, mydriatics, chronic complications—cataracts, glaucoma, and CNVM	36

INFLAMMATORY CHORIORETINOPATHIES (For other "White Dot Syndromes" see table 59-3)

Differential Diagnosis	Historical Features	Key Findings	Treatment	Chapter Number
Multiple evanescent white dot syndrome	Young (20–50), female, photopsias, typically unilateral, can involve other eye, can be recurrent	GVF—Enlarged blind spot, Minimal vitritis, Fl. Angio—"wreath sign", characteristic RPE changes in fovea in chronic cases	Self limited, rarely corticosteroids	36
APMPPE	Young (20–40), M = F, viral prodrome, bilateral, acute visual loss	No vitritis, creamy, white plaque-like retinal lesions	Self limited, rare chronic RPE changes	36
Birdshot retinochoroidopathy	Floaters, vision loss, chronic, later onset (>40), nyctalopia	Multifocal, creamy, yellow lesions in choroid in periphery, CME on Fl. Angio, +HLA-A29–90%, vitritis, diminished ERG	Corticosteroids	36

AIDS ASSOCIATED RETINITIS

AIDS-associated retinitis	Floaters, painless sudden to subacute visual loss, CD4 <100	CMV retinitis—"pizza-pie" retinal necrosis along vessels, periphlebitis, ± hemorrhages, progressive in weeks	Foscarnet, ganciclovir, or combination (IV, intravitreal, implant)	38
	CD4 <100 Extraocular zoster, ?herpetic	Progressive outer retinal necrosis—PORN—Outer retinitis, punctate white spots that become confluent peripherally, classic foveal lesions, progressive in days	Foscarnet + ganciclovir	

OCULOPLASTIC

PROPTOSIS IN CHILDREN

Differential Diagnosis	Historical Features	Key Findings	Treatment	Chapter Number
Orbital Cellulitis	Pain, fever, lid swelling, hx sinus disease, tooth extraction, trauma	Decreased vision proptosis, and motility, ±increased WBC, fever, sinus opacification on X-ray	IV antibiotics, later oral antibiotics, surgical drainage of abscess	25
Infantile hemangioma	Onset soon after birth, increase with crying, "strawberry birthmarks"	Strawberry birthmarks, amblyopia, mechanical ptosis, astigmatism	Observation intralesional steroids for induced astigmatism, occlusion of visual axis or amblyopia	25
Lymphangioma	First decade of life, proptosis due to bleeding, may increase in size with URI	Multilobulated lesion on CT, blood cysts, massive proptosis with bleed, optic nerve compression	Cold compresses, observe, drain if optic nerve compression, CO^2 laser surgical debridement only severe cases.	25
Plexiform Neurofibroma	History Neurofibromatosis, painless lateral lid mass	Café-au-lait spots, pulsatile exophthalmos, S-shaped lid deformity, absent greater wing sphenoid on CT "bag of worms" on palpation	Surgical debulking, difficult due to infiltrative nature	25
Optic Nerve Glioma	First decade, painless, proptosis, slow growth neurofibromatosis, visual loss may not be recognized	Optic nerve tumor on CT, optic atrophy Firm to retropulse Poor VA, +MG pupil	Observe, radiation surgery if chiasm threatened, neurosurgery	8
Rhabdomyosarcoma	Rapid onset painless, proptosis, median age 7–8 years, even infancy Ptosis (33%)	Tumor usually in superior orbit, globe displacement, normal WBC, Lid edema biopsy ± stricted muscle	Biopsy ASAP, irradiation and chemotherapy; prognosis good if tumor confined to orbit	25
Metastatic neuroblastoma	Rapid onset proptosis in young child, eyelid discoloration	Eyelid ecchymosis, opsoclonus Horner's abdominal mass, bony destruction on CT, increased urine VMA, diaphoresis tachycardia	Biopsy ASAP, irradiation and chemotherapy; prognosis generally poor	25
Orbital Pseudotumor	Rapid onset proptosis, malaise, constitutional symptoms, often bilateral	Inflammatory signs, eosinophilia, iritis, localized or diffuse inflammatory mass on CT	Steroids, low dose irradiation	25

Differential Diagnosis	Historical Features	Key Findings	Treatment	Chapter Number
Histiocytosis X Eosinophilic granuloma (Hand-Schüller-Christian)	Palpable mass Tender Rash Runny nose Fedver Subacute	Firm mass CT—lytic bone lesion Diabetes insipidus Palpable lymph nodes	Excision Radiation Chem Tx	25
Dermoid cyst	Slow growth Diplopia May have acute inflammation	Rubbery mass Proptosis with mastication (if temporal wall involved) CT—cyst with bone scalloping	Excision	25
Leukemia (chloroma)	Rapid growth Fever Initable	Avail proptosis Firm Blood Chem—elevated WDG CT—diffuse orbital mass	ChemTx	25

LACRIMAL GLAND TUMORS

Dacryoadenitis bacterial and viral	Painful swelling, fever, lid erythema, conjunctival discharge	S-shaped lid deformity, suppuration, increased WBC, fever, lymphadenopathy	Bacterial—antibiotics; viral—observe	25
Pseudotumor (idiopathic inflammation)	Abrupt onset of pain, swelling, injection; may be bilateral	S-shaped lid deformity, tenderness, mass on CT molds to adjacent structures and enhances	Biopsy Corticosteroids low Dose irradiation	25
Pleomorphic adenoma (benign mixed tumor)	Slow growing, painless, firm mass; second to fifth decades, symptoms often present more than 1 year	Well-circumscribed, round to oval mass on CT with with bony excavation/ expansion; globe displaced down and in; no inflammatory signs	No biopsy, complete excision, keep pseudo-capsule intact	25
Adenoid cystic carcinoma	Painful, firm mass; diplopia, globe displacement; onset 4th decade, symptoms often present less than 1 year	Infiltrating poorly circumscribed mass with bony destruction on CT, calcification, perineural invasion	Biopsy, exenteration after biopsy confirmation with removal of involved bone; prognosis generally poor	25
Lymphoma	Painless, slow-growing mass, minimal proptosis and globe displacement, may be bilateral, older age group	Molds to globe and orbital bones on CT, low reflective on ECHO, salmon-colored subconjunctival component	Biopsy, systemic work-up, radiation if localized, chemotherapy if systemic	25

OPTICS AND REFRACTION

DECREASE DISTANCE VISION

Differential Diagnosis	Historical Features	Key Findings	Treatment	Chapter Number
Myopia	Gradual increase during adolescence Must rule out diabetes or cataract if rapid change in older age group	High "K" readings or long eye or both	Provide full optical Rx Evaluate blood Glucose or cataract if indicated	3
Astigmatism	Gradual change from "with the rule" to "against the rule". Lid lesions and pterygia can induce changes	"K" readings usually aligned with refractive error	Full correction Moderate changes in power	3
Absolute Hyperopia	Decreased near vision is worse. Rapid increase possibly due to macular edema	Flat "K" readings short eye, or both	Full non-cycloplegic refraction Retinal evaluation if rapid change	3

DECREASED NEAR VISION

Differential Diagnosis	Historical Features	Key Findings	Treatment	Chapter Number
Hyperopia	Distance vision occasionally affected also Discomfort with loss of place reading	Low "K" readings and/or short eye 3	Full hyperopic noncylcoplegic correction	3
Presbyopia	Affects patients over age 40, hyperopes sooner, and myopes later	Decrease in ability to change focus for near work (reduced accommodative amplitude)	Near (or reading correction) or multifocal	3
Accomodative insufficiency	Rare onset age 6 to teens	Decrease accommodation unknown etiology	Bifocals	3

RETINA

VITREOUS HEMORRHAGE

Differential Diagnosis	Historical Features	Key Findings	Treatment	Chapter Number
Proliferative diabetic retinopathy	Established history of diabetes mellitus, acute onset of dark streaks, floaters	Fibrovascular proliferations in posterior pole, vitreous attached at disk by ultrasound	Panretinal photocoagulation, vitrectomy when indicated	60
Retinal tear	Floaters, photopsias	Posterior vitreous detachment, vitreous pigment cells	Cryopexy or photocoagulation of tear, vitreous hemorrhage usually clears spontaneously	61
Branch retinal vein occlusion	Diminished vision months previously, hypertension or atherosclerotic disease	Sectoral capillary nonperfusion, collateral vessels, neovascular proliferation	Scatter photocoagulation to areas of nonperfusion if neovascularization present, vitrectomy if nonclearing	60
Trauma	Blunt or penetrating injury to the eye, more frequent in young men	Laceration of the globe, orbital fracture	Extensive search for globe rupture or foreign body	64
Shaken baby syndrome	Inconsistencies in history, bony fractures in different stages of healing	Sub-, intra-, and preretinal hemorrhages, intracranial hemorrhage, giant retinal tear	Early vitrectomy if amblyopia is risked	64
Valsalva retinopathy	Acute rise in intra-abdominal or thoracic pressure associated with straining	Preretinal hemorrhage often near disk	Exclude subarachnoid hemorrhage (Terson's syndrome), usually clears spontaneously	64
Any neovascularization	Sickle cell, collagen-vascular diseases, Eales' disease, FEVR	Retinal neovascularization	Photocoagulation or cryotherapy to areas of ischemia	60

RETINAL DETACHMENT (CHILD)

Differential Diagnosis	Historical Features	Key Findings	Treatment	Chapter Number
Retinopathy of prematurity	Less than 28 weeks gestation, birth weight under 1000 g, oxygen administration, twin	Retrolental mass, tractional retinal elevation, peripheral retinal trough	Scleral buckling for Stage 4, vitrectomy for Stage 5	22
Retinoblastoma	Leukocoria, strabismus, family history in 5%, uni- or bilateral	Solitary or multiple fleshy retinal tumors, may grow intravitreal or subretinal, normal size eye	External beam irradiation or enucleation, if bilateral rule out pinealoma	22
Coats' disease	Leukocoria, strabismus, unilateral, no family history	Yellow exudative retinal detachment	Triple freeze cryotherapy, photocoagulation, or vitrectomy with endolaser	60

Differential Diagnosis	Historical Features	Key Findings	Treatment	Chapter Number
Familial exudative vitreoretinopathy	Autosomal dominant inheritance, bilateral, pseudoexotropia	Avascular border in temporal periphery, peripheral proliferative retinopathy, retinal folds, tractional retinal detachment, subretinal and intraretinal exudation	Vitrectomy	56
Incontinentia pigmenti	Usually females, maternal abortions, characteristic skin lesions at birth	Peripheral fibrovascular proliferation associated with a peripheral avascular zone, dental anomalies (65%), CNS involvement (30%)	Vitrectomy	56
Norrie's disease	Family history, only males, present at birth, bilateral	Retinal fold, PHPV, mental retardation (60%), impaired hearing (30%)	Genetic counseling, vitreous surgery unsuccessful	56
Shaken baby syndrome	Inconsistencies in history, bony fractures in different stages of healing	Sub-, intra-, and preretinal hemorrhages, intracranial hemorrhage, giant retinal tear	Early vitrectomy if amblyopia is risked	64

CHOROIDAL MASS (ADULT)

Differential Diagnosis	Historical Features	Key Findings	Treatment	Chapter Number
Choroidal detachment	Hypotony, inflammation, trauma, surgical wound leak	Smooth, dark, dome-shaped, may extend anteriorly to scleral spur, serous or hemorrhagic by ultrasound	Observation, oral corticosteroids, surgical drainage if "kissing"	62
Metastatic carcinoma	Diminished vision, lung or breast cancer diagnosed or occult, may be bilateral	Bullous, exudative RD with underlying yellow choroidal mass	Palliative external beam irradiation	62
Malignant melanoma	Asymptomatic or diminished vision, lenticular astigmatism or glaucoma, unilateral	Brown or amelanotic dome-shaped mass, lipofuscin pigment, may be mushroom-shaped if extends through Bruch's membrane	Observation, episcleral plaque irradiation, enucleation, proton beam irradiation, surgical resection	62
Hemangioma	Metamorphopsia, diminished central vision, unilateral	Mildly elevated orange lesion with indistinct margins	Grid laser photocoagulation over tumor if associated with subretinal fluid threatening the macula	62

Differential Diagnosis	Historical Features	Key Findings	Treatment	Chapter Number
Osteoma	Metamorphopsia, adolescent or young adult females	Yellow-white mildly elevated peripapillary lesion with sharp borders	Observation, photocoagulation if choroidal neovascularization develops	62

CHOROIDAL NEOVASCULAR MEMBRANES

Differential Diagnosis	Historical Features	Key Findings	Treatment	Chapter Number
Presumed ocular histoplasmosis syndrome	Ohio-Mississippi valley resident	Punched-out chorioretinal lesions, juxtapapillary atrophy, disciform macular scars, no vitreous inflammation	Photocoagulation vs. surgical excision	34, 59
Age-related macular degeneration	Older patient complaining of metamorphopsia, central scotoma	Soft drusen, geographic atrophy, disciform scars may be present in either eye	Photocoagulation of juxtafoveal or extrafoveal lesions, surgical excision under study	59
Angioid streaks	Association with Paget's disease, pseudoxanthoma elasticum, Ehler-Danlos, sickle cell disease	Breaks in Bruch's membrane	Safety glasses; Photocoagulation for CNVM, but recurrence common	59
Pathologic myopia	High myopia (usually > −6 D)	Thin, atrophic RPE; staphyloma, lacquer cracks	Safety glasses; Photocoagulation for CNVM, but recurrence common	59
Serpiginous choroidopathy	Painless blurring of vision, recurrent episodes	Peripapillary areas of choriocapillaris atrophy spreading centrifugally	Laser photocoagulation	34, 59
Multifocal choroiditis and panuveitis	Young, healthy, myopic females; acute vision loss with photopsias and scotomas	Vitritis, anterior uveitis, multiple small lesions at level of RPE or choriocapillaris	Local and systemic steroids	59

NEOVASCULARIZATION OF THE RETINA

Differential Diagnosis	Historical Features	Key Findings	Treatment	Chapter Number
Proliferative diabetic retinopathy (common)	Diabetes mellitus	Dot-blot hemorrhages in posterior pole, can have vitreous hemorrhage	Panretinal photocoagulation if high-risk characteristics present	60
Sickle cell	Sickle disease (SS, SC, S-thal)	Black sunbursts, salmon patches, sea-fans, comma-shaped conjunctival vessels	Panretinal photocoagulation or cryotherapy	60
Central/branch retinal vein occlusion (common)	3 months after loss of vision	severe ischemia and capillary nonperfusion on IVFA, flame-shaped hemorrhages, cotton wool spots	Scatter photocoagulation of affected quadrant	60

Differential Diagnosis	Historical Features	Key Findings	Treatment	Chapter Number
Vasculitis	Systemic vasculitic disease (especially systemic lupus erythematosus)	Sheathed vessels	Prednisone, systemic immunosuppression, photocoagulation	60
Eales' disease (rare)	Young, healthy adults	Vascular sheathing, peripheral nonperfusion, neovascularization along border of perfused and avascular retina	Photocoagulation of nonperfused retina	60
Familial exudative vitreoretinopathy (rare)	Autosomal dominant	Incomplete vascularization of peripheral retina, neovascularization at border, fibrovascular proliferation, intraretinal and subretinal exudates	Photocoagulation or cryotherapy of nonperfused retina	56
Talc retinopathy (rare)	Intravenous drug abuse	Small, white, refractile emboli in perifoveal capillaries, branch retinal artery occlusions		59

STRABISMUS

ESOTROPIA

Differential Diagnosis	Historical Features	Key Findings	Treatment	Chapter Number
Infantile esotropia (congenital ET)	Onset prior to 6 months of age.	Constant large angle esotropia (greater than 30 PD). Associated motor anomalies include: dissociated vertical deviation, inferior oblique overaction, latent nystagmus, OKN asymmetry. Amblyopia is common and associated with strong fixation preference for one eye.	Occlusion therapy for amblyopia if present. Prescribe full hypermetropic correction if greater than +2.50. Strabismus surgery (bilateral medial rectus recession).	17
Accommodative esotropia	Onset between infancy and adulthood, but most commonly presents between 2 and 5 years of age.	Starts as an intermittent esodeviation and progresses to a constant tropia. Tends to be a variable angle usually greater at near. Hypertropia usually greater than +2.00. May have high ACA ratio with or without hypermetropia.	Prescribe full hypermetropic correction. Prescribe bifocal plus add if single vision glasses corrects distance (<8 PD) but ET at near (>8 PD). Surgery is indicated if the distance deviation is not corrected (<8 PD) (partially accommodative esotropia). Phospholine iodine is a temporary treatment but optical correction is preferred.	17
Duane's syndrome Type I	Congenital onset, face turn opposite to Duane's Eye.	Ipsilateral limitation of abduction, with lid fissure widening on attempted abduction and narrowing on adduction. Usually unilateral with an ipsilateral face turn: Goldenhar's syndrome and maternal use of Thalidomide.	Surgery indicated to correct face turn. Ipsilateral medial rectus recession.	20
Divergence insufficiency	Acquired usually after 1 year of age.	Esotropia greater in the distance than near. Often associated with sixth nerve mild paresis. MRI of head important to rule out neurological etiology.	Strabismus surgery, Recession of medial rectus muscle OU. Neuroimaging	17

Differential Diagnosis	Historical Features	Key Findings	Treatment	Page Number
Neurologic Causes (Acquired ET) Consider myasthenia, sixth nerve palsy, hydrocephalus, Moebius' syndrome, Arnold-Chiari malformation.	Acquired in infancy through adulthood.	Variable angle esotropia usually with limited abduction, and often a divergence insufficiency pattern.	Neuroimaging (head MRI), Tensilon test and neurologic evaluation is indicated. Treat neurologic disease, then consider strabismus surgery.	9
Congenital fibrosis syndrome (strabismus fixes)	Congenital	Congenitally fibrotic and tight medial rectus muscle. May be unilateral or bilateral. Limited abduction with positive forced ductions. Other extraocular muscles may be involved, ptosis may be present.	Strabismus surgery (recession of tight medial rectus muscle).	20
Cyclic esotropia	Usually after 2 years of age.	May be associated with mild hypermetropia. Esodeviation occurs in a rhythmic pattern, (e.g., every other day, every third day). On straight days, patient has excellent fusion and stereopsis. When tropic patients usually suppress.	Strabismus surgery for full deviation on tropic day (bilateral medial rectus recessions).	17

EXOTROPIA

Differential Diagnosis	Historical Features	Key Findings	Treatment	Page Number
Intermittent Exotropia *Common*	Usually after 2 years of age.	Intermittent deviation, high grade stereopsis when fusing, suppression when tropic. Amblyopia unusual.	Part time occlusion of dominant eye. Over minus if myopic. Strabismus surgery (lateral rectus recession OU).	18
Convergence Insufficiency *Common*	After 5 years of age usually presenting in young adults.	Asthenopia and reading fatigue most common, diplopia unusual. Poor fusional convergence. Rarely associated with accommodative insufficiency. Remote near point of convergence. Base out prism convergence less than 20 PD.	Orthoptic exercises primary treatment (pencil push ups, base out prism exercises).	18
Sensory Exotropia *Common*	After visual loss.	Ipsilateral vision loss. Variable angle XT.	Strabismus surgery (ipsilateral lateral rectus recession and medial rectus resection).	18

Differential Diagnosis	Historical Features	Key Findings	Treatment	Chapter Number
Duane's Type III or rarely Type II	Congenital	Limited abduction and adduction Duane's eye in abduction (type III). Contralateral face turn. May be associated with an upshoot and a downshoot on attempted adduction. Lid fissure narrowing on attempted adduction and lid fissure widening on abduction.	Strabismus surgery (ipsilateral lateral rectus recession). Consider lateral rectus recession with Y-split if there is significant upshoot and downshoot.	20
Dissociated horizontal deviation (DHD)	Exotropia usually occurs after previous surgery for congenital esotropia.	Slow exo-drift on cover test, may have coexisting esotropia.	Strabismus surgery (ipsilateral lateral rectus recession).	20
Slipped or lost medial rectus muscle.	Progressive exotropia after medial rectus surgery.	Limited adduction with lid fissure widening on attempted adduction. May occur after poterygium removal.	Retrieval of lost medial rectus muscle. Horizontal transposition of ½ SR and IR (Hummelsheim) with ipsilateral lateral rectus recession.	20
Neurological Disease *Myasthenia gravis, chronic progressive external ophthalmoplegia, acquired third nerve palsy (brain tumor)*	Acquired in infancy to adulthood.	Diplopia, limited adduction. Tension test, ECG, Neuroimaging (MRI), Neurologic evaluation.	Specific for neurologic disease	9
Congenital exotropia	First 6 months of life.	Large angle, constant exotropia, often associated with congenital neurologic disorders or cranial synostosis	Strabismus surgery (lateral rectus recession OU).	20
Congenital third nerve Palsy	Congenital	Ptosis, hypotropia and exotropia (eye down and out), may fuse with a contralateral face turn and chin elevation. Limited adduction, supraduction and infraduction, with Ipsilateral superior oblique overaction. Pupils are often spared.	Strabismus surgery (ipsilateral lateral rectus recession, medial rectus resection and superior oblique weakening procedure). Ptosis repair but be conservative if Bell's phenomenon absent.	20

Differential Diagnosis	Historical Features	Key Findings	Treatment	Chapter Number
HYPERTROPIA				
Congenital superior oblique palsy	Congenital, but is usually diagnosed in childhood or even late adulthood.	Often unilateral or asymmetric bilateral. Ipsilateral hyper-deviation increases with ipsilateral head tilt. Compensatory contralateral head tilt. Large vertical fusional vergence amplitudes. Inferior oblique overaction with superior oblique underaction, V-pattern. Usually no diplopia, no subjective extorsion, but objective extorsion on fundus exam. Facial asymmetry, and lax superior oblique tendon in some cases.	Conservative observation or Strabismus surgery. 1. Ipsilateral inferior oblique recession (hyper less than 10 PD) 2. Ipsilateral inferior oblique recession with contralateral inferior rectus recession (hyper greater than or equal to 10 PD). 3. Ipsilateral superior oblique tuck (if SO is underacting and the SO tendon is lax).	19
Traumatic superior oblique palsy	Acquired after closed head trauma.	Usually bilateral, may be asymmetric. Small ipsilateral hypertropia with poor vertical fusion amplitudes. Vertical-extorsional diplopia. Esotropia in downgaze (arrow "V" pattern). Superior oblique underaction, inferior oblique overaction usually bilateral. Positive head tilt test RH 2 tilt right, LH 2 tilt left.	Strabismus surgery Harato Ito for extorsion. Inferior oblique recession if obliques overacting. Superior oblique tuck for significant superior oblique under-action.	19
Primary inferior oblique overaction	Usually after 2 years of age.	Usually bilateral associated with congenital ET. No diplopia, V-pattern (Y sub-type), hyper increases to opposite side gaze, negative head tilt test, no subjective torsion but objective extorsion on fundus exam.	Inferior oblique weakening procedure (e.g., inferior oblique recession with anteriorization, myectomy).	19
Dissociated vertical deviation (DVD)	Usually after 2 years of age.	Usually bilateral associated with congenital esotropia. Hyperdeviation without contralateral hypodeviation. Often a latent deviation which is manifest when the patient is fatigued, or the eye is covered. Three components elevation, abduction, extorsion. No diplopia.	Ipsilateral superior rectus recessions large (usually bilateral but may be asymmetric).	20

Differential Diagnosis	Historical Features	Key Findings	Treatment	Chapter Number
Primary superior oblique overaction	Recognized after 2 years of age.	Usually bilateral. Superior oblique overaction with or without inferior oblique underaction. A-pattern (lambda subtype), negative head tilt test, right hypotropia in left gaze, left hypotropia in right gaze. May be associated with exotropia and chin depression to allow fusion.	Superior oblique weakening procedure (superior oblique tenotomy or superior oblique silicone expander), In fusing patients (e.g., intermittent exotropia with SOOA and A-pattern) avoid tenotomy, Use SO silicone expander and/or infraplaced lateral rectus OU.	19
Double elevator palsy	At birth.	Hypodeviation associated with limited elevation in abduction and adduction, ptosis common, may fuse with chin elevation, 70% have inferior rectus restriction positive forced ductions, 30% have true superior rectus inferior oblique palsy.	Tight inferior rectus: recess ipsilateral inferior rectus True palsy: partial tendon (Hummelshiem or Jensen) or full tendon (Knapp tendon transposition of MR and LR superiorly).	20
Brown's syndrome	At birth for true congenital Brown's syndrome. May be acquired.	Usually unilateral. May be acquired secondary to inflammation or superior nasal mass. Limited elevation in adduction, positive forced ductions. No significant superior oblique overaction and no significant A-pattern.	Superior oblique weakening procedure SO silicone tendon expander preferred procedure, or SO tenotomy with or without an ipsilateral inferior oblique recession).	20
Graves' ophthalmopathy	Acquired in adulthood.	Hypotropia with restricted elevation associated with positive forced ductions. Esotropia commonly coexists. Proptosis and lid lag. Enlarged rectus muscles on orbital MRI or CT scans.	Strabismus surgery after acute inflammitory phase and after orbital decompression surgery. Recession of inferior rectus muscle (aim for slight under-correction as late overcorrection is common).	9
Floor fracture	After blunt trauma to orbit.	Hypotropia with restricted elevation and positive forced ductions. Enophthalmos, hypesthesia of cheek. CT scan of orbit shows floor fracture.	Strabismus surgery after repair of orbital floor fracture. IR recession for hypotropia. If IR underaction is present, small resection of ipsilateral inferior rectus and small recession contralateral inferior rectus.	26

Differential Diagnosis	Historical Features	Key Findings	Treatment	Chapter Number
Retrobulbar injection into inferior rectus muscle	After retrobulbar injection usually for cataract surgery in elderly patient.	Initial IR paresis, then secondary contracture of ipsilateral IR with ipsilateral hypotropia. Ipsilateral IR may "overact" resulting in a hypotropia which increases in downgaze. Positive forced ductions, tight ipsilateral inferior rectus. Orbital imaging may show enlarged inferior rectus muscle.	Ipsilateral inferior rectus recession.	20
Neurologic disorders third nerve palsy, myasthenia gravis, chronic progressive external ophthalmoplegia.	Acquired usually in adulthood.	Hyperdeviation often with limited ductions. Diplopia	Specific for neurologic disease. Tensilon test, Neuroimaging (MRI). Neurologic evaluation	9
Inferior oblique palsy *Rare*	Usually congenital but can be acquired associated with closed head trauma or localized cerebral vascular disease.	Limited elevation in adduction, negative forced ductions, significant superior oblique overaction, and A-pattern.	Ipsilateral superior oblique weakening procedure (SO silicone tendon expander or SO tenotomy) with contralateral superior rectus recession.	19

Orbital and Ocular Anatomy

Section Editor: Bradley N. Lemke

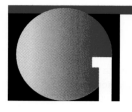

Orbital and Ocular Anatomy

Bryan S. Sires, Bradley N. Lemke, Marilyn C. Kincaid

■ ORBITAL OSTEOLOGY

Orbital Bones

The spatial configuration and relationships of the orbits are best understood by examining a human skull (Figures 1–1 and 1–2). The shape of the anterior orbit resembles a four-sided pyramid that becomes three-sided near the apex. The adult lateral orbital walls are approximately 90° from each other, or 45° from the sagittal midline plane. The divergent axis of each orbit is half of 45° or 22.5° (Fig. 1–2). In contrast, medial walls are parallel (35). The two medial walls of the orbits are 2.5 cm apart; they are 4.5 to 5.0 cm long from the orbital rim anteriorly to the orbital apex posteriorly. The eyes tend to diverge in accordance with their bony surroundings as seen with acquired visual loss, general anesthesia, or in death.

Seven bones comprise the orbit. They have an integral relationship with the nasolacrimal canal and paranasal sinuses to be discussed later. The bones in alphabetical order are the ethmoid, frontal, lacrimal, maxillary, palatine, sphenoid and zygomatic (Fig. 1–1). Each one has a specific relation to one or more of the various walls which comprise the orbit.

Orbital Rim

The adult orbital rim is the anterior opening to the orbit and has a rectangular configuration with a horizontal dimension of 40–45 mm, and a vertical dimension of 30–35 mm (Fig. 1–1). The widest dimension is about 1 cm posterior to the rim, which corresponds to the equator of the globe. The lateral and inferolateral orbital rim is formed by the zygomatic bone. It serves as an orbital protector that can withstand significant trauma without fracturing. When fractured, step-offs may be felt at either the zygomaticomaxillary or zygomaticofrontal sutures. The medial aspect of the inferior rim is made up by the maxillary bone which joins the zygoma at the zygomaticomaxillary suture. Just medial to and below this suture is the infraorbital foramen which encloses the infraorbital nerve. The maxillary bone narrows medially as it turns superiorly to meet the maxillary process of the frontal bone. The frontal bone encompasses the superior orbital margin and extends laterally and medially to form portions of these borders. The medial superior rim contains an indentation, the supraorbital notch. Medially between the superior orbits is the smooth glabellar region. Laterally, the frontal bone meets the zygoma at the zygomaticofrontal suture.

The medial orbital rim is complicated by the nasolacrimal drainage system. The lacrimal drainage sac resides in the lacrimal fossa between the anterior and posterior lacrimal crests. The anterior crest, continuous with the inferior rim, is part of the maxillary bone, while the posterior crest is lacrimal bone and is continuous with the superior orbital rim. Thus, the definable orbital rim has been likened to a single coil of a spiral (62) with overlap at the lacrimal fossa. Anatomic anterior-posterior variation of the suture location between the maxillary and lacrimal bones leads to variable caliber of the lacrimal fossa and variable thickness of the bone.

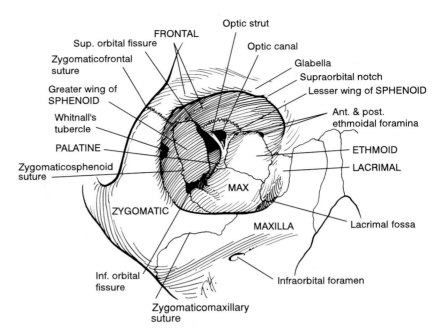

Figure 1–1.
Anterior view of the orbital skeleton and foramina.
The walls are composed of seven bones: sphenoid,
frontal, zygomatic, maxillary, palatine, ethmoid,
and lacrimal.

Orbital Walls

The orbital walls are embryologically derived from neural crest cells. Ossification is completed by birth with the exception of the orbital apex. All orbital bones are membranous with the exception of the lesser sphenoid which has an endochondral cartilaginous intermediate. Membranous bone is derived from mesenchymal cells differentiating directly into osteoblasts while endochondral bone is created from a cartilaginous anlage at a metaphyseal interface.

The triangular *orbital roof* is mainly formed by the orbital plate of the frontal bone. Typically, the roof is strong and rarely succumbs to blunt ocular trauma. The orbital roof is 3 mm thick posteriorly and is thinnest just behind the superior rim anteriorly. Posteriorly, the roof remains flat and receives a contribution from the lesser wing of the sphenoid bone. The meningeal foramen can be found near the suture between the frontal and the sphenoid bones. It conducts a lacrimal artery communication with the external carotid. The optic foramen in the orbital apex pierces the lesser wing of the sphenoid bone at a 22.5° angle from the midline (Fig 1–2.) The trochlear fossa is found in the superior anteromedial orbit while the lacrimal gland fossa is seen superiolaterally just above the frontozygomatic suture line.

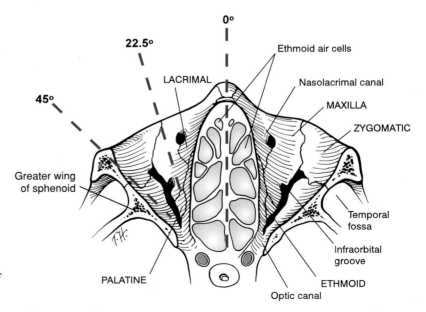

Figure 1–2.
Axial section through the orbits superior to the floor.
Medial walls are nearly parallel to the midsagittal plane
(0°) while the lateral walls diverge at 45 degrees, the
orbital axis is 22.5° divergent from midline.

The *lateral orbital wall* is bounded by the superior and inferior orbital fissures. Posteriorly, the inferior orbital fissure communicates with the pterygopalatine and infratemporal fossae. The greater wing of the sphenoid is alone in forming the posterior aspect of the lateral wall while anteriorly it is met by the zygoma and the zygomatic process of the frontal bone. The vertically oriented zygomaticosphenoid suture is a convenient breaking point for bone removal during a lateral orbitotomy. Just inside the lateral orbital rim is the lateral orbital *tubercle of Whitnall* (Fig. 1–1) where the lateral canthal ligament, lateral rectus check ligament, lateral horn of the levator, Lockwood's suspensory ligament of the eye, orbital septum, and lacrimal fascia attach (61). Whitnall's tubercle is usually the location for reattachment of tissues in the lateral tarsal strip or other lateral canthal tightening procedures.

The *orbital floor* is the shortest of the orbital walls and is shaped like an equilateral triangle. Most of the floor is composed of the orbital plate of the maxillary bone with a small contribution from the palatine bone posteriorly and the zygoma anterolaterally. The infraorbital groove arises in the orbital portion of the maxillary bone. The intracranial portion is described in the section on the orbital apex below. As it passes anteriorly, the groove becomes a canal within the maxillary bone. The infraorbital canal eventually opens through the infraorbital foramen on the anterior face of the maxilla. The infraorbital groove, canal, and foramen transmit the maxillary division of the trigeminal nerve (cranial nerve V). In childhood, the infraorbital foramen is situated immediately below the orbital rim, but as the face grows, the foramen migrates 6–10 mm below the rim. The infraorbital groove starts 2.5 to 3.0 cm posterior to the inferior orbital rim. *Blowout fractures* typically involve the medial orbital floor where the bone is thinnest. Anesthesia of the cheek secondary to trauma to the maxillary division of cranial nerve V can be caused by a fracture that disrupts the infraorbital canal.

The *medial orbital wall* is the thinnest (0.2 to 0.4 mm) and smallest. The medial wall is 4.5 to 5.0 cm in length. The ethmoid bone makes up most of the medial wall with contributions from the anterior lacrimal crest of the maxillary bone, and the posterior lacrimal crest of lacrimal bone. The medial wall thickens posteriorly near the body of the sphenoid and anteriorly near the lacrimal crests and fossa. The ethmoid bone is pneumatized (ethmoid air cells) with honeycomb-patterned bullae which act as a supportive structure (Fig. 1–2). The thinnest portion, the *lamina papyracea,* can be easily breached by inflammatory and neoplastic processes originating in the ethmoid air cells as well as by surgical dissection and trauma. The anterior and posterior ethmoidal foramina are located along the frontoethmoidal suture 20 and 35 mm posterior to the anterior lacrimal crest, respectively. These foramina convey branches of the ophthalmic artery and the nasocilliary nerve. Also, these foramina mark the horizontal level of the cribiform plate which is of critical importance during surgical decompression of the medial wall.

Orbital Apex

The orbital apex is an extremely complex anatomic region within a limited amount of space. This results from the narrowing of the bony walls and the large number of structures passing through it, including the exit of the venous channels, the entrance of the arterial vessels, numerous nerves, and the origin of five out of six extraocular muscles and the superior levator muscle (all but inferior oblique) (Fig. 1–3). The *superior orbital fissure* (2.2 cm long) is a variable transverse slit between the greater and lesser wings of the sphenoids. The superior portion of the superior orbital fissure is usually narrow and is where the lacrimal, frontal (sensory nerves) and trochlear nerve (motor nerve) enter the orbit. Structures which pass through the inferior portion of the superior orbital fissure include the superior and inferior divisions of cranial nerve III, cranial nerve VI, the ophthalmic branch of cranial nerve V (nasociliary), sympathetic nerve fibers, and the superior orbital vein. The middle meningeal artery anastomosis with the ophthalmic artery may enter here, if not through its own foramen at the frontosphenoid suture.

Enlargement of the superior orbital fissure may be the result of pathologic processes including aneurysm, meningioma, chordoma, pituitary adenoma or orbital apex tumors (48). Idiopathic inflammation of the superior orbital fissure and apex can lead to painful ophthalmoplegia known as *Tolosa Hunt syndrome*. The ophthalmoplegia is caused by inflammation of the extraocular muscle nerves while the pain is induced by inflammatory involvement of the ophthalmic division of the trigeminal nerve. Outflow obstruction of the venous channels can induce stasis edema of the lids and orbital contents resulting in proptosis of the globe.

Medial to the superior orbital fissure lies the optic foramen, which conveys the optic nerve and the ophthalmic artery with surrounding sympathetic plexus. The optic canal attains adult dimensions by age three and typically exhibits symmetry within the individual. In the adult the *optic canal* is 8–10 mm long and the optic foramen measures about 6.0 mm in diameter. Optic foramen enlargement of 7.0 mm or larger is commonly seen with optic nerve gliomas. The inferior root of the lesser wing of the sphenoid bone, and the optic strut, separates the optic foramen from the superior fissure (Fig. 1–1). This thin optic strut forming the lateral and inferior border of the optic canal is subject to deformation due to the pathologic processes just mentioned.

The *inferior orbital fissure* (2 cm long) is a bony defect between the orbital floor and the lateral wall in the pos-

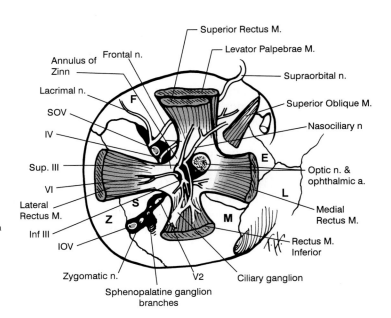

Figure 1–3.
The orbital apex with structures passing through the superior and inferior orbital fissure and the optic canal. Structures passing through the superior orbital fissure include the lacrimal nerve (sensory, V1), nasociliary nerve (sensory, V1), frontal nerve (sensory, V1), abducens nerve (VI), trochlear nerve (IV), inferior division of the oculomotor nerve (Inf III), superior division of the oculomotor nerve (Sup III), and the superior ophthalmic vein (SOV). The optic nerve passes through the optic canal with the ophthalmic artery. The zygomatic nerve, maxillary division of cranial nerve V (V2), sphenopalatine ganglion branches, and the inferior orbital vein pass through the inferior orbital fissure.

terior orbit. It is bounded by the sphenoid, maxillary, and palatine bones. The axis of the fissure is an anterior projection of the optic foramen, which deviates 38° laterally from the midsagittal plane. This fissure is an important surgical landmark since it is the posterior limit of a subperiosteal dissection along the orbital floor, and is about 20 mm posterior to the anterior orbital rim. Posterior to the infraorbital fissure the foramen rotundum pierces the greater sphenoid wing carrying the maxillary division of cranial nerve V toward the orbit. The internal maxillary artery arrives with the maxillary nerve and they become the infraorbital artery and nerve as they enter the infraorbital groove. The inferior orbital fissure also transmits the zygomatic nerve (sensory nerve), branches of the sphenopalatine ganglion (parasympathetic nerve to the lacrimal gland) and venous blood via the inferior orbital vein to the pterygoid plexus.

Annulus of Zinn

The *annulus of Zinn* is a tendinous ring that spans the optic foramen and the superior orbital fissure in the apex. The four rectus muscles arise from the annulus of Zinn (Fig. 1–3).

Nose and Paranasal Sinuses

Understanding sinus anatomy allows recognition of the surgical relationships to the orbital spaces along with understanding sinus function. The bony plates of the orbital roof, floor, and medial wall are intimately related to the nasal cavity. The frontal, maxillary, ethmoid, and sphenoid bones are pneumatized by paranasal sinuses arising from and contiguous with the nasal cavity.

The nose functions as a filtering, moisturizing air port, and a collector of sinus secretions. The nasal cav-

ity mucosa is lined by pseudostratified, ciliated columnar epithelium with copious goblet cells. The vascular mucoperiosteum of the nose is carried into the sinuses where densely populated cilia rhythmically beat mucus toward the ostium. The internal lateral nasal wall is thrown into three horizontal ridges termed turbinates, with the resultant spaces below each given corresponding names (Fig. 1–4). The inferior turbinate, a bone unto itself, arises anterior to the other turbinates and is the largest. When the external nares are dilated by a nasal speculum the inferior turbinate and the inferior meatus can be visualized by tilting the blades to look along the nasal floor. The inferior turbinate attaches to the medial aspect of the maxillary bone, while the more posterior middle, superior and the sometimes-present supreme turbinates are outcroppings of the ethmoid bone. The *nasolacrimal duct* is partially formed by and drains under the inferior turbinate (Fig. 1–5) while the anterior and middle ethmoid, frontal, and maxillary sinuses drain under the middle tubinate. The anterior and middle ethmoid air cells drain under the middle turbinate. The posterior ethmoid sinuses drain in the superior meatus. Variability exists and the previous two sinuses can be found to drain under the middle meatus.

The maxillary sinus is the largest of the paranasal sinuses. The sinus roof is the orbital floor. It is thin medially where it is most likely to fracture and thickens laterally along the course of the infraorbital canal. The medial wall of the maxillary sinus opposes the nasal cavity. The bony nasolacrimal canal lies within the medial wall anteriorly. The lateral wall of the sinus is also thin and subject to fracture with zygomatic displacement.

The ethmoid sinus is divided into anterior, middle and posterior regions based on its development relative to the middle turbinate. The anterior cells are smaller with smaller ostia and therefore more subject to occlusion from inflammation. Two important structures pro-

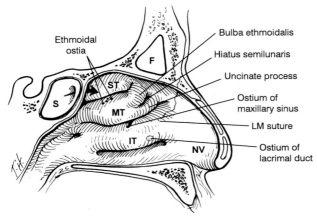

Figure 1–4.
Sagittal view of the endonasal space. Each meatal region is named for the turbinate that lies above. Superior turbinate (ST), maxillary sinus ostium, middle turbinate (MT), nasal vestibule (NV), inferior turbinate (IT), ostium of the nasal lacrimal duct, sphenoid sinus (S), hiatus semilunaris, frontal sinus (F), and uncinate process. LM = lacrimal maxillary.

ject vertically from the ethmoid bone. The crista galli superiorly bisects the cribiform plate and continues inferiorly as the vomer. The ethmoid sinuses are the most exuberant in their growth pattern and can pneumatize the frontal, sphenoid, palatine, and lacrimal bones. Three to 15 air cells expand from each lateral border of the cribiform plate. Convolutions on the medial aspect of each air cell mass form the middle, superior and supreme (if present) turbinates.

The frontal sinuses are found in the anterior, inferior, and medial aspects of the frontal bone. Development is not complete until adulthood. The sinuses can develop asymmetrically and vary in size and shape with greater development in the male. The two sinuses are separated in the midline by the intersinus septum. The frontal sinus is particularly prone to mucocele formation (50).

The sphenoid sinus also continues to develop until adulthood. A midline septum divides the sinus into asymmetric parts. Ethmoid air cells that articulate with

Figure 1–5a.
Nasolacrimal excretory system with a portion of the maxillary bone removed. The nasolacrimal duct can be seen emptying under the inferior turbinate in the lateral nose.

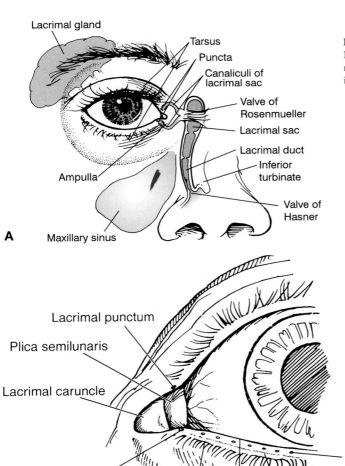

Figure 1–5b.
Drawing of medial canthal area showing lacrimal caruncle, lacrimal punctum orifice of meibomian glands and gray line. Note that the gray line is just anterior to the meibomian gland orifices.

the anterior sphenoid bone may actually pneumatize the sphenoid and are called Onadi cells. When the sphenoid sinus body is nearly replaced by air cells, only a thin layer of bone, periosteum and mucous epithe- lium separate the respiratory tract from the internal carotid, cavernous sinus and cranial nerve V. Thus, sphenoid sinusitis can be devastating and early treat- ment is imperative.

■ EYELIDS

Relation to the Face

The eyelids represent specialized structures of the face designed to protect, moisten, and cleanse the ocular surfaces (Figures 1–6 and 1–7).

Eyebrow

The eyebrow represents a specialized area where the frontalis muscle and the orbicularis muscle planes in- terdigitate (Fig. 1–6) (35). Frontalis muscle contraction elevates the eyebrow, while forced orbicularis contrac- tion causes depression. The bilateral corrugator super- ciliaris muscles arise from the superomedial orbital mar- gin and extend superiorly and laterally to insert in the muscle and skin of the medial eyebrow. Corrugator con- traction creates a depression over the medial eyebrow and depresses it toward the midline. The procerus mus- cle overlying the glabella is continuous with the frontalis. Contraction of the procerus lowers the central forehead and results in a horizontal crease in the glabel- lar region. The eyebrow skin is thick, and contain a dense subcutaneous fibroadipose layer. Large hair folli- cles are present with associated sweat and sebaceous glands.

Over the forehead, the galea aponeurotica encases the frontalis muscle (Fig. 1–7a). The superficial galea anteriorly separates the skin/subcutaneous layer from the frontalis muscle while the deep galea is posteriorly interspersed between the frontalis muscle and the pe- riosteum of the frontal bone. Inferiorly, over the supe- rior orbital rim, the posterior galea divides once again in order to envelope the eyebrow fat pad (Figures 1–8 and 1–9). The posterior deep galea has firm attach- ments to the supraorbital ridge of the frontal bone. These attachments are less dense laterally and this in part explains why *eyebrow ptosis* (drooping of brow) oc- curs first in the lateral region (34). Anteriorly, the frontalis muscle fibers interdigitate with the orbicularis oculi muscle.

Malar Region

The malar region, commonly known as the cheek, has distinct cutaneous boundaries. The medial extent is lim- ited by the base of the nose and the nasolabial fold while the superior limits are demarcated by skin folds. The curvilinear superior demarcation consists of the nasoju- gal fold which runs from the medial canthal area infer- olaterally and is continuous with the malar crease which turns superolaterally toward the lateral canthus. The malar crease is the junction between the orbicularis muscle and the malar fat. These creases also form the in- ferior border of the lower eyelid, and are created by the orbitomalar ligament connecting the SMAS (see below)

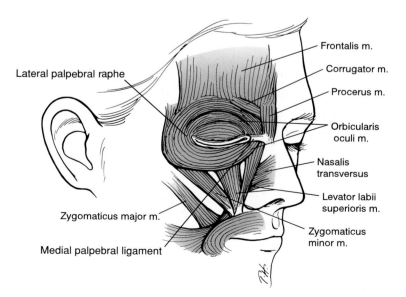

Frontalis m.

Corrugator m.

Procerus m.

Orbicularis oculi m.

Nasalis transversus

Levator labii superioris m.

Zygomaticus minor m.

Lateral palpebral raphe

Zygomaticus major m.

Medial palpebral ligament

Figure 1–6.
Muscles of the superficial face associated with facial expression. These muscles are innervated by different branches of the facial nerve (motor, VII). The orbicularis muscle produces eyelid closure.

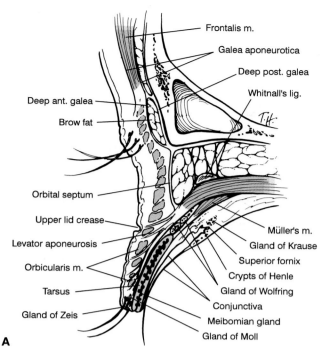

A

- Frontalis m.
- Galea aponeurotica
- Deep post. galea
- Whitnall's lig.
- Deep ant. galea
- Brow fat
- Orbital septum
- Upper lid crease
- Levator aponeurosis
- Orbicularis m.
- Tarsus
- Gland of Zeis
- Müller's m.
- Gland of Krause
- Superior fornix
- Crypts of Henle
- Gland of Wolfring
- Conjunctiva
- Meibomian gland
- Gland of Moll

Figure 1–7a.
Sagittal section of the upper lid containing the various tear secreting glands along with the eyebrow and the superior fornix. The basal secretory tear glands reside near the surface of the posterior eyelid, in addition to the eyelid margin and the superior fornix.

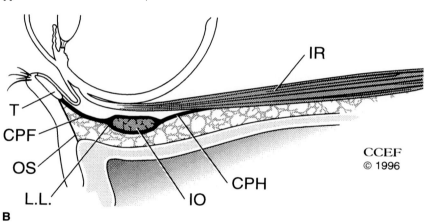

B

- IR
- T
- CPF
- OS
- L.L.
- IO
- CPH
- CCEF
- © 1996

Figure 1–7b.
Sagittal section of the lower lid showing the lower lid retractors. The capsule palpebral fascia (CPF) extends from the tarsus (T) to the inferior oblique muscle (IO). The capsule palperabral head (CPH) extends from the inferior rectus muscle (IR) to envelop the inferior oblique muscle. The fascia at the anterior junction of the capsule palpebral fascia and capsule palpebral head is termed Lockwood's suspensory ligament. The *inferior tarsal muscle* which is not shown is a very diaphanous muscle which is found within the lower lid retractors (CPF and CPH). Orbital septum (OS) is seen extending from the tarsus to the orbital rim.

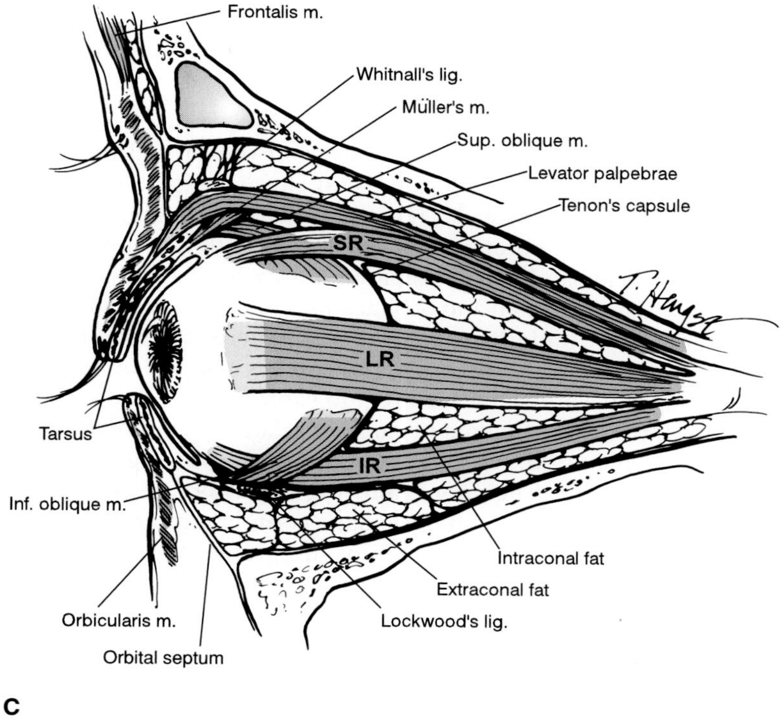

Figure 1–7c.
Sagittal section of the eyebrow, upper and lower eyelid, as well as the globe and the extraocular muscles within the orbit.

C

- Frontalis m.
- Whitnall's lig.
- Müller's m.
- Sup. oblique m.
- Levator palpebrae
- Tenon's capsule
- SR
- LR
- IR
- Tarsus
- Inf. oblique m.
- Orbicularis m.
- Orbital septum
- Lockwood's lig.
- Extraconal fat
- Intraconal fat

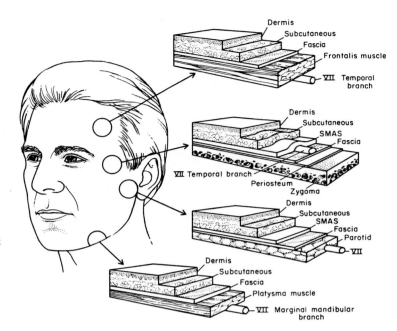

Figure 1–8.
Cross-sectional anatomy of facial soft tissue layers. Note that the SMAS is a mid-face structure. The facial nerve (motor) runs through this region and is at risk of being cut during facial surgery. Modified from May M, Sobol SM, Mester SJ: Laryngoscope In: Summers BK, Siegle RJ: Facial cutaneous reconstructive surgery: Facial flaps. J Am Acad Dermatol 1993;29:918.

to the inferior orbital rim. Eyelid edema extends inferiorly to, but usually not below these folds. The inferomedial border of the malar region is called the nasolabial fold; it runs from the ala of the nose to the angle of the mouth in a linear direction. This fold is created by fibrous adhesions to the maxillary bone and is the inferior border of the malar fat pad (65). The angular vessels run within this fold. The lateral extent of the malar region is the preauricular region.

The bony aspects of the malar region include components of the maxillary and zygomatic bones. Laterally the zygomatic bone forms the zygomatic arch along with its frontal process and anterior aspect where it interfaces with the maxilla. Anteriorly, the malar region overlies the anterior superior aspect of the maxilla (61).

Superficial Musculoaponeurotic System

The superficial musculoaponeurotic system (SMAS) is a soft tissue layer deep to the skin and subcutaneous layers that envelopes the head, with regional variations in its connections to the skin and to the underlying skeletal apparatus (Fig. 1–8). The SMAS is anatomically complex in the ocular region and serves to support the soft tissues of the malar, zygomatic arch and parotid regions. This discrete fascial layer was described in 1974 and functions to support and divide the subcutaneous fat into two distinct layers (39). Its clinical importance relates to its function as a dissection plane for face lifts (facial rhytidectomy) and its clinical relationship to the eyelids and brow.

The lateral extent of the SMAS is the parotid gland fascia (16) while medially it extends to the orbicularis

oculi and the nasolabial fold. The orbicularis oculi muscle, is a local SMAS modification, covers the orbital aperture while inserting within the orbital rim in a complex fashion. The fibers close to the lid margin are fine and densely distributed while the peripheral fibers are coarse and loosely distributed. The central fibers encircle the palpebral fissure in a parallel and concentric fashion, while the lateral fibers splaying tangentially may be important in the creation of the horizontal skin wrinkles at the lateral canthus. Superiorly, the orbicularis oculi lies in direct contact with the dermis and represent the only facial location where the SMAS is not covered by the septated fatty subcutaneous layer.

Orbicularis Muscle

The orbicularis muscle (protractor muscle) is the superficial muscle plane covering the orbital opening, and is responsible for eyelid closure (Fig. 1–6). There are three muscular regions: pretarsal, preseptal, and orbital. The pretarsal orbicularis is tightly adherent to the tarsus and can be separated only by sharp dissection. The preseptal and orbital components are less adherent to the underlying tissues except where they are attached to bone. The preseptal portion lies over the orbital septum while the orbital region extends beyond the orbital rim. Attachments occur at the lateral palpebral raphe (at lateral canthus), the supraorbital ridge, medial palpebral ligament, and the malar crease inferiorly. Gentle, unforced orbicularis contraction results in eyelid closure through use of the pretarsal and preseptal components. With forceful eyelid closure, there is increased function and centripetal overriding of the pre-

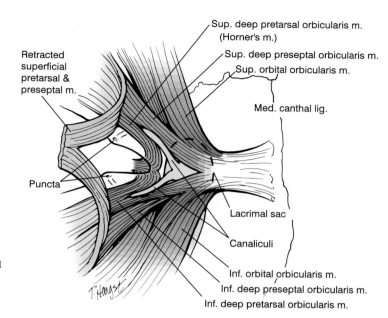

Retracted
superficial
pretarsal &
preseptal m.

Sup. deep pretarsal orbicularis m.
(Horner's m.)

Sup. deep preseptal orbicularis m.

Sup. orbital orbicularis m.

Med. canthal lig.

Puncta

Lacrimal sac

Canaliculi

Inf. orbital orbicularis m.

Inf. deep preseptal orbicularis m.

Inf. deep pretarsal orbicularis m.

Figure 1–9.
Medial canthal ligament attachments encircling the lacrimal sac (dotted line). Eyelid closure causes the lower lid to move toward the nasolacrimal sac, thereby compressing the sac and forcing tears into the nose. Opening of the eyelids cause negative pressure in the nasolacrimal sac which draws tears into it from the palpebral fissure.

septal and the orbital components. *Riolan's muscle* is a small part of the orbicularis muscle found along the eyelid margin. It is separated from the pretarsal fibers by the eyelash follicles. This strip of orbicularis muscle represents the *eyelid margin* grayline (Fig. 1–5B) (63).

Medially, the deep orbicularis insertions are complicated by the anatomy of the nasolacrimal excretory system (Fig 1–9). Pretarsal and preseptal orbicularis muscles have insertions deep to the medial orbital rim, which allow a posterior and medial pull on the eyelids. The deep pretarsal heads insert on the posterior lacrimal crest and lacrimal fascia, while the deep preseptal fibers (*Horner's muscle*) insert more peripherally on the lacrimal fascia. The *medial and lateral canthal ligaments* are fibrous connections from the medial and lateral tarsus to the orbital rims, respectively. The medial canthal ligament has two limbs that extend from the medial tarsus. The superficial limb connects to the frontal process of the maxilla and the frontal bone. The deep limb of the medial canthal ligament inserts across the lacrimal fascia posteriorly to the posterior lacrimal crest. The deep fibers serve as the anterior border of the deep pretarsal muscles (Horner's muscle).

At the lateral canthus, the superficial preseptal and orbital orbicularis fibers pass uninterrupted across the orbital rim and attach on the deep underside to the zygoma along a horizontal line termed the *lateral palpebral raphe*. The deep pretarsal muscle inserts about 4 mm deep within the lateral orbit to the lateral palpebral raphe at the *lateral orbital tubercle* (*Whitnall's tubercle*). The lateral canthal ligament also connects the lateral tarsus to the lateral orbital tubercle. Other insertions to

the lateral orbital tubercle include the orbital septum, the lateral levator horn, the lacrimal gland fascia, Whitnall's ligament, Lockwood's ligament, and the lateral rectus check ligament.

Lacrimal Pump

Understanding the function of the medial deep pretarsal orbicularis muscle is accomplished by understanding the complex anatomy (Figures 1–5 and 1–9). The path for tears to travel from the eye into the nose begins at the punctum, a 2 mm vertical channel, and continues into the horizontal canaliculus toward the nose. The upper and lower canaliculi drain either via a common canaliculus or directly into the lacrimal sac. The relationship of these structures to the orbicularis muscle provides functional drainage of tears. The posterior insertion of the deep pretarsal orbicularis muscle along the lacrimal fascia and the posterior lacrimal crest provides a posterior anchor which opposes the eyelids to the convex globe. Contraction of the muscle draws the eyelids (mainly the lower) medially and posteriorly. This compresses the nasolacrimal sac and forces tears into the nose. The *valve of Rosenmueller* is located at the junction of the canaliculi and sacrimal Sac (Fig. 1–5A) and deters retrograde flow from the sac back towards the eye. Upon opening the eyes, the resultant lateral pull on the lacrimal diaphragm results in a negative pressure in the lacrimal sac that draws the tears from the canaliculi toward the sac. Additional tear movement is created by the pretarsal muscle which encases the lacrimal ampullae at the medial extents of the tarsal plates. The fluid in them is pushed toward the sac by the muscle compression and shortening. This phenomenon has been termed the lacrimal pump. Any weakening of the eyelid muscles can cause *epiphora* because of an ineffective lacrimal pump, despite normal punctum position. Increased laxity, caused by elongation of the tarsus or the medial or lateral canthal ligaments, can result in frank ectropion (See chapter 24).

Eyelid Lamellae

Skin

Eyelid skin histologically consists of two layers: epidermis (keratinized squamous epithelium), and the dermis. The epidermis is replete with the usual five layers found in skin in other regions of the body. The layers from superficial to deep are the stratum corneum, the stratum lucidum, the stratum granulosum, the stratum malpighii, and the stratum germinativum. The dermis is the inner layer and the major constituent is the structural protein, collagen. The eyelid dermis is thin leading to minimal scarring following surgery or trauma but this makes it difficult to match for lid skin grafts. Sebaceous glands, hair follicles, apocrine units and eccrine sweat glands reside in the dermis.

In both the upper and lower eyelids, the pretarsal tissues are firmly adherent to the underlying tissues, compared to the preseptal tissues which are more loosely attached, creating a potential space for fluid accumulation. The upper eyelid crease reflects the attachment of the levator aponeurosis to the pretarsal orbicularis fibers and skin at the superior border of the tarsus (Fig. 1–7A). The upper eyelid crease is more inferior in Asians due to the fusion of the orbital septum with levator aponeurosis between the lid margin and the superior border of the tarsus. This anatomic difference also allows the preaponeurotic fat to occupy a position more inferiorly and anteriorly in the upper eyelid which creates a fuller appearing upper eyelid skin fold in Asians. The skin just superior to the upper eyelid crease is the superior eyelid skin fold. The lower eyelid crease is less well defined compared to that of the upper eyelid. The commissures are the junction points between the upper and lower eyelids where they meet laterally and medially, whereas the medial and lateral canthi are the angles formed by the eyelids at the commissures.

The skin of the eyelids is thin and subjected to constant movement with each blink. Thus, the laxity that occurs with age is not unexpected. The upper eyelid skin fold assumes a greater proportion of area with the loss of age-related skin elasticity.

Wound healing of the skin of the eyelid is rapid secondary to the rich vascular blood supply. This is also beneficial in minimizing infection following trauma or surgery.

Subcutaneous Layer

The subcutaneous layer is a variable mixture of lobules of fat cells separated by fibrous septa composed of collagen and blood vessels. Subcutaneous fat is sparse in the preorbital and preseptal region and absent beneath the pretarsal skin, leading to minimal scarring.

Eyelid Muscles

The muscles of the eyelids are divided into two groups according to their function. The first group closes the eyelids and are termed protractors; the second group opens the eyelids and are called the retractors (Figures 1–6, 1–7a, and 1–7b).

The *orbicularis oculi muscle* is the protractor of the eyelids (see p. 10, Orbicularis muscle above). Contraction of this muscle narrows the palpebral fissure and contributes to the *lacrimal pump*. It is innervated by cranial nerve VII (motor). The skin, the subcutaneous layer and the orbicularis oculi muscle constitute the *anterior surgical lamellae* of the eyelid.

The retractors of the eyelids widen the palpebral fissure upon contraction (Fig. 1–7). The upper eyelid retractors are the *levator palpebrae* muscle, continuous with its aponeurosis, and the sympathetically innervated superior tarsal muscle called *Müller's muscle*. In the lower eyelid the retractors are extensions of the inferior rectus muscle termed the *capsulopalpebral fascia, capsulopalpebral head,* and the *inferior tarsal muscle* (Fig 1–7b) (21). The developed levator palpebrae and Müller's muscle provide great vertical mobility to the upper eyelid. With blinking, the lower eyelid does not move appreciably in the vertical direction, but rather nasally. The extensions to the lower eyelid from the inferior rectus are smaller and serve to depress the eyelid several millimeters in downgaze to avoid obstruction of the vision.

The origin of the levator muscle arises from the lesser wing of the sphenoid bone above the annulus of Zinn (Figures 1–1 and 1–3). The origin is lateral to the origin of the superior oblique and superior to the superior rectus. The levator travels anteriorly along the superior orbit with the supraorbital artery and the frontal and supratrochlear nerves. The superior rectus muscle lies beneath the levator, upon which it rests. These muscles can be easily divided except where they are attached along their medial edge by a fascial connection. Both muscles are innervated by the superior division of cranial nerve III which enters the muscles about 12 mm anterior to the orbital apex. The innervation of all the extraocular muscles is on the bulbar aspect at the junction of the posterior one-third and the anterior two-thirds.

Just behind the superior orbital rim a fibrous transverse condensation attaches superiorly to the edges of the widening levator. The fibrous condensation is the superior transverse ligament (*Whitnall's ligament*) which extends from the fascia of the trochlea across laterally to the lacrimal gland capsule and the lateral orbital tubercle (frontal process zygoma). It has been referred to as a support ligament of the upper eyelid and a check ligament of the levator because it limits the posterior pull of the muscle. At the superior transverse ligament, the levator changes from a fleshy muscle posteriorly to a fibrous aponeurotic sheath (*levator aponeurosis*) anteriorly. The superior transverse ligament has recently been shown on MRI scanning to cause a superior hitch in the course of the levator in its function as a swinging suspender of that structure (15).

The *levator aponeurosis* is 14–20 mm in length and divides into anterior and posterior components as it approaches the tarsus. The anterior component is composed of fine aponeurotic lamellae that insert into the connective tissue strands between the pretarsal orbicularis muscle bundles (Fig. 1–7A) (56). The upper eyelid crease is created by the uppermost of these attachments. Levator aponeurotic disinsertion is the primary cause of *acquired senile or traumatic ptosis*. The lid crease becomes elevated with the disinsertion of these anterior levator aponeurotic insertional fibers. The terminal fibers exhibit a high degree of elasticity which are known to fracture with aging. The posterior component of the aponeurosis inserts firmly onto the anterior surface of the lower one-third of the tarsus. The firmest attachment is about 3 mm above the eyelid margin with less firm attachments superiorly.

In addition to the tarsal insertions, the levator aponeurosis expands into a broad, fibrous sheet which inserts into the lateral aspect of the orbital rim. This occurs behind the medial and lateral commissures of the eye. The commissures are the junction points between the upper and lower eyelids where they meet medially and laterally. The *canthi* are the angles formed by the eyelids at these commissures. The osseous insertions are termed the *medial and lateral horns* of the levator. The levator horns are situated inferior to the extremities of the Whitnall's transverse suspensory ligament and the two structures can be confused during surgery. The lateral horn is a strong, fibrous band that incompletely divides the lacrimal gland into two lobes. It continues inferiorly to insert on the lateral orbital tubercle and to the lateral canthal ligament. The medial horn is thin and filmy as it passes around the traversing superior oblique tendon and inferiorly to reach the medial canthal ligament and the posterior lacrimal crest. This insertion is less dense medially allowing greater mobility of the medial aspect of the upper lid.

The *superior tarsal muscle* of *Müller* arises from the underside of the levator muscle about 14 mm above the superior tarsal border. It inserts on the posterior aspect of the superior tarsal border and is easily separated from the levator except at the origin. The space between the levator and Müller's muscle is called the postaponeurotic space. Disruption of sympathetic innervation to Müller's muscle results in 2 mm of Horner's blepharoptosis. Müller's muscle is firmly adherent to the conjunctiva especially at the superior tarsal border. The peripheral palpebral arterial arcade is located at the superior tarsal border adjacent to Müller's muscle.

Lower eyelid depression in downgaze represents the extent of vertical movement of the lower lid. This motor action is secondary to palpebral extensions from the inferior rectus muscle. The inferior rectus muscle sends off a capsulopalpebral head that splits to encompass the inferior oblique muscle (Fig. 1–7B). The external inferior part of the split is a thin fibrous layer while the bulbar portion thickens and contains smooth muscle cells. These two layers fuse anterior to the inferior oblique muscle to form the suspensory *ligament of Lockwood* (22). Lockwood's suspensory ligament is a hammock-like structure extending to the medial and lateral orbital walls. This structure often will support the globe following maxillectomy with removal of the orbital floor as long as the attachments are not disturbed. This ligament is responsible for maintaining globe position relative to the orbit. The capsulopalpebral fascia's innermost head inserts to Tenon's fascia and the conjunctival cul-de-sac, and the outermost head penetrates the orbital septum 4 mm below the tarsus then terminates in the orbicularis and skin. Recession of the inferior rectus muscle results in lower eyelid retraction if these attachments are not severed.

Posterior Orbicularis Fascia

The fascia of the orbit can be divided into three parts that include the fascia covering the globe (*Tenon's fascia*), the extraocular muscle coverings (*intermuscular septum*) and the *check ligament* extensions of the extraocular muscle fascia that reach to the surrounding bone and eyelids. This discussion will be limited to the latter two components with emphasis on the relationship to the eyelids. The Tenon's bulbar fascia will be discussed in the globe section.

Each extraocular muscle sheath sends extensions to the orbital walls. Anteriorly they become prominent and are designated as check ligaments. The medial and lateral rectus check ligaments are the best developed. The lateral check ligament is the strongest and inserts on the posterior aspect of *Whitnall's lateral orbital tubercle* with minor contributions to the lateral conjunctival fornix and to the lateral orbital septum. The medial check ligament inserts on the lacrimal bone behind the posterior lacrimal crest and to the medial orbital septum, caruncle, and plica semilunaris. The superior rectus muscle sheath coalesces anteriorly with that of the levator palpebral superioris muscle (36). The *superior transverse ligament* (*Whitnall's ligament*) functions as a superior check ligament by resisting further elevation of the upper lid and suspends the levator muscle. The fused inferior rectus and inferior oblique muscle sheaths have fascial attachments to the inferior periorbita for possible checking function.

Orbital Septum

The orbit lies behind the orbital septum, which is the deepest layer of the superficial fascia covering the orbital opening (Fig. 1–7). Medially, the septum covers the posterior aspect of Horner's muscle as it inserts on the posterior lacrimal crest. At the lateral canthus, the septum attaches to the lateral orbital rim.

The septum inserts on the inferior tarsus after joining the lower eyelid retractors 4 to 5 mm below this structure. The superior orbital septum does not gain access to the superior tarsal plate due to the intervening levator aponeurosis. The septum inserts on the aponeurosis about 10 mm above the superior eyelid margin. A considerable amount of variation in the septum exists between individuals. With age, the septum attenuates, allowing orbital fat to herniate forward.

During surgical dissection the septum can be identified by tugging on it and feeling a firm attachment to the orbital rim. The septum is routinely violated during levator surgery and blepharoplasty. The preaponeurotic fat is located immediately posterior to the septum.

Preseptal cellulitis is an infectious process anterior to the septum whereas an orbital cellulitis is an infection posterior to the septum involving the orbital contents (see Chapter 25).

Tarsal Plates

The tarsal plates are firm dense fibrous connective tissue structures (not cartilage) that provide the eyelids with a strong structural integrity. The lid marginal aspect of the tarsal plate is nearly flat while the tarsal edge opposite the margin tapers convexly away from the margin. The upper eyelid tarsus is about 10 mm in vertical dimension centrally while the lower eyelid tarsus has a vertical height of about 4 mm. The disparity in their dimensions reflects their contribution in covering the globe anteriorly. The tarsal plates have fibrous extensions that emanate from their medial and lateral aspects which connect to the orbital rims and are called "canthal ligaments". The orbicularis is densely fixed to the entire anterior surface of the inferior tarsal plate. In the upper lid, the situation is different because of the intervening levator aponeurosis insertion in the upper lid. The levator is connected to the orbicularis muscle by an elastic fiber network (56). A small region of the anterior inferior aspect of the tarsus in the upper eyelid is affixed

to the orbicularis muscle by the same elastic fiber network. At the lid crease, the elastic fiber network penetrates the orbicularis muscle to attach directly to the skin thereby creating the crease. The posterior aspects of all tarsal plates are lined by firmly adherent conjunctiva that continues to the mucocutaneous junction (grey line) (63).

Lacrimal and Accessory Glands

The eyelids contain several specialized glands that secrete components for the tear layer (Fig. 1–7a). The tear layer consists 3 components, 1. surface oils secreted by the *Meibomian, Moll* and *Zeis glands*, 2. aqueous part that is produced by the main lacrimal gland and the accessory lacrimal glands of *Krause* and *Wolfring*, and 3. basal mucinous layer produced by the conjunctival *goblet cells*. The tear layer acts as a protective and lubricating mechanism for the eye along with being the first refractive medium of the eye.

The glands responsible for the *lipid layer* are the meibomian glands, the glands of Zeis and the glands of Moll. This layer is responsible for limiting the amount of evaporation of the aqueous layer. It is about 0.1 microns thick. The *meibomian gland* is a branched acinar gland containing a long central duct extending the vertical height of the tarsal plate. The ductal epithelium is keratinized. The glands number approximately 25 in the upper tarsus and 10 in the lower tarsus and are of the sebaceous type. The orifices of these glands are located just anterior to the mucocutaneous junction (Fig. 1–5B). The meibomian glands expand in height, width and diameter along with tarsal plate growth. The *gland of Zeis* are also sebaceous glands that empty into each of the follicles of the cilia. The cilia number approximately 100 in the upper lid and 50 in the lower lid. Sebaceous glands (Meibomian and Zeis) are holocrine in nature which signifies excretion of the fat content along with the entire cell as they turn over. In contrast, the *gland of Moll* is an apocrine spiral sweat gland that secretes a fatty component with only the pinched off apical portion of each cell. This gland terminates on either the eyelid margin, a sebaceous gland, or a ciliary follicle.

The *aqueous-producing glands* have two functional varieties. Some divide these glands into basic secretors and reflex secretors. The accessory lacrimal *glands of Krause* (fornix) and *Wolfring* (superior tarsal border) are believed to be basic secretors along with the mucin and oil glands. The accessory lacrimal glands located in both the upper and lower lids have been thought to provide the aqueous component of the tear layer under ordinary condition (26). The accessory lacrimal glands of Krause and Wolfring are architecturally similar to the main lacrimal gland. The orbital and palpebral lobes of the main lacrimal gland were thought to participate in reflex tearing but removal of them can produce *kerato-*

conjunctivitis sicca even with normal accessory lacrimal glands. Many tests of volume production and composition of tears exist. Commonly used clinical determinations can be done by performing Schirmer tests and tear breakup times. The aqueous layer is typically about 6 microns thick.

The main *lacrimal gland* is a bean-shaped structure located in the superior temporal orbit (Fig. 1–5). It resides in the shallow lacrimal fossa in the frontal bone. The gland is divided into two lobes, orbital and palpebral, by the lateral horn of the levator aponeurosis and the underlying Müller's muscle. Division of the two lobes is incomplete with a posterior attachment between them. The orbital lobe conforms to a space between the orbital wall and the globe. This lobe is bound by the orbital septum and the preaponeurotic fat pad in front, the orbital fat posteriorly, medially by the superior and lateral rectus intermuscular septum and laterally by bone. The palpebral lobe lies below the levator aponeurosis. It is separated from the conjunctiva only medially where Müller's muscle intervenes. The gland is supported by the conjunctiva, the intermuscular septum, the lacrimal fascia connected to Whitnall's ligament and by the lateral horn of the aponeurosis. Secretory ducts from the lacrimal gland drain into the superotemporal conjunctival fornix. The orbital lobe secretory ducts pass through the parenchyma of the palpebral lobe or remain tightly bound to its capsule. Histologically, the acini are made up of a basal myoepithelial cell layer with inner columnar secretory cells. The columnar cells produce the aqueous component that is pushed by the myoepithelial cells toward the ducts for expression onto the ocular surface.

The arterial blood supply of the lacrimal gland is from the lacrimal branch of the ophthalmic artery. This artery passes through the gland to also provide the blood supply to the upper and lower temporal lids. The lacrimal vein follows a similar course as the artery and drains into the superior ophthalmic vein.

The innervation of the lacrimal gland is from cranial nerves V (trigeminal) and VII (facial) as well as from the superior cervical ganglion sympathetics. The lacrimal nerve (cranial nerve V_1) supplies the sensory component of the conjunctiva and skin around the lacrimal gland and carries postganglionic parasympathetic fibers for reflex lacrimation. Higher level control of lacrimation comes from descending autonomic pathways from the hypothalamus (emotional crying) and the olfactory system (tearing to smell) to the lacrimal nucleus. Irritation of the conjunctiva or cornea causes reflex lacrimation as afferent sensory pathways from the ophthalmic and maxillary divisions of the trigeminal nerve stimulate the trigeminal sensory nuclei which in turn stimulate the lacrimal nucleus (pons) by way of internuncial neurons. The efferent preganglion fibers from the lacrimal nucleus join the nervus intermedius (sensory root of cranial nerve VII). They exit the pons and pass into the internal auditory canal, through the geniculate ganglion in the petrous pyramid and forward as the greater superficial petrosal nerve. This nerve enters the vidian canal and joins the deep petrosal nerve to become the *vidian nerve*. This enters and synapses in the sphenopalatine ganglion then passes to the infraorbital nerve (V_2) which gives off postganglionic fibers to the lacrimal nerve. The lacrimal nerve (V_1) is sensory in nature but provides the main secretomotor function. The sympathetics are thought to stimulate basal secretion. *Crocodile tears* is tearing on gustatory stimulation caused by aberent innervation of the lacrimal gland by the nerve to the salivary glands. It is usually secondary to facial nerve injury and misdirection of salivary fibers to the greater superficial petrosal nerve.

Lid Nerve Supply

The innervation of the eyelids includes the facial nerve (motor), the oculomotor nerve (motor), the ophthalmic and maxillary divisions of the trigeminal nerve (sensory) and the sympathetics from the superior cervical ganglion.

The facial nerve (VII) exits the pons to enter the temporal bone at the internal acoustic meatus along with the sensory nervus intermedius and the acoustic nerve. It leaves via the facial canal posterior to the styloid process at the stylomastoid foramen. It passes anteriorly to the parotid gland where it divides numerous times. The five main divisions include the temporal, zygomatic, buccal, mandibular and the cervical (Fig. 1–10). The orbicularis is served by the temporal, zygomatic, and buccal divisions with extensive interdigitation between them. The nerve lies beneath the orbicularis and the other muscles of the superficial plane that it serves. The procerus innervation (motor nerve from C.N. VII) passes inferior to the eye before it ascends adjacent to the nose, while the corrugator nerve (motor nerve from C.N. VII) may pass either below or above the eye. The procerus and corrugator muscles serve facial expression of the central brow region. Damage to the central facial nerve or to the temporal or zygomatic branches may result in lagophthalmos with resultant ocular drying, infection, and ultimately corneal perforation.

The superior division of the oculomotor nerve (III) supplies the levator to retract the upper eyelid. The inferior division innervates the capsulopalpebral fascia that acts to retract the lower eyelid.

Two sensory branches of the trigeminal nerve (V) pass through the orbit from the trigeminal ganglion to reach the face. The ophthalmic and maxillary nerves supply the cutaneous branches to the eyelids. There is overlap along the naso-orbital valley and the lateral canthus. The ophthalmic nerve innervates the ipsilateral

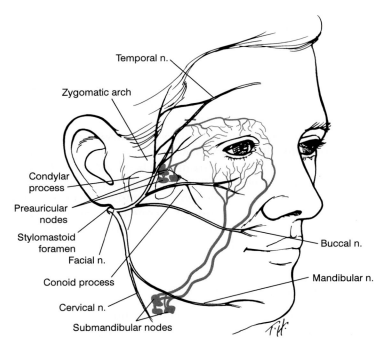

Temporal n.

Zygomatic arch

Condylar process

Preauricular nodes

Stylomastoid foramen

Facial n.

Conoid process

Cervical n.

Submandibular nodes

Buccal n.

Mandibular n.

Figure 1–10.
The distribution of the five branches of the peripheral facial nerve and their association to the facial skeleton. Also, note the superficial distribution of the lymphatic drainage from the periorbital region and associated lymph nodes. From Basic Science and Clinical Science. San Francisco: American Academy of Ophthalmology, 1993, booklet #7.

scalp, forehead, upper eyelid and the medial and lateral canthi. The maxillary nerve innervates the ipsilateral temporal scalp, lateral canthus, the lower eyelid, malar region, the nasolabial fold, and the upper lip.

The sympathetic nerves supply the superior (*Müller's muscle*) and inferior tarsal muscles. Disruption of the superior cervical sympathetic chain results in *Horner's syndrome* causing an upper lid blepharoptosis, slight elevation of the lower eyelid (*reverse ptosis*) and a miotic pupil. The upper lid ptosis is typically 2 mm secondary to loss of sympathetic tone to Müller muscle side. The pathway of the sympathetics is via the oculomotor nerve, the divisions of the orbital arteries and along the trigeminal branches.

Eyelid Circulation

The arterial blood supply of the eyelids is derived from the internal and external carotid arteries. Ultimately these two arterial systems have several anastomoses in and around the eyelids (Fig. 1–11).

The external carotid artery supplies the facial artery, transverse facial artery, and superficial temple artery which supply the medial, inferior temporal, and superior temporal aspect of the lids respectively. The facial artery courses superior-nasally crossing the mandible diagonally to become the angular artery as it lies between the nose and the lower lid. The angular artery is quite superficial at the medial canthus and perforates the orbital septum just superiorly to the medial canthal ligament to anastomosis with branches of the ophthalmic artery. The superficial temporal artery is important in

the diagnosis of giant cell arteritis as it is the most common site for arterial biopsy used to verify the diagnosis. Periocular cutaneous contributions of the internal carotid artery via the ophthalmic artery include the lacrimal artery, supraorbital artery, supratrochlear artery and the medial palpebral arteries. The lacrimal artery branches into the zygomaticofacial artery. These deep orbital vessels which are derived from the ophthalmic artery surface to anastomose with the superficial temporal artery, transverse facial artery and angular artery all which come from external carotid artery.

The main arteries of the upper eyelids are the marginal and peripheral tarsal arcades. These arcades are derived from deep anastomoses between the lacrimal branches and the medial palpebral artery. The marginal arcade lies on the anterior tarsal surface near the eyelid margin and must be respected during reconstructive tarsal procedures. The peripheral arcade lies on the superior aspect of the tarsus. The peripheral arcade supplies the superior conjunctival fornix and communicates with the anterior ciliary arteries near the limbus.

The lower eyelid has a lesser developed double inferior marginal arcade which connects with zygomatical facial artery, medial palpebral artery and a branch of the superficial temporal artery. The rich blood supply to the upper and lower lid accounts for the dramatic bleeding which occurs following an eyelid laceration. Because of the various anastomoses and vascular arcades, bleeding can be difficult to stop and requires immediate direct pressure.

The venous system is formed by anastomoses between the superficial and deep orbital systems. The main superficial venous structure is the facial vein. It arises from the medial eyebrow as a confluence of the frontal and supraorbital veins. Along the medial canthus the facial vein is called the angular vein. The angular vein forms important anastomes to the superior orbital vein within the orbit via the supraorbital vein. This is the route superficial infections follow to cause *cavernous sinus thrombosis*. The supraorbital vein forms a deep preauricular plexus lateral to the lateral canthus beneath the orbicularis and joins the superficial temporal vein. The facial vein follows the same course to the artery, but it is more superficial and lateral. Another superficial to deep communication exists between the facial vein and the pterygoid plexus via the deep facial vein. The pterygoid plexus communicates with the cavernous sinus through branches traversing the inferior orbital fissure to the inferior orbital vein.

Eyelid Lymphatic Drainage

The lymphatic system of the eyelids occurs via a medial and lateral system that drain to the submandibular and superficial preauricular nodes, respectively (Fig. 1–10). The preauricular nodes can then drain into the deeper cervical nodes. The importance of the lymphatic anatomy is helpful in diagnosis of infections and the spread of neoplasms. Recently, lymphatics have been identified within the monkey lacrimal gland, extraocular muscles, orbital apex, and the optic nerve arachnoid (53).

■ CONJUNCTIVA

The conjunctiva is a mucosal lining of the eye and the inside of the eyelids. There are four areas of the conjunctiva. They include the palpebral (tarsal) conjunctiva that covers the inside of the lid, the bulbar conjunctiva that covers the globe, fornix conjunctiva which is redundant in a V shape and connects the palpebral to the bulbar conjuctiva (conjunctional cul-de-sac), and the limbal conjunctiva that forms a border between the cornea and the limbus. In the upper lid, the palpebral portion of the conjunctiva continues to the superior fornix applied to the Müller's muscle. Just above the tarsus, the conjunctiva and Müller's muscle are tightly bound but become less so posteriorly. In the lower lid, the conjunctiva is easily elevated from the inferior lid retractors without difficulty until the inferior fornix is reached. The superior reflection of the palpebral conjunctiva is about 13 mm from the open eyelid margin and 20 to 25 mm with the eye closed. The inferior fornix reflection remains 9 to 10 mm from the lower eyelid margin because the lower eyelid does not significantly elevate with closure (54). The bulbar conjunctiva overlying the globe is loosely adherent to the underlying Tenon's fascia until it approaches the corneoscleral limbus, where it is tightly bound, and fuses with Tenon's.

Deep to the conjunctival epithelium is the substantia propria which is a thick yet loose connective tissue that contains numerous cell types. These cells include fi-

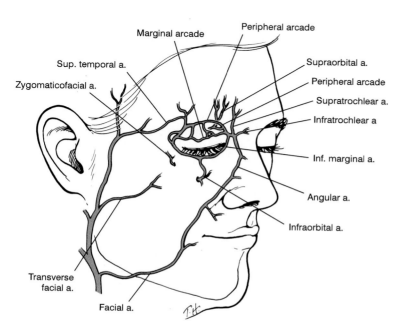

Figure 1–11.
The superficial arteries of the face and the palpebral regions. Note the redundancy of the blood supply to the eyelids from the facial and carotid arterial systems.

broblasts, polymorphonuclear leukocytes, lymphocytes, plasma cells and germinal lymphoid follicles.

Histologically, the conjunctiva is a nonkeratinizing squamous epithelium. It forms the posterior layer of the eyelids (palpebral conjunctiva)—extends into the fornices before acutely changing direction to cover the anterior aspect of the globe (bulbar conjunctiva) up to the limbus. In a few areas, the overlying conjunctiva is firmly attached to underlying structures by fine fibrous anchoring strands. This occurs at the bulbar limbus and the tarsus. There normally exist small blood vessels that extend in and among these fine fibrous strands. All four rectus muscles contribute connective tissue septa that form suspensory ligaments to create the 360° conjunctival fornix.

The mucus secreted by the *goblet cells* of the conjunctiva is one of three components found in the tear layer. Mucus-containing goblet cells are found in highest concentration in the fornices, the lid margin, the limbus and the plica semilunaris. Mucus acts as an interface between the hydrophobic corneal epithelium and the hydrophilic aqueous tear layer and is responsible for proper wetting of the corneal surface. Corneal drying occurs despite adequate aqueous film in conditions that destroy conjunctival goblet cells. The plica semilunaris is located in the nasal conjunctiva within the palpebral fissure. Just medial to the plica is the caruncle (Fig. 1–5B). The *caruncle* is a stratified squamous epithelium containing sebaceous glands, hair follicles and accessory lacrimal glands within the stroma.

The normal conjunctiva acts as a physical and immunological barrier to invasion by exogenous substances including microorganisms. The layers of the conjunctiva consists of the surface epithelium and the substantia propria. The normal human conjunctiva contains an extraordinary number of different cell types. Besides the surface epithelial cells and fibroblasts in the substantia propria, there are numerous infiltrative inflammatory cells, including lymphocytes, plasma cells, neutrophils and fixed-tissue mast cells. Many of these cell types are involved in phagocytosis and in processing antigen for its elimination. Epithelial cells have been found to participate in phagocytosis and to possess acid hydrolase containing lysosomes similar to white cells for foreign material degradation.

■ EYEBALL

The eyeball is a fluid-filled sphere (Fig. 1–12). The structural wall of the eye consists of the cornea anteriorly with a radius of curvature of approximately 8 mm and sclera posteriorly with a radius of approximately 12 mm. The eye is not perfectly round as it is slightly elongated and flattened. The anterior posterior diameter measures approximately 24 mm, vertical diameter 23 mm and the horizontal diameter approximately 23.5 mm. The shape of the globe is maintained by hydrolic pressure of approximately 10–20 mm mercury. Intraocular pressures over 22 mm increase the risk for optic nerve damage which is the basis for glaucoma. The eye can be divided into two chambers, the anterior chamber which is anterior to the iris plane and posterior chamber which is structured posterior to the iris. The optic nerve is located nasal to the fovea centralis which is the visual center of the eye. The ora serrata marks the end of the retina and the beginning of the pars plana and ciliary body. The location of the ora serrata corresponds to the insertion site of the four rectus muscles. The eye is protected by the bony orbit and cushioned by the surrounding orbital fat.

■ CORNEA/SCLERA

Cornea

The cornea is an amazing biological structure because of its optical properties which allow the transmission of light energy. This is possible because the collagen that makes up the cornea has a high degree of order. The normal transparent cornea does not contain blood vessels. Aqueous humor from the anterior chamber and surface tears provide nutrients and oxygen. Blood vessels at the limbal zone provide some nourishment to the peripheral cornea. These limbal vessels are the source of corneal inflammatory cells and inflammatory mediators. Because the central cornea is avascular, it is relatively "immune privileged" which is why there is a high success rate for corneal transplants (penetrating keratoplasty). Since the central cornea is avascular, it heals very slowly (1). Corneal sutures must be left in place for several months. The smooth curvature of the cornea is the major focusing element of the eye and it provides approximately ⅔rds of the eye's 60 diopters of converging power. The three main layers of the cornea include the epithelium, the stroma, and the endothelium. Corneal ultrastructure helps in explaining how it functions and maintains itself in a normal physiological condition. The cornea is innervated by sensory nerves from the ophthalmic division of the trigeminal nerve mostly by way of long ciliary nerves that penetrate the sclera just posterior to the limbus. These nerves can be visual-

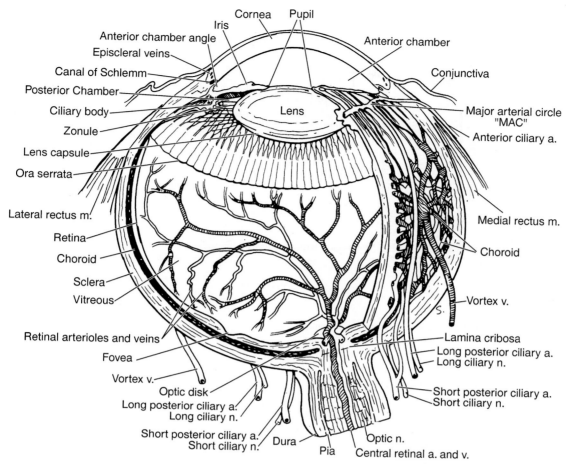

Figure 1–12.
Drawing of eye showing important anatomical structures of the eye.

ized at the slit lamp as thin radial lines best seen near the limbus. Terminal branches pierce Bowman's membrane to innervate the epithelium forming the intraepithelial plexus. The cornea is a very sensitive organ and disruption of the corneal epithelium (corneal abrasion) results in one of the most severe forms of pain. The cornea is responsible for approximately two-thirds of the eye's 60 diopters of converging power.

Corneal Epithelium

The human nonkeratinized, stratified squamous corneal epithelium is comprised of three layers; 1) surface cells, 2) wing cells, and 3) basal cells (columnar) (Fig. 1–13). Two to three layers of wing cells sit on top of a single layer of basal columnar cells. They are separated from the underlying connective tissue by an epithelial basement membrane (basal lamina). The epithelial basement membrane, like other basement membranes, is composed of collagen type IV. The collagen is capable of self-assembly into biological networks that provide a substrate for cellular attachment directed by various extracellular matrix proteins. The wing cells are described

in this manner because of their thin lateral extensions. Towards the corneal surface, these wing cells become extremely long and thin. The apical surface of the surface cells are extremely irregular with microvilli, but the corneal tear film makes the surface optically smooth. These cells are attached to one another by multiple desmosomes and migrate together to the surface where they are shed into the tear film. The basal cells are attached to the basement membrane by hemidesmosomes. Mitosis of the basal cells leads to new wing and surface cells. *Recurrent corneal erosions* may occur because of poor functioning hemidesmosomes secondary to prior trauma or metabolic product accumulation caused by a corneal degeneration or dystrophy. Histiocytes, lymphocytes, macrophages, and pigmented melanocytes may reside in the corneal epithelium, and they are primarily located in the peripheral cornea near the limbus where there is a blood supply.

The corneal epithelium provides a protective barrier by selectively allowing nonpolar molecules to pass through it secondary to the lipophilic content of the plasma membrane. This is in contrast to the corneal stroma which allows the passage of polar molecules (hy-

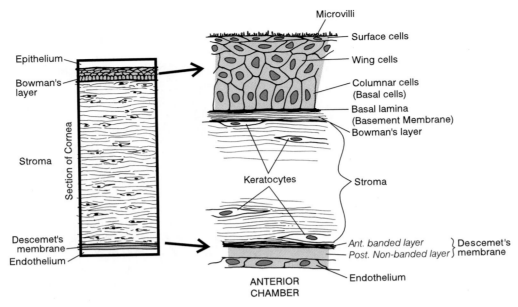

Figure 1–13.
Diagrammatic representation of the corneal ultrastructure through all five layers.

drophilic). This is the basis of why different drugs penetrate the cornea at different rates.

Damage to the corneal epithelium (*corneal abrasion*) is repaired by rapid resurfacing of the debrided corneal stroma by epithelial cells. Within the first six hours, a single layer of basal epithelial cells at the wound margin becomes mobile by releasing their hemidesmosomal attachments to the basement, and slide to cover the defective membrane (10). Actin assembly and disassembly provide the cytoskeletal locomotive support for the sliding epithelial cells. Fibronectin is the major extracellular matrix protein, providing a permanent attachment to basement membrane via binding to collagen type IV and the proteoglycan heparin sulfate (45). When resurfacing is complete, the epithelium reattaches to the basement membrane by newly made hemidesmosomes and the anchoring collagen type VII. These molecules are thought to span Bowman's layer, thereby linking the corneal epithelium to the stroma.

Bowman's Layer

Bowman's layer (membrane) is an acellular layer of the anterior corneal stroma just posterior to the basement membrane of the epithelium. It is made up of unorganized collagen fibers and glycosaminoglycans providing plasticity and structural support. It has an overall thickness of 8 to 14 microns constituting about 2% of the total corneal thickness and is not a true basement membrane. The posterior border merges with the corneal stroma. Following injury, Bowman's membrane is not replaced and if violated will lead to scar opacification.

Corneal Stroma

The corneal stroma is the major component of the cornea constituting 90% of the thickness or about 500 microns. Collagen type I, a predominantly fibrous protein with high tensile strength and low extensibility, is the main corneal stromal biomolecule. The collagen fibrils within the corneal stroma are regularly spaced and of uniform diameter. The fibrils have a macroperiodicity of 640 angstroms and are similar to typical collagen. They lie in wide thin sheets called lamellae. About 200 lamellae are stacked and make up the stroma. In the anterior third of the stroma, these lamellae are obliquely orientated while the posterior two-thirds of the stromal lamellae are parallel to the surface. This explains the relative ease of a deeper corneal stromal lamellar surgical dissection. Stromal transparency has been attributed to this architectural spacing. Disruption of the lamellae, such as edema, leads to an opaque cornea and decreased visual acuity capability (38). Other collagen types in the cornea stroma include III, V, and VI (41). Collagen type III is associated with fetal tissue and repair processes, while collagen type V plays a role in collagen fibril diameter regulation. Collagen type VI regulates the organization of the corneal lamellar structure. Stromal proteoglycans also have a role in collagen fibril spacing, in addition to being closely associated with the collagen fibrils. Proteoglycans are molecules made up of glycosaminoglycans attached to core proteins. Glycosaminoglycans are serially linked carbohydrate dimers. Keratin sulfate and chondroitin/dermatan sulfate are the main glycosaminoglycans found in the corneal stroma. Imbalances in the quantity of these molecules have been implicated in the pathogenesis of macular corneal dystrophy and corneal ectasias such as *keratoconus* and *pellucid marginal degeneration* (14).

The main cell of the corneal stroma is the *keratocyte* which is responsible for synthesizing and placing down the new collagen/proteoglycan matrix under normal basal metabolic conditions. There is constant synthesis and degradation of these biomolecules. In certain diseased states, such as *keratolysis,* the degradation process out-paces synthesis leading to thinning of the corneal stroma. Metalloproteinases, such as collagenase, degrade the biomolecules of the corneal stroma. Recent interest in metalloproteinase inhibitors has led to a new family of drugs for various corneal diseases.

The keratocyte is a fairly stable cell demonstrating minimal mitotic activity in a normal state. However, following injury the keratocytes undergo proliferation, migration, and a phenotypic change. It appears that the keratocytes are under the influence of factors produced by the epithelium following injury. The keratocytes adjacent to the wound repopulate the defect and undergo a change in morphology to one of a myofibroblast. This transformed cell type can bridge the defect and reapproximate the margins through inherent smooth muscle contractile properties. These cells also secrete collagens and glycoproteins. The newly created extracellular matrix is quite disorganized with resulting opacification. Remodeling occurs over several months but not to the previous uninterrupted state. The collagen spacing in the lamellae is altered due to a larger than normal collagen fiber size and a change in the size and distribution of the proteoglycans. The proteoglycans are larger with a greater proportion of chondroitin/dermatan sulfate glycosaminoglycan and negligible amounts of keratin sulfate. Over time these changes approach but do not attain the uninterrupted state, thereby resulting in an opaque stromal scar and decreased vision (8, 9).

Descemet's membrane

Descemet's membrane, the basement membrane of the corneal endothelium, is a periodic acid-Schiff (PAS)-positive structure of unusual thickness. An accumulation of material in this basement membrane leads to increased thickness with age. In a child the average thickness is 3 to 4 microns while in an adult it is 10 to 12 microns. There are two distinct regions morphologically. The anterior banded zone is present from birth while the posterior nonbanded zone is laid down throughout the lifetime of an individual. Excrescences of Descemet's membrane occur in the peripheral cornea in the elderly called *Hassall-Henle warts.* In the central cornea, autosomal dominant *Fuchs endothelial dystrophy* leads to excrescences called *guttae.*

Corneal Endothelium

Corneal endothelial cells are derived from neural crest cells. They are hexagonal cells and play an important role in active transport and deturgescence of the normal corneal stroma. Adjacent cells interlock through tortuous interdigitations and tight junctions. The endothelium act as a permeability barrier between the aqueous humor and the corneal stroma and serves as a pump to dehydrate the stroma. This energy-dependent process pumps fluid across the endothelial apical plasma membrane into the aqueous humor. Oxygen is provided by the aqueous for the endothelial pump mechanisms. Four pumping transport mechanisms exist and include sodium-potassium ATPase pump, sodium-hydrogen ATPase pump, diffusion, and a carbonic anhydrase system. Injury to the endothelium from a variety of causes leads to edema and opacification. Loss of a significant number of endothelial cells from trauma or degeneration results in a defective pump mechanism, inviving of aqueous (corneal edema), and loss of corneal clarity. Human corneal endothelial cells are almost totally amitotic soon after birth, thus, so once these cells are lost they do not regenerate and can only be replaced by corneal transplantation. These cells have limited regenerative capacity but are able to migrate and enlarge in order to cover a greater surface area. Endothelial cells are able to slide over fibronectin along Descemet's membrane to cover defects. With age, there is gradual attrition of endothelial cells as at birth there are approximately 3,500 to 4,000 cells per millimeter square, whereas there are only 1,400 to 2,500 cells per square per square millimeter in adults. The critical cell density below which corneal edema occurs is approximately 400 to 700 cells per square millimeter. Endothelial cell count (density) and morphology can be used as an indicator of the "health" of the cornea. Retrocorneal fibrous membranes are believed to be caused by endothelial cells which have undergone fibrous metaplasia secondary to a damaging insult.

Corneal Topography

The basic anatomic aspects previously discussed account for the physical dimensions of the cornea which play a significant role in determining the topography of the anterior corneal surface. Advances in keratorefractive surgery have been possible because of corneal topographical analysis and is an important tool for diagnosis and therapy (32).

The cornea is not a uniformly thick structure (Fig. 1–14). The central cornea is approximately 500 microns thick with a trend toward peripheral thickening. The average thickness at the limbus is about 1200 microns. The difference in thickness is secondary to the differ-

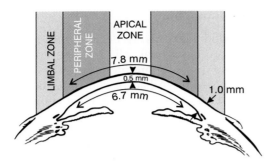

Figure 1–14.
Cross-section through the central cornea with increasing thickness toward the peripheral cornea. The three topographic zones are marked above. The different anterior and posterior radii of curvatures for this normal cornea account for the variable thickness, thinner centrally, thicker in periphery.

Arbitrarily, the corneal surface can be divided into three zones and include the apical, peripheral, and limbal (Fig. 1–14) zone (49). Precise borders do not exist, but each helps us to understand the overall functional capabilities of the cornea.

The central or apical area does not have a uniform definition. However, it is known that this area normally has the least amount of dioptric power variability. Some definitions include that the amount of curvature in this area does not change by more than one diopter. In an ideal cornea, the apical zone would approach perfect sphericity. In reality, most young people have sphero cylindrical lenses with *"with the rule" astigmatism*. This means that the vertical meridian is steeper while the horizontal meridian is the flatter. This corneal shape has been attributed to the contribution of the lid and its interaction with the ocular surface.

The peripheral zone is the area peripheral to the apical zone and extends to the center border of the limbus. Topographically, the usual tendency is for this region to undergo progressive flattening. The overall result is an aspheric surface (48). The peripheral zone is important in contact lens fitting and with regard to keratorefractive surgery.

ences in the curvature of radius of the anterior and posterior corneal surfaces. The average anterior surface radius of curvature is approximately 7.8 mm while the posterior surface is about 6.7 mm (55). The difference between the anterior and posterior radii of curvature affords an average of 43 diopters of convergence lens power. In reality, the air-tear film interface is responsible for this power. Since the tear film conforms to the anterior corneal surface, the two are one and the same. Also, this surface is the main topographical determinant of the ocular optical system and the lens contributes about one-third of the total refractive power of the eye. Corneal thickness, radius of curvature, and the surface regularity directly affect the corneal topography.

The final region is the limbal zone and is the transition from the cornea to the sclera. Generally, the cornea has a steeper radius of curvature than the sclera, there is an apparent sulcus at this interface (55). This region is important because it is affected by peripheral corneal thinning diseases and is the site of numerous surgical procedures.

The *surgical limbus* is about 2 mm wide and is divided into two equal regions (Fig. 1–15). They include the an-

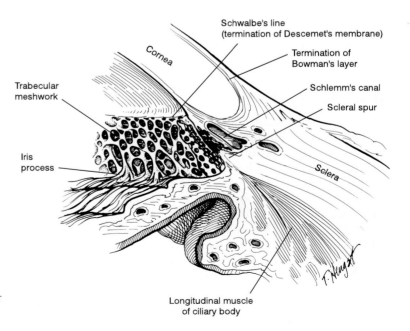

Figure 1–15.
Anatomy of the surgical limbus. The region encompasses the space from Schwalbe's line anteriorly to the scleral spur posteriorly.

terior bluish gray zone overlying the clear cornea extending between the termination of Bowman's layer and Descemet's membrane (Schwalbe s line) and secondly, a posterior white zone extending from Schwalbe's line to the scleral spur.

Sclera

The sclera covers the posterior 80% of the globe's surface. Unlike the corneal collagen, scleral collagen fibrils vary in size and shape. They have a tendency to taper at their ends and are not continuous fibers as in the cornea. The scleral collagen fibrils range from 1000–1600 angstroms in diameter. The opaque white character of the sclera is markedly different from the transparent cornea and is the result of the sclera having a greater water content amongst the nonuniformly oriented variably sized collagen fibers. The sclera is also composed of proteoglycans and fibroblasts.

Three potential openings exist in the scleral surface for other anatomic structures including the cornea, optic nerve, and the emissaria. The rectus muscle tendons insert into the outer scleral collagen. Tenon's capsule and the bulbar conjunctiva join to make firm attachments at the limbus and drape over the sclera and the rectus muscles. The sclera has variable thickness with the thinnest location being just posterior to the rectus muscle insertions (0.3 mm) and the thickest at the posterior pole (1.0 mm). During strabismus surgery and scleral buckle procedures care must be taken when placing scleral sutures because of the extreme thinness of the tissues and possible perforation. *Blunt trauma* can lead to *scleral rupture* in thin areas. These include a meridional arc parallel to the equator but opposite to the impact site, the equator (thickness 0.4–0.5 mm), nasal to the superior oblique tendon insertion, the lamina cribosa-scleral interface, and behind the rectus muscle insertions. However, the superonasal quadrant near the limbus is the most frequent site of scleral rupture.

The sclera is basically avascular except for the episcleral vessels and the intrascleral plexus just posterior to the limbus. Because it is relatively avascular, the sclera is slow healing after a laceration and requires months before obtaining normal strength. Episclera consists of a dense, vascular connective tissue that blends with the superficial stroma deep and the conjunctiva and Tenon's capsule superficially. Emissaria are channels for the passage of the arteries, veins and ciliary nerves. Choroidal malignant melanoma can migrate out of the eye via direct extension through these emissaria. The sclera receives sensory innervation from the ciliary nerves with short ciliary nerves supplying posterior sclera and two long ciliary nerves supplying the anterior sclera. The sclera is not as sensitive as the cornea; however, scleral inflammation (scleritis) will produce a dull aching pain.

■ ANTERIOR CHAMBER

Aqueous Humor Composition/Function

The aqueous humor is the fluid substance that fills the volume of the anterior chamber. The liquid humor can be thought of as a blood substitute for the avascular lens, cornea and trabecular meshwork. It provides a continuous flow of oxygen and the necessary nutrients through the anterior and posterior chambers for these tissues while at the same time removing their waste products. This fluid is an optically clear medium, allowing the unimpeded transmission of light along the visual pathway. In order to perform this optical function properly, the aqueous humor is devoid of all blood cell components and greater than 99% of the plasma proteins. The presence of either any cell type or protein in the anterior chamber results in clinically evident *anterior chamber cell* or *anterior chamber flare*, respectively.

Aqueous humor formation and composition has been studied for decades and has led to a better understanding of the normal state and various pathologic conditions (6). The nonpigmented epithelium of the ciliary body processes is responsible for producing aqueous humor by active secretion of solutes into the posterior chamber (28).

There are four mechanisms for the production of aqueous. They are diffusion, active secretion, ultrafiltration and carbonic anhydrase activity (Fig. 1–16). Tight junctions (zonulae occludentes) between the nonpigmented cells prevents random diffusion of nutrients into the posterior chamber and is a prerequisite for active secretion and maintenance of the blood-aqueous barrier. During the secretion of aqueous, nutrients from the ciliary process capillaries pass through several anatomic layers in the ciliary body. In order, they include the capillary endothelium and its basement membrane, the basement membrane and the cells of the pigmented epithelium, and finally alongside the nonpigmented epithelial cells and through their basement membrane into the posterior chamber. The active solute pump sets up a concentration gradient that forces an osmotic flow of water into the posterior chamber. Sodium has the central role and is secreted by an energy dependant sodium/potassium-adenosine triphosphatase (ATP) pump found in the nonpig-

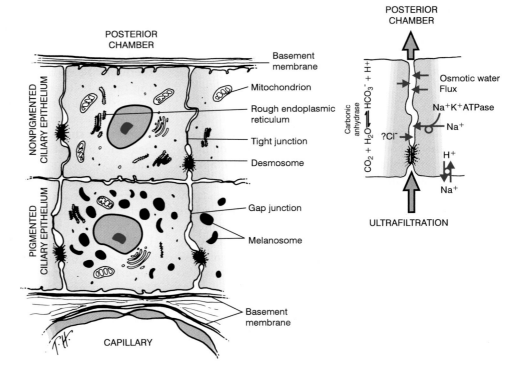

Figure 1–16.
Physiology of Aqueous Production at Ciliary Process. Diagrammatic representation of the apex to apex interface of the nonpigmented and pigmented epithelial cells. The mechanisms for aqueous humor production by the nonpigmented epithelium is shown in the inset on the right.

mented ciliary epithelial cells (47). The carbonic anhydrase system is also a form of active transport. The carbonic *anhydrase inhibitor, acetazolamide,* has been used clinically to lower intraocular pressure. It prevents the formation of bicarbonate and hydrogen from water and carbon dioxide. Three theories exist to explain the linkage between this drug and lower intraocular pressure: (1) inhibition of carbonic anhydrase causes a decrease in bicarbonate available for movement with sodium to the aqueous side to maintain neutrality; (2) a change in intracellular pH may inhibit the active transport pump; and/or (3) decreased production of hydrogen ions decreases the hydrogen/sodium exchange and reduces the intracellular sodium available for transport into the intercellular channel, decreasing active transport.

The composition of the aqueous depends on the nature of the freshly produced fluid, the subsequent passive and active solute exchange across the various interfacing tissues it bathes, and the rate of exit from the eye (Table 1–1) (3). Inorganic and organic ions, carbohydrates, glutathione and urea, amino acids and proteins, oxygen, carbon dioxide and water are the major ingredients found in the aqueous humor. The aqueous is slightly hyperosmotic to plasma and may be higher near the surface of the nonpigmented ciliary epithelium. No difference in osmolarity has been found between samples from the anterior and posterior chambers.

Inorganic cation concentrations, such as sodium, potassium, magnesium, iron, copper, and zinc in the aqueous are similar to those in the plasma. However,

calcium is present at only half the plasma level. The major anions of the aqueous humor include chloride and bicarbonate and can vary by as much as 30% above and below the levels found in the plasma. The relative proportions of carbon dioxide and bicarbonate determine the pH of the aqueous humor which ranges from 7.5–7.6.

Organic anions such as lactate and ascorbate can be found in the aqueous humor. The aqueous concentration of lactate is always higher than that of the plasma. It enters the posterior chamber readily across the ciliary epithelium but does not tend to accumulate there. The metabolism of glucose by various tissues including the ciliary epithelium, retina, lens, and cornea, contributes significantly to the lactate content of the aqueous. The presence of ascorbate is possibly the most interesting constituent of the aqueous since it is found in concentrations ten to fifty times higher than in the plasma. The function of ascorbate in the eye remains speculative and includes functions such as antioxidation, regulation of collagen synthesis in the trabecular meshwork for normal outflow, and absorption of damaging ultraviolet radiation.

The aqueous concentration of glucose is only about 80% of that found in the plasma. The rate of entry of glucose into the posterior chamber is much more rapid than would be predicted from consideration of its size and lipid solubility. This suggests that its ability to pass across the ciliary epithelium occurs by facilitated diffusion. A specific carrier is probably involved but no evi-

TABLE 1–1.

Aqueous Humor Concentrations of the Inorganic and
Organic Constituents in Either Monkey or Man (5)

	Concentration		
Inorganic Substances	**Anterior Aqueous**	**Posterior Aqueous**	**Plasma**
Bicarbonate (μmol/ml)	20.2	—	27.5
Chloride (μmol/ml)	131.3	—	115.0
Calcium (μmol/ml)	2.5	2.5	4.9
Hydrogen ion (pH)	7.49	—	—
Magnesium (μmol/ml)	1.2	1.3	1.2
Oxygen (mm Hg)	53	—	—
Phosphate (μmol/ml)	0.62	—	1.11
Potassium (μmol/ml)	3.6	4.1	4.2
Sodium (μmol/ml)	152	—	148

Organic Substances			
Ascorbate (μmol/ml)	1.06	—	0.04
Citrate (μmol/ml)	0.12	—	—
Creatinine (μmol/ml)	0.04	—	0.03
Glucose (μmol/ml)	2.8	—	5.9
Hyaluronate (μg/ml)	1.1	—	—
Lactate (μmol/ml)	4.5	—	1.9
Protein (mg/100 ml)	13.5	—	—
Urea (μmol/ml)	6.1	—	7.3

dence exists for an active transport mechanism. Insulin has not been demonstrated to affect the rate of entry of glucose into the anterior chamber. Glucose can diffuse into the cornea. The concentration in the corneal endothelium and the extracellular space is about half that of the aqueous.

The relative amounts of amino acids in the anterior chamber vary widely secondary to variously proposed amino acid transport systems. These systems include specific mechanisms for the transport of neutral, basic, and acidic amino acids and urea, but have not been well defined. In addition to the proposed active transport system for urea, passive diffusion across all biological membranes can occur secondary to its low molecular weight. Urea concentration in the aqueous humor is about 80–90% of that in the plasma.

Glutathione is an important anabolic tripeptide with a reactive sulfhydryl group with reducing power. The concentration in the aqueous is deceptively high compared to that found in the plasma because in the blood it is virtually all contained or sequestered within the red blood cells. The aqueous glutathione is derived by diffusion from blood, active transport in the ciliary epithelium and by loss from the lens and cornea.

The aqueous protein concentration differs from plasma in that there is an almost complete absence of protein in the aqueous. The usual aqueous contains about 0.02 grams of protein per 100 ml, compared to the usual plasma concentration of 7 grams of protein per 100 ml. The blood-aqueous barrier normally limits the protein of aqueous humor to less than 1% of its plasma concentration. The aqueous protein composition differs from that of the plasma. The lower-molecular-weight proteins, like albumin and beta-globulins, are more prominent in the normal aqueous compared to the heavy-molecular-weight proteins like lipoproteins and immunoglobulins. Basically, the aqueous:plasma ratios for various proteins are inversely proportional to the molecular weight of the proteins (11). Thus, the blood-aqueous barrier behaves as a semiporous membrane with a pore radius of about 105 microns. However, this relationship does not hold true in the environment of inflammation. In patients with uveitis, the blood-aqueous barrier breaks down and the aqueous humor concentration of protein increases to levels greater than 1 gram of protein per 100 ml. The effect is that the aqueous humor protein concentration approaches that of the plasma. Normally, the primary aqueous does not clot, but with the massive influx of plasminogen with its activator, a plasmoid aqueous results with loss of the anterior chamber convection current. Plasminogen is contained in the primary aqueous in significant amounts and may play a role to keep it free of fibrin. Secondary (diseased) aqueous contains significant amounts of all the major components of coagulation and fibrinolysis. In addition, ascorbic acid concentrations actually decrease as do the concentrations of amino acids. This is the result of increased fluid flow and more exchange across the damaged epithelium without an increase in secretion. The concentration of glucose is essentially unchanged. With stabilization of the blood-aqueous barrier and the presence of fibrinolytic enzymes, the aqueous returns to its usual state. These fibrinolytic enzymes have also been postulated to play a role in the maintenance of outflow resistance.

Immunoglobulin levels in the aqueous have been characterized and show that IgG is found in highest concentration. During *uveitis,* the IgG levels increase along with detectable amounts of IgM and IgA. Complement can also be found in minute levels in the normal aqueous humor.

The alpha and gamma lens crystallins are found in the aqueous humor in small amounts in eyes with clear lenses. However, the concentration increases in eyes with cataractous changes indicating that protein leaks through intact lens capsule and epithelium and may create subclinical state of *phacolytic glaucoma.*

Aqueous humor protein levels may be altered in the presence of intraocular malignancies and may be diagnostically helpful. Retinoblastoma causes an increase in the globulin content whereas nonmalignant states usually cause a decrease. *Lactate dehydrogenase (LDH)* is found in only small amounts in normal aqueous humor. The aqueous:plasma ratio of LDH is reported to be greater than 1.50 in patients with *retinoblastoma* while in other diseased states the ratio is typically less than 0.60 (57). The proposed source of aqueous LDH is from dying cells and the release of the cytosolic enzymes. LDH is not disease specific and can be found in *Coats' disease.* However, *enolase* levels in the aqueous and plasma may be of assistance in diagnosis of retinoblastoma and ocular melanoma.

Other substances found in the aqueous include lipids, hyaluronic acid, sialic acid, trivalent chromium ions, vitamin B_{12}, endogenous corticosteroids, and monoamine metabolites. The significance of their presence is not known.

One of the first structures to interact with the newly produced aqueous humor is the *vitreous humor.* The vitreous humor is a gel consisting of collagen fibers bound by hyaluronic acid. About 98% of this gel is water so low that molecular weight substances such as ions, glucose, and amino acids can diffuse unimpeded into and out of the vitreous cavity.

The *crystalline lens* normally takes up amino acids from the aqueous humor. These amino acids are used to synthesize lens-specific proteins such as crystallins. However, if aqueous humor concentration of amino acids is low, the lens may act as a reservoir and release amino acids back into the anterior chamber. Removal of the lens results in an increase in anterior chamber glucose content and a decrease in lactic acid. This is secondary to lower metabolic demand. Therefore, the lens is capable of altering the concentrations of glucose, amino acids, and other solutes in the anterior chamber.

Solute exchange between the aqueous humor and the cornea has a significant role in normal corneal metabolism. The cornea receives most of its oxygen supply via the atmosphere; however, the thicker peripheral cornea receives some nutritional needs from the limbal vasculature. Oxygen is present in the aqueous humor at a partial pressure of about 55 mm Hg, about one-third the atmospheric concentration. The central cornea derives its glucose supply from the circulating aqueous with a high glucose concentration in the anterior chamber compared to the posterior chamber. The reverse is true for the by-product lactic acid. Amino acids entering the cornea do so probably by diffusion. The corneal endothelium functions as a fluid pump to maintain a clear deturgesced state. Approximately 10 microliters/hour of fluid is pumped back into the aqueous by the corneal endothelium. This is a small contribution to aqueous humor formation since the normal aqueous humor production rate is about 150 microliters/hour.

Trabecular Meshwork

After the aqueous enters the anterior chamber via the pupillary aperture, it exits the eye mostly through the trabecular meshwork but some leaves by the uveoscleral path (20). The trabecular meshwork lies in the limbal region of the anterior chamber angle. In cross-section, it has a triangular shape with its base located posteriorly between the scleral spur and ciliary body and its apex located at Schwalbe's line (Fig. 1–17). At first it appears confusing because the outflow apparatus is derived from various structures including cornea, sclera ciliary body, and iris. The trabecular meshwork consists of a series of parallel layers of thin connective tissue stacked upon one another. The lamellae are perforated by various sized pores which result in a criss-cross pattern of overlapping connective tissue trabeculae. This is a one-way valve as fluid can leave the eye but fluid can not enter from the trabecular meshwork. The extracellular matrix of the trabecular beams is composed of a central core of collagen types I and III and an outer cortical zone of types III, IV, and V with heparin sulfate proteoglycan, fibronectin, and laminin for cellular attachment sites. Each trabecula is lined by a monolayer of endothelium. These cells contain a series of gap junctions that tightly bind adjacent endothelial cells to each other. The apex of the trabecular meshwork consists of three to five layers of trabeculae while the base is composed of as many as 15 to 20 layers.

The trabecular meshwork is divided into three distinct regions. They include the uveal portion, the corneoscleral meshwork, and the juxtacanalicular region (See Chapter 42). The uveal meshwork is the innermost layer and borders the anterior chamber. It is cord-like with pigment granule-containing endothelial cells which can be visualized on gonioscopy. The corneoscleral meshwork is external to the uveal meshwork and accounts for most of the region while the juxtacanalicular region is a thin strip bordering the endothelial lining of *Schlemm's canal.* The canal of Schlemm resembles a lymphatic vessel, being formed by a monolayer of nonfenestrated endothelium with tight junctions. The corneoscleral meshwork has a laminar pattern with a single row of endothelial cells containing multiple pinocytotic vesicles.

The principle resistance to aqueous flow out of the eye is produced in the trabecular meshwork. The resistance rises as the pores of the trabecular meshwork decrease in size from the uveal meshwork across the corneoscleral region to the juxtacanalicular tissue (Fig. 1–17). Thus, the juxtacanalicular tissue is the area of highest resistance to aqueous outflow in the normal eye. Glycosaminoglycans and glycoproteins are the main constituents of the juxtanalicular tissue and this tissue is covered on the Schlemm's canal side by a monolayer of juxtacanalicular cells. The passages are 1.5 microns in

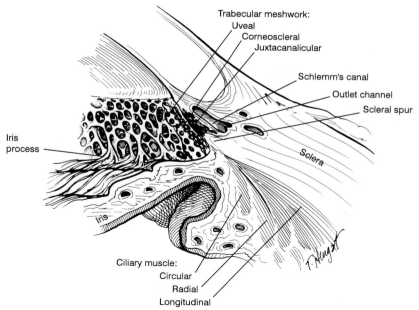

Trabecular meshwork:
Uveal
Corneoscleral
Juxtacanalicular

Schlemm's canal
Outlet channel
Scleral spur

Sclera

Iris process

Iris

Ciliary muscle:
Circular
Radial
Longitudinal

Figure 1–17.

Anatomic features of the anterior chamber angle and the trabecular meshwork. In cross-section, the trabecular meshwork has a triangular shape. Parallel, perforated laminae of trabecular tissue are greatest in number posteriorly at the base of the triangle and fuse together anteriorly to reduce the number of laminae (apex of triangle). In addition, there are zones of the trabecular meshwork from inside out including the uveal portion, corneoscleral region, and the juxtacanalicular zone. Aqueous humor flows through the narrowing perforations in the laminae to eventually enter Schlemm's canal.

diameter through which aqueous flows. The juxtacanalicular cells produce giant vacuoles which protrude into the lumen of Schlemm's canal. It has been proposed that these vacuoles serve as an active pathway for aqueous flow. Once the aqueous reaches *Schlemm's canal* it flows via the collector channels into the episcleral veins. Flow is related to the *episcleral venous pressure* which is normally 8–12 mmHg. For example, in disease states such as *Sturge-Weber* and *neurofibromatosis,* the episcleral venous pressure can be elevated and results in decreased outflow and an increase in the intraocular pressure. Twenty to 30 endothelial-lined conduits exit Schlemm's canal radially and they make up the collector channels. Rarely, during gonioscopy, visible laminar flow of aqueous into a vein can be seen along with an adjacent layering of the blood and clear aqueous fluid.

Aqueous is able to escape from the eye by two mechanisms. The first is pressure dependent while the other is pressure independent. The pressure dependent system has aqueous leaving via the trabecular meshwork and outflow increases as the IOP increases. The resistance to flow in the trabecular meshwork plays a role in *open angle glaucoma* and indicates increased resistance to flow occurring in the narrow channels of the juxtacanalicular meshwork. This may be related to a change in the extracellular matrix, particularly an increase in the sulfated proteoglycans.

The *uveoscleral outflow* path works by bulk flow of aqueous through the ciliary body, and is removed by the bloodstream or by seepage of the fluid through the scleral wall and into the surrounding orbital tissues (3). This has been measured to occur with a constant flow rate, is pressure independent, is not energy dependant, and accounts for up to 20% of aqueous outflow.

■ UVEA: IRIS, CILIARY BODY, CHOROID

The *uveal tract* is a densely pigmented, vascular layer between the sclera on the outside and the retina on the inside. The uvea is firmly attached to the sclera at the scleral spur, the exits of the vortex veins, and the optic disc. These sites are severed during evisceration. The uvea is also subdivided into three anatomic compartments which include the iris, ciliary body, and the choroid. The main function of the uveal tract is one of nutrition.

The choriocapillaris, the highest blood flow system in the body, provides vascular support to the metabolically demanding retinal pigment epithelium, and rods and cones of the sensory retina, while aqueous humor from the ciliary body supplies the nourishment to the lens and other anterior segment structures. In addition, the musculature of the iris controls pupillary diameter as a means to regulate the amount of light allowed into the eye. Light regulation is homeostatic for attaining the highest level of visual acuity along with being protective to the retina by limiting the amount of damaging light rays. The ciliary body muscle is also able to alter the lens shape to provide accommodation and may have a role in intraocular pressure maintenance. Longitudinal muscle contraction may affect aqueous outflow because of an attachment to the scleral spur anteriorly. Pilocarpine causes contraction of the longitudinal muscle, pulls on scleral spur, stretches trabecular meshwork, thus increases aqueous outflow and reduces intraocular pressure (IOP).

Iris

The *iris* is the most anterior portion of the uveal tract and is thickest near the central collarette and thinnest peripherally at the iris root. Disruption at the iris root is an *iridodialysis*. The iris is responsible for the "color" of the eye. The color is dependent upon the pigmentation of the anterior border layer and deep stroma and the presence of stromal melanocytes (Fig. 1–18). A lightly pigmented iris appears blue while a heavily pigmented iris is said to be brown. The pigmented epithelium is continuous with the nonpigmented epithelium of the ciliary body and the neurosensory retina. This epithelium allows only incident light to pass into the eye through the pupil and minimizes the amount of reflected light that has entered the eye. The anterior 75% of the iris is a vascular stroma and provides nutrition to the anterior segment of the eye. The peripheral iris blood vessels are radial to the central pupil but become concentric around the pupil. These vessels emanate from the major arterial circle in the ciliary body (Fig. 1–20). Essentially the iris is a musculovascular diaphragm with a cental opening, the pupil (2).

The *major arterial circle* is formed by the posterior ciliary vessels along with *the anterior ciliary vessels* coming from the rectus muscles (Fig. 1–20). All rectus muscles send off two branches, with the exception of the lateral rectus which transmits only one branch. Tributaries from the major arterial circle send the radial branches to the lesser arterial circle in the iris collarette as described above. The vessel walls are relatively thick so pupillary dilation or contraction does not lead to kinking of the vessels and nutritional compromise of the iris. The vessels are nonfenestrated and are surrounded by a thick adventitial connective tissue which explains why fluorescein is relatively impermeable on iris angiography except for lightly pigmented iris (blue eyes).

The iris contains two antagonistic muscles which control the pupillary response. The sphincter iridis and the dilator pupillae are derived from the neuroectoderm. The pupillary excursion can change quite dramatically because of the interaction of these two mus-

cles (59). The iris sphincter is able to shorten to 87% of its total length by the contraction of the iris sphincter muscle fibers running in a circular band surrounding the pupil. This muscle has fibrous connections to the iris stroma and the iris dilator muscle in various sections throughout the 360-degree circumference, which is why a focally transected sphincter is still able to function. The dilator muscle of the iris is a thin long band of radial fibers and is continuous with the ciliary body pigment epithelium and the retinal pigment epithelium. The iris muscles are innervated by the autonomic nervous system. Sympathetic fibers control the dilator muscle and parasympathetic fibers act upon the sphincter muscle.

The anterior border of the iris contains multiple

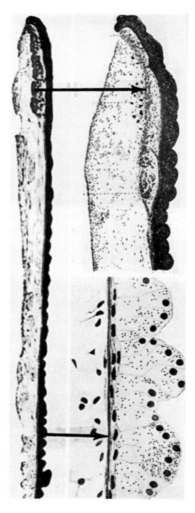

Figure 1–18.
Histologic cross section of an iris. The upper arrow points to the sphincter muscle with the lower arrow pointing to the dilator muscle. Note that the stroma is made up of connective tissue primarily. From Saltzmann M. Anatomy and histology of the human eyeball. Chicago: The University of Chicago Press, 1912.

crevices and crypts between the vascular radiations. This surface is not covered by a continuous layer of cells but rather by an irregular arrangement of condensed neural crest connective tissue which merges with the ciliary body. The aqueous humor is able to flow freely through the iris stroma which consists of collagen, mucopolysaccharide, melanocytes and nonpigmented cells.

Ciliary Body

The *ciliary body* is located between the iris and the ora serrata of the retina (Fig. 1–19). The unique morphology of this structure is necessary for the specialized functions of accomodation, regulation of outflow facility, and production of aqueous humor (40). The ciliary body is triangular in cross-section with the apex directed posteriorly toward the ora serrata and the base giving rise to the iris. It is attached to the sclera near the base by an insertion into the scleral spur. The ciliary body is commonly divided into two sections (2). The anterior portion is the pars plicata and the posterior segment is the pars plana (Figures 1–19 and 1–25). The zonules attach primarily in the valleys of the ciliary processes of the pars plicata but also along the pars plana and even the anterior aspect of the retina. Ciliary body contraction causes an anterior shift and reduces the tension on the ciliary zonules to allow the elastic lens to increase its curvature (becomes more spherical), and produce accommodation. These landmarks are also important in the surgical intervention of the posterior pole. Surgery to reduce aqueous production (cryotherapy for glaucoma) from the pars plicata is directed at 2 to 3 mm posterior to the limbus, while surgical access to the vitreous is via the pars plana approach, 3.5 to 6 mm from the limbus, in order to avoid damage to the lens anteriorly and the retina posteriorly.

The *pars plicata* features about 75 ciliary processes. These provide a large surface area for secretory function. These 2 mm-long vascularized connective tissue fronds start at the posterior aspect of the iris root and project into the posterior chamber. The space between the anterior ciliary processes and the posterior surface of the iris is the ciliary sulcus. Two layers of epithelium, nonpigmented secretory cells and pigmented cells cover the processes. They are arranged apex to apex so the nonpigmented epithelium and its basement membrane face the vitreous and lens, and the pigmented epithelium and its basement membrane face the ciliary body stroma. Aqueous humor formation is performed by an energy-dependent secretory process (see page 23). The blood-aqueous barrier is formed by zonulae occludentes near the apical intercellular border of the nonpigmented epithelium.

The *pars plana* extends from the posterior border of the ciliary processes to the ora serrata. It is covered by

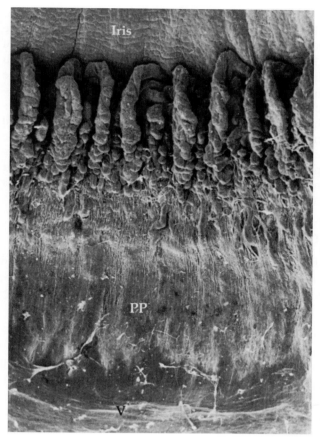

Figure 1–19.

A scanning electron micrograph of the lateral wall of the posterior chamber with the lens and zonules removed. Both the major and minor ciliary processes blend with the pars plana (PP) posteriorly. This is also the region of the vitreous base (V). (×42). From Ritch R, Shields MB, Krupin T: The Glaucomas. St Louis: Mosby, 1989.

the continuous layer of double epithelium from the pars plicata. The nonpigmented epithelium flattens gradually as it extends posteriorly to blend into the sensory retina. The pigmented layer of the pars plana blends posteriorly into the pigmented epithelium of the retina.

The *blood supply of the ciliary body* is similar to that of the *iris* (Fig. 1–20). The *anterior ciliary arteries* and the *long posterior ciliary arteries* make contributions to the marginal capillary system of the ciliary body (40). Anterior and posterior arterioles from the major arteriole circle provide the diffuse inner and outer capillaries. The anterior system is generally more numerous in capillaries and more dilated than the posterior system. The whole system is set up to shunt blood to different locations, depending upon the required function. Shunting of blood to completely bypass the ciliary body is also possible. Blood is drained from this region by the choroidal veins into the *vortex vein* system.

Three bands of *ciliary muscles* are located between the ciliary processes and sclera (Fig. 1–17). There are longitudinal, radial, and circular muscle fibers. Most of the muscle is made up of the longitudinal fibers which insert on the scleral spur. The radial muscles arise in the midportion of the ciliary body while the circular muscles line the innermost portion. The ciliary muscles behave like smooth muscle fibers. Both myelinated and nonmyelinated nerve fibers have been observed in the ciliary body. The main innervation is from the parasympathetic fibers from cranial nerve III (oculomotor nerve). Sympathetic fibers have been seen but their function is not well understood.

Choroid

The choroid is a 0.25 mm. vascular structure with dense pigmentation (uvea). The choroid consists of three vascular layers: 1. choriocapillaris (capillary layer in apposition to Brook's membrane), 2. Sattler's layer (middle layer of medium size vessels), and 3. Haller's layer (outer layer of large caliber vessels). The Sattler's, and Haller's layers are intertwined and are not fenestrated as is the choriocapillaris. The choroid also consists of melanocytes, fibroblasts, ganglion cells, and a variety of inflammatory cells.

The *choroid* extends from the ora serrata to the optic nerve and is sandwiched between the sclera and retina. There is a smooth transition from ciliary body stroma to choroid. The choroid has a spongy black appearance. It is the posterior portion of the uvea and it has an extraordinary blood flow rate. About 70% of the globe's blood is found in *choriocapillaris,* the smallest caliber choroidal vessels (18), however, they are the largest capillaries in the body. The choroidal functions include nourishing the retinal pigment epithelium and retina (external to the outer aspect of the inner nuclear layer), heat dissipation, and the production of visual pigment.

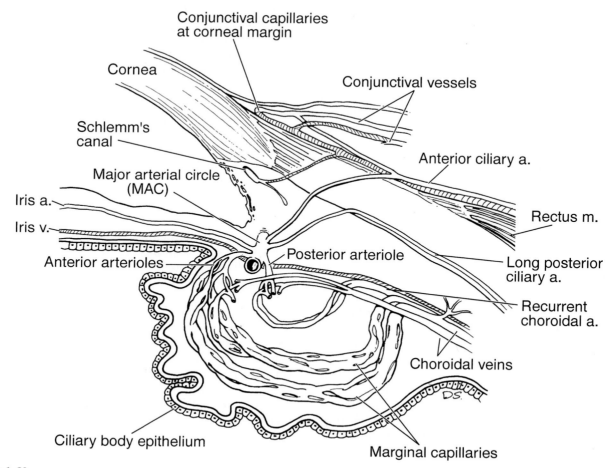

Figure 1–20.

A schematic representation of the ciliary process microvasculature. This illustrates the anterior and posterior arteriolar supplies from the major arterial circle (MAC). Interprocess connections are circled, arrows indicate their relationship to the choroidal veins proving possible shunts around the ciliary processes. From Ritch R, Shields MB, Krupin T: The Glaucomas. St Louis: Mosby, 1989, p. 82.

The exception is in the foveal zone where the sole vascular supply to the retina is the choriocapillaris. The choriocapillaris ends peripherally at the ora serrata, just posterior to the pars plana.

The choroidal vasculature is unusual since the arteries do not run parallel to the veins. The *ophthalmic artery* divides into the medial and lateral *posterior ciliary arteries.* These vessels then divide into one *long posterior ciliary artery* and a variable number of *short posterior ciliary arteries* (Fig. 1–12). The two long posterior ciliary arteries pierce the sclera about 4 mm from the optic nerve (Fig. 1–35A) and travel anteriorly via the suprachoroidal space to their branch point near the ora serrata. Rupturing these arteries leads to a *suprachoroidal hemorrhage.* At this point, about four branches reverse course to run posterior to the equator. The two long posterior arteries supply approximately 50% of the anterior segment circulation. The 15 to 20 short posterior ciliary arteries pierce the sclera around the optic nerve (Fig. 1–35A) and also run in the suprachoroidal space before entering the peripapillary choroid. These branch immediately and supply the posterior choriocapillaris up to the equator. The *anterior ciliary arteries* described earlier also make a contribution to the choriocapillaris in addition to the iris and ciliary body. About 8 to 12 branches pass through the ciliary body to connect to the anterior choricapillaris. Venous drainage is mainly via the *vortex veinuses* system, which drains into the superior and inferior *ophthalmic veins.* Most of the blood passes through the cavernous sinus while some goes through the pterygoid plexus.

Choroidal blood flow is regulated by the autonomic nervous system. The innervation of the choroid is supplied by about 20 *short posterior ciliary nerves.* Both the sympathetic and the parasympathetic systems innervate the vasculature, but only the sympathetic system has an autoregulatory effect on blood flow. The high blood flow may also maintain a constant retinal temperature.

The suprachoroidal space is a potential space between the sclera and choroid. The *lamina fusca* is the connective tissue layer of the inner pigmented sclera that interfaces with the large vessels of the choroidal stroma. The darkly pigmented appearance is secondary to the large number of melanocytes present. This zone also consistes of collagen and elastic fibers, fibrocytes, ganglion cells, and nerve plexuses. This transition zone is approximately 30 microns thick. The only blood vessels present in this region are the ones that randomly pass through. Serous effusions and hemorrhages can occur in this space secondary to hypotony and inflammation.

The unusually rapid transformation from arteriole to capillary leading to the choriocapillaris enables the *choriocapillaris* to perform its functions. The capillaries are large in diameter (up to 40 to 60 microns) with thin walls. They are uniplanar beneath the retinal pigment epithelium. Unlike other capillaries in the systemic circulation, the choriocapillaris allows the passage of several erythrocytes at one time. Multiple fenestrations with diaphragms are mostly present on the internal aspect of the vessel wall, facing the retinal pigment epithelium. The blood-ocular barrier for this vascular system exists at the level of the retinal pigment epithelium. The fenestrations assist in the diffusion of metabolites. In fact, fluorescein molecules are seen to leak early on angiography and produce a mosaic pattern corresponding to the vascular architecture of the choriocapillaris. The lobular pattern is in the posterior pole and is made up of a central precapillary arteriole that becomes the capillary network and then empties into a peripheral postcapillary venule (Figures 1–12 and 1–21). This allows rapid blood flow, acting as a heat diffuser to protect the macula from heat generated by light interacting with the retina. There are various regional pattern differences (Fig. 1–21) (64). The above pattern explains why the blood flow is most rapid in this region. In the equatorial region, the capillaries act as a more direct interface between the arterioles and the venules and create a spindle shape. In the periphery, the capillaries are a direct route and form right angles between the arterioles and the venules. This creates a characteristic ladder appearance. The nuclei of the endothelial cells line up on the external aspect of the vessels, leaving minimal room for fenestrations. Connective tissue and nerves are seen in the spaces between the capillaries.

The innermost layer of the choroid is the PAS-positive *Bruch's membrane,* which is a true basement membrane (Figures 1–26 and 1–27). The PAS staining increases with age along with an increase in thickness. In a child, it is 2 microns thick centrally and in the adult, it is 2 to 4 microns thick. Peripherally, it is typically thinner. At the electron microscopic level, five distinct layers make up Bruch's membrane. From inside to outside, they include the basement membrane of the retinal pigment epithelium, the inner collagenous zone, the elastic fiber area, the outer collagenous zone, and the basement membrane of the choriocapillaris endothelium. This series of connective tissue sheets is highly permeable to fluorescein.

■ LENS

The lens refracts divergent rays of light so they are uniformly focused on the retina, providing maximal visual acuity. Moreover, it has the capacity for variable focusing for an infinite number of object distances. This is in stark contrast to the cornea, which has no ability to variably focus. The lens and cornea are able to transmit

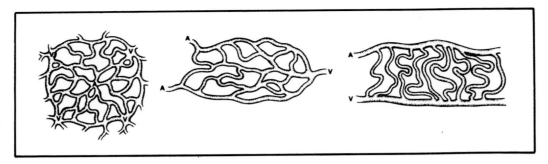

Figure 1–21.
Lobular pattern of posterior choriocapillaris (left), spindle pattern of equatorial choriocapillaris (center), and ladder pattern of peripheral choriocapillaris (right). (A) arterioles; (V) venules. Yoneya S, Tso, MOM: Angioarchitecture of the human choroid. Arch Ophthalmol 1987;105:681–687.

light because of their transparent properties but the manner of maintenance between the two structures is quite different. The cornea constantly pumps fluid across a semipermeable membrane while the lens has a highly ordered extracellular matrix created by a uniform cell with a specialized internal content.

The lens is an asymmetric biconvex structure in the posterior chamber directly behind the pupil and iris. It lacks innervation and has a regressed hyaloid vascular system from fetal life. Lens dimensions include an anterior-posterior diameter of 4 to 5 mm which varies prior to the age 40 and is more constant with presbyopia. Accommodation allows for variable lens thickness caused by tension and relaxation of the interfacing zonules with the ciliary body processes.

The zonules exit from the crypts between the ciliary processes and insert into the equatorial lens capsule in an anterior and posterior bundle (Fig. 1–22). The space between these bundles and peripheral to the equator of the lens is the *canal of Hannover*. The *canal of Petit* is the space between the posterior bundle of zonules and the anterior vitreous cortex (Fig. 1–25). The zonule fibers resemble vitreous collagen fibers in their physical diameter but they are much more tightly packed, resist collagenase, and are solublized by chymotrypsin. Their amino acid composition more closely resembles elastin than collagen. Perhaps they are related to the microfibrils of elastic tissue. Recently, fibrillin has been localized to the zonules, lens capsule, ciliary processes and lamina cribrosa (60). Its elastic property and important location may play a significant role in accommodation. Pathologically, the presence of fibrillin could explain why ectopia lentis occurs in *Marfan* patients along with the aneurysmal dilations of the aorta. The aneurysms occur as the result of an abnormality in the elastic layer of large blood vessels where fibrillin is found. Loss of

this elastic property may also account for presbyopia (lack of accommodation with age) (27).

The lens structure is the direct result of embryonic development of the invaginating surface epithelium into a lens placode and an understanding of its development will simplify the anatomy. The epithelium is pinched off to complete invagination, resulting in a lens vesicle. The vesicle is an inside-out hollow ball of lens epithelial cells with their apices pointed inward and their basal sides outward. The cuboidal cells elongate and are then terminally differentiated into primary lens fiber cells. This structure is then referred as the *embryonic nucleus*. The lens stem cells are located in a narrow band just anterior to the equator. These cells undergo mitotic division in this germinative zone and throughout life become multiple layers of fiber-like cells referred to as secondary fiber cells (also see Embryology Chapter 2, p. 64 to 66). At birth there are about 1.5 million fibers but by age 80, there are 3.5 million fibers on the average (33). As younger fibers are formed, the nuclei of the deeper, older cells migrate to the anterior equatorial surface to create the lens bow. Eventually, the nuclei and cytoplasmic organelles disappear. The initial secondary fiber cells meet at the *Y-shaped sutures*. The anterior suture is upright while the posterior one is upside-down. This is commonly called the *fetal nucleus* and can be visualized directly under the capsule at birth. Subsequent cells from later generations form irregular stellate structures that are less readily visible by biomicroscopy. This transition clinically is seen as the boundary between the nucleus and the cortex. All primary and secondary fiber cells are retained and metabolically supported for a lifetime. If these cells fail to be preserved, then various pathologic processes can be encountered.

The lens *epithelium* is a single layer of cuboidal cells (Fig. 1–23). They extend to the equator where they be-

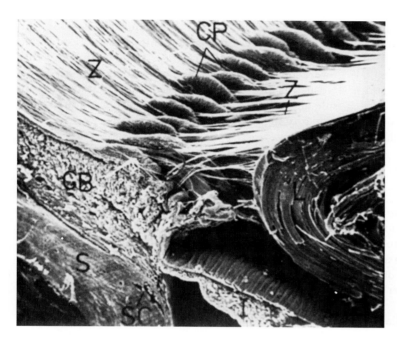

Figure 1–22.
Scanning electron micrograph of the accommodative apparatus. Zonules (Z), ciliary processes (CP), iris (I), ciliary body (CB), sclera (S), lens (L), and Schlemm's canal (SC). From Rohen SC: Invest Ophthalmol Vis Sci 1979;18:136.

gin their differentiation into fiber cells. The cells lie on their basement membrane and interdigitate with each other. Zonulae occludentes join the adjacent lens fibers together. The lens capsule is a transparent PAS-positive elastic basement membrane, the product of the lens epithelium. Up to age 35, the entire capsule is uniformly thick but later it is altered. It becomes significantly thicker anteriorly throughout life as the result of deposition while there is concomitant posterior thinning because of compression. The lens epithelial cells are probably responsible for secondary posterior capsule opacification after extracapsular cataract surgery.

The normal adult lens is 65% water and 35% protein. The delicate balance between these constituents is responsible for the maintenance of transparency. The proteins were originally divided into two groups, the soluble crystallins and the insoluble albuminoid fraction. The crystallins are subdivided by molecular weight and electrophoretic mobility. Albuminoid is about 12.5% of the total protein fraction while alpha, beta and gamma crystallins make up 31.7, 55.4 and 1.5% of the total protein content, respectively (44).

The alpha-crystallin is the largest molecule of the three crystallines and also has a very close relationship to the albuminoid group. The proportion of alpha-crystallin is highest in the cortex of the young but decreases with age. By contrast, albuminoid is highest in the nucleus and continues to accumulate. With time there is a conversion of the ratio with progressively more albuminoid and less alpha-crystallin. In fact, the conversion is the result of direct transformation of alpha-crystallin into albuminoid.

A chaperone role has been postulated for alpha-crys-

tallin (25). Denaturation of any of the lens proteins will have detrimental effect on transparency. When proteins denature, they aggregate and form large insoluble particles. Cells in the lens are unique in that they have no mechanism for protein regeneration of new normal product. Once a lens cell proceeds with its terminal differentiation, this reparative function is lost. The aggregation of denatured protein means loss of transparency. Alpha-crystallin has been shown to play a role in the suppression of protein aggregation and even the refolding

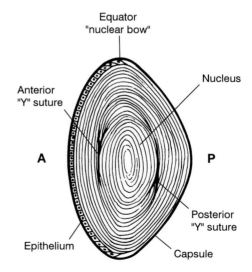

Figure 1–23.
Gross and ultrastructural representation of the lens and its components. Note the Y sutures between the junction of the nuclear and cortical components.

or renaturation of denatured proteins. Its decline in content in the aged implies a significant role in *cataractogenesis* as the result of increased protein denaturation and aggregation.

Glutathione and ascorbic acid are also present in unusually high amounts in the lens. Glutathione is continuously formed in the lens and the reduced form may play a role in hydrogen transport for oxidative metabolism. The loss of anabolic enzymes for glutathione synthesis have been shown to be responsible for human *subcapsular cataracts* (46), confirming that several mechanisms exist for cataract generation. Ascorbic acid is in the highest concentration under the capsule and may also participate in hydrogen donation in oxidative metabolism.

■ VITREOUS BODY

The vitreous is a transparent structure that fills the posterior eye and allows light to pass without obstruction. It is located posterior to the lens and anterior to the retina. It fills the center of the eye and makes up a volume of about 4 ml which constitutes about 80% of the globe. This is the largest ocular structure but perhaps the least understood (51, 58).

The main constituents of the vitreous are collagen, hyaluronic acid, and water. Their interaction is important in understanding the function of this structure. Water is responsible for this structure's transparent characteristics and accounts for 99% of the volume by weight, while 1% is solid content. Collagen type II is the major structural protein but shows minor variations in amino acid content and secondary carbohydrate modifications when compared to the cartilaginous type II collagen. The close similarities of these two type II collagen molecules leads one to conclude that the vitreous has a mechanical role similar to cartilage. The vitreous scaffold may play a role in the protection of the inner eye by minimizing movement and by creating an outward stabilizing force on the retina for optimal function. Collagen type IX is also present in the vitreous as well as cartilage but there is a small difference in the size between the two variably located molecules. The function of type IX has not been well worked out to date.

Hyaluronic acid is a glycosaminoglycan and is named because of its discovery in the clear colorless vitreous ("hyalos" means glass in Greek). Glycosaminoglycans are repeating units of disaccharides which are linked to a core protein resulting in proteoglycans, which are high in content in the vitreous. These molecules typically bind with collagen, and in the case of the vitreous, the interaction is quite tenacious. This results in a lightly cross-linked polymer structure. In the vitreous, hyaluronic acid is the cross-linking element for the collagen molecules and is able to hold an extremely large volume of water relative to its weight (Fig. 1–24). Documenting changes in the relationship between these two molecules has led to the understanding of various pathological states, including vitreous liquefaction and posterior vitreous detachments. Syneretic cavities have been found to be depleted of collagen with no other significant difference in biochemical make-up from normal vitreous.

Water is the main component of the vitreous and it fills nearly most of the remaining space left behind by the hyaluronic acid and collagen. The polar nature of water also allows for significant interaction to occur with the glycoprotein scaffold. The alignment of the water produces a gelatinous material. This structure minimizes light scatter so the gelatin is transparent for optimal visual function.

This hydrated network is the product of the residing cells called hyalocytes. These cells have been shown to produce large amounts of hyaluronic acid, particularly in the cortical vitreous near the interface with the retina. The amount of hyaluronic acid adjacent to the posterior surface of the lens is significantly reduced. Hyalocytes have also been shown to produce collagen and various other enzymes for construction of its surrounding environment. Other vitreous components, such as salts, glucose and its waste products, vitamins, lipids and nitrogenous molecules, are present because of the metabolism of these cells. Ascorbic acid is evenly distributed throughout the vitreous and has been shown to absorb ultraviolet light. In essence, the vitreous acts as a depository for various substances involved in its maintenance and does so by playing a role in the movement and homeostasis of these intraocular solutes and solvents. Control of this transport is regulated in part by the molecular sieve characteristics of the vitreous gel which tends to allow smaller molecules easier access like a gel filtration column. The energy produced by the hyalocytes from glucose is needed to manufacture the extracellular matrix and to perform a basal phagocytic function. Under conditions of stress and inflammation, these cells catabolically alter their surrounding biochemical environment.

The vitreous cortex is the peripheral outer shell of the vitreous. It consists of the anterior vitreous cortex and the posterior vitreous cortex. Collagen type IV, along with linking glycoproteins such as laminin, is responsible for the strong interaction with the internal limiting membrane of the retina. The interaction occurs anteriorly from the pars plana to involve the entire

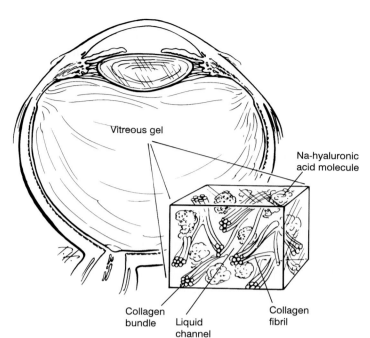

Figure 1–24.
Ultrastructure of the human vitreous. Collagen fibrils are present with bundles of parallel collagen fibrils in cross-section (arrow). The enlarged schematic diagram also pictures the vitreous ultrastructure, depicting the association of the hyaluronic acid molecules with the collagen fibrils.

retina posteriorly. The *vitreous base* has an exceptionally strong attachment both anterior and posterior to the ora serrata (Fig. 1–25). The vitreal collagen fibers insert directly into the basal lamina without an intervening linker component creating a strong weld. The vitreous is also firmly attached to the area around the optic nerve. The only region not inserted into the basal lamina is anterior to the peripheral anterior hyaloid face. This region includes the zonules and the posterior

chamber aqueous humor. It is similar to the synovial surface of a joint and helps to explain why similar inflammatory diseases may affect both locations. Centrally, the anterior hyaloid face has an adhesion to the posterior peripheral lens capsule and is called the *hyaloideocapsular (Wiegert's) ligament*. There is a tendency for this structure to break down during midlife, which facilitates surgical vitrectomy in older patients. Central to this structure and posterior to the posterior lens cap-

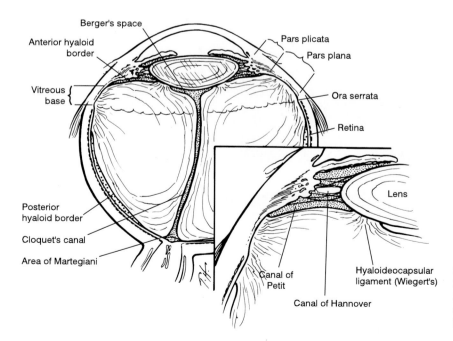

Figure 1–25.
Representation of the gross vitreous anatomy. Note the defined organization of the gel with respect to other intraocular structures despite it having an amorphous quality.

sule is *Berger's space* which narrows to become *Cloquet's canal* as it approaches the optic nerve (Fig. 1–25). This canal is the location of the embryonic hyaloid vasculature and the primary vitreous. In the human vitreous, there are fine, parallel fibers, which run in an anterior-posterior direction. The fibers arise in the vitreous base and travel in a circumferential fashion to the vitreous cortex while the central fibers run parallel to Cloquet's canal. The secondary vitreous makes up most of the adult vitreous and contains channels throughout the substance. The channels probably play a role in the transport of various substances. The zonules constitute the tertiary vitreous, which is a misnomer since they originate from the ciliary body.

■ RETINA

The retina is a highly organized structure made up of alternating layers of cell bodies and synaptic processes (Fig. 1–26). Besides capturing light and transducing it to a pattern of neural activity for transmission to the brain, the retina also carries out numerous other functions in processing this information. These functions include the processing of the light energy into "on and off" channels, color processing, contrast enhancement, and feature detection. The retinal ganglion cells are the final common pathway for visual information travelling through their axoms from the retina to the brain. The above functions are performed by the receptive-field properties of the retinal ganglion cells.

Retinal Topography

A brief overview of the stratification of the retinal structure demonstrates that the rod and cone photoreceptors are located at the distal or outer edge of the retina (31) (Fig. 1–27). The fenestrated external limiting membrane is made up of the attachment sites of adjacent photoreceptors and Müller cells (Fig. 1–27). The outer segments of the photoreceptors contain light-sensitive pigments that reside within stacked disc membranes (Fig. 1–30). The outer portions of the photoreceptors are surrounded by processes of the retinal pigment epithelial cells as well as a specialized extracellular matrix. Both play a role in the function of the photoreceptors.

The proximal ends of the photoreceptors synapse with bipolar cells and horizontal cells. The horizontal cells are the interneurons of the outer retina and create a feedback loop onto the photoreceptor terminals. This region of synapsing cells is called the outer plexiform layer (Fig. 1–27). In the macula (Fig. 1–28), the outer plexiform layer is thicker secondary to the rods and

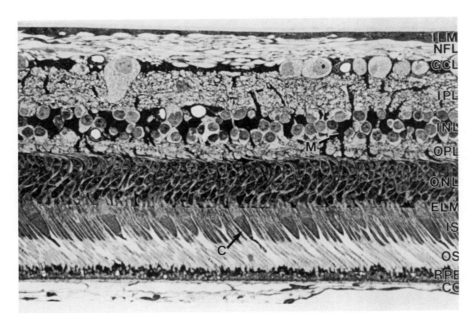

Figure 1–26.
A light micrograph of a section through a monkey retina. Several cell and synaptic layers can be identified: ILM, inner limiting membrane; NFL, nerve fiber layer; GCL, ganglion cell layer; IPL, inner plexiform layer; INL, inner nuclear layer; M, Müller cells; OPL, outer plexiform layer; ONL, outer nuclear layer; ELM, external limiting membrane; IS, photoreceptor inner segments; OS, photoreceptor outer segments; RPE, retinal pigment epithelium; and CC, choriocapillaris. Note that the cones (C) are scattered but more prominent than the numerous thin rods. From Ryan SR et al: Retina 2e. St Louis: Mosby, 1994, p 38.

cones becoming more oblique in orientation as they deviate from the fovea. This layer is known as the fiber *layer of Henle*. At the foveola, the fiber layer of Henle lies almost parallel to the nerve fiber layer, explaining the star pattern of accumulated lipid or blood products in this region.

The bipolar cells relay information from the photoreceptors to the inner plexiform layer where they contact amacrine and ganglion cells. Amacrine cells are the interneurons of the inner retina and they make contacts by synapsing with other amacrine cells, ganglion cells, and feeding back onto bipolar cells. This region is the inner plexiform layer. These cells provide directional selectivity and feedforward inhibition of the ganglion cells. The nuclei of the bipolar, Müller, horizontal and amacrine cells constitute the inner nuclear layer.

The final common pathway for the receptive field are the ganglion cells, whose axons project to the lateral geniculate nucleus. The ganglion cells receive their synaptic input from the bipolar and amacrine cells. The axons of the ganglion cells form the nerve fiber layer. They become myelinated after passing through the lamina cribosa of the optic nerve.

The internal limiting membrane is a true membrane and is made from the footplates of Müller cells. The internal limiting membrane attaches to the smooth basal lamina of the retina that interfaces with the vitreous. This internal limiting basement membrane is continuous with the basement membrane of the nonpigmented ciliary epithelium.

The overall direction of the cells and their processes in the retina allow the discrimination of the layer where an exudate or blood product accumulates in a pathological process. The middle and outer retinal elements are perpendicular to the plane of the retinal pigment epithelial cells but the inner retinal elements are parallel. Blood in the outer layer creates round blots while the blood in the inner layers produces flame-shaped patterns.

The *macula* is regarded clinically as the area within the retinal vascular arcades (Fig. 1–28). However, the histological definition is a region where more than one layer of the ganglion cells are found. The center of the macula lies 4.5 mm temporal and slightly inferior to the center of the optic nerve. The macula is about 6 mm in diameter and extends nasally from the fovea, almost reaching the optic disc. The fovea is a 1.5 mm diameter area in the center of the macula. The foveal borders are indistinct peripherally, but centrally there is a depression called the foveola. Only photoreceptors, glial cells, and Müller cells are present in this area. The foveal avascular zone is a capillary-free zone and is bounded in an intermediate location between the foveola and the fovea. The diameter of this region is 250 to 600 microns. The macula lutea, or yellow spot, is a gross anatomic description of a yellow reflex and is probably the result of either carotenoid or xanthophil pigment in this region.

The retina equator is peripheral to the macula, and refers to an equatorial plane of the globe. The equator can be identified externally and internally by its proximity to the vortex veins. Externally the equator is about 8 mm anterior to the superior vortex veins, and 6 mm anterior to the inferior vortex veins. Internally the retinal equator is located approximately 5 mm anterior to the superior vortex vein and 4 mm anterior to the inferior vortex veins. The retinal distance is shorter because the vortex veins tunnel through the sclera in a posterior to anterior direction. The equator is approximately 12 mm posterior to the corneal limbus.

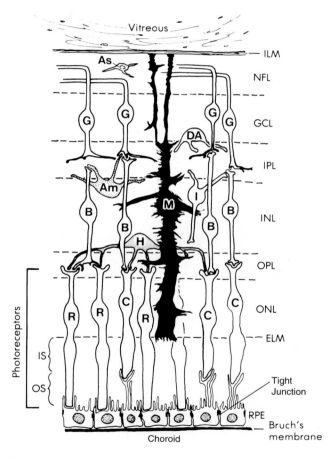

Figure 1–27.
Schematic diagram of the cell types and histologic layers in the human retina. Retinal layers are labelled as in Figure 1–26. Also shown are Bruch's membrane and the edge of the vitreous. The basic relationship between rod (R) and cone (C) photoreceptors as well as bipolar (B), horizontal (H), amacine (Am), inner plexiform cell (I), and ganglion (G) neurons are depicted. The Müller cell (M) extends almost the entire width of the retina. Astrocytes (As) are found primarily in the nerve fiber layer (NFL). Modified from Dowling JE, Boycott BB: In: Ryan, et al: Retina, 2/e. St Louis: Mosby, 1994.

Figure 1–28a.
The anatomic macula containing the fovea and foveola within the geometric center of the macula. The lower portion shows a cross-section of the macular region depression. From Shields MB: A Study Guide for Glaucoma. Baltimore: Williams & Wilkins, 1982.

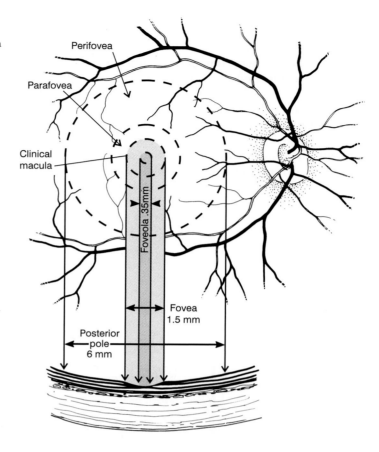

A

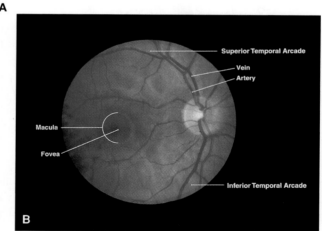

Figure 1–28b.
Clinical fundus photograph showing normal optic disc macula and retina vessels. The macula is surrounded by the temporal retinal vascular arcade. The clinical macula is relatively ill-defined and represents the area inside the temporal arcade which can be seen by the circular light reflex.

The ora serrata is the boundary point between the retina and the pars plana. Externally, the ora serrata is 6 mm from the limbus nasally and 7 mm temporally. A clinically convenient landmark is the insertion of the medial rectus nasally and the lateral rectus insertion temporally. The retinal vaculature ends in loops before reaching the ora serrata. Thus, this region is a "watershed" zone between the anterior and posterior vascular systems and may explain why peripheral retinal degen-

erations commonly occur in this area. The retina in this area is markedly attenuated with malformed photoreceptors and cystic structures.

Macula Versus Periphery (42)

Receptor Distribution . The density of the 6,000,000 cones is maximal in the fovea, which contains approximately 10% of the entire retinal cone population. The cone density across the rest of the retina decreases rapidly outside the macular region. The 0.1 mm central region of the 1.5 mm fovea, *the foveal pit,* is free of cells at its base with the exception of red and green cones. The central two degrees of the visual angle is free of blue cones. This area is the thinnest retina (0.1 mm). (The papillomacular bundle is the area of thickest retina between the optic nerve and the macula [0.23 mm]. Glial cells and Müller cells have been identified in this region. The grain density of the foveal cones accounts for the upper limits of visual acuity since it closely matches the minimum resolvable visual angle. Beyond the macula the cone density is fairly constant but asymmetric with greater densities nasally than temporally.

The 120 million rods are distributed unevenly across the retina with the exception of a complete void of rods within 0.25 mm of the fovea. Peripheral to this rod-free zone, the number of rods rapidly increases with maximum densities at 18 degrees temporally and 23 degrees nasally.

Ganglion Cells. The macula is characterized by a ganglion layer that is more than one cell layer thick. The fovea is surrounded by the parafoveal ridge, which consists of a heaped up layer of ganglion cells and inner nuclear layer cells displaced away from the fovea. Changes in the ganglion cell layer thickness are most striking when comparing the parafoveal region, where the layer may be six cells thick, to the peripheral retina, where the layer is only one cell thick.

The axons of the ganglion cells that constitute the nerve fiber layer have distinct patterns as they approach the optic disc (Fig. 1–29). The fibers nasal to the disc follow a straight course to the disc similar to spokes on a wheel. The temporal fibers, except those of the papillomacular bundle, follow a variable curvilinear course. Most of the superior, temporal, and inferior foveal fibers take an arcuate pattern to the optic disc. The median raphe is a watershed zone extending temporal from the fovea and it is from this structure that fibers are directed either in a superior or inferior direction. Peripheral temporal fibers arch above and below the temporal foveal fibers, significantly increasing the thickness of the nerve fiber layer in these areas.

At the optic nerve margin, the nerve fibers are collected into bundles by the surrounding Müller fibers. These can be seen as radiating stripes on ophthalmoscopy near the nerve head where the bundles are thick. Also, the bundles contain fibers of widely varying lengths at the margin of the optic disc. Short fibers originate near the nerve head and are superficial while the long fibers from the periphery are deep (Fig. 1–28). This demonstrates a horizontal and vertical

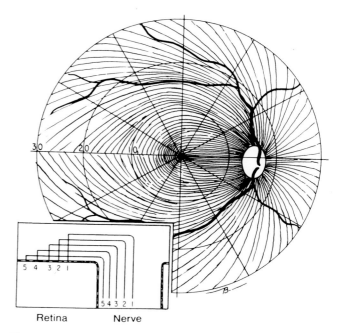

Figure 1–29.
Anatomy of retinal nerve fiber distribution. Inset depicts a cross-sectional view of axonal arrangements. Peripheral fibers run closer to the choroid and exit in the peripheral optic nerve while fibers starting closer to the optic nerve are positioned closer to the vitreous and occupy a more central nerve position.

nerve fiber bundle organization of substantial complexity.

Neurosensory Retina (4)

Photoreceptors. Photoreceptors consist of two basic types and are distinguished by light intensity function, color discrimination, and visual acuity sensitivity. *Rods* mediate scotopic, black and white, low resolution vision while *cones* provide photopic, color, high resolution vision. All photoreceptors have an outer segment that contains visual pigment, an inner segment for metabolic functions, a nucleus, and a synaptic terminal (Fig. 1–30). The inner and outer segments are connected by a cytoplasmic bridge called a cilium. Rods are cylindrical in shape while cones taper from the inner to the outer segment. The rod synaptic terminal, a spherule, is small, while the cone has a large synaptic terminal called a pedicle. Exceptions exist, such as the foveal cones which actually have a cylindrical shape.

The outer segment of the photoreceptor is the site of phototransduction, where light energy is converted into an electrochemical signal. Both rods and cones contain an elaborate system of stacked discs which arise from the invaginations in the cell's plasma membrane. A continuous process of outer segment renewal occurs with disintegation of the apical surface. The debris is re-

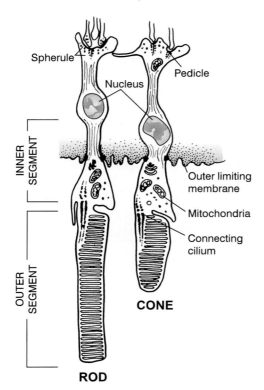

Figure 1–30.
Depiction of the ultrastructural cellular components of the rod and cone photoreceptor cells. The inner segments are characterized by many mitochondria, Golgi complexes, and ribosomes. The outer segments are made up of stacked discs. From Hageman GS, Johnson LV: J Comp Neurol 1986;249:482. Reprinted with permission of Alan R. Liss, Inc.

moved by adjacent retinal pigment epithelial cell phagocytosis. Thus, as old discs are removed, they are replaced by new discs at the base with constant turnover. Photopigments reside within the discs and are oriented to maximize their interaction with quanta of light. The physiology of these photopigments is discussed later.

The inner segment is connected to the outer segment by a specialized cilium. The retinal cilium has nine pairs of microtubules with no central pair. This differs from motile cilia. The ellipsoid portion of the inner segment contains a dense aggregation of mitochondria, where as the myoid part contains the Golgi complex with vesicular components including free and membrane-bound ribosomes. The nucleus and large quantities of glycogen are also located in the wider myoid portion of the inner segment.

The *interphotoreceptor matrix (IPRM)* lies between the apex of the neural retina and the retinal pigmented epithelium (RPE) (Fig. 1–31B). It also surrounds the outer segments and the ellipsoid portion of the inner segments of the photoreceptor. The interphotoreceptor retinol binding protein is a soluble glycoprotein made by the photoreceptors that mediates the transport of the vitamin A derivative, retinol, between the RPE and photoreceptors. Peculiar to the IPRM is its biochemical composition (24). Collagen is conspicuously absent and no known attachment factors, such as fibronectin or laminin, are found. Up to 80 proteins are contained within the matrix along with a variety of sugars. Chondroitin-4-sulfate proteoglycan is widely distributed throughout the retina while chondroitin-6-sulfate proteoglycan is associated with the cone photoreceptors. These molecules may act as insulation for the outer segments or even a facilitating role between the RPE and the photoreceptors.

Interneurons (Fig. 1–27). The interneuron cell bodies constitute the inner nuclear cell layer and consist of the bipolar, horizontal and amacrine cells (4). The bipolar cells primarily occupy the middle and inner thirds of this layer and extend synaptic processes in both directions. The horizontal cells are located near the outer nuclear layer and send their synaptic processes there; the amacrine cells have an analogous relationship to the inner nuclear layer.

Bipolar Cells

Functionally, bipolar cells are divided into two types, which are distinguished by a varied response to different types of photoreceptor neurotransmitters. The depolarizing center bipolar cells depolarize to central illumination and the hyperpolarizing center bipolar cells hyperpolarize to center illumination. Both cell types make connections with ganglion cells (Fig. 1–27).

Morphologically, three types of bipolar cells are recognized. One type is exclusively related to the rods while the other two are related to the cones but make two different types of connections with the cones. The connection types are either invaginating or flat. The invaginating bipolar cell corresponds to the depolarizing cell function and the flat bipolar cell functions in a hyperpolarizing manner. Both play a role in the generation of the ON or OFF responses to light in the retina.

Midget bipolar cells are another cell type related to the cones of the macular region and play a role in high visual acuity. They are responsible for maximum sensitivity and have only a single contact with the cone terminal while the average rod-related bipolar cell contacts as many as 45 rod terminals.

Horizontal Cells

Horizontal cells, like amacrine cells, are local-circuit neurons. These cells possess short or no axons and interact extensively with adjacent cells. Horizontal and

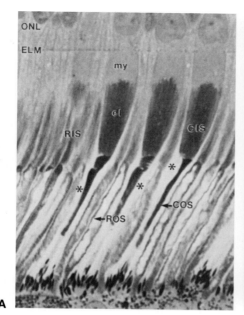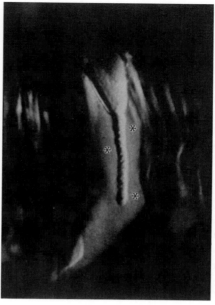

Figure 1–31.

Light micrograph of a central monkey retina thick section. A, The cone outer segments (COS) and inner segments (CIS) are readily distinguished from the rod outer (ROS) and inner (RIS) segments. Distinct regions of the interphotoreceptor matrix surround the COS and CIS (asterisks). ONL, outer nuclear layer; ELM, external limiting membrane; RPE, retinal pigment epithelium. (×2000) (B) Fluorescent light micrograph of a monkey retina demonstrating the distinct cylindric domains of the interphotoreceptor matrix (IPRM) MY (asterisks) that ensheath the cone photoreceptor inner and outer segments. EL = ellipsoid region of the inner segment of the cone which has dense mitochondria, and MY = myoid which contains Golgi complex and ribosomes. Reprinted from Hagerman GS and Johnson LV: Journal Comp Neurol 249:482, 1986. Ryan SJ et al: Retina 2e. St Louis: Mosby 1994. p. 39.

amacrine cell processes modulate and transform visual information that is ultimately conveyed to the brain.

In the central retina, horizontal cells are postsynaptic to 6 to 12 cones while in the periphery it may be as high as 50 cones per horizontal cell. Again, like the bipolar cells, the circuitry of the horizontal cells is designed to increase sensitivity and ultimately visual acuity in the region of the macula.

Two morphologically distinct horizontal cells exist. Type I cells have stout dendrites that contact only cones and a single axon which has an extensive contact with only rods. This provides a control point to modify the signal according to the type of photoreceptor input and biofeedback to the rods or cones dependent on photopic or scotopic input. Type II cells contact only cones with slim dendritic branches and a short axon.

Amacrine Cells

The amacrine cell bodies occupy the innermost portion of the inner nuclear layer and function as local circuit neurons. Their long processes contact the dendrites of bipolar, ganglion, interplexiform and other amacrine cells. Amacrine cells have also been found to reside in the ganglion cell layer. Amacrine cells are characterized by the degree of stratification of their processes; for example, unistratified, bistratified, or multistratified if the

multiple branches of the main process interact in one, two, or multiple levels, respectively. More recently they have been classified according to neurotransmitter type and up to 30 different types of amacrine cells have been discovered using this classification.

Interplexiform Cells

Interplexiform cells were discovered about 15 years agos as a distinct class of neurons. The cell bodies are located at the inner border of the inner nuclear layer; however, the processes from these cells extend to both the inner and outer plexiform layers. In the outer plexiform layer, the interplexiform cell is only presynaptic to the bipolar and horizontal cells while in the inner nuclear layer, it is both presynaptic and postsynaptic. Two different populations of these cells can be distinguished according to neurotransmitter type. Gamma-amino butyric acid (GABA)-positive processes of interplexiform cells project to the outer plexiform layer while tyrosine hydroxylase-positive interplexiform cell processes terminate in the inner plexiform layer.

Ganglion Cells. Ganglion cells transmit processed retinal information down their axons. The axons of the ganglion cells travels by way of the optic nerve, from the inner retinal nerve fiber layer to the post-chiasmal lateral geniculate body. Ganglion cell classification has no consensus, other than being based on a morphological scheme. Currently three schemes exist with some similarities. The nomenclature used for each scheme is species-specific as devised for the cat, monkey, and human.

M-Cells. The M type ganglion cells are sparse with large dendritic trees. They function by having a concentric center-surround receptive field. They function similarly to the Y cell found in the cat retina in being sensitive to movement. This allows the edge of an object to be distinguished at the retinal level.

P-Cells. The P type ganglion cells are X cells in the cat. Functionally, they are sensitive to high spatial frequencies, and fine detail. These cells also function as the color discrimination and integration center for the three primary color sensitive cones.

W-Cells. This is a heterogeneous group of ganglion cells that respond to brightness rather than contrast.

Plexiform Layer. Outer Plexiform Layer. The outer plexiform layer is made up of the interconnections between the photoreceptor synaptic bodies and the horizontal and bipolar cells. The outer plexiform layer is where horizontal dendrites and bipolar cell dendrites connect with the cone terminal pediculus and the rod terminal spherules (Fig. 1–30). The synaptic processes of a cone is termed a triad. The central processes in cone triads are derived from a corresponding bipolar cell. Dendrites from other bipolar cells make superficial contacts that are peripheral to the central processes, and each macular cone has at least 15–25 dendritic contacts.

Rod spherule terminals are innervated by horizontal cells and a rod bipolar cell. Since the rod receptive fields are larger than the cone receptive fields, one rod bipolar cell serves at least 33 rod spherules. Interphotoreceptor cell and interhorizontal cell contacts also prevail in the outer plexiform layer (Fig. 1–30).

Inner Plexiform Layer. The synaptic contacts in the inner plexiform layer are more complex than those of the outer plexiform layer because more contacts are made between a larger number of different cell types. Most of the synapses are made by either bipolar cells or amacrine cells. The bipolar terminals contact the amacrine cell processes and the ganglion cell dendrites.

Abundant synapses between amacrine cells and other cells are seen within the inner plexiform layer. However, two unusual synaptic complexes exist involving amacrine cells. First, many bipolar terminals interact with amacrine cells that make a nearby synapse back onto the terminal of the bipolar terminal to provide feedback. Another arrangement is a series of synapses, providing local interactions amongst the amacrine cells.

This is accomplished by one amacrine process synapsing on an adjacent amacrine process and so on.

Retinal Circulation. The retinal circulation emanates from the optic nerve head and supplies the inner retina from the inner aspect of the inner nuclear layer to the nerve fiber layer (13). The choroid supplies the outer layers of the retina including the outer aspect of the inner nuclear layer. The central retinal artery lies nasal to the central retinal vein within the nerve head. The arteries are narrower and straighter than the adjacent veins. The nasal arcade vessels radiate directly from the nerve head while the temporal arcade vessels arch above and below the macula in an arcuate pattern similar to the nerve fiber layer (Fig. 1–28). Cilioretinal vessels may pass directly from the temporal optic disc toward the macula. Arteries usually pass over veins at arteriovenous crossings, with greatest frequency in the superior temporal quadrant. This accounts for the increased frequency of branch retinal vein occlusions in this vicinity. Large vessels may penetrate into the inner plexiform layer but only capillaries are found in the inner nuclear layer. However, the main capillary bed of the retina is found in the nerve fiber-ganglion cell layers in addition to the inner nuclear layer.

No nervous system control exists for the retinal circulation. The retinal vasculature is controlled by a non-nervous mechanism, mainly the intrinsic tissue oxygen level. Tissue homeostasis requires a constant oxygen level and retinal perfusion pressure.

Glial Cells of the Retina. Three main classes of retinal glia exist and include the Müller cells, astrocytes, and microglia (43). Oligodendrocytes are evident around myelinated nerve fibers in the optic nerve and are analogous with the peripheral nerve Schwann cells. These cells provide structural and nutritional support.

Müller Cells. The Müller cell is the most prominent retinal cell, making up the internal limiting membrane and spanning to the external limiting membrane. The cell bodies are located in the internal nuclear layer among those of the amacrine and bipolar cells (Fig. 1–27). These cells probably play a role in the orientation, displacement, and positioning of neurons during development.

In the nuclear layers, lateral processes from the Müller cells form a honeycomb around the various cell bodies. These lateral processes intervene between most small vascular components and other neuronal processes.

In the outer retina, cell junctions between Müller cell processes and photoreceptors form the highly fenestrated external limiting membrane. This is not a true membrane. In the peripheral retina, the external limiting membrane fuses with the pigment epithelium at the ora serrata.

The Müller cell machinery is distinctive and consists of abundant glial fibrils, glycogen granules, and smooth endoplasmic reticulum. These cells also contain large quantities of lactate dehydrogenase, indicative of their role in retinal carbohydrate metabolism. These cells also play a role in potassium homeostasis and neurotransmitter degradation.

Astrocytes. Retinal astrocytes are similar to central nervous system astrocytes in their support of neural tissue. In the retina, they reside in the nerve fiber layer where their number is proportional to the thickness of the layer. Two types of astrocytes exist, elongate and stellate. Elongate astrocytes do not contact blood vessels while the stellate astrocytes have limited interaction. The exact function of these cells is not entirely clear. Speculation exists concerning a neuronal insulation function and a synergistic gliotic role with retinal pigment epithelial and Müller cells.

Microglia. The microglia tend to be flat cells and are most common in the inner plexiform layer. They can occur in the outer plexiform layer and have been confused with horizontal cells without axons. The cell bodies are slender with a few thick basal processes and many short blunt spines.

These cells are derived from mesoderm and may arise from pericytes of blood vessels. They have a phagocytic role and are activated in retinal pathologic conditions.

Retinal Pigment Epithelium. Retinal pigment epithelium (RPE) has a very specialized organization, including polygonal shape, tight junctions, apical microvilli, and basal plasma membrane invaginations, for specific functions (24). The functions of this highly organized cell include the absorption of scattered light through the presence of melanin granules, heat exchange, maintenance of the blood-retinal barrier, synthesis of the interphotoreceptor matrix, degradation of phagocytosed outer segment debris, photoreceptor outer segment renewal, retinol uptake, and active transport.

Blood Retinal Barrier and Transport. Selective transport of nutrients from the choriocapillaris to the outer retina is the result of the RPE between these two layers. Tight junctions between the RPE cells prevent the diffusion of small molecules and metabolites required by the outer retina and are obtained only by an exchange across the RPE cells. The apical microvilli and the basal cell membrane invaginations increase the surface area for nutrient and waste transport.

The tight junctions are series of lateral intercellular adhesions called junctional complexes. Zonulae occludentes and zonulae adherentes actually form the barrier. The former structure is fused plasma membrane which forms a circular band between adjacent cells. The latter structure is similar to a desmosome in cross-section.

RPE-Photoreceptor Interface
Phagocytosis. Several studies have demonstrated that the tips of rod outer segments are shed and phagocytized by the RPE (24). The number of phagosomes in the RPE is driven by the light cycle. The largest number of RPE phagosomes are seen 1–3 hours after the onset of light when the previously active rods become quiescent and just after dark when the cones become less active. The hormone melatonin has been shown to control disc shedding as a result of the light-dark cycle. This orderly shedding of the photoreceptor provides a means to renew the parts of the visual membrane apparatus.

Two distinct phagocytic processes in the RPE cells exist. These include a slow, nonspecific processing of foreign material and a rapid, specific uptake of shed photoreceptor outer segments. The latter process is initiated by binding of the photoreceptor fragments to the RPE apical microvilli that interdigitate with outer segments. After binding, invagination of the RPE plasma membrane occurs around the plasma membrane of the outer segment. Next, the outer segment is ingested leading to a phagosome. This process occurs because of a reorganization of the microfilaments in the microvilli.

The phagosomes are then transported to the basal portion of the cell by a microtubule-mediated transport system. This is an energy-dependent process. Finally, the phagosomes fuse with lysosomes that contain enzymes to completely degrade the membrane-bound proteins. Aging and pathological conditions may cause deficiencies in the degradation with the formation of lipofuscin granules. The role of lipofuscin granules in disease is not entirely clear.

Photoreceptor Renewal. Photoreceptor renewal is a complex process whereby protein and lipid from the inner segment of the photoreceptor continuously migrate toward the outer segment where they are assembled into new discs or dispersed within the cell for homeostatic function.

The renewal process has been worked out primarily for the rod photoreceptor (5). Using autoradiography, an injection of radioactive amino acids was followed over time (Fig. 1–32). The radioactivity was isolated to the Golgi complex of the inner segment where secondary carbohydrate modification takes place. These vesicles then migrate in about two hours to the connecting cilium and fuse with the plasma membrane. A band of radioactivity is observed at the most basal portion of the outer segment. Over the next several weeks, the band moves apically until it reaches the tips of the rod outer segments. The amino acids have been shown to be incorporated into opsin and once in the discs, rhodopsin is made with the incorporation of 11-cis-retinaldehyde (see below). This same general pattern holds

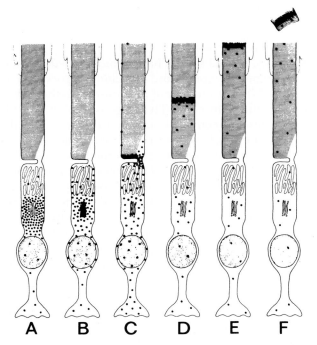

Figure 1–32.
Illustration of the rod photoreceptor outer segment disc membrane renewal including membrane assembly, detachment, and phagocytosis. Radioactive amino acids are incorporated into nascent proteins in the inner segment (A). The proteins are transported to the Golgi apparatus (B) for modification. Opsin is then transported to the apical plasma membrane of the inner segment and assembled to form the new basal outer segment discs (C). With time the radioactive discs are displaced the length of the outer segment (D and E). Finally they are shed from the outer segment and phagocytized by the retinal pigment epithelium. From Young RW: Invest Ophthalmol 1976;15:700–725.

true for the lipids used in the photoreceptor membranes. The lipids are made in the smooth endoplasmic reticulum of the inner segment. Both the newly synthesized opsin and lipid form a vesicle that is transported to the base of the growing outer segment. The lipid, however, is not transported to the apical cell in a discrete band; but diffuses throughout the entire outer segment.

Photochemical Physiology. Absorption of a photon by a visual pigment is the initial event in the visual excitation chain (17). The visual pigment for rod cells is called rhodopsin. Rhodopsin is attached in a single molecular layer to the outer segment discs of the rods. Rhodopsin is composed of two parts, vitamin A aldehyde (11-cis-retinal), and opsin (protein). The light absorbing molecule is vitamin A aldehyde and the protein opsin acts to secure the vitamin A aldehyde to the outer segment disc. Upon stimulation with light, the vitamin A aldehyde changes from the cis to trans form and is released from the visual pigment protein opsin. The trans form of vitamin A aldehyde is straighter than the cis form which results in an unfolding of the protein (Fig.

1–33). Rhodopsin is firmly imbedded in the lipid layer of the outer segment and is stabilized by fatty acids of the lipid layer. Photon excitation of the 11-cis retinal is termed bleaching. The actual bleaching cascade takes less than a millisecond and goes through eight intermediate steps (Fig. 1–34). The most important intermediate of rhodopsin is metarhodopsin since it actually initiates visual excitation. The ultimate breakdown products of metarhodopsin are all-trans-retinal and opsin.

The all-trans-retinal must be reisomerized and combined with opsin to form a regenerated visual pigment (rhodopsin). Vitamin A comes from three sources including the circulation from the liver, ingested outer segment material (phagosomes), and visual pigment in the photoreceptors. Rhodopsin is regenerated by the conversion of all-trans-retinal (aldehyde) to all-trans-retinol (alcohol) by the enzyme retinol dehydrogenase in the outer segments. All trans-retinol (alcohol) is then transported to the RPE where it is isomerized to 11-cis-retinol by retinoid isomerase. The 11-cis-retinol is then returned to the outer segments where it is oxidized to 11-cis-retinal (aldehyde) and then recombined with opsin to form rhodopsin. Rhodopsin is specific to the rod photoreceptor, and has a peak absorption of light at a wavelength of about 500 nm.

Cone cell visual pigment is very similar to the rhodopsin of rods. There are three types of cone photoliable visual pigments that absorb specific wavelengths of light. Cones are, therefore, designated by their sensitivity to a specific wavelength of light and the three types of cones are: blue (short wave length approximately 450

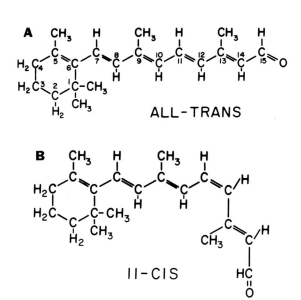

Figure 1–33.
The chemical structures of (A) all-trans-retinaldehyde and (B) cis-retinaldehyde. From Anderson RE: Biochemistry of the Eye. San Francisco: American Academy of Ophthalmology. 1983;190.

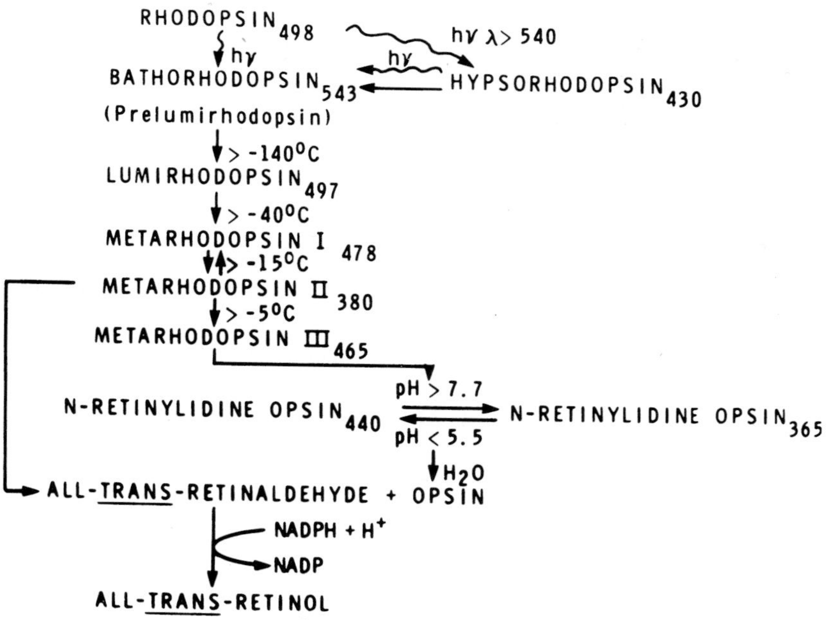

```
RHODOPSIN₄₉₈        hν λ> 540
     ⟩ hν      hν
BATHORHODOPSIN₅₄₃ ← HYPSORHODOPSIN₄₃₀
(Prelumirhodopsin)
     ↓ > -140°C
LUMIRHODOPSIN₄₉₇
     ↓ > -40°C
METARHODOPSIN I ₄₇₈
     ↓↑ > -15°C
METARHODOPSIN II ₃₈₀
     ↓ > -5°C
METARHODOPSIN III ₄₆₅
                    pH > 7.7
N-RETINYLIDINE OPSIN₄₄₀ ⇌ N-RETINYLIDINE OPSIN₃₆₅
                    pH < 5.5
                    ↓ H₂O
ALL-TRANS-RETINALDEHYDE + OPSIN
           ↓— NADPH + H⁺
           ↓→ NADP
ALL-TRANS-RETINOL
```

Figure 1–34.
The rhodopsin bleaching sequence. From Anderson RE: Biochemistry of the Eye. San Francisco: American Academy of Ophthalmology. 1983;190.

mm), green (middle wavelength approximately 530 nm), and red (long wavelength approximately 565 nm). The sensitivity of each cone cell to a particular wavelength is determined by the specific type of visual protein (opsin). Cone opsins are called iodopsin.

Selective wavelength absorption by the cones is only a crude initiation step for the color vision processing. Color receptive fields exist and allow the visual cortex to recognize action potentials which ultimately provide the entire color spectrum. The P-type ganglion cell provides the integration of the color information from the three distinct color cones before proceeding to the occipital lobe for final interpretation.

■ ORBITAL FIBROADIPOSE SYSTEM

Periorbita

The periorbita is a variably adherent and highly innervated fibrous layer that covers the bones of the orbit. This is analogous to other bones in the body which are covered by a similar layer called the periosteum. The periorbita has several firm attachment points in the orbit including the suture lines, the foramina, the fissures, the arcus marginalis (orbital rim), and the lacrimal crest. At other locations, the periorbita can be lifted from the bone with relative ease, both for the surgeon getting exposure to the bone or by accumulations of blood or pus. The periorbita adjacent to the orbital rim is a dense layer while the layer next to the orbital contents is more loosely packed. The periorbita is extensively vacularized with interconnections so no vascular borders exists. Innervation is supplied by twigs from the regional branches of the intraorbital trigeminal nerve (V_1/V_2, sensory).

Both the optic foramen and the superior orbital fissure periorbita are thick and continuous with the dura mater posteriorly. Therefore, surgery or trauma posteriorly may result in cerebrospinal fluid leaks. The periorbita is also continuous with the bones of the sphenopalatine and temporal fossae through the inferior orbital fissure.

Anteriorly, the periorbita is continuous with the periosteum of the frontal, zygomatic, maxillary, and nasal bones. From the region of the arcus marginalis, it is continuous with the orbital septum.

The lacrimal fascia is an extension of the periorbita. It covers the lacrimal sac between the anterior and posterior lacrimal crests while the periorbita proper covers the lacrimal fossa. In essence, these two structures envelope the lacrimal sac.

Septa

The fibrous tissue organization within the orbit has classically been described in terms of gross anatomy dissection findings (30). The orbit has been divided into three regions including the extraperiosteal, the extraconal and the intraconal spaces. The extraconal and intraconal spaces are separated by the rectus muscles and intermuscular septa (Fig. 1–7C). These septa are more dense in the anterior orbit, leading to difficult dissection. They are formed by radially orientated fibrovascular connective tissue which acts as bridges between the muscles and the periorbita. In addition, these septa connect and provide support to all of the intraorbital structures. This creates highly complex surgical spaces despite leading to anatomic uniformity of the tissue relationships. The orbital fat is divided into lobules by the connective tissue septa which surrounds all orbital structures. Thus, fractures and trauma to the orbit with resultant altered connective tissue architecture account for the varied clinical results (50).

Muscle Sheaths

The extraocular muscles are ensheathed in muscular fascia which also stretch between the muscles. These sheaths of connective tissues have been referred to the intermuscular septa—however they have a complex conformation. These fascial coverings are thin posteriorly but become much denser anteriorly. The fascial membranes connect to the orbital walls external to the muscle cone and to the fibrous septa dividing the intraconal fat. The two sides of the muscular fascia vary in thickness with the bulbar side being thinner while the thicker external aspect forms the check ligaments for the rectus muscles. The fascia contains scattered smooth muscle fibers that are innervated by the sympathetic nervous system.

A definite connection exists between the muscles and their fascia over the anterior one-third of their lengths. This is especially true where the fascia of the muscles inserts onto the globe. This explains why movement persists after an enucleation when the muscles have not been reinserted to an implant. The inability of the muscles to retract deep into the posterior orbit provide some movement to the anteriorly placed implant.

Check ligaments are orbital wall extensions from extraocular muscle sheaths which become prominent anteriorly and on the external surface of the muscles. Originally it was thought that these structures limited the excursion of the extraocular muscles. However, these fascial sheaths neither "check" the motion of the globe nor are they true ligaments. They function primarily as support structures for the globe and the surrounding tissues. The best developed check ligaments are those of the horizontal muscles because of their major support of the globe against gravity in the orbit. The lateral rectus check ligament is the strongest and inserts on the posterior aspect of Whitnall's lateral orbital tubercle with minor contributions to the lateral conjunctival fornix and lateral orbital septum. The medial rectus check ligament inserts on several points including the bone just posterior to the posterior lacrimal crest, medial orbital septum, caruncle, and the plica semilunaris. The superior rectus muscle sheath blends with the sheath of the levator palpebral superioris muscle. The superior transverse Whitnall's ligament has been postulated to serve as the superior check ligament serving as a fulcrum for upper lid excursion. The fused sheaths of the inferior oblique and inferior rectus muscles propagate fascial connections to the inferior periorbita for some checking function.

Tenon's Capsule

Tenon's capsule, also known as the fascia bulbi, is a fibrous membrane that extends anteriorly from the posterior aspect of the globe at the optic nerve to fuse with the conjunctiva 2 to 3 mm posterior to the limbus. The optic nerve is attached to Tenon's capsule as it passes through the fascia. It is thickest anteriorly and thins posteriorly over the globe. Anterior to the equator, Tenon's capsule extends forward over the extraocular muscles and divides them from the extraconal structures such as orbital fat. It is closely applied over the globe but may be lifted off to reveal a fine netlike structure. The resultant potential space is called Tenon's space. Externally, it joins the network of fibrous septa dividing the lobules of orbital fat. Posterior to the equator, Tenon's capsule is a fibrous condensation with the extraocular muscles passing external to the recti muscles, separating the intraconal orbital fat from the sclera. Violation of Tenon's capsule in this location exposes the intraconal orbital fat to the sclera, muscle, intermuscular membrane and/or conjunctiva which results in adhesions and can limit globe motility. Tenon's capsule is penetrated by various nerves, vessels, and all six extraocular muscles to reach the globe anteriorly. Orbital implants used after enucleation are placed within this fibrous space.

Lockwood's Suspensory Ligament

A hammock-like structure has been described extending between the medial and lateral orbital walls from the fused fascia of the inferior rectus and inferior oblique muscles (37). The capsulopalpebral fascia extends from the inferior oblique to tarsus and surrounds the inferior oblique to fuse to the suspensory ligament of Lockwood (Fig. 1–7B). The capsulopalpebral head extends from the inferior rectus to the inferior oblique to join with Lockwood's ligament.

Orbital Fat

The orbital fat occupies the remainder of the space in the orbit that is not filled with fascia, globe, muscles, nerves, vessels, and glandular structures (29). Anteriorly, the fat is fibrous while being lobular posteriorly due to the decreased density of a fibrous scaffold. The fat is a cushion that stabilizes and supports the globe and allows it a wide range of motion. Fat adherence to the sclera following surgical or accidental trauma to Tenon's capsule can result in restriction of eye movement and strabismus (See Fig. 20–4).

Behind the orbital septum in the upper lid lies the

yellow preaponeurotic fat pad. Medial to this and inferior to the trochlea lies the medial fat pad, which is firm and white. Removal of this fat pad during blepharoplasty usually requires placement of a deep anesthetic in the medial orbit. The close relationship of the medial fat pad to the trochlea and the medial palpebral artery requires careful attention when operating in this region.

The orbital fat in the inferior orbit is divided into three compartments (7). The medial third of the fat is divided from the central third by the inferior oblique muscle. An arcuate expansion of the inferior oblique muscle sheath travelling inferotemporally toward the orbital floor divides the lateral fat pad from the central fat. The inferior orbital fat provides an excellent landmark for the transconjunctival approach. The dissection remains anterior to the orbital fat and septum to reach the orbital floor and rim.

■ EXTRAOCULAR MUSCLES

The extraocular muscles are the orbital structures responsible for eye movement and alignment (Fig. 1–7C) (52). All extraocular muscles arise from the orbital apex, except for the inferior oblique, which originates just posterior to the lacrimal fossa (Fig. 1–3). The superior portion of the annulus of Zinn is called the upper tendon of Lockwood while the inferior portion of the ring is called the lower tendon of Zinn. There are four *rectus muscles* that course straight from the annulus of Zinn to the globe. The superior rectus and the medial rectus originate from the superior tendon and the inferior rectus and the lateral rectus originate from the inferior tendon. The levator and the superior oblique muscles arise from the periosteum of the lesser wing of the sphenoid superior and medial to the annulus of Zinn. Posteriorly, the annulus is connected to dura while medially and laterally it attaches to the lesser and greater wings of the sphenoid, respectively.

The extraocular muscles are a specialized form of skeletal muscle. Two distinct muscle fiber types exist in order to carry out diverse functions. The feldenstruktur muscle fiber is a slow tonic type able to carry out smooth pursuit movements while the fibrillenstruktur muscle fiber is adapted for fast movement consistent with saccadic movements. All rectus muscles are innervated from the intraconal side at the posterior $\frac{2}{3}$ of the muscles.

The extraocular muscles grow in childhood as the orbit and eye enlarge. Interestingly, the angular relationship of the muscles to the eye remains constant. The horizontal recti reach a length of about 40 mm while the superior rectus is slightly longer and the inferior rectus is slightly shorter. The medial rectus has the greatest mass and the superior rectus the least. The insertions of the recti muscles progressively increase their distance from the corneal limbus in a clockwise fashion for the right eye and counter-clockwise fashion for the left eye. The medial rectus is closest and the superior rectus is the farthest. This anatomic relationship is termed the *spiral of Tillaux* (Fig. 1–35B). Significant variation may occur between individuals. Recession of the rectus muscles tends to produce proptosis and resection enophthalmus. The oblique muscles insert on the posterior lateral aspect of the globe (Fig. 1–35). For further discussion of vertical rectus and oblique muscles see Chapter 14 and Figure 14–1. Table 14–1 summarizes the anatomy of the extraocular muscles.

Medial Rectus

The medial rectus remains close to the medial orbital wall until it reaches the anterior third of its course when it angles medially to insert on the eye about 5.5 mm from the limbus (Fig. 14–1A). It has the greatest mass of the recti, perhaps because of the constant need to maintain the eye in primary position despite the 22° divergent orbital axis (Fig. 1–2). The sole action of this muscle is to adduct the eye (nasal turn). It is innervated by the inferior division of the third cranial nerve. Important structures adjacent to the medial rectus include the nasociliary nerve and the ophthalmic artery which are just superior. The blood supply is provided by the inferior muscular branch of the ophthalmic artery. The medial rectus is the one horizontal muscle without an attachment to an oblique muscle. If dissinserted during surgery it will retract posteriorly and be lost (see Chapter 20).

Inferior Rectus

The inferior rectus muscle lies adjacent to the posterior orbital floor in the area of the palatine bone. As it advances anteriorly, it tends to elevate away from the floor and follows the dimensions of the globe. The space between the muscle and the anterior orbital floor is filled with orbital fat. The inferior rectus inserts about 6.5 mm from the limbus. Its main action is depression of the globe but also can extort and adduct the globe as secondary functions. Fibrous septa have been shown to radiate to the inferior periorbita. Incarceration of this tissue alone in an orbital floor fracture may restrict this muscle. The inferior oblique muscle travels inferior to the inferior rectus muscle and their conjoined fascia forms the suspensory ligament of Lockwood. Recession of the inferior rectus causes lower lid retraction. The large inferior division of the third nerve innervates both the inferior oblique and travels anterior to the lateral

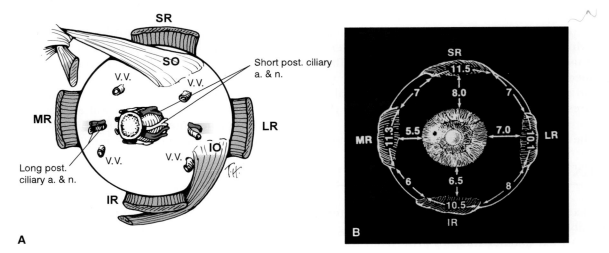

Figure 1–35a.
Drawing of the posterior globe. The optic nerve and the surrounding vessels and nerves is seen. (VV), vortex veins. The short posterior ciliary arteries and nerves encompass the optic nerve while the long posterior ciliary arteries and nerves are a small distance from the nerve on the horizontal meridian. The extraocular muscles are also depicted: SR, superior rectus; LR, lateral rectus; IR, inferior rectus; MR, medial rectus; SO, superior oblique; and IO, inferior oblique. **Figure 1–35b.** Drawing of the four rectus muscles and their location in relationship to each other and the corneal limbus. Note the medial rectus (MR) is closest to the limbus and the superior rectus (SR) furthest from the limbus. The muscle insertions are approximately 10 mm wide and the muscles are separated by approximately 7 mm. Each of the rectus muscles has two anterior ciliary arteries associated with it except for the lateral rectus (LR) which has a single artery (ciliary arteries not shown). Inferior rectus muscle (IR).

border of the inferior rectus. This muscle is vascularized by the inferior muscular branch of the ophthalmic artery.

Lateral Rectus

The lateral rectus is the only extraocular rectus muscle near the orbital apex not juxtaposed to the optic nerve. It is connected to the main portion of the annulus of Zinn by both the superior tendon of Lockwood and the lower tendon of Zinn. These tendons pass over the superior orbital fissure creating a passageway for the superior and inferior divisions of the third nerve, the abducens nerve and the nasociliary nerve. As the lateral rectus is followed anteriorly it still remains separated from the optic nerve by the ciliary ganglion, the nasociliary nerve and ophthalmic artery, which are embedded in the loose intraconal fat. The lateral rectus has fibrous connections to the inferior oblique muscle which inserts at its inferior border. The blood supply is primarily from the lacrimal artery. Anteriorly in the orbit, the lacrimal gland with attendant artery and nerve are just superior with fat intervening along the lateral orbital wall. The muscle inserts 7 mm from the limbus. The sole action of this muscle is abduction. This rectus muscle has the longest arc of contact (12 mm) to the globe for all recti muscles. The other recti muscles have an arc of contact of 7 mm. The reason is because the orbit projects in a divergent manner and the globe is straight in the sagittal plane. Therefore, the muscle wraps itself around the globe more in order to reach its insertion.

Superior Rectus

The superior rectus has a significant relationship with the levator of the upper eyelid which lies immediately above it. Recession of the superior rectus can cause upper lid retraction unless the connecting fibers are removed. These two muscles arise from the same mesoblastic mass and account for the fusion of these two muscles at the medial border. The nasociliary nerve and ophthalmic artery track medially and superiorly as they pass anteriorly from the superior orbital fissure. They eventually pass beneath the superior rectus. The superior rectus must also angle laterally to reach the eye in a similar manner to the lateral rectus. This helps explain the secondary functions of adduction and incyclotortion. The primary action is elevation. A larger contribution of elevation occurs when the eye is abducted. (In adduction, a significant contribution of elevation comes from the inferior oblique.) Of the four recti muscles, the superior rectus inserts the greatest distance from the limbus. On the average this distance is 7.7 to 8.0 mm. The superior oblique tendon courses under the superior rectus and there are check ligaments between these structures. This muscle is innervated by the superior division of the third cranial nerve. The vascular supply is by the superior muscular branch of the ophthalmic artery.

Superior Oblique

The superior oblique muscle is the roundest extraocular muscle and has the longest tendon. It originates in the orbital apex superior and medial to the annulus of Zinn. The muscle courses 32 mm from the apex in an anterior direction closely applied to the superomedial wall of the orbit. Beneath the superior oblique are the terminal branches of the nasociliary nerves and ophthalmic artery which separate it from the medial rectus. As the muscle approaches the trochlea (10mm posterior), it narrows into a 1–2 mm diameter tendon to allow smooth nonrestricted movement through the trochlea. The tendon is about 25 mm in length, the longest extraocular tendon. The functional origin of the superior oblique is the trochlea. The tendon passes through the trochlea and makes a 52° angle posteriorly, laterally, and inferiorly to the globe (Fig. 14–1B). The tendon passes underneath the superior rectus and fans out to insert on the posterior lateral surface of the eye (Figs. 1–35A and 14–1c). The variable insertion is 10–11 mm in length along a posterior, lateral convex line along the temporal border of the superior rectus. The superior oblique is innervated by cranial nerve IV (trochlea) and the muscle actions include depression, intortion, and abduction. The superior oblique muscle is vascularized by the superior muscular branch of the ophthalmic artery like the superior rectus muscle.

Trochlea

The *trochlea* is located in the shallow trochlear fossa on the anteromedial orbital roof (Fig. 14–C). It consists of a crescent-shaped cartilage suspended from the periorbita (23). Between the cartilage and the superior oblique tendon is a bursa-like structure. The presumed function is to reduce friction. The periorbita to which the trochlea is attached can be carefully elevated from the bone by the surgeon and replaced; even so, there may be alterations to the muscular function postoperatively.

Inferior Oblique

The inferior oblique is the only extraocular muscle that does not arise from the orbital apex, but instead from the lateral border of the lacrimal fossa. The muscle travels in a similar direction to the reflected superior oblique tendon, although somewhat more divergent from the medial wall (Fig. 14–1A). The insertion of the inferior oblique onto the globe is posterior to the equator and in the inferotemporal quadrant. The insertion is in close proximity to the macula (2.2 mm inferior and lateral). The length of this muscle is about 37 mm. In contrast to the superior oblique tendon being the longest extraocular tendon, the 1-mm inferior oblique tendon is the shortest. The tendon and even muscle fibers have been shown to enter the sclera at the insertion. However, the arc of contact with the globe is 15 mm and is larger than any other extraocular muscle. The inferior oblique is innervated by the inferior division of cranial nerve III and the muscle's function is elevation, extorsion, and abduction. The vascular supply is provided by the inferior muscular branch of the ophthalmic artery and the infraorbital artery. The suspensory ligament of the globe is formed in part by the fascia of the inferior oblique along with the fascia from the inferior rectus.

Levator Palpebrae Superioris/Müller's Muscle

A detailed description of the anatomy of this muscle is provided in the eyelid section (see Pages 12 and 13, Chapter 27).

■ ORBITAL NERVES

Optic Nerve

The optic nerve represent a peripheral brain tract. It is the only cranial nerve supported by neuroglial cells and bathed in cerebrospinal fluid within a meningeal covering. The optic nerve travels through various anatomic regions in order to go from the eye to the optic chiasm (Fig. 1–36). The entire course of the visual fibers in order is intraocular (1 mm), intraorbital (30 mm), intracanalicular (6 mm), intracranial (10 mm), chiasmatic, optic tract, ganglionic (synapse), optic radiation, and occipital cortex.

The distance from the posterior globe to the orbital apex is about 20 mm. The portion just posterior to the globe has a thin covering of Tenon's capsule. Since the intraorbital portion of the optic nerve is 30 mm, the remaining slack results in a gentle S-shaped configuration. This anatomic configuration explains how the optic nerve can artifactually appear to be transected on axial cuts on computed tomography of the orbits, since tortuosity of the nerve in a superior or inferior direction may leave it out of the plane of imaging. However, this degree of play in the nerve allows free movement of the globe under physiologic states and affords a margin of safety in various proptotic states. The intraorbital optic nerve is surrounded and cushioned by large lobules of

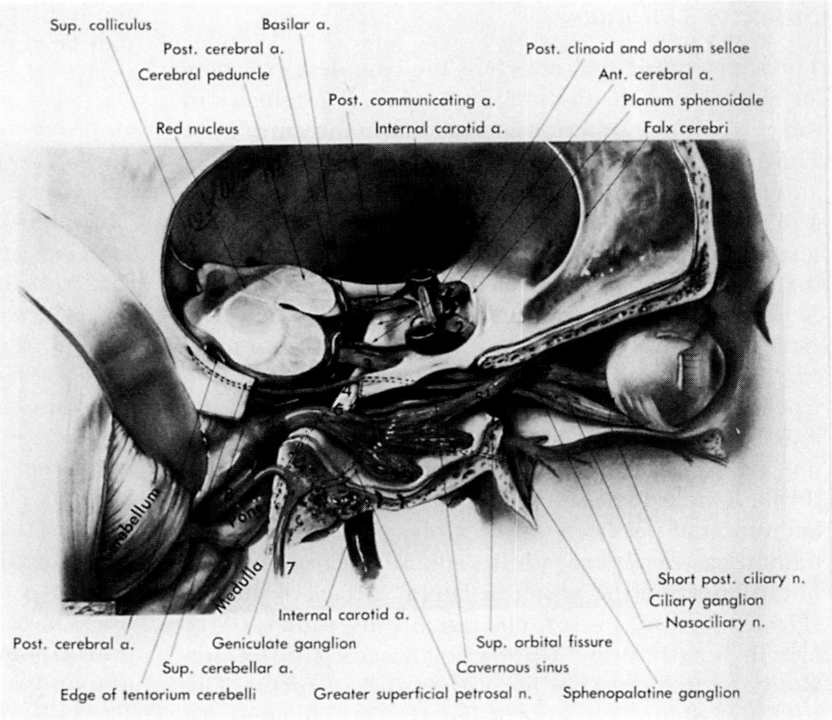

Figure 1–36.
Representation of the cranial nerves in the region of the midbrain, middle fossa, cavernous sinus, and orbital apex. A portion of the tentorial ridge is removed to demonstrate the course of the trochlear nerve (4). The cerebellum is retracted to show the posterior fossa. The midbrain is in cross-section at the level of the superior colliculi and the red nuclei. (2) optic nerve and chiasm; (3) oculomotor nerve; (5) trigeminal nerve [51, ophthalmic division; 52, maxillary division; 53, mandibular division]; (6) abducens nerve; (7) facial nerve; (8) acoustic nerve. Glaser JS: Neuro-ophthalmology. 2e. Philadelphia: JB Lippincott, 1990;365.

intraconal fat, which allows freedom of movement. The nerve is covered by pia, arachnoid, and dura. The dura thickens near the optic canal and fuses with the periorbita of the canal (19). This close anatomic relationship accounts for traumatic optic neuropathy within the canal caused by shearing of small vessels, hemorrhage and edema which compress the optic nerve. The cerebrospinal fluid surrounding the optic nerve communicates freely with the fluid bathing the midbrain, explaining instances of sudden respiratory arrest following retrobulbar injection (12).

The axons found within the optic nerve arise from the ganglion cell layer of the retina and course through the scleral cribiform plate (*lamina cribrosa*). The lamina cribrosa is the point where myelination of the optic nerve stops and unmyelinated retinal nerve fibers begin. The diameter of the intraocular portion of the optic nerve is 1–2 mm but it expands to 3–4 mm, just posterior to the *lamina cribrosa*. This is secondary to myelination of the nerve fibers and supporting neuroglial cells. The nerve exits the globe about 3 mm medial and 1 mm below the posterior pole.

The *central retinal artery*, a branch of the ophthalmic artery, enters inferomedially about 10 mm behind the globe. The rest of the anterior optic nerve is supplied by collateral branches via the posterior ciliary circulation and the pia-arachnoid plexus (22). The optic chiasm is supplied by the anterior cerebral and internal carotid arteries.

Sensory

The *trigeminal nerve (cranial nerve V)* supplies the sensory component to the globe and orbit. The ophthalmic and maxillary divisions of the sensory trigeminal nerve enter the orbit and pass through to supply the superior two-thirds of the face. The deeper structures below the cutaneous distribution are likewise innervated.

The ophthalmic division enters the orbit through the superior fissure as three branches—the lacrimal, frontal, and nasociliary nerves. The lacrimal nerve is the smallest branch and is located most laterally in the superior orbital fissure. It joins the lacrimal artery to pass superotemporally to the posterior aspect of the lacrimal gland. It then divides into the superior and inferior branches. The superior branch supplies the gland, conjunctiva, and the lateral upper eyelid. The inferior branch supplies the gland and has overlap with the zygomaticotemporal nerve. The frontal branch of the trigeminal nerve passes beneath the periorbita and divides anteriorly in the orbit to form the supratrochlear branch and the larger supraorbital branch. The nasociliary branch of the ophthalmic division is the only one that passes through the annulus of Zinn. As it passes anterior through the orbit from the apex, it crosses over the optic nerve with the ophthalmic artery to lie between the superior oblique and the medial rectus muscles. The nasociliary nerve gives off a sensory root to the ciliary ganglion, two or three long posterior ciliary nerves to the globe, the anterior ethmoidal nerve, and a terminal infratrochlear branch. The anterior ethmoidal nerve terminates as the external nasal nerve which supplies the skin of the tip of the nose. Herpes zoster ophthalmicus almost always also involves the skin on the tip of the nose (*Hutchinson's sign*).

The maxillary division of the trigeminal nerve enters the orbit posteriorly through the inferior orbital fissure from the sphenomaxillary fossa. The nerve travels along the orbital floor and parallels the medial wall in the newborn but becomes slightly convex laterally with expansion of the maxillary sinus in the adult. Along the floor, it enters the infraorbital groove and then the infraorbital canal to emerge from the infraorbital foramen. Several branches form in the sphenomaxillary fossa including the zygomatic, sphenopalatine, and the posterosuperior alveolar branches. The middle and anterior superior alveolar branches arise in the infraorbital canal. The infraorbital nerve supplies sensation to the nose, cheek, and upper lip. Orbital floor fracture usually results in anesthesia of the ipsilateral cheek. The trigeminal nerve also provides proprioceptive sensation to the branches of the third, fourth, and sixth nerves while in the cavernous sinus. Also, it provides anastomosis with the facial nerve peripherally beneath the superficial muscle plane.

Motor

The *oculomotor nerve (cranial nerve III)* originates as a nucleus located in the periaqueductal gray matter of the rostral mesencephalon below the aqueduct at the level of the superior colliculi. The inferior rectus, inferior oblique and the medial rectus subnuclei have uncrossed projections while the superior rectus subnucleus has crossed projections. The subnuclei of the levator palpebrae superioris are midline and have bilateral projections similar to the visceral nucleus mediating parasympathetic innervation to the pupil. Therefore, central pathology of the central third nucleus is manifest as bilateral ptosis and pupillary involvement along with possible contralateral elevation deficit involving the superior rectus.

The oculomotor neurons leave the nuclear complex and pass ventrally through the red nucleus and the medial portion of each cerebral peduncle to exit in the interpeduncular space. After leaving the brainstem, the nerve passes between the posterior cerebral and superior cerebellar arteries. It passes lateral and parallel to the posterior communicating artery of the circle of Willis. Aneurysms, tumors, or meningitis in this region manifest with pupillary involvement and pain in the great majority of cases. As the third nerve passes under the tentorial edge, it is prone to compression from uncal herniation and trauma.

Upon entering the cavernous sinus, the third nerve runs dorsal to the fourth nerve in the lateral wall of the sinus. In the anterior cavernous sinus, the third nerve divides into a superior and an inferior branch. The superior branch innervates the superior rectus and the levator palpebrae superioris muscles. The inferior branch innervates the medial rectus, inferior oblique, and inferior rectus, in addition to the parasympathetic fibers to the ciliary ganglion which eventually innervate the iris sphincter and ciliary body. The branches enter the orbit through the annulus separated by the nasociliary nerve.

The superior branch arises within the muscle cone to reach the superior rectus on its medial side about 15 mm from the orbital apex. Fibers terminate in the levator palpebrae superioris by passing medial to the medial rectus in the majority of cases as opposed to through the medial rectus.

The inferior branch travels underneath the optic nerve to innervate the medial and inferior rectus muscles. The large terminal branch to the inferior oblique passes anteriorly and is closely associated with the lateral border of the inferior rectus. The terminal branch also gives off a parasympathetic twig to the ciliary ganglion above.

The *trochlear nerve (cranial nerve IV)* arises in cells within the periaqueductal gray matter under the aqueduct of Sylvius caudal to and continuous with the oculomotor nucleus. The medial longitudinal fasciculus passes inferolateral to the trochlear nucleus. The axons of the fourth nerve pass dorsal to the aqueduct and decussate completely in the anterior medullary velum. The axons leave the brainstem on the dorsal surface just caudal to the inferior colliculus. The nerve then passes forward around the brainstem to run under the free edge of the tentorium passing between the posterior cerebral and superior cerebellar arteries. The long course within the subarachnoid space makes it especially subject to damage from closed head injuries involving contrecoup forces. Head trauma usually causes bilateral superior oblique palsies because the two nerves exit the brainstem close together (2 to 3 mm apart). It pierces the dura to enter the cavernous sinus, running in the lateral wall on each side. It enters the orbit through the superior orbital fissure but temporal to the annulus of Zinn and travels to innervate the superior oblique muscle and innervates the muscle on the outside as opposed to the other extraocular muscles. The path is outside the muscle cone therefore the superior oblique continues to function after a retrobulbar block.

The *abducens nerve (cranial nerve VI)* arises in a collection of motor cells situated in the floor of the fourth ventricle (sixth nerve nucleus). The facial nerve fasciculus loops over the top of the abducens nucleus forming the genu of the facial nerve. The fibers that emerge as the abducens nerve, exit the brainstem at the pontomedullary junction. After leaving the brainstem, the abducens nerve runs up along the clivus and passes between the pons and the anterior inferior cerebellar artery before penetrating the dura. Penetration of the dura occurs at a variable distance below the posterior clinoid processes about 10 cm below the crest of the petrous bone. It then passes beneath the petroclinoid ligament (Gruber's) and through Durello's canal. This area is susceptible to traumatic injury from head trauma. The abducens nerve then enters the cavernous sinus and has a relatively unprotected position within the sinus unlike cranial nerves III, IV, and V which are in the lateral walls. Within the cavernous sinus the abducens is joined briefly by sympathetic branches which pass to branches of the first division of the trigeminal nerve and onto the iris dilator. Rarely, intracavernous sinus pathology may cause a postganglionic *Horner's syndrome with a lateral rectus paresis.* As the nerve enters the orbit through the superior orbital fissure and the annulus of Zinn, it lies between the optic nerve and the lateral rectus muscle. The abducens terminates by innervating the lateral rectus muscle on the inner surface at the posterior third of the muscle (see also Chapter 9).

Autonomic

The *sympathetic nerve* supply to the orbit allows for pupillary dilation, function of the smooth muscles of the eyelids, and vasoconstriction. These fibers probably originate in the posterior hypothalamus. They descend uncrossed to terminate in the interomediolateral cell column of the spinal cord at levels C8 to T2, called the ciliospinal center of Budge. Pupillomotor fibers exit the spinal cord at T1 and then enter the cervical sympathetic chain at the inferior cervical ganglion. The fibers ascend to synapse in the superior cervical ganglion. The postganglionic fibers travel with the internal carotid to enter the cranium. In the cavernous sinus these fibers join either the first division of the trigeminal nerve or the sixth nerve before jumping to the trigeminal nerve. Sympathetic fibers reach the ciliary body and the iris dilator muscle via the nasociliary nerve and the long ciliary nerves.

The *parasympathetic* efferent supply originates in the midbrain adjacent to the third nerve. The fibers are initially located on the superior surface of the third nerve but as the nerve travels forward in the subarachnoid space and cavernous sinus, the pupillary fibers move down around the outside of the nerve to enter the inferior division. The fibers finally synapse in the ciliary ganglion and postganglionic fibers are then distributed to the iris sphincter and ciliary body by the short ciliary nerves.

Parasympathetic innervation of the lacrimal gland is a complex maze and involves several cranial nerves. Parasympathetic fibers for lacrimation and salivation from the superior salvitory nucleus and sensory functions from the solitary nucleus form the nervus intermedius. This nerve joins the facial nerve motor fibers before exiting the brainstem at the pontomedullary junction. Next, these nerves enter the fallopian canal through the internal auditory canal along with the auditory nerve (VIII). At the geniculate ganglion level the fibers destined for the lacrimal gland leave the facial nerve and traverse the vidian and greater superficial petrosal nerve. The nerve fibers reach postganglionic fibers in the sphenopalatine ganglion and send parasympathetic innervation to the lacrimal gland by the maxillary division (V2) of the trigeminal nerve and the lacrimal nerve.

■ REFERENCES

1. Assil KK and Quantock AJ: Wound healing in response to keratorefractive surgery. Surv Ophthalmol, 1993:38: 289–302.
2. Barsky D: Anatomy of the uveal tract—In Tasman W, Jaeger EA (eds): Duane's Clinical Ophthalmology. Philadelphia JB Lippincott, 1990:1–10.
3. Bill A: Conventional and uveoscleral drainage of aqueous humor in the cynomolgus monkey (Macaca irus) at normal and high intraocular pressure. Exp Eye Res, 1966: 5:45–56.
4. Blanks JC: Morphology of the retina. In Ryan SJ (ed): Retina. St. Louis: CV Mosby, 1994:37–53.
5. Bok D: Retinal photoreceptor disc shedding and pigment epithelium phagocytosis, In Ryan SJ (ed): Retina, edition 2. St. Louis CV Mosby, 1994:81–94.
6. Caprioli J: The ciliary epithelia and aqueous humor—In Hart WM (ed): Adler's Physiology of the Eye, edition 9. St. Louis CV Mosby Year Book, 1992:228–247.
7. Castanares S: Blepharoplasty for herniated intraorbital fat: antomical basis for a new approach. Plast Reconstr Surg, 1951:8:46–58.
8. Cintron C, Hassinger LC, Kublin CL, Cannon DJ: Biochemical and ultrastructural changes in collagen during corneal wound healing. J Ultrastruct Res—1978:65:13–22.
9. Cintron C, Covington HI and Kublin CL: Morphologic analyses of proteoglycans in rabbit corneal scars. Invest Ophthalmol Vis Sci, 1990:31:1789–1798.
10. Crosson CE: Cellular changes following epithelial abrasion—In Beuerman RW et al (eds): Healing Process in the Cornea. London, Gulf Publishing, 1989:3–15.
11. Dernouchamps JP: The proteins of the aqeous humor. Doc Ophthalmol, 1982:53:193–200.
12. Drysdale DB: Experimental subdural retrobulbar injection of anesthesia. Ann Ophthalmol, 1984:16:716–719.
13. Ernest JT: Retinal circulation, In Ryan SJ (ed): Retina. St. Louis, CV Mosby, 1994:72–75.
14. Funderburgh JL, Funderburgh ML, Rodrigues MM, Krachmer JH, Conrad GW: Altered antigenicity of keratan

sulfate proteoglycan in selected corneal diseases. Invest Ophthalmol Vis Sci, 1990:31:419–428.

15. Goldberg RA, Wu JC, Jesmanowicz A, and Hyde JS: Eyelid anatomy revisited: dynamic high-resolution magnetic resonance images of Whitnall's ligament and upper eyelid structures with the use of a surface coil. Arch Ophthalmol, 1992:110:1598–1600.

16. Gosain AK, Yousif NJ, Madiedo G, Larson DL, Matloub HS, and Sanger, JR: Surgical anatomy of the SMAS: a reinvestigation. Plast Reconstr Surg, 1993:92:1254–1265.

17. Gouras P and Charles S: Physiology of the retina, In Tasman W, Jaeger EA (eds): Duane's Clinical Ophthalmology. Philadelphia, JB Lippincott, 1993:1–13.

18. Guyer DR, Schachat AP, and Green WR: The choroid: structural considerations. In: Ryan SJ (ed): Retina, edition 2. St. Louis, CV Mosby, 1994:18–31.

19. Habel MS and Maniscalco JE: Surgical relations of the orbit and optic nerve: an anatomical study under magnification. Ann Plast Surg, 1980:4:265.

20. Hart WM: Intraocular pressure, In Hart, WM (ed): Adler's Physiology of the Eye. St. Louis, Mosby Year Book, 1992:248–267.

21. Hawes MJ and Dortzbach RK: The microscopic anatomy of the lower eyelid retractors. Arch Ophthalmol, 1982:100:1313–1318.

22. Hayreh SS: The ophthalmic artery. III. branches. Br J Ophthalmolk, 1962:46:212.

23. Helveston EM, Merriam WW, Ellis FD, Shellhamer RH, Gosling GC: The trochlea: a study of the anatomy and physiology. Ophthalmology, 1982:89:124–133.

24. Hewitt AT and Adler R: The retinal pigment epithelium and the interphotoreceptor matrix: structure and specialized functions. In: Ryan SJ (ed): Retina, edition 2. St. Louis: CV Mosby, 1994:58–71.

25. Horwitz J: The function of alpha-crystalline. Invest Ophthalmol Vis Sci, 1993:34:10–22.

26. Jones LT: The lacrimal secretory system and its treatment. Am J Ophthalmol, 1966:62:47–60.

27. Kaufman PL: Accomodation and presbyopia: neuromuscular and biophysical aspects. In Hart WM (ed): Adler's Physiology of the Eye, edition 9. St. Louis: Mosby Year Book, 1992:391–411.

28. Kinsey VE: Ion movement in the eye. Circulation, 1960:21:968–976.

29. Kikkawa DO and Lemke BN: Orbital and eyelid anatomy. In Dortzbach RK (ed): Ophthalmic Plastic Surgery: prevention and management of complications. New York: Raven Press, 1994:1–29.

30. Koorneef L: Orbital septae: anatomy and function. Ophthalmology, 1979:86:876–885.

31. Kozart DM: Anatomic Correlates of the Retina. In Tasman W and Jaeger EA (eds): Duane's Clinical Ophthalmology Philadelphia: JB Lippincott, 1990:3(1):1–18.

32. Kraff CR and Robin JB: Normal corneal topography. In Schanzlin DJ and Robin JB (eds): Corneal Topography: Measuring and modifying the cornea. New York: Springer-Verlag, 1992:33–38.

33. Kruszak JR: Embryology and anatomy of the lens. In Tasman W and Jaeger EA (eds): Duane's Clinical Ophthalmology. Philadelphia: JB Lippincott, 1990:1(71A):1–9.

34. Lemke BN and Stasior OG: The anatomy of eyebrow ptosis. Arch Ophthalmol, 1982:100:981–986.

35. Lemke BN: Anatomy of ocular adnexa and orbit. In Smith BC (ed): Ophthalmic Plastic and Reconstructive Surgery. St Louis: CV Mosby, 1987:3–74.

36. Lemke BN, Stasior OG, and Rosenberg PN: The surgical relations of the levator palpebrae superioris muscle. Ophthal Plast Reconstr Surg, 1988:4:25–30.

37. Lockwood CB: The anatomy of the muscles, ligaments, and fascia of the orbit, including an account of the capsule of tenon, the check ligaments of recti, and of the suspensory ligament of the eye. J Anat Physiol, 1886;20:1.

38. Maurice DM: The structure and transparency of the cornea. J Physiol (Lond), 1957:136:263–286.

39. Mitz V and Peyronie M: The superficial musculo-aponeurotic system (SMAS) in the parotid and cheek area. Plast Reconstr Surg, 1976:58:80–88.

40. Morrison JC, Van Buskirk EM, and Freddo, TF: Anatomy, microcirculation, and ultrastructure of the ciliary body. In Ritch R, Shields MB, and Krupin T (eds): The Glaucomas. St. Louis, CV Mosby, 1989:75–88.

41. Nimni ME: Collagen, Vols I-III, Boca Raton, CRC Press, 1988.

42. Ogden TE: Topography of the retina. In Ryan SJ (ed): Retina. St. Louis, CV Mosby, 1994:32–36.

43. Ogden TE: Glia of the retina. In Ryan SJ (ed): Retina, edition 2. St. Louis, CV Mosby, 1994:54–57.

44. Olson L: Anatomy and embyology of the lens. In Tasman W and Jaeger EA (eds): Duane's Clinical Ophthalmology. Philadelphia: JB Lippincott, 1990:1(71):1–8.

45. Pierschbacher MD, Ruoslahti E: Cell attachment activity of fibronectin can be duplicated by small synthetic fragments of the molecule. Nature, 1984:309:30.

46. Rathbun WB, Schmidt AJ, Holleschau: Activity loss of glutathione synthesis enzymes associated with human subcapsular cataract. Invest Ophthalmol Vis Sci, 1993:34:2049–2054.

47. Riley MV, Kishida K: ATPases of ciliary epithelium:cellular and subcellular distribution and probable role in secretion of aqueous humor. Exp Eye Res, 1986:42:559–572.

48. Rischbieth RHC, Bull JWD: The significance of enlargement of the superior orbital fissure. Br J Radiol, 1958:31:125–135.

49. Rowsey JJ: Corneal Topography. In Dabezies OH (ed): Contact Lenses: The CLAO guide to basic science and clinical practice. Boston: Little, Brown, 1984:4.1–4.8.

50. Rootman J: Diseases of the orbit. Philadelphia: JB Lippincott, 1988:3–18.

51. Sebag J: The vitreous. In Hart WM (ed): Adler's Physiology of the Eye, edition 9. St. Louis, Mosby Year Book, 1992:268–347.

52. Sherman DD and Lemke BN: Orbital anatomy and its clinical applications. In Tasman W (ed): Duane's Clincal Ophthalmology. Philadelphia: JB Lippincott, 1992:1–26.

53. Sherman DD, Gonnering RS, Wallow IHL, et al: Identification of orbital lymphatics: enzyme histochemical light microscopic and electron microscopic studies. Ophthal Plast Reconstr Surg, 1993;9:153–169.

54. Shovlin JP, Lemke BN, and Dortzbach RK: The anatomy of the suspensory apparatus of the conjunctival fornix. Thesis research presented to the American Society of Ophthalmic Plastic and Reconstructive Surgery, Chicago, IL, November, 1993.

55. Smith TW: Corneal Topography. Documenta Ophthalmologica, 1977:43:249–276.

56. Stasior GO, Lemke BN, Wallow IH, Dortzbach RK: Levator Aponeurosis Elastic Fiber Network. Ophthal Plast Reconstr Surg, 1993;9:1–10.

57. Swartz M, Herbst R, and Goldberg M: Aqueous humor lactic acid dehydrogenase in retinoblastoma. Am J Ophthalmol, 1974:4:612–616.

58. Tasman W: The vitreous. In Tasman W and Jaeger EA (eds): Duane's Clinical Ophthalmolgy. Philadelphia, JB Lippincott, 1990:(3(38):1–18.

59. Thompson HS: The pupil. In Hart WM (ed): Adler's Physiology of the Eye, edition 9. St. Louis—Mosby Year Book, 1992:311–328.

60. Wheatley HM, Flowers BE, Maumenee IH, Azar D, Whittum-Hudson J, and Traboulsi EI: Immunohistochemical localization of fibrillin in human ocular tissues. Invest Ophthalmol Vis Sci, 1994:35:1446.

61. Whitnall SE: On the tubercle of the malar bone and on the lateral attachments of the tarsal plates. J Anat Physiol, 1911:45:426–432.

62. Whitnall SE: Anatomy of the human orbit. London: Oxford University Press, 1932.

63. Wulc AE, Dryden RM and Khatchaturian T: Where is the gray line. Arch Ophthalmol, 1987:105:1092–1098.

64. Yoneya S and Tso MOM: Angioarchitecture of the human choroid. Arch Ophthalmol, 1987:105:681–687.

65. Yousif NJ, Gosain A, Matloub HS, Sanger JR, Madiedo G, Larson DL: The nasolabial fold: an anatomic and histologic reappraisal. Plast Reconstr Surg, 1994:93:60–69.

II Embryology and Eye Development

Section Editor: Kenneth W. Wright

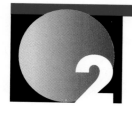

Embryology and Eye Development

Kenneth W. Wright

I. FORMATION OF THREE GERM LAYERS

The ovum and sperm unite within the fallopian tube and after fertilization, cellular mitosis occurs producing a solid sphere of 12 to 16 cells called the morula. Approximately six days after fertilization, fluid accumulates within the cell mass to form a central cavity, transforming the solid mass into a cyst, termed the blastocyst which penetrates the uterine mucosa. Cells at one end of the blastocyst proliferate and form two layers, the epiblast and hypoblast, which together are called the embryoblast. These two cellular layers bridge the central cavity of the blastocyst forming two separate cavities, the amniotic cavity above, and the yolk sac below. During the second week of gestation, the embryoblast transforms into a trilaminar embryo in a process called *gastrulation* (Fig. 2–1). The middle layer of cells is formed as central epiblast cells divide and invaginate between the epiblast and hypoblast. The primitive streak represents the area of invaginating epiblast cells (Fig. 2–1). Invaginating epiblast cells replace the hypoblast cells to form the endoderm. This process of gastrulation results in three definitive germ layers: ectoderm (surface and neural), mesoderm and endoderm, all which are derived from primitive epiblast cells (Fig. 2–2). Towards the end of gastrulation, the cephalic ectoderm expands to form the neural plate (Figures 2–2 and 2–3). A groove forms in the center of the neural plate termed the neural groove. The ectoderm of the neural plate further differentiates into surface ectoderm (periphery) and neural ectoderm (centrally) (Fig. 2–2). Note that throughout the figures, tissues tinted with red indicate cells derived from neural ectoderm (except "Y" sutures Fig. 2–14).

The process of gastrulation proceeds from a cranial to caudal direction, continuing through the fourth week of gestation. Neural ectoderm is located centrally along the neural groove while surface ectoderm is lateral to the neural groove (Figures 2–2 and 2–3). The expanding cephalic ectoderm forms bilateral elevations termed the neural folds which eventually develop into the head and brain. As the neural groove and neural folds develop, paraxial mesoderm in the center of the embryo increases in size and segment into somites towards the end of the fourth week of gestation (Fig. 2–4). The ridges of the neural groove approach each other and fuse over the top of the neural groove, creating a central lumen, the neural tube. Fusion of the neural groove progresses in both a caudal and cephalad direction. This process of fusion results in internalization of neural ectoderm, producing an embryo covered by surface ectoderm. The first sign of the developing eye is seen at 22 days gestation as two optic sulci or optic pits which occur in the neural ectoderm of the neural folds (Fig. 2–5). The optic sulci develop from the inside the neural groove and subsequently migrate towards the surface ectoderm (see development of optic vesicle and cup on p. 60).

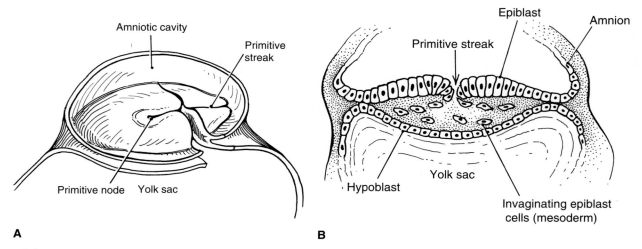

A   **B**

Figure 2–1.
Diagram at the second week of gestation showing the formation of a trilaminar embryo and the process of gastrulation. A, The top view or ventral view of the embryo including primitive node and primitive streak. B, Cross-section showing gastrulation with invagination of epiblast cells, which spread between the epiblast and hypoblast.

■ II. NEURAL CREST CELLS, MESODERM, AND MESENCHYME

During the process of neural fold elevation and fusion, a specialized population of mesenchymal cells, the neural crest cells, migrate from the junction of the neural ectoderm and surface ectoderm (Fig. 2–5). These neural crest cells contribute to the development of major ocular structures which include the cornea stroma, iris stroma, ciliary muscle, choroid, sclera, orbital cartilage and orbital bone. At one time, the mesoderm (middle embryonic layer) was thought to be the origin of most of the ocular and adnexal tissues. Now it is known that neu-

ral crest cells are the precursors for most of the ocular structures and mesoderm plays a relatively small role, contributing to striated muscle of the extraocular muscles and vascular endothelium. The term mesenchyme is a broad term for embryonic connective tissue—tissue

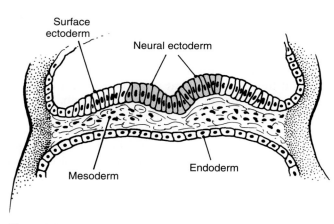

Figure 2–2.
Diagram of a seventeen-day-old embryo showing the three definitive germ layers: ectoderm, mesoderm, and endoderm. The ectoderm further differentiates into surface ectoderm (clear cells) and neural ectoderm (red cells). Note that throughout the diagrams the red tinted cells represent tissue derived from neural ectoderm.

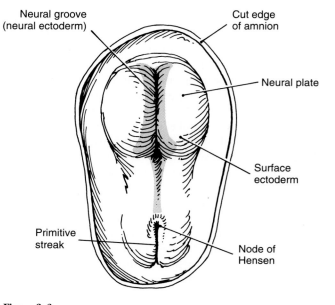

Figure 2–3.
Diagram of an eighteen-day old embryo showing formation of the neural plate at the cephalic end of the embryo. Note the formation of the neural groove which is lined with neural ectoderm.

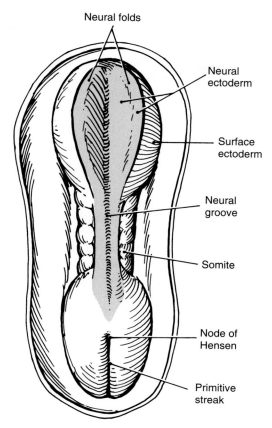

Neural folds

Neural
ectoderm

Surface
ectoderm

Neural
groove

Somite

Node of
Hensen

Primitive
streak

Figure 2–4.
Diagram of a nineteen-day-old embryo showing neural folds on each side of the central neural groove. Neural ectoderm lines the neural groove and surface ectoderm is located lateral to the neural fold. The neural folds progressively come together and zipper close, thus internalizing the neural groove and neural ectoderm.

TABLE 2–1
Embryonic Origins of Ocular Structures

Neural Ectoderm	Neural Crest
(Optic Cup)	(mesenchyme)
Neural retina	Trabecular meshwork
Retinal pigment epithelium	Stroma of iris, ciliary body
Posterior iris epithelium	Choroid and Sclera
Sphincter and dilator pupillae	Ciliary muscles
Bi-layered ciliary epithelium	Corneal stroma keratocytes and endothelium
Optic nerve	Perivascular connective tissue and smooth muscle cells
	Meninges of optic nerve
	Orbital cartilage and bone
	Connective tissue of the extrinsic ocular muscles

Surface Ectoderm	Mesoderm
(Epithelium)	(Muscle and Vascular Endothelium)
Lens	Extrinsic ocular myoblasts (extraocular muscles)
Corneal and conjunctival epithelium	Vascular endothelia, including Schlemm's canal
Lacrimal gland	Endothelium of choriocapillaris
Lid epidermis	Blood
Cilia	Temporal portion of sclera
Epithelium of adnexa glands	

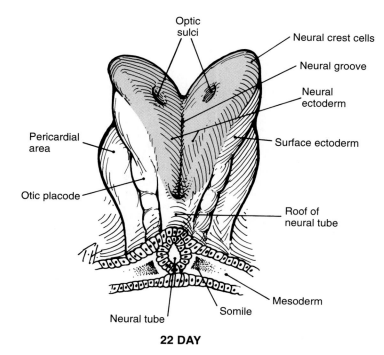

Optic
sulci

Neural crest cells

Neural groove

Neural
ectoderm

Surface ectoderm

Roof of
neural tube

Mesoderm

Somile

Neural tube

Pericardial
area

Otic placode

22 DAY

Figure 2–5.
Diagram of a twenty-two-day-old embryo showing cephalic development. Note that the neural groove has partially closed, and the closed tube is called the neural tube. Optic sulci are seen on the neural ectoderm side of the enlarging neural folds, and will grow out toward the surface ectoderm. Optic sulci are the first evidence of the eye, and eventually become the sensory retina, RPE, and optic nerve (neural ectoderm). The neural folds continue to come together in a caudal to cephalad direction. Neural crest cells develop along the junction of the surface ectoderm and neural ectoderm.

that will develop into the structural framework of the body. In the head and neck, most mesenchyme is derived from neural crest cells. The trunk and extremities, however, develop from mesenchyme which comes from mesoderm located in somites. There are approximately 40 somites which develop into connective tissue, cartilage, muscle, and bone for the trunk and extremities. Somitomeres are smaller somites in the cephalic area, and these are mesodermal in origin and give rise to the myoblasts of the extraocular muscle and vascular endothelium around the eye. Table 2–1 lists the embryonic tissue origin of ocular structures.

■ III. DEVELOPMENT OF OPTICAL VESICLE AND OPTIC CUP

The neural folds progressively dilate and undergo neural segmentation into specific parts of the brain, i.e., forebrain (prosencephalon), midbrain (mesencephalon), and hindbrain (rhombencephalon) (Fig. 2–6A). The eye develops from the forebrain beginning as optic sulci which are invaginations of the neural ectoderm (Fig. 2–6A). As the optic sulci enlarge moving towards the surface ectoderm of the forebrain, the two forebrain vesicles approach each other to fuse, thus internalizing the neural ectoderm and completing closure of the anterior neuropore (Fig. 2–6B). Closure of the anterior neuropore with fusion of the forebrain creates the enclosed optic vesicles (Fig. 2–6B). This transformation of the optic sulcus into the optic vesicle occurs at the end of the fourth week of gestation. Note that the optic vesicle is comprised of a single cell layer of neural ectoderm (Fig. 2–7). The optic vesicle forms connections to the overlying surface ectoderm but there is no direct cell-to-cell contact. Connections between the surface ectoderm and the neural ectoderm of the optic vesicle stimulates thickening of the local surface ectoderm and formation of the lens placode. The optic stalk is a narrowing of the optic vesicle towards the midline of the embryo which eventually develops into the optic

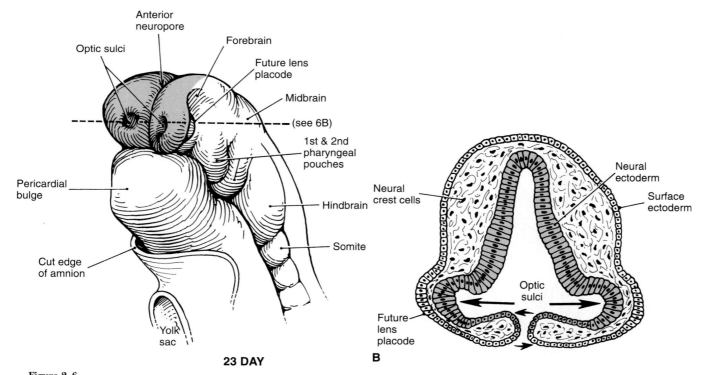

Figure 2–6.
A, Diagram of a twenty-four-day-old embryo showing early eye development. The optic sulci produce a bulge of the surface ectoderm. The dotted line through the optic sulci show the area of cross-section for Figure 2–6B. Note at this stage the anterior neural pore is still open. Cross-section at the level of the dotted line in Figure 2–6A showing the process of fusion of the anterior neural pore which internalizes the neural ectoderm. As the forebrain fuses the optic sulci push laterally so the neural ectoderm comes in contact with the surface ectoderm producing a bulge in the area of the future lens placode.

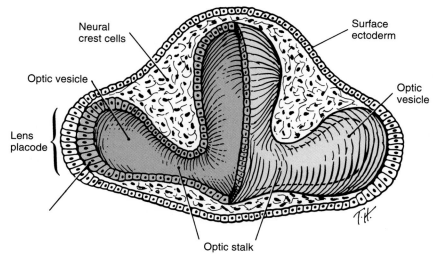

Figure 2–7.
At 27 days' gestation, the anterior neural pore is closed and two optic vessicles have formed. The neural ectoderm of the optic vessicle connects with the surface ectoderm which initiates the development of the lens placode. The optic stalks are present and represent the future optic nerves.

nerve. Neural crest cells migrate around the optic vesicle and eventually give rise to virtually all the connective tissue structures of the eye and orbit.

The lens placode invaginates into the optic vesicle. As the lens placode invaginates, the neural ectoderm of the optic vesicle also invaginates, folding onto itself so the optic vesicle collapses (Fig. 2–8). This invagination of the neural ectoderm creates a double layer of neural ectoderm which is termed the optic cup (Fig. 2–9). The inner layer of the optic cup will develop into the neurosensory retina while the outer layer will develop into the retinal pigment epithelium. Note that the inferior aspect of the optic cup is open because the invagination of the optic cup occurs in an eccentric manner. The open fissure is located inferior and slightly nasal, and is

called either the optic fissure, fetal fissure, embryonic fissure, or choroidal fissure.

The mesenchymal tissue of primarily neural crest origin fills the optic fissure and surrounds the optic cup. At the end of the first month of gestation, the hyaloid artery develops from the mesenchyme in the optic fissure. The lens vesicle pinches off and detaches from the surface ectoderm to become completely internalized at the beginning of the second month gestation. The hyaloid artery extends anteriorly towards the developing lens vesicle and is part of the primary vitreous (Fig. 2–10). The optic fissure begins its closure at the equator of the eye around the seventh week of gestation. Closure of the optic fissure continues in an anterior and posterior direction and is completed by the end of the sev-

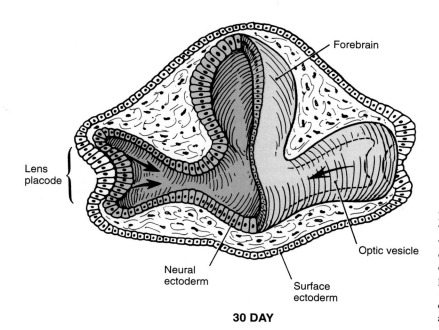

30 DAY

Figure 2–8.
The lens placode invaginates collapsing the optic vesicle and creating a double layer of neural ectoderm. This double layer of neural ectoderm will develop into the optic cup consisting of retinal pigment epithelium (outer layer) and sensory retina (inner layer). Note that with this folding of the neural ectoderm the apices of the neural ectoderm are in apposition.

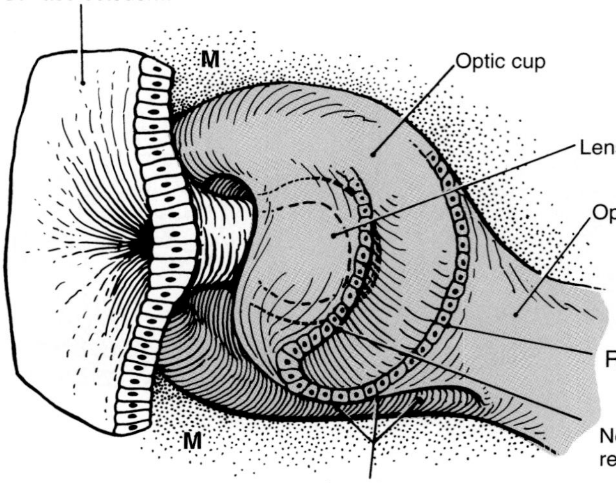

Figure 2–9.
At approximately 32 days' gestation, the lens placode has developed into a spherical structure, the lens vesicle. The lens vesicle is enveloped by the optic cup except for the area of the optic fissure located inferiorly. The optic cup consists of two layers of neural ectoderm with the outer layer developing into the retinal pigment epithelium and the inner layer into the neurosensory retina.

enth week. Closure of the optic cup allows establishment of intraocular pressure and is critical for the establishment of a normal sized eye. Abnormal closure of the optic fissure results in a small eye (see coloboma below).

As the optic fissure closes posteriorly, the hyaloid artery becomes enclosed within the newly formed optic nerve. At the stage of optic fissure closure, the primitive neurosensory retina and pigment epithelium are in apposition, the optic nerve is developing with the central hyaloid vessel, and the lens separates from the cornea, thus forming a primitive anterior chamber (Fig. 2–11).

Mesenchymal cells under the surface ectoderm are derived from neural crest cells and they form the corneal endothelium, corneal stroma and anterior iris stroma. The surface ectoderm develops into the corneal epithelium. Neural crest cell derived mesenchymal tissue around the developing retina develops into the choroid and sclera. Mesenchymal tissue of mesodermal origin accumulates to form myoblasts and eventually develops into the extraocular muscles. Inside the optic cup, the hyaloid artery branches to envelope the developing lens, and this network of vessels posterior to the lens forms the primary vitreous (Fig. 2–11). The develop-

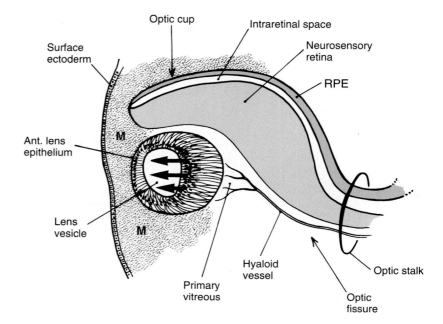

Figure 2–10.
At 36 days' gestation, the lens vesicle has separated from the surface ectoderm. A hyaloid vessel is seen in the optic fissure along with the primary vitreous just posterior to the lens vesicle. The inner layer of the optic cup thickens developing into the neural sensory retina. Mesenchyme (M) derived from neural crest cells surrounds the optic cup, lens, and lens vesicle.

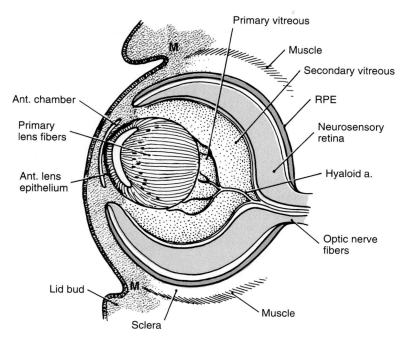

Figure 2–11.

Drawing at the end of the 7 week gestation showing development of the primary lens fibers from posterior epithelial cells, early formation of the anterior chamber, and closure of the optic fissure. Note mesenchyme M, of neural crest origin, fills the spaces between the lens, optic cup, and surface ectoderm. In the figure note that a primitive anterior chamber is being formed, there is primary vitreous posterior to the lens in the area of the hyaloid artery branches, with a secondary vitreous peripheral to the primary vitreous. Sclera is being formed by mesenchyme derived from neural crest cells, primitive extraocular muscles are being formed from mesoderm, and early lid buds are forming. Surface ectoderm lines the exterior of the developing eye and eyelids.

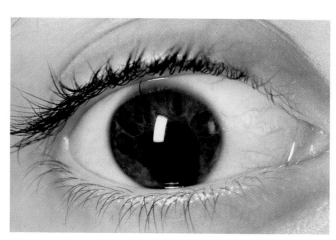

Figure 2–12.

Photograph of a typical iris coloboma with a keyhole pupil located inferiorly, and slightly nasally at approximately 5 o'clock position. The eye is slightly small.

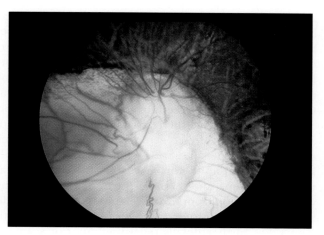

Figure 2–13.

Photograph of an optic nerve coloboma. Notice that the optic nerve is disrupted and the retinal vessels are splayed out and disorganized. Inferiorly the white area represents a choroidal coloboma. Choroidal colobomas are typically found inferiorly.

ment of specific structures of the eye is described in more detail below. Table 2–1 lists the embryological origin of specific ocular tissues.

Colobomas

Colobomas represent abnormal optic cup closure and are often associated with microphthalmia (Fig. 2–12). Colobomas are found along the optic fissure—and are typically located inferiorly, just nasal to the 6:00-o'clock position. Colobomas can occur anywhere along the optic fissure line and can involve the iris, choroid, or optic nerve (Fig. 2–13). The optic fissure closes at the equator first so most colobomas are either anterior (iris coloboma) or posterior (optic nerve coloboma) to the equator. Posterior colobomas are often associated with microphthalmia as delayed fissure closure results in delayed increased intraocular pressure. Systemic anomalies and syndromes may be associated with colobomas including those listed in Table 2–2.

Colobomatous microphthalmia with cyst is a rare anomaly consisting of a microphthalmic eye and an ipsilateral lower lid cyst. The eye may be so small it can be misdiagnosed as anophthalmia (total lack of eye development). It may be bilateral or asymmetric with a severely microphthalmic eye on one side and a localized coloboma of the fellow eye.

TABLE 2–2

CHARGE Syndrome—*C*olobomatous microphthalmia, *H*eart defect, *A*tresia choanal, *R*etarded growth, *G*enital hypoplasia, *E*ar anomalies (deafness).
Basal encephalocele—Associated with optic nerve colobomas.
Meckel's syndrome—colobomatous microphthalmia, occipital encephalocele, heart defect renal and hepatic disease.
Lenz's syndrome—colobomatous microphthalmia.
Rubinstein-Taybi syndrome—coloboma, cataract, ptosis, mental retardation, broad fingers and toes, short stature, cardiac and renal anomalies.
Basal cell nevus syndrome—iris coloboma, cataract, hypertelorism, multiple basal cell nevi over torso (prone to carcinoma), mental retardation
Cat's eye syndrome—colobomatous microphthalmia, anal atresia, preauricular skin tags, abnormality chromosome 22.
Trisomy 13—microphthalmia, corneal opacities, cataracts, retinal dyplasia, cardiovascular anomalies, polycystic kidney, polydactyly of hands and feet, central nervous system anomalies, death in infancy usually by age one year.

■ IV. LENS DEVELOPMENT

The lens develops from surface ectoderm which is in apposition to the apex of the optic vesicle (Fig. 2–7). Adhesions between the optic vesicle and the overlying surface ectoderm result in changes in the surface ectoderm to form the lens placode. The lens placode invaginates into the optic cup—and forms the lens vesicle (Figures 2–8 and 2–9). The size of the lens vesicle is determined by the size of the lens placode (the area of contact between the optic vesicle (neural ectoderm) and the surface ectoderm). Separation of the lens vesicle from surface ectoderm involves cellular necrosis and basement membrane breakdown, accompanied by active migration of epithelial cells. Teratogens can cause induction of a small lens vesicle which fails to undergo normal separation from the surface ectoderm. Anterior chamber cleavage syndromes (anterior segment dysgenesis) with keratolenticular adhesions may result from faulty keratolenticular separation. Milder forms of abnormal lens vesicle separation from surface ectoderm would include anterior polar capsular cataracts and anterior lenticonus. For further details regarding anterior segment dysgenesis, see Iris and iridocorneal angle development below.

The lens vesicle consists of a single layer of epithelial cells with the apices directed inwards toward the center of the hollow sphere. The base of the epithelial cells produce a basal lamina on the surface of the lens vesicle that develops into the lens capsule. Posterior epithelial cells lengthen to fill the lumen of the lens vesicle (Fig. 2–10). These posterior lens epithelial cells lose their nuclei, lose organelles, and become optically translucent as they develop into *primary lens fibers* (Fig. 2–11). The stimulus for the posterior epithelial cells to elongate and differentiate into primary lens fibers comes from the primitive retina. Chick eye experiments have shown that rotation of the lens vesicle results in elongation of the lens epithelial cells nearest the primitive retina. Primary lens fibers make up the *embryonic nucleus,* which in the mature lens, is the central round slightly dark sphere inside the larger fetal nucleus (Fig. 2–14). Primary lens fibers are oriented horizontally in a linear parallel fashion and there are no Y-sutures within the embryonic nucleus. The cells lining the anterior aspect of the developing lens remain cuboidal and become the permanent anterior lens epithelium (Figures 2–11 and 2–14).

Anterior epithelial cells give rise to *secondary lens fibers* after completion of the embryonic nucleus. Central anterior epithelial cells migrate to the lens periphery where they elongate, lose their nucleus and differentiate into secondary lens fibers. The secondary lens fibers course around the embryonic nucleus (which is

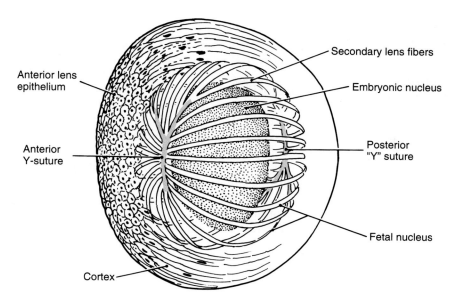

Anterior lens epithelium

Secondary lens fibers

Embryonic nucleus

Anterior Y-suture

Posterior "Y" suture

Fetal nucleus

Cortex

Figure 2–14.
A neonatal crystalline lens. Note that the anterior "Y" suture is upright and the posterior "Y" suture is inverted. The "Y" sutures represent the ends of the secondary lens fibers which span from the anterior to posterior pole of the fetal nucleus. The "Y" sutures delineate the fetal nucleus from the surrounding lens cortex. Anterior epithelial cells continue to produce cortical material postnatally.

derived from posterior epithelium) arching in an anterior and posterior direction and form the *fetal nucleus*. Secondary lens fibers have blunt tips, so when they meet at the anterior and posterior poles of the lens, they form a faint adherence or suture which takes the form of a Y shape. The anterior Y-suture is oriented upright and the posterior Y-suture is inverted (Fig. 2–14). *Cortical lens fibers* form around the fetal nucleus from continued mitotic activity of anterior epithelial cells. In contrast to secondary lens fibers of the fetal nucleus, cortical lens fibers have tapered ends and do not form a Y-suture. Clinically, one can identify the fetal nucleus as that part of the central lens which is inside the Y-sutures. Infantile cataracts which are inside or involve the

Y-sutures are considered congenital, whereas cortical cataracts peripheral to the Y-sutures are considered acquired (usually lamellar cataracts). This distinction has exceptions as cortical cataracts secondarily can spread into the nucleus, and nuclear cataracts can spread into the cortex. At birth, most of the lens is made up of embryonic and fetal nuclear fibers with minimal mature lens cortex.

The process of lens development requires significant nutrition and this is supplied by the hyaloid vessels. The hyaloid artery is a branch of the primitive ophthalmic artery which first enters the eye through the open optic fissure (Fig. 2–10). After closure of the optic fissure, the hyaloid vessels become incorporated into

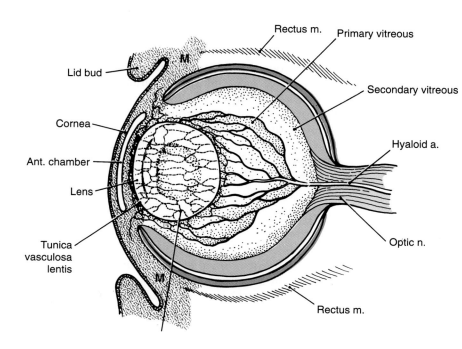

Rectus m.

Primary vitreous

Lid bud

Secondary vitreous

Cornea

Ant. chamber

Lens

Tunica vasculosa lentis

Hyaloid a.

Optic n.

Rectus m.

Figure 2–15.
Ocular development at 2 months shows extensive development of the hyaloid vascular system including the tunica vasculosa lentis. Note that the anterior aspect of the tunica vasculosa lentis forms the pupillary membrane. The primary vitreous is the retrolental area vascularized by the hyaloid vessels. The secondary vitreous is avascular and peripheral to the primary vitreous. The cornea is forming as the anterior chamber elongates.

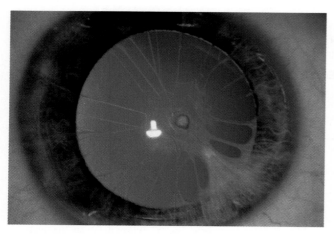

Figure 2–16.
Photograph of persistent pupillary membranes with anterior polar cataract.

enchyme that overlie the anterior lens capsule forms the pupillary membrane. At approximately nine weeks gestation the hyaloid vasculature reaches its greatest development (Fig. 2–15), then regresses by approximately the third to fourth month of gestation (Fig. 2–17). Incomplete regression of hyaloid vasculature can lead to various clinical findings. *Mittendorf's dot* is a small area of fibrosis on the posterior capsule, measuring no more than 2 mm and located just nasal to the posterior pole of the lens. Often there is a small ghost vessel which emanates off the optic nerve to connect with the Mittendorf's dot. Mittendorf's dot represents incomplete regression of the hyaloid artery. Mittendorf's dot rarely, if ever, interferes with visual acuity. A more severe abnormality of regression of the posterior hyaloid vasculature is *persistent hyperplastic primary vitreous* (PHPV) (see p. 328, Fig. 21–6). Incomplete regression of the tunica vasculosa lentis produces the clinical finding of *persistent pupillary membranes* (Fig. 2–16). Persistent pupillary membranes may be associated with an anterior polar cataract—however, in most cases pupillary membranes do not interfere with visual acuity.

the center of the optic nerve (Fig. 2–11). The hyaloid artery divides into many branches (*primary vitreous*), which surrounds the developing lens forming the tunica vasculosa lentis. The vessel network and mes-

■ V. VITREOUS DEVELOPMENT

The development of the vitreous is closely related to the development and regression of the hyaloid vasculature. At approximately five weeks' gestation, the *primary vitreous* forms from mesenchymal cells (neural crest cell origin) located just posterior to the developing lens—and hyaloid vessels (Fig. 2–10). As the fetal fissure closes, the *secondary vitreous* forms circumferentially around the primary vitreous (Fig. 2–11). The secondary vitreous is made up of primitive hyalocytes, compact collagenous fibrillar material, and small amounts of hyaluronic acid. The volume of the secondary vitreous expands as primitive hyalocytes produce collagen fibrils. *Tertiary vitreous* forms at the equator of the lens in the area of the developing ciliary body. Collagen fibers of the tertiary vitreous condense to form the vitreous base and primitive lens zonules in the area of the developing ciliary processes (Fig. 2–17). These primitive fibers are called the marginal *bundle of Drualt* which forms the lens zonules.

By the fourth month of gestation, the primary vitreous and hyaloid vessels start to atrophy, forming a clear central zone termed *Cloquet's canal* (Fig. 2–17). Cloquet's canal is seen clinically as the central clear zone emanating from the optic nerve to the posterior capsule and it represents a remnant of the primary vitreous. The anterior aspect of the primary vitreous continues to regress, however, and an attachment forms between the vitreous and posterior lens capsule termed the capsulohyaloidal ligament or *Wiegert's ligament*. Wiegert's ligament slowly dissipates postnatally and is virtually non-existent by 30 to 40 years of age. Children and infants have an intact Wiegert's ligament which makes intracapsular cataract surgery at high risk for vitreous loss. At birth, most of the posterior vitreous consists of secondary vitreous which has cleared, with the vitreous base and zonules representing tertiary vitreous.

■ VI. CORNEA, IRIS AND ANGLE DEVELOPMENT

As the optic fissure closes at the seventh week of gestation, the primitive lens separates from anterior mesenchyme to form a shallow cleft which is the primitive anterior chamber (Fig. 2–11). This mesenchymal tissue anterior to the lens is derived from neural crest cells and

gives rise to the corneal endothelium, corneal stroma, the anterior iris stroma, the ciliary muscle and most of the structures of the iridocorneal angle. The surface of the developing cornea is lined with surface ectoderm which gives rise to the corneal epithelium. The anterior

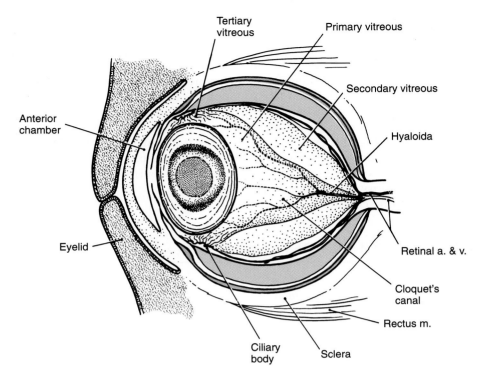

Figure 2–17.
At 3½ months' gestation, the anterior aspect of the developing retinal pigment epithelium differentiates into the iris pigment epithelium and moves anteriorly to form the primitive iris. Mesenchyme of neural crest origin forms the iris stroma. The tertiary vitreous is located between the equator of the lens and the anterior aspect of the developing retina. This is where the lens zonules will form. The thicker red structure represents the neurosensory retina and the outer, thinner red structure represents the retinal pigment epithelium. At this stage, the eyelid buds are fused. The sclera and extraocular muscles can be identified. The corneal epithelium has separated from the epithelium of the eyelids.

corneal stroma, just underlying the surface ectoderm condenses to form Bowman's layer. Layer is derived from neural crest cells, not surface ectoderm, and it is not a true basement membrane of the corneal epithelium. Neural crest cells are also the precursors to the corneal endothelium and corneal stroma including keratocytes that secrete type 1 collagen and fibronectin. The endothelium becomes confluent during the fourth month of gestation, developing zonulae occludentes. Intact epithelium plays an important role in the dehydration of the corneal stroma. Descemet's membrane forms as a true basement membrane for the endothelium at approximately six months' gestation and by this time the cornea is relatively transparent.

The pigmented and non-pigmented epithelium of the iris and ciliary body develop from the anterior aspect of the optic cup which is derived from neural ectoderm (Fig. 2–17). The apices of the pigmented epithelium are directed towards the center of the eye while the apices of nonpigmented epithelium are directed outward. Thus, the orientation of the pigmented and non-pigmented epithelial cells are apex to apex. This orientation comes from the fact that optic cup invagination folds neural ectoderm apex to apex (Fig. 2–8). Mesenchymal tissue (neural crest origin) anterior to the iris pigmented epithelium develops into the iris stroma.

The ciliary body develops as neural ectoderm of the anterior optic cup folds, and underlying mesenchyme differentiates into the ciliary muscles. Vesicles appear within the ciliary epithelial cells in the area of the ciliary processes at approximately four-and-a-half months, which represents the first production of aqueous humor.

The iridocorneal angle develops as anterior mesenchyme separates in the area of the developing iris (Fig. 2–17). Necrosis, phagocytosis and remodeling occurs in the area of the angle to produce clefts or the primitive trabecular meshwork. Differential growth results in a posterior movement of the iris and ciliary body relative to the developing trabecular meshwork, which results in deepening of the anterior chamber, and exposure of the trabecular meshwork to the anterior chamber. Failure of angle maturation including persistence of mesenchymal tissue (*Barkan's membrane*) and failure of posterior migration of the iris and ciliary body, may contribute to *congenital glaucoma.*

Anterior Segment Dysgenesis

Abnormalities of anterior segment development give rise to many well-known clinical entities. Anterior segment dysgenesis syndromes include *posterior embryotoxon*—(anterior displacement of Schwalbe's line), *Axenfeld's anomaly* (anterior displacement of Schwalbe's line associated with peripheral iris strands connecting to Schwalbe's line), *Peters's anomaly* (central corneal opacity with absence of Descemet's membrane and endothelium in the area of the opacity), and *Rieger's anomaly* (iris stroma hypoplasia with iridocorneal fibrous attachments). Congenital glaucoma is frequently associated with anterior segment dysgenesis syndromes. Since most of the structures involved with anterior segment dysgenesis are of neural crest origin, some have labeled these conditions as *ocular neurocristopathies*. This term seems appropriate when one considers the other non-ocular anomalies which occur in association with anterior segment dysgenesis syndromes. Rieger's syndrome, for example, is associated with craniofacial connective tissue disorders and abnormal teeth. Remember that neural crest cells are the predominant cell population of the developing craniofacial region.

Other anomalies of anterior segment formation include *corneal plana* (congenitally flat cornea), *sclerocornea* (indistinct corneal/sclera junction with sclera extending anteriorly), and *ectopia lentis et pupillae* in which there is eccentric location of both the lens and the pupil.

■ VII. CHOROID AND SCLERA DEVELOPMENT

The choroid and sclera develop from mesenchymal tissue of neural crest origin which is peripheral to the optic cup. Sclera forms from condensed mesenchymal tissue which is continuous with the cornea. Condensation of the mesenchymal tissue into sclera progresses posteriorly towards the optic nerve. By approximately three months gestation, the sclera extends to the optic nerve (Fig. 2–17). Posteriorly, mesenchymal cells penetrate the optic nerve to form the lamina cribrosa.

The choroid develops from mesenchymal tissue of neural crest cell origin and from mesodermal mesenchyme as in the choroid there are many endothelial blood spaces that are of mesodermal origin. The endothelial blood spaces organize into the embryonic choriocapillaris by approximately two months' gestation. The choriocapillaris develops on the outer surface of the retinal pigment epithelium. At approximately four months' gestation the choriocapillaris connects with short posterior arteries and joins with the four vortex veins.

■ VIII. RETINAL DEVELOPMENT

The retina develops from the optic cup which is a double layer of neural ectoderm. The neurosensory retina develops from the inner non-pigmented layer while the retinal pigment epithelium (RPE) develops from the outer pigmented layer of the optic cup (Figures 2–9 and 2–10). Note that anteriorly the pigmented and non-pigmented layer of the optic cup forms the pigmented and non-pigmented epithelium of the pars plana, ciliary body, and iris (Fig. 2–17). Because of invagination of the optic vesicle to form the optic cup (Figures 2–8 and 2–9), the apices of the non-pigmented layer are directed outward and face the apices of the outer pigmented layer which are directed inward. Thus, as in the case of the ciliary epithelium, the apices of the two cell layers of the optic cup are in direct contact. Initially, primitive RPE cells are columnar, but within approximately one month, they evolve into a single layer of cuboidal cells that contain pigment granules. By approximately six weeks' gestation, the choriocapillaris is starting to form and Bruch's membrane, the basal lamina of the RPE, is present. The RPE cells take on a hexagonal shape and develop microvilli which interdigitate with photoreceptors from the sensory retina at approximately four months' gestation.

The neurosensory retina which develops from the inner, non-pigmented layer of the optic cup, differentiates into an outer nuclear zone and an inner marginal zone (anuclear) at one month gestation. Cells within the nuclear zone proliferate and migrate into the outer marginal zone, thus creating inner and outer neuroblastic layers. The inner neuroblastic layer is the first to differentiate, giving rise to a primitive nerve fiber layer. Cell differentiation progresses from the inner to outer layers of the neurosensory retina and from central to peripheral retina. The nerve fiber layer courses from developing ganglion cells to the optic nerve. Retinal cell division and mitosis have almost totally ceased by 15 weeks' gestation and further retinal development continues through differentiation of existing cells and refinement of synaptic connections. Müller, amacrine, and horizontal cells come from the neuroblastic layer while bipolar cells and photoreceptors mature last in the outermost zone of the retina. Macular differentiation occurs relatively late; the first sign is the presence of rows of ganglion cells and immature cones that accumulate in the central macular area. Around the seventh month gestation, the fovea is formed as the ganglion cells and inner layers of the retina spread out to form a central macular depression. Cones in the foveal area elongate and are directed horizontally to form the foveal depression. Changes in the foveal area continue, even after birth. The fovea at birth is fairly well developed and consists of a single row of ganglion cells, a row of bipolar cells, and the horizontal outer plexiform layer of Henle. Only after several months' postpartum do the ganglion and bipolar cells completely vacate the fovea centralis.

The retinal vasculature develops from a branch of the fetal ophthalmic artery which in turn is a branch of the internal carotid artery. The ophthalmic artery becomes entrapped in the optic cup as the optic fissure closes. The ophthalmic artery branches to form the hyaloid vasculature. Part of the hyaloid vasculature, the hyaloid artery within the optic stalk, develops into the central retinal artery. Gradually, branches of the hyaloid artery atrophy and regress. By the fourth month of gestation, regression of the hyaloid vasculature is complete. The central retinal artery and retinal vasculature persists. Incomplete regression of the hyaloid vasculature can lead to persistent hyperplastic primary vitreous or, in a milder form, *Bergmeister's papilla*. Bergmeister's papilla is a small stalk emanating from the optic nerve a few millimeters into the vitreous. It represents a remnant of hyaloid vasculature with glial fibrosis. The retinal vessels develop simultaneously as the hyaloid vasculature regresses. Mesenchymal cells from the wall of the hyaloid vein at the optic nerve form buds which invade the nerve fiber layer at approximately four months' gestation. Solid cords of mesenchymal cells within the outer layers of the retina canalize and contain red blood cells by approximately five months' gestation. The central retinal artery grows peripherally from the optic nerve to form the temporal and nasal retinal arcades. By five months' gestation, the retinal arcades have progressed to the equator of the eye and the long and short posterior ciliary arteries become functional. The retinal arteries continue to grow and reach the nasal ora serrata first and the temporal ora serrata last. Thus, a newborn infant will have immature temporal retina without complete vascularization. This explains why *retinopathy of prematurity* is more severe and more frequently found involving the temporal retina than the nasal retina. Retinal endothelial cell growth has been shown to be stimulated by low oxygen tension and inhibited by high oxygen tension (1, 2). One theory regarding the etiology of retinopathy of prematurity is that there is an initial increase in oxygen tension in premature infants placed on supplemental oxygen which inhibits the development of peripheral capillary networks. This lack of a peripheral capillary network results in retinal hypoxia and abnormal peripheral vasculature. Relative retinal hypoxia results in secondary endothelial cell growth and neovascularization (3). (Also see Chapter 22)

■ IX. OPTIC NERVE DEVELOPMENT

The optic nerve develops from the optic stalk which is the posterior extension of the optic cup. The optic stalk is of neural ectoderm origin. The ophthalmic artery becomes enclosed within the optic stalk when the optic cup closes. The hyaloid vessels emerge from the developing optic nerve and extend towards the lens. A glial cell sheath forms around the hyaloid artery. Other glial cells migrate into the optic nerve and form the optic disc. Glial cells that contribute to the optic nerve and the lamina cribrosa come from the inner layer, or nonpigmented layer, of the optic stalk (Figures 2–7, 2–9, and 2–10). Mesenchymal cells (neural crest cell origin) migrate into the nerve and help to form the lamina cribrosa. The optic nerve shifts nasally as the temporal aspect of the eye enlarges during the third months' gestation. The anatomical border between the optic nerve and retina is termed the tissue of Kuhnt, and this tissue is derived from glial tissue (neural ectoderm) and from mesenchyme (neural crest cell origin). At approximately seven months' gestation, myelinization of the optic nerve starts, originating at the chiasm and progressing towards the eye. Myelinization normally stops at the lamina cribrosa at approximately one month after birth. Myelinization of the optic nerve continues postnatally; at birth the myelin layer is thin and reaches its normal thickness in late childhood. The clinical finding of *myelinated optic disc* and *retinal fibers* is a result of myelinization that passes through an intact lamina cribrosa and involves the disc and nerve fiber layer of the retina (5). *Myelinated retinal nerve fibers* are often associated with high myopia and amblyopia. The amblyopia in these patients usually responds well to treatment. Significant refractive errors should be corrected along with occlusion therapy as indicated even if the macula is involved with myelinization (6).

■ X. EXTRAOCULAR MUSCLE

Extraocular muscles are derived from mesoderm in somitomeres which first appear at approximately six weeks' gestation (Fig. 2–11). Muscle growth and differentiation occur simultaneously along the course of the muscle rather than a posterior to anterior pattern of growth and development (4).

■ XI. EYELIDS

Eyelids develop from surface ectoderm and neural crest cell mesenchyme. The surface ectoderm gives rise to the epidermis, cilia and conjunctival epithelium. Deeper structures are derived from neural crest cell mesenchyme including the dermis and tarsus. The orbicularis and levator eyelid muscles are derived from mesoderm, as are the extraocular muscles of the eye. Eyelid buds can be seen by approximately seven weeks' gestation (Fig. 2–11). Eyelid buds develop from mesenchymal accumulations called the frontal nasal (upper lid) and maxillary (lower lid) processes. These processes grow together, and the upper and lower lids fuse at approximately 12 weeks (Fig. 2–17). Eyelid glands and cilia develop by approximately seven months' gestation and the eyelids gradually separate at the end of the six months' gestation.

Cryptophthalmos is a failure of the eyelids to differentiate and separate. The lid skin is adherent to the cornea and conjunctiva and covers the eye without a lid fissure opening, lashes, or normal tarsal structures.

Ankyloblepharon is fusion of the upper and lower eyelid margins, either completely or partially.

Euryblepharon is a congenitaly lax lower lid with downward displacement of the temporal aspect of the lower lids. This may be seen in Down's syndrome and can cause corneal exposure.

Epiblepharon is a redundant fold of lower lid skin that rotates the lid margin inward as the lashes are in contact with the cornea. Spontaneous resolution usually occurs by 2 to 3 years of age. If it does not resolve or if the cornea decompensates, surgical excision of the redundant skin fold is indicated.

Lid colobomas are a congenital defect of the eyelid that usually involves the upper lid. They are not related to abnormal closure of the optic fissure as is the case for uveal colobomas and optic nerve colobomas. A lid notch or a total absence of the lid may be present, and the remaining lid tissue may be adherent to the cornea or conjunctiva.

Phakomatous choristoma of the lower lid is an ectopic location of surface ectoderm in the lower eyelid that differentiates into a crystalline lens. Remember the lens normally comes from surface ectoderm. This is a rare cause of a lower lid mass.

Dermoid Cysts

Dermoids are choristomas and represent rests or inclusions of epidermal and dermal tissues, which are often deep to the surface epithelium. Abnormalities of surface ectoderm invagination, neural crest cell migration and mesenchymal differentiation probably contribute to the formation of dermoids and dermolipomas. Abnormal retention of surface ectoderm is the most likely cause of dermoids. Cysts can contain fat, hair, epithelium, and/or sebaceous secretions. Dermoids occur at the limbus (limbal dermoid, Fig. 2–18), lateral canthal conjunctiva (*dermolipoma*) and subcutaneously around or in the orbit (*subcutaneous dermoid*). Dermoids are usually localized along bony sutures often attached superior temporally.

Limbal dermoids may occur in association with Goldenhar syndrome or occur in isolation without an associated systemic disease. In some cases corneal astigmatism will cause amblyopia. Surgical removal consists of a superficial keratectomy unless the lesion involves the deep corneal stroma, in which case a lamellar graft may be needed. Secondary scarring may be a late postoperative complication—and give the appearance of recurrence of the dermoid.

Ectodermal Dysplasia

There are multiple types of ectodermal dysplasia but the general characteristics include abnormal teeth, hair, nails and decreased sweating. There may be absence of one or more digits (ectrodactyly). Ocular findings include atresia of the lacrimal drainage system, hypertelorism, large epicanthal folds, severe blepharitis, dry eyes, keratitis and photophobia. There is actually a normal production of aqueous tears; however, the tear film is unstable because of meibomian gland dysfunction. The keratitis may be secondary to the meibomian gland blepharitis, tear film abnormalities or may be a primary problem associated with the ectodermal dysplasia.

■ REFERENCES

1. Ashton T, Tripathi B, Knight G: Effect of oxygen on the developing retinal vessels of the rabbit. I. Anatomy and development of the retinal vessels of the rabbit. Exp Eye Res 1972;14:214.
2. Ashton T, Tripathi B, Knight G: Effect of oxygen on the developing retinal vessels of the rabbit. II. In vivo experiments. Exp Eye Res 1972;14:221.
3. Patz A: Current concepts of the effects of oxygen on the developing retina. Curr Eye Res 1984;3:159–163.
4. Sevel D: Reappraisal of the origin of human extraocular muscles. Ophthalmol 1981;88:1330.
5. Straatsma BR, Foos RY, Heckenlively JR, Taylor GN: Myelinated retinal nerve fibers. Am J Ophthalmol 1981;91:25–38.
6. Summers CG, Romig L, Lavoie JD: Unexpected good results after therapy for anisometropic amblyopia associated with unilateral peripapillary myelinated nerve fibers. J Pediatr Ophthal Strabismus 1991;28(3):134–136.

III Optics and Refraction

Section Editor: Donald N. Schwartz

"Essential" Optics Formulas

- **Snell's Law:**

  $$n_1 \cdot \sin \theta_1 = n_2 \cdot \sin \theta_2$$

  where: n_1 = index of refraction of first medium,
  n_2 = index of refraction of second medium,
  θ_1, θ_2 = angles of incidence and refraction, respectively

- **Lens Power Calculation:**

  $$D = \frac{100 \ cm}{f}$$

  where: D = lens power (diopters), f = focal length (cm)

- **Vergence Formula:**

  $$U + D = V$$

  where: U = object vergence (diopters), D = lens power (diopters),
  V = image vergence (diopters)

- **Prentice's Rule:** (lens induced prism)

  $$PD = h \cdot D$$

  where: PD = deviation (prism diopters), h = distance from optical center (cm),
  D = lens power (diopters)

- **Power of a Spherical Refracting Surface:**

  $$D = \frac{n_2 - n_1}{r}$$

  where: D = power (diopters), n_1, n_2 = indices of refraction, r = radius of curvature (m)

- **Power of a Thin Lens in a Second Media:**

  $$\frac{D_{lens \ in \ second \ media}}{D_{lens \ in \ first \ media}} = \frac{n_{lens} - n_{second \ media}}{n_{lens} - n_{original \ media}}$$

  where: D = power (diopters), n = indices of refraction

- **Reflecting power of Spherical Mirror:**

  $$D = \frac{100}{f} = \frac{200}{r}$$

  where: D = power (diopters), f = focal length (cm), r = radius of curvature (cm)

- **Effective Lens Power:** (power of lens when acting at a different distance)

  $$D_2 = \frac{D_1}{1 - s \cdot D_1}$$

  where: D_1 = lens power, old position, D_2 = lens power, new position (diopters)

- **Magnification of Distant Object:** (simple magnifer, reference distance = 25 cm)

  $$M = \frac{D}{4}$$

  where: D = lens power (diopters), s = difference in lens postion (m),
  s is negative if lens moved forward

- **Transcerse (Linear or Lateral) Magnification:**

  $$M_{lateral} = \frac{image \ height}{object \ height} = \frac{image \ distance}{object \ distance} = \frac{U}{V}$$

  where: U = object vergence (diopters),
  V = image vergence (diopters)

- **Axial (Depth) Magnification:**

  $$M_{axial} = M_{lateral}^2$$

- **Magnification of Telescope:**

  $$M_{telescope} = \frac{D_{eyepiece}}{D_{objective}}$$

  where: D = power of objective and eyepeice lenses (diopters)

- **Accomodation Through Telescope:**

  $$Total \ Accomodation = Normal \ accomodation \ required \cdot M_{telescope}^2$$

- **IOL Power Calculation:**

  $$D = A - 2.5 \cdot (axial \ length) - 0.9 \cdot (average \ K \ reading)$$

  where: D = IOL power (diopters),
  A = "A" constant, specific for each type of IOL

- **Retinal Image Size:** (based on schematic eye)

  $$\frac{retinal \ image \ size \ (mm)}{17 \ mm} = \frac{object \ size \ (cm)}{distance \ eye \ (cm)}$$

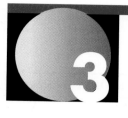

3 Optics and Refraction

Donald N. Schwartz, Than-Lan Quan

The distinguishing characteristic of the visual system is its function to focus incident visible radiation and use this focused image to form a perception. At the initiation of this complex series of events is the formation of a useable image by the eye, focused on the retina. Critical to every point along the way of this image formation is the branch of the physical sciences of optics. It is with this concern that optics is approached along with its more immediate clinical representation of refraction. The formation of an image by the eye, whether in focus with accommodation relaxed (emmetropia) or out of focus (ametropia) is the same process. The problem of ametropia is, arguably, the most common prob-lem that an ophthalmologist will encounter. The recognition of the refractive status of the eye and its correction, or better amelioration, with lenses is the area commonly referred to as refraction.

From a practical perspective, an ophthalmologist frequently must prove skills to a patient. Before a patient allows significant medical or surgical treatment by his/her physician, the skill in correcting optical problems is certainly one facet that the patient will remember. Rightly or wrongly, the ability to correct refractive errors may be used as one guide in the selection of a physician for future medical or surgical care.

■ PHYSICAL OPTICS

Light energy has two aspects: wave—when it passes through air or a vacuum; and particle or photons—when it is being absorbed or when it is being generated in a light source.

Wave Theory

The wave theory of light, first proposed by Christian Huygens (13) in the 1600s and later popularized by Young and Maxwell, deals with light as a form of radiant energy. Light is a form of electromagnetic energy with the following electromagnetic properties (Fig. 3–1):

Wavelength (λ): distance between crests
Amplitude (A): the height of the crests
Frequency (v): the number of crests that pass a fixed point per second

The wavelengths of visible light occupy a small portion of the entire electromagnetic spectrum, mainly be-tween 400 and 700 nm. The boundaries are not precise, and under certain conditions, the eye can detect light well into the infrared and ultraviolet range. Indeed, recent aphakes, without the ultraviolet (UV) absorption of the crystalline lens, may see well below 400 nm and may complain of bluish tints.

Wavelength (λ) and frequency (v) traveling through a medium are related by the following equation, where v is the velocity of light in the medium (Table 3–1):

$$v = v\lambda$$

The velocity of light in a vacuum (c) is a fundamental constant of nature and is approximately 3.00×10^{10} cm/sec. When light passes through a medium other than a vacuum, its velocity (v) is reduced. This velocity is inversely related to the index of refraction (n) of the medium which is expressed as the ratio:

$$n = \frac{c}{v}$$

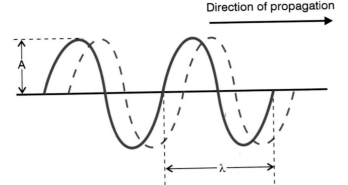

Direction of propagation

Figure 3–1.
Wave theory. A amplitude, λ wavelength.
Dotted waveform represents propagation of wave front.

TABLE 3–1
Common Refractive Indices

Medium	Index of Refraction
Air	1.00
Aqueous	1.33
Crystalline lens	1.42
Cornea	1.37
Glass	1.49
Plastic	1.52

of the velocity of light in a vacuum to that in the medium.

The frequency of light does not change on traveling through such a medium, but the wavelength λ_m is shortened (30), as governed by the relationship:

$$\frac{\lambda}{\lambda_m} = \frac{c}{v} = n$$

Photon (Particle) Aspects of Light

When light interacts with matter, energy is emitted or absorbed. Max Planck, a German physicist of the 1800s, postulated that this energy is packaged in discrete units or quanta (6). The energy content (E) of a quantum is, however, not constant, but varies with the frequency (v) of the light. This energy (E) is determined:

$$E = hv$$

where

v = frequency of light
h = Planck's constant (6.6254×10^{-27} erg sec)

Interference

Interference occurs when two light waves from the same source are brought together (Fig. 3–2A). Interference is best observed when the light is monochromatic (i.e., when light is composed of a single or narrow band of wavelengths).

Constructive interference occurs when the crests coincide (in phase). *Destructive interference* occurs when the crest of one wave coincides with the trough of the other (180° out of phase). Destructive interference is complete when the two waves have exactly the same amplitude.

Interference allows antireflection coatings to be designed to enhance destructive interference and nullify reflected light, thereby allowing all incident light to be transmitted through a lens (See Fig. 3–2B).

Coherence

Coherence measures the ability of two light waves to produce interference. An example of coherent light is laser energy.

Spatial coherence indicates the ability of two separate portions of the wave to produce interference (points P & Q). *Temporal coherence* measures the ability of a beam to interfere with another portion of itself (points P & R) (See Fig. 3–2A).

Polarization

The orientation of light is random. This is analogous to swinging a jump-rope in all directions. Polarization is a filtering process which eliminates the randomly directed waves, allowing only waves with the same orientation to pass through the filter. This would be analogous to passing the jump-rope through a picket fence. The rope could be swung in all directions, but only those waves aligned with the picket fence would pass through. Two polarizing filters set in the same orientation will allow light to pass, but if turned 90° to each other, the light will be blocked by the second filter. This polarization occurs in specific controlled circumstances, but it also occurs with reflection from a surface where light becomes plane polarized. It is this property that allows polarizing "sunglasses" to reduce reflected light glare, particularly from the surface of water.

Diffraction

Diffraction is a change in the direction of the light wave as it encounters an obstruction, an aperture, or other irregularity in the medium. The shorter the wavelength, the less it is diffracted. Diffraction sets a limit on visual acuity when the pupil size is less than about 2.5 mm (for the emmetrope). Smaller pupils may result in significant decrease in acuity, which may require pupil enlargement. The image formed on the retina from a distant small source has the form of a circular blur circle surrounded by brighter and darker rings that fade out at the edges, the center of which is called the *Airy disc* (17). The minimum resolvable distance between two light sources is approximately equal to the radius of this Airy disc. Diffractive optics are used in some intraocular lenses and contact lenses.

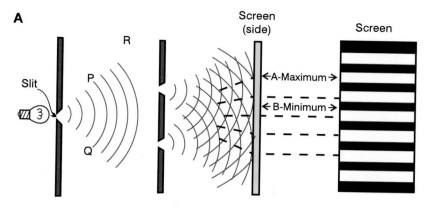

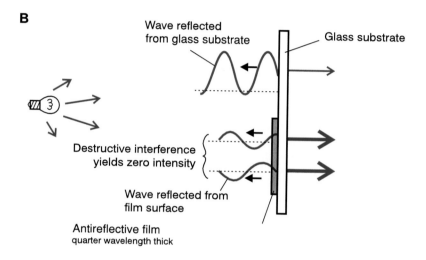

A - Constructive interference
B - Destructive interference

Destructive interference
yields zero intensity

Wave reflected from
film surface

Antireflective film
quarter wavelength thick

Figure 3–2.

A, Light from the bulb passes through the first slit creating a point source of light. The second screen generates two point sources of light. These two point sources of light interact to produce constructive and destructive interference. Where two peaks or two troughs coincide, the effect is additive and produces constructive interference. This produces a bright band on the screen (A-maximum). When peak and trough waves interact, they neutralize each other causing destructive interference which produces a black band on the screen (B-minimum).

B, Top wave shows light striking glass substrate without anti-reflective film. Black arrow represents light reflected back (NOT transmitted) which causes glare. Bottom two waveforms represent light passing through glass with antireflective (AR) film. The film is one quarter thickness of the incoming light wavelength. A small portion of the light is reflected off the surface of the AR film, and; some of the light passes through the AR film and is reflected off the glass. Since this light reflecting off of the glass travels twice through the AR film, it becomes one half wavelength or 180° out of phase with the light reflected off the surface of the AR film. This results in destructive interference which reduces glare. Note that the troughs and peaks of the lower two reflected waves coincide.

■ GEOMETRIC OPTICS

Geometric optics treats light as rays and deals with image properties of lenses and mirrors.

Point Sources, Rays, Pencils and Beams of Light

A *point source* is a luminous body from which light emerges equally in all directions in an infinite number of light *rays* (Fig. 3–3). When these light rays are limited by an aperture, the selected group of rays then form a *pencil of light rays. Beams of light* are made up of pencils of light rays from an *extended source*, a composite of many point sources.

Refraction of Light at Interfaces
Snell's Law

Rays of light, when moving from media of one optical density (refractive index) to another, are changed in di-

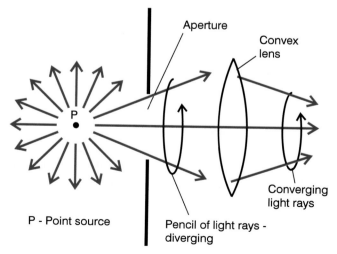

P - Point source

Figure 3–3.
Divergence and convergence of light rays.

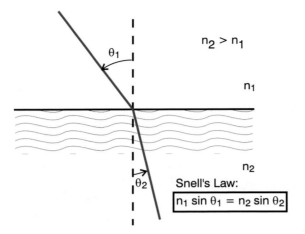

Figure 3–4.
Snell's Law.

rection. The amount of this effect, *refraction,* follows Snell's Law. The refracted ray lies in the plane of incidence, and the sine of the angle of refraction bears a constant ratio to the sine of the angle of incidence.

The amount of bending is determined by Snell's Law (Fig. 3–4):

$$n_1 \sin\theta_1 = n_2 \sin\theta_2$$

where

θ_1 = angle of incidence
θ_2 = angle of refraction
n_1 = index of refraction of the first medium
n_2 = index of refraction of the second medium

(θ_1 and θ_2 are measured from the normal to the surface at the point of incidence).

By inference, a ray striking the surface of a refracting medium perpendicularly will change velocity but not be refracted since sine of 0 is 1. As light travels from a medium with a lower refractive index to that of a higher refractive index, it is bent toward the normal.

Critical Angle and Total Internal Reflection

The phenomenon of internal reflection *only* occurs when light passes from a medium of greater refractive index to that of lesser refractive index. Light is bent *away* from the normal as it passes from a medium of greater refractive index to that of lesser refractive index. An angle of incidence is possible to encounter that causes the light to be bent and be retained within the higher refractive index medium, *total internal reflection.* This specific angle is the *critical angle* (Fig. 3–5).

As angle θ_1 increases, so does angle θ_2. When angle θ_1 reaches a magnitude such that angle θ_2 will be 90° (perpendicular) to the normal, it is then called the critical angle, θ_c.

If θ_2 is now increased further, the light ray will not escape from the medium, and the phenomenon of *total internal reflection* takes place.

$$n_1 \sin\theta_c = n_2 \sin 90°$$

and

$$\sin\theta_c = \frac{n_2}{n_1}$$

The properties of the critical angle and internal reflection are useful in optical appications such as fiber optic tubules. Total internal reflection at the corneal surface is the principle behind the goniolens and its ability to allow a view of the anterior chamber angle (6).

Prismatic Deviation

The rays emanating from object X will be bent appropriately as they leave the water medium as dictated by Snell's law. However, to the examiner viewing from an angle, the rays seem to originate from a point X′ that is not as deep in the water as the original point X (Fig. 3–6).

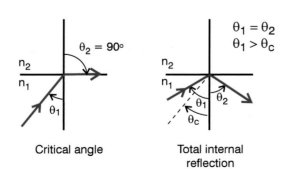

Figure 3–5.
Critical angle. Total internal reflection.

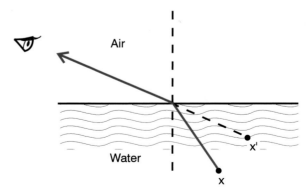

Figure 3–6.
Prismatic deviation.

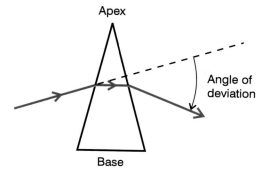

Figure 3–7.
Ophthalmic prism.

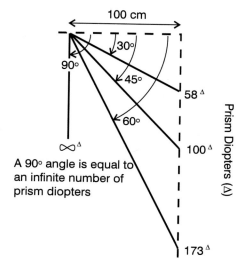

Figure 3–9.
Relationship of prism diopter to degrees.

Ophthalmic Prisms

A prism is essentially two angulated plane refracting surfaces. It displaces, as well as deviates, light rays (Fig. 3–7).

The effect of a prism on light waves is analogous to a line of soldiers marching through a triangular section of sand. The soldiers march more slowly through the sand. Those soldiers at the base of the triangle take longer to traverse than those at the apex. The difference in exit times causes the line of soldiers to "bend" toward the base. Light passes more slowly through prism material (glass or plastic) than through air. Therefore light passing through the apex of the prism exits before the light passing through the base. This bends the light towards the base of the prism.

The total angle of deviation is the sum of the deviations produced at each of the faces. The angle of minimum deviation occurs where there is equal bending at the two surfaces (6).

Prism Diopter

The power of a prism is measured in "prism diopters" (Δ) and is defined as the amount of displacement in centimeters of a light ray passing through the prism, measured 100 cm from the prism (Fig. 3–8).

For small angles under 100 PD (45°), the degrees of deviation are approximately half the number of PDs (Fig. 3–9). In reality, the relationship is not a linear but rather a trigonometric one (1).

Calibration of Prism

Most prisms are calibrated in the Prentice position (17), with one face of the prism perpendicular to the light rays (Fig. 3–10). All bending of light then effectively occurs at the opposite face. This is how prisms in spectacles are measured. The back surface is placed against the nosecone of the lensometer.

Orthoptic prisms made of glass are calibrated in the Prentice position; hence they are best held with the back surface perpendicular to the visual axis.

Plastic prisms and prism bars made of plastic are, on the other hand, calibrated by the angle of minimum deviation. They are best held with the rear surface parallel to the frontal plane (23).

"Stacking" of prisms with bases aligned in the same direction does not give a simple addition of powers; it is best to split the prisms between the two eyes. It is, however, acceptable to add or "stack" vertical and horizontal prisms together.

Displacement of Images by Prisms

When a prism is placed in the path of converging light rays, the rays will be bent toward the base of the prism. Hence, *real images* (see page 81 and Fig. 3–16) formed

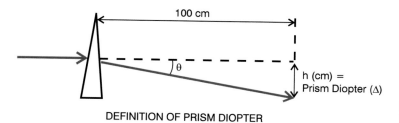

DEFINITION OF PRISM DIOPTER

Figure 3–8.
Definition of prism diopter.

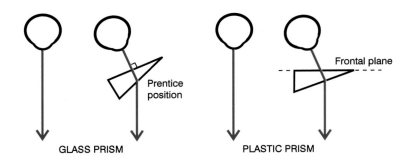

Figure 3–10.
Calibration of glass and plastic prisms.

by these converging light rays also will be displaced toward the *base* of the prism (Fig. 3–11A).

If one looks through a prism at an object, the object will appear to be displaced toward the apex of the prism (Fig. 3–11B). This displaced image is actually a *virtual image.*

This is the basis for using prisms in the alternate cover test for neutralization of eye movements in strabismus. The neutralizing prism always has the apex in the direction of the eye deviation (see Fig. 14–12).

Vector Addition of Prisms

Because a prism has both an apex and a base, it has a specific orientation, or vector. To order an oblique prism, it is important to specify properly the direction of the base and the angle of deviation.

Prismatic deviations in different directions are additive by ordinary vector addition (Fig. 3–12). Hence, an oblique prism can be created by combining a horizontal and a vertical prism.

Lens Vergence

Vergence is a measure of the amount of spreading (divergence) or coming together (convergence) of light rays from a single source (Fig. 3-13). A vergence can be measured at any distance from a light source. Light rays coming from a point source in nature will diverge. Converging light can only be produced by an optical system. Rays close to the light source are more divergent than the rays encountered far from the point source. Light from the sun for example is almost parallel with little divergence. At any point along the light path, vergence is defined as the reciprocal of the distance in meters (d) from the point source.

This value is measured in diopter (D) units.

$$\text{Vergence formula} \quad D = \frac{1}{d \; \text{(meters)}}$$

In Figure 3–13, the "point of focus" represents the point light source for diverging light (red arrows to the right). Note that at a distance of 50 cm ($d = \frac{1}{2}$m), light has a divergence equal to 2D. By convention divergence is expressed by a negative number, therefore at 50 cm, the vergence would be -2D. Convergence is expressed as a positive number. Red lines to the left of "point of focus" represent converging light which comes together at the "point of focus". Note that at 33 cm the vergence is $+3$D. Remember to convert all distances to meters when using the vergence formula. Parallel light has zero vergence as 1/infinity approaches zero. For purposes of clinical practice, we consider light from a source greater than 6 m (20 ft) as parallel (vergence = $\frac{1}{6}$ D or 0.1667D). (We can assume that rays coming from a distant light source such as the sun would have essentially zero vergence by the time they reach the earth.)

Lens Power Formula. Lenses impart a change in vergence to light. A converging lens adds plus vergence to light,

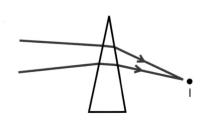

A - Real image displaced toward the base

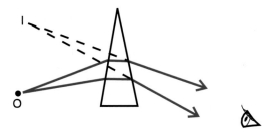

B - Virtual image displaced toward the apex

Figure 3–11.
A, Real image (I) displacement towards base. **B,** virtual image (I) observed towards apex (O = object).

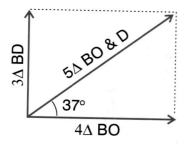

Figure 3–12.
Vector addition of prisms.

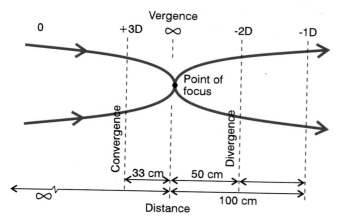

Figure 3–13.
Vergence graph.

and a diverging lens adds minus vergence to light. The amount of vergence added to the light is defined as the power of the lens.

The basic lens formula is as follows:

$$U + D = V$$

All variables express vergence in diopters

U = vergence of light entering the lens (object)
D = power of the lens
V = vergence of light leaving the lens (image)

The object and image distances from the lens can be calculated as the reciprocals of the respective vergence (U or V).

Example: Where is the image of an object located 25 cm from a +5.00 D lens? (See Fig. 3–14)

$$U = -\frac{1}{0.25m} = -4.00 \text{ Diopters}$$

(minus indicates diverging rays)

$$\begin{aligned} V &= U + D \\ &= -4.00 + 5.00 \\ &= +1.00D \end{aligned}$$

A plus or convex lens acts as two prisms base to base, while a minus or concave lens acts like two prisms apex to apex (see Fig. 3–15–A). Lens powers must always be written with a + or − sign. The image is therefore 1 meter to the right of the lens.

Prismatic Effects of Lenses (Prentice's Rule). A ray passing through the center of the lens is not deviated, however a ray that passes through a part of the lens away from the center (optical axis), is deviated according to Prentice's rule (Fig. 3–15A). The amount of this prism deviation (Δ) is proportional to both the power of the lens (D) and the distance from the optical axis (h) in centimeters (Fig. 3–15B).

$$\Delta = hD$$

Conjugate Points, Conjugate Planes. *Conjugate points* are the two points of an optical system where an object placed at one point will be imaged at the other point. For example, in Fig. 3–16A the object (O) and image (I) are conjugate points. There is an infinite number of conjugate points in an optical system. A group of object points can form an object plane. Like conjugate points an object plane will be focused by a lens system to form an image plane.

Real Versus Virtual Objects and Images. Object rays exist only on the incoming side of an optical system, and image rays exist only the outgoing side of an optical system. By convention, the rays are drawn coming from the left toward the right (Fig. 3–16).

Object and image spaces, however, exist on either side of the optical system. An object or image is *real* if it is located on the same side as its respective rays and is *virtual* if it is on the opposite side. Virtual objects and images are located by extensions of the respective rays through the lens system.

Object-Image Movement. It was discussed previously that there is an infinite number of conjugate points in an optical system. Hence, as the object is moved along the optical axis, the image also moves (Fig. 3–17).

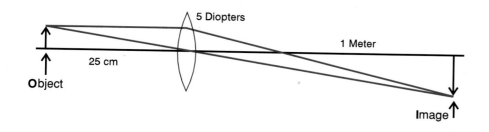

Figure 3–14.
Illustration of example.

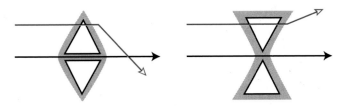

Figure 3–15A.

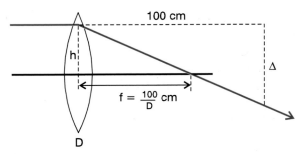

Figure 3–15B.
Prentice's rule.

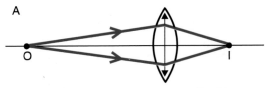

Real Object   Real Image

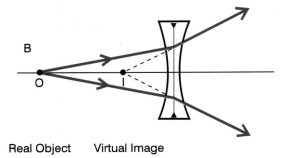

Real Object   Virtual Image

The image always moves in the same direction as the object relative to the lens.

Multiple Lens Systems. The basic vergence relationship still applies for multiple lens systems. In this case, the image space for the first lens becomes the object space for the second lens, and the image space for the second lens then becomes the object space for the third lens and so on. (See also telescopes: Figs 3–25 and 3–26.)

Focal Points and Focal Lengths. Each lens has two focal points (Fig. 3–18). The *primary focal point* (F_1) is the point at which the object must be placed to create an image at infinity. That is, such that the emerging image rays from the lens are parallel. The *secondary focal point* (F_2) is the image point created by the lens when the object is located at infinity. That is, when the incoming object rays are parallel.

The *focal lengths* (primary and secondary) are the distances from the center of an ideally thin lens to each of

C

Virtual Object
Real Image

Figure 3–16.
Real and virtual images and objects.

its focal points. For an ideally thin lens, the primary and secondary focal lengths are the same. The value, measured in meters, is the reciprocal of the dioptric power of the lens. Simplistically, the nodal point is the optical center of a lens, and light passing through the nodal point emerges undeviated.

Ray Tracing

Images formed by lenses can be located along the optical axis by either applying the vergence formula or by

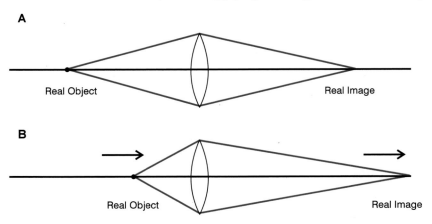

Figure 3–17.
Object-image movement. The image always moves in the same direction as the object.

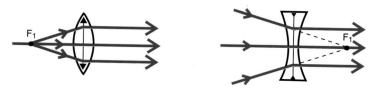

PRIMARY FOCAL POINT

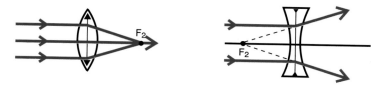

SECONDARY FOCAL POINT

Figure 3–18.
Primary (F_1) and secondary (F_2) focal points.

ray tracing. The optical axis is a line that connects the centers of curvature of the front and back surfaces of the lens. Even though the numerical distance is more accurately determined using the vergence formula, the size and orientation of the image are better represented by ray tracing.

An ideally thin lens has a nodal point located at the center of the lens. The central ray (ray 1) (Fig. 3–19) passes through this point and is thereby undeviated in its passage through the lens. Ray 2 passing through the primary focal point F_1 emerges from the lens parallel to the axis. And ray 3 entering the lens parallel to the axis must pass through the F_2, the secondary focal point. The intersection of these three principal rays determine the location of the image.

Using the central ray, it is also evident that if the image is on the opposite side of the lens from the object, it will be inverted with respect to the object. If it is on the same side of the lens as the object, it will be erect.

Thick Lenses

Biconvex and Biconcave Lenses. Only an ideal thin lens can be described by its optical center and the two focal points. Most ordinary lens with thickness must be described by six cardinal points: two focal points, two principal points, and two nodal points. For practical purposes (when the media on both sides of a lens have the same refractive index) the principal points and the nodal points are the same. The planes perpendicular to the optic axis at the focal points and principal points are called focal planes and principal planes, respectively (Fig. 3–20).

The principles of ray tracing can still be applied to a thick lens with some modifications.

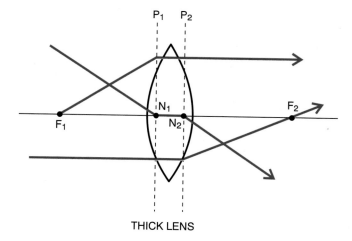

THICK LENS

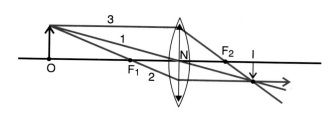

Figure 3–19.
Ray tracing. To find the location, orientation, and size of the image for object "O" three principal rays are drawn (red lines). Ray 1 passes through the nodal point of the lens and is undeviated. Ray 2 passes through the primary focal point (F_1) and emerges parallel to the optical axis. Note that the primary focal point (F_1) would be located $1/2$m to the left of a +2D lens. Ray 3 approaches the lens parallel to the optical axis (zero vergence) and is refracted through the secondary focal point (F_2). Note, for a +2D lens the secondary focal point (F_2) would be located $1/2$m to the right of the lens.

Figure 3–20.
Ray tracing in a thick lens. P_1 and P_2 are principal planes perpendicular to their corresponding nodal points N_1, N_2 (same as principal points). The refracting power of P_1 is determined by the curvature of the front (left) of the lens, and the power of P_2 is determined by the curvature of the back (right). The primary focal point of the lens, F_1, is an average of the powers of P_1 and P_2, as is the secondary focal point, F_2. Ray coming from F_1 (primary focal point) is refracted by P_1 and P_2 to produce a ray parallel to the optical axis. A parallel ray is refracted by P_1 and P_2 to pass through the secondary focal point, F_2.

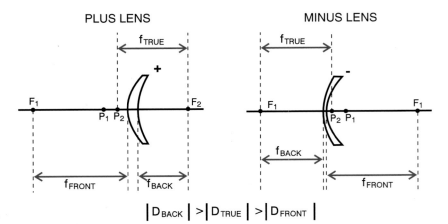

Figure 3–21.
True power vs. vertex power.

$$|D_{BACK}| > |D_{TRUE}| > |D_{FRONT}|$$

The principal planes will act as refracting surfaces. An object ray passing through the primary focal point will emerge from the primary principal plane parallel to the optical axis. An object ray parallel to the axis will emerge from the secondary principal plane converging toward the secondary focal point.

The central ray heading toward the primary nodal point will emerge from the secondary nodal point parallel to its original direction.

The focal lengths are measured from the principal planes, not from the lens surfaces.

The nodal points always coincide with the principal planes if the refractive media on either side of the lens are the same. If the refractive media are different, as in the case of the eye, the nodal points will shift toward the side of the medium with the higher refractive index.

True Power versus Vertex Power. The true power of a lens is always measured in reference to the principal planes (Fig. 3–21). However, the locations of these planes are not always readily available. For spectacle lenses, the power must then be measured in reference to the surfaces of the lens. A lens has two refractive surfaces, the front and the back surfaces. The front vertex (lens curvature) power is measured in reference to the vertex of the front surface. The front vertex power is the reciprocal of the distance from the front surface to its primary focal point. The back vertex power, on the other hand, is measured in reference to the vertex of the back surface and is the reciprocal of the distance from the back surface of the lens to its secondary focal point. The higher the vertex power the closer the focal point is to the lens.

Front and back vertex powers are identical for an equiconvex or equiconcave lens, but modern ophthalmic lenses are generally meniscus shaped. These lenses are deeply curved so as to remain equidistant from the eye in various fields of gaze. If the anterior curve is steeper, then it would be a convergent (or plus) lens. If the posterior curve is steeper, then it would be a divergent (or minus) lens.

Plus meniscus lenses displace the principal planes anteriorly and minus meniscus lenses displace the principal planes posteriorly. For both plus and minus meniscus lenses, the back vertex power is always greater than the true power, which in turn is greater than the front vertex power.

The *lensometer* (also called the lensmeter) measures the back vertex power of a lens. The lensometer works on the Bandal principles consisting of an afocal telescope, a standard lens, and a movable illuminated target. The lens to be measured is placed at the lensometer aperture, which is located at the secondary focal point of the standard lens, located between this lens and the telescope. The mires are seen through a lens system or combination system of lenses. Because the standard lens focal point is known, the distance needed to move the target to the changed focal point due to the unknown lens gives the power. It is linearly proportional to the vertex power of the lens.

Behavior of Light Inside Refractive Media

Refraction by a Single Spherical Surface

Power of a Spherical Refracting Surface. So far, we have approached the lens as one refractive unit. However, each lens surface has its own refractive power. The power of a spherical refractive surface with different refractive media on either sides is determined as:

$$D = \frac{n_1 - n_2}{r}$$

where

$n_1 - n_2$ = difference in refractive indices
r = radius of curvature (meters) and may have either + or − value.

The sign of the power is determined by the following simple convention: within an imaginary rectangle enclosing the surface, if the medium with the higher refractive index is convex, then the surface has a plus (con-

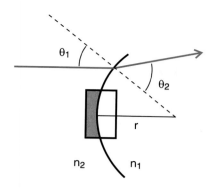

Figure 3–22.
Refraction at a spherical surface. N₁ and N₂ represent two media (optical) with different indices of refraction. "r" represents the radius of curvature for media n₁. In this example, because n₁ is less than n₂, the light ray is bent away from the normal (diverged). Note that the shaded area of the rectangle (with the higher refractive index) has a concave shape (minus lens). θ₁ is smaller than θ₂ thus the light is diverging.

verging) power. If, on the other hand, it is concave, then the surface has minus (diverging) power (Fig. 3–22).

Example: What is the refractive power of the back of the cornea, given that the indices of refraction are 1.37 and 1.33 for the cornea and aqueous respectively. The radius of the cornea is 7 mm.

$$D_{cornea} = -\frac{1.33 - 1.37}{0.007} = -5.7D$$

The back surface of the cornea has a diverging power because the corneal stroma, which has a higher refractive index than the aqueous, is concave relative to the aqueous.

Reduced Vergence. If light travels through different refractive media, such as into the eye where light has to pass from air to vitreous, object and image vergences will necessarily be influenced by the different refractive indices. In such cases, the basic vergence relationship still applies, provided the general definition of vergence is used, which includes the index of refraction of the different media.

$$U + D = V$$

with

$$U = \frac{n_1}{u}$$

$$V = \frac{n_2}{v}$$

where

n_1 = refractive index of object space
n_2 = refractive index of image space
u = distance of object from refractive surface
v = distance of image from refractive surface

Hence:

$$\frac{n_1}{u} + \frac{(n_1 - n_2)}{r} = \frac{n_2}{v}$$

$$\frac{n_1}{u} + D = \frac{n_2}{v}$$

$$U + D = V$$

Example: Where is the image of an object placed 20 cm from a spherical surface with radius of curvature of 5 cm separating air from glass, given the indices of refraction of air and glass are 1.0 and 1.5, respectively.

$$U = \frac{n_1}{u} = -\frac{1.0}{0.2} = -5D$$

This is negative indicating the light is diverging from the object.

$$D = \frac{1.5 - 1.0}{0.05} = \frac{0.50}{0.05} = +10D$$

This is positive now indicating converging rays after passing through the optical surface.

$$V = U + D = -5 + 10 = 5 = \frac{n_2}{v}$$

$$v = 0.33m$$

The image is located $0.33m$ to the right of the surface in glass medium.

Power of a Thin Lens Immersed in a Medium (Other than Air). A lens' dioptric power is in reality the sum of the dioptric powers of its two refractive surfaces.

$$D_{lens} = D_{front\ surface} + D_{back\ surface}$$

$$\frac{n_2 - n_1}{r_1} + \frac{n_1 - n_2}{r_2}$$

then

$$\frac{n_2 - n_1}{\dfrac{1}{r_1} - \dfrac{1}{r_2}}$$

where

n_1 = refractive index of the medium
n_2 = refractive index of the lens
r_1 = radius of curvature (m) of the front surface
r_2 = radius of curvature (m) of the back surface

We can see that the power of the lens is proportionate to the difference in the refractive indices between the lens and the medium in which it is immersed (since r_1 and r_2 are constant for a given lens). This formula can be simplified as below.

Example: if the power of an intraocular lens is +20 D (as measured in aqueous), what would the power be

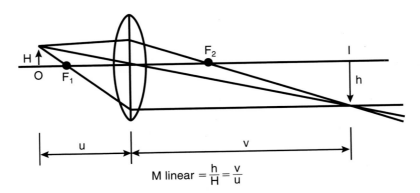

$$M \text{ linear} = \frac{h}{H} = \frac{v}{u}$$

Figure 3–23.
Linear magnification.

if measured in air? Given the refractive indices are 1.49 for the plastic lens, 1.33 for aqueous, and 1.00 for air.

$$\frac{D_{\text{air}}}{D_{\text{aqueous}}} = \frac{(n_{\text{IOL}} - n_{\text{AIR}})}{(n_{\text{IOL}} - n_{\text{aqueous}})}$$

$$\frac{D_{\text{air}}}{+20D} = \frac{(1.49 - 1.00)}{(1.49 - 1.33)}$$

$$D_{\text{air}} = +61D$$

Magnification

Linear magnification refers to devices that project an image onto a film or a screen (camera or projectors). Angular magnification refers to a visual instrument that a person can look through (telescope or microscope).

Linear Magnification. Linear magnification, also called transverse or lateral magnification, is the ratio of the image height (h) relative to the object height (H) (Fig. 3–23). By similar triangles, this is also the ratio of the respective distances from the lens.

$$M_{\text{LATERAL}} = \text{magnification} = \frac{\text{Im. height}}{\text{ob. height}} = \frac{h}{H}$$

$$= \frac{\text{Im. distance}}{\text{ob. distance}} = \frac{v}{u} = \text{(power in diopters)}$$

where

U = object vergence
V = image vergence

If lateral magnification is negative (indicating that the vergences of the object and image are of opposite signs), then the image is on the opposite side of the lens from the object and will be inverted with respect to the object, and vice versa.

The indirect ophthalmoscope provides an example of lateral magnification. A condensing lens is placed in front of the patient's eye to allow pencils of light from the patient's peripheral retina to be brought into focus. This lens diameter and distance from the patient's eye determine the field of view. This lens places the patient's pupil and the examiner's pupil at conjugate planes. The image created is real and inverted. The linear magnification may be expressed as the ratio of the power of the patient's eye (60D) to the power of the condensing lens.

For example, a +20D condensing lens produces 60D/20D or 3× magnification.

$$\text{Lateral magnification} = \frac{60D}{20D} = 3\times \text{mag}$$

Angular Magnification. Linear magnification is not useful when dealing with objects or images at infinity. In these cases, the lateral magnification is either zero or infinitely large. In visual optics, it is more useful to deal with the apparent object and image sizes as appreciated by the eye.

An object or image has a certain fixed size, but it will appear larger or smaller if the observer moves closer or

Figure 3–24.
Angular magnification. Straight red line represents object light ray with no lens, passing through the nodal point of the eye. The black line that passes through the nodal point has been refracted by the lens. The ratio between θ lens and θ no lens is the angular magnification.

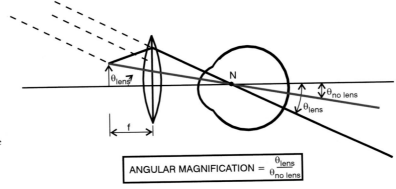

$$\text{ANGULAR MAGNIFICATION} = \frac{\theta_{\text{lens}}}{\theta_{\text{no lens}}}$$

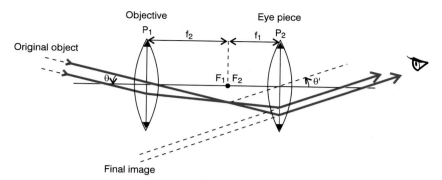

Figure 3–25.
Astronomical telescope. Image inverted.

farther away. In this case the angle subtended by the object or image varies according to its distance from the eye. This angle may be increased by a lens system (Fig. 3–24). Angular magnification is the basis behind Low Vision aids. It allows the spreading of the optical image over a greater number of photoreceptors (17).

$$M_{angular} = \frac{\angle \text{subtended by the image produced by the lens system}}{\angle \text{subtended by the object without the lens system}}$$

$$M_{angular} = \frac{\theta_{lens}}{\theta_{no\ lens}}$$

A simple magnifier is a plus lens used to effectively increase the angle subtended by a near object, usually placed at its focal point. When the object is placed at the primary focal point of a lens system, the image will be at infinity (definition of primary focal point). The visual angle subtended at the retina, θ_{lens}, remains constant regardless of the distance of the object-lens system from the eye, since all rays emerging from the lens are parallel. $\theta_{no\ lens}$, however, changes with the object distance from the eye. Angular magnification, hence, also changes. A reference point must thus be chosen. The reference angle subtended by the object alone without the system is arbitrarily chosen to be that subtended by the object if it were placed at a distance 25 cm from the eye.

$$M_{reference} = \frac{\theta_{lens}}{\theta_{reference}} = \frac{\tan^{-1}(obj/f)}{\tan^{-1}(obj/25cm)} \cong \frac{25cm}{f} = \frac{D}{4}$$

where

D = power of lens in diopters
M_{ref} = magnification compared with image viewed at 25 cm

It should be noted the 1/4 m is only the chosen standard distance. If another distance d (in meters) is used as the reference distance, then the magnification of a simple magnifier would simply be $(D) \times (d)$.

For example, the direct ophthalmoscope simply illuminates the retina and allows us to use the patient's own optical system as a simple magnifier. Since dioptric power of an emmetropic eye is roughly 60 D, the angular magnification of fundus detail is 60/4 or 15×. The

optic nerve then would appear 15 times larger through the ophthalmoscope than it would look if situated 25 cm from the examiner's eye with the cornea and lens removed.

Axial Magnification. Axial magnification is the ratio of the image depth to the object depth as measured along the optical axis. It is actually the ratio of the axial image shift to the axial object shift. This is proportional to the square of the linear magnification.

$$M_{axial} = (M_{lateral})^2$$

Lens Systems

Telescopes. Telescopes receive incident parallel rays and discharge them at a new angle to produce angular magnification. They are usually created using two lenses, the eyepiece and the objective. The objective forms a small image of a distant object, and the eyepiece is then used to "look" at the image formed by the objective. In other words, these lenses are placed such that the primary focal point of the eyepiece coincides with the secondary focal point of the objective.

There are two types of telescopes, astronomical and Galilean.

Astronomical Telescope. The astronomical telescope consists of two plus (converging) lenses and forms an inverted image (Fig. 3–25). The lenses are positioned such that the secondary focal point of one lens coincides with the primary focal point of the other. An easy way to remember that an astronomical telescope produces an inverted image is when looking at a star (through an astronomical telescope) it does not matter if the image is upright or not.

The optical system of the slit lamp is a modified astronomical telescope (that is instead of only two plus lenses, the objective is composed of a series of lenses to reduce aberration). The final image is therefore real and inverted with respect to the object. Prisms are then placed between the objective and the eyepiece to reinvert the image. The magnification provided by the slit lamp can be obtained by using different objectives, different eyepieces, or by adding a Galilean telescope sys-

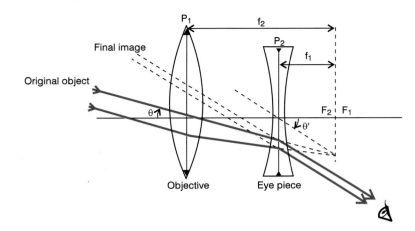

Figure 3–26.
Galilean telescope. Image erect.

tem between the objective and the eyepiece. The indirect ophthalmoscope is another example of an astronomical telescope.

Galilean Telescope. The Galilean telescope and the principles of its operation are important in ophthalmic optics and the correction of refractive error. In Galilean telescopes, the objective is a plus lens while the eyepiece is a minus lens. The lenses are positioned such that the secondary focal point of the plus lens coincides with the primary focal point of the minus lens. It forms an upright image (Fig. 3–26).

Magnification. The magnification given by telescopes:

$$M_{\text{telescope}} = \frac{\theta'}{\theta} = \frac{f_{\text{obj}}}{f_{\text{eye}}} = \frac{D_{\text{eyepiece}}}{D_{\text{objective}}}$$

Surgical Loupe. Certain high-power surgical loupes are astronomical telescopes with image-inverting prisms. These are called expanded field telescopes. The basic surgical loupes are however Galilean telescopes with an "add" to correct for the working distance (standard telescopes were originally designed for objects at an infinite distance). The add is usually combined with the objective as one lens. This add only allows for focusing at near without using accommodation and provides little if any magnification.

Accommodation Through a Telescope. The amount of accommodation through a telescope is given by the following formula:

Total Accommodation =
Accommodative Stimulus × $(M_{\text{telescope}})^2$

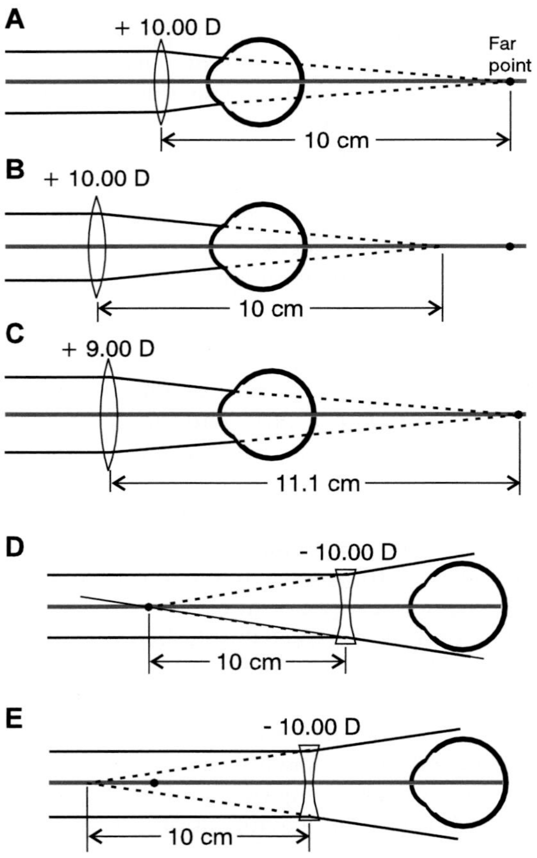

Figure 3–27.
Lens effectivity.
A: This is a hypermetropic eye (+10D refractive error), the far point is behind the retina. Here, the +10D lens focuses light onto the far point, correcting the hypermetropia.
B: Same hypermetropic eye as A, but the +10D lens is moved away from the eye. Note that the light is now focused in front of the far point. Because the lens has been moved away from the eye, its effective power has been increased. The patient is now over-corrected (lens induced myopia).
C: A weaker (less plus) lens at this new location will bring light into focus at the far point. Moving the lens forward allows a greater distance for the light to converge into focus thus increasing the effective lens power.
D: This is a −10D myope, the far point is in front of the eye.
E: Moving the −10D lens forward also moves the focal point in front of the far point, reducing the effective (minus) power.

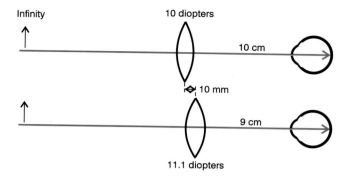

Figure 3–28.
Effectivity (example).

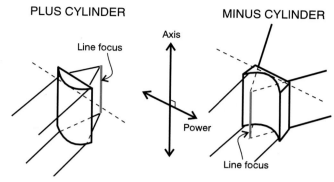

Figure 3–29.
Plano cylinder lens. **NOTE: Cylinder Power is 90° away from its axis.** In this diagram, cylinder axis is at 90° (vertical) while power is at 180° (horizontal).

Example: What is the accommodation required to view an object 50 cm from a 3× telescope?

$$Ta = 2D \times (3)^2 = 18D$$

It is of interest to note that if we introduce a +2D lens in front of the objective, effectively creating a surgical loupe, then the normal accommodation would be zero and no accommodation would be needed through the telescope.

Lens Effectivity

Although the power of a lens is constant, its effect on an optical system depends on its location with respect to the remaining elements of the optical system. To bring parallel rays into focus at a particular point, different lenses of different powers may be used, depending on their location with respect to this particular point.

This principle is important when considering the location of a lens with respect to the eye.

For plus lenses (Fig. 3–27), moving a plus lens forward (away from the eye) will increase its effective power. The power should therefore be decreased if it is to maintain the same effectiveness on the eye. For minus lenses, the opposite is true. Moving a minus lens forward will decrease its effective power (since effective plus power is added). Or it may more easily be remembered that moving any lens away from the eye increases its plus power. The power should therefore be increased to maintain the proper effectiveness on the eye.

Example: a +10 D lens is moved 10 mm backward from its original position (Fig. 3–28). How does its effective power change? What power would the lens have to be to maintain the proper distance correction?

Moving a plus lens backward, toward the eye, decreases its effective power. Hence, a stronger plus lens must be used to maintain the same effectiveness. In this case, we need a stronger plus lens of +11.1 D at the new location, to maintain the same focus in the eye.

The power of the lens needed at the new location (D_n) can be calculated using the following formula:

$$D_n = \frac{D_o}{1 - dD_o}$$

where

D_o = original lens power
d = difference in location (in meters)
   d is $(-)$ if the lens is moved forward
   and $(+)$ if it is moved backward.

Lens effectivity becomes clinically significant when dealing with aphakia and contact lenses with powers greater than 4 D.

Astigmatic Lenses

Unlike a spherical lens, which has the same surface radius of curvature and, therefore, the same refractive power in all meridians, astigmatic lenses have different surface radii at different meridians. The refractive power varies from meridian to meridian, with the extreme values always 90° apart. An astigmatic surface cannot bring an image into sharp single point focus.

Planocylindrical Lenses. The simplest astigmatic surface is a cylindrical one (Fig. 3–29). It can be appreciated by considering the cut surface of a cylinder. A cylindrical lens can be either plus or minus.

Each lens has maximum power in the meridian perpendicular to the axis of the cylinder. Parallel rays incident on the lens surface will form an image line parallel to the axis. A plus lens will form a real focal line, whereas a minus lens will form a virtual one.

The Maddox rod, a useful optical tool, is a set of parallel high-powered cylindrical lenses used to form a line image from a point source. The image formed by the Maddox rod is real and parallel to the axis of the cylinder. (See also Maddox Rod in horizontal phoria measurements).

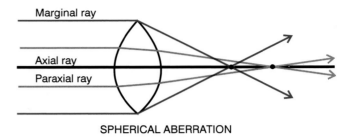

Figure 3–31.
Spherical aberration.

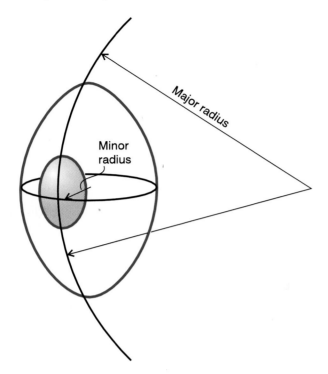

Figure 3–30.
Spherocylindrical lens.

Spherocylindrical Lenses. Most spectacle lenses are spherocylindrical (Fig. 3–30) or toroidal. They look like a slice from the side of a barrel or football.

The power cross (see lens power notation) helps to illustrate the power present in the meridians (axes) of the lens.

Lens Aberrations

Chromatic Aberrations. Lights of different wavelengths travel through the same medium at different velocities. This causes polychromatic white light to be separated into its component colors upon refraction by a lens. Blue rays of shorter wavelength are refracted more strongly, and therefore come to a focus closer to the lens than the longer red rays. In the eye, the interval between visible blue light and red light is 1.25D. If focused on yellow light, we are approximately 0.87D myopic for blue light and 0.37D hyperopic for red. Chromatic aberration is the principle behind the Duochrome test. An achromatic lens is a combination of a convex and a concave lens of different refractive indices that reduce color dispersion and chromatic aberration.

Monochromatic Aberrations

Spherical Aberration. Spherical aberration exists when peripheral rays strike a spherical surface (Fig. 3–31). Peripheral rays are refracted more strongly than paraxial rays and come into focus closer to the lens. This can be reduced by changing the lens to a planoconvex or meniscus shape. In spectacles, spherical aberration also can be reduced by grinding less power into the lens at the periphery. This type of lens is aspheric.

A dilated pupil will allow maximal aberration and induces a slight degree of myopia. A miotic pupil reduces spherical aberration and provides a clearer image. Spherical aberration is also lessened in the eye by the crystalline lens having a higher refractive index in the nucleus than in the cortex.

The peripheral cornea, with a decreasing radius of curvature, also decreases spherical aberration.

Curvature of Field. Any lens will focus light rays from an extended linear object onto a curved image plane. This curved image plane is called the *Petzval surface*.[17] It is curved toward the edges of a plus lens (*pin cushion distortion*) and away from the edges of a minus lens (*barrel distortion*). This effect increases with the power of the lens. It is of interest that the curve of the retina closely approximates the Petzval surface of the eye's optics.

Distortion. Distortion is produced by unequal magnification over the field of view. If peripheral magnification is greater than axial magnification, *pincushion* distortion is produced. If the reverse is true, then *barrel* distortion ensues. Distortion is influenced not only by the type of lens but also by the position of the aperture "stop," which is the opening limiting the number and position of the light rays that will form the final image. An aperture stop located in front of a plus lens will create a barrel distortion, while the same aperture stop located behind the same lens will create a pincushion distortion. An aperture between the lenses of a system reduces distortion, making it *orthoscopic*.

Astigmatism of Oblique Incidence and Pantoscopic Tilt. Oblique astigmatism occurs when light rays strike a lens at an oblique angle or if the object is located off the optical axis. The refracted rays do not come to a point but rather form a *conoid of Sturm* (see also astigmatism in

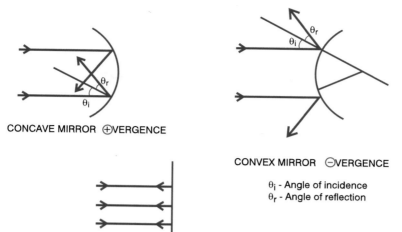

Figure 3–32.
Mirror vergence.

CONCAVE MIRROR ⊕VERGENCE

CONVEX MIRROR ⊖VERGENCE

θ_i - Angle of incidence
θ_r - Angle of reflection

PLANE MIRROR — NO VERGENCE

Ophthalmic Optics), an interval of focus from anterior (strongest power) to posterior (weakest power). Hence, an astigmatic image is created when rays are obliquely incident on a spherical surface.

Tilting a spherical lens also creates the same effect called *pantoscopic tilt*. The axis of the induced cylinder is always in the meridian around which the lens is pivoted, and the amount of astigmatism induced is dependent on the degree of tilt (proportional to the tangent of the angle of tilt) and power of the lens. Not only is a cylinder induced with tilting, the power of the sphere is also increased by an amount equal to $1/3\sin^2\theta$ (with θ being the angle of tilt).

This tilting-induced effect has practical consequences. Spectacles are fit with a small amount of *Pantoscopic tilt*. This tilt of the lower part of the lens closer to the face than the upper part of the lens allows a more perpendicular line of sight, through the lens, when one is looking down to read. Too much or too little of this tilt induces unwanted astigmatism.

To gain more minus power through their lenses, myopes would tilt their spectacles and at the same time slide them closer to their eyes. Conversely, hyperopes would slide the spectacles away from their eyes and down the nose to gain more effective power in addition to tilting.

Reflection

Law of Reflection. When light rays strike a surface with negligible permeability to light, they are bounced off the surface or reflected. The "laws of reflection" mandate that the angle of reflection is always equal to the angle of incidence (both measured from the normal to the reflecting surface). The incident and reflected rays remain in the same plane. Mirrors are smooth surfaces that reflect light. They can add vergence to light (con-

vex or concave mirrors) (Fig. 3–32) or simply reverse the direction of light (plane mirror).

The reflected rays can form an image in much the same way as refracted rays can. The only difference is that, because mirrors reverse the direction of light, the image space is now reversed (i.e., the image space is on the same side as the object space). The basic vergence relationship $U + D = V$, can still be applied to mirrors. *Real images* formed by converging light rays will have plus vergence and be on the *same side* as the object. *Virtual images* formed by extension of diverging light will have *minus vergence* and be on the *side opposite* the object.

Reflecting Power of a Mirror. The reflecting power is the amount of vergence added to a pencil of light rays by the mirror. It is related to the radius of curvature of the mirror by this simple equation:

$$D = 1/f = \frac{2}{r}$$

where D = reflecting power in diopters
f = focal length in meters
r = radius of curvature in m
since $f = r/2$

By convention, r is positive for concave mirrors (since plus vergence is added) and negative for convex mirrors. Only the surface of the mirror is involved in reflection; the reflecting power is not influenced by the index of refraction of the mirror.

Ray Tracing for Mirrors. Ray tracing principles can be conveniently used to find the character and position of the image (Fig. 3–33). The following rules apply:

- Spherical mirrors only have one focal point (F)
- Incident ray parallel to the axis will be reflected through the focal point (Ray 1).

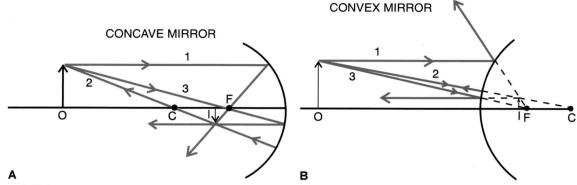

Figure 3–33A.
A, Concave mirror ray tracing. **B,** Convex mirror ray tracing. Note: the focal point (F) is located halfway between the center of curvature (C) and the surface of the mirror. Another expression of the reflecting power of a mirror formula is F = ¹/₂ r (radius).

- An incident ray passing through the center of curvature of the mirror will be reflected back upon itself (Ray 2).
- Incident rays passing through the focal point will be reflected parallel to the axis (Ray 3).

Magnification. As with lenses, magnification is the ratio of the image size to the object size, and is proportional to the respective distances of the image and object from the mirror.

$$M = \frac{\text{IMAGE distance}}{\text{OBJECT distance}} = \frac{U}{V} = \frac{v}{u}$$

A positive magnification signifies an erect image, and a negative magnification signifies an inverted image.

Plane Mirror. Plane mirrors add no vergence to the reflected light, but simply reverse its direction.

Example: An object is located 50 cm to the left of a plane mirror. Where will its image be located?

The object has a vergence U of −2.00 D (−1/0.5 m)

The reflecting power of a plane mirror $D = 0$ ($D = r/2$ and for a plane mirror, $r = 0$)

Hence, applying the vergence formula:

$$V = U + D$$
$$V = -2.0 \text{ D} + 0 \text{ D}$$
$$V = 1/v = -50 \text{ cm}$$

With minus vergence, the image is formed by diverging rays. It, therefore, must be virtual and is located 50 cm on the side opposite to the object (or to the right of the mirror). It also is erect. Plane mirrors always create virtual and erect images of the same size as the object.

Spherical Mirror. Spherical mirrors add vergence to light in addition to reversing its direction. *Concave mirrors* add plus vergence to light and have positive power. *Convex mirrors* add minus vergence and have negative power.

Example 1: an object is located 50 cm to the left of a concave mirror with a radius of 20 cm. Where is the image located?

$$U = -\frac{1}{0.5m} = -2.00D$$

$$D = \frac{2}{r} = \frac{2}{0.2m} = +10.0D$$

Therefore $V = -2.00 + 10.00 = +8.00$ D

It is a real image (with plus vergence) and is located at 12.5 cm to the left of the mirror (image space is the same as object space with mirrors).

$$M = \frac{U}{V} = \frac{-2.00}{+8.00} = -0.25$$

The image is thus minified and inverted.

Example 2: An object is located at the same distance as example 1 but before a convex mirror of the same radius.

$$U = -2.00 \text{ D}$$
$$D = -10.00 \text{ D}$$
$$V = U + D = -12.00 \text{ D}$$
$$v = 1/V = -8.3 \text{ cm}$$
$$M = U/V = -2.0/-12.0 = 1/6 = +0.167$$

The image is virtual, erect, and minified and is located 8.3 cm to the right of the mirror.

A concave mirror can create a real or virtual image that can be magnified or minified, erect or inverted, depending on the location of the object with respect to the focal point of the mirror. A convex mirror, however, always creates a virtual, erect, and minified image.

An example of a convex mirror commonly found in ophthalmology is the surface of the cornea. A keratometer is an instrument that projects lights onto the corneal surface and by using the images formed allows determination of the radius of curvature of the cornea and thereby its refractive power.

The traditional manual keratometer uses reflection of an illuminated target that is projected onto a small area of the cornea. The size of the reflected image (first Purkinje-Sanson image) relative to the size of the object (mires of keratometer) allows calculation of the radius of curvature of the cornea. More recent and more accurate determination of the curvature(s) of the entire corneal surface is provided by corneal topography.

Purkinje Puzzlement

Purkinje Sanson Images: These are four reflected images from the eye. The first Purkinje image is the reflection off the front surface of the cornea. The second Purkinje im-age is the reflection off the back surface of the cornea. The third and fourth Purkinje images are reflections off the anterior and posterior surfaces of the crystalline lens respectively. The anterior lens acts as a convex mirror, forming a virtual image. The posterior lens acts as a con-cave mirror forming a real image of a distant object.

Purkinje Shift. This represents the change in spectral sensitivity of the retina. Under photopic (light) condi-tion, the retina is most sensitive to light at 555nm wave-length. Under scotopic (dark) conditions, the maxi-mum sensitivity shifts to light at 510nm wavelength.

Purkinje Image/Figure. This is an entopic phe-nomenon of vision. A bright light (such as a slit lamp beam) moving across the retina will allow the patient to see the shadow created by their retinal blood vessels onto their retina.

■ OPHTHALMIC OPTICS

Schematic and Reduced Eyes

The total optical power of the eye is slightly less than 60D. The cornea accounts for approximately two-thirds of this power and the lens almost one-third, but smaller amounts are derived from interfaces within the globe. For practical purposes, the optical system can be simpli-fied to a *schematic eye* (9) as described by Gullstrand, which illustrates the *Cardinal points* (8) of the eye. These are comprised of the primary and secondary focal points, the principal points, and the nodal points of the eye. Because the principal points and the nodal points are so close (0.254 mm separating each pair in the pha-kic eye), very little inaccuracy results in using a more sim-plified or *reduced eye* (Fig. 3–34). The reduced eye (or ac-tually called the "simplified eye" by Donders) treats the entire optical system of the eye as if all refraction oc-curred at a single refracting surface. In this phakic power

reduced schematic eye (4), the following values were es-tablished:

1. Radius of curvature 5.73 mm
2. Anterior focal length −17.05 mm
3. Posterior focal length 22.78 mm.
4. Nodal point 5.65 mm behind the anterior corneal surface
5. The power is +58.6 D
6. Nodal point from retina is 17.00 mm

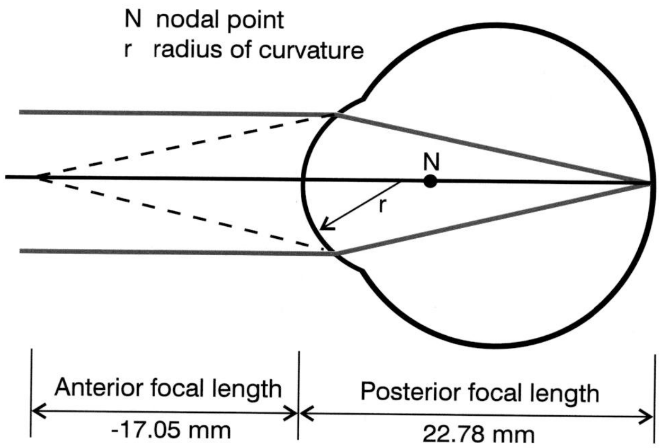

Conjugate foci are two points on the visual axis where an object placed at one point will be imaged at the other and vice versa. Here the far point and the retina may be considered as conjugate foci. The *far point* for any eye is that point which is conjugate with the fovea; if the far point is at optical infinity, the eye is *emmetropic*. In this case of optical harmony, the opti-cal power and the axial length are matched so that the image is brought into focus on the retina. Departures from this situation are called *refractive errors* or *ametropia*.

Retinal Image Size

Based on the reduced schematic eye, it becomes easy to calculate the size of a retinal image of a known object, such as a Snellen letter.

Since light rays passing through the nodal point of the schematic eye are not deviated, the retinal image size and the object size are directly proportional based on their respective distances from the eye.

The distance to the object is measured from the cornea, since the additional distance to the nodal point is negligible.

N nodal point
r radius of curvature

Anterior focal length
-17.05 mm

Posterior focal length
22.78 mm

Figure 3–34.
Reduced schematic eye.

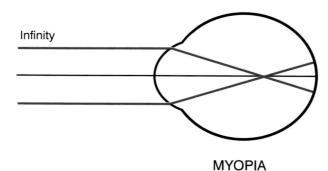

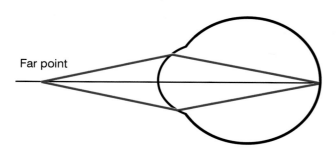

Figure 3–35.
Top: Myopia, parallel light focuses in front of retina.
Bottom: Object at far point in focus on retina.

Example: What is the retinal size of 1.0 cm Snellen letter viewed at a distance of 6 m?

$$\frac{\text{Retinal size (mm)}}{17 \text{ mm (nodal point to retina)}} =$$

$$\frac{\text{letter height (mm)}}{\text{distance from the eye (mm)}}$$

$$\text{Retinal size (mm)} = \left(\frac{10 \text{ mm}}{6000 \text{ mm}}\right) \times 17 \text{ mm} = 0.0283 \text{ mm}$$

Myopia and Hyperopia

If the optical system is too powerful for the length of the eye or if the length is too long for the optical system, the rays will be brought into focus in front of the retina, in the vitreous humor. This situation is *myopia* (Fig. 3–35).

If, conversely, the optical power of the eye is too weak for the length so that the image would be in focus behind the retina (with accommodation relaxed), this is called *hyperopia* (Fig. 3–36).

Astigmatism

Myopia and hyperopia are spherical refractive errors. The surface of the cornea acts as a sphere, and the other optical components of the eye also act with equal power in all meridians. Where there is a variability in the power of the eye in various meridians, or axes, there is *astigmatism* (Fig. 3–37). Commonly, this is demonstrated by

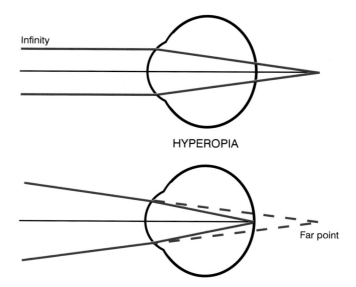

Figure 3–36.
Top: Hyperopia, parallel light in focus behind the retina.
Bottom: Far point behind retina. Positive vergence from a lens will focus rays on retina.

comparing the surface effect of a basketball with a football. Rays are affected equally by the perfectly round sphere basketball shape. Those rays passing through the football shape are affected differently depending on whether they are refracted by the longer or shorter curvature. The shorter, smaller radius of curvature will refract rays into focus more anteriorly than the longer radius of curvature. Astigmatism results in a prolonged interval of focus, rather than a point. This interval is called the *interval of Sturm* (intervalle focal or Brennstrecke). It extends from the anterior-most focal position to the posterior-most position. At each end, the rays are brought into a line of focus rather than a point focus. Only one axis is in focus at a time, and these line ends of this interval represent the most and the least focal power of the eye. If one were to observe the images at the end of this interval, one would see a focused line at each end. These lines would be 90° apart. As one moved

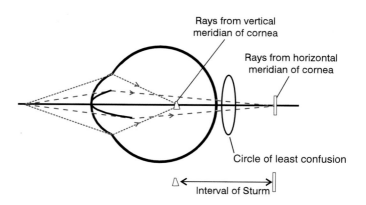

Figure 3–37.
Astigmatism and interval of sturm.

ASTIGMATISM

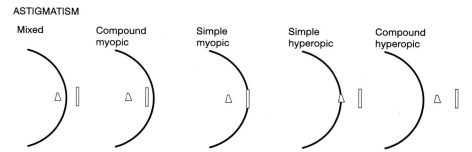

Figure 3–38.
Types of astigmatism.

from one end to the other, one would find an ellipse of focus, the axis of which corresponds to the closer line. Near the center of this interval is encountered the *circle of least confusion*. If a patient has astigmatism, and is able, with accommodation, to move the interval of Sturm to its clearest position, he/she typically will position this circle of least confusion on the retina. This interval would thereby straddle the retina. This type of astigmatism is mixed astigmatism. The other various possible positions of the interval of Sturm relative to the retina give rise to other types of astigmatism: *compound myopic, simple myopic* (with the posterior end of the interval on the retina), *simple hyperopic* (the anterior end on the retina), and *compound hyperopic astigmatism* (Fig. 3–38).

Lens Power Notation

The power of a lens typically is written in 0.25 diopter (D) increments. Occasionally, 0.125 powers are written. The notation for ophthalmic lenses *always* includes a "+" or "−." The sphere portion is written first, combined with the astigmatic or cylinder portion and its axis.

Example: −1.75 D Sph + 1.00 D Cyl axis 180°
This is typically shortened to −1.75 + 1.00 × 180

This represents a negative, or −1.75 D spherical (DS) lens combined with a +1.00 D cylinder with an axis of 180°. An axis notation is written in increasing degree demarcation from 1°, counterclockwise through 45°, 90°, 135°, and to 180°. By convention, 0°, or horizontal, is always written as 180°.

This *same* lens also may be written in minus cylinder form:

$$- 0.75 - 1.00 \times 90$$

A lens *power cross* diagram (5) (Fig. 3–39) gives a pictorial representation of the location and amount of power of the lens. If one looks at a *power cross* diagram of this lens, one may see that in the vertical direction or at 90° the power is −0.75 diopters. The power at 180° is −1.75 diopters. It must be remembered that the axis location is 90° away from the location of the power.

The actual grind creating the cylinder may be determined by the use of the Geneva Lens Clock. Turning this gauge on the surface of the lens allows determination of the actual power and/or the presence of more than one curvature of the surface.

The same lens may be described as plus cylinder or minus cylinder, there is a rapid way of converting the written notation from plus cylinder to minus cylinder

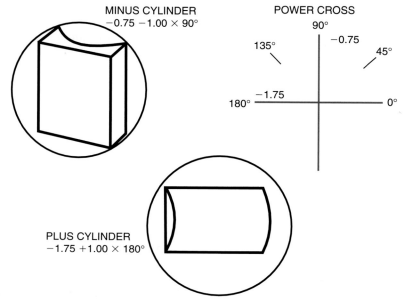

MINUS CYLINDER
−0.75 −1.00 × 90°

POWER CROSS
90°
135°
−0.75
45°
180° —— −1.75 —— 0°

PLUS CYLINDER
−1.75 +1.00 × 180°

Figure 3–39.
Power cross diagram (red)
and spherocylindrical lenses.

and vice-versa. The steps to convert the lens power from minus to plus cylinder and vice versa are:

1. Add, algebraically, the power of the sphere to the cylinder.
2. Convert the sign of the cylinder to the opposite sign.
3. Change the axis by 90 degrees.

   Example: $-1.75 + 1.00 \times 180$

1. Addition gives total of -0.75 DS.
2. conversion of the sign $\longrightarrow$ now -1.00 cylinder
3. conversion of the axis $\longrightarrow$ now axis 90

   Now written $-0.75 -1.00 \times 90$

Spherical Equivalent

The spherical equivalent (*S.E.*) of a spherical lens is simply that spherical lens power. For sphero-cylindrical lenses, the spherical equivalent may be determined by taking the spherical component and adding, algebraically, to it one-half of the cylinder. This sum is the spherical equivalent. For example: the S.E. of the lens $+3.00$ (D.Sph) is $+3.00$. The spherical equivalent of $+2.00 +1.00 \times 90$ is $+2.50$. (note that the axis becomes irrelevant). The S.E. of $-1.00 +4.00 \times 180$ is $+1.00$. The spherical equivalent would offer the best correction for a patient with astigmatism where sphero-cylindrical lenses were unavailable.

■ REFRACTION

Refraction as is commonly referred to in ophthalmology is the clinical application of optics to quantify the patient's ametropia and the lenses necessary to correct this error (24).

This *refractive error* may be determined by various methods, but these methods may be divided into two main classes: objective and subjective. The objective methods are employed when patients are unable to co-operate or respond to questions, i.e. mental ability, infants, language problems, etc. The subjective techniques are used when the patient is able to cooperate with the examiner to indicate differences in vision through various lens choices.

Vertex distance

Vertex distance is defined as the distance from the anterior surface of the cornea to the back surface of the lens. For practical purposes it is measured with eyelids closed. It becomes clinically significant for prescriptions of more than five diopters (plus or minus). This is a practice application of lens effectivity.

Retinoscopy

Retinoscopy (12) (earlier called skiascopy, or measurement of a shadow) is used in the objective portion of the

refraction to serve as the starting point for subjective refinement or sometimes to serve as the final *refractive* correction. As long ago as 1862, Bowman called attention to the rotation of the mirror used in ophthalmoscopy to bring out characteristics of irregular astigmatism. Donders, in 1864 attributed "...the discovery of regular astigmatism of the cornea ... by using the mirror of the ophthalmoscope ..."

The streak retinoscope has been designed (originally by Jack Copeland by serendipity) (2) to allow the examiner to project a light onto the retina of the patient and to observe specific attributes of this reflected light. The two components of retinoscopy are the projection system (Fig. 3–40) and the observation system. The projection system employs a light source which is varied from divergent rays to convergent rays by lenses or mirrors. The source of this light is typically a bulb filament which projects as a line or streak. This light enters the patient's eye and passes through the optical system onto the retina (8). This illuminated area of the retina then serves as the object source of light, which is observed by the examiner. The optical system of the patient's eye then projects this retinal light to the patient's far point.

The far point of the emmetropic eye is at optical infinity. The myopic eye has its far point somewhere between the patient and infinity. The hyperopic eye has a far point somewhere between the eye and negative in-

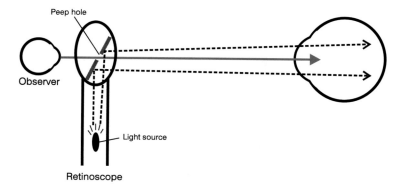

Figure 3–40.
Retinoscope projection system.

finity, or in essence, from behind the patient's eye to infinity.

The relationship of the far point of the eye and the position of the examiner is the basis of retinoscopy (Fig. 3–41). The view of the retinal light source, its qualities and movement allows the examiner to determine his/her position relative to the far point of the patient.

If one performs retinoscopy at the far point of an eye, the reflex from the retina fills the entire pupil with a rapid light flash as the retinoscope light sweeps across the patient's eye (Fig. 3–45). This light reflex has infinite speed across the pupil, so fast in fact that it is not possible to determine from which direction it begins and where it ends. The flash fills the entire pupil space with light even though the original source is a thin linear filament.

If retinoscopy is performed from somewhere between the patient and the patient's far point, the movement of the reflex seen in the pupil is characteristically *with motion* (Fig. 3–42). This with motion means that the actual motion of the retinoscope beam across the patient's face and eye is in the same direction as the reflex seen from within the eye. Three attributes: speed, intensity, and fullness of the image help to indicate the distance from the far point of the examiner. As the far point is approached, the intensity, speed and fullness of

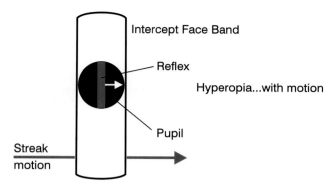

Figure 3–42.
Hyperopia–"with motion."

the image increase. Conversely, as one examines farther from the farpoint the image becomes dimmer, the speed slower and the fullness decreases to allow better visibility of the filament.

The opposite reflex of *with motion* is *against motion.* This situation occurs when there is myopia and the examiner is located beyond the far point of the patient. As the retinoscope beam passes across the patient's pupil, the movement of the brief reflex is seen to move in the opposite direction (Fig. 3–43).

A

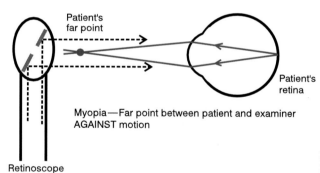

Myopia—Far point between patient and examiner
AGAINST motion

Figure 3–41A.
Retinoscope–myopia.

B

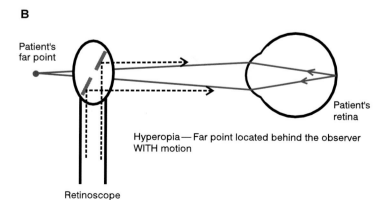

Hyperopia—Far point located behind the observer
WITH motion

Figure 3–41B.
Retinoscope–hyperopia.

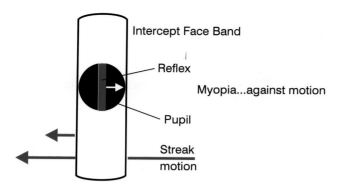

Figure 3–43.
Myopia–"against motion."

It may be difficult to determine exactly when the point of neutrality is reached. Against motion (Fig. 3–43) is more difficult to judge than with motion, particularly when almost at neutrality.

Estimation techniques for myopia and hyperopia and ophthalmoscopic retinoscopy (27) allow for more advanced utilization of this brilliantly conceived refracting instrument.

Retinoscopy Technique

The technique for refraction and retinoscopy in this text assumes the use of plus cylinder refractors. The technique is generally the same for minus cylinder refractors, but small differences will be noted where applicable.

The distance is usually about 66 cm (1.5 diopters) from the retinoscope to the patient's eye. This distance is called the working distance and must be accounted for later in the lens power.

The retinoscopy beam is projected onto the faceplate of the refractor and then moved across the patient's pupil in a sweeping motion across the refractor. To begin, the filament axis is aligned either vertically (90 degrees) or horizontally (180 degrees). If the axis of the beam is 90 degrees, the beam is swept from side to

side, and the axis under evaluation is 90 degrees. Conversely, if the axis of the beam is 180 degrees, the beam is swept up and down (vertically), and the axis being evaluated is 180 degrees. The axis may be turned to any position by the knob controlled by the forefinger and determined by the axis of astigmatism of the patient. It is the reflected beam seen at the pupil that demands our attention for the remainder of retinoscopy.

Optics of Retinoscopy

The optics involved in retinoscopy must be kept in mind during its performance. As the first sweep is made across the patient's pupil with or against motion may be appreciated (Fig. 3–42). At this point we add plus lenses to neutralize with motion or minus lenses to neutralize against. We wish to reach, with the addition of spherical lenses, the optical condition of simple hyperopic astigmatism (*for the plus cylinder refractor*). This optical situation is appreciated as having incident light brought into focus with some rays in focus on the retina and others that would be in focus behind the retina. The interval of Sturm is thereby positioned with its anterior end on the retina. The astigmatic axis is appreciated as a discontinuity of the axis of the projected retinoscopy light and that returning from the patient (Fig. 3–44). These must be aligned by rotating the projected beam to match the axis of that of the patient. Once simple hyperopic astigmatism is reached with spheres, the interval of Sturm can then be collapsed using plus cylindrical lenses. Cylindrical lenses have their predominant optical effect on light rays in one axis. It should be noted that with minus cylinder refractors, simple myopic astigmatism is reached with spheres, and then minus cylinders are used to collapse the interval of Sturm.

Working Distance

Retinoscopy is performed at a working distance typically 66 cm in front of the patient (1.5 diopters). Therefore 1.5 diopters of minus power must eventually

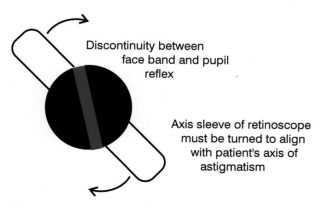

Figure 3–44.
Astigmatism. Discontinuity of pupil reflex.

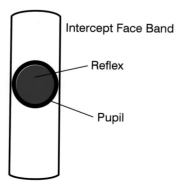

Figure 3–45.
Neutrality. Pupil filled with infinitely fast reflex.

be added to the refractor to move the far point to infinity and compensate for this optical situation. If there were no lenses required to neutralize the patient, this would mean that the patient's far point was exactly at 66 cm and he/she would be a 1.5 diopter myope (Fig. 3–45).

Scheme of Retinoscopy

1. Refractor aligned with proper PD
2. Patient with unobstructed view of a large non-accommodative target.
3. Position with right eyes (examiner's and patient's), right hand, right sides.
4. Other hand positioned on refractor lens wheel with arm position determining working distance.
5. Dim ambient light to enlarge pupils.
6. Few passes to determine overall *"with"* or *"against"* motion
7. Add spheres to reach simple hyperopic astigmatism (in plus cylinder refractors), one axis neutral and the other located 90 degrees away has "with" motion.
8. Axis located with most "with" motion.
9. Plus cylinder added in axis until "with" is neutralized.
10. Working distance removed (subtract 1.50 D).
11. Go on to the other eye ... left eyes, left hand, left side.

Automated Refractors

Automated refractors are available which operate to give either objective or subjective findings. Their use is expanding as their accuracy is improving.

Manifest Refraction

Manifest refraction is the portion of the examination that allows the examiner to refine the objective findings based on patient response. The patient is shown choices of lenses, and encouraged to select the lens that is "clearer". Great attention must be given to the words selected in instructing the patient as to exactly what is required.

The subjective nature of this portion of the examination creates a significant challenge for patient management. This portion of the test has many overlays in patient response to authority, truthfulness of the patient, decisiveness, and the patient wishing to please the examiner at the expense of accurate observation. The speed at which the lenses are presented may be too fast, or too slow. The inflection in the examiner's voice may inadvertently encourage a certain choice. The lack of a clear choice for the patient inevitably occurs towards the final portion of the examination, and the patient usually feels that the final lens may not be correct as a result of this ambiguous selection process. Too few choices causes the patient to feel that not enough attention is given to detail; too many choices results in frustration and waning attention to the selection.

The endpoint of retinoscopy may serve as the beginning for subjective refraction. Alternatively, the patient's old prescription may be placed in the refractor if reasonable vision is achieved with these lenses. The two most frequently used methods for subjective refraction involve the use of the astigmatic clock dial and the Jackson cross cylinder.

Astigmatic Clock Dial

Theory. Spherical lenses cause rays in every axis to be focused equally (Fig. 3–46). A plus lens added in front of an eye causes all rays to be brought into focus more anteriorly. A minus sphere causes rays to be focused more posteriorly in all axes. Cylindrical lenses have a different property, for they affect rays in one axis predominantly. A cylindrical lens, if placed with its axis at 90 degrees has an effect on rays which strike the lens in the horizontal plane. Those rays in the vertical plane pass through the lens unchanged. If one imagines a stack of rays (like pancakes) in horizontal orientation passing through a plus cylinder lens axis 90 degrees, it could be seen that each horizontal plane would form a point focus behind the cylinder lens. These point foci would form a vertical line. Therefore a cylindrical lens has its effect on light perpendicular to its axis, but forms an image parallel to its axis. Furthermore, if such a cylinder were to increase in power, the vertical line focus formed behind the lens would move anterior. It is understood then that a plus

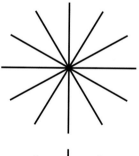

Astigmatism Clock Dial

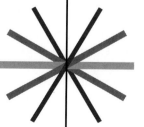

Clock dial seen by "fogged" patient with astigmatism

12:00 clearest: 3:00–9:00 blurred simple myopic astigmatism "With the Rule"
+ cylinder axis 90°
    or
− cylinder axis 180°

Figure 3–46.
Astigmatic clock dial.

cylinder lens axis 90 degrees, if increased in power, will cause its vertical line focus to move anteriorly. Any cylinder placed with its axis in alignment with the orientation of focused rays on the retina may be used to manipulate these rays, plus to move them anteriorly and minus to move them posteriorly.

Method. The astigmatic clock dial, or sunburst target, is used to determine first the axis of astigmatism and secondly the amount of astigmatism. The patient views the target monocularly, with no correction in the lens blank. Plus sphere lenses are added in front of the eye until the target is blurred or "fogged". This fogging is critical to the test, for it causes accommodation to be relaxed. It also creates a condition of myopia or compound myopic astigmatism. The manipulation of the Interval of Sturm so that all the rays are focused anterior to the retina (compound myopic astigmatism) allows the examiner to control the test. Creation of the "fog" creates a situation where accommodation is relaxed, for if the patient accommodates, the target will simply become even more blurred. The "fogged" target is evaluated by the patient. Under these conditions, the entire Interval of Sturm is anterior to the retina. The closest rays to the retina will be seen clearer than the more anterior rays. The axis of astigmatism can be determined by aligning the cylinder axis marker of the refractor with the clearer rays (with plus cylinder refractors). For example if the patient indicates that the lines as indicated on a clock dial are clearer from 12:00 to 6:00, the axis is then set at 90 degrees, coinciding with this vertical axis. If the clearer lines were 3:00 to 9:00 then the axis would be set at 180; if oblique, the axis would still be aligned with the oblique clock hours preferred by the patient. The Interval of Sturm is then collapsed using plus cylinder lenses to bring the posterior end up to the anterior end of the Interval. Once the Interval of Sturm is collapsed into a point focus, the lines are then all seen equally foggy. This point focus is then moved back to the retina with the use of minus sphere lenses.

With a minus cylinder refractor, the concept remains the same, but the type and axis of the lenses are different. In the "fogged" situation, the most posterior portion of the Interval of Sturm remains the clearest axis. Using the minus cylinder allows the examiner to collapse the anterior end of the Interval backwards. What must be appreciated here is that the axis which is the clearest to the patient must be exactly 90 degrees from the axis that the examiner manipulates with the minus cylinder. In other words, the examiner aligns the minus cylinder axis perpendicular to the line that the patient reports as clearest. The minus cylinder is then increased, compensating with + sphere to maintain the Spherical Equivalent, (see Spherical Equivalent) until all lines are equal.

Highlights of Astigmatic Dial Refraction

1. Monocular test
2. Fogging of +1.00 to +1.50 diopters
3. Ask the patient "which line is clearest" as on a clock dial.
4. In plus cylinder refractors, line up the cylinder parallel to the line seen clearest by the patient. In minus cylinder refractors, line up the axis perpendicular to the line seen clearest by the patient.
5. Add cylinder until all lines are equally blurred. After each 0.50 cylinder added, compensate with opposite sign sphere to maintain the spherical equivalent.
6. The fogging sphere is then gradually reduced to best acuity.

Jackson Cross Cylinder Technique

A special condition exists with certain lenses such as −1.00 +2.00 × 180, for the *Spherical Equivalent of such a lens is* 0. This type of lens is used in the *Jackson* (12) cross cylinder, for the property of a lens with a spherical equivalent of 0 is very useful. The cross cylinder technique is probably used more often than the astigmatic dial.

Theory. The technique is based on maintaining the spherical equivalent in the same position relative to the retina, but using a spherocylindrical lens in different axis orientations to determine the refractive error. The concept is elegant and brilliant in its ability to manipulate the interval of Sturm by expansion and contraction without affecting its position relative to the retina. The position of the interval is such that the circle of least confusion is placed on the retina with spherical lenses. The ability of the patient to appreciate a clearer image when the interval of Sturm is contracted compared with when it is expanded is the basis for this test. Alignment of the cross cylinder is performed first to determine the position of the axis of the patient's cylinder. Once the axis is found, the alignment of the cross cylinder is shifted to determine the amount.

Method. For the Jackson cross cylinder technique, the best target to use is a Snellen line of letters two or three lines larger than the best visual acuity allows (Fig. 3–47). The eyes are examined separately, with only the eye being examined open to look at the target, the other occluded.

The patient is instructed to observe the line of letters. Careful instructions to the patient, at this point, are critical to this test. The patient is told, "I will be showing you two lenses as you look at the line of letters. Please tell me which lens makes the line of letters clearer. At times neither lens will be very clear, but tell me which one is better. At times they may look about the same, please tell me

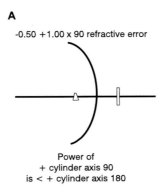

A

-0.50 +1.00 x 90 refractive error

Power of
+ cylinder axis 90
is < + cylinder axis 180

B Jackson cross cylinder

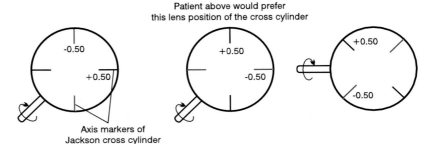

Patient above would prefer
this lens position of the cross cylinder

Figure 3–47.
Jackson cross cylinder.

Axis markers of
Jackson cross cylinder

if they do, but try to tell me which is clearer if you can." These instructions are critical, for what the patient is about to do can be very frustrating. The patient must be aware, and assured, that choices between two blurry lenses that look almost exactly the same will give the examiner proper information to prescribe the correct lens. The examiner is attempting to reach an endpoint where the choices between lenses is equal. This is unsettling to the patient unless forewarned.

Cross Cylinder Without Initial Astigmatism Correction

The best spherical equivalent is used to allow best acuity. This places the circle of least confusion on the retina. An additional plus 0.50 D is added to verify that the target becomes blurred and that the patient is not undercorrected. It is then removed. This first method allows us to find the presence of a measurable amount of astigmatism, refine the axis, and then find the amount. Initial presentation allows determination if there is measurable astigmatism in axis 90 or 180. The cross cylinder is placed in front of the eye to be tested. The Jackson cross cylinder is placed so that when "flipped" the axis marker will move from 90 to 180 or vise versa. If the patient states that neither is substantially better than the other, there is no significant with the rule or against the rule astigmatism. "With the rule" astigmatism is corrected with plus cylinder axis 90° or minus cylinder correction axis 180°. "Against the Rule" astigmatism is corrected by plus cylinder at 180° or minus cylinder at axis 90°. The axis alignment is now

changed to flip between axis 45 and 135. Again, the patient is offered a choice.

Wherever the patient prefers one more than the other, 0.25 D of cylinder is added aligned with the preferred axis. The patient is then given the opportunity to reject this added cylinder or to choose more until 0.50 cylinder is present.

Refinement of Cylinder

With the cylinder in place from the approach above, or beginning with the cylinder found by retinoscopy, refinement of both the axis and then the amount are begun.

Axis

Once it has been determined that there is a measurable amount of astigmatism, the axis must be refined with the straddling position of the Jackson cross cylinder. Refinement of the axis uses a bracketing technique, where progressively smaller changes in axis are presented as the patients actual cylinder axis is approached. The straddling choices present the patient with choices 45° on either side of the preliminary axis with the patient's preference determining the direction of refinement. The method places the cross cylinder so that the cylinder axis markers are exactly 45° on each side of the cylinder axis marker of the refractor. The patient is then given a choice, as the cross cylinder is flipped, as to the clearer image. The image will be clearer as it approaches the patient's true astigmatic axis. According to the patient's selection, the flip cylinder and the refractor cylinder are rotated in the direction of the clearer image. The endpoint is that where the patient is unable to see a difference in clarity between the two choices. This endpoint occurs where the refractor cylinder axis is aligned with the patient's actual astigmatic error axis and the flip cylinder plus and minus notations straddle the refractor axis. Once the axis is refined, the amount of cylinder may be determined.

Amount

As the amount of cylinder is being refined, one may view the process as a bartering or "selling" cylinder to the patient. The cross cylinder is positioned so that the power of the cross cylinder is aligned with the patient's cylinder. The patient is given the choice as the cross cylinder is flipped to accept more cylinder or reject the present amount of cylinder. The process is continued with the patient accepting or rejecting cylinder amounts until the lens choices presented appear equal to the patient. As the cylinder in the refractor is changed more than 0.50 D, the sphere must be compensated in the opposite direction to maintain the same spherical equivalent. In plus cylinder refraction, for every +1.00 D cylinder increase, reduce the sphere by 0.50 D.

Once the process of astigmatism correction is completed, the sphere is rechecked for best visual acuity with the least amount of minus sphere (or most amount of plus) tolerated.

Highlights of Jackson Cross Cylinder Refraction Technique

1. Monocular test
2. Target viewed without fog beginning with either
   a. best spherical equivalent
   b. retinoscopy findings
   c. previous spectacle correction in refractor
3. Maximum plus sphere added to #2 that allows best acuity
4. Target used is two or three lines worse than best acuity
5. Find axis of cylinder first
   a. Find presence of cylinder using cross cylinder
   b. Refine cylinder from retinoscopy
6. Find power in cylinder
   Remember to compensate with 0.25 sphere for each 0.50 cylinder change
7. Refine sphere

Balance

Once the individual eye findings have been maximized in acuity, it is important to balance the eyes to be sure that the two eyes have equal accommodative stimuli. As

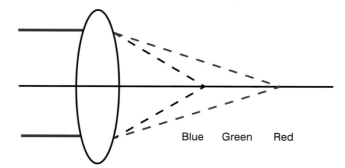

Figure 3–48.
Duochrome test.

the subjective refraction process above is followed, it should be realized that accommodation is neither held in check with the Jackson cross cylinder technique, nor is there any assurance that if accommodation has been active, it has been used equally with each eye. Balance techniques may use prism dissociation, polaroid, and others, but have as a common principle that fusion is disrupted and the patient compares the images from each eye simultaneously. Fogging is used to control accommodation.

The technique of prism dissociation is begun with the best correction before each eye. A 6 base down prism is placed before one eye. Plus lenses of 1.00 D to 1.25 D are added simultaneously to both eyes to induce fogging, thereby relaxing accommodation. The target used is typically the 20/80 or 20/100 line of letters. The patient is asked to determine which of the two images is clearer. Additional plus lenses are added to the clearer image until the two images are most nearly equal; this is the endpoint. The prism is then removed. The target is changed to the best line of acuity previously seen monocularly. Then plus lenses are reduced simultaneously before each eye until best acuity is reached. Care must be taken not to reduce the plus power too far. If one continues to remove plus (add minus) lenses beyond the removal of the fogging lens, accommodation is stimulated and the patient usually comments that the target is quite clear but smaller.

Duochrome Test

The duochrome test is used to help determine the endpoint in refraction where the best acuity lens is uncertain, or as a check test for the endpoint (Fig. 3–48). Although some may claim to use it as a balance test, its use on a monocular basis does not control accommodation. The underlying principle is that of chromatic aberration of the eye, where shorter wavelength rays are brought into focus anterior to longer wavelength light rays. At the desired endpoint, where the yellow or central position of the spectrum rays are exactly in focus on the retina, the red would be behind the retina and the green (or blue) would be in focus in front of the retina. When the duochrome slide, presenting letters on green and red backgrounds side by side is seen to be in equal focus, the yellow rays must be focused on the retina. If the red (longer wavelength) background letters are in better focus, the entire spectrum must be anterior to the retina. Minus lenses must be added to move the focal point posteriorly and reach the endpoint. Hence the mneumonic: RAMGAP—Red Add Minus Green Add Plus. Appropriate lenses are added to give equal clarity to the red and green sides (or just slightly better clarity to red to "crowd Plus"). The test is performed binocularly in a room as dark as possible. The darkness helps to enlarge the pupil and accentuate the chromatic aberration effect.

Phoria Measurements

Horizontal Phorias (See Chapter 14)

The visual axis is the line that connects the fovea with the object of gaze that passes through the nodal point of the eye. A *heterophoria* is a latent misalignment of the visual axes of the patient. It becomes apparent when fusion is broken. A *heterotropia* is the manifest misalignment of the visual axes. The measurement of a phoria is the determination of the relative positions of the two visual axes. These measurements are performed with the patient's best distance correction.

Risley Prism

The Risley prism (Fig. 3–49) is actually two equal prisms placed one in front of the other. As the measuring knob is turned, the relative orientation of the bases of the prisms change. At one extreme, the bases are aligned one on top of the other, and the total prism power is the sum of the two prisms. When the prisms are rotated within the Risley prism ring 180° and the bases are exactly opposite each other, the total prism power is 0.

The Risley prism is used either in conjunction with a Maddox rod or another Risley prism to determine the direction and amount of heterophoria. Fusion must be broken by either prism dissociation (a second Risley prism) or image incompatibility (Maddox rod); then the measuring Risley prism is used to measure the amount of heterophoria.

Fusion is typically broken with a 6 base down prism in front of one eye. The patient is directed to observe this upper image while the lower image is slowly moved back and forth with the measuring Risley prism in front of the other eye until the two images are aligned thus measuring the patient's phoria.

Maddox Rod

The Maddox rod is used to break fusion by creating disparate images that eliminate fusional cues. The Maddox rod is actually a tight group of parallel cylinders. When one looks through these very high power cylinders at a single point light source, a streak of light is seen by the observer (Fig. 3–50). When the rod is placed with the cylinders axis 180°, or horizontal, a vertical streak of light is seen. How is this possible? The cylinders are of such high power that their focal plane is so close to the rod lenses that the rays become so divergent that they are not clearly visualized. The image is formed so close to the lens and thereby too divergent at the eye to be focused; the observer will then see the virtual image, which is a line perpendicular to the axes of the cylinders located at the plane of the object point (23). The only rays that are able to be observed and focused, therefore, are rays that are parallel to the cylinder axes. The highly divergent rays create a vertical blur whereas the rays parallel to the axes allow accurate horizontal images of the point light stacked one on another, thus a vertical line, or streak, is seen.

Horizontal Phorias. The horizontal Maddox rod is typically placed before the left eye. A point source of light or "muscle light" is used as the target. The Risley prism is placed over the right eye with the "0" at 90°, allowing base out and base in measurements. One definite disadvantage of the Maddox rod method is the lack of control over accommodative convergence, for the target is a light and not a letter on which to maintain focus.

Figure 3–49.
Balance. Prism dissociation. Base down prism in front of left eye dissociates this patient with a horizontal phoria causing vertical diplopia and manifesting the horizontal phoria. A Risley prism oriented horizontally in front of the right eye is adjusted to neutralize the horizontal deviation so the arrows are aligned vertically as seen in the circle at the right of the figure (patient's view).

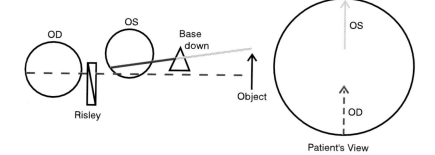

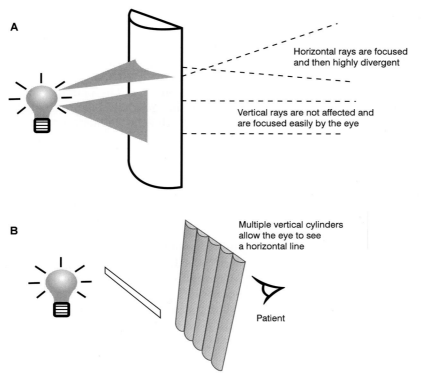

Figure 3–50.
Maddox rod.

Vertical Phorias. Measurement is performed with two Risley prisms. The target is a single letter from the 20/40 or 20/50 line. Prism dissociation is accomplished with a 10Δ to 12Δ base in prism in front of one eye. This type and amount of prism is required to create horizontal dissociation, for convergence can overcome very large amounts of base out prism; horizontal separation is necessary to measure vertical phorias. The target is a single letter as with horizontal phorias. The measuring Risley prism is oriented to allow base up and base down readings before the other eye. The patient is instructed to observe when the moving letter is exactly the same level as the other.

Vertical phorias can also be measured with the Maddox rod oriented to create a horizontal streak (rods vertical). The error induced by accommodative convergence in measuring horizontal phorias with a Maddox rod is not present when measuring vertical orientations.

Binocular Vergences

Although a patient may, on examination, be found to have a significant phoria, the ability to compensate for this deviation will determine whether there are associated symptoms and whether the prescription of prism is necessary (Fig. 3–51). The measurement of these disjunctive movements, convergence of the eyes (positive vergence) or divergence of the eyes (negative vergence) is performed with two Risley prisms (see fusional vergence, ch. 14). The prisms are positioned before each

eye with the prism bases in the same direction (either out, or in) for horizontal duction measurement. Measuring vertical ductions requires only one prism. It is positioned to read base up or base down. As prism power is increased and presented to the patient, the eyes will turn toward the prism apices to maintain fusion. An increase in base out prism will cause an eye to turn in towards the prism apex. With both eyes turning in, this base out prism stimulates and ultimately allows measurement of convergence.

The convergence movement initially is stimulated by fusional demands, with disparate images causing fusional convergence. As the base out prism is increased, there is a point where fusional convergence is exhausted. At this point further increases in base out

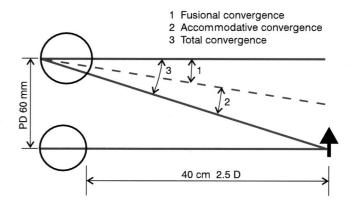

Figure 3–51.
Binocular vergences.

prism can cause diplopia, or accommodative convergence. A subconscious choice is made between seeing a double clear image (diplopia) or using accommodative convergence and seeing a single, blurry image. A single blurred image is more acceptable, and therefore the added accommodative convergence allows a greater amount of convergence as measured by the prisms. The total convergence is thus the sum of the fusional convergence and the accommodative convergence.

The term *positive relative convergence* is used to describe a measurement of convergence movement of the eyes with accommodation held fixed. *Negative relative convergence* is a measurement of divergence movements of the eyes with accommodation held fixed. Because accommodation is held fixed when these tests are performed (usually at near testing distances), these measurements in effect represent fusional reserves. It is the fusional portion of convergence that is critical in evaluating the adequacy of the compensatory duction.

Method of Testing Vergences

Risley prisms are placed base out before each eye to measure convergence. For fusional divergence, base in prism is added before each eye. When measuring distance fusional divergence, it should be noted that there will be no blur point before diplopia results. This lack of blur represents the appropriate prescription for distance vision with all accommodation relaxed.

Vertical vergences may be measured with a prism before one eye set for base up and base down readings. An appropriate target would be a single 20/40 letter. Break and recovery of fusion are noted in each direction (vergence amplitudes, see Chap. 14).

Prescribing Prism

Prescriptions of prism greater than 10 PD total is unusual. The added weight, peripheral optical distortion and decreased cosmetic effect all create secondary problems. Fresnel plastic press-on prisms offer a partial solution, but these often have the disadvantage of visible vertical or horizontal ridges on the lenses.

The patient's symptoms of asthenopia, frontal headaches, temporal headaches, intermittent diplopia, repetitive reading of the same line of letters, and so forth, point to difficulty with maintaining fusion and poor compensatory capacity. The phoria and the compensatory duction allow us to determine the appropriate prism to incorporate in the prescription. The presence of symptoms allows us to determine the appropriateness of prescribing prism. Underlying considerations with prism prescriptions suggest that conservative changes are tolerated better by patients. The least prism to alleviate symptoms is the appropriate amount.

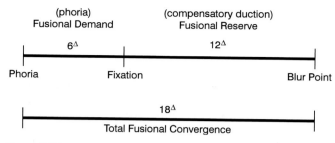

Figure 3–52.
(example 1).

Sheard (25) has developed a mathematical model to determine the appropriate amount of prism to alleviate symptoms: (1) the *total fusional convergence* must be equal to *at least three* times the phoria; (2) the *compensatory duction* must be *twice* the phoria (Fig. 3–52).

Prism prescription = ⅔ phoria—⅓ compensatory duction

These criteria are represented mathematically as the equation above. If the amount is greater than 0, then that amount of prism is prescribed.

Ex. 1. 6 prism diopters of exophoria
18 prism diopters of Total Fusional Convergence

(therefore 12 Prism Diopters of compensatory duction)

⅔ phoria − ⅓ compensatory duction

⅔ (6) − ⅓ (12) =
4   −   4 =   0

Ex. 2. 9 prism diopters of exophoria
21 prism diopters Total Fusional Convergence
(12 Prism diopters of compensatory duction)

⅔ (9) − ⅓ (12) =
6   −   4 =   +2

Therefore, 2 PD total would be prescribed, split between the two lenses. Because the phoria is exophoria, the direction prescribed would be base in.

It should be clear that in the above examples that the phoria, or deviation, was exophoria. If prism is *prescribed*, it is base in prism. The compensatory duction, or the ability to overcome the phoria is convergence. The *measurement of this compensatory duction*, convergence, is performed with base out prisms.

Prescribing for vertical phorias also is done when symptoms justify it. A frequent method to determine the amount to prescribe is: one half the difference between the base down to break and the base up to break is the amount prescribed.

Ex. 1. Measurement with Risley before the OS.
Hyperphoria is found OS

Base down to break   4 Base down
Base up to break   2 Base up

$$\frac{4-2}{2} = \begin{array}{l} \text{1 Base down total} \\ \text{1/2 Base down in OS} \\ \text{1/2 Base up in OD} \end{array}$$

A prism is produced by having the lens surface ground on a bias (on an angle). The optician calculates and places the lens blank appropriately to create the prism. Another way of creating prism is by purposefully decentering the lenses to create prism (see Prentice's Rule).

Example: A ray passing through a 6.00 D lens 4 mm from the optic axis will have 2.4 PD of prism deviation.

Such a deviation is helpful if needed by the patient. Thus, appropriate decentration of this amount can create prism to correct for symptomatic phorias. However, if a lens is decentered from appropriate alignment with the patient's interpupillary distance (IPD), the induced prism may cause symptoms of fatigue and possibly diplopia.

Presbyopia

Presbyopia is the physiologic decrease in accommodation that occurs with advancing age. Accommodative amplitude decreases from birth; presbyopia is said to begin when the near point has receded beyond 22 cm. As one continues to require clear vision for near point tasks, the inability to change focus from distance to near vision requires a separate corrective power lens for each distance. Various optical methods of ameliorating this problem will be discussed later.

Accommodative Amplitude

Various researchers (including Donders) in the early part of this century have determined the "normals" of accommodative amplitude expected by age (Table 3–2).

TABLE 3–2
Table of Accommodative Amplitudes[23]

Age	Amplitude of Accommodation (Diopters)	Nearpoint for Emmetrope (cm)
10	14.0	7.0
15	12.0	8.3
20	10.0	10.0
25	8.5	11.7
30	7.0	14.2
35	5.5	18.2
40	4.5	22.2
45	3.5	28.5
50	2.5	40.0
55	1.75	57.0
60	1.00	100.0
65	0.50	200.0
70	0.25	400.0
75	0.0	Infinity

TABLE 3–3
Preliminary Near Adds

Age	Add at 13 Inches	Add at 16 Inches
40	+1.25	+1.00
45	+1.50	+1.25
48	+1.75	+1.50
50	+2.00	+1.75
55	+2.25	+2.00
60	+2.50	+2.25
65	+2.75	+2.50

Determination of Add

The comfortable correction for near centered tasks depends on a number of factors beyond accommodative amplitude: the distance that is required to be clear, the length of the patients arms, the cultural biases regarding multifocal lenses, the underlying refractive error, etc. The difference between the power of the distance prescription and the power of the near prescription is called the add. Patients typically accept a prescription for near tasks which allows for the maintenance of 50% accommodative amplitude in reserve.

Age Table of Preliminary Adds

By knowing the patient's age and working distance, one can estimate a preliminary bifocal add power from the table (Table 3–3).

Although accommodative amplitudes may vary between the two eyes, many practitioners routinely perform tests to determine near point adds binocularly.

The adds from Table 3–3 may be used to determine the total near prescription and placed in a trial frame. The range of clearest vision is then modified, if needed, to correspond to the patient's near work distance. Increasing plus power allows a closer and shorter range; reducing plus allows a longer and further clear range.

As with other changes in prescription, moderation in changing the amount of bifocal adds is a major touchstone for patient satisfaction. It is safer to make a moderate change than a severe change, for even though optically appropriate, patient adaptation to the old prescription distance will affect proper use of the new corrective lenses. Patients will rarely seek a change in prescription for changes in near adds of less than 0.50 D. Conversely, if a change of more than 1.00 D has occurred, the patient typically would have needed and sought help sooner.

Myopia

Myopia is from the Greek term that translates to "I close." This term reflects the universal tendency for patients with myopia to squint their eyes to decrease the pupillary aperture to allow clearer vision. The decrease in the pupillary aperture reduces rays that are not axial or paraxial thereby reducing the blur spot on the retina.

Classification

Refractive myopia occurs when the power of the optical system (corneal curvature and lens power) is too strong for the length of the eye. Axial myopia is when the length of the eye is too long for the optical system. Axial myopia or a long eye is determined with axial A-scan ultrasound to be longer than 24.5 mm. Usually there is some of each component. The visual acuity can be corrected to 20/20 with appropriate concave, or minus, lenses. Simple myopia is further categorized into low myopia less than 2 D, moderate myopia from 2 to 6 D, and high myopia above 6 D.

Etiology

Myopia usually follows an autosomal-dominant inheritance pattern. There has been a periodic debate as to the influence of the environment in the development of myopia. Helmholtz, in his *Treatise on Physiologic Optics,* stated that myopia was due to exposure to small objects during near vision use. In 1864, Donders stated the same conclusion.

Studies of Japanese school children found that during the years of World War II, when school work was significantly curtailed, myopia was substantially less than the years just before and after the war.

Young, in evaluating incidence of myopia by comparing students from fourth grade to graduate school, found a respective incidence of 6 to 50%. He also found a significantly higher incidence in honor students, but there was no correlation to intelligence quotient. This relationship strongly suggested that excessive near work was a factor. Decreasing the tonic ciliary contraction by the use of cycloplegics (29) has been advocated as a means of decreasing the progression of myopia. The medication necessary along with its attendant side effects and the need for concurrent bifocal spectacles makes this treatment controversial.

More recent work with form, but not illumination, deprivation in monkeys (20, 28), other mammals, and even chickens indicates a relationship with a poor ocular image and increased myopia. Dopamine (26) has recently been implicated in the biochemical process relating retinal visual responses to signals that regulate scleral growth and globe enlargement.

Pathologic Myopia

This myopia is also called "progressive" or "degenerative" or previously "malignant myopia." Associated with this type of myopia is a significantly increased tendency towards ocular pathology. The posterior pole is primarily involved with decreased central vision. There is a thinning of the sclera and elongation of the posterior pole. Atrophy of the choroid occurs beginning with the smaller vessels of the choriocapillaris. Complications also involve breaks in Descemet's membrane, liquefaction of the vitreous, central retinal atrophy (Fuchs' spot), and retinal detachment. In England, it is the most common cause of legal blindness in the 40- to 60-year age group.

Treatment

In the 19th century, insufficient illumination was periodically believed to be either the cause or the cure for myopia. Physical effort, manual labor, or gymnastics were attacked as causing myopia, and there were advocates of forbidding such activities to decrease myopia. Because close work has been associated with myopia, periodically there had been calls for changes in school curricula to allow education mediated by sound and touch rather than sight (7).

Surgical treatment to alleviate or prevent myopia have included tenotomy of various extraocular muscles, subconjunctival injections, and/or intravenous use of saline, eserine, or pilocarpine. Other techniques have included ocular compression or ocular "rolling." Atropine to eliminate ciliary spasm and the use of bifocals to decrease accommodative stimulus have their advocates. Today, most ophthalmologists believe that these techniques do not work or that the treatment is worse than the problem.

Other contemporary management techniques for myopia include the use of spectacles, contact lenses, scleral reinforcing surgery, clear lens lensectomy, negative power intraocular lenses, intrastromal corneal devices, and various keratorefractive procedures.

Myopia is treated with the optical goal of providing the least minus power to allow the best distance visual acuity. Decreasing the best distance correction in a prepresbyope to allow better near vision, monovision contact lens use, and other specific situations occur infrequently and require individualization of distance correction.

Hyperopia

Hyperopia (also called hypermetropia) is that optical condition where, when accommodation is relaxed, rays of light from infinity would come to focus behind the retina. The power of the optical system of the eye is too weak for the axial length of the eye. Either the length of the eye is too short, axial hyperopia, or the optical system is too weak, refractive hyperopia. Mixtures of the two types is common. Axial hyperopia, with a short eye (less than 22.00 mm) is correlated with narrow anterior chambers and esostrabismic deviations.

The clinical classification of hyperopia (from Duke-Elder) is helpful in understanding the evaluation and prescription of corrective lenses.

Total hyperopia is the sum of the latent hyperopia and the manifest hyperopia.

Latent hyperopia is that hyperopia that is completely corrected by, or masked by, accommodation. It becomes manifest when accommodation amplitude is decreased in presbyopia. Using a cyloplegic will allow it to be uncovered.

Manifest hyperopia is that hyperopia that is found during refraction without a cycloplegic. It is the combination of facultative hyperopia and absolute hyperopia.

Facultative hyperopia is compensated by accommodation. It can be relaxed and uncovered with plus lenses. A patient with facultative hyperopia may have 20/20 vision uncorrected and maintain 20/20 vision as plus lenses are slowly increased to the limits of the facultative portion as accommodation is relaxed.

Absolute hyperopia is that portion of hyperopia that the patient is unable to compensate for with accommodation. Because the patient is unable to compensate for this amount, the vision will be blurred.

Example: A 50-year-old patient has distance visual acuity uncorrected of 20/40. He accepts +1.00 D of plus power to increase his acuity to 20/20 (absolute hyperopia). He takes an additional +1.00 D (facultative hyperopia), which he gradually accepts until his vision begins to blur. After administration of a cycloplegic agent, he accepts another +1.00 D (latent hyperopia).

Symptoms of Hyperopia

Patients with hyperopia typically complain about near vision tasks. Headaches, particularly frontal, temporal, and periocular are common. Reading the same line over again and problems with tracking may occur. Many of the same symptoms that occur with esophoria occur with uncorrected hyperopia. Indeed excess accommodative convergence secondary to the increased accommodative demands at near is seen frequently with hyperopia. Accommodative spasms can cause blur and considerable discomfort. Blurred distance vision occurs with hyperopia (absolute). Particularly at night, with decreased distance cues available, even the patient with only facultative hyperopia may experience blurred vision.

Correction of Hyperopia

The absolute portion must be corrected with + sphere lenses to allow best acuity. Giving more plus prescrip-

tion will correct for the facultative, and this should be done with careful instruction to the patient that there will probably be some time to adjust to the glasses. It should be realized that a newly corrected hyperope has been using accommodation to see at distance vision before the use of glasses. It will take time to relax this tonic accommodation, and, until this happens, the patient will experience blurred distance vision. With this in mind some practitioners will prescribe 50 to 75% of the manifest hyperopia to allow easier adjustment.

In cases of esophoria, and particularly accommodative esotropia, full hyperopic correction should be given including the latent portion. It is critical to correct all latent hypermetropia before esotropia.

In children without symptoms, hyperopia up to +3.00 D may go uncorrected unless an esodeviation is present. During teenage years, +1.00 to +3.00 D should be corrected with a prescription for near work. As the eye ages, the facultative portion becomes absolute and must be corrected fully.

Astigmatism

Astigmatism is from the Greek stigma, or point; astigma or without a point describes the lack of a point focus.

Astigmatism is caused for the most part by a difference in curvatures in the various meridians of the cornea. Other optical components of the ocular refractive system can add to the corneal component of astigmatism.

Regular astigmatism occurs when the meridians of highest and lowest refractive power are perpendicular to each other and fully correctable by spherocylindrical lenses (see also retinoscopy and interval of Sturm). Irregular astigmatism usually occurs with corneal pathology (i.e., keratoconus or scarring). This is difficult to correct with spectacles, but contact lenses or corneal surgery may offer a better solution.

"With the rule" astigmatism occurs when the curvature at 90° (axis 180°) is greater than the curvature at 180° (axis 90°). *"Against the rule"* astigmatism is the opposite situation. In with the rule astigmatism, the axis of the higher curvature is 180, thereby effecting the rays focused in a horizontal line. These rays will therefore be at the anterior end of the interval of Sturm. Typically, there is a progression of with the rule gradually shifting to against the rule astigmatism with age. An aging decrease in the tightness of the lids is believed to account for this shift. There is also a symmetry to astigmatism such that if one eye is with the rule, usually the other is with the rule. In situations of oblique astigmatism the axes are usually found to be in a mirror image of one another. Because of this mirror image symmetry, if one were to add the sum of the axes of astigmatism the total would be close to 180.

Prescribing for Astigmatism

A first prescription for astigmatism may be difficult for the patient to adapt to. With the rule and against the rule astigmatism can make the patient feel a few inches shorter or taller. Spatial distortions are particularly true of oblique axis astigmatism. Even the door frames and walls may appear to be curved. Because of the distortions that some people encounter with oblique cylinders, some practitioners tend to prescribe the axis not as found, but biased toward horizontal or vertical. This shifting of the axis may allow easier adjustment to the prescription, but it is at the expense of acuity. A marked prescription change in the axis typically causes a difficult adjustment for the patient. It is best to minimize such changes. If the prescriber takes the time to counsel patients about expected distortion, this may preempt patient complaints, loss of confidence, and dissatisfaction.

Aphakia

Historical

Although aphakia (unnamed until Donders coined this term in the 19th century) is much less common than before intraocular lenses were developed, it will be encountered by today's practitioners. As early as 1623, Benito Daza de Valdez of Spain advocated the use of high-power spectacle lenses in aphakia. Later, in 1856, Helmholtz elucidated the optics of aphakia. Aphakia was so troublesome that Landoldt (17) in 1886 was moved to write "... enucleation simplifies so many things. Aphakic vision is so complicated..."!

An appreciation of the difficulties encountered by the aphakic patient will give some important insight into optical considerations in general and a greater appreciation of the importance of the intraocular lens. One way for the practitioner to simulate the effects of aphakia is to wear −11.00 (or greater) D contact lenses and compensatory corrective + spectacle lenses in a trial frame.

Optics

If one considers the Gullstrand schematic eye, the total power is 58.64 D, and the corneal power is 43.05 D. By removing the lens, we thereby reduce the power by 15.59 D. A +10.00 D lens approximately 10 mm anterior to the cornea corrects this ametropia.

The position of a high power lens can have a substantial effect on the power of the lens in the system. As a lens is moved anteriorly, the relative plus power increases, or conversely, a weaker plus lens placed in the spectacle plane can replace a stronger lens from the intraocular or corneal position. There is a different effectivity of the lens power depending on its relative position. The movement and positioning of such a lens is not uncommon with aphakic patients. Movement of the glasses by slipping/or poor adjustment can mean substantial changes in power; on many occasions, the change in refraction found by the examiner is less than that obtained by the patient in moving the lens down his/her nose.

Aberrations

Spherical Aberration. Many aberrations occur as a result of using such high-power lenses in front of the eye. Spherical aberration occurs because of the increased refraction of peripheral rays compared with paraxial rays which brings them into focus anterior to the focal point of the axial rays. In addition, there is an inherent astigmatism created by oblique rays through such thick lenses resulting in the "pin cushion" distortion seen with high plus lenses. The use of aspheric lenses decreases these aberrations by varying the power over the surface of the lens. Instead of a spherical, constant power, the power drops off toward the periphery.

Chromatic Aberration. This is due to differences in refraction over the visible spectrum of light. The shorter wavelength light is refracted more than the longer wavelength light. This phenomenon is evident with prisms. Toward the edge of such a high-power plus lens, prism power of more than 20 PD is common.

Magnification occurs with aphakic optical correction. In an emmetropia phakic eye (58.6 D of power) the anterior focal point would be 17.04 mm in front of the cornea. By decreasing the optical power of the eye by removing the lens (15 D), the anterior focal point recedes to 23 mm. The image and object distances are proportional to the focal lengths of the power of the optical system. Therefore the ratio would be 17:23 or 1:1.36 or a magnification of 36%.

False Depth Perception, False Projection, and Swim. False depth perception is almost entirely due to the magnification experienced by the patient with aphakic spectacles. As one throughout life has adapted to objects that appear a certain size at a certain distance, a sudden change in size of objects is not acceptable. One "knows" the size of a coffee cup that one has used for years. Because this cup has not changed size and yet appears larger, the only logical perceptual reason is that it must be closer.

As one views objects through the peripheral portion of a high plus aphakic lens, it is recalled that prism is induced that will create a false location of the image. This is in addition to the size and/or distance problem noted above. Besides these difficulties, the movement of images occurs with rapid eye movements creating against motion. This against motion means that there is perceived motion of the image in the opposite direction of the patient's eye movement.

Ring Scotoma. As the lens power increases, there is a point at which peripheral rays are deviated so much by the induced prism that they are unable to enter the pupil. Central rays enter the pupil. Peripheral rays beyond the spectacle edge enter the pupil, but there is a midperipheral band of rays that do not enter the pupil. These rays form a ring-shaped scotoma when evaluated on a perimeter.

As the patient finds objects appearing and disappearing when they pass though the ring scotoma area of the lens, the effect is similar to a jack-in-the-box. People and objects will jump in and out of the field of vision, creating a disconcerting situation.

Besides the monocular problems as noted above, binocular vision is hampered by any small deviation in the fit of spectacles, which can cause power changes and/or vertical prism. In addition, it should be appreciated that the lenses themselves increase convergence required for near work. As an object moves closer to the patient's face, the rays that enter the eyes from this object necessarily pass through more nasal portions of the lenses. The nasal portion acts as a significant base out prism inducing and requiring increased convergence to maintain fusion.

Underlying principles to decrease the problems noted above are to use an aspheric lens of the thinnest edge thickness and the smallest size compatible with proper frame fit.

Considerations for the Final Prescription

The prescription must correct insufficient vision at distance, near, or discomfort, or any combination of these. Usually the distance prescription is the subjective finding or the retinoscopy finding. If there is no presbyopia, this is also usually sufficient for near.

There are certain situations that may dictate that the prescription is different from the subjective findings. *Anisometropia* is that situation where there is a significant power difference between the eyes. Greater than 3 D of spherical equivalent power difference typically creates symptoms. *Aniseikonia,* a difference in image size, is one cause of symptoms associated with anisometropia. Although magnification differences of up to 5% are tolerated, fusion becomes quite difficult. The evaluation and correction of aniseikonia test the ingenuity of the examiner and optician. Increasing the anterior base curve of the lens, the distance from the eye (vertex distance) and the thickness of the lens all create an increase in magnification.

Vertical prism induced by viewing through the lower part of the lens, as in a multifocal, is another problem that must be addressed with an anisometropic prescription. The different power distance prescription lenses will create different vertical prisms that have the potential for creating asthenopia and even diplopia. Prentice's rule shows us the vertical deviation created looking through the reading add (Power difference between the lenses multiplied by the distance in centimeters from the optical center). At approximately 3.00 D of difference, the vertical prism is such that a compensation is required. Either the use of a separate single vision reading lens, which allows near vision through the optical center, is used, or a "slab-off" is ground to compensate for the prism. The slab-off is a bicentric grind of the anterior surface of the more minus lens to create base up prism without changing the power. Other methods using special bifocal segments are also sometimes incorporated into the prescription.

In situations of anisometropia, it is important to be certain of the final balance, for it may indicate that the amount of anisometropia is less than was found in monocular testing. Try to maintain the same spherical equivalent power difference between the eyes as was comfortably worn before.

Prism Prescription

The use of prisms, once begun, almost always continues. There may be a tendency for the patient to adapt to and require greater and greater amounts. Moderation in any change of prism is usually tolerated better than large changes. Prism can be ground into the prescription, but it also may be purposefully induced by decentering the optical centers of the lenses away from the interpupillary distance (IPD). Higher power lenses are necessary to create significant prism by decentration. Decreased weight and increased cosmesis are gains in providing prism by decentration.

Significant Phorias

Distance Esophoria. Use as much plus power as the patient can tolerate. If there is a residual amount, and fusional divergence is small, base out prism is indicated.

Near Esophoria (Accommodative Convergence Excess). The AC/A ratio relates the amount of accommodative convergence (AC) in PD stimulated by each D of accommodative stimulus (A). If the AC/A is high, a bifocal would be indicated, for decreasing accommodative stimulus would decrease the convergence excess. Also use as much plus power as can be tolerated.

Distance Exophoria. Correct with as much minus as tolerated. In younger patients with high accommodative amplitude, overcorrecting with minus may be helpful. Base in prism is readily accepted, but a trial of base out exercises may be helpful to increase convergence amplitude.

Near Exophoria. Prescribe as much minus as possible. If the positive relative convergence is inadequate, base in prism is indicated.

Multifocals

A decision must be made, when accommodative amplitude has decreased, to correct the near distance with a separate power than that for distance vision. Associated with this decision is the method of correction; multiple pairs of lenses or multifocal lenses.

One Pair or Multiples. The emmetropic presbyope may be corrected with a single vision reading lens or 50% eye lenses. Great care must be given to explaining the decrease in distance vision that will be encountered with the use of full reading glasses. It is helpful to place the reading lens in a trial frame to allow the patient to look across the room. Even this demonstration may be insufficient to convince the patient of the inconvenience of single vision reading lenses. A plano multifocal with a large reading area may be appropriate for a patient who spends a great deal of time with tasks at a desk or reading distance. Use of a progressive lens allows superior cosmesis at the expense of the size of the reading area.

The ametropic presbyope may be corrected with a pair of single vision lenses for near, which may give better optical service if there is a very high refractive error. Reading through the periphery of the lens unfortunately increases the aberrations. If the patient is myopic and barely presbyopic, some practitioners prefer to decrease the distance prescription by 0.50 D to allow another year or so of single vision lens use.

In some instances, single vision lenses may serve the needs better than multifocals. These include:

When there is a marked difference between the near and the distance phorias (i.e., convergence excess).

In the presence of an "A" or "V" pattern (see strabismus).

In senile divergence insufficiency.

In significant degrees of anisometropia using two pair of single vision lenses allows the patient to look through the optical centers eliminating the induced vertical prism through the periphery.

There are two main types of multifocal lenses, depending on whether the lens is of one piece of the same refractive index material (one piece) or a lens with a separate refractive index add fused onto the main distance portion (fused).

A one-piece multifocal lens creates various powers by different curvatures on the anterior or posterior lens surface. Examples would be the "Executive" or the "Ultex" series. The progressive lenses and blended multifocal lenses are made in this same way.

Fused multifocal lenses have a smooth surface on the anterior lens surface with the power created by the difference in refractive indices and the difference in curvature at the fusion interface. Examples would be flat-top and round-top multifocals.

Progressive multifocal lenses are becoming more popular. They have a substantial cosmetic advantage over the multifocals that have visible lines. They also have advantages of clear vision at multiple distances. Presently their main disadvantage is a midperipheral distortion, which is inherent in their production. It is most noticeable when the patient turns his/her head. Most patients can adapt to this distortion. The exact position of the IPD is more critical in fitting this type of lens than any other.

Image Jump and Object Displacement. Two optical problems that are noted as one looks from the distance portion to the reading portion of a multifocal lens are image jump and object displacement (Fig. 3–53).

Image jump. This is because a minus lens induces base down prism through the lower aspect of the lens while a flat-top bifocal induces base up prism. A plus lens induces base up prism through the lower aspect of the lens while the round-top or ultex bifocal add induces base down prism. The combination of these opposing prisms

Figure 3–53.
Image jump and object displacement. **A:** Ultex bifocal. The optical center is at the bottom of the lens (actually even below the lens). Side view shows the base down prism effect of this add on a plano lens. **B:** Flat top bifocal. The optical center is at the top of the add. Side view shows there is a base-up prism effect on a plano lens. **C:** Executive bifocal. The optical center is at the top of the bifocal add. View shows the base up prism effect of this add. **D:** A minus lens showing base down prism effect, and object displacement when viewing through the lower aspect of the lens. **E:** Flat top bifocal on minus lens. The minus lens induces base down prism and the flat top induces base up prism. These prisms cancel each other and there is minimal object displacement. **F:** Ultex bifocal on minus lens. The minus lens induces base down prism and the ultex add also induces base down prism. The effect of these prisms are additive and there is maximum object displacement.

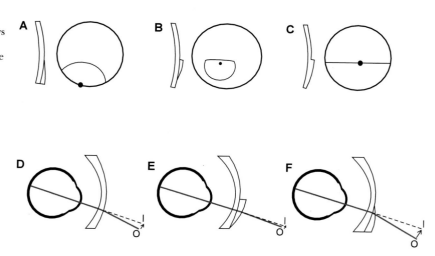

TABLE 3–4
Glasses Complaints—Trouble Shooting

Symptom	Problem	Remedy
A. Headache	1. Prescription not formulated properly	*. Check original examination Rx against the lens power and the prescription pad
	2. PD off	*. Check PD against the optical centers
	3. Lens aberration	*. Check for this flaw on Lensometer and have lens remade
	4. Too much minus prescribed	*. Re-examine, rebalance, cycloplegic exam
	5. Frame too tight	*. Larger frame
B. Distance vision blur	1. Rx too strong or too weak or cylinder axis off.	* Recheck original exam findings vs. glasses. Check for transcription error *. Check for change in prescription such as exam error or diabetes or vertex distance where glasses are actually fitting.
	2. Multifocal component fits too high	*. recheck seg height
C. Visual discomfort	1. PD not accurate	*. recheck PD
	2. Base Curve difference from previous glasses	*. check base curve vs. old Rx base curve
	3. Frame adjustments off	*. check pantoscopic angle *. check face form
	4. Lens size difference	*. compare to previous size lens
D. Diplopia	1. Excess or insufficient prism	*. recheck phorias *. check PD and optical centers *. check for vertical prism
	2. Excess of minus	*. re-balance *. cycloplegia
E. Horizontal or vertical lines not straight	1. New astigmatism Rx.	*. Reassure *. May need to decrease cylinder, or decrease obliquity of axis
	2. Lens size larger than old lens.	*. Reassure *. May need to redo to smaller size
F. Distortion	1. Poor quality lens	*. Rx redo
	2. Lens power wrong	*. Check Rx vs. exam findings
	3. Frame not fitting well	*. check pantoscopic *. check face form
G. Holds reading material too close, or too far	1. Near Rx too strong, or too weak	*. check distance lens power first
	2. Add position, size, height	*. check add power, shape and position *. early cataracts
H. Blur at intermediate distance	1. May need trifocal or progressive lens	*. check distance Rx *. check specific task distance

result in minimal object displacement. The amount of prism induced is dependent on the location of the optical center of the bifocal segment with respect to the top of the segment. A round-top segment would produce more base down prism than a flat-top because of the greater distance to the optical center of the segment.

Object displacement is a result of the total prismatic power resulting from the combination of both the distance prescription and the near add. If they are the same direction and hence additive, object displacement will be greater. If they are the opposite direction, this will decrease the amount of object displacement. A flat top bifocal add with a minus (concave) distance prescription (Fig. 3–53E) or a round-top with a plus (convex) distance prescription have the least object displacement.

Troubleshooting

Problems with Glasses. There will be times when patients will return with prescription in hand, unable to comfortably wear that which was prescribed. Many of the complaints simply require reassurance. This is particularly true when large changes in power or new cylinder prescription are required. It is best to minimize such changes, but if such changes are required, one should prepare patients for expected difficulty in adjustment. If the prescriber indicates a potential problem, the patient will be impressed by the prescriber's foresight. If the patient is not forewarned, the prescriber is perceived as trying to explain away an error. (Table 3–4.)

■ CONTACT LENSES

Historical

The earliest idea of using an apparatus in contact with the eye to change, or neutralize, the optical effect of the cornea is attributed to Leonardo da Vinci (10) at the beginning of the 16th century. Kevin Touhy (12), in manufacturing the contact lens out of Polymethylmethacrylate (PMMA) plastic, began the modern era of contact lens fitting. The lens was fit to the cornea, almost the same overall diameter of the cornea, but flatter than the flattest keratometry finding. A smaller corneal lens with a fit approximating the corneal curvature was the next advance, occurring in the 1950s and 1960s.

The next change in direction involved using hydrogel materials, and in 1964 (14), hydroxyethyl methacrylate (HEMA) was adapted from Czechoslovakia for use in the United States. Various advances in manufacturing techniques and processes occurred during the 1960s through today. Changes in material, water content, thickness, oxygen transmission, and other parameters have allowed lenses now to be disposable and used for extended periods without removal. Toric lenses, multifocal lenses, and cosmetic lenses have allowed use of contact lenses for larger potential patient bases.

The advances in technology and material for rigid lenses have progressed in parallel to the more flexible lenses, but due to more immediate patient comfort with the softer material, rigid lenses have not seen similar popularity.

Lens Parameters

Fitting techniques for the various lenses must be approached with a knowledge of basic terminology of the lenses (3). The various materials require specific fitting methods. These methods of fitting require varying specific contact lens parameters to allow the most comfortable and physiologic fit (Fig. 3–54).

The general terms for contact lens measurements are seen in this diagram.

Base Curve

The central posterior curve, which forms the optical zone (OZ), is ground, or formed, to approximate the central corneal curvature. This radius of curvature is measured in millimeters.

Corresponding to this measurement in millimeters is a corneal curvature measurement, or K reading, determined by keratometry or corneal topography.

Example: 7.34 mm = 46.00 D K

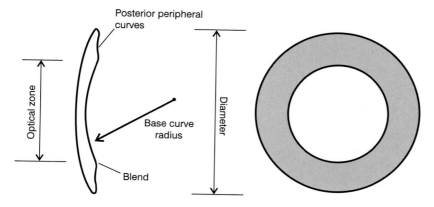

Figure 3–54.
Contact lens dimensions.

Power

As with spectacle lenses, the contact lens (rigid lenses) power may be determined in D with a lensometer. A back or front vertex power is measured depending on the specific lens type.

Example: −5.25 D sphere

Diameter

The greatest measurement across the total lens surface. The measurement is in 0.1-mm increments.

Example: Diameter = 8.4 mm

Optic Zone

That portion of overall diameter, measured in 0.1-mm increments, that has the base curve of the lens and/or is responsible for the effective power of the lens. It is the total diameter minus the peripheral curves.

Example: Optic zone (OZ) = 6.2 mm

Center Thickness

The center thickness is measured in 0.01-mm increments. It is found at the optical center of the lens.

Example: Center thickness (CT) = 0.10 mm

Peripheral Curves

As the lens curvature approaches the edge, flatter curves are blended progressively from the base curve outward. The number of these curves varies from lens to lens. Typically with an apical clearance fit of a lens, the peripheral curves actually touch the cornea; these must be finished and blended smoothly to avoid corneal damage.

Edge

The edge of the lens must be thin enough to avoid constant sensation and dislodging by the lids, but thick enough to avoid injury to the corneal epithelium and to allow easier removal. It should provide some minimal standoff to allow tear exchange to occur. Edge shape is best evaluated by the shadowgraph or Radiuscope techniques.

Fitting Considerations for Rigid Lenses

Although there are a multitude of lens materials, there are two general types of lenses, rigid and flexible. For purposes of this discussion, the rigid lenses are considered such if they cannot be folded without breaking or creasing.

There are a number of competing forces that must be considered when fitting a rigid lens. Knowledge of these forces and relationships is important in an initial fit and critical in determining changes in lens configuration to make a lens fit better.

Fitting a rigid lens primarily depends on the relationship between the base curve of the lens and the flatter curve of the cornea. As the base curve of the contact lens becomes steeper than the corneal curvature, the fit becomes tighter. Conversely, as the contact lens becomes flatter, the fit becomes looser. As the overall diameter of a high minus lens increases, the edge thickness increases. The increase in edge thickness tends to cause the upper lid to hold it more firmly and move the lens higher.

Fitting Techniques for a Nonflexible Lens

The fitting techniques to follow pertain to gas-permeable lenses as opposed to PMMA lenses, for fewer and fewer PMMA lenses are being fit (3). Typically the PMMA lenses must be fit smaller to allow better tear flow for metabolic reasons.

The ideal method of fitting a contact lens involves:

1. obtaining the spectacle refraction
2. noting the spectacle plane (vertex distance)
3. taking K readings (or other corneal topography readings)
4. converting the spectacle lens power to the expected contact lens power
5. determining the appropriate base curve and contact lens parameters
6. placing this theoretical lens on the eye as a trial fit
7. modifying the fit based on the appearance of the trial lens.

Power Conversion

The distance spectacle refraction is determined in the usual manner. If a plus cylinder refraction has been performed, it is then changed to a minus cylinder lens notation.

Example: $-5.00 + 2.00 \times 90°$ becomes $-3.00 -2.00 \times 180°$

Conversion to minus cylinder is important because of the relationship of the base curve of the contact lens to the astigmatic corneal surface. The anterior contact lens surface becomes the new refracting surface of the eye; an astigmatic spectacle refraction is dramatically changed. If all the astigmatism is due to corneal toricity, the patient is able to be fit with a spherical contact lens. Behind this contact lens, a minus cylinder "tear lens" will be created; the anterior tear surface will match the base curve of the contact lens, and the back surface of the tear lens will conform to the anterior corneal surface thereby negating its power.

As the spectacle lens power increases greater than 4.00 D, the change in effective power in moving from the spectacle plane to the cornea becomes important. Although vertex distance conversion tables are available, they typically assume a spectacle plane distance of 12 mm. Using the formula for effectivity we can calculate the contact lens power:

$$D_c = \frac{D_s}{1 - d(D_s)}$$

D_c = Contact lens power
D_s = Spectacle lens power
d = distance of spectacle plane to cornea in meters

Example 1: Spectacle power −6.50 D sphere

12 mm spectacle plane

$$Dc = \frac{-6.50}{1 - 0.012\,(-6.50)}$$

then

$$Dc = \frac{-6.50}{1 - (-0.078)}$$

$$= \frac{-6.50}{1.078} = -6.029$$

The most appropriate contact lens would be −6.00 D.

Base Curve

These determinations are typically based on the keratometry findings, and in particular the flatter of the K readings. Lenses are fit "flatter than K," "steeper than K," or "on" this K reading. Factors that determine the type of fit relative to "K" are the amount of corneal toricity and the size of the lens. As the corneal toricity increases, the lens is fit "steeper" and as the lens is fit smaller, the lens is fit "steeper."

Example: K = 43.00 D at 180 / 42.00 D at 90

The flatter K is 42.00 D with the power at 90 (axis 180). Corneal astigmatism in this eye is 1.00 D.

TABLE 3–5

Corneal Toricity	Lens Diameters		
	9.7 mm	9.2 mm	8.7 mm
0.0 TO 0.50	0.50 flatter	0.25 flatter	on flat K
0.75 TO 1.25	0.25 flatter	on flat K	0.25 steeper
1.50 TO 2.00	on flat K	0.25 steeper	0.50 steeper
2.25 TO 2.75	0.25 steeper	0.50 steeper	0.75 steeper
3.00 TO 3.50	0.50 steeper	0.75 steeper	1.00 steeper

If the spectacle refraction for this eye was −3.00 + 1.00 axis 90 converting to minus cylinder—2.00 −1.00 axis 180. Therefore, the total astigmatism of the eye is accounted for completely by the corneal toricity. If the eye were fit with a spherical lens, the astigmatism would be compensated for completely by the tear lens.

The base curve of the lens is dependent on the overall diameter of the lens and the corneal toricity. Table 3–5 helps to illustrate typical fitting situations relative to the base and steeper or flatter K reading. It must be remembered that when fitting steeper, or flatter than K, a corresponding change in lens power must be used to compensate for the tear lens created.

The diameter of the lens must allow complete coverage of the pupil, in dim illumination, with the optical zone. A lens with diameter of 9.2 mm is usually sufficient to provide coverage.

Trial Lenses

Trial lens evaluation allows the theoretical good fit determined above to be analyzed and modified. This evaluation involves observing the movement of the lens during a blink cycle and the use of fluorescein dye to observe the tear lake under the lens.

Lens position during the blink should allow the upper lens edge to approach the superior limbus. Position at this location decreases lens edge awareness and minimizes lens movement.

If the lens is riding low, increasing the diameter and increasing the base curve (flattening the lens) will allow higher positioning.

Evaluation of the fluorescein pattern allows determination of the areas of lens clearance and touch. As the dye glows light green when illuminated by cobalt blue light, the increased intensity of glow indicates greater tear accumulation. Where there is no tear film, where the lens touches the cornea, the appearance is black, from an absence of fluorescein glow. Typically an RPG lens is best fit with mild apical clearance (a soft glow centrally) or alignment with a slight peripheral clearance pattern.

Over-refraction over the trial contact lens allows a refinement of the prescription. Although the theoretical contact lens design should allow best acuity, variables in residual astigmatism and other factors may result in a trial lens that could be improved. Besides marginal improvements because of the factors noted, an over-refraction over a high power contact lens allows refinement using low power lenses with less inherent aberration.

Modification of the lens based on the above analysis is performed to maximize the prescription and to improve the optical and physiologic fit.

Soft (Flexible) Contact Lenses

At least 30 different manufacturers presently make flexible hydrophilic contact lenses. Manufacturing techniques include lathe cutting, spin casting, and injection molding. Each of these types of lenses has specific fitting characteristics. The oxygen permeability is affected by lens design and by the specific material used in the lens fabrication. The size of the lens, base curve, and thickness all play a part in the fitting characteristics of each type of lens.

Fitting the Soft Contact Lens

The K readings are not as critical in fitting soft lenses as they are in fitting rigid lenses, but they are helpful.

Diameter of the lens is selected based on the corneal diameter, visible iris diameter and pupil size. Usually the lens is selected that is about 1.5 mm larger than the visible iris diameter.

Base curve selection is initially determined by the diameter and modified based on K readings. The larger the lens diameter, the flatter the lens is fit. Lenses of approximately 13 mm diameter are fit 0.5 mm flatter than K. As the lens diameter increases, the lens is fit progressively flatter than K.

Evaluation of the movement of the lens on the eye is critical to choosing and/or modifying lens parameters. With a blink, a good fitting soft lens should move from 0.5 mm to 1.0 mm. Lens movement can be decreased by fitting steeper and increased by fitting flatter.

Alterations in corneal metabolism, increase in temperature, and decrease in oxygen available to the cornea occur with the use of extended wear contact lenses. A significant increase in the risk of keratitis is present when these lenses are worn for extended periods (see section on keratitis, Ch. 51).

Other Specialized Contact Lenses

Management of Astigmatism

When there is residual astigmatism, not ameliorated with a spherical contact lens, there are two general methods of correction.

When there is substantial corneal toricity causing residual astigmatism, then use a back surface toric base curve lens to allow stabilization. When this lens is fit aligned to the corneal toricity, the anterior surface curve of the contact lens is then able to be modified to correct for the residual astigmatism. This lens is a bitoric contact lens.

When there is significant residual astigmatism, without substantial corneal toricity, a lens may be fitted which is weighted by prism ballast to avoid rotation. This is because, usually there are 10° to 15° of rotation of the contact lens with each blink. This rotation must be overcome to allow correction of the astigmatism.

Presbyopia Management

When a patient has successfully worn contact lenses and reaches presbyopia, there are a few strategies that may be used to allow good vision at all needed distances.

Monovision. The use of single vision contact lenses allows the dominant eye to use the distance vision contact lens; the nondominant eye is then fit with a lens incorporating the near prescription. It is helpful to demonstrate this effect to the patient by using a trial frame with the appropriate lenses in place, for when simply described and not demonstrated, the patient is rarely enthusiastic.

Distance Contact Lenses and Reading Spectacles. Use of the distance contact lens and reading spectacles is a reasonable alternative with high distance prescription and intolerance to other correction methods.

Multifocal Contact Lenses. (Fig. 3–55) Multifocal contact lenses offer an alternative method for providing a near add. Patient selection is very important with this type of lens. Usually these lenses are more successfully worn by patients who have worn contact lenses for many years, as this allows only a change in a type of lens as opposed to using this lens as an initial fit. Patients who require higher-power distance lenses also typically are more successful, for there is greater motivation.

These lenses have been designed to allow near and distance vision sections of the lens. When the lens has different zones, they are of two main types. A large near add zone is located at the bottom of the lens. This is truncated to be held in place by the lower lid as the eye rotates down to read. The near add is provided in an annulus form so that the central portion is the distance prescription and the peripheral portion of the lens is the near add.

Other multifocal contact lens designs use asphericity or Fresnel zone plate diffraction to allow various lens powers at once (see Fig. 3–55). The Fresnel zone plate has as its basic optical principal, the use of diffraction to form multiple images, distance and near, at the same time. The rings are spaced so that light from each adjacent ring is exactly one wavelength greater than that of the next smaller ring. Positioning and pupil placement

Figure 3–55.
Diagram of three configurations for a multi-focal contact lens with the shaded area representing the add configuration. On the left is the add decentered inferiorly, in the center is a doughnut configuration, and on the right is the Fresnel or concentric ring configuration.

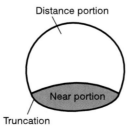

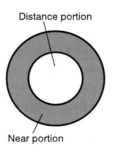

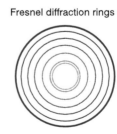

problems are decreased with this type of lens, but there is loss of contrast. Because of this loss of contrast due to multiple images, vision in dim or marginal illumination is decreased.

Other Special Purpose Lens Types
Cosmetic Lenses

These lenses are used for changing the apparent color of the eye. These may be used for concealing cosmetic defects, corneal scars, and so forth, or simply to change one's eye color.

Bandage Lenses

These soft lenses are used therapeutically to help various corneal disease processes, or as an adjunct for the delivery of certain medications.

Intrastromal Corneal Lenses

Investigational at this time, these lenses, implanted within the corneal stroma, alter the corneal curvature to change the refractive power of the eye.

■ INTRAOCULAR LENSES

Historical

Widely held to be one of the most important advances in ophthalmic surgery, the intraocular lens (IOL) was conceived of, at least, during the 18th century. The first reported implantation of a glass lens after removal of a cataract occurred in 1795 by Casaamata (19). The modern era of IOLs was initiated and developed in Britain during World War II. Harold Ridley, MD, first began implanting IOLs at the time of cataract surgery in 1949. The concept at that time, as now, was that replacement of the power of the eye lost because of cataract surgery should be placed within the posterior chamber after an extracapsular extraction. This surgery was "designed to cure aphakia and was not simply to make cataract glasses unnecessary." (22) (See section on Aphakia.) Although the first IOL operation eventually allowed visual acuity of 20/60, the refractive error that ensued was −18.00 −6.00 axis 120.

Optical Considerations

Magnification comparisons of a phakic eye to the aphakic eye when corrected with spectacles shows that aphakic spectacles cause approximately a 25% enlargement of the image. Contact lenses account for an increased image size of 6 to 7%, which is just at the limit of tolerance for aniseikonia. Using anterior chamber lenses decreases the magnification difference to 1.5%, and the magnification difference disappears when an IOL is placed within the capsule bag compared to the phakic eye.

Power Considerations

Various formulas and equations have been developed to allow the determination of the appropriate IOL power. The factors that must be taken into account in determining the lens power are keratometry readings, axial length of the eye, location of the IOL, and specific optical properties of the lens type.

Keratometry Readings

The K readings indicate the optical power of the cornea. They may be taken in the standard manner. Although steepest and flattest K are determined, the axis is not critical. With toric IOLs, the axis determination will become important.

Length of the Eye

A-Scan biometry ultrasound measurements routinely are performed to determine the length of the eye from the corneal surface to the retina along the visual axis. The speed of the ultra sound through the eye will vary depending on the presence or absence of the crystalline lens or an IOL. Speed of the ultrasound is also affected by the percentage of the eye that is fluid (longer eyes have a larger proportion of fluid) and the thickness of the crystalline lens. Another variability is the pressure exerted on the cornea during the measurement. Ossonig immersion techniques have been shown to produce an axial length measurement that is 0.26 mm longer than the more commonly used applanation techniques. Typically multiple measurements are obtained. Averaging these readings decreases the potential for error.

Location of the Lens

Placement of the IOL within the capsular bag is generally considered to be the optimal position to decrease optical magnification and minimize physiologic disruption within the globe. The distance of the IOL from the cornea, anterior chamber depth (ACD), will vary from lens to lens and even from surgeon to surgeon. The first generation of theoretical formulas used an empirically derived constant to calculate the appropriate IOL power.

Later, regression formulas were derived which replaced the ACD with an A-constant that was specific for each IOL. An example of this type is the SRK (21) formula, written:

$$P = A + BL + CK$$

where

P = power of IOL for emmetropia
L = axial length
K = average K readings (D)
A = constant derived from postoperative refractions
B = constant (−2.5); C = constant (−0.9).

Because of increasingly inaccurate lens power calculations in very short (less than 22 mm) and very long (more than 26mm) eyes, second generation IOL formulas replaced the constant ACD with a variable ACD dependent on axial length.

Further refinement of formulas, the third generation formulas, such as Holliday, SRKII, and Binkhorst, varied the ACD as a function of both axial length and of corneal curvature.

Formulas are becoming more and more sophisticated to account for the more difficult problems of very short and very long eyes. Each formula has its supporters and statistical proof of accuracy. It should be kept in mind that K reading errors or errors in the measurement of axial length are *more important* than the errors resulting from variability between the five IOL power prediction formulas (15).

Lens Types

Placement of the lens, in the anterior chamber, in the capsular bag, or anterior to the capsule will define, to a large degree, the power to be used. The lens material (PMMA, silicon, acrylic, and so forth), and hence its refractive index, will have an effect on the power and placement of the lens. The position of the haptics and their angulation will change the location of the lens and therefore the effective power.

Multifocal IOLs are presently manufactured in a number of configurations: a central near add portion encircled by a peripheral distance section, a central distance and mid portion near surrounded by a distance portion, a lens using diffraction optics, and a foldable lens using aspheric optics. Usually the near add power is selected to be approximately 3.00 D greater than the distance portion. Multifocal lenses offer the promise of a postcataract surgery patient being able to do without glasses completely, but in order to achieve this goal, the

IOL power must be exact and there must be little if any postoperative astigmatism. Unfortunately, at this time multifocal lenses have a decrease in contrast compared to single vision IOLs (18).

The lens power choice allows the ophthalmologist to decide, with the patient, what the refractive error will be postoperatively. Many ophthalmologists strive for a mild amount of myopia, about −0.50. This amount is chosen with an understanding that the calculation of the power may not be perfect. If the patient ends up −0.50, the patient will be able to function quite well at distance without correction and even some near tasks without correction. If a calculation or measurement error varies 0.50 D either side from this −0.50, the patient will be either emmetropia or still mildly myopic and still able to function fairly well. This strategy works well with a patient with little or no underlying refractive error; it fails with a patient who has a large refractive error. If the nonoperated eye retains its substantial refractive error, anisometropia of more than 3.00 D may cause vertical prism problems through spectacle bifocal adds. With larger refractive errors, the first eye may be designed toward emmetropia, but within 3 D of the remaining eye. The second eye, when needing surgery may then be designed even further towards emmetropia than the first. In patients who have been myopic for many years, attempts at emmetropia, while gratifying from a lens design and selection perspective, may be met with disappointment by the patient. A myopic patient who had taken for granted reading without correction, waking and seeing a wristwatch without correction, is frequently unhappy even with a demonstration that proves that distance visual acuity is 20/20 without correction. These patients would be best served by retaining some myopia in their intraocular lens design.

Other Intraocular Lens Uses

Severe refractive errors may be corrected by placement of an IOL in the anterior chamber in front of the normal crystalline lens. At the present time, such lenses are limited to use in myopia of greater than −6.00 D (11).

In cases of concurrent cataract and macular degeneration, the use of a standard intraocular lens with a high-power negative central portion may give some benefit. The peripheral portion serves in the standard manner, but the central portion serves as an intraocular ocular portion of a telescopic visual aid. Placing the ocular portion of a telescopic aid within the eye has the potential for increasing the optical quality compared to a wholly external low vision aid. This "teledioptric" IOL is under investigation.

■ REFRACTIVE SURGERY

The subject of refractive surgery is beyond the scope of this section. Interest continues to grow in improving techniques and technology. Most of this surgery involves reshaping the cornea by incisional means (i.e., radial keratotomy and automated lamellar keratectomy) or laser ablation (i.e., photorefractive keratectomy), or both incisional and laser (with modification of lamellar keratectomy) or thermal collagen shrinkage techniques. As noted above, the use of IOLs in phakic patients and the use of intrastromal implants have stimulated interest. (See Chap. 52 on corneal surgery).

■ LOW VISION

Visual impairment, low vision, or low visual acuity refers to a decrease in correctable acuity from average or standard norms of vision. "A partially sighted person is one who, with conventional corrections, is not able to perform vision tasks needed for vocational, avocational, or social needs." (16) A decrease in function may be minor or severe, depending on the remaining vision and the needs of the patient. Many underlying pathologies can account for the decrease in vision, but the field of low vision is involved with using optical and nonoptical methods to enhance the visual abilities of these patients. The decrease in vision may be either in acuity or visual field or a combination of the two. The method of determination of the appropriate visual aid or apparatus is beyond the scope of this section.

Simple optical aids of high plus lenses and/or hand-held magnifiers serve for the large majority of low vision patients. Increasing the plus power of spectacle lenses allows an increase in magnification, but this gain is at the expense of a decreased working distance and a decreased depth of field. Hand held magnifiers allow a more comfortable working distance. Most commonly these lenses are in the range of 5 to 12 D.

$$\text{Magnifying power } (\times) = \frac{\text{Equivalent power (diopters)}}{4}$$

More complicated systems using telescopic optics allow better distance vision for the low vision patient. Usually the Galilean telescope is used to give a magnified, enlarged image. It consists of a concave ocular lens and a convex objective lens. When used for distance vision it is afocal, but it can be used for near and intermediate distances when combined with appropriate plus lenses. Typical telescopic aids have a magnification of 2 to 6×. An increase in magnification advantage is decreased by aberration, decreasing field of vision, and increase in weight.

■ REFERENCES

1. American Academy of Ophthalmology. Basic and Clinical Science Course. Vol. 2. 1990–1991.
2. Corboy John M. The Retinoscopy Book: A Manual for Beginners. 1979.
3. Dohenny Eye Institute Basic Contact Lens Fitting Manual.
4. Donders FC. On the Anomalies of Accommodation and Refraction of the Eye. Translated by William Daniel Moore, 1952. London: The New Sydenham Society, 1864.
5. Druiff Guy E. Refraction: A Simple and Concise Treatise on Practical Sight Testing. London: Anglo-American Optical Company, 1911.
6. Duane TD, Jaeger EA (eds). Clinical Ophthalmology. Volume 1. Philadelphia: Harper & Row, 1990.
7. Duke-Elder S. System of Ophthalmology. Ophthalmic Optics and Refraction. St Louis: Mosby, 1991.
8. Hartridge G. The Refraction of the Eye, A Manual for Students. 16th edition. Philadelphia: P. Blakeston's Sons, 1919.
9. Helmholtz H. Treatise on Physiologic Optics. Volume 1. New York: Dover, 1924.
10. Hofstetter H, Graham R. Leonardo and Contact Lenses. Am J Optometry 1953;30:41–44.
11. Holladay J. Refractive Power Calculations for Intraocular Lenses in the Phakic Eye. Am J Opthalmol 1993;116:63–66.
12. Jackson E. Skiascopy and Its Practicle Application to the Study of Refraction. 4th Edition. Denver, Colorado: Herrick Book and Stationery, 1905.
13. Jenkins, White. Fundamentals of Optics. 3rd Edition. New York: McGraw-Hill, 1957.
14. Lowther G., Snyder C. Contact Lenses, Procedures and

Techniques. 2nd Edition. Boston: Butterworth-Heine-mann, 1992.

15. McEwen JR, Massengill RK, Friedel SD. Effect of Keratometry and axial length measurement errors on primary implant power calculations. J Cataract Refract Surg 1990;16:61–70.

16. Mehr E, Jose R. School of Optometry at University of California at Berkeley. In: Faye E (ed.). Low Vision. Springfield, Illinois: Charles C Thomas, 1975.

17. Michaels D. Visual Optics and Refraction: A Clinical Approach. 3rd Edition. St Louis: Mosby, 1985.

18. Miller D. In: Maxwell WA, Nordan LT (eds.). Current Concepts of Multifocal Intraocular Lenses. Thorofare, New Jersey: Slack, 1991.

19. Nordlohne ME. The Intraocular Implant Lens: Development and Results with Special Reference to the Bindhorst Lens. In: Apple D, Mamalis N, Olson R, Kincaid M. Intraocular Lenses, Evolution, Designs, Complications, and Pathology. Baltimore: Williams & Wilkins, 1989.

20. Raviola E, Weisel T. An Animal Model of Myopia. NEJM 1985;1609–1615.

21. Retzlaff J. A New Intraocular Lens Calculation Formula. Am Intra-Ocular Implant Soc J 1980;6:148–152.

22. Ridley H. In: Apple D, Mamalis N, Olson R, Kincaid M. Intraocular Lenses, Evolution, Designs, Complications, and Pathology. Baltimore: Williams & Wilkins, 1989.

23. Rubin ML. Optics for Clinicians. Florida: Triad Scientific Publishers, 1971.

24. Safir A. Refraction and Clinical Optics. New York: Harper & Row, 1980.

25. Sheard C. Prescription of Prisms. Am J Optometry 1934;11:364–378.

26. Stone R, Ton Lin P, Iuvone M, Laties A. Myopia and the Control of Eye Growth. Chichester: CIBA Foundation Symposium #155, 1990;45–62.

27. Weinstock, Wirtschafter J. A Decision-Oriented Manual of Retinoscopy. Springfield, Illinois: Charles C Thomas, 1976.

28. Weisel TN, Raviola E. Myopia and Eye Enlargement after Neonatal Lid Fusion in Monkeys. Nature 1977;266:66–68.

29. Yen M-Y, Liu J-H, Kao S-C, Shiao H-H. Comparison of the Effect of Atropine and Cyclopentolate on Myopia. Ann Opthalmol 1989;21:180–187.

30. Yves L. Light Colour and Vision. London: Chapman and Hall 1957.

IV Neuro-ophthalmology

Section Editor: Edward G. Buckley

4 Neuro-ophthalmology Examination

Timothy J. Martin

The essential components of the neuro-ophthalmology examination will be presented. Some specialized examination techniques will be discussed in more detail in the sections devoted to specific disorders. Additional excellent general resources are included in the bibliography (1–4, 10, 18).

■ A. HISTORY

A directed, thorough history is the most important part of a neuro-ophthalmology examination. Frequently, the diagnosis (or at least a refined differential diagnosis) is evident from the history alone.

It is often difficult for a patient to accurately describe a visual complaint. For example, "blurry vision" or "can't focus" may mean a visual field defect or diplopia. The patient with a homonymous hemianopic visual field event may insist that the problem occurred in only one eye—the side of the visual field loss. Long-standing unilateral visual loss may have been acutely "discovered" when the sound eye was momentarily covered. "Dizziness" may be oscillopsia (ie, unstable moving vision caused by acquired nystagmus) or vertigo. "Sinus" and "migraine" are labels that patients give to every conceivable type of pain.

Historical details concerning the character of visual loss are especially important in patients with transient events, since subsequent visual testing may offer few clues. Transient visual loss may last seconds (transient visual obscurations from papilledema), a few minutes (amaurosis fugax from embolic disease), 15–20 minutes (migraine-related visual events), or hours (ocular causes such as dry eye). When multiple events have occurred, the frequency, variability, possible inciting fac-

tors (such as hot bath or sauna in Uhthoff's phenomenon), and actions that produce relief must be ascertained. The patient with episodic visual phenomena should be told what to observe during future attacks.

The *course* of persistent vision loss may be sudden and unchanging (anterior ischemic optic neuropathy); may worsen gradually over months (compressive lesions, cataract) or over days (optic neuritis); may decline in abrupt steps (vascular causes, optic disc drusen) or "like a curtain" (retinal embolic events); or may show recovery (optic neuritis, neuroretinitis).

Associated visual phenomena can include photopsias (retinal disorders, "big blind spot" syndromes), scintillating scotomas (migraine), hallucinations (Charles Bonnet phenomenon: vivid "release" hallucinations in a blind hemi-field), floaters (vitreoretinal disease), or color aberrations (digoxin toxicity).

Accompanying ophthalmic signs and symptoms must be sought, such as eye pain or redness, diplopia, or ptosis. Visual events temporally associated with neurologic symptoms such as dizziness, vertigo, and confusion suggest insufficiency of the posterior cerebral circulation. Headache typically follows the visual aura in classical migraine.

Complex disturbances of higher cortical function

may simply be summarized by patients as "not seeing too well." Visual agnosia (seeing but not recognizing) may be generalized, or it may be limited, as in patients who have difficulty recognizing faces (prosopagnosia). Simultanagnosia (inability to recognize a whole picture from its parts), central achromatopsia, palinopsia (pathologic persistence and reappearance of images) and central polyopia are other examples of higher cortical dysfunction (10).

As with visual loss, understanding the time course of *diplopia* is frequently diagnostic. Diplopic symptoms may be of sudden (vascular events) or gradual (compression) onset, constant or intermittent, variable, or fatigue-related (myasthenia gravis). Symptoms may be related to position of gaze (cranial nerve paresis) or alleviated with a specific head position (fourth cranial nerve palsy). The two images may be oriented horizontally (sixth cranial nerve palsy), vertically or obliquely (third or fourth cranial nerve palsy), or tilted (fourth cranial nerve palsy). The double vision may be worse at distance than near (sixth cranial nerve palsy). Important accompanying symptoms include proptosis (orbital diseases), pain (ischemia or aneurysm), ptosis and anisocoria (third cranial nerve paresis), or symptoms of brainstem or hemispheric dysfunction. Constitutional symptoms (giant cell arteritis), and weakness (myasthenia) may offer important clues.

Diplopia that disappears when either eye is covered is clearly "binocular," and it results from a misalignment of the visual axis between the two eyes. Monocular double vision frequently results from lenticular or corneal disease. Generally, the second image is of lesser quality, and will disappear when testing with a pinhole. Less commonly it can be of central cerebral origin, or reported by patients with functional disorders (9).

Important characteristics of *pain* in the *head* or *orbit* include location (scalp tenderness in arteritis), character (deep, boring, sharp), intensity, time profile, accompanying symptoms (scintillations, nausea, vomiting as in migraine), variability, triggering factors, and relief efforts. Pain with eye movement is frequently associated with visual loss from optic neuritis. Scalp tenderness and jaw claudication may accompany ischemic optic neuropathy or acute cranial neuropathies from giant cell arteritis. The lancinating facial pain of trigeminal neuralgia is often severe, but short lived, and may be associated with touching specific facial "trigger" zones.

■ B. EXAMINATION OF THE AFFERENT VISUAL SYSTEM: MEASURING "VISION"

Visual Acuity

The greatest variability in measurement of visual acuity (Fig. 4–1) is introduced by the examiner's technique (2). Since many patients simply refuse to read if the letters are not perfectly clear, the examiner must "push" the patient, encouraging him or her to read smaller and smaller lines.

Much can be learned by observing how a patient reads a visual acuity chart. The patient with a homonymous visual field defect frequently reads only half the letters in a line. The patient with severe visual field constriction needs plenty of time to find the chart, but may read 20/20 after this initial struggle.

A thorough refraction is required to find the best-corrected visual acuity. Although "pinhole" acuity is a helpful tool in identifying refractive errors, it is no substitute for a manifest refraction.

Contrast Sensitivity Testing

Many patients with visual disorders may perform reasonably well on high-contrast tasks (such as Snellen acuity), but complain bitterly of their inability to function in the "real world." A variety of clinical contrast sensitivity tests have been developed to measure discriminatory function at various contrast levels (2, 14) (see Fig. 4–2).

Brightness Testing

The patient who has recovered from a unilateral optic neuropathy may note a decrease in the brightness of light compared to the normal eye, despite a relatively normal visual acuity and visual field. A subjective measure of relative brightness can be obtained by having the patient observe a light source or white object with each eye, and asking "If this amount of light is worth a dollar (light in the better eye), then how much is this worth in cents (light in the affected eye)?" Simultaneous binocular comparison, neutral density filters, or crossed polarized filters can be used to measure differences in interocular brightness (11, 17).

Photostress Testing

A bright light directed at the macula will bleach the photopigments, and the subject will have a transient scotoma, often with after-images. The normal retina can generally recover in less than a minute, depending on the intensity and duration of the photostress. Patients

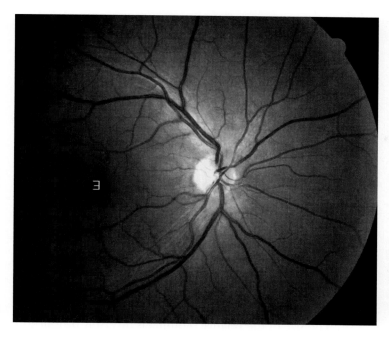

Figure 4–1.
A representation of the retinal image (inverted) formed by the 20/400 "E" is superimposed on this sixty-degree photograph of a normal fundus. The 20/400 "E" is less than two degrees in angular diameter. Thus, Snellen acuity testing evaluates only a tiny (but very significant) fraction of retinal area.

with macular disease (macular edema, age-related macular degeneration) take longer to recover than patients with optic nerve disorders. Each eye is tested separately. The patient looks directly into a bright light source (the indirect ophthalmoscope) for 10 seconds. The examiner then determines the number of seconds until the patient can read within one line of his or her (pre-stress) visual acuity. Normal patients require less than a minute for recovery, and both eyes generally recover in about the same amount of time (5).

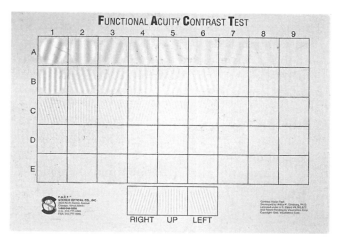

Figure 4–2.
Functional Acuity Contrast Test (Stereo Optical Co., Inc, Chicago Illinois; reproduced with permission from Visumetrics Corp). The patient looks at each contrast sensitivity grating, and is asked whether the bars are oriented to the right, to the left, or straight up and down. Each row represents a different spatial frequency (bar size), with decreasing contrast. A contrast threshold is thus obtained for five different spatial frequencies. This information is often plotted as a curve, comparing contrast threshold to spatial frequency.

The Amsler grid (Fig. 4–3) requires patients to evaluate the absence (scotoma) or irregularity (metamorphopsia) of a line grid covering the central 20 degrees of the visual field while looking at a fixation dot. Although this grid is most frequently used to detect and follow metamorphopsia in age-related macular degeneration, it is useful in both retinal and optic nerve disease. The sensitivity of this test may be greatly increased when cross-polarizing glasses are used to decrease illumination (22).

Color Vision Testing

The terminology used in describing congenital color vision defects is cumbersome but logical. The cone pigment in question is named by a root word: protan is red (color vision disorder of the first kind); deuteran is green; tritan is blue. A given cone pigment may be deficient (suffix- omaly) or entirely absent (suffix- opia). Thus, protanopia is a congenital condition in which there is a complete absence of red cone pigments, and deuteranomaly describes the relative lack of green sensitive pigments. Patients who maintain some degree of cone function usually have good visual acuity.

Virtually all clinical tests of color vision were originally designed to detect the congenital "pure," single-color pigment defects. The use of *isochromatic plates* is based on the principle that subjects with protan and deutran defects cannot distinguish between certain colors, and thus are unable to see a letter, number, or shape hidden in a matrix of colored dots. The *Farnsworth-Munsell 100-hue test* (Fig. 4–4) requires the subject to order a sequence of colored disks. Grading schemes allow determination of an error axis, which

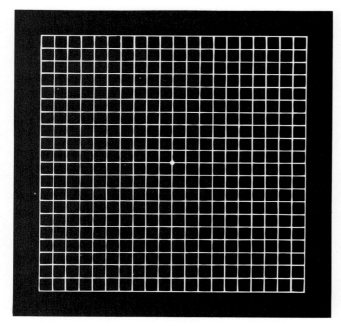

Figure 4–3.
The Amsler grid is held at a normal reading distance and viewed monocularly in best near correction (actual grid size is a 10 cm square). The patient is asked to look directly at the center dot, and is asked a series of questions regarding the sharpness and regularity of the grid lines. It can easily be performed by the patient at home to monitor metamorphopsia from macular degeneration or central scotomas.

may coincide with known protan, deuteran, or tritan error axes. The *Nagel anomaloscope* allows relative quantitation of red and green cone deficiencies by measuring the intensity of red and green light a subject needs in order to match a yellow target.

Many acquired disorders of the retina or optic nerve may alter the perception of color before gross deficits can be detected with acuity or perimetry testing. However, these acquired disorders are far less "pure" than congenital disorders of color vision, since they affect all three cone pigment systems and the rods to variable and unpredictable extents. These color deficiencies only rarely follow a specific pattern or axis on the color tests, although it has been observed that macular problems tend to cause loss of blue/yellow color discrimination, while optic nerve defects tend to result in red/green defects (8). Despite the shortcomings, the tests are frequently used clinically to detect and follow acquired optic nerve disease (6, 16). Comparing color saturation (with red bottle cap) remains a relatively sensitive, easily performed color test.

Visual Fields Testing

Visual Field General Terms

The visual field represents the peripheral extent of vision. Nasally, the visual field extends approximately 60°, temporally 90°, superiorly 50°, and inferiorly 70°. The optic disc produces a blind spot which is 5° in diameter and is located 15° temporal to central fixation. The optic disc is actually nasal to the fovea, but projects a scotoma to the temporal field. Sensitivity is most acute in the central visual field (corresponding to foveal vision), and diminishes as one moves peripherally. One can plot out the sensitivity of the visual field by visual field testing (see Glaucoma section Chapter 43).

Various terms are used to describe defects in the visual field. A scotoma is a defect in the visual field. An *absolute scotoma* is when no stimulus is perceived in the effective field, no matter how intense the stimulus. A *relative scotoma* is an area of diminished sensitivity, but intense stimului, (bigger and brighter) will be perceived in this area. A relative scotoma will be missed by a large bright stimuli, however it will be identified by a dimmer and smaller stimuli. Thus, the size and shape of a relative scotoma depends on the intensity of the stimulus. The size of the relative scotoma is inversely proportionally to the intensity of the stimulus. Scotomas can also be classified as to location and to morphology.

Types of Visual Field Defects

Central: involves central visual field and fixation.

Paracentral: central fixation is preserved, but the scotoma closely approaches central fixation.

Cecocentral: extends from central fixation to the blind spot.

Arcuate: follows the nerve fiber layer and appears as an arc directed toward the blind spot. This scotoma respects the horizontal meridian as do the axons of the ganglion cells.

Altitudinal: involves two horizontal quadrants but respects the horizontal meridian (superior altitudinal defect versus inferior altitudinal defect).

Quadrantanopia: involves one quadrant of the visual field (e.g. superior temporal quadrantanopia).

Heminopia: a visual field defect which respects the vertical midline and involves the superior and inferior quadrants (nasal hemianopia or temporal hemianopia).

Bilateral Visual Field Defects

Homonymous: a visual field defect which involves the same side of visual space in both eyes. For example, a right homonymous hemianopsia would be a scotoma of the right visual field in both eyes (ie, temporal hemianopia of the right eye and nasal hemianopia of the left eye).

Congruity: indicates how symmetrical the visual field defects are between fellow eyes.

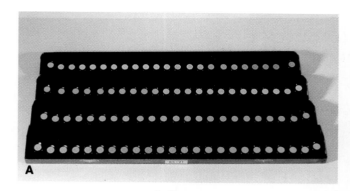

A

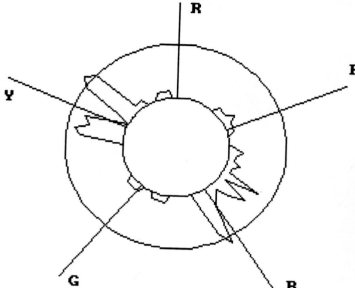

B

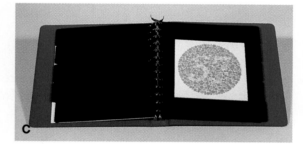

C

Figure 4–4.
Color Tests. A. The Farnsworth-Munsell 100-hue test (FM100). The subject is required to order the color caps in each tray. Standardized lighting and patient supervision are required. B. Test scoring produces a plot that shows where in the color wheel errors were made, often producing a characteristic axis of color confusion. The total error score is a single number, which may be more helpful in following acquired color vision deficits. This plot illustrates a tritan defect (blue, yellow). C, Pseudo-isochromatic Plates (Richmond Products, Boca Raton, Florida). Color-plate tests are easier to perform and take far less time than the FM100, but they lack sensitivity and specificity in acquired color vision deficits. Generally, total errors are reported, but errors on specific plates may help to diagnose congenital color vision disorders.

Computerized perimetry (Fig. 5–A, B) instruments test predetermined points in the visual field with a variety of light-stimulus intensities. Patient responses interactively direct the computer software to determine the light intensity threshold for a given static point in the visual field. This method has the advantage of producing reproducible, quantifiable maps of the visual field, which then can be analyzed statistically (13).

The *Goldmann perimeter* (Fig. 4–5, C, D) is a mechanical device that allows movement of calibrated lights in and out of the patient's seeing visual field to produce a map of the patient's kinetic visual field. With Goldmann perimetry, the perimetrist, rather than a computer, determines the strategy for testing and thus can interact with the patient on a human level. In tangent screen testing, the examiner moves white discs of calibrated size on a flat, black background to map the central visual field (7).

Confrontation visual field (Fig. 4–5, E) testing compares two strategic portions of the visual field on either side of the horizontal or the vertical meridian. First, each eye is tested individually by having the patient fixate on the examiner's nose. The examiner's hands are placed in the right and left superior quadrants of the patient's visual field, testing across the vertical meridian (to detect chiasmal and retrochiasmal disorders). The patient is asked to compare the two hands and to note which hand appears fuzzier, blurrier, or dimmer. The test is then performed in the lower quadrants. Next, the horizontal meridian (important in optic nerve-related visual field loss) can be tested in similar fashion (with the examiner's hands pointing in opposite directions above and below the meridian). The other eye is tested, and then both eyes are tested together to inspect for homonymous visual field loss. Another method asks the patient to "mimic" the number of extended fingers on the examiner's two hands.

Using two red objects (or a single one moved between positions) may increase the sensitivity of confrontation perimetry, especially when defining a central scotoma. In this test the patient looks directly at a red object on the examiner's nose and is asked to compare its color to that of an identical red object at various positions in the paracentral visual field (4, 21).

The *relative afferent pupillary defect* (RAPD) is an objective comparison of the visual integrity of the

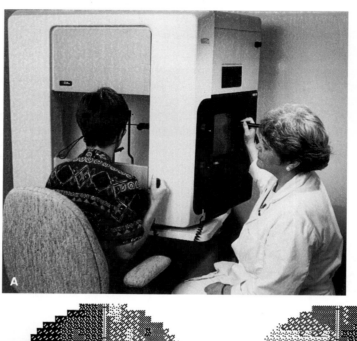

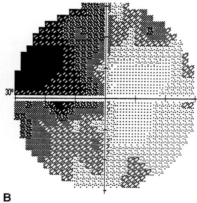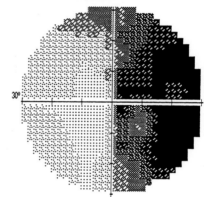

Figure 4–5.
The technique and documentation of a variety of perimetric methods are demonstrated. A. The Humphrey Field Analyzer automated perimeter. As the patient fixates on a central target, the computer directs a spot of light on the perimeter bowl for a brief period of time. The patient responds by pushing a hand-held button, if the light is seen. The patient's response helps to direct the test to determine threshold values. B. The result is a computer printout that maps the visual field, compares the data to normals, and assesses the reliability of the patient's performance. This patient has bilateral temporal visual field defects from a lesion in the chiasm. C. The Goldmann perimeter. A perimetrist directs the test, monitors and encourages the patient to maintain fixation, and records the patient's response. This versatile machine is highly dependent on the skill of the perimetrist.
(continued on next page)

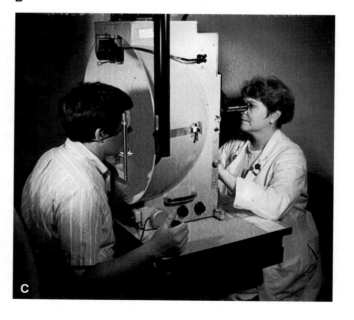

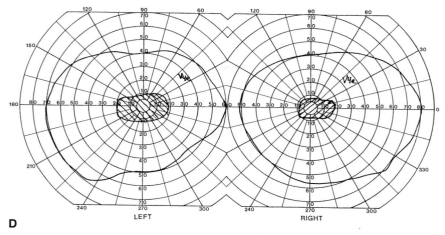

D

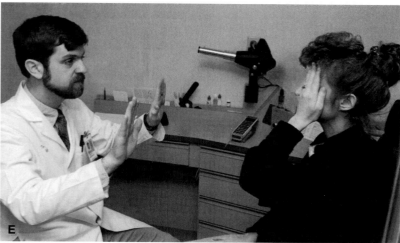

E

Figure 4–5. *(continued)*
D. The resulting map of kinetic perimetry is essentially a contour map of the "hill of vision." This patient has a normal peripheral visual field, but bilateral dense cecocentral scotomas from alcohol/nutritional optic neuropathy. E. Confrontation visual field testing uses the examiner's hands, red targets, or even the examiner's face, to have the patient compare two areas of the visual field. The results are highly dependent on the examiner and patient and are not standardized. However, the simplicity and versatility of this method make it an extraordinarily powerful tool.

two eyes and is one of the most important tools in neuro-ophthalmology to detect optic nerve disease (19). See Chapter 11 (Pupils) for the technique and interpretation.

■ C. EXAMINATION OF THE EFFERENT VISUAL SYSTEM:

Eyelid

Asymmetry of the eyelids should be approached with the same caution as anisocoria—it isn't always obvious which eye is the abnormal one. Eyelid retraction can occur in Grave's disease of the orbit, in mid-brain disorders, or secondary to efforts to overcome a contralateral ptosis (see ptosis section).

Examination of ptosis should include a measurement of upper lid height, levator excursion, upper lid crease, and of lower lid malposition ("up-side-down" ptosis in patients with oculosympathetic paresis).

Pupils

(See Chapter 11). Afferent pupillary defects present as anisocoria—a difference in the right and left pupillary sizes. Anisocoria is never due to loss of vision—relative pupillary size is not affected even if one eye is normal and the other is blind. Anisocoria is an efferent problem stemming from unequal of sympathetic or parasympathetic ocular innervation, or from iris abnormalities (20). (See Chapter 9.)

Ocular Motility

Horizontal versions are observed to locate weakness or slowness of the adducting eye (intranuclear ophthalmoplegia), abducting eye (abducens nerve deficit), or both (gaze paresis) (9).

Movements in the primary vertical plane (straight up and down) will give information about vertical gaze disturbances (dorsal midbrain syndrome, third and fourth nerve palsy) or orbital disease (Graves' orbitopathy). Following the examiner's target is essentially a pursuit function; saccades must be tested separately by having the patient look quickly from one target to another in the desired plane.

The patient's report of which positions produce diplopia, and the severity of the diplopia in those positions, is a helpful addition to the examiner's observations. Dissociating the two eyes with a red lens (or Maddox rod) over the right eye and asking, "Are the red and white lights further apart looking here to the right, or when I move them to the left?" helps the patient report his or her observations. A maddox rod before both eyes (double maddox rod) allows estimation of ocular torsion (superior oblique palsy).

Optokinetic nystagmus (OKN) testing (see Chapter 6) is performed by presenting the patient with moving black and white bars on a rotating drum or strip. Brief ocular pursuit movements are induced in the direction of the stimulus motion, with short saccades occurring in the opposite direction to re-fixate on the stimulus. The horizontal response may be abnormal in patients with congenital nystagmus, parietal lobe lesions, or saccadic abnormalities. Patients with functional visual loss claiming total blindness can be shown to have at least some vision if they respond to this reflex stimulus (18).

■ D. OTHER SPECIALIZED EXAMINATIONS

Sensory components of the *trigeminal nerve* (V) may be tested with a cotton tip applicator with the end pulled to a fine point. The threads are lightly brushed against the inferior cornea of each eye (*before* any eye drops are given). The intensity of the patient's blink response, and the subjective sensation between the two eyes is compared. With the patient's eyes closed, the wisp of cotton is then used to compare sensation between the right and left cheek and brow. Pain pathways may be tested in a similar manner with a pin, or by breaking the stick of the applicator obliquely to create a sharp wooden point (*not* for corneal testing). Motor components may be evaluated by comparing the bulk of the right and left masseter muscles when the patient is gritting his or her teeth. The strength of the pterygoid muscles is evaluated by lateral jaw movements against resistance.

Weakness and asymmetry of the motor portion of the *facial nerve* (VII) may be evident as the examiner observes the patient during the history. Orbicularis function can be tested by observing the speed, completeness, and symmetry of blinking. Comparing the degree of lash rotation in forced eye closure, or observing attempts to open the eyes in forced eye closure is also helpful. Lower facial function is tested by having the patient show the teeth (forced smile)—or pucker. When unilateral lower facial weakness is present, having the patient raise the brows to wrinkle the forehead may show involvement of the upper face as well, suggesting a

peripheral rather than a central disorder of the facial nerve. Abnormalities in taste, deficiencies of lacrimation and salivation, and hyperacusis may be identified in the history, but are difficult to test accurately without specialized equipment.

Aberrant regeneration (see Chapter 9: Eye Movements) following facial nerve paresis may manifest as involuntary twitching of lower facial muscle on voluntary eye closure (common following Bell's palsy). Miswiring between the fifth and seventh cranial nerves may result in "*crocodile tears*" (lacrimation with jaw movement) or jaw-winking (ptosis synchronous with jaw movement).

Disorders of facial nerve *over-activity* include orbicularis myokymia (unilateral orbicularis), essential blepharospasm (bilateral orbicularis) and hemifacial spasm (unilateral upper and lower facial muscles) (12).

Dysfunction of the *vestibuloacoustic nerve* (cranial nerve VIII) may cause decreased hearing or vestibular dysfunction. Evaluation of this nerve becomes important in the examination of patients with sixth or seventh cranial nerve dysfunction (cerebellopontine angle lesion). Although sophisticated hearing tests are beyond the expertise of the ophthalmologist, the patient's right and left hearing can be compared to each other, and to the examiner's hearing with a softly ticking watch or tuning fork. Vestibular dysfunction may be manifest as vertigo, as oscillopsia in the history, or as nystagmus on examination.

■ E. EXAMINATION OF THE COMATOSE PATIENT

The evaluation of *comatose patients* must rely entirely on examination by inspection, or by elicitation of physiologic reflexes. The general size of both pupils may be influenced by medications, toxins, or brainstem disease. The presence of an anisocoria may reveal third

cranial nerve dysfunction (uncal herniation), oculosympathetic paresis, ocular trauma, or previous eye surgery. Ocular movements may be induced by oculocephalic reflexes (doll's head maneuver) if the patient's condition/injury permits, or by bedside warm and cold caloric irrigation (see Chapter 6: Nystagmus). Inspection of the anterior segment of the eye may require a portable slit lamp. Although the fundus examination is vital (e.g., to diagnose Terson's syndrome, malignant hypertension, papilledema), the eye should be dilated only after careful documentation of the pupillary testing (see above). Always inform the nursing staff and the patient's other physicians when the pupils have been dilated. Short-acting drops are preferred since the pupillary examination is helpful in following the neurological status of the comatose patient (15) (Table 4–1).

TABLE 4–1
Ocular Signs in Coma

Level of Impairment	Extraocular Movement				Pupils	
	Rest Position	Doll's Head	Cold Calorics	Defective System	Size	Reactivity
Unilateral hemispheral	Tonic deviation toward lesion	Intact*	Intact*	Fronto-mesencephalic (saccadic)	In hemispheral disease, pupillary signs are inconstant and usually of little help. In coma, pupil is usually small but reactive.	
Bilateral or diffuse hemispheral	Straight†/divergent; slow disconjugate wandering	Intact*	Tonic phase only	Bilateral fronto-mesencephalic		
Metabolic, including drugs						
Light	Straight†/divergent	Intact*/diminished	Intact*/diminished	(Above)	Small	Reactive
Deep	Slow disconjugate wandering or fixed	Absent	Absent	Brainstem reticular		
Midbrain	Straight† or skew; ±III	Horizontal only; adduction lag	Horizontal only; adduction lag; ±skew	Rostral mesencephalic vertical gaze	Mid-dilated; ±III	Fixed
Pons	Straight† or deviated opposite lesion; ±skew; ±bobbing	May fail to one/both sides; ±internuclear; ±VI	May fail to one/both sides; ±internuclear; ±VI	Pontine paramedian reticular	Pinpoint	Reactive
Cerebellum‡						
Early	Deviated opposite lesion; gaze palsy toward lesion	Normal or diminished toward side of gaze palsy	Normal or diminished toward side of gaze palsy	?	(Normal)	
Late	± Skew	Diminished/absent toward side of gaze palsy	Diminished/absent toward side of gaze palsy		Pinpoint	Reactive

* Bilaterally intact doll's head or caloric deviations preclude the possibility of severe pontine lesions. (The onset of reflex paralysis of eye movements in the course of coma is considered a sign of secondary brainstem hemorrhages.)

† In coma, eyes directed straight have no localizing value.

‡ The syndrome of acute cerebellar hemorrhage consists of occipital headache, ataxia, vertigo, conjugate gaze palsy, and progressive lethargy.

From Glaser JS (editor): Neuro-Opthalmology. 2nd ed. Philadelphia: J.B. Lippincott Co., 1990, p. 59.

■ F. FUNCTIONAL VISUAL LOSS

Patients who insist that they have a visual deficit despite evidence to the contrary are said to have "functional" visual loss. Although a few of these patients may be exaggerating milder "real" deficits, most have completely normal vision. Such patients represent a broad spectrum, ranging from innocent, anxious patients who make no conscious effort to deceive ("hysterics"), to patients who consciously scheme for secondary gain—often to collect disability benefits ("malingerers"). Fortunately, it is not the ophthalmologist's task to judge a patient's motives, but to simply report the facts of the examination to the patient and to authorized parties.

The examiner must be familiar with methods designed to "trick" the patient into disclosing his or her real visual abilities; not so that the examiner can confront the patient, but primarily to reassure the patient, and thus prevent needless extensive investigation into imaginary disorders.

Visual acuity should be tested by starting with the 20/10 or 20/15 line, or the smallest lines available. Once the patient begins to recognize some characters, he or she may be persuaded to read smaller lines when the phoropter ("magnifying binoculars") is placed in front of the eyes, with trivial changes from the current refraction announced as "even more magnification."

If a patient with suspected functional visual loss complains of poor vision in only one eye, the examiner can use the phoropter to make it less clear to the patient which eye is being tested. In this situation, both eyes view the Snellen chart through their best correction in the phoropter. The examiner announces that they will now test the "good" eye: The largest test letters are revealed first, and as the patient progresses to smaller lines, the "good" eye is blurred (fogging) with progressive plus lenses. When the patient has read the smallest possible line (for example, 20/30), the "bad" eye is occluded to determine the best possible acuity that can be achieved in the fogged eye (perhaps only 20/200), thereby demonstrating a visual acuity of at least 20/30 in the eye of complaint.

Tests of stereoacuity (such as the Titmus fly test) may allow documentation of good binocular vision, since the patient is generally unaware of the physiology (or implications) of good stereopsis. Stereoacuity of 40 arc seconds requires visual acuity of at least 20/25 OU.

After the eyes are dilated, the patient may be persuaded that the larger pupils will let more light in and thus will perform better at the phoropter or in visual field testing. After pupillary dilation, the Potential Acuity Meter (PAM) can be used to project the Snellen chart directly onto the macula. The examiner tells the patient that because of his or her difficulty in seeing the standard chart, a device will be used that projects the letters directly on the brain tissue (true statement), bypassing most of the eye (also true), and that even legally blind people can see the smallest letters with this new technology (true for at least some cataract patients with vision of 20/200 or less). Very few functional patients can resist reading the smallest possible line.

In patients claiming "total blindness," an optokinetic stimulus or a moving mirror may induce corresponding eye movement, thereby confirming at least some vision. A threatening gesture to induce a blink, or an emotionally charged stimulus (such as written profanity) to produce a response has been advocated by some sources.

In functional patients, it is much easier to prove normal visual acuity than to show that the visual fields are normal. This is because it is virtually impossible to perform perimetry without the patient being aware of which eye is being tested. Some functional patients may cooperate and perform a normal visual field examination if they are persuaded that dilating the eye will greatly expand the visual field, or if it is suggested that people with very poor central vision compensate with "supernormal" side vision. Frequently, the examiner can only show that the patient's visual field test results are nonphysiologic or inconsistent. Physiologic consistency of marked peripheral visual field constriction (the most common "functional" visual field) can be noted by performing tangent screen perimetry at two different distances with appropriate relative targets. For example, a 10-degree visual field at one meter should "expand" to twice the size when the patient is tested at two meters (be sure also to double the size of the target). Patients who produce the same size field (tunnel visual field) or a smaller field—have demonstrated a nonphysiologic finding. Some patients with a monocular visual complaint will produce a hemifield defect when tested with both eyes open, but a normal, full visual field in the better eye.

Careful detection and/or measurement of the relative afferent pupillary defect (RAPD) is of vital importance in patients suspected of feigning visual loss. In patients with monocular complaints, documentation of a normal visual acuity and field in the sound eye, normal bilateral eye examination, and the lack of an RAPD is compelling evidence that a significant visual defect is unlikely in the eye of complaint. Electroretinography can objectively document relative health of the retina, but it does not test optic nerve function. Visual Evoked Potential testing is helpful if it is normal, but abnormal results can be produced by inattention, lack of accommodation, or failure to fixate on the alternating checkerboard pattern.

There is never a reason for the examiner to maliciously "confront" the patient proven to have functional visual loss. The patient (and the family if present) is presented with the good news that the examination showed the eyes and brain to be capable of normal vision and full recovery, and that a full report supporting this finding would be forthcoming. Patients near the hysterical end of the spectrum will benefit from reassurance, and those who are truly malingering will find it hard to argue with good news.

■ REFERENCES

1. Burde RM, Savino PJ, Trobe JD: Clinical Decisions in Neuro-ophthalmology, ed 2. St. Louis—CV Mosby Co, 1992.
2. Frisén L: Clinical Tests of Vision. New York—Raven Press, 1990.
3. Glaser JS: Neuro-opthalmologic examination: General considerations and special techniques. In Glaser JS (editor); Neuro-Ophthalmology. Philadelphia: JB Lippincott Company, 1990, pp. 37–60.
4. Glaser JS, Goodwin JA: Neuro-opthalmologic examination: The visual sensory system. In Glaser JS (editor); Neuro-ophthalmology. Philadelphia—JB Lippincott Company, 1990, pp. 9–36.
5. Glaser JS, Savino PJ, Sumers KD, McDonald SA, Knighton RW: The photostress recovery test in the clinical assessment of visual function. Am J Ophthalmol 83:255–260, 1977.
6. Hart WM, Jr.: Acquired dyschromatopsias. Surv Ophthalmol 32:10–31, 1987.
7. Keltner JL, Johnson CA: Automated and manual perimetry—A six-year overview. Special emphasis on neuro-ophthalmic problems. Ophthalmology 91:68–85, 1984.
8. Kollner—H: Die Stoungen des Farbensinnes. Ihre Klinische Bedeutung und ihre Diagnose. Berlin, Karger, 1912.
9. Leigh RJ, Zee DS: The Neurology of Eye Movements. Philadelphia—FA Davis Co, 1991, pp. 293–530.
10. Lepore FE: The neuro-ophthalmologic case history: Elucidating the symptoms. In Glaser JS (editor); Neuro-ophthalmology. Philadelphia—JB Lippincott Company, 1990, pp. 1–7.
11. Martin TJ, Robison GD—IV: Instrument for measuring relative brightness perception. AJO 1994;117:625–631.
12. May M, Galetta S: The facial nerve, in Duane TD, Jager EA (editors): Clinical Ophthalmology, Vol 2, chapter 8. Philadelphia, JB Lippincott Co, 1988, pp 30–31.
13. Mills RP: Automated perimetry in neuro-ophthalmology. Internat Ophthalmol Clin 31(4):51–70, 1991.
14. Pelli DG, Robson JG, Wilkins AJ: The design of a new letter chart for measuring contrast sensitivity. Clin Vision Sci 2:187–190, 1988.
15. Plum F, Posner JB: The diagnosis of stupor and coma, 3rd ed. Philadelphia—FA Davis, 1980.
16. Pokorny J, Smith VC, Verriest G, et al: Congenital and Acquired Color Vision Defects. New York—Grune & Stratton, 1979.
17. Sadun AA, Lessell S: Brightness-sense and optic nerve disease. Arch Ophthalmol 103:39–43, 1985.
18. Slamovits TL, Hedges TR III, Kupersmith MJ, Newman NJ, Sadun AA, Sedwick LA: Basic and Clinical Science Course 1994–1995, Section 5, Neuro-Ophthalmology. San Francisco—American Academy of Ophthalmology, 1994.
19. Thompson HS, Corbett JJ, Cox TA: How to measure the afferent pupillary defect. Surv Ophthalmol 26:39–42, 1981.
20. Thompson HS, Kardon RH: Clinical importance of pupillary inequality. In Focal Points: Clinical Modules for Ophthalmologists. San Francisco—American Academy of Ophthalmology, vol 10, 1992, pp 1–12.
21. Trobe JD, Acosta PC, Krischer JP, Trick GL: Confrontation visual field techniques in the detection of anterior visual pathway lesions. Ann Neurol 10:28–34, 1981.
22. Wall M, Sadun AA: Threshold Amsler grid testing: Cross-polarizing lenses enhance yield. Arch Ophthalmol 104:520–523, 1986.

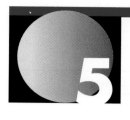

5 Neuro-Anatomy of the Sensory Visual System

Edward G. Buckley

The visual sensory system begins with the retinal ganglion cells and ends in the occipital lobe at the striate cortex, remaining in a relatively horizontal plane, anterior to posterior, as it transverses the brain (Fig. 5–1). Since the information which is transmitted by the optic nerve, chiasm, optic radiations, and visual cortex is very different and highly organized, abnormalities in visual function can usually be attributed to a specific area in the brain enabling accurate anatomical localization (Table 5–1).

■ EMBRYOLOGY

The visual sensory system is formed early in the embryo and begins at the 1.5–2 mm (three week) stage when the optic vesical begins to form. The precursor to the optic nerve forms as a proximal constriction, the optic stock, between the optic vesicle and the prosencephalon at the 4 mm (four week) embryonic stage (5). During the 18–25 mm embryonic stage, fascicles of the ganglion cell axons grow from the developing retina into the optic stock. At a gestational age of approximately 50 days the optic nerve contains a full compliment of retinal ganglion cell axons. At the end of the second month of gestation, the two optic nerves unite in the floor of the diencephalon forming the optic chiasm with a partial decussation of fibers (7). Myelin is added to the nerve beginning at the optic chiasm in the 23rd week of gestation and progresses toward the lamina cribosa completing its journey by 4–6 weeks after birth.

■ RETINA

The process of converting light to neuro-images begins in the highly complex cellular structure of the retina. While photoreceptors (rods and cones) are the elements of the retina that are sensitive to light, there are numerous other cell types which begin the process of modifying and end-coding the signal even before it reaches the ganglion cell. Different types of ganglion cells continue this process by selectively transmitting specific visual information such as acuity, color, contrast, and movement detection. The large Alpha *ganglion cells* transmit information about motion detection while the smaller Beta *ganglion cells* transmit information about color and contrast. This type of differentiation in function continues throughout the visual sensory system.

A spacial as well as functional segregation also exists throughout the visual system (6). Nerve fibers from retinal ganglion cells which respond to a specific portion of

TABLE 5–1
Ophthalmic Signs from Visual Pathway Lesions

Lesion	Vision	Pupil	Visual Field Defects
Optic Disc	Normal or decreased	Ipsilateral afferent defect	Central scotoma, altitudinal, arcuate
Optic Nerve	Decreased	Ipsilateral afferent defect	Central scotoma, altitudinal, hemianopic wedge
Chiasm	Normal or decreased	Normal or afferent defect	Bitemporal, junctional, binasal
Optic Tract	Normal	Contralateral afferent defect	Hemianopia
Lateral Geniculate	Normal	Normal	Homonymous congruous sectorial defects
Optic Radiations	Normal	Normal	Homonymous quadrantopia or hemianopia
Occipital Cortex	Normal	Normal	Homonymous congruous hemianopia or quadrantopia, bilateral altitudinal, checkerboard, monocular crescent

the visual field remain anatomically segregated throughout the visual system. A "retinotopic" representation occurs with the superior visual field projected onto the inferior retina and the nasal field onto the temporal retina. This inverted relationship continues in the optic nerves, chiasm, radiations and visual cortex (Fig. 5–2). At the retinal level, the division is centered around the fovea such that the nasal visual field is represented by retinal ganglion cells temporal to the fovea and the temporal visual field is represented by ganglion cells nasal to the fovea. A line from the optic disc to the fovea separates the superior and inferior projections. The ar-

rangement changes somewhat as the fibers travel posteriorly (Fig. 5–3).

The fovea, which is a specialized area of the retina consisting primarily of cones, has a photoreceptor to ganglion cell ratio approaching one to one. These ganglion cell axons travel directly to the optic nerve in the papillomacular bundle which comprises approximately 60–70% of the fibers traveling in the optic nerve. So as not to degrade the visual image, the remaining fibers detour around the macular area and travel in an arcuate course above and below the papillomacular bundle making retinal and optic disc lesions easily identifiable by visual field testing.

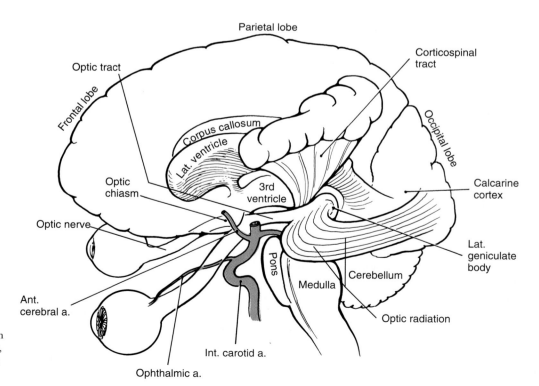

Figure 5–1.
The *afferent visual system.* Because of the close relationship of the visual system to other intracranial structures, lesions in these areas can often be easily localized.

OPTIC DISC

The optic disc is the exit site of all retinal ganglion cell axons. It is located 3.5 mm nasal to the fovea and is approximately 1.7 mm in vertical diameter and 1.5 mm in horizontal diameter. There are no photoreceptors overlying the disc. On visual field testing it is projected into the temporal visual field as an absolute scotoma approximately 15 degrees from fixation. There is a central depression of variable width and depth which is called the "optic cup". The normal ratio of cup diameter to disc diameter is approximately .03. The retinal axons pass through a fenestrated connective tissue called the lamina cribrosa. Here axonal bundles become compartmentalized and are surrounded by glial tissue (myelinated).

The blood supply to the optic disc comes from the *circle of Zinn-Haller*. It receives blood from three sources, the short posterior ciliary arteries, the choroidal vessels, and the pial vessels that supply the outer surface of the optic nerve.

OPTIC NERVE

The optic nerve can be divided into four distinct segments (3). The intraocular portion (the optic disc) is non-myelinated and approximately one millimeter in length. Immediately behind the sclera, the orbital portion of the nerve axons become myelinated. Since the optic nerve is really a central nervous system tract, myelin is formed by oligodendrocytes as opposed to Schwann cells which perform this function in peripheral nerves. In addition, the optic nerve is susceptible to the same diseases as other central nervous system tracts such as multiple sclerosis. The nerve is also surrounded by three layers of meninges; the pia, arachnoid, and dura mater. The subarachnoid space contains cerebrospinal fluid, is continuous with the intracranial subarachnoid space, and extends into the posterior one-half of the scleral thickness where it is separated from the vitreous cavity by a thin layer of scleral fibers. The combination of myelination and meningeal sheaths results in enlargement of the nerve from 1.5 mm to 3–4 mm in diameter as it exits the globe (10).

The intraorbital portion of the optic nerve is approximately 30 mm in length (4). Since the distance from the posterior aspect of the globe to the orbital apex is only 20 mm, there is a considerable amount of redundancy which causes the nerve to take an S-shaped configuration. This extra length allows for ocular movement and approximately 8–9 mm of axial proptosis without injury to the nerve. The intraorbital portion of the optic nerve is surrounded by the posterior ciliary arteries and nerves. The central retinal artery enters the nerve inferior and medially about 15 mm behind the globe.

At the orbital apex the optic nerve enters the bony optic canal and is surrounded by the Annulus of Zinn which is composed of the tendinous origins of the superior, medial, and inferior rectus muscles. Along with the optic nerve, the canal contains the ophthalmic artery. The optic canal measures 5–7 mm in length and runs posteriorly and medially forming an angle of approximately 35 degrees with the mid-sagittal plane. As the optic nerve exits the canal posteriorly it passes through a fold of dura which is fixed to the periostium of the bone making it particularly susceptible to traumatic injury. In addition, small tumors or ophthalmic artery aneurysms in this location can result in severe visual loss.

The intracranial segment of the optic nerve measures approximately 15 mm in length and courses posteriorly and medially, ascending at an angle of approximately 45 degrees to the horizontal plane. Superiorly is the inferior surface of the frontal lobes and the anterior cerebral and anterior communicating arteries. Inferiorly is the intracavernous portion of the internal carotid artery. Aneurysms arising from any of these vessels may compress the nerve in this region.

The optic nerve axons retain a similar spacial orientation as those in the retina. Those fibers serving the superior retina remain superior and those from the medial retina remain medial. The macula fibers which constitute a large portion of the optic nerve are located centrally.

OPTIC CHIASM

The optic nerves converge just above the sella turcica to form a structure called the optic chiasm (because it is shaped like the Greek letter "Chi"). The fibers originating from the nasal half of each retina cross in the chiasm to join the temporal retinal fibers from the contralateral optic nerve to form the optic tracts (Fig.

5–1). Thus the nasal retinal fibers from the right eye join the temporal retinal fibers from the left eye to form the left optic tract which contains visual information exclusively from the right hemifield (Figs. 5–2 and 5–3). Since the nasal retina represents the larger temporal visual field (53% of the nerve) there are more crossed than uncrossed fibers in the chiasm. Fibers that originate in the inferior retina remain inferior in the optic nerve and optic chiasm. Inferior nasal fibers (serving superior temporal visual field) cross in the anterior portion of the chiasm and loop into the terminal portion of the opposite optic nerve before proceeding into the contralateral optic tract (*Wilbrand's knee*) (Figures 5–2 and 5–3). The superior nasal fibers cross in the posterior notch of the chiasm and join with the contralateral superior temporal fibers beyond the chiasm

in the medial side of the tract. The macular fibers are predominantly posterior and superior in the chiasm.

The optic chiasm measures 13 mm (10–20 mm) in transverse diameter, 8 mm (4–13 mm) in anterior posterior extent and is 3–5 mm thick. It lies above the sphenoid bone and the dorsum sellae (2). It is separated from the diaphragma sellae and pituitary gland by a distance of up to 10 mm. Lesions of the pituitary gland often have to be quite large before actually compressing the optic chiasm. The optic chiasm is contiguous with the floor of the third ventricle and is often compressed by ventricular tumors or hydrocephalus. Its position over the dorsum sellae can vary considerably in the anterior/posterior direction.

A few fibers have been shown to exit from the dorsal surface of the optic chiasm and enter directly into the

Figure 5–2.
A schematic of the visual afferent system. Sections A–F illustrate the retinotopic arrangement of the nerve fibers as they travel from the optic nerve to the occipital lobe. Superior fibers tend to remain superior except in the tract and lateral geniculate where they rotate medially. Sections 1–9 illustrate typical visual field defects secondary to a lesion at the numbered location. Lesions located at the chiasm or more posterior result in bilateral visual field defects. Section #3 involves Wilbrand's knee from the opposite optic nerve (also see Fig. 5–3). The more posterior the lesion the more "congruous" the field defect. (M = macula, I = inferior, S = superior, T = temporal, N = nasal, Hypoth = Hypothalmus).

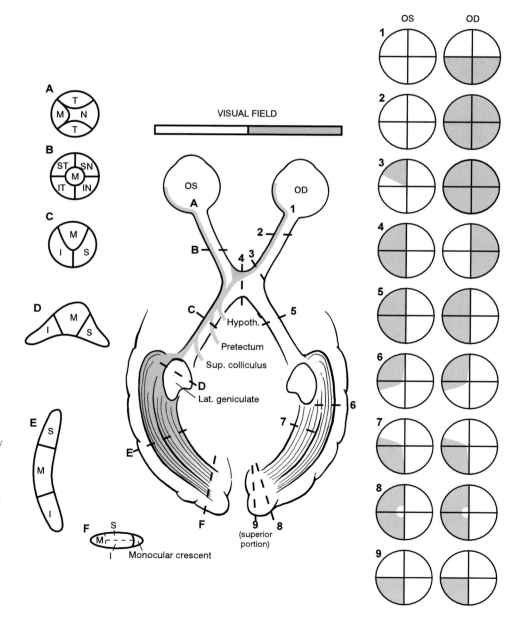

hypothalamus to terminate in the supra-chiasmatic nucleus or the supra-optic nucleus of the hypothalamus (8). These pathways provide the visual information necessary to produce the *circadian control* of the neuro endocrine system (Fig. 5–2) (9).

■ OPTIC TRACTS

The optic tracts contain visual information from the same visual hemisphere of each eye. The left optic tract contains information from the right visual hemifield of each eye, and the right optic tract contains information from the left hemifield. The tract begins at the posterior notch of the chiasm and proceeds posteriorly and laterally around the cerebral peduncle. The fibers terminate in the ipsilateral lateral geniculate nucleus. A group of axons leave the tract and proceed to the superior colliculus and the pretectum of the rostral mesencephalon. These fibers represent the afferent limb of the pupillomotor reflex (Figures 5–1, 5–2, and 5–3).

The retinotopic configuration is slightly different in the tract than elsewhere. As similar visual field fibers begin to join in the anterior tract, the inferior retinal fibers are located laterally and the superior retinal fibers are located medially. This represents approximately a 90 degree rotation medially from the normal position elsewhere in the visual system (Fig. 5–1). The nerve fibers from the corresponding retinal elements are not closely aligned at this stage. Tract lesions will characteristically cause an incongruous homonymous hemianopsia. In addition, because the cell bodies are located in the retina, optic atrophy may occur.

■ LATERAL GENICULATE NUCLEUS

Fibers that originate from the retinal ganglion cells synapse at the lateral geniculate nucleus with cells whose axons will eventually terminate in the occipital cortex at the lateral geniculate nucleus (Fig. 5–1). Neurons of the lateral geniculate nucleus form six layers. Ipsilateral retinal ganglion cells synapse in layers 2, 3, and 5, while contralateral retinal fibers synapse in layers 1, 4, and 6 (Fig. 5–4). As in the optic tract, a 90 degree medial rotation occurs so that nerve fibers from the superior retina lie medially while nerve fibers from the inferior retina lie laterally. As the fibers leave the lateral geniculate, a lateral rotation occurs so that superior and inferior retinal fibers again lie superior and inferior in the optic radiations and cerebral cortex.

Retinal *alpha and beta ganglion* cells terminate in different layers of the lateral geniculate nucleus. The large alpha cells terminate in the *magnocellular* layers 1 and 2, and are responsible for motion detection, stereopsis, and low spacial frequency contrast sensitivity. The smaller beta cells terminate in the *parvicellular* layers 3, 4, 5, and 6, and are responsible for fine spacial resolution and color vision. The information conveyed by the magnocellular and parvicellular layers of the lateral geniculate nucleus remain segregated in the occipital striate cortex and is directed to different regions within the extra striate cortex.

■ OPTIC RADIATIONS

Fibers from the lateral part (inferior fibers) of the lateral geniculate nucleus are directed inferiorly and forward to sweep around the anterior tip of the temporal horn of the lateral ventricle. The most anterior/inferior fiber fascicle forms a bend (*Meyer's loop*) containing fibers that represent the inferior retinal quadrants (contralateral superior visual field). This loop is located approximately 4 cm caudal to the anterior pole of the temporal lobe. This configuration of the anterior portion of the visual radiations explains the tendency for superior homonymous quadranopic field defects with anterior temporal lobe lesions. Fibers from the medial portion of the lateral geniculate nucleus (superior retinal fibers) take a more direct, non-looping course to the occipital lobe. In the parietal lobe the radiation fibers course around the occipital horn of the lateral ventricle.

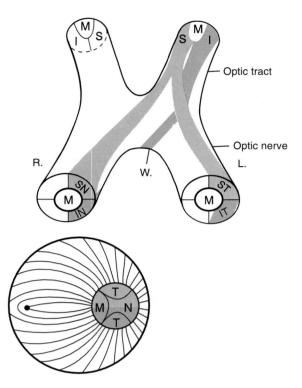

Figure 5–3.

Nerve fiber anatomy of optic chiasm. Nerve fibers receiving
information from similar visual field areas join together at the
chiasm. The superior nasal fibers from the right optic nerve join the
superior temporal fibers from the left optic nerve to form the
superior fibers of the optic tract. The inferior nasal fibers of the
right optic nerve detour into the left optic nerve before joining the
inferior temporal fibers W = (Wilbrand's knee). A lesion of the left
optic nerve at this location can cause a right superior temporal field
defect. (Junctional visual field defect. See Fig. 5–2, #3) Superior
fibers shown in grey, inferior fibers shown in red. (M = macula, S =
superior, I = inferior, N = nasal, T = temporal, R = right, L = left.)

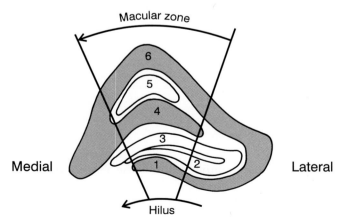

Figure 5–4.

A left lateral geniculate nucleus mid-coronal section. The retinal
projections from the ipsilateral optic nerve join in layers 2, 3, 5.
Those from the contralateral optic nerve join in sections 1, 4, 6.
Note the extensive macular representation.

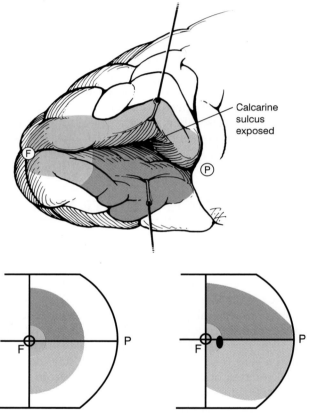

Figure 5–5.

Calcarine fissure left occipital lobe. A schematic showing the visual
field regions and their location in the calcarine cortex. More
posterior areas (grey) subserve the macula and make up
approximately 50% of the cortex. The foveal projections are on the
posterior surface of the occipital lobe (F). The peripheral visual field
areas are shown in red. Note that the upper field is represented in
the inferior calcarine strip and the lower field in the superior strip.
The temporal field of the right eye extends further than that of the
left. This monocular temporal crescent of the right eye is
represented at the most anterior portion of the calcarine cortex (P).

OCCIPITAL LOBE (STRIATE CORTEX)

The vision areas in the occipital cortex are made up of the *striate cortex* (Brodmann's Area 17), the parastriate cortex (Area 18) and the peristriate cortex (Area 19). The fibers from the optic radiations terminate in the striate cortex which is located along the inter-hemispheric surface above and below the calcarine fissure of the occipital lobe. Superior retinal fibers terminate in the upper calcarine strip and inferior retinal fibers terminate in the lower calcarine strip. The most posterior portion of the striate cortex is devoted to macular function which extends onto the lateral surface of the occipital lobe. The more anterior portions represent peripheral retina with the most anterior portion representing the monocular temporal crescent (Fig. 5–5). Cells in this area receive input solely from the peripheral nasal retina of the contralateral eye. Lesions in this area, therefore, can result in only monocular visual field loss or in an *incongruous (different field loss pattern in each eye) homonymous hemianopsia*. Because the striate cortex is divided into superior and inferior divisions as well as left and right, discreet lesions can result in *quadranopic visual field defects* which are quite similar in both eyes (*congruous*).

Visual information is transferred to the association Areas 18 and 19 for interpretation and processing. Area 18 sends information to the sensory motor pathways which are responsible for ipsilateral smooth pursuit eye movements. In addition, connections are made to the contralateral area 18 through the corpus callosum to integrate the two halves of the visual field. Final visual analysis is performed in the dominant parietal lobe (usually left hemisphere). A lesion interrupting the interconnections between the hemispheres and located on the dominant side can result in a "disconnection" *syndrome*. As an example, a patient who is left hemisphere dominant can have a lesion in the anterior portion of the left occipital lobe which interrupts the connecting fibers from area 18 on the right. Objects presented into the intact left visual field may not be recognized due to this "disconnection" between the right occipital lobe and the left hemisphere visual intergration area. A larger lesion may result in a complete right homonymous hemianopsia with the patient exhibiting alexia, agnosia, or agraphia in the remaining intact left visual field.

VASCULAR SUPPLY

The orbital portion of the optic nerve is supplied by the ophthalmic artery as well as small branches from the internal carotid, anterior cerebral, and anterior communicating arteries (1). The *optic chiasm* is supplied superiorly from the anterior cerebral artery and inferiorly from the internal carotid, posterior communicating, and posterior cerebral arteries. The *optic tract* is supplied by branches of the posterior cerebral artery and precommunicating portions of the anterior cerebral arteries. A branch of the middle cerebral artery and the anterior choroidal artery also supplies the optic tract.

The *lateral geniculate body* is supplied by the anterior thalamic branches of the posterior cerebral artery, anterior choroidal artery, and a portion of the posterior choroidal artery. The *optic radiations* are supplied by branches of the anterior choroidal, middle cerebral, and posterior cerebral arteries. *Calcarine fissure* is supplied mainly by the posterior cerebral artery with the occipital tip receiving a branch from the middle cerebral artery. This dual blood supply to the visual cortical area forms the basis for "macular sparing" than can occur in occipital lobe lesions.

REFERENCES

1. Anderson DR: Vascular supply of the optic nerve of primates. Am J Ophthalmol—1970:70:341.
2. Dutton JJ: Atlas of clinical and surgical orbital anatomy W.B. Saunders, Philadelphia, 1994.
3. Glaser JL: Neuro-ophthalmology. J.B. Lippincott Co. Philadelphia, 1990:61–81.
4. Hayreh SS: Anatomy and physiology of the optic nerve head. Trans Am Acad Ophthalmol Otolaryngol—1974:78:240–254.
5. Lemire R, Loeser J, Leech R, et al.: Normal and abnormal development of the human nervous system. In: The Optic System. Harper and Row, New York, 1975:196–205.
6. Livingstone M, Hubel D: Segregation of form, color, movement and depth. Anatomy, physiology and perception. Science—1988:240;740.
7. Rhodes RH: Development of the optic nerve. In: Jakobiec, FA (ed) Ocular anatomy, embryology and teratology. Philadelphia. Harper and Row, 1982:601–649.

8. Sadun AA, Johnson BM, Schaecheter JD: Neuroanatomy of the human visual system. Part III: Three retinal projections to the hypothalamus. Neuro Ophthalmology—1986:6:371–379.

9. Sadun AA, Schaecheter JD, Smith L: A retinohypothalmic pathway in man: light mediation of circadian rhythms. Brain Res—1984:302:371–377.

10. Sergott RC, Cohen MS, Bosley TM, et al.: The role of optic nerve sheath fenestration in management of anterior ischemic optic neuropathy. Arch Ophthalmol—1990:108: 1064–1065.

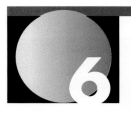

6 Neuro-imaging Techniques

Edward G. Buckley

■ MAGNETIC RESONANCE IMAGING

Magnetic resonance imaging (MRI) has become increasingly important in the diagnosis of diseases of the central nervous system (5). Its ability to give multi-slice imaging in virtually any plane of orientation and even three dimensional imaging has significantly advanced our ability for non-invasive assessment of the central nervous system. The process is based on the behavior of the hydrogen nucleus, the positively charged proton, in a magnetic field (6). When placed in a powerful magnetic field, the proton assumes an alignment with respect to the field either with or against the direction. When radio frequency energy is applied, protons aligned with the magnetic field absorb the energy and reverse their direction. The protons subsequently release the absorbed energy and in doing so produce a voltage (the magnetic resonance signal) which can be measured by a radio antennae. This antennae can surround the patient or be placed on a specific surface (surface coil). The major measurements used to construct the MRI image include:

1. *T1 relaxation time* (longitudinal or spin lattice relaxation time): as the nuclei return to the lower energy state (relax), energy is lost by interaction with the surrounding lattice or environment.
2. *T2 relaxation time* (transverse or spin/spin relaxation time)—this refers to the loss of energy that occurs because of the interaction with other nuclei aligned with the magnetic field.
3. Proton density.

T1 and T2 values are intrinsic to a given tissue. The images can be weighted to any of these parameters by varying the pulse sequence, the interval between repetitions of the pulse sequence, and the interval between radio frequency excitation and the measurement of the magnetic resonance signal (echo time). The scan images are pictorial representations of the spacial distribution of mobile protons. Contrast on scan images depends on the density of mobile protons in tissues and the relaxation times. One major weakness of magnetic resonance imaging in orbital work is its failure to image bone. Bone contains *slow moving* protons and appears black on magnetic resonance scans.

The most common scanning method utilized is the spin echo technique (2). With this technique one can obtain either T1 or T2 weighted images. To obtain a T1 weighted image requires approximately two minutes of scan time. The T1 value reflects the amount of water content within the tissue (7) (Fig. 6–1). Water has a longer T1 value than lipid. The imaging of the brain's grey and white matter is possible because of a difference in relative amounts of lipid and water in these tissues (1). On T1 weighted images, cerebral spinal fluid, aqueous, and vitreous appear dark and fat appears bright (Table 6–1).

The T2 value is in part dependent on the amount of molecular motion in tissue. In solids a T2 Time is always much shorter than a T1, but in liquids a T2 Time can be almost equal. In T2 weighted images, aqueous and vitreous are bright and fat is dark (Fig. 6–2). Air, cortical bone and calcium give no signal at all and appear black (Table 2). Anatomical detail is usually better seen on T1 weighted images. T2 weighted images tend to be more useful for showing abnormalities such as demyelinating plaques, tumors, and infarctions. Gadolinium-Diethylene Thiamine Pentacetic acid is useful as an intra-

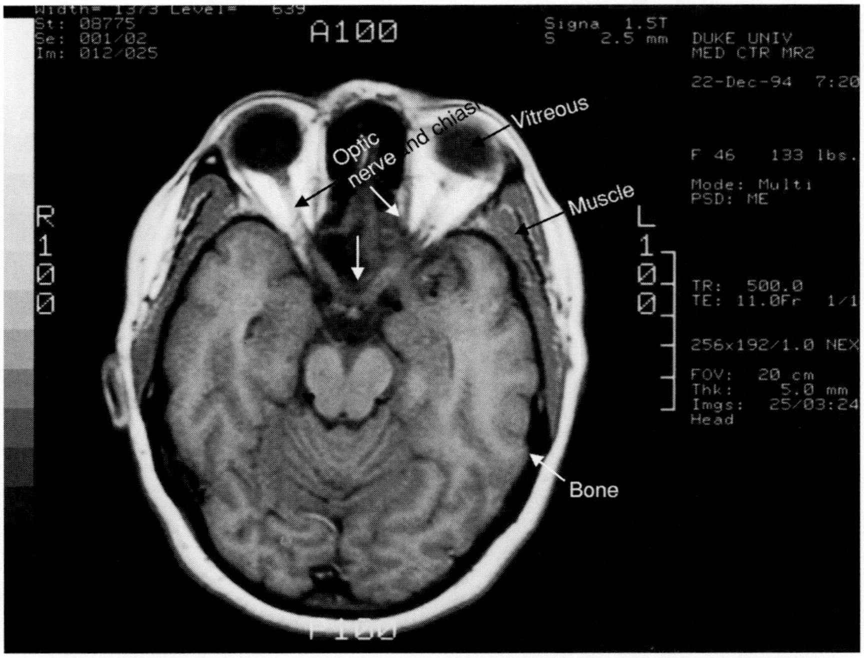

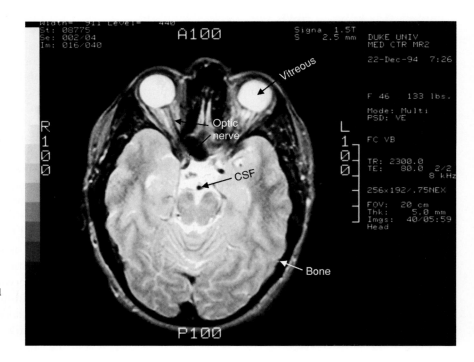

Figure 6–1.
T-1 weighted axial MRI scan of the head and ocular structures. Note that the vitreous blood and cerebral spinal fluid are all dark. Arrows illustrate the outline of the optic nerves and chiasm. The bone is not imaged on MRI scans and appears black. Whitish outline is actually skin and subcutaneous fat.

Figure 6–2.
T-2 weighted axial MRI scan of the head and ocular structures. Vitreous, cerebral spinal fluid, and blood are all white. Arrows show course of optic nerve in the orbit. Bones appear black.

venous contrast agent and highlight areas of blood brain barrier breakdown with a hyperintense signal on T1 weighted scans (4). Contrast enhancement also increases the signal intensity of well profused extra-axial lesions or those with slow blood flow such as the cavernous sinus.

A rapidly developing technology is MRI angiography (5). By using different parameters, blood appears as increased signal intensity without injection of contrast medium. Computer reconstruction results in three dimensional images that can be viewed on multiple projections. With continued improvements, MRI angiography may replace invasive cerebral angiography in many cases (8).

TABLE 6–1
Relative Signal Intensity on T-1 and T-2 Weighted MRI Scan

Tissue	T-1 Weighted	T-2 Weighted	Tissue	T-1 Weighted	T-2 Weighted
Brain			Cyst	Very Dark	Very Bright
white matter	Bright	Mod. Dark	Tissue enhanced with gadolinium		
gray matter	Mod. Dark	Bright	Low concentration	Very bright	Bright
CSF	Very Dark	Very Bright	High concentration	Mod. Dark	Very Dark
MS plaque	Dark	Bright	Muscle	Dark	Dark
Infarct	Dark	Bright	Hematoma		
Tumor	Dark	Bright	Acute	Mod. Dark	Dark
Abscess	Dark	Bright	Subacute	Bright rim	Bright
Water	Very Dark	Very Bright	Chronic	Dark rim ± bright center	Dark rim ± bright center
Fat	Bright	Dark			
Cortical Bone	Dark	Dark			
Air	Dark	Dark			

Adapted from Edelman et al (2) and Slamovits (4).

ADVANTAGES/DISADVANTAGES

The main advantages of MRI scanning are its ability to obtain high quality images in any plane. Since the presence of bone does not interfere with imaging (as in CT scanning), areas of high bone content such as the posterior fossa and cavernous sinus can be well defined. MRI is also useful for vascular malformations and aneurysms. Contrast MRI has become exceedingly useful in detecting multiple sclerosis (Table 6–2) (9).

A major disadvantage to MRI scanning is its long scan time and tight patient compartment which is especially bothersome to claustrophobic patients. MRI scanning is contraindicated in patients who have significant metallic appliances and cardiac pacemakers or if there is a question of an intraocular metallic foreign body.

TABLE 6–2
Preferred Imaging Techniques in Neuro-Ophthalmology

Location/Disease	CT Scan	MRI	Location/Disease	CT Scan	MRI
Ocular			Posterior fossa		+
Retinoblastoma	+		Intracerebral		
Melanoma		+	Tumor		+
Coats disease		+	Infections		+
Foreign bodies	+		Multiple sclerosis		+
Orbit	+		Infarction		+
Orbital Mass	+		Hematoma		
Optic Nerve Tumors	+		Acute	+	
Meningioma	+		Chronic		+
Glioma	+	+	Hydrocephalus		+
Thyroid Myopathy	+		Vascular disease		
Fractures	+		AV malformation	+	+
Intrasellar (microadenomas)			Aneurysm		
Suprasellar	+	+	Sinus Thrombosis	+	+
Chiasmal lesion		+	Dural Fistula	+	
Cavernous sinus		+	Congenital Malformation		+

Modified from Smith, JL and Quencer, RM: Neuroimaging, J. Clin. Neuroophthalmol, 7:97, 1987.

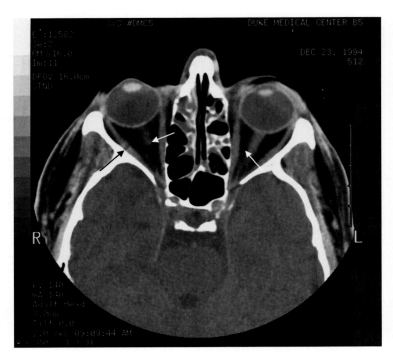

Figure 6–3.
Axial CT scan of the orbits. Note that ocular structures are seen in fine detail and extraocular muscles (dark arrow) and optic nerve (open arrow) are imaged easily. Contiguous sinus disease is easily identified and bony abnormalities are well imaged.

■ COMPUTERIZED TOMOGRAPHY

Computerized tomography (CT) scanning became widely available in the early 1970's. Tomographic x-ray images were computerized and then regenerated using algorithms which resulted in a two dimensional image. These images allowed identification of soft tissue structures which were difficult to appreciate using standard x-ray techniques (Fig. 6–3). Multiple scans could be obtained allowing superior diagnosis of intracranial diseases. Axial and coronal scans are performed directly and sagittal images are computer generated from the axial scans. CT scanned images can provide detail with a spacial resolution of $1 \times 1 \times 1.5$ mm^3. Injection of Iodinated intravenous dye improves the imaging of blood brain barrier breakdown areas associated with mass lesions, inflammation, infarcts, or demyelination. These enhanced CT scans are preferable unless the patient has a history of contrast allergy or renal insufficiency, or unless the scans are being obtained for localization of a foreign body. Pretreatment with steroids can be used in patients with a known allergic history. A patient undergoing a CT scan is exposed to approximately 2–3 rads. This is a dose similar to two chest x-rays or two orbital series of skull x-rays.

■ ADVANTAGES/DISADVANTAGES

The major advantage of CT scanning is its ability to image bone and adjacent soft tissue structures. CT scanning is preferred for orbital abnormalities because orbital fat provides excellent contrast from the other orbital structures. CT scanning is also useful in localizing metallic foreign bodies and is the only imaging technique available when significant metallic objects or appliances are present. CT scanning can detect calcium which is helpful in identifying such tumors as retinoblastoma or craniopharyngioma. Because of its ability to image bone it can be very helpful in identifying skull and facial fractures as well as for localization of intraocular foreign bodies (Table 6–2).

The main disadvantage of CT scans includes poor contrast between different soft tissues, artifacts from metallic objects, and the lack of direct sagittal scanning capability in the sagittal plane (Slamovitz).

■ POSITRON EMISSION TOMOGRAPHY (PET)

PET is a sensitive method of non invasively quantitating the physiology and biochemistry of the body. The moment to moment changes in the concentration of a radiopharmaceutical can be measured. Thus the kinetics of transport metabolism can be evaluated by modeling methods. The process is based on the existence of radionuclides of carbon nitrogen and oxygen as well as other elements. When the nucleus of one of these elements has fewer neutrons than protons, there is a tendency for a proton to become a neutron and this transformation results in the release of a positron. The positron interacts with an electron causing the release of energy in the form of high energy photons. These photons are converted into an electrical signal and the distribution of this activity is calculated by tomographic reconstruction procedures similar to those used in CT scanning (2).

■ REFERENCES

1. Brent-Zawadzki M: Magnetic resonance imaging of the brain. Radiology—1988:166:1–10.
2. Budinger TF, Drenzo SE, Huesman RH: Instrumentation for positron emission tomography. Ann Neurol 15 (suppl), 1984:535–543.
3. Council on scientific affairs magnetic resonance imaging of the central nervous system. JAMA—1988:259:1211–1222.
4. Edelman RR, Kleefield J, Wentz KU, Atkinson DJ: Basic principles of magnetic resonance imaging. In: Edelman RR, Hesselink JR (eds): Clinical magnetic resonance imaging. Philadelphia: W.B. Saunders, 1990:16.
5. Edelman RR, Mattle HP, Atkinson DJ, et al.: Magnetic resonance angiography. Am J Roentgenol—1990:154: 937–946.
6. Edelman RR, Warach S: Magnetic resonance imaging (first of two parts). NJM—1993:328:708–715.
7. Hupp S, Kline L: Magnetic resonance imaging of the optic chiasm. Survey of Ophthalmol—1991:36:207–216.
8. Jay WM: Advances in magnetic resonance imaging. Am J Ophthalmol—1989;108:592–596.
9. Slamovits TL, Gardner TA: Neuroimaging in neuro ophthalmology. Ophthalmol—1988:96:555–568.

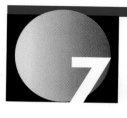

7 Optic Nerve Abnormalities

Steven Awner

I. Anomalous Optic Nerves

Drusen

Drusen (German, crystal) of the optic nerve head are recognized by the clinical appearance of an irregularly raised disc with a lobular surface in an otherwise healthy, asymptomatic individual. The disc may appear elevated with blurred margins, and nodular, glistening structures may be visible (Fig. 7–1). Using the red-free (green) filter on the direct ophthalmoscope, autofluorescence may be observed. Unlike early disc edema, there is no opacification of the peripapillary nerve fiber layer. Spontaneous venous pulsations are usually present, as well as anomalous branching of the retinal vessels, absence of disc hyperemia (capillary dilatation), and absence of venous engorgement. The central cup may be absent, but the vessels are not obscured crossing the disc margin and unlike papilledema, there are no peripapillary hemorrhages of exudates.

There is no leakage on fluorescein angiography differentiating this from early disc edema (1). Ancillary tests such as B-scan ultrasonography or CT scanning can reveal calcification in older children, however, these exams are not necessary to make the diagnosis. While most cases are idiopathic, association with acquired ocular diseases such as retinitis pigmentosa (54), angioid streaks, optic atrophy, vascular occlusions, hypertensive retinopathy, and chronic papilledema have been reported (1).

Usually inapparent during early life, drusen typi-cally enlarge with time and emerge to the disc surface during the teenage years. Approximately 75% are bilateral (1). Examination of family members can be productive, as drusen are sometimes inherited in an autosomal-dominant fashion with variable expressivity. Optic nerve drusen have only been described in Caucasian patients (1).

Drusen are the result of axonal degeneration and are composed of acellular concentric laminations which become calcified (67). Rarely, peripheral visual field loss and anterior ischemic optic neuropathy with retention of normal central visual acuity can occur with deep drusen that cause compression of nerve fibers (46, 60).

Optic Nerve Hypoplasia

Optic nerve hypoplasia is a rare nonprogressive congenital anomaly affecting one or both optic nerves and characterized by a decreased number of axons. Optic nerve hypoplasia is the most common developmental anomaly of the optic nerve and is important to recognize because of the potential for associated developmental and neuroendocrine problems.

Pathogenesis

Optic nerve hypoplasia usually occurs when an insult to the visual pathway transpires before development is completed (20, 47). Evidence suggests that the normal

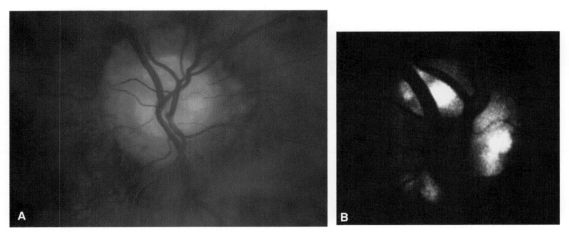

Figure 7–1.
Optic nerve drusen. Left, Pseudopapilledema appearance, note globular, calcific structures visible on disc surface, and absence of central cup. Right: Autofluorescence. Obtained using exciter filter and barrier filter. (Courtesy of Peter Buch, CRA.)

topographical development of the visual system progresses by selective regression of supernumerary axons (53). This process may be carried to an extreme resulting in hypoplastic nerve(s) (74). Teratogenic factors have been implicated, including phenytoin, quinine, lysergic acid diethylamide (LSD), phencyclidine (PCP), alcohol (50% of fetal alcohol syndrome), and possibly maternal diabetes and intrauterine cytomegalovirus (CMV) (74).

Clinical Manifestations

The child with bilateral optic nerve hypoplasia (approximately 60% of cases) usually presents with decreased vi-

sion and nystagmus. Unilateral or asymmetric bilateral cases often present with strabismus and amblyopia. Visual potential is determined by the integrity of the papillo-macular bundle and does not correlate with the overall size of the disc.

The classic appearance is a small gray optic disc surrounded by a yellow halo of hypopigmentation due to peripapillary retinal pigment epithelial and choroidal absence (the "double ring" sign) (Fig. 7–2) (72). The optic nerves may appear nearly normal in size with margins that are often sharply defined due to loss of axons in contrast to the normal disc which has slightly blurred nasal and superior margins. The retinal vessels are usually of normal caliber although their pattern at the disc

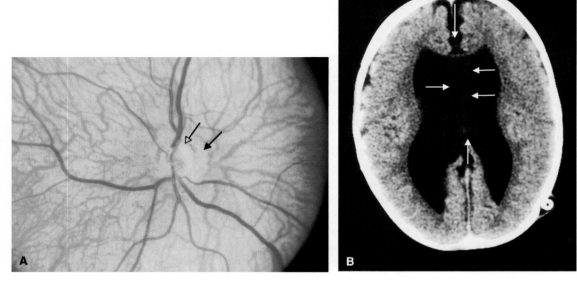

Figure 7–2a.
2a. Optic nerve hypoplasia. Notice the double-ring sign due to small optic disc (open arrow) within normal scleral canal (closed arrow).
2b. Septo-optic dysplasia. Axial CT scan demonstrates absence of septum pellucidum and hypoplasia of the corpus callosum (arrows).

can be very abnormal (40). Pupillary responses to light are usually sluggish or absent. In asymmetric bilateral or unilateral cases, an afferent pupil defect can be detected. Visual field testing performed in older patients has demonstrated generalized constriction, altitudinal, and bitemporal hemianopic defects (40). A unique type of optic nerve hypoplasia has been described in cases with maternal diabetes. It involves segmental hypoplasia of the superior disc with inferior altitudinal visual field defects (51).

Optic nerve hypoplasia is frequently associated with multiple CNS malformations. A common presentation is the triad of nystagmus, poor vision, and short stature: *Septo-optic dysplasia* (SOD) or *"de Morsier's Syndrome"* (55). The associated intracranial deficits include absence of the septum pellucidum, partial or complete agenesis of the corpus callosum, dysplasia of the anterior third ventricle (Holoprosencephaly), and bilateral optic nerve hypoplasia (Fig. 7–2b). The structural defects can be associated with significant hypothalamic-pituitary axis abnormalities. Endocrine abnormalities may also occur in patients with optic nerve hypoplasia but without midline craniofacial anomalies (63) (Table 7–1).

The findings of posterior pituitary ectopia and cerebral hemispheric abnormalities on MRI are highly predictive of pituitary hormone and neurodevelopmental deficits (12).

General management recommendations include neuroimaging, endocrine evaluation, and a trial of occlusion therapy in unilateral or asymmetric bilateral cases for strabismic amblyopia.

Optic Disc Colobomas

Ocular coloboma is a common ocular malformation which refers to a developmental defect in the internal structure of the eye. It can occur as an isolated finding in an otherwise healthy individual or as part of a complex malformation syndrome. Ocular colobomas can present as an optic disc, retinochoroidal or iris anomaly and can be autosomal dominant.

TABLE 7–1
Optic Nerve Hypoplasia: Associated Endocrinologic Abnormalities

---

Growth hormone deficiency
Congenital hypothyroidism
   a) prolonged hyperbilirubinemia (neonatal jaundice)
Diabetes insipidus
Infantile hypoglycemia
   a) neonatal seizures or coma
Hyperprolactinemia
Sexual precocity
Hypoadrenalism

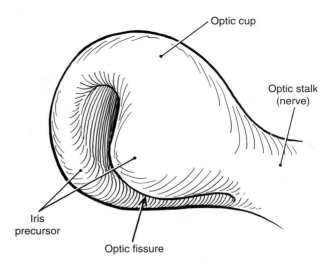

Figure 7–3.
Developing eye. Embryonal fissure located inferiorly.

Pathogenesis

Colobomas result from failure of the embryonic fissure to properly close. The embryonic fissure is the opening along the inferior aspect of the developing eye through which mesodermal tissue enters the globe (Fig. 7–3). Closure normally begins at the midpoint of the fissure at approximately five to six weeks and extends proximally and distally. Failure of closure of the proximal end results in optic disc coloboma. Multiple secondary ocular malformations may accompany colobomas presumably due to neuroectodermal induction anomalies. The peripapillary retina may be dysplastic and there may be ectopic choroidal development into cartilage, bone, muscle or fat (1).

Clinical Manifestations

The colobomatous disc is an enlarged, excavated, sharply demarcated defect with normal retinal vessels appearing at the margin of the excavation. The location of the excavation is always centered inferiorly, reflecting its embryologic origins (1, 52). An associated staphyloma of the inferior choroid and retina may be present. The retinal vessels may course around the adjacent chorioretinal coloboma or pass directly over the defect (Fig. 7–4).

When the coloboma is isolated to the disc, vision may be normal unless the defect involves the macula or microphthalmia is present (1). Serous macular detachments can occur from isolated optic disc colobomas. Colobomas can be unilateral or bilateral, and asymmetric microphthalmos may be associated with coloboma and/or with a colobomatous cyst. Unilateral optic disc colobomas can present with strabismus, decreased vision, amblyopia, or microphthalmos. *Fuchs' coloboma* or inferior crescent is a partial coloboma involving the in-

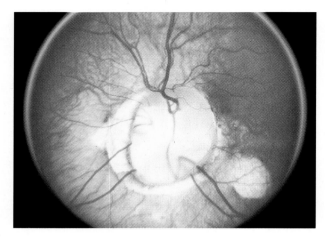

Figure 7–4.
Optic disc coloboma. Excavation of nerve inferiorly with normal retinal vessels.

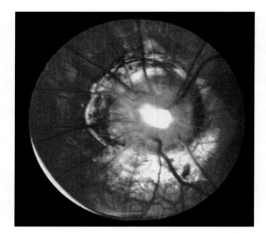

Figure 7–5.
Morning-Glory disc anomaly. Enlarged disc with central glial tuft and retinal vessels coursing radially. Peripapillary pigmentary disturbance is also noted.

ferior aspect of the optic nerve head and is generally an incidental finding in an otherwise normal eye.

An important systemic syndrome associated with optic disc colobomas is the *CHARGE association* (*C*oloboma, *H*eart defects, choanal *A*tresia, *R*etarded growth and development, *G*enital hypoplasia, and *E*ar anomalies) (16). A chromosomal abnormality should be considered when colobomas occur in patients with multiple congenital anomalies, mental retardation, or growth failure (16). Associated central nervous system abnormalities such as basal encephalocele can occur and neuroimaging should be considered, especially in bilateral cases.

Morning-Glory Disc Anomaly

The morning-glory disc anomaly is a rare congenital excavated lesion involving the optic disc. The morning-glory disc is embryologically unrelated to optic disc coloboma and is so named because of its resemblance to the morning glory flower (36). The morning-glory disc is situated within a funnel-shaped staphylomatous excavation involving the nerve and peripapillary retina (Fig. 7-5). The retinal vessels are abnormal, appearing at the peripheral disc and coursing over the elevated pink rim in a radial fashion (1, 36, 52). Pulsatile opening and closing of the disc excavation during fundus photography has been observed and may be related to fluctuation of fluid between the subarachnoid and subretinal space (52). Pollock hypothesized that the morning glory syndrome represents an anomalous persistence of the posterior cavity of the primitive optic cup which produces a funnel-shaped enlargement of the distal optic stalk where it joins the optic cup. The glial and vascular abnormalities occur at a later stage of development (52).

Clinical Manifestations

Most cases are unilateral presenting with strabismus and poor vision (20/200 to finger counting). Bilateral cases

tend to have better acuity (9). Females are affected twice as often as males and most cases occur in Caucasians (52). Visual field testing typically reveals a central scotoma with preserved peripheral fields (9).

Follow up is important to monitor for development of nonrhegmatogenous retinal detachment which occurs in 38% of eyes. Basal encephaloceles may accompany morning-glory syndrome. Midline defects such as hypertelorism, cleft lip or cleft palate should alert the practitioner to investigate further with craniofacial evaluation and neuroimaging (21, 33).

Myelinated Retinal Nerve Fibers

Myelination (Medullation) of the optic disc and superficial retinal nerve fiber layer is a benign developmental anomaly. Myelination of the visual pathways normally begins in the lateral geniculate body during mid-gestation and proceeds peripherally along the optic tracts, chiasm and nerves. By full term or in the immediate postnatal period, myelination normally halts at the lamina cribosa. Continued myelin deposition produces a flat white, striated appearance of the nerve fibers over the disc and adjacent retinal surface (1, 14). A feathery edge is usually noted and the lesion follows the arcuate pattern of the normal nerve fiber layer. There is no surrounding retinal pigment epithelial disturbance. Myelinated nerve fibers have occasionally been noted in the peripheral retina separated from the optic disc by normal retina (Fig. 7–6).

Clinical Manifestations

Myelinated nerve fibers are noted in males twice as often as females and occur unilaterally in 80% of cases. Visual acuity is generally unaffected but if decreased, high myopia and macular hypoplasia should be suspected. Enlargement of the blind spot or an arcuate

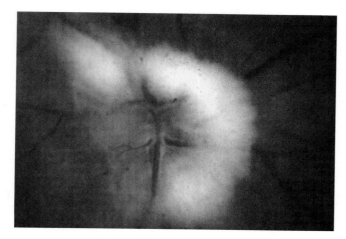

Figure 7–6.
Myelinated retinal nerve fibers.

scotoma corresponding to the affected retina may be noted (1). The condition is nonprogressive once identified and treatment should be directed to any associated anisometropic amblyopia. Myelination adjacent to the disc can give the appearance of pseudo disc edema (Table 7–2).

Pigmented Optic Disc

Congenital gray pigmentation of the optic nerve occurs in premature infants with delayed visual maturation, infants with ocular albinism and in isolated chromosomal abnormalities (partial trisomy 10q syndrome). The gray appearance of these discs is a transient phenomenon lasting for several months and is not caused by melanin deposition. The disappearance of the gray discoloration is attributed to an optical effect that normalizes with early development. Another group of patients have gray discs due to melanin deposition within or on the surface of the disc. This rare condition has been reported in a chromosomal abnormality (interstitial deletion of chromosome 17) and in Aicardi's syndrome (66). Visual potential is normal unless concordant disc anomalies such as hypoplasia are present (14). Acquired pigment of the disc can occur by deposition of blood products following vitreal hemorrhage or retinal detachment. Other

TABLE 7–2
Pseudopapilledema

> Optic disc elevated
> Margins blurred
> No opacification of nerve fiber layer
> Central cup absent
> Anomalous branching of retinal vessels
> No disc hyperemia
> No vessel enlargement
> Spontaneous venous pulsations usually present
> No peripapillary hemorrhages or exudates

pigmented optic nerve lesions include melanocytoma—and juxtapapillary choroidal melanomas (1).

Optic Pits

An optic pit is a congenital anomaly of the optic nerve consisting of a focal depression usually present on the temporal disc (Fig. 7–7). It occurs sporadically at a frequency of 1:11,000 births (39) with no sexual or racial predilection. The involved eye has an enlarged optic nerve (megalopapilla) in 80% of unilateral cases (1). Bilateral optic nerve pits are seen in 15% of cases and several eyes have been documented to have multiple pits within them. It can occupy between 0.1 to 0.7 disc diameters. The majority are located temporally (approximately 60%), ⅓ are located centrally and the remainder can occur at any other site on the disc (14).

Optic pits have been associated with serous detachments of the retina and macula. The retinal elevation is usually tear-drop shaped and can extend temporally from the disc margin to the macula. Multiple small yellow subretinal spots may be visible. The elevation is usually shallow and has been observed to fluctuate in size with time (14). Vision can be decreased or blurred with metamorphopsia. Multiple therapeutic modalities have been tried including retinal laser photocoagulation along the temporal disc margin with variable success. Controversy exists as to the etiology of the serous fluid. Hypotheses include liquefied vitreous from a posterior vitreous detachment (PVD) leaking into the pit or communication of cerebrospinal fluid (CSF) from the subarachnoid space (1, 14). Fluorescein angiography does help differentiate this entity from central serous retinopathy (14).

The Congenital Tilted Disc

This rare anomaly has been recognized by various names, including Fuchs' coloboma, congenital crescent, conus,

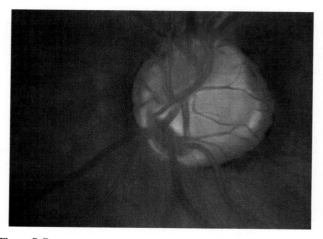

Figure 7–7.
Optic pit. (Courtesy of James D. Reynolds, MD.)

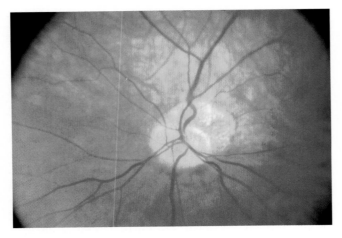

Figure 7–8.
Congenital tilted disc syndrome.

dysversion of the optic nerve head, and situs inversus. The inferior crescent appearance is caused by a D-shaped scleral opening which is smaller than the round retinal aperture at the optic nerve head (Fig. 7–8) (17). Neurosensory retina courses over the sclera without underlying retinal pigment epithelium or choroid accentuating the depressed inferior edge of the disc as compared to the crowded appearance of the superior disc.

The congenital tilted disc syndrome is nonprogressive and seen equally in male and female patients. There are no known associated systemic or neurologic diseases (1). Vision may be mildly reduced and a supero-temporal visual field defect corresponds to the loss of axons inferonasally. With bilateral tilted discs, bitemporal hemianopsias that do not respect the vertical midline may occur and need to be distinguished from true intracranial disease (73).

II. *Optic Neuropathies*

Optic Disc Edema

Definition

Optic disc edema is a diffuse or focal swelling of the optic nerve head caused by many ocular and systemic conditions. *Papilledema* is defined as bilateral (often asymmetric) optic disc edema due to raised intracranial pressure. Unilateral disc edema is usually associated with ocular or orbital processes while bilateral disc edema is due to intracranial or systemic diseases (Table 7–4). Early (acute) papilledema does not cause significant visual dysfunction.

Neuroimaging is urgently obtained in most cases of true papilledema. If an intracranial mass lesion is excluded and the ventricles are found to be normal or small in size, lumbar puncture should be performed to confirm the diagnosis.

TABLE 7–3
Differential Diagnosis of Pseudopapilledema

> Optic disc drusen
> Myelinated nerve fibers
> Persistence of Bergmeister's papilla
> Hyperopia
> Optic neuritis
> Epipapillary hamartomas and tumors

TABLE 7–4
Etiology of Disc Edema

Unilateral Disc Edema
  Optic Neuritis
  Anterior Ischemic Optic Neuropathy
  Ocular Hypotony (after surgery, trauma, uveitis)
  Glaucoma
  Central Retinal Vein Occlusion
  Intraorbital Tumors
  Optic Nerve Sheath Meningioma and Glioma
  Inflammation
    Syphilitic
    Neuroretinitis
  Carotid—cavernous sinus fistula
Bilateral Disc Edema (Papilledema)
  Mass lesions (neoplasms)
  Obstructive hydrocephalus
  Intracranial bleeding/hematoma
    1. Traumatic head injury (subarachnoid hemorrhage)
    2. Aneurysmal rupture
    3. Arteria-venous malformations (AVM)
  Venous outflow obstruction
    1. Venous sinus thrombosis
    2. Hypercoagulable states
    3. Mastoiditis
    4. Bilateral radical neck dissection
    5. Superior Vena Cava syndrome
  Previous inflammation (meningitis)
  Leptomeningeal cancer
  Idiopathic (pseudotumor cerebri)

Pathogenesis

The mechanism of papilledema is controversial. As intracranial cerebrospinal fluid (CSF) pressure increases, there also is a rise in the perioptic CSF pressure of the intraorbital optic nerve sheath. This compresses the optic nerve and blocks axoplasmic flow with initial intra-axonal edema. There is subsequent venous engorgement with extracellular edema, hemorrhage and exudate. The rate of rise and degree of elevation in intracranial pressure determines the rate of development of papilledema. A sudden rise of intracranial pressure (ICP) by a subarachnoid hemorrhage may produce papilledema rapidly (within hours) and with greater severity than does a slow elevation of ICP, which may take one week for clinical papilledema to be evident. The rate of regression of papilledema likewise reflects the chronicity of the disc edema; rapid regression of early papilledema occurs more quickly than does regression of fully developed or chronic papilledema, even with rapid lowering of ICP.

Clinical Manifestations

Papilledema is associated with transient visual obscurations lasting seconds and less frequently, with diplopia from abducens nerve palsy. In the early phases of papilledema, the vision is normal with mild blind spot enlargement on visual field testing. Chronic papilledema causes permanent visual loss with diminished acuity and visual field, brightness desaturation, dyschromatopsia, diminished pupillary responses, and eventual optic atrophy and blindness.

Nonspecific symptoms may include headache, nausea, vomiting, and neck stiffness; these accompany elevated intracranial pressure of any cause.

Ophthalmoscopically, papilledema is categorized into early, fully developed, and chronic stages. The earliest funduscopic change is thickening of the nerve fiber layer on the optic disc, obscuring the underlying retinal vessels (at first inferiorly, then superiorly, nasally, and lastly temporally). Using the red-free filter on the direct ophthalmoscope, one can observe loss of the peripapillary superficial light reflexes (28). The disc appears hyperemic due to capillary dilatation—occasional splinter nerve fiber layer hemorrhages are seen and the central physiologic cup is preserved. Spontaneous venous pulsations are absent when intracranial pressure is greater than 200 mm H_2O (71), however, they are not present in 20% of the normal population (41).

Acute, fully developed papilledema demonstrates elevation of the disc, enlarged veins, a larger number of splinter hemorrhages, and cotton wool spots (Fig. 7–9). In severe cases, circumferential retinal folds or striae appear, and choroidal folds may be visible. Hard exudates may be seen around the disc or in a half star shape radiating from the nasal macula due to the fan-shaped nerve fiber layer of the macula. Retinal hemorrhages may dissect to the subhyaloid or vitreous spaces.

Chronic papilledema has loss of the physiologic cup with marked obscuration of the peripapillary vessels and disc elevation giving a "champagne cork" appearance. Chronic papilledema can persist for months to years without loss of vision. Eventually disc swelling diminishes due to loss of retinal axons, with sheathed and narrowed retinal veins. Once atrophic, the optic discs are incapable of further swelling due to the lack of axons.

Pathology

The pallid swelling of disc edema results from a blockage of orthograde axoplasmic transport with dilatation

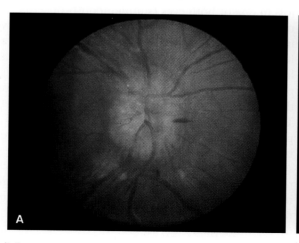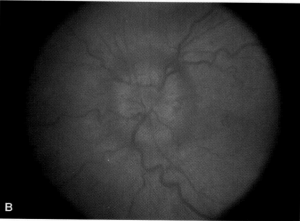

Figure 7–9.
Papilledema. **9a.** Fully developed papilledema with disc elevation, hyperemia, edematous nerve fiber layer, loss of central cup and splinter hemorrhages. **9b,** Papilledema with peripapillary subretinal hemorrhage and "champagne cork" appearance.

of ganglion cell axons. There is destruction, swelling, and fragmentation of the nerve fibers on the optic disc as well as the finding of "cytoid bodies." Electron microscopy demonstrates intracellular accumulation of mitochondria and axoplasmic debris at the site of axonal stasis (43, 68). This represents a non-specific response to anoxic injury of the nerve fibers. Elevation of the disc laterally displaces the peripapillary sensory retina causing blind spot enlargement on visual field testing.

Pseudotumor Cerebri

Pseudotumor cerebri (PTC) or *idiopathic intracranial hypertension* is a diagnosis made once intracranial mass lesions and other common causes of elevated intracranial pressure are excluded. The CSF pressure is elevated above 250 mm H_2O with normal fluid constituents.

The "typical" patient profile is a young, obese woman between 20 and 40 years of age. Recent weight gain is often an accompanying feature as is the hormonal changes of pregnancy and oral contraceptive use. A variety of drugs and endocrinologic disturbances have been implicated as etiologic factors in the development of PTC (Table 7–5). Empty sella syndrome is often present as well. PTC can occur in children, with equal gender frequency, and can be devastating visually

TABLE 7–5
Causes of Pseudotumor Cerebri

Endocrine
Hypothyroidism
Hyperthyroidism
Hypoparathyroidism
Adrenal insufficiency
Renal insufficiency
Exogenous growth hormone
Drug
Corticosteroid use/withdrawal
Vitamin A
Tetracycline
Lithium carbonate
Nalidixic acid
Phenytoin
Indomethacin
Nitrofurantoin
Oral contraceptives
Amiodarone
Sulfa
Other
Sarcoidosis
Systemic lupus erythematosis
Pregnancy
Iron deficiency anemia
Obesity

due to delay in diagnosis and treatment. Patients may present with abducens nerve palsy without other focal neurologic signs.

Treatment

Routine neuro-ophthalmic follow up is vital in patients with pseudotumor cerebri to prevent permanent visual loss. In adults, visual field evaluation to monitor nerve fiber layer damage is mandatory as insidious visual field loss may occur. Patients often seek medical attention for their symptoms of headache and transient obscurations of vision. Initial treatment consists of weight loss, elimination of any precipitating agents, and medication. Carbonic anhydrase inhibitors (acetazolamide or methazolamide) are started initially with furosemide or steroids adjunctively. However, corticosteroids may contribute to the elevation of intracranial pressure or raise the intraocular pressure. In children, the natural history of pseudotumor cerebri may be more progressive and visually damaging. Some practitioners recommend urgent therapy with intravenous steroids followed by a slow taper over several months monitoring the ophthalmoscopic appearance and visual function.

If progressive visual field loss occurs despite conservative medical therapy, surgical decompression is warranted. The two most utilized techniques are optic nerve sheath decompression (13) and lumbar-peritoneal shunting. Fenestration of a single optic nerve sheath in the more affected eye via a medial orbital approach will prevent further loss of vision, occasionally allow resolution of disc edema bilaterally and provide relief from headaches. Lumbar-peritoneal shunts are useful for patients with severe, intractable headaches.

Optic Neuritis

Optic neuritis is the rapid development of acute visual loss in one or both eyes (simultaneously or sequentially) usually due to acute demyelination of the optic nerves or inflammation. It usually occurs presents in young adulthood between the ages of 18 and 45 and within days may lead to severe loss of vision. Anterior optic neuritis (papillitis) (one-third of patients) occurs with blurring of the disc margin, hyperemia and elevation of the disc. There are no venous engorgement and minimal peripapillary hemorrhages (Fig. 7–10). Posterior or retrobulbar optic neuritis (two-thirds of patients) has the same symptomatology with a normal-appearing disc and retina. Other associated signs of optic nerve dysfunction include an afferent pupil defect, visual field loss, brightness desaturation, decreased contrast sensitivity, and dyschromatopsia. Pain on eye movement is very characteristic, occurring in 90% of patients with 40% experiencing pain before visual symptoms. (Table 7–6) (3, 50).

TABLE 7–6
Differentiation of Blurred Disc Margins

	Papilledema	Ischemic Optic Neuropathy	Optic Neuritis
Symptoms	Transient obscurations of vision, headache, emesis focal neurologic signs	None, painless, if arteritic constitutional symptoms	Pain with eye movement, acute loss of vision, metamorphopsia
Visual Acuity	Normal, late visual loss (optic atrophy)	Normal to 20/200 (non-arteritic) Less than 20/200 (arteritic)	20/20 to hand motions
Visual Field	Normal, enlarged blind spot	Altitudinal, arcuate, central	Generalized depression, altitudinal, central
Pupils	Normal	Afferent pupil defect	Afferent pupil defect
Fundus	Bilateral disc swelling, peripapillary hemorrhages, cotton wool spots	Pallid swelling, occasional CRAO* in arteritic	Papillitis (⅓) Retrobulbar (⅔)
Other	Always bilateral, may be asymmetric	Arteritic (over 50 years) bilateral in days to weeks, non-arteritic	White matter plaques on MRI
Age	Any age	40–60 years	Usually 15–50 years
Treatment	Rule-out neurosurgical emergency, lower intracranial pressure (ICP)	Check ESR, temporal artery biopsy & steroids if arteritic	Steroids for neurologic events, monocular patient, bilateral
Outcome	Good, if ICP lower, optic atrophy possible	Stable visual loss 25-40% fellow eyes affected	Generally good recovery in several weeks

	Pseudo Disc Edema (congenitally anomalous)	Compressive Optic Neuropathy	Toxic Optic Neuropathy
Symptoms	Asymptomatic	Variable proptosis, insidious visual loss	Painless, insidious bilateral central loss
Visual Acuity	Normal	Normal to NLP	Diminished 20/30—NLP
Visual Field	Possible enlarged blind spot arcuate	Variable defects, peripheral constriction	Ceco-central scotomas
Pupils	Normal	Afferent pupil defect	Possible afferent pupil defect
Fundus	Disc elevated, anomalous vessels, no central cup, hemorrhages or exudates	Normal optociliary shunts, choroidal folds	Normal, optic atrophy
Other	Usually unilateral	Ptosis, motility disturbance, usually unilateral	Neurologic symptoms
Age	Any age		20–60 years
Treatment	Observation	Neuroimaging	Remove offending agent, replace dietary deficiencies
Outcome	Normal	Variable	Reversible early

* CRAO = Central Retinal Artery Occlusion

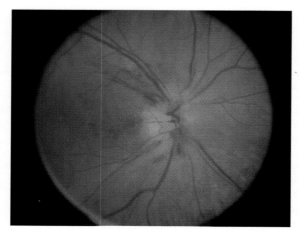

Figure 7–10.
Leber's hereditary optic neuropathy. Features include circumpapillary telangiectatic microangiopathy, disc hyperemia, "pseudoedema" (swelling of peripapillary nerve fiber layer), dilation, and tortuosity of retinal vessels. (Courtesy of Stephen C. Pollock, MD.)

The natural history of optic neuritis is recovery of vision with mild residual deficits noticeable to the patient including metamorphopsia—and decreased contrast sensitivity. A small central scotoma may persist and the optic disc may be pale temporally following an attack of papillitis. Some patients do not recover vision.

In adults, the most common cause of optic neuritis is idiopathic demyelination. Auto-immune disease (i.e., systemic lupus erythematosus), inflammatory lesions such as syphilis, sinusitis, viral causes (measles, mumps, chicken pox, infectious mononucleosis, herpes zoster, and immunizations), vasculitis, uveitis, exogenous drugs and toxins need to be considered. In children, optic neuritis is usually a post-viral, bilateral papillitis with more severe visual loss (20/200).

Devic's disease or neuromyelitis optica is the occurrence of bilateral optic neuritis followed by transverse myelitis days to weeks subsequently.

Multiple visual field defects occur including generalized depression, altitudinal defects, and central scotomas (35, 50). Almost 50% of visual fields are abnormal in the uninvolved fellow eye (6).

In the otherwise healthy patient with typical optic neuritis, rigorous laboratory evaluation is not productive (50). Examination of the cerebrospinal may show a mild lymphocytosis and protein elevation.

Treatment

Intravenous steroids have been shown to speed the return of visual function and may be indicated in bilateral severe visual loss, monocular patients, or in cases where there is a need for binocularity (occupational). If an MRI brain scan (obtained within eight days of onset) is suggestive of multiple sclerosis (greater than two white matter, high intensity, enhancing lesions), IV steroid therapy should be considered as treatment as it may decrease the frequency of subsequent neuorologic events (3–5). Children respond dramatically to intravenous steroids with prompt recovery of vision in most cases.

Prognosis

If visual improvement does not start within the first three weeks—or worsens following completion of steroid therapy, investigation for other etiologies such as compressive optic nerve lesions, vasculitis, sarcoidosis, syphilis, and Lyme disease should be pursued. Optic neuritis recurs in 15–30% of patients (4, 57).

There is a subsequent risk for developing multiple sclerosis (MS) in 74% of women and 34% of men with uncomplicated optic neuritis (57). A positive family history, female gender, younger age, white race and any prior non-specific neurologic symptoms (including prior optic neuritis) are associated with increased risk of MS.

Optic Disc Vasculitis

Optic disc vasculitis (big blind spot syndrome, papillophlebitis) is a rare unilateral optic neuropathy considered a mild form of central vein occlusion. Characterized by marked optic disc edema, retinal venous dilation, tortuosity, and peripapillary retinal hemorrhages, with mild visual dysfunction. Screening for autoimmune diseases such as systemic lupus erythematosus, Sjögren's syndrome and ulcerative colitis should be considered. Treatment with steroids has been effective, although visual recovery is variable (30).

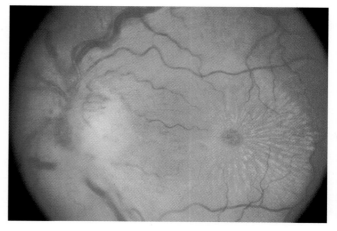

Figure 7–11.
Nonarteritic ischemic optic neuropathy (NAION).

Neuroretinitis

Neuroretinitis (Leber's idiopathic stellate neuroretinitis) is an acute optic neuropathy with disc swelling, peripapillary and macular lipid hard exudates in a star pattern, and vitreous cells (Fig. 7–11). It is a self-limited, systemic inflammatory disease that often follows a viral illness in patients younger than 50 years of age.

Infectious agents such as cat scratch fever (*Bartonella henselae* and *B. quintana*), influenza, mumps, chicken pox, tuberculosis, and leptospirosis have been implicated. The clinical course is usually benign, although permanent visual loss can occur. A VDRL and FTA-ABS should be performed to exclude neurosyphilis (18, 42). Treatment with systemic steroids has not been shown to be effective.

■ HEREDITARY OPTIC ATROPHY

Dominant Optic Atrophy

Must be considered in any child with insidious bilateral loss of central vision. Characteristically this usually begins before the age of 10 years—is bilateral but it can be asymmetrical. The visual loss is usually mild and ranges from 20/25 to 20/100. Visual fields show a subtle central or cecocentral scotoma with normal peripheral isopters. Color vision testing reveals a tritan or generalized dyschromatopsia. The temporal optic disc is pale with an area of triangular excavation. Inheritance is autosomal-dominant although family pedigrees are hard to elicit. Long-term prognosis is good with visual function rarely reduced to the 20/200 level. Differential diagnosis includes nutritional optic neuropathy, demyelinating disease, macular dystrophies, glaucoma, and other hereditary optic atrophies.

Recessive Optic Atrophy

A rare form of bilateral severe visual loss seen in children before the ages of five. Nystagmus is present in approximately half the patients. Funduscopic exam reveals a pale optic disc with vascular attenuation of the type characteristically seen in retinal degenerations. Electroretinographic testing, however, is normal. Other systemic abnormalities such as mental retardation, spasticity, hypertonia, and cerebellar ataxia can occur (*Behr's syndrome*).

Leber's Hereditary Optic Neuropathy (LHON)

A maternally inherited disease characterized by acute or subacute bilateral loss of central vision. Recent advances in monocular genetics have confirmed several primary mitochondrial DNA (mtDNA) point mutations at nucleotide positions 11778 (most common), 3460, and 14484 causing defective oxidative phosphorylation (32,

33). LHON is characterized by progressive bilateral (sequential or simultaneous) severe, painless central vision loss to the 20/200 level or worse, with acquired red/green dyschromatopsia, and central or cecocentral scotomas in otherwise healthy patients (usually male) in their second to fourth decade of life. Recovery of vision has been reported in 4–37% of patients, with the best prognosis in the 14484 mutation. The classic fundus picture consists of a triad of circumpapillary telangiectatic microangiopathy, pseudoedema of the disc, and absence of fluorescein staining. (Fig. 7–12) There is an association between LHON and the cardiac pre-excitation arrhythmia syndromes of Wolff-Parkinson-White. Molecular genetic analysis of mtDNA from leukocytes is currently available and the finding of a primary mutation is virtually pathognomonic for the disease. Currently there is no effective treatment.

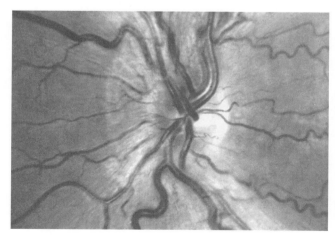

Figure 7–12.
Neuroretinitis. Note papillitis (optic disc swelling) and macular star formation due to lipid exudation from disc into Henle's nerve fiber layer.

■ NONARTERITIC ISCHEMIC OPTIC NEUROPATHY (NAION)

Pathogenesis

NAION is due to posterior ciliary artery insufficiency which causes relative ischemia to the prelaminar disc. The edematous axons compress the capillary and venous circulation, initiating a cycle of ischemia and axonal swelling which causes infarction of the nerve fibers and subsequent symptoms of optic nerve dysfunction (15).

Clinical Manifestations

NAION affects men and women in their fifth and sixth decade, with a slight male preponderance (1.5M:1F). Sudden painless visual loss is usually apparent upon awakening (8); although some studies contradict this as-

sertion (58). Vision can range from 20/20 to no light perception (NLP) but generally is better than 20/100. Patients most often exhibit inferior altitudinal visual field loss, although nerve fiber layer arcuate defects, generalized constriction or cecocentral scotomas are seen as well (26). Ophthalmoscopically, the disc usually exhibits pallid swelling in a sectorial or diffuse pattern (pathognomonic) (Fig. 7–13). Hyperemia of the disc may occur acutely. Lack of optic nerve abnormalities should make the diagnosis of NAION suspect, however, posterior ischemic optic neuropathy (PION) has been reported with hypotensive episodes (24). Optic atrophy and retinal arteriolar narrowing are constant late features (Table 7–6).

The visual loss is usually irreversible. Progressive stepwise deterioration in acuity and visual field may occur after six weeks (37). Spontaneous recovery has been

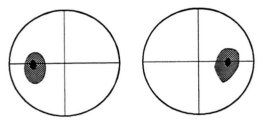

A. Bilateral Enlarged Blind Spots

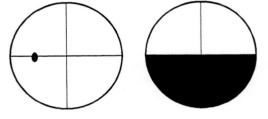

D. Altitudinal Defect OD

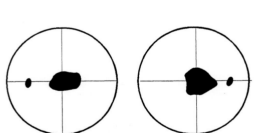

B. Bilateral Central Scotomas

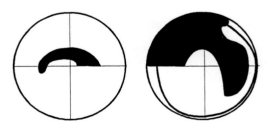

E. Arcuate Scotoma OU with Nasal Step

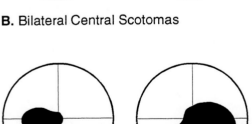

C. Bilateral Cecocentral Scotomas

Figure 7–13.
Visual field defects in optic nerve diseases.

noted (2) and recurrences in the same eye also may rarely occur months to years later (7, 11).

The fellow eye may be affected in up to 25–40% of patients (8, 61), with young diabetic males being at highest risk (8).

Laboratory

No definitive ancillary tests confirm the diagnosis of NAION. A Westergren erythrocyte sedimentation rate (ESR) is recommended in all patients over the age of 50 years to rule out temporal arteritis. General medical evaluation to monitor blood pressure and blood glucose levels is recommended.

Treatment

No form of treatment has been shown to improve the visual function in NAION (30, 62).

■ ARTERITIC ISCHEMIC OPTIC NEUROPATHY (GIANT CELL ARTERITIS)

A disease afflicting the elderly, its prevalence increases markedly from the sixth decade (33/100,000 population) through eighth decades (844/100,000 population) of life (22). Sudden, painless, and profound visual loss (count fingers to no light perception) (10, 56) occurs with "chalk-white" edema of the optic nerve. Perimetry commonly demonstrates central scotomas, inferior altitudinal, or inferior nasal defects. Females are affected three times as often as males (29). Bilateral presentation is common and concomitant central retinal artery occlusion or ciliary artery occlusion are well known (25).

Careful questioning for systemic symptoms of *temporal arteritis* such as headache, low grade fever, loss of appetite, malaise, jaw claudication, myalgia, arthralgia, tenderness upon brushing hair, or weight loss may help confirm the diagnosis. Tenderness over the temporal artery is common and the vessel may be pulseless. Abrupt loss of vision in the fellow eye may occur within days to weeks (69).

Laboratory and Treatment

The most useful laboratory test is the Westergren ESR. The ESR normally increases with age (divide the age plus ten by two in females and the age by two in males to calculate the upper limit of the normal ESR) (44) and is abnormal if greater than 35 mm/hr. Aspirin and nonsteroidal anti-inflammatory medications can artificially reduce the ESR. Prompt therapy with high-dose systemic steroids is crucial. The elderly are susceptible to the systemic complications of steroids (exacerbation of blood glucose control, weight gain, gastric bleeding, myocardial infarction, aseptic necrosis of the hip, etc.) and treatment is usually carried on for a minimum of six months to one year. A temporal artery biopsy should be obtained to confirm the diagnosis. Biopsy negative temporal arteritis has been reported, and biopsy of the contralateral side may be indicated if the ipsilateral biopsy is negative to establish the diagnosis (45). Serial sectioning is often required by the pathologist due to "skip" lesions.

Pathology

Pathologic examination of the temporal artery reveals fragmentation of the internal elastic lamina and inflammation with giant cell infiltrates of the tunica media of the artery. The ocular pathology reveals greatest involvement of the optic nerve at or just posterior to the lamina cribosa, with degeneration of the nerve, fibrosis, loss of myelin, and generalized loss of retinal ganglion cells (27).

■ TOXIC OPTIC NEUROPATHY

Bilateral, insidious loss of central vision with other signs of optic nerve dysfunction (bilateral cecocentral scotomas, dyschromatopsia) must be evaluated for nutritional deficiency, exogenous drug use, excessive alcohol and tobacco use (Table 7–6). Nutritional amblyopia, previously known as "*tobacco-alcohol amblyopia*," has been associated with diets poor in vitamin B complex, folic acid, and thiamine. Hematologic evaluation for pernicious anemia is recommended. Visual loss is usually reversible with dietary changes, B-complex vitamin supplementation, intramuscular thiamine, folate, and tobacco cessation (as indicated) if begun before optic atrophy develops. Bilateral atrophy of the papillomacular bundle has been noted pathologically (59).

The most commonly cited agents responsible for dose-dependent, occasionally reversible bilateral optic neuropathy are the anti-tuberculous agents *ethambutol* (recommended maintenance dose is 15 mg/kg/day) and *isoniazid* (addition of pyridoxine, vitamin B6, 25 to 100 mg per day may reduce toxicity). Another anti-infective agent, *chloramphenicol*, may cause reversible optic nerve toxicity at doses of 1000 mg per day. Digitalis may cause reversible toxicity as well as the oral hypoglycemic agents chlorpropamide and tolbutamide.

Chloroquine, disulfirum (Antabuse), and D-penicillamine also have potential optic nerve toxicity. Methanol intoxication causes severe, permanent loss of vision with disc edema. Halogenated hydroxyquinolones (Entero-vioform, Diodoquin, and Clioquinol) can cause a neurologic syndrome of subacute myelo-optic neuropathy (SMON).

SARCOID OPTIC NEUROPATHY

The optic nerve is the second most commonly affected cranial nerve in sarcoidosis after the facial nerve. Optic nerve involvement occurs in approximately 5% of ocular cases and can be the presenting sign of systemic granulomatous disease. Vision can be affected abruptly with acuity ranging from 20/20 to no light perception. Granulomas of the nerve head are the commonest form; other manifestations include disc edema, retrobulbar neuropathy, and optic atrophy due to elevated intracranial pressure or compression. Other ocular signs of granulomatous inflammation may be present including vitreous cells, retinal periphlebitis, chorioretinitis, choroidal granulomas, and iritis. Systemically, pulmonary and dermatologic signs and symptoms may precede or follow ocular disease.

Histopathologic confirmation is considered by some to be mandatory for diagnosis, however, clinical suspicion and focused testing may obviate blind biopsies. Chest x-ray and serologic tests for angiotensin converting enzyme (ACE), serum lysozyme, calcium, and erythrocyte sedimentation rate are useful. Gallium scanning may demonstrate increased uptake in the lacrimal and parotid glands, hilar regions and liver. Fluorescein angiography can show disc leakage and periphlebitis. Investigation for infectious optic neuropathies should be performed. Anergy to skin testing with Candida, mumps and Trichophyton control antigens is an ancillary sign of altered delayed type hypersensitivity and may be performed in conjunction with tuberculin skin tests. A short course of systemic corticosteroid therapy may be helpful although spontaneous recovery is possible. Since central nervous system involvement can occur in one-third of patients with posterior segment sarcoid, neuroimaging should be obtained.

INFECTIOUS OPTIC NEUROPATHY

Several congenital and acquired infectious diseases can affect the optic nerve with infiltration of the arachnoid sheath or parenchyma and cause papillitis, disc edema, ischemic optic neuropathy and secondary optic atrophy. The diagnostic workup of any optic neuropathy includes evaluation for these infectious agents.

Syphilis (Treponema pallidum) is the most common of the infectious optic neuropathies and can present acutely with optic disc edema from nerve sheath infiltration (optic perineuritis) which may have blind spot enlargement only or as optic neuritis or neuroretinitis with visual dysfunction. Papilledema may occur in secondary syphilis from chronic arachnoiditis with hydrocephalus. Tertiary syphilis can present with ischemic optic neuropathy, elevated ESR and giant cells on temporal artery biopsy simulating temporal arteritis. Congenital infection usually manifests as a chorioretinitis. Retinal arteriolar attenuation, sheathing and obliteration with slowly progressive optic atrophy may occur in tertiary syphilis. Serologic testing using the VDRL and FTA-Abs serum antibody tests should be performed. CSF evaluation for neurosyphilis with VDRL is recommended. Treatment is with high dose parenteral penicillin.

Lyme optic neuropathy is rare and is due to the spirochete Borrelia burgdorferi. Occurrence in an endemic area with a history of the characteristic skin rash (erythema migrans), a preceding flulike illness and other systemic symptoms (arthritidis, cardiomyopathy) are useful ancillary features. Bell's palsy (peripheral facial nerve) is the most common cranial nerve involved. Optic neuritis may be associated with intraocular inflammation, encephalomyopathy, neuroretinitis. Papilledema has been described in patients with intracranial disease. Optic atrophy may be a late sequela. Neurologic consultation and CSF examination for pleocytosis should be considered. Like syphilis, any ocular structure is susceptible to involvement. Indirect immunofluorescence antibody (IFA) and enzyme-linked immunosorbent assays (ELISA) serologic testing is available; false-positive results may occur with syphilis, relapsing fever, leptospirosis, infectious mononucleosis and collagen-vascular diseases.

Tuberculosis (TB), like syphilis, may affect any part of the eye including the optic nerve. Infection is always present systemically, usually involving the meninges or lungs. TB meningitis peaks around age 5, with a retrobulbar optic neuritis which may result in no light perception vision. Optic neuritis is associated with choroidal tubercles and widespread disease. Papilledema is rarely encountered.

Toxoplasmosis and **toxocariasis** can cause an inflammatory papillitis. Optic atrophy may result from chorioretinal lesions or from papilledema found in intracranial toxoplasmosis.

Human immunodeficiency virus (HIV) may be a cause of optic neuropathy. HIV-associated optic neuropathies include **cytomegalovirus (CMV)** papillitis, syphilis, and herpesvirus acute retinal necrosis.

■ RADIATION OPTIC NEUROPAHTY

Radiation therapy for ocular (melanoma, retinoblastoma) and periocular (CNS, sinus, orbital) conditions may result in delayed radiation-induced vascular damage to the retina and optic nerve. Doses less than 7000 rads total delivered at less than 200 rad/day are considered safe. However, concomitant microvascular disease (ie, diabetes mellitus) or chemotherapy may increase the susceptibility of the optic nerve to this rare entity. Clinically, patients may present with amaurosis fugax and visual loss accompanied by ophthalmoscopic signs of disc swelling, peripapillary hard exudates, hemorrhages and subretinal fluid. These symptoms begin approximately 12 months following local radiation

(cobalt-60 plaques) and 19 months after external beam irradiation. The latency is presumably due to ischemic damage. Cotton-wool spots are also common and fluorescein angiogram demonstrates capillary nonperfusion of the disc. Disc swelling usually clears after several months with resultant optic atrophy due to ischemic demyelination with obliterative endarteritis. Irreversible visual loss to count fingers or worse vision occurs in most patients. There is no proven therapy, yet, spontaneous improvement has been reported. The use of hyperbaric oxygen therapy to reverse the visual loss and prevent involvement of the fellow eye has met with limited success in small groups of patients.

■ REFERENCES

1. Apple DJ, Rabb MF, Walsh PM: Congenital anomalies of the optic disc. Surv Ophthalmol—1982;27:3–41.
2. Barrett DA, Glaser JS, Schatz NJ, Winterkorn JMS: Spontaneous recovery of vision in progressive anterior ischemic optic neuropathy. J Clin Neuro-ophthalmol—1992;12:219–225.
3. Beck RW, Cleary PA, Anderson MA, et al.: A randomized, controlled trial of corticosteroids in the treatment of acute optic neuritis. N Engl J Med—1992;326:581–588.
4. Beck RW, Cleary PA: The Optic Neuritis Study Group: Optic Neuritis Treatment Trial: One year follow-up results. Arch Ophthalmol—1993;111:773–775.
5. Beck RW, Cleary PA, Trobe JD, et al.: The effect of corticosteroids for acute optic neuritis on the subsequent development of multiple sclerosis. N Engl J Med—1993;329:1764–1769.
6. Beck RW, Kupersmith MJ, Cleary PA, Katz B, The Optic Neuritis Study Group: Fellow eye abnormalities in acute unilateral optic neuritis: Experience of the optic neuritis treatment trial. Ophthalmol—1993;100:691–698.
7. Beck RW, Savino PJ, Schatz NJ, Smith CH, Sergott R: Anterior ischemic optic neuropathy: Recurrent episodes in the same eye. Brit J Ophthalmol—1983;67:705–709.
8. Beri M, Klugman MR, Kohler JA, Hayreh SS: Anterior ischemic optic neuropathy VII: incidence of bilaterality and various influencing factors. Ophthalmol—1987;94:1020–1028.
9. Beyer WB, Quencer RM, Osher RH: Morning glory syndrome: A functional analysis including fluorescein angiography, ultrasonography, and computerized tomography. Ophthalmol—1982;89:1362–1367.
10. Boghen DR, Glaser JS: Ischaemic optic neuropathy: The clinical profile and natural history. Brain—1975;98:689–708.
11. Borchert M, Lessell S: Progressive and recurrent nonarteritic anterior ischemic optic neuropathy. Am J Ophthalmol—1988;106:443–449.
12. Brodsky MC, Glasier CM: Optic nerve hypoplasia: Clinical significance of associated central nervous system abnormalities on magnetic resonance imaging. Arch Ophthalmol—1993;111:66–74.
13. Brourman ND, Spoor TC, Ramocki JM: Optic nerve sheath decompression for pseudotumor cerebri. Arch Ophthalmol—1988;106:1378–1383.
14. Brown GC, Tasman WS: Congenital anomalies of the optic disc. New York Grune and Stratton, 1983; pp 97–126, 178–183, 207–212, 263–265.
15. Burde RM: Optic disc risk factors for nonarteritic anterior ischemic optic neuropathy. Am J Ophthalmol—1993;116:759–764.
16. Chestler RJ, France TD: Ocular findings in CHARGE syndrome: Six case reports and a review. Ophthalmology—1988;95:1613–1619.
17. Dorrell D: The tilted disc. Brit J Ophthalmol—1978;62:16–20.

18. Dreyer RF, Hopen G, Gan DM, Smith JL: Leber's idiopathic stellate neuroretinitis. Arch Ophthalmol—1984; 102:1140–1145.

19. DuBois LG, Feldon SE: Evidence for a metabolic trigger for Leber's hereditary optic neuropathy: A case report. J Clin Neuro-ophthalmol—1992;12:15–16.

20. Frisen L, Holmegaard L: Spectrum of optic nerve hypoplasia. Br J Ophthalmol—1978;62:7–15.

21. Goldhammer Y, Smith JL: Optic nerve anomalies in basal encephalocele. Arch Ophthalmol—1975;93:115–118.

22. Hauser WA, Ferguson RH, Holley KE: Temporal arteritis in Rochester, Minnesota, 1951–1967. Mayo Clin Proc—1971;46:597–602.

23. Hayreh SS: Pathogenesis of oedema of the optic disc (papilloedema): A preliminary report. Brit J Ophthalmol—1964;48:522–543.

24. Hayreh SS: Anterior ischemic optic neuropathy: Clinical features and pathogenesis of post-hemorrhagic amaurosis. Ophthalmology—1987;94:1488–1502.

25. Hayreh SS: Anterior ischemic optic neuropathy: Differentiation of arteritic from non-arteritic type and its management. Eye—1990;4:25–41.

26. Hayreh SS, Podhajsky P: Visual field defects in anterior ischemic optic neuropathy. Docum Ophthalm Proc Series—1979;19:53–71.

27. Henkind P, Charles NC, Pearson J: Histopathology of ischemic optic neuropathy. Am J Ophthalmol—1970;69: 78–90.

28. Hoyt WF, Knight CL: Comparison of congenital disc blurring and incipient papilledema in red-free light-a photographic study. Invest Ophthalmol—1973;12:241–247.

29. Huston KA, Hunder GG, Lie JT, Kennedy RH: Temporal arteritis: a 25-year epidemiological, clinical, and pathological study. Ann Intern Med—1978;88:162–167.

30. Ischemic Optic Neuropathy Decompression Trial Research Group: Optic Nerve Decompression Surgery for Nonarteritic Anterior Ischemic Optic Neuropathy (NAION) is not effective and may be harmful. JAMA–1995;273:625–632.

31. Jabs DA, Miller NR, Newman SA, Johnson MA, Stevens MB: Optic neuropathy in systemic lupus erythematosus. Arch Ophthalmol—1986;104:564–568.

32. Johns DR, Heher KL, Miller NR, Smith KH: Leber's hereditary optic neuropathy: Clinical manifestations of the 14484 mutation. Arch Ophthalmol—1993;111: 495–498.

33. Johns DR, Smith KH, Miller NR: Leber's hereditary optic neuropathy: Clinical manifestations of the 3460 mutation. Arch Ophthalmol—1992;110:1577–1581.

34. Keltner JL: Optic nerve sheath decompression. Arch Ophthalmol—1988;106:1365–1369.

35. Keltner JL, Johnson CA, Spurr JO, Beck RW, Optic Neuritis Study Group: Baseline visual field profile of optic neuritis: The experience of the Optic Neuritis Treatment Trial. Arch Ophthalmol—1993;111:231–234.

36. Kindler P: Morning glory syndrome: unusual congenital optic disc anomaly. Am J Ophthalmol—1970;69:376–384.

37. Kline LB: Progression of visual defects in ischemic optic neuropathy. Am J Ophthalmol—1988;106:199–203.

38. Koenig SB, Naidich TP, Lissner G: The morning glory syndrome associated with sphenoidal encephalocele. Ophthalmol—1982;89:1368–1373.

39. Kranenburg EW: Crater-like holes in the optic disc and central serous retinopathy. Arch Ophthalmol—1960;64: 912–928.

40. Lambert SR, Hoyt CS, Narahara MM: Optic nerve hypoplasia. Surv Ophthalmol—1987;32:1–9.

41. Lorentzen SE: Incidence of spontaneous venous pulsations in the retina. Acta Ophthalmol—1970;48:765–776.

42. Maitland CG, Miller NR: Neuroretinitis. Arch Ophthalmol—1984;102:1146–1150.

43. McLeod D: Retinal ischemia, disc swelling, and axoplasmic transport. Br J Ophthalmol—1978;62:591–594.

44. Miller A, Green M: Simple rule for calculating normal erythrocyte sedimentation rate. Br Med J—1983;286:266.

45. Miller GR, Smith JL: Ischemic optic neuropathy. Am J Ophthalmol—1966;62:103–115.

46. Moody TA, Irvine AR, Cahn PH, et al: Sudden visual field constriction associated with optic disc drusen. J Clin Neuro-Ophthalmol—1993;13:8–13.

47. Mosier MA, Lieberman MF, Green WR, Knox DL: Hypoplasia of the optic nerve. Arch Ophthalmol—1978;96: 1437–1442.

48. Mullaney J: Curious colobomata. Trans Ophthalmol Soc UK—1977;97:517–522.

49. Nikoskelainen E, Hoyt WF, Nummelin K: Ophthalmoscopic findings in Leber's hereditary optic neuropathy: II. The fundus findings in the affected family members. Arch Ophthalmol—1983;101:1059–1068.

50. Optic Neuritis Study Group: The clinical profile of optic neuritis: Experience of the Optic Neuritis Treatment Trial. Arch Ophthalmol—1991;109:1673–1678.

51. Peterson RA, Walton DS: Optic nerve hypoplasia with good visual acuity and visual field defects. Arch Ophthalmol—1977;95:254–258.

52. Pollock S: The morning glory disc anomaly: Contractile movement, classification, and embryogensis. Documenta Ophthalmologica—1987;65:439–460.

53. Provis JM, Van Driel D, Billson FA, Russel P: Human fetal optic nerve: Overproduction and elimination of retinal axons during development. J Comp Neurol—1985;238: 92–100.

54. Puck A, Tso MOM, Fishman GA: Drusen of the optic nerve associated with retinitis pigmentosa. Arch Ophthalmol—1985;103:231–234.

55. Reeves DL: Congenital absence of the septum pellucidum. Bull Johns Hopkins Hospital—1941;69:61–71.

56. Repka MX, Savino PJ, Schatz NJ, Sergott RC: Clinical profile and long-term implications of anterior ischemic optic neuropathy. Am J Ophthalmol—1983;96:478–483.

57. Rizzo JF, Lessell S: Risk of developing multiple sclerosis after uncomplicated optic neuritis: A long-term prospective study. Neurology—1988;38:185–190.

58. Rizzo JF, Lessell S: Optic neuritis and ischemic optic neuropathy: Overlapping clinical profiles. Arch Ophthalmol— 1991;109:1668–1672.

59. Rizzo JF, Lessell S: Tobacco amblyopia. Am J Ophthalmol—1993;116:84–87.

60. Rucker CW: Defects in visual fields produced by hyaline bodies in the optic disks. Arch Ophthalmol—1944;32: 56–59.

61. Sawle GV, James CB, Ross Russell RW: The natural history of non-arteritic anterior ischemic optic neuropathy. J Neurol Neurosurg Psych—1990;53:830–833.

62. Sergott R, Cohen MS, Bosley TM, Savino PJ: Optic nerve decompression may improve the progressive form of nonarteritic ischemic optic neuropathy. Arch Ophthalmol—1989;107:1743–1754.

63. Skarf B, Hoyt CS: Optic nerve hypoplasia in children: Association with anomalies of the endocrine and CNS. Arch Ophthalmol—1984;102:62–67.

64. Smith JL, Hoyt WF, Susac JO: Ocular fundus in acute Leber optic neuropathy. Arch Ophthalmol—1973;90:349–354.

65. Stone EM, Newman NJ, Miller NR, et al.: Visual recovery in patients with Leber's hereditary optic neuropathy and the 11778 mutation. J Clin Neuro-Ophthalmol—1992;12:10–14.

66. Taylor D: Pediatric Ophthalmology. Blackwell, 1990; p. 441.

67. Tso MOM: Pathology and pathogenesis of drusen of the optic nervehead. Ophthalmol—1981;88:1066–1079.

68. Tso MOM, Fine BS: Electron microscopic study of human papilledema. Am J Ophthalmol—1976;82:424–434.

69. Wagener HP, Hollenhorst RW: The ocular lesions of temporal arteritis. Am J Ophthalmol—1958;45:617–630.

70. Wallace DC, Singh G, Lott MT, et al.: Mitochondrial DNA mutation associated with Leber's hereditary optic neuropathy. Science—1988;242:1427–1430.

71. Walsh TJ, Garden J, Gallagher B: Obliteration of retinal venous pulsations. Am J Ophthalmol—1969;67:954–956.

72. Walton DS, Robb RM: Optic nerve hypoplasia: a report of 20 cases. Arch Ophthalmol—1970;84:572–578.

73. Young SE, Walsh FB, Knox DL: The tilted disc syndrome. Am J Ophthalmol—1976;82:16–23.

74. Zeki SM, Dutton GN: Optic nerve hypoplasia in children. Br J Ophthalmol—1990;74:300–304.

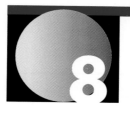

8 Visual Pathway Disorders

John M. DeVaro

■ A. OPTIC NERVE DISORDERS

Optic Glioma

Optic gliomas present in two very different forms: the benign juvenile pilocytic astrocytoma in children and the rare malignant glioblastoma in adults. These tumors are contrasted in Table 8–1.

Clinical Manifestations

Optic gliomas are most common in children under ten years of age. They represent two-thirds of all primary optic nerve tumors and <5% of all intracranial tumors. Their reported association with neurofibromatosis has varied widely (10–70%) (4). Conversely, up to 15% of patients with NF 1, and none with NF 2, will have optic gliomas (11). Onset of symptoms may be sudden with rapid loss of vision and headache, but in general growth is insidious. Proptosis is indicative of intraorbital tumor. Visual field defects may be chiasmal in nature, but follow no standard pattern. The tumors are histopathologically benign, but malignant in function secondary to compression effect, especially with more posterior involvement. Here, diabetes insipidus and the *diencephalic syndrome* can result. This latter condition includes failure to thrive after a period of normal growth, hyperactivity and euphoria, skin pallor, hypotension, and hypoglycemia (Fig. 8–1).

Chiasmal gliomas are more common than the isolated orbital type. They may present to the ophthalmologist for evaluation of unilateral/bilateral visual loss, strabismus, "amblyopia," optic atrophy/disc hypoplasia, or nystagmus. The nystagmus can be difficult to differentiate from the more benign *spasmus nutans*, resulting in delayed diagnosis of the tumor. Important signs to search for include optic atrophy, increased intracranial pressure with hydrocephalus, and poor feeding secondary to diencephalic syndrome.

The rare malignant optic glioma occurs most often in middle-aged males. It is marked by pain, disc edema, and rapid visual loss mimicking optic neuritis. Transient improvement can occur with corticosteroid therapy. Prognosis is poor. Tumor appears to spread by subpial and dural routes. Death can occur within months. No effective treatment is known. Current palliative efforts include a combination of radiotherapy and chemotherapy.

Meningioma

After pituitary tumors, meningiomas are the most common neural tumor to have neuro-ophthalmologic manifestations. They have a widespread distribution throughout the central nervous system. Essentially benign encapsulated tumors possessing a favorable surgical outcome where possible, they are the most common in middle-aged women and are rare below the age of twenty. Pregnancy can promote growth of the tumor and accelerate the progression of visual loss. There is a higher incidence of neurofibromatosis in patients with meningioma (4). Three types of meningioma which often present with visual pathway involvement are optic nerve sheath, tuberculum sellae, and sphenoid wing meningiomas.

Clinical Manifestations

Optic nerve sheath meningiomas are the second most common optic nerve tumor, but represent only 1% of all

TABLE 8–1
Primary gliomas of nerve and chiasm (7)

	Childhood	Adulthood
Age at onset of symptoms	4 to 8 years	Middle age
Presentation	Visual defects, proptosis	Rapid, severe unilateral visual loss; mimics optic neuritis
Clinical course	Relatively stable, nonprogressive	Rapid bilateral visual deterioration; other intracranial signs
Prognosis	Compatible with long life	Death within months to 2 years
Neurofibromatosis	Related in 20–40% of cases	No relationship
Histology	Non-invasive, pilocytic astrocytoma	Invasive, malignant astrocytoma (glioblastoma); may metastasize

meningiomas. They can produce slowly progressive loss of visual acuity and field, dyschromatopsia, and an afferent pupil defect. Visual field defects include cecocentral scotoma, generalized depression, and peripheral constriction. Mild proptosis and disc edema with venous congestion are relative early signs. The classic triad of visual loss, optic atrophy, and optociliary shunt vessels is seen infrequently. Intracranial extension may rarely occur (Fig. 8–2a).

Parasellar meningiomas often present with a chronic non-specific headache. These lesions are often not diagnosed until significant visual loss has occurred, making initial presentation to the ophthalmologist rather common. Visual field loss is often first monocular, slowly progressing to a markedly asymmetric binocular deficit resulting from slow advancement of the tumor across the tuberculum to the contralateral optic nerve or chiasm. One or both optic dics may be pale, and optociliary shunt vessels are seen (Figures 8–2b and 8–2c). *Sphenoid wing meningiomas* may become quite large and invasive prior to diagnosis (Fig. 8–2d). A large subfrontal meningioma may compress one optic nerve (causing ipsilateral optic atrophy), and the foramen of Monro (causing hydrocephalus and contralateral papilledema), resulting in the rare *Foster-Kennedy syndrome.*

Radiologic Studies

On CT scan, the classic finding of an optic nerve sheath meningioma is tubular enlargement of the optic nerve with a "railroad tract" sign on axial images and a "double ring sign" on coronals images due to involvement of the nerve sheath around the nerve. This finding differentiates the tumor from optic nerve glioma, where tumor infiltrates the nerve itself and grows in a subdural fashion compressing the subarachnoid space (Fig. 8–3). Calcification occasionally occurs and also allows differentiation from optic nerve glioma. The use of fat saturation (suppression) and gadolinium-DTPA enhancement techniques are improving the ability of MRI to evaluate intracanalicular extension.

With intracranial meningioma, CT scanning will re-

veal a calcified, contrast-enhancing mass with surrounding hyperostosis of adjacent bone, but is inferior to the multiplanar imaging capabilities of MRI in assessing suprasellar or intrasellar extension, postsurgical changes, and vascular displacement or encapsulation. There is a grainy appearance on MRI secondary to calcification and tumor heterogeneity. Angiography is an important tool in evaluating tumor vascularity prior to neurosurgical intervention. As MR angiography techniques improve, they may obviate the need for pre-operative arteriography (13).

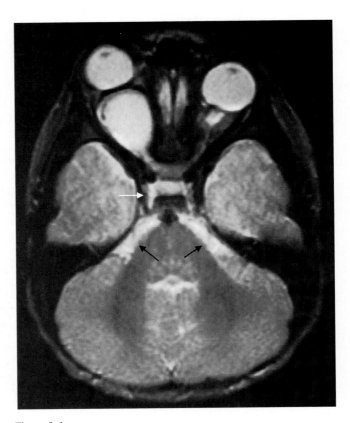

Figure 8–1.
MRI scan of a patient with a right optic nerve glioma. Note the extensive involvement of the contralateral optic nerve, the chiasm (black arrow), and the optic tracts (white arrows).

Treatment

Meningiomas are benign tumors; clinical observation is often warranted prior to invasive therapy. Patients should be monitored closely for signs of progressive neurologic deficit (e.g. loss of vision, visual field deficit, ocular motility disturbance) or impending neurologic compromise (e.g. herniation). For obvious reasons, optic nerve sheath meningiomas are more often treated conservatively. As they are not very radiosensitive, the preferred treatment of intracranial meningiomas is neurosurgical removal or debulking. When total exci-

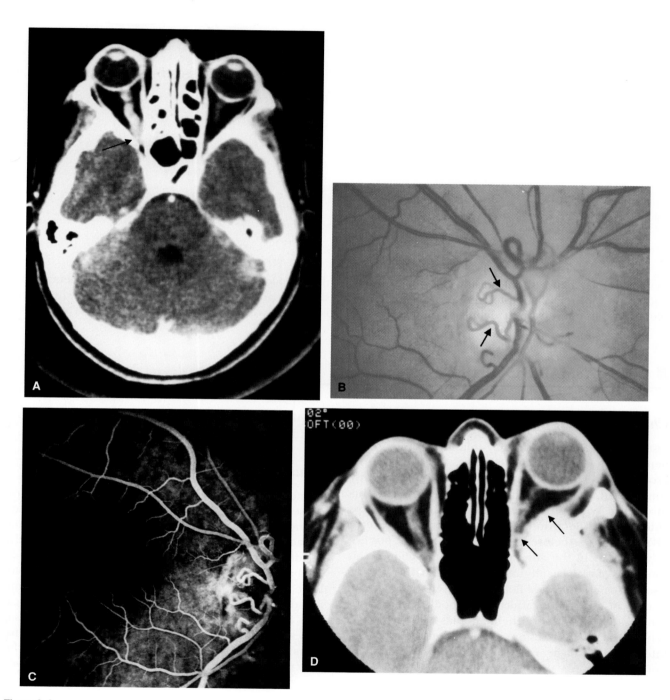

Figure 8–2.
Meningiomas: a. CT scan of a right optic nerve sheath meningioma. Note extension into the optic canal (arrow). b. Optociliary shunt vessels in same patient (arrows). c. Fluorescein angiogram of optociliary shunt vessels. Note absence of fluorescein leakage. d. Sphenoid wing meningioma. Note invasion into orbit and optic canal (arrows).

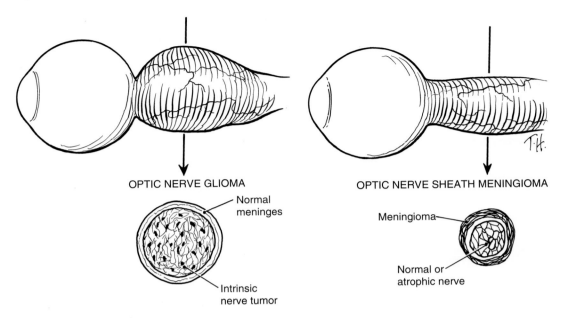

OPTIC NERVE GLIOMA

OPTIC NERVE SHEATH MENINGIOMA

Normal meninges

Intrinsic nerve tumor

Meningioma

Normal or atrophic nerve

Figure 8–3.
Comparison of the characteristics of optic glioma and optic nerve sheath meningioma.

sion is possible, a cure should result. Postoperative radiotherapy appears to at least increase the recurrence-free interval in conservatively debulked tumors. Radiotherapy alone is an alternative when the patient is considered a poor surgical candidate, especially when there is extensive involvement of bone or major arteries.

■ B. CHIASMAL DISORDERS

Chiasmal Visual Field Defects

Visual field defects produced by chiasmal lesions are dependent on its anatomic location, the direction of growth, and whether nerve fibers are being directly compressed, or being pushed against contiguous structures (12). Within the chiasm, infero-nasal fibers cross anteriorly and loop into the contralateral optic nerve (*Wilbrand's knee*) before resuming their course posteriorly. Lesions in the anterior angle of the chiasm can cause loss of visual acuity and visual field in one eye and a supero-temporal visual field defect in the other (junctional scotoma). Those affecting the body of the chiasm can produce bitemporal hemianopias without loss of central visual acuity. Lesions in the posterior chiasm can interrupt the crossing macular fibers resulting in bitemporal hemianopic scotomata (Fig. 8–4). Other conditions can mimic bitemporal hemianopias, including tilted optic discs, papilledema (with enlarged blind spots), nasal retinal lesions (colobomas, sector retinitis pigmentosa, chorioretinal scars), and redundant overhanging upper lid tissue. A differential diagnosis and a comparison of the clinical presentation of various chiasmal lesions are provided in Tables 8–2 and 8–3, respectively.

Pituitary Adenoma

Tumors of the pituitary gland are the most common cause of chiasmal visual field defects in adults. Pituitary adenomas comprise 12–15% of clinically symptomatic intracranial tumors. Autopsy studies have reported the incidence of asymptomatic pituitary adenomas to be as high as 20–27%, with a large number staining on histologic section for prolactin (7). They are defined as microadenomas if they are confined to the sella and measure 10 mm or less in diameter, and macroadenomas if they are greater than 10 mm. Occasionally, pituitary tumors are associated with other endocrine tumors in the pancreas and parathyroid gland (*multiple endocrine neoplasia, type I*).

Clinical Manifestations

Symptomatic adenomas occur most commonly in the fourth to the seventh decades. Nonocular findings may

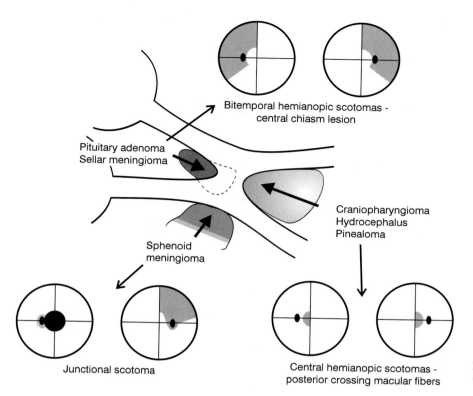

Bitemporal hemianopic scotomas - central chiasm lesion

Pituitary adenoma
Sellar meningioma

Craniopharyngioma
Hydrocephalus
Pinealoma

Sphenoid
meningioma

Junctional scotoma

Central hemianopic scotomas - posterior crossing macular fibers

Figure 8–4.
Chiasmal visual field defects.

TABLE 8–2
Differential diagnosis of chiasmal lesions (12)

Neoplastic mass lesions
  Pituitary adenoma
  Craniopharyngioma
  Meningioma
  Glioma (optic nerve, chiasm, hypothalmus)
  Dysgerminoma
  Chordoma
  Nasopharyngeal carcinoma
  Metastasis
Non-neoplastic mass lesions
  Aneurysm
  Sphenoid sinus mucocele
  Fibrous dysplasia
  Arachnoid cyst
  Histiocytosis X (Langerhans histiocytosis)
  Rathke's cleft cyst
Vascular/Inflammatory/Other
  Granulomatous disease (sarcoid, tuberculosis, fungal)
  Vasculitis (systemic lupus erythematosus); ischemic
  Syphilis
  Pituitary abscess
  Trauma
  Radiation necrosis

TABLE 8–3
Parachiasmal Lesions: Clinical Clues (12)

Clinical Finding	Suspected Lesion
Precocious puberty	Dysgerminoma
	Fibrous dysplasia
Hypopituitarism	Adenoma
	Hypothalmic glioma
	Craniopharyngioma
Personality changes	Craniopharyngioma
	Frontal meningioma
Sudden blindness	Pituitary apoplexy
	Aneurysm
Diabetes insipidus	Hypothalmic glioma
	Hystiocytosis X
Ophthalmoplegia	Nasopharyngeal carcinoma
	Chordoma
	Invasive adenoma
Normal enhanced CT	Arachnoid cyst
	Nonmass lesions
Diencephalic syndrome	Glioma
Calcification	Craniopharyngioma
	Meningioma
	Aneurysm
	Chordoma

include chronic headache (in more than two-thirds of patients), fatigue, loss of libido, impotence or amenorrhea, galactorrhea or gynecomastia, sexual hair change, or other signs of gonadal, thyroidal, or adrenal insufficiency.

Secretory adenomas usually become symptomatic earlier in their clinical course than non-secretors, and thus tend to be smaller in size at the time of presentation. In a 1000-case series reported by Wilson in 1984, over 77% were secretory, with prolactin being the most common, followed by growth hormone, adrenocorticotropin, and thyroid stimulating hormone (15). Nonsecretors are usually null cell adenomas.

Ocular signs include loss of vision, visual field, and ocular motility disorders. Hollenhorst and Younge reported a 1973 Mayo Clinic series in which 42% of patients with pituitary adenomas initially presented with visual loss (8). With the increasing use of neuroimaging and sensitive hormonal assays, this number is decreasing while the incidence of neuroendocrine presentations rises.

Visual field loss varies with the anatomy of the lesion. Asymmetry is common, with greater loss of visual acuity and an afferent pupillary defect on the side of greater visual field compromise. More posterior chiasmal compression is marked by optic tract involvement and incongruous hemianopias. Rarely, arcuate Bjerrum scotomas can be found and be confused with glaucoma.

Prolactinomas and Bromocriptine

Prolactinomas are the most common type of pituitary adenoma. They are more common in women, where they present with amenorrhea and galactorrhea. Men present with loss of libido, impotence, gynecomastia, galactorrhea, and hypopituitarism. Serum prolactin is elevated well above the normal range of 200 ng/ml, and rises with tumor size. These tumors can respond to medical treatment with *bromocriptine,* an ergot derivative and dopamine agonist. This drug has been shown to reduce prolactin secretion, reduce the size of approximately 80% of microadenomas, and reverse visual field defects. To a lesser extent, it can lower growth hormone levels in acromegaly and has shown some effect in non-prolactin secretors. However, larger tumors do not respond as well, cystic necrosis can develop, and prompt tumor regrowth can occur when dosage is stopped. The use of preoperative bromocriptine to reduce the size of macroadenomas larger than 2 cm prior to neurosurgical removal has proved helpful.

Pituitary Apoplexy

During pregnancy, pituitary adenomas can enlarge, sometimes secondary to pituitary apoplexy, a potentially lethal condition. Therefore, acute onset of headache, visual loss, multiple ocular motor nerve palsies, and facial pain or numbness should prompt CT or MRI of the brain to rule out enlargement of the sella tursica. Lumbar puncture findings of subarachnoid blood may also prove helpful. Pregnant women with a growing pituitary lesion may be most safely delivered by Ceasarian section to avoid apoplexy during labor and delivery. High-dose corticosteroid therapy is the first therapeutic maneuver in pituitary apoplexy.

Radiologic Studies

Pituitary adenomas are best evaluated by MRI, which, with its multiplanar imaging capability, can best demonstrate the anatomic location of intrasellar and suprasellar masses (Fig. 8–5). Large tumors may be associated with enlargement of the sella turcica. These bony changes are better demonstrated on CT scan, but overall MRI is the procedure of choice. Intralesional cyst formation, hemorrhage, and empty sella syndrome are often easily detected on MRI. It should be noted, however, that some pituitary microadenomas may be missed with radiologic imaging, even in the presence of clinical manifestations such as Cushing's disease (9, 13, 14).

Treatment

Pituitary tumors may be removed surgically, often by a microsurgical transsphenoidal approach. This tech-

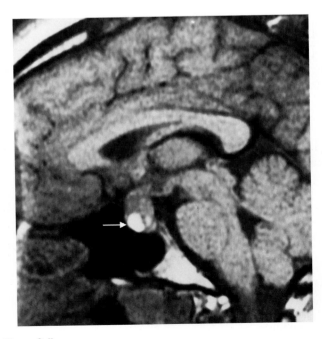

Figure 8–5.
MRI scan of a pituitary adenoma arising from anterior lobe of pituitary gland with intralesional hemorrhage (arrow). (Courtesy of Linda G. Leithe, MD, Durham, NC).

nique allows adequate decompression of the chiasm with low morbidity (2.3%) and mortality (0.4%) (2). Treatment is indicated for loss of visual acuity or field, or endocrine dysfunction. Improvement in vision can occur after neurosurgical decompression of the chiasmal environment is achieved. Most visual recovery will occur within 3 to 4 months post-operatively and is somewhat dependent on the duration of visual morbidity and the degree of optic nerve pallor. The role of radiation therapy for pituitary adenoma remains controversial but can prove helpful when extrasellar extension of tumor into the anterior and middle cranial fossa makes a transsphenoidal approach less effective. Recurrence of visual loss after surgical, medical, or radiation therapy may be due to tumor regrowth, arachnoidal adhesions and progressive empty sella syndrome, or delayed radiation necrosis.

Craniopharyngioma

Characteristically becoming symptomatic between the ages of 10 and 25 years, this is a group of tumors arising from nests of squamous epithilial cells that are remnants of Rathke's pouch. They represent up to 13% of all intracranial tumors of childhood (1). Craniopharyngiomas can be solid, cystic, or a combination of the two. Cysts contain a thick viscous material comprised of degenerated and necrotic blood, epithelium, and cholesterol crystals. Dystrophic calcification of the debris can be seen in over 80% of childhood tumors.

Clinical Manifestations

Craniopharyngiomas are more common in the first two decades of life, but there is a second peak of incidence in the fifth to seventh decades. Signs and symptoms vary with the age of the patient, site of the tumor, and rate of growth.

In children under fifteen, visual disturbance and headache (from increased inracranial pressure) are most frequent. Early visual deterioration is often missed unless severe bilateral impairment or headache, vomiting and changes in behavior prompt investigation. Papilledema (65%) and optic atrophy (60%) are common (7). Pituitary deficiency, with or without diabetes insipidus, delayed sexual development, and growth retardation, obesity, and somnolence secondary to hypothalmic compromise can occur. Cranial nerve palsies, either by direct pressure on the nerves or by increased intracranial pressure, can occur. Acquired *see-saw nystagmus* and bitemporal hemianopias resulting from large parasellar tumors expanding within the third ventricle are a hallmark of childhood craniopharyngioma. Less common findings include premature sexual development, extrapyramidal signs, cerebellar ataxia, and orthostatic hypotension. An occasional paradoxical pupillary response to light has been reported.

Particularly in older patients, an unusual feature of craniopharyngiomas is the finding of relatively normal optic discs in association with extensive visual deficit. Papilledema is less common, and about one third will demonstrate some problem with mentation (1). Occult endocrine dysfunction can be noted later. With a suprasellar lesion, asymmetric chiasmal visual field defects are prominent, with a bitemporal hemianopia being most common. Optic tract involvement can produce a homonymous pattern with reduced visual acuity.

Radiologic Studies

Diagnosis is made by clinical findings and radiologic scanning (Fig. 8–6). Some craniopharyngiomas can escape initial radiologic detection by possessing a radiodensity similar to surrounding brain tissue. Later, calcification of parts of the tumor facilitates its detection. In general, CT best detects calcific changes, while MRI best delineates tumor heterogeneity and cyst formation (cyst contents are bright on T1 images secondary to blood and high protein content), as well as the involvement of the surrounding optic chiasm, third ventricle, and intracavernous carotid arteries.

Treatment

While preferred therapy is controversial, options include total excision, evacuation of the cyst contents and removal of the cyst wall, biopsy followed by radiotherapy, or a combination of surgery and radiation. Neuro-

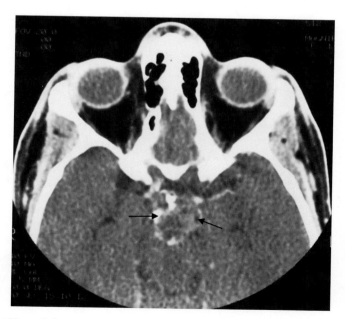

Figure 8–6.
CT scan of a suprasellar craniopharyngioma. Note the calcification (white arrow) and cyst formation (black arrow).

surgical approach is generally by craniotomy, but if the tumor is subdiaphragmatic or has a large cystic component, a transsphenoidal approach can be employed. Total extirpation is very difficult to achieve. Since serious visual, endocrine, and neurologic complications can result from aggressive surgery, some prefer conservative surgery followed by radiotherapy (2). Recurrences usually present in the first 2 years, but may be delayed by more aggressive resections. In most cases, life-time endocrine replacement is anticipated.

■ RETROCHIASMAL LESIONS

Visual field defects due to retrochiasmal lesions tend to occur on the same side of the visual space in each eye (homonymous hemianopia). Incomplete homonymous visual field defects are examined for the degree of similarity or congruity. The further posterior the lesion, the more congruous the defect, for nerve fibers from corresponding retinal elements in each eye become more closely aligned as they progress posteriorly along the visual pathways. Hemianopias of retrochiasmal origin are notable for 1) their respect of the vertical midline—and 2) normal visual acuity, even in the presence of complete fixation-splitting homonymous hemianopias. Unless the posterior notch of the chiasm is involved, visual acuity is usually spared. The visual field defect that originates from a retrochiasmal lesion is related to the point of fixation and not to the blind spot.

Optic Tract

Isolated lesions of the optic tract or lateral geniculate nucleus are rare, and are more likely to be secondary to large mass lesions involving the chiasm (e.g. pituitary adenoma, internal carotid artery aneurysm, craniopharyngioma, optic glioma). The optic tracts are in closer proximity to and more vulnerable to sellar processes in prefixed chiasms. Intrinsic brain tumors, trauma, and demyelinative lesions can also involve the optic tract.

Total interruption of the tract produces a complete, fixation-splitting contralateral homonymous hemianopia. As this defect can result from any retrochiasmal lesion, perimetry is non-localizing. However, bilateral optic atrophy of retrochiasmal origin (temporal atro-

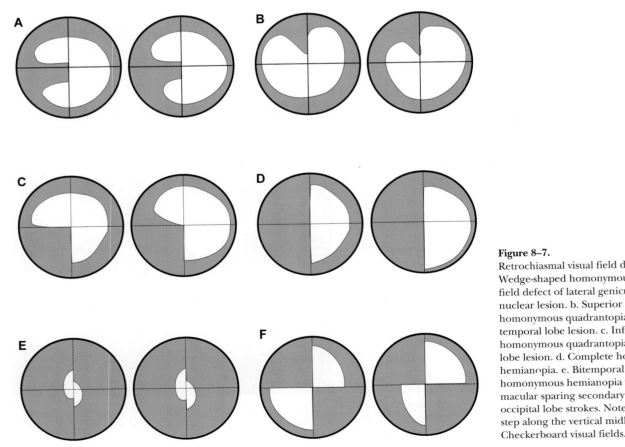

Figure 8–7.
Retrochiasmal visual field defects: a. Wedge-shaped homonymous visual field defect of lateral geniculate nuclear lesion. b. Superior homonymous quadrantopia of temporal lobe lesion. c. Inferior homonymous quadrantopia of parietal lobe lesion. d. Complete homonymous hemianopia. e. Bitemporal homonymous hemianopia with macular sparing secondary to bilateral occipital lobe strokes. Note the vertical step along the vertical midline. f. Checkerboard visual fields.

phy of the ipsilateral optic disc and bow-tie configuration atrophy of the nasal and temporal portions of the contralateral disc) can only occur in lesions of the optic tract or lateral geniculate nucleus.

Afferent pupillary defects can occur. As more than half (60%) of afferent pupillary fibers decussate at the chiasm, the APD tends to occur contralateral to the side of lesion. In general, differential diagnosis, radiologic evaluation, and treatment are similar to those for chiasmal lesions.

Lateral Geniculate Nucleus

Total destruction of the lateral geniculate nucleus results in a non-localizing, complete, fixation-splitting, contralateral homonymous hemianopia. However, the visual field defect which localizes a lesion to the lateral geniculate nucleus is a wedge-shaped homonymous defect (Fig. 8–7a). As afferent pupillary fibers exit the optic tract anterior to the lateral geniculate nucleus, afferent pupillary defects are not encountered.

The lateral geniculate nucleus posesses a dual vascular supply: the distal anterior choroidal branch of the internal carotid artery and the lateral choroidal branch of the posterior cerebral artery. Occlusion of the former may cause homonymous loss of upper and lower sectors of the visual field (keyhole defect) with corresponding sectoral optic atrophy, while occlusion of the latter may cause homonymous horizontal sectoranopia and sectoral optic atrophy (5, 6, 10).

Because of the proximity of the lateral geniculate nucleus to the internal capsule and thalamus, hemiparesis and hemisensory loss can occur, especially in the scenario of invasion by intrinsic brain tumor, but also with infarction, arteriovenous malformation, and trauma. Suspicion of infarction warrants evaluation for embolism and vasculitis.

Optic Radiations

Since axons from the ganglion cells of the retina terminate in the lateral geniculate nucleus, lesions beyond this structure do not result in optic disc pallor. Temporal and parietal lobe lesions are often associated with multiple neurologic defecits—and are usually secondary to tumors. Isolated visual loss is rare. Conversely, occipital lobe lesions are usually vascular (hypoperfusion, thrombosis, embolism) and account for as much as 89% of cases of isolated homonymous visual field loss in patients over 50 years of age (10).

Temporal Lobe

The inferior fibers of the optic radiations, corresponding to the superior aspect of the contralateral half of the visual field, course anteriorly into the temporal lobe to form Meyer's loop. Here they pass the internal capsule and the temporal isthmus, in the territory of the anterior choroidal artery. Temporal lobe lesions produce a relatively incongruous visual field defect, because fibers serving homologous points in the visual field of the two eyes are not adjacent. Deficits are usually denser above (Fig. 8–7b) and can be associated with seizures, feelings of déjà-vu, and formed ictal hallucinations (e.g. familiar faces). A lesion in a dominant temporal lobe may cause aphasia and contralateral motor paresis. A nondominant lesion can produce hemianesthesia and loss of body recognition.

Parietal Lobe

In the parietal lobe, the fibers of the optic radiation become more compact and their arrangement more homologous. Lesions here tend to produce deficits that are relatively more congruous and either complete or denser below (e.g. inferior quadrantopia, Fig. 8–7c). Parietal lobe lesions may produce hemiparesis, visual perceptual difficulties, agnosias, right-left confusion, acalculia, optokinetic nystagmus asymmetry, and spasticity of conjugate gaze.

Asymmetric horizontal *optokinetic nystagmus* (OKN) is characteristic of parietal lobe lesions. Note that as the parieto-occipital lobe/PPRF complex controls the ipsilateral slow pursuit component, a deficit will be seen when the OKN stimulus is moved in the direction of the damaged parietal lobe. Generally, a normal OKN response in the presence of a homonymous hemianopia decreases the likelihood of a parietal lesion. However, since the more medial aspects of the parietal lobe are supplied by branches of the anterior cerebral artery, OKN responses can be normal and symmetric after occlusions of the posterior or middle cerebral artery.

Cogan observed that in unilateral parietal lobe lesions, attempts to produce the Bell's phenomenon will result in tonic deviation of the eyes to the side opposite the parietal lobe lesion. This phenomenon, termed *spasticity of conjugate gaze*, is less commonly seen in temporal and occipital lesions (3).

Occipital Lobe

Homonymous visual field defects from occipital lesions are extremely congruous, whether they are hemianopic or involve a lesser area of field (Fig. 8–7d). It should be noted that lack of congruity in general rules out an occipital lobe defect, while the contrary is not true, i.e., congruous homonymous visual field defects may occur from lesions anywhere along the retrochiasmal pathways. In addition to vascular infarction and hypoperfusion, other causes of occipital lobe injury include neoplasm (meningioma, metastasis, glioma), congenital (porencephaly, arteriovenous malformation), traumatic, and toxic.

Certain phenomena are noted in occipital lobe lesions:

Macular sparing: Some occipital hemianopias preserve an area around central fixation. There are two possible mechanisms: a watershed zone between branches of the middle and posterior cerebral arteries may provide a dual vascular supply in the event that one supply is occluded; or, intermixing of ipsi- and contralateral fibers may provide a dual nerve supply to both sides of the occipital cortex.

Bilateral homonymous hemianopia with macular sparing (key hole field): Careful examination of what appears to be a tubular field will reveal a vertical step along the vertical midline (Fig. 8–7c).

Temporal crescent syndrome: Fibers representing the nasal retina synapse more anteriorly along the interhemispheric fissure, and can be spared in certain occipital strokes, causing preservation of a temporal crescent of field. Less frequently, this is the only portion of the visual cortex damaged, resulting in loss of this temporal crescent. This can lead to confusion in assessing the degree of congruity.

Checkerboard field: Bilateral sectorinopias, superior on one side and inferior on the contralateral side. For example, a left superior quadrantopia combined with a right inferior quadrantopia (Fig. 8–7f).

Cortical blindness: A rare syndrome of total blindness due to bilateral occipital lobe lesions, with preservation of pupillary responses and normal fundi. Most commonly due to bilateral occipital infarction, either simultaneous or consecutive. Can be associated with denial of blindness and fabrication of an imaginary visual environment *(Anton's syndrome).*

Riddoch phenomenon: Most prominent in retrogeniculate lesions, involves the perception of moving but not static targets.

Unformed visual hallucinations: Unlike the formed hallucinations associated with temporal lobe disease (c.f.), lesions of the visual cortex usually cause unformed visual hallucinations.

■ REFERENCES

1. Burde RM, Savino PJ, Trobe JD: Clinical Decisions in Neuro-Ophthalmology. St. Louis: CV Mosby Company, 1985, p. 338.

2. Capo H, Kupersmith MJ: Efficacy and complications of radiotherapy of anterior visual pathway tumors. Neurologic Clinics—1991:9(1):179–203.

3. Cogan DG: Neurologic significance of lateral conjugate deviation of the eyes on forced closure of the lids. Arch Ophthalmol—1948;62:694.

4. Dutton JJ: Gliomas of the anterior visual pathway. Surv Ophthalmol—1994;38:427–452.

5. Frisén L, Holmegaard L, Rosenkrantz M: Sectorial optic atrophy and homonymous field defects in two patients with partial lesions of the lateral geniculate nucleus. J Neurol Neurosurg Psychiatry—1978:41:374.

6. Frisén L: Quadruple sectoranopia and sectorial optic atrophy. A syndrome of the distal anterior choroidal artery. J Neurol Neurosurg Psychiatry—1979:42:590.

7. Glaser JS: Topical diagnosis: the optic chiasm. In: Tasman W and Jaeger EA (eds): Duane's Clinical Ophthalmology. Philadelphia: JB Lippincott Company—1993;2(6):1–39.

8. Hollenhorst RW, Younge BR: Ocular manifestations produced by adenomas of the pituitary gland: analysis of 1000 cases. In: Kohler PO and Ross GT (eds): Diagnosis and Treatment of Pituitary Tumors. New York: American Elsevier Publishing Company, 1973: p 53.

9. Hupp SL, Kline LB: Magnetic resonance imaging of the optic chiasm. Survey of Ophthalmology—1991:36(3):207–216.

10. Lessell S, Lessell IM, Glaser JS: Topical diagnosis: retrochiasmal visual pathways and higher cortical function. In: Tasman W and Jaeger EA (eds): Duane's Clinical Ophthalmology. Philadelphia: JB Lippincott Company, 1993;2(7):1–24.

11. Mulvihill JJ, Parry DM, Sherman JL, et al: Neurofibromatosis 1 (Recklinghausen Disease) and Neurofibromatosis 2 (Bilateral Acoustic Neurofibromatosis). Ann Intern Med—1990:113:39–52.

12. Newman SA: Diagnosis and treatment of chiasmal lesions. In: Smith RE, Frueh BR, Hoyt CS, et al. (eds): Focal Points 1987: Clinical Modules for Ophthalmologists. American Academy of Ophthalmology—1987:5(1):1–11.

13. Ramsey RG: Neuroradiology. Philadelphia: WB Saunders Company, 1994, 1034.

14. Slamovits TL, Gardner TA: Neuroimaging in neuro-ophthalmology. Ophthalmology—1989:96(4):555–568.

15. Wilson CB: A decade of pituitary microsurgery: The Herbert Olivecrona lecture. Journal of Neurosurgery—1984:61:814.

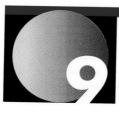

9 Eye Movement Disorders

Edward G. Buckley

Classification of eye movement disorders by the anatomical location of the abnormality aids in the clinical diagnosis. The four main areas are brain (supranuclear disorders), cranial nerve, neuromuscular junction, and muscle.

■ SUPRANUCLEAR CONTROL OF EYE MOVEMENTS

Saccadic System

Saccades are rapid conjugate eye movements with a peak velocity of 100 to 700 degrees per second lasting from 50 to 100 milliseconds which are used to quickly locate an object. Interestingly, visual function is suppressed during the saccadic movement (2). Saccadic eye movements can occur during sleep (rapid eye movement (REM) sleep) but these movements are slightly slower than those made while awake.

Saccadic eye movements originate in the primary frontal eye fields (FEF) (Broadman's area 8) and the superior colliculus (SC). Both regions project to the contralateral paramedian pontine reticular formation (PPRF, horizontal saccades) and the rostral interstitial nucleus of the medial longitudinal fasciculus (riMLF, vertical saccades) (Fig. 9–1). The FEF and SC represent parallel pathways for triggering saccades since damage to both is necessary for defects in voluntary saccadic eye movements. *Burst* cells in the PPRF and riMLF initiate the fast movement and are controlled by Pause cells which serve to stabilize the eyes after fast movement. Vertical saccades require simultaneous activity in both frontal eye fields or both superior calliculus (Fig. 9–2).

Smooth Pursuit System

Once an object has been "localized", continued fixation is maintained by slower conjugate eye movements termed smooth *pursuit*. Moving targets can usually be pursued accurately when the velocity is less than 50 degrees per second. Proprioception or even just the "perception" of movement can elicit a smooth pursuit eye movement.

The neuroanatomical pathways for the smooth pursuit system are not clearly defined. The visual cortex at the occipital-parieto-temporal junction is responsible for initiating ipsilateral smooth pursuit of targets. The pathway from this area to the brainstem is uncertain and the major route appears to be deep in the parietal lobe. The pathways terminate in a group of nuclei located in the dorsal lateral area of the pons (dorsal lateral pontine nuclei, DLPN), which in turn project to the ipsilateral cerebellum (flocculus and anterior vermis). The connections from the cerebellum to the ocular motor nuclei appear to be similar to those used by the vestibular system (see Fig. 10–5). The vertical pursuit pathways also involve the cerebellum in the region of the dentate nucleus—and travel to the ocular motor nuclei via the MLF.

Vergence Eye Movements

When an object is moving toward or away from the observer, the eyes must move in dissimilar (disconjugate) directions, either divergent or convergent. These *vergence* movements are typically slow and are stimulated by retinal blur or retinal disparity which elicit accom-

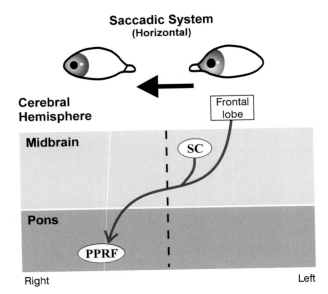

Figure 9–1.
Horizontal saccadic system. Horizontal saccades are initiated in the contralateral frontal lobe. A fast eye movement to the right (illustrated above) is initiated in the left frontal lobe and left superior colliculus. A signal is conveyed to the right parapontine reticular formation (PPRF) for initiation of fast eye movement to the right. (See Figure 9–3A).

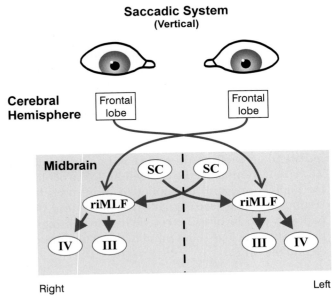

Figure 9–2.
Vertical saccadic system. Vertical saccadic eye movements require bilateral frontal lobe and superior colliculus (SC) stimulation. A signal is conveyed to the rostral interstitial nucleus of the MLF (riMLF)—and then to the corresponding third nerve nucleus. (See Figure 9–3).

modative or fusional efforts. As with saccades, visual suppression occurs during vergence movements (18).

The cortical pathways that control convergence and divergence are unknown. The pre-motor locations for these movements are located in the pretectal area above the third nerve nucleus.

Oculomotor Apraxia

Oculomotor apraxia is an abnormality in the *horizontal* saccade and smooth pursuit motor systems characterized by normal random and visually evoked saccades but inability to move the eyes to command. The congenital form is accompanied by head thrusts which are used to change fixation from one target to another. Eyelid closure often occurs at the beginning of the head thrust to break fixation with the old target. As the child becomes older, the degree and excursion of head thrust decreases and, by adulthood, it is virtually eliminated. Patients with acquired oculomotor apraxia use blinks to break the fixation reflex and then turn their head toward the new fixation point. Vertical eye movements may be affected, but this is rare and there is retention of random saccadic horizontal movements. On optokinetic testing the fast phase of the optokinetic response is absent and the eyes are slowly driven toward the direction of the drum rotation. The location of the lesion in congenital oculomotor apraxia is unknown but when acquired it is usually caused by bilateral lesions in the supranuclear gaze pathways originating from the frontal lobes. It can be familial and has been associated with hypoplasia of the corpus callosum, hypoplasia of the cerebellum, and brainstem neoplasm (1, 3, 37).

Vertical Gaze Palsies

Vertical gaze palsies are almost always caused by lesions in the rostral midbrain near the area of the rostral interstitial nucleus of the MLF (riMLF). These lesions must either be bilateral or involve the crossing posterior commissure fibers (see Fig. 9–3). The medial portion of the riMLF is mainly devoted to down gaze whereas the lateral portion subserves up gaze. The lateral fibers course medially in the nucleus and cross in the posterior commissure before traveling in the MLF. Bilateral medial riMLF lesions can produce isolated down gaze palsies whereas a lesion in the posterior commissure can produce both up and down gaze paralysis. There have been case reports of a single unilateral lesion resulting in vertical gaze palsy (9).

Dorsal Midbrain Syndrome (Parinaud's)

Compressive lesions of the dorsal midbrain at the level of the posterior commissure can result in paralysis of up

Vertical Gaze Pathways

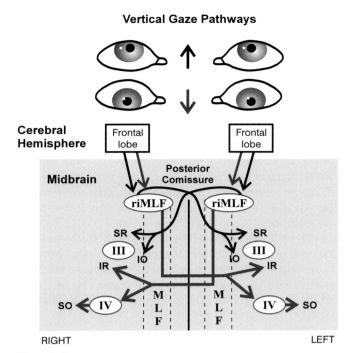

Figure 9–3.
Vertical gaze pathways. Vertical gaze is initiated by bilateral frontal lobe stimulation. The final common pathway is the rostral interstitial nucleus of the medial longitudinal fasciculus (riMLF). The lateral riMLF is responsible for up gaze with bilateral signals sent to both superior recti and inferior oblique. These fibers cross in the posterior commissure. Down gaze is initiated in the medial portion of the riMLF where signals are sent to the third and fourth nerve nuclei via the medial longitudinal fasciculus (MLF). (III=third nerve nucleus, IV=fourth nerve nucleus, SR=superior rectus, IO=inferior oblique, IR=inferior rectus, SO=superior oblique).

gaze, lid retraction which is exaggerated on attempted up gaze (Collier's sign), light-near dissociation, (pupils that constrict better with accommodation than with bright light), paralysis of convergence, paralysis of accommodation, (and convergence-retraction nystagmus best seen on attempted up gaze) (Parinaud's syndrome). Down-gaze may be limited and a skew deviation may occur with the higher eye on the side of the lesion. The eyes may be tonically deviated downward ("setting sun" sign). This type of downward deviation can occur in otherwise healthy neonates but in these children the eyes can easily be moved above the horizontal midline with the doll's head maneuver (10). The most common etiologies of Parinaud's syndrome are pineal tumors, hydrocephalus, and hemorrhage.

Progressive Supranuclear Palsy

Progressive supranuclear palsy is a degenerative disorder which is manifest by progressive ophthalmoplegia, pseudo-bulbar palsy, dysarthria, Parkinson-like symptoms, hyperreflexia, and dementia (14). The ophthal-

moplegia usually begins with limitation of downward gaze, followed by upward gaze, and eventually, complete ophthalmoplegia. Initially, oculo-cephalic responses are intact and the eyes can be moved into different gaze positions using the doll's head maneuver (34). The pathologic changes consist of loss of nerve cells and neuro-fibrillary tangles (different from Alzheimer's syndrome) which mainly involve neurons with relative sparing of axons and tracks. Involvement of the midbrain tegmentum and rostral interstitial nucleus of the MLF are necessary for ophthalmoplegia. The dementia which occurs often makes the individual unaware of their oculomotor limitations. There is no treatment for the disorder and it usually progresses to death within a few years (14).

Vestibular Eye Movements

Vestibular initiated eye movements occur after stimulation of the semicircular canals and the otolith organs. The signal is relayed to the ipsilateral vestibular nucleus where excitatory and inhibitory signals are sent to the oculomotor nuclei. Excitatory horizontal signals are transmitted to the *contralateral* sixth nerve nucleus directing the eyes (to initiate a conjugate eye movement) away from the stimulated ear using the same pathway as voluntary horizontal conjugate eye movements (see Fig. 10–5). Vertical and torsional excitatory signals travel by way of the medial longitudinal fasciculus (MLF) and the brachium conjunctivum to the *contralateral* oculomotor and trochlear nerve nuclei.

Horizontal Gaze Center (Paramedian Pontine Reticular Formation, PPRF)

The *voluntary* horizontal gaze center (PPRF) receives inputs from the contralateral superior colliculus (SC) and frontal eye fields (FEF) and projects directly to the abducens nerve nucleus which is in close proximity (see Fig. 9–4). Interneurons from the abducens nucleus travel via the contralateral MLF to stimulate the medial rectus. Voluntary gaze to the left (i.e., left lateral, right medial rectus) is initiated from the left PPRF. The PPRF does not play a significant role in the initiation of eye movements from vestibular stimulation or for smooth pursuit as these project directly to the abducens nucleus (4, 8). Therefore, it is possible to have a lesion in the PPRF which would result in an ipsilateral gaze paralysis but with intact vestibulo-ocular movements (doll's head, calorics) (8). Because the pathway for horizontal gaze relies on the internuclear neurons which originate in the ipsilateral abducens nucleus, a lesion of the sixth nerve nucleus produces an ipsilateral gaze palsy. A gaze palsy with ipsilateral facial weakness is most likely a le-

Horizontal Gaze Center

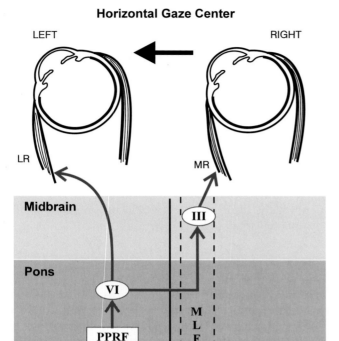

Figure 9–4.
Horizontal gaze center. The final common pathway for horizontal gaze begins at the parapontine reticular formation (PPRF). From here a signal is conveyed to the sixth nerve nucleus (VI) which controls the ipsilateral lateral rectus (LR). An internuclear connection to the contralateral third nerve nucleus is made by an interneuron which travels in the medial longitudinal fasciculus (MLF). The third nerve then sends a signal to the medial rectus, thus coordinating the left and right eye on left gaze.

sion of the sixth nerve nucleus as opposed to a PPRF lesion because of the close proximity of the VII nerve fibers which loop around the nucleus (35).

Acute unilateral hemispheric lesions which involve basal ganglion, thalamic, and upper brainstem areas can result in a *contralateral* gaze palsy. Pursuit is jerky toward the side of the lesion and absent to the contralateral side. With time, the gaze palsy becomes a saccadic palsy and typically resolves. A horizontal gaze palsy can also occur from an ipsilateral cerebellar infarct.

Internuclear Ophthalmoplegia (INO)

The medial longitudinal fasciculus extends from the mid-thoracic cord to the rostral midbrain and is the major interneuronal pathway between the oculomotor nuclei. One of its functions is to connect the abducens nuclei with the contralateral third nucleus enabling conjugate horizontal gaze. A unilateral lesion in the MLF between the abducens and oculomotor nucleus results in failure of the ipsilateral medial rectus to adduct

on horizontal gaze. Thus, a right MLF lesion results in failure of the right medial rectus to adduct on attempted left gaze (Fig. 9–5). Nystagmus of the contralateral abducting eye is a common finding and occurs as a result of excessive innervation to the normal lateral rectus muscle (a consequence of Hering's law of equal innervation to yoke muscles) (38). The most common cause of internuclear ophthalmoplegia (INO) in young adults is demyelinating disease, especially if the INO is bilateral, and occlusive vascular disease in older individuals. A variety of other etiologies have been reported including tumors, inflammation, carcinomatous meningitis, Arnold-Chiari malformation, and spinal cerebellar degeneration.

The WEBINO syndrome (*Wall-E*yed *B*ilateral INO) 20 is an unusual form of bilateral internuclear ophthalmoplegia which results in a large exotropia (20). The reason for the exotropia is unclear but it may be due to a bilateral lesion in the MLF very close to the medial rec-

Internuclear Ophthalmopelgia (INO)

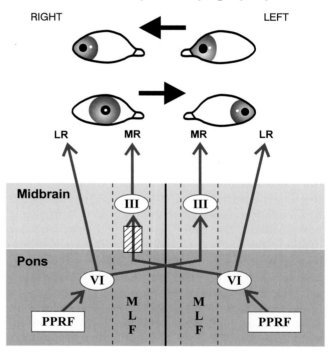

Figure 9–5.
Right internuclear ophthalmoplegia. A schematic illustrating the lesion responsible for a right internuclear ophthalmoplegia. Note that a lesion in the right medial longitudinal fasciculus (MLF) disconnects the left lateral rectus from the right medial rectus. Hence, on attempted left gaze the right eye does not adduct. Normal right gaze remains intact. (LR=lateral rectus, MR=medial rectus, PPRF=parapontine reticular formation, VI=sixth nerve nucleus, III=third nerve nucleus).

C. Miller Fisher "1 ½" Syndrome

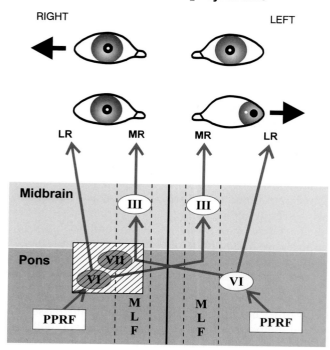

Figure 9–6.
C. Miller Fisher 1½ syndrome. A lesion in the right pons can result in a right gaze palsy and internuclear ophthalmoplegia.

tus subnucleus. Skew deviation and vertical nystagmus may also be present.

"One and A Half" (C. Miller Fisher) Syndrome

A highly localizing eye movement disorder can occur from a lesion in the pons involving the PPRF, sixth nerve nucleus, and the ipsilateral MLF. Such a lesion causes an ipsilateral gaze palsy with an inability of both eyes to look toward the side of the lesion (the one) and an ipsilateral medial rectus paralysis due to involvement of the ipsilateral medial longitudinal fasciculus (the half) (Fig. 9–6). The only horizontal eye movement remaining is abduction of the contralateral eye due to the intact contralateral sixth nerve nucleus. An ipsilateral facial nerve paralysis may also occur due to involvement of the seventh nerve fascicle as it loops around the sixth nerve nucleus. The etiology is usually an infarction, multiple sclerosis, arteriovenous (AV) malformation, or a posterior fossa tumor (30).

Skew Deviation

Skew deviation is a vertical strabismus of small size (less than 10 prism diopters) which is not localizable to any

vertical extraocular muscle. It is associated with significant brainstem or cerebellar injury and the hypotropic eye is usually ipsilateral to the side of the predominant brainstem lesion (12). The deviation is usually comitant (equal in all fields of gaze) but when incomitant tends to mimic an inferior rectus weakness. Lesions associated with skew deviations may occur in the midbrain, pons, or medulla.

Cerebellar Abnormalities

The cerebellum plays an intricate part in the overall integrity of all eye movements with numerous connections to the gaze centers, vestibular nuclei, and oculomotor nuclei. Abnormalities in the cerebellum result in a wide variety of ocular motility disturbances (Table 9–1). Specific cerebellar eye signs are difficult to recognize because disorders of the cerebellum frequently involve the brainstem (tumor, Arnold-Chiari malformation, multiple sclerosis, vascular disease). Saccadic dysmetria (which manifests as seccadic overshooting) appears to be caused by damage to the cerebellar dorsal vermis and fastigial nuclei while most of the other cerebellar signs are caused by damage to parts of the flocculus (vestibulo-cerebellum) (21).

TABLE 9–1
Cerebellar System Eye Signs

Cogwheel (saccadic) pursuit movements
Hypometric saccades
Horizontal gaze palsy or paresis
Slow saccades
Skew deviation
Slowed upward gaze
Square-wave jerks
Macro square-wave jerks
Macro saccadic oscillations
Nystagmus
   Horizontal gaze-evoked and paretic (unilateral or bilateral)
   Upbeat
   Downbeat
   Positional
   Rebound
   Acquired pendular
Ocular dysmetria
Ocular flutter
Opsoclonus
Ocular myoclonus

■ CRANIAL NERVE DYSFUNCTION

Oculomotor Nerve Palsy

The oculomotor nerve is responsible for elevation (superior rectus, inferior oblique), adduction (medial rectus), and depression (inferior rectus). It also provides innervation to the levator muscle to elevate the lid and parasympathetic innervation to the pupil causing constriction. A complete oculomotor nerve palsy results in ptosis, pupillary dilation, and the eye resting in the down and out position (Fig. 9–7).

Anatomy/Clinical Syndromes (Table 9–2)

Nucleus. The third nerve nucleus is located at the level of the superior colliculus, just ventral to the cerebral aqueduct near the midline of the rostral midbrain and is composed of numerous sub-nuclei (Fig. 9–8). The medial rectus, inferior rectus, and inferior oblique subnucleus project ipsilaterally while the superior rectus subnucleus projects contralaterally. Both levator muscles are innervated by a single midline central caudal nucleus. The Edinger-Westphal nucleus provides parasympathetic innervation to both pupils (Fig. 11–1). Because of this unique anatomical configuration, certain clinical presentations are diagnostic of a nuclear le-

sion (Table 9–3). For example, a patient with bilateral ptosis, *left* superior rectus weakness and *right* inferior rectus, medial rectus and inferior oblique weakness has a lesion in the right third nerve nucleus.

Fasciculus. The oculomotor neurons leave the nuclear complex and pass ventrally through the red nucleus and the cerebral peduncle (Fig. 9–9). Lesions in the red nucleus result in third nerve palsy, contralateral ataxia and intension tremor (*Benedikt's syndrome*) while lesions in the cerebral peduncle involve the cortical spinal tracts which result in third nerve palsy and contralateral hemiplegia (*Weber's syndrome*). Most oculomotor brainstem injuries are due to ischemia (30).

Interpeduncular

The third nerve leaves the brainstem and passes between the posterior cerebral and superior cerebellar arteries traveling infero-lateral but parallel to the posterior communicating artery (PCA) and medial to the edge of the tentorium. Here the nerve is vulnerable to damage from transtentorial herniation, trauma, meningitis, and compression from an aneurysm of the poste-

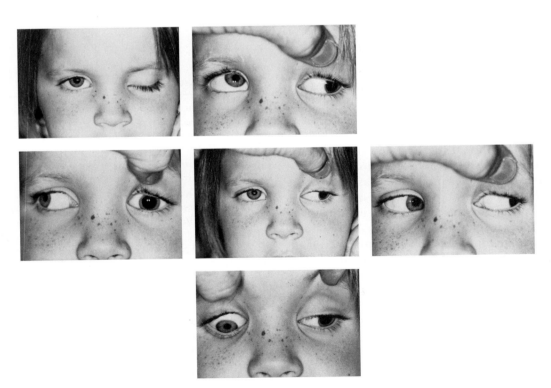

Figure 9–7.
Left third nerve palsy. Patient with a left third nerve palsy illustrating inability to adduct, elevate, or depress the left eye. Note complete ptosis and dilated pupil on the left.

TABLE 9–2
Etiology of Oculomotor Nerve Palsies

	Oculomotor (III)	Trochlear (IV)	Abducens (VI)
Nuclear	Infarction	Infarction	Infarction
	Tumor (mets)	Tumor (rare)	Demyelination
Interpeduncular	Aneurysm	Trauma	Trauma
	Ischemia (diabetic)	Ischemia (diabetic)	Ischemia (diabetic)
	Meningitis	Tumor (rare)	Tumor (CPA) (acoustic neuroma, meningioma, clivis chordoma, nasophar. ca.)
			Meningitis
			ICP
Cavernous Sinus	Fistula (Carotid, dural)	Inflammation (Tolosa-Hunt)	Inflammation (Tolosa-Hunt)
	Aneurysm	Aneurysm Tumor (same)	Aneurysm Tumor (same)
	Tumor (Menigioma, pituitary, sphenoid sinus ca., metastatic)		
	Infection (Mucormycosis, Herpes zoster	Infection (same)	Infection (same)
Orbit	Trauma	Trauma	Trauma
	Infection	Infection	Infection
	Pseudotumor		Pseudotumor
Misc.	Polyneuritis	Congenital ENT,	Viral
	Migraine	neurosurgical procedures	Petrous ridge inflammation
	Cyclic		

rior communicating artery or extra-axial tumor. Pupillary involvement is an early sign of a lesion in this location because of the superficial, dorsal-medial location of the pupillomotor fibers (Table 9–4). While pupillary involvement is seen in approximately 95% of cases due to a posterior communicating artery aneurysm at the junction of the internal carotid, a normal pupil does not completely exclude the possibility of aneurysm (23). However, pupillary sparing isolated third nerve palsies caused by aneurysms usually have only partial motility dysfunction (33). An acute complete oculomotor palsy with fixed pupil even when microvascular disease is pre-

sent, is an indication for further neuroradiologic imaging (30). Pupillary dilation can also be the first sign of an ipsilateral expanding supratentorial mass with compression of the oculomotor nerve against the petroclinoid ligament. Progression of tentorial herniation rapidly leads to other oculomotor nerve signs (11).

Cavernous Sinus. The oculomotor nerve travels in the cavernous sinus superiorly in the lateral wall (Fig. 9–10). It is in close proximity to the trochlear nerve, abducens nerve, oculosympathetics, and the first division of the trigeminal nerve. Disease processes in this region usu-

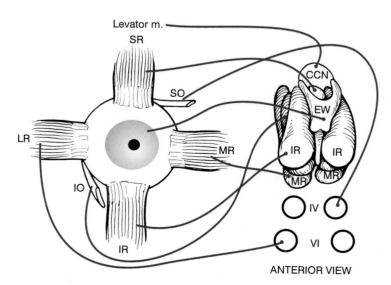

Figure 9–8.
Eye muscle innervation. A schematic showing the nuclear innervation of the extraocular muscles. Note that the superior rectus (SR) and superior oblique (SO) are innervated by contralateral cranial nuclei. Both pupils, which are innervated by the Edinger Westfal nucleus (EW), and the levator, which is innervated by the central caudal nucleus (CCN) receive input from a single nucleus.

TABLE 9–3
Third Nerve Palsy Nuclear Lesions

1. Conditions that cannot represent nuclear lesions
   a. Unilateral external ophthalomoplegia (with or without pupil involvement) associated with normal contralateral superior rectus function
   b. Unilateral internal ophthalmoplegia
   c. Unilateral ptosis
2. Conditions that may be nuclear
   a. Bilateral total third nerve palsy
   b. Bilateral ptosis
   c. Bilateral internal ophthalmoplegia
   d. Bilateral medial rectus palsy
   e. Isolated single muscle involvement (except levator and superior rectus)
3. Obligatory nuclear lesions
   a. Unilateral third nerve palsy with contralateral superior rectus and bilateral partial ptosis
   b. Bilateral third nerve palsy (with or without internal ophthalmoplegia) associated with spared levator function

ally affect more than one of these nerves. Etiologies include neoplasm, aneurysm, thrombosis, carotid cavernous sinus fistula, pituitary apoplexy, granulomatous inflammation (Tolosa Hunt syndrome), infection (herpes zoster), and ischemia. Third nerve palsies due to lesions in the cavernous sinus tend to be partial, only involving some of the extraocular muscles and have a tendency to appear to spare the pupil, in some cases because of co-existing sympathetic paresis (pseudosparing). The oculomotor nerve splits into a *superior division* (superior rectus, levator) and *inferior division* (medial rectus, inferior rectus, inferior oblique, (parasympathetic fibers to ciliary body and pupil)) somewhere between the anterior cavernous sinus and the orbital apex.

Orbital. Lesions within the orbit that produce oculomotor nerve palsies are usually associated with visual loss, other cranial nerve dysfunction, and proptosis. If an oculomotor dysfunction does occur from an orbital lesion it is usually incomplete due to the separation of the nerve into superior and inferior divisions. The most common cause of intraorbital involvement of the third nerve is trauma with occasional involvement by viral infections and tumors. Lesions at the orbital apex can be difficult to separate from those in the anterior cavernous sinus.

Oculomotor Palsy

Patients with an isolated oculomotor palsy can present in a variety of ways (Table 9–4). Remember, the pupilary fibers are superficial in location. Third nerve palsies that are caused by ischemia from microvascular disease tend to affect the deep fibers (oculomotor fibers) more

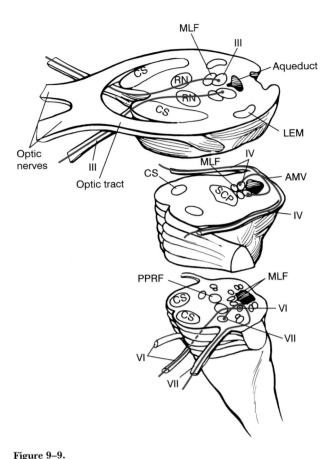

Figure 9–9.
Oculomotor brainstem anatomy. Top section: Oculomotor nerve (III). Note the relationship of the oculomotor nerve to the red nucleus (RN) and cortical spinal tracts (CS). Lesions in the red nucleus result in a third nerve palsy plus ipsilateral intention tremor (Benedikt's syndrome) while lesions in the cortical spinal tract result in third nerve palsies with contralateral hemiparesis (Weber's syndrome). Middle section: *Trochlear nerve* (IV). The fourth nerve is the only cranial nerve to exit posteriorly. It crosses in the anterior medullary vellum (AMV). Lesions in this area can result in bilateral fourth nerve palsies. Bottom section: *Abducens nerve* (VI). The sixth nerve is in close proximity to many brainstem nuclei. Of special importance is the facial nerve which loops around the sixth nerve nucleus before exiting. Also in close proximity are the horizontal gaze center (PPRF) and the medial longitudinal fasciculus (MLF). Lesions in this area can result in gaze palsies, internuclear ophthalmoplegias, and ipsilateral facial paralysis.

and peripheral (pupillary fibers) tend to be spared. Compressive lesions, however, usually affect the peripheral fibers earlier than central fiber. The most common presentation is the sudden onset of painful ophthalmoplegia with *pupillary sparing*. The pain may be quite severe and may precede the ophthalmoplegia by days or it may accompany the onset of ptosis or diplopia as a mild brow pain or headache. It is usually in the middle aged to elderly patient with diabetes and/or hypertension and is secondary to a microvascular insult. The ophthalmoplegia may be partial and complete recovery usually occurs by three months. Initial evaluation should in-

TABLE 9–4
"Isolated" Third Nerve Palsy Dangerosity Ranking

MOST	

D A N G E R O U S	• Complete—plus pupil
	   Probable aneurysm—Internal carotid/posterior communicating
	• Complete—plus partial pupil
	   Possible aneurysm—Internal carotid/posterior cerebral artery, cavernous sinus
	• Incomplete—pupil spared
	   Rare aneurysm
	      Superior cerebellar—posterior cerebral
	      Cavernous sinus
	   Mass—Cavernous sinus, Orbit

LEAST	• Complete—pupil spared Microvascular—Diabetes, Hypertension

TABLE 9–5
Etiology of Superior Oblique Paresis

Trauma	Collagen vascular diseases
Congenital	systemic lupus
Vascular disorders	polymyalgia rheumatica
diabetes	temporal arteritis
hypertension	Toxic substances
aneurysms	lead poisoning
arteriovenous malformations	quinoline poisoning
migraine	vitamin deficiency
Inflammatory disorders	alcohol
acute meningitis	Neoplasms
tuberculous meningitis	glioma
sarcoidosis	meningioma
syphilis	pituitary tumors
encephalomyelitis	schwannoma
Guillain-Barre syndrome	pinealoma
herpes zoster ophthalmocus	metastatic
botulism	Neuromuscular disorders
diphtheria	myasthenia gravis

Buckley, EG: Fourth nerve palsies. in Neuro-Ophthalmological Disorders, ed. Tusa, RL and Newman, SA. Dekker, New York, 1995.

clude a thorough examination to rule out other neurologic abnormalities, testing for diabetes, and a sedimentation rate to rule out temporal arteritis. If the ophthalmoplegia does not improve after eight to ten weeks then neuro-imaging should be considered. A second presentation is a *pupillary sparing* third nerve palsy with *no pain*. While this can also be due to microvascular disease, it is important to also consider a myopathy or a neuromuscular junction abnormality (myasthenia). The sudden onset of a *painful* third nerve palsy with *pupillary involvement* (immediate or developing over several days) should be evaluated for posterior communicating artery aneurysm. Magnetic resonance angiography may detect a small aneurysm but conventional angiography may still be necessary. Patients who manifest *incomplete* oculomotor palsy with *pupillary sparing*, particularly if the inferior division has been spared, should have angiography because of the high probability of having a compressive lesion at the superior cerebellar-posterior cerebral artery junction or in the cavernous sinus (6, 33). The last group are those patients who have a *complete* oculomotor palsy with *partial pupillary* involvement.

A small group of patients with this "relative pupillary sparing" have been found to have aneurysms. Angiography should be considered unless they have clear cut vasculopathic findings (33).

Childhood Oculomotor Nerve Palsy

Congenital oculomotor nerve palsy is considered an isolated disorder and usually results from birth trauma or developmental anomaly. Oculomotor synkinesis often occurs on the affected side (7). A small subgroup of patients with congenital oculomotor palsy have superimposed episodic contraction of some of the muscles supplied by the third nerve (*cyclic oculomotor palsy*). Typically there is lid elevation, miosis, adduction, and increased accommodation lasting approximately ten to thirty sec-

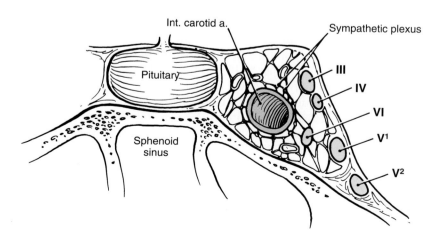

Figure 9–10.
Left cavernous sinus. A schematic illustrating structures present in the cavernous sinus. Cranial nerves III, IV, and V all lie against the lateral wall. The sixth nerve (VI) and the sympathetics are in close proximity to the internal carotid artery. Aneurysms of the carotid artery can cause an ipsilateral sixth nerve palsy with a Horner's syndrome. Abnormalities of the pituitary gland and a sphenoid sinus can impact on the cavernous sinus.

onds. Cycles reoccur about every two minutes even during sleep. Voluntary gaze efforts may influence the duration and intensity of the cycles in some cases. This unusual motility disorder usually persists throughout life. Patients do not require workup unless there is evidence of another progressive neurologic deficit (17, 24). Acquired oculomotor nerve palsy in childhood is usually associated with other signs of neurologic or systemic disease. The majority are traumatic, but may also be caused by *migraine,* meningitis, infection, or vaccination (9).

Aberrant Regeneration (Oculomotor Synkinesis)

Aberrant regeneration of the oculomotor nerve is characterized by elevation of the upper lid on attempted adduction or depression of the eye, retraction of the globe on attempted depression or elevation of the eye, and constriction of the pupil on attempted adduction or depression (Fig. 9–11). Aberrant regeneration has been observed in congenital third nerve palsies, in palsies secondary to tumors, aneurysms, and trauma, but *not* following ischemic ophthalmoplegia or demyelinated syndromes. Primary aberrant regeneration (aberrant regeneration without a preceding paralytic phase)—has been described with meningiomas and internal carotid artery aneurysms (28). The precise mechanism of aberrant regeneration is unknown but it is most likely due to a misdirection of regenerating motor axons within an injured oculomotor nerve. Alternative theories include ephaptic transmission (axon-axon cross-talk) and synaptic reorganization of the oculomotor nucleus following retrograde axonal degeneration (15).

Treatment of Third Nerve Palsies. The treatment of third nerve palsies is complicated because so many of the extraocular muscles are dysfunctional. Complete third nerve palsies should be approached with extreme caution since restoration of normal extraocular movement is impossible. The goals of surgery for partial palsies are to align the eyes in the primary position and in down gaze while retaining as much horizontal and vertical movement as possible. This will often necessitate both horizontal and vertical muscle surgery, usually involving both eyes. In addition to standard rectus muscle recessions and resections, transposition procedures, superior oblique tendon relocation, and faden operations are often necessary. Ptosis surgery and pharmacologic management of the pupil may also be required.

Fourth Nerve Palsies (Table 9–2)

Anatomy

The fourth cranial nerve is unique in that it is the only cranial nerve to exit dorsally from the brainstem. The

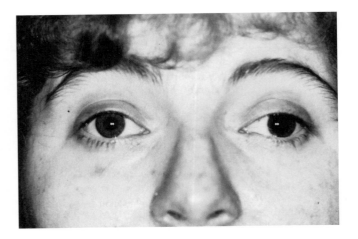
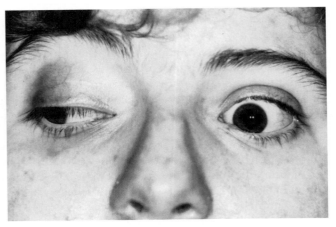

Figure 9–11.
Aberrant regeneration. Patient with a left third nerve palsy. TOP: Patient in the primary position. BOTTOM: Patient looking down and to the right. Note elevation of the lid on attempted down gaze. Aberrant regeneration is seen commonly after trauma and tumor involvement of the third nerve. It is never seen after ischemia.

nucleus is at the level of the inferior colliculus just inferior to the third nerve nuclear complex. The nerve exits posteriorly, crosses to the opposite side in the *anterior medullary velum* which is located near the fourth ventricle (Fig. 9–9). (Injuries in this region result in *bilateral* fourth nerve palsies.) It continues anteriorly in the subarachnoid space entering the cavernous sinus just below the oculomotor nerve and travels anteriorly in the lateral wall (Fig. 9–10), entering the superior orbital fissure *outside* the Annulus of Zinn to supply the superior oblique muscle. The superior oblique muscle is *contralaterally* innervated since the *left* fourth nerve nucleus supplies innervation to the *right* superior oblique muscle (Figs. 9–8, 9–9).

Clinical Characteristics

Patients with unilateral fourth nerve palsies complain of vertical and torsional diplopia. The diplopia is worse on

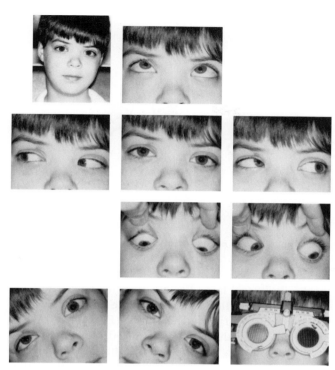

Figure 9–12.
Right fourth nerve palsy. Patient demonstrating characteristic findings of a right fourth nerve palsy which consists of a right hyperdeviation worse on left gaze and right head tilt. Bottom right photo demonstrates excyclotorsion by double maddox rod testing. Upper left hand photo shows characteristic left head tilt.

esotropia, and marked incyclotorsion (>10 degrees) (32) (Fig. 9–13). It can be difficult to recognize a fourth nerve palsy because ocular rotations are often "look" normal. The "three step test" is useful in documenting an isolated vertical muscle palsy. The characteristics of a fourth nerve palsy using the "three step test" are shown in Fig. 9–14.

Isolated Fourth Nerve Palsy

The most common cause of an isolated fourth nerve palsy is trauma (Table 9–5). The magnitude of the head trauma need not be severe but fourth nerve palsies associated with *minor* head trauma can be the result of undiagnosed intracranial tumors. An isolated fourth nerve palsy after *significant* head trauma requires no further radiologic evaluation. Usually vertical diplopia with a significant cyclotorsional component is due to bilateral fourth nerve injury.

Most other isolated fourth nerve palsies are felt to be congenital or microvascular. The etiology of congenital fourth nerve palsies is unknown. Patients usually become symptomatic in their third or fourth decades, had a head tilt present as a child or adolescent, have a history of increasing difficulties over many years, and, on examination, have large vertical fusional amplitudes (greater than 10–15 prism diopters—normal <4 prism diopters). The presence of a head tilt in photographs many years prior to the onset of the diplopia favors a long-standing benign condition.

Microvascular fourth nerve palsies occur in older individuals in the seventh and eighth decades. These usually result in small vertical deviations but the patients are very symptomatic because they lack vertical fusional amplitudes. As with other causes of neurologic microvascular disease, the workup is limited and involves a

gaze away from the involved superior oblique muscle and the patient may manifest a head tilt to the opposite side to eliminate diplopia (Fig. 9–12). Patients with *bilateral* fourth nerve palsies will often develop a chin tuck position since the eyes are usually straight in up gaze, have a large "V" pattern (esotropia worse in down gaze)

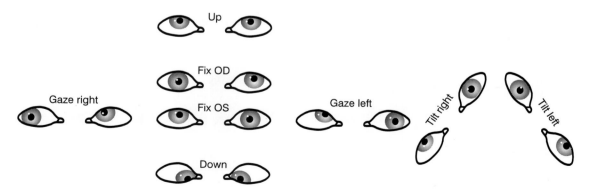

Figure 9–13.
Bilateral superior oblique palsy. A schematic illustrating motility pattern. Note large "V" pattern and alternating hyperdeviations on lateral gaze and head tilt.

Right Superior Oblique Palsy

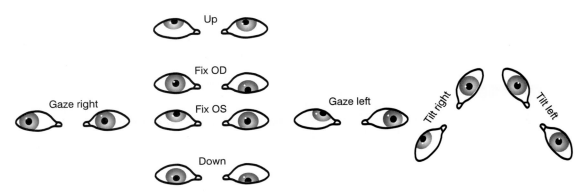

Figure 9–14.
Right superior oblique palsy. A schematic illustrating the "Park's three-step" for a right superior oblique palsy. Note the patient exhibits a right hyperdeviation worse on gaze left and right head tilt.

search for hypertension, diabetes, and vascular inflammatory disorders such as temporal arteritis.

A fourth nerve palsy is *rarely* a sign of intracranial neoplasms. The most common primary brain tumor involving the fourth nerve is a glioma of the cerebellum or midbrain. In data compiled from 318 patients with oculomotor nerve palsies from neoplasms, only 14 patients (4.4%) had fourth nerve involvement (19, 25, 26). An isolated fourth nerve palsy was the first sign of metastatic disease in only one case (19).

Treatment of Fourth Nerve Palsies

The treatment of diplopia associated with fourth nerve palsies depends on the etiology and the duration of symptoms. Many acquired fourth nerve palsies secondary to trauma or microvascular disease will spontaneously resolve by 3–4 months. In these situations prisms or monocular patching are helpful in eliminating symptoms. In patients with persistent vertical diplopia, strabismus surgery can be performed.

Sixth Nerve (Abducens) Palsy

Sixth nerve palsies are the most common of the oculomotor nerve palsies. Clinically it presents as a paralysis

of the ipsilateral lateral rectus muscle which results in an abduction deficit toward the side of the lesion, esotropia, and horizontal diplopia (Fig. 9–15). While most patients with an acute acquired esotropia have a sixth nerve palsy, a thorough ophthalmic and neurologic evaluation is necessary to eliminate the other causes of abduction deficits (Table 9–6).

Anatomy/Clinical Syndromes (Table 9–2)

Nucleus. The sixth nerve nucleus is located in the pons near the midline ventral to the fourth ventricle and the aqueduct of sylvus. It is in close association to the seventh nerve nucleus and the seventh nerve fascicle loops around the abducens nucleus before exiting from the brainstem (see Fig. 9–9). A nuclear sixth nerve lesion usually results in absent horizontal gaze toward the side of the lesion (due to disruption of the interneurons to the contralateral medial rectus subnucleus) and an ipsilateral peripheral facial nerve palsy.

Fasciculus. The fibers of the sixth nerve nucleus exit ventral medially and pass laterally to exit the brainstem at the ponto medullary junction. Lesions in the dorsal pons (*Folville's syndrome*) result in ipsilateral abduction

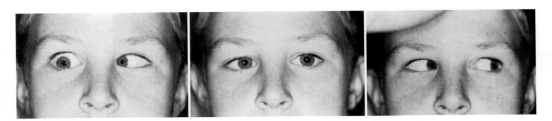

Figure 9–15.
Right sixth nerve palsy. Patient demonstrates an inability to abduct the right eye. An esotropia is present in the primary position. There is no abnormality on gaze left.

TABLE 9–6
Causes of Abduction Deficits

Sixth nerve palsies
Graves' myopathy (fibrotic medial rectus)
Myasthenia
Orbital inflammatory pseudotumor
Orbital trauma (medial rectus entrapment)
Congenital defects (Duane, Mobius)
''Convergence spasm''

---

weakness (or gaze palsy if abducens nucleus is involved), ipsilateral facial weakness and analgesia, ipsilateral peripheral deafness, loss of taste from the anterior two-thirds of the tongue, and ipsilateral Horner's syndrome. Lesions of the ventral pons (*Millard-Gubler syndrome*) produce in addition to the above signs, a contralateral hemiplegia from involvement of the corticospinal tract. Such brainstem injuries are usually the result of ischemia (anterior inferior cerebellar artery or paramedian perforating arteries), demyelination, or tumor.

Peripheral Nerve. After leaving the brainstem, the sixth nerve courses upward, passing between the pons and the anterior inferior cerebellar artery before penetrating the dura overlying the clivus. Because of its fixed attachment to the dura at this point, it is susceptible to stretching injuries from increased intracranial pressure which cause downward displacement of the brainstem. Unilateral or bilateral sixth nerve paralysis are a frequent finding of increased intracranial pressure along with headache, nausea, vomiting, and papilledema. Sixth nerve palsies can also result after lumbar puncture, lumbar peritoneal shunts, and contrast myelography by a similar mechanism. Tumors such as chordomas and nasopharyngeal carcinoma often involve the sixth nerve at this location.

Before the sixth nerve enters the cavernous sinus it passes through the *inferior petrous sinus* and underneath the petroclinoid ligament (*Droello's canal*). At this location it is susceptible to irritation and inflammation of the mastoid or petrous bone from otitis media which can produce ipsilateral sixth nerve palsy, facial weakness, pain in the distribution of the ophthalmic division of the trigeminal nerve, and decreased tearing (*Gradenigo's syndrome*).

Unilateral or bilateral sixth and seventh nerve palsies can occur following head trauma due to basilar skull fractures which involve the petrous bone. Leakage of blood or spinal fluid from the external ear or ecchy- mosis of the mastoid area (*Battle's sign*) is evidence of a basal skull fracture.

Intercavernous Sinus. In the cavernous sinus, the sixth nerve courses anteriorly and laterally around the carotid artery and medial and parallel to the ophthalmic division of the trigeminal nerve. The branch of the carotid sympathetics join the nerve briefly before traveling with the first branch of the trigeminal nerve. The abducens nerve is not attached to the lateral wall of the cavernous sinus as are the third and fourth nerves. Lesions of the cavernous sinus often involve more than one cranial nerve, however, isolated sixth nerve palsies frequently occur with carotid cavernous fistulas, intercavernous aneurysms, and cavernous sinus thrombosis (4). A painful isolated sixth nerve palsy should be evaluated for intercavernous aneurysm and a chronic sixth nerve palsy may be the only sign of an intercavernous meningioma. An ipsilateral Horner's syndrome with an isolated sixth nerve palsy indicates a lesion in the cavernous sinus due to carotid artery aneurysm or neoplasm (5).

Isolated Sixth Nerve Palsy

Isolated sixth nerve palsies can occur from microvascular disease secondary to hypertension, diabetes, and rarely from temporal arteritis. If a workup for these disorders is negative, further radiologic evaluation is not necessary unless other cranial nerves become involved, there is associated ocular or facial pain, or improvement fails to occur after three or four months. Twenty-five percent of chronic sixth nerve palsies have been found to be due to tumor or aneurysms (27). Isolated sixth nerve palsies in children are usually of post-viral origin, either secondary to upper respiratory illness or immunization. A workup in this age group should rule out middle ear infection and sinus disease. Recurrent sixth nerve palsies can occur in children and are usually benign (36).

Treatment of Sixth Nerve Palsies

Acute traumatic or microvascular sixth nerve palsies usually require no treatment and will resolve spontaneously in two to three months. Contracture of the medial rectus during the paralysis can be prevented by the use of botulinum toxin injections into the ipsilateral medial rectus. This therapeutic maneuver should not be used in situations where the etiology of the sixth nerve palsy is in doubt. Strabismus surgery if necessary is often quite successful.

■ NEUROMUSCULAR JUNCTION ABNORMALITIES

Myasthenia Gravis

Myasthenia gravis is an autoimmune disorder of neuromuscular transmission caused by antibody formation to the post synaptic acetylcholine receptors of skeletal muscle endplates. The exact cause of the autoimmune activity is unknown but abnormalities in the thymus may be responsible for stimulating the humoral immune system. Approximately 10% of patients with myasthenia have been found to have thymomas.

The most commonly affected muscles are the levator, extraocular muscles, orbicularis oculi, triceps, quadriceps, and tongue (31). Ocular muscle involvement eventually occurs in 90% of all patients and is the initial complaint in 50–75%. Fifty to 70% of the patients with only ocular symptoms progress to generalized myasthenia within two years while 20% remain purely ocular.

A variable ptosis is the hallmark of ocular myasthenia gravis and often begins with a unilateral ptosis noted only on fatigue or at the end of the day. It may be associated with contralateral upper lid retraction which occurs because of Herring's law of equal innervation. Clinically, the ptosis can be exaggerated by sustained up gaze or repeated eyelid closure. Another useful sign is elicited by having the patient rapidly redirect their eyes from down gaze to the primary position. When performing this maneuver, the lids will overshoot upward and then slowly settle to the ptotic position (*Cogan's lid twitch sign*).

Extraocular muscle involvement can occur with or without ptosis. It can mimic any of the extraocular muscle palsies and can vary from a simple weakness of adduction of one eye (pseudo internuclear ophthalmoplegia) to a complete external ophthalmoplegia (Table 9–7). The pupils and accommodation are not involved.

A Tensilon test can be used to confirm the diagnosis of myasthenia gravis. Most myasthenics will show some improvement following the intravenous injection of edrophonium (Tensilon), a fast acting anti-cholinesterase. A negative Tensilon test does not rule out the diagnosis of myasthenia, especially in chronic ocular myasthenia.

An alternative to Tensilon is the use of intramuscular Prostigmine (.02 mg per kilogram not to exceed 1.5 mg mixed with atropine injected as a mixture into one of the deltoid muscles). This is particularly useful in patients with diplopia but without ptosis and in children who will not tolerate IV drug administration. Ocular motility assessment is made 30–45 minutes after intermuscular injection.

Other diagnostic tests for myasthenia include electromyography, anti-acetylcholine receptor antibody titers, and MRI of the mediastinum (thymoma). Tests of thyroid function and for collagen vascular disease should also be performed.

Treatment of myasthenia gravis is based on increasing the amount of neurotransmitter or decreasing the immune response to the muscle receptor. Pyridostigmine (Mestinon) is a long acting anti-cholinesterase

TABLE 9–7
Ocular Motility Defects

	Graves' Ophthalmopathy	Myasthenia	Ocular Myopathy (PEO)	Combined III, IV, VI
Course	Chronic + history of dysthyroidism	Acute, intermittent, then chronic	Slowly progressive	Acute
Bilateral	Usually but asymetrical	Usually, often asymetrical	Always	Rarely
Pain	No; Foreign body sensation	No	No	Variable
Diplopia	Variable	Yes	No	Yes
Pupils	Normal	Normal	Normal	Normal except for III
Lids	Retraction	Ptosis	Ptosis	Ptosis (III only)
Tensilon	Negative	Positive	Negative	Negative
Forced duction	Positive	Negative	Variable	Negative
Other signs	Lid retraction, scleral injection, proptosis, lid edema	Ptosis, fatigability, orbicularis weakness	Ptosis, orbicularis weakness, temporalis wasting, retinal pigment abnormality	Varies depending on location of lesion, facial weakness, trigeminal anesthesia, decreased hearing, arm, leg weakness

which makes more acetylcholine available to the receptors. It requires frequent administration (4–5 times/day) and has a high incidence of gastrointestinal side effects. Corticosteroids suppress the immune response and decrease receptor antibody production. Other therapeutic options include thymectomy, cyto- toxic drugs, and plasmapheresis. Purely ocular myasthenia can be refractive to treatment and may require combination therapy. Ptosis and strabismus surgery have been effective in those patients unresponsive to other modalities.

■ OCULAR MYOPATHIES

Dysthyroid Myopathy (Graves' Disease)

Thyroid myopathy is a condition which produces enlargement of the extraocular muscles resulting in restrictive strabismus, proptosis, lid retraction, and in some individuals, optic nerve compression with loss of vision. It is encountered in all age groups but is most common in the middle ages from 20–50 and almost never occurs below the age of 15 years. The motility disorder and thyroid condition are only loosely related and ocular problems can occur in patients with any thyroid state.

The exact mechanism for the enlargement of the extraocular muscles is unknown. Pathologic examination reveals lymphocytic and plasmocytic infiltration with edema and fibrosis. Investigators have demonstrated the presence of antibodies against eye muscle antigens in patients with Graves' ophthalmopathy (29).

Typically the muscle enlargement begins slowly and often the patient only complains of mild diplopia, usually in the morning, which improves several hours after wakening. There may be increased congestion in and around the eyes with mild lower lid edema and con- junctival injection (Fig. 9–16). If the process is symmetrical, diplopia may not occur until late. The inferior rectus is the most frequently involved muscle followed by the medial and, only rarely, the superior rectus. The lateral rectus is almost never involved in this process. Patients will usually complain of vertical double vision which is worse on up gaze due to a tight and fibrotic inferior rectus muscle. Another common presentation is that of a pseudo sixth nerve palsy due to a tight medial rectus muscle limiting abduction (Fig. 9–16). The clinical suspicion of restrictive strabismus can be confirmed using the forced duction test. In subtle cases, spontaneous lid retraction (stare) or lid lag on down gaze may be observable (4). The conjunctival vessels overlying the muscle insertions are often tortuous and dilated.

The clinical course of thyroid eye disease is quite variable. Some patients exhibit only mild motility disturbances which resolve spontaneously over several months to a year. Other individuals will take a more fulminant course with massive enlargement of the extraocular muscles, extensive proptosis, and severe diplopia. The process eventually "burns out," leaving the patient with either partial or total resolution of the

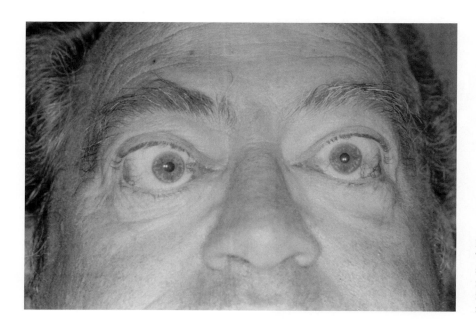

Figure 9–16.
Thyroid myopathy. Note marked proptosis and lid retraction. Esotropia is present. The most common extraocular muscle involvement is the inferior and medial rectus.

extraocular muscle involvement. As a general rule, the more restrictive the process during the acute phase, the less likely it will completely resolve. Patients who are suspected of having thyroid myopathy should be evaluated with CT or MRI scanning. Enlarged extraocular muscles are easily seen with this technique and a particular pattern of enlargement of the muscle belly helps distinguish thyroid myopathy from inflammatory disorders which tend to enlarge the muscle at the insertion (Fig. 9–17). The finding of enlarged extraocular muscles bilaterally is almost pathognomonic for Grave's ophthalmopathy. Other disorders which produce large extraocular muscles include myositis, tumor infiltration, lymphoma, orbital venous congestion, and trichinosis. In addition to neuroradiologic investigation, laboratory evaluation of thyroid function is important and should include T3, T4, TSH, and T3-Resin uptake (free T4 index). The majority of patients with euthyroid Grave's disease demonstrate an autonomous thyroid gland that has escaped the normal feedback regulatory control of circulating thyrotropin (TSH). After administration of intravenous TRH, the TSH level normally increases within 30 minutes. Markedly decreased or absent TSH response to TRH confirms the presence of thyroid dysfunction in the presence of normal hormonal levels (TRH stimulation test).

The treatment for thyroid eye disease is limited to symptomatic relief during the acute phase unless optic nerve compression or severe proptosis occurs. Under those circumstances systemic steroids, low dose orbital radiation, or orbital decompression may be necessary. Steroids and radiation are not useful in managing the diplopia. Botulinum toxin has been found to be useful

TABLE 9–8

Manifestation of the Kearns-Sayre-Daroff Syndrome ("Ophthalmoplegia Plus")

Cardinal manifestations
  External ophthalmoplegia with onset in childhood
  Retinal pigmentary degeneration
  Cardiac conduction defects
  Elevated cerebrospinal fluid protein
  Abnormal muscle mitochondria
  Spongiform encephalopathy, including brain stem
  Negative family history
Associated manifestations
  Short stature
  Neurologic
    Deafness
    Cerebellar ataxia
    Mild corticospinal tract signs
    "Descending" myopathy of face and limbs
    Subnormal intelligence
    Slowed electroencephalogram
    Aseptic meningitis (by history)
    Demyelinating radiculopathy
    Decreased ventilatory drive
    Hyperglycemic acidotic coma/death
  Endocrine
    Diabetes mellitus
    Hypogonadism
    Hypoparathyroidism
    Growth hormone deficiency
    Adrenal dysfunction
  Skeletal and dental anomalies
  Corneal edema

Glaser, JS, and Bachynski, B: Infranuclear disorders of eye movement. In: Glaser, JS (ed), Neuro-ophthalmology. Philadelphia, J.B. Lippincott Co., 1990; p. 402.

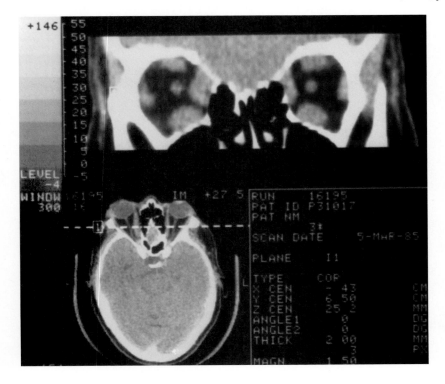

Figure 9–17.
CT scan of thyroid myopathy. Note enlargement of all the extraocular muscles especially the inferior and medial rectus.

in providing symptomatic relief in patients with small angle vertical or horizontal deviations. Strabismus and lid surgery should be deferred until the condition is stable for at least six months and the patient's thyroid status has been normalized.

Mitochondrial Cytopathies (Chronic Progressive External Ophthalmoplegia)

Chronic progressive external ophthalmoplegia (CPEO) consists of slowly progressive bilateral ptosis and inability to move the eyes. There is accompanying weakness of the orbicularis oculi but the pupils are spared. CPEO may be a part of degenerative disorders of the nervous system such as spinal cerebellar degeneration and hereditary ataxia, deficiency states such as abetalipoproteinemia (Basen-Kornzweig disease), or it may be a primary manifestation of mitochondrial dysfunction. In these patients, in addition to a limitation of ocular movement, there is often associated other ocular, neurologic, and systemic abnormalities.

The primary defect in patients with CPEO appears to be in the mitochondria of skeletal muscle and other tissues. Muscle biopsies treated with a modified trichrome stain under light microscopy reveal "ragged red fibers," which are felt to be clumps of degenerative mitochondria. The exact metabolic defect is unknown. Both autosomal dominant and maternal inheritance of CPEO have been identified (22).

Ptosis is usually the first sign and may precede the ophthalmoplegia by years. It is usually bilateral but can be asymmetric early in the disease. Often the ptosis will be severe enough to result in a head tilt position. The ophthalmoplegia is bilateral and patients usually do not notice diplopia until the motility disturbance becomes severe. Downward movements are relatively intact compared to upward and horizontal movements but most cases eventually proceed to complete ophthalmoplegia.

The *Kearns Sayre syndrome* is a special form of CPEO that has multi system involvement Table 9–8. It usually presents before age 20 with bilateral ophthalmoplegia and a pigmentary retinopathy, characterized by a "salt and pepper" appearance of the posterior pole but normal ERG. Of particular importance are the cardiac conduction abnormalities which occur in these patients. Complete heart block may cause sudden death and may occur early in the course of the disease. These patients must be followed with sequential ECG's.

The differential diagnosis of CPEO includes chronic ocular myasthenia, dysthyroid myopathy, brainstem dysfunction with gaze palsies, progressive supranuclear palsy, Parkinsonism, and oculopharyngeal dystrophy.

There is no specific therapy for CPEO. If diplopia develops strabismus surgery can be performed. Ptosis surgery should be approached with caution because of the poor Bell's phenomena and risks of corneal exposure. In patients with cardiac abnormalities, a pacemaker may be lifesaving.

Oculopharyngeal Dystrophy

Oculopharyngeal dystrophy is characterized by progressive external ophthalmoplegia, ptosis, wasting of the temporalis muscle, and involvement of the pharyngeal muscles. It has been traced to Quebec where a large number of French Canadians are affected. It is inherited as an autosomal dominant trait and becomes manifest after age 40. There is no abnormality of the mitochondria on muscle biopsy, though there are degenerative changes which can be present with variable involvement of the lids, pharyngeal muscles, and extraocular muscles.

Idiopathic Myositis

Patients with orbital myositis have the acute onset of diplopia, orbital pain, focal or diffuse conjunctival injection with chemosis, and proptosis. It can be unilateral or bilateral and can involve one or more of the extraocular muscles. It usually involves young individuals and can be isolated or recurrent. It can also occur with systemic disorders characterized by collagen vascular disease or granulomatous inflammation. CT will reveal the enlargement of the extraocular muscles which extends to the muscle insertion. Biopsy of the involved muscle shows lymphocytic infiltration. Biopsies, however, should be avoided as they tend to worsen the clinical situation. Corticosteroids are the mainstay of treatment and the response is usually dramatic with lessening of the pain within 24 hours and marked improvement in ocular motility by 48 hours. A slow steroid taper is necessary in order to avoid recurrence.

Myotonic Dystrophy

Myotonic dystrophy is an autosomal dominant muscular dystrophy which is accompanied by dystrophic changes in testicle, lenses, skin, hair, and brain. Myotonia is persistent contracture of muscle fibers when they should be relaxed. It is felt to be a disorder of the muscle membrane and has a characteristic electromyographic response (sounds like a bomber). The disease begins in the hands and usually it progresses to the face and then limbs. A characteristic facial expression arises because of atrophy and dysfunction of the facial muscles (myopathic facies). Frontal baldness also occurs because of skin abnormality. Ocular findings include ptosis, external ophthalmoplegia, cataracts, miotic pupils, and retinal degeneration. The ophthalmoplegia may mimic progressive external ophthalmoplegia or may just consist of slowed eye movements. The most common ocular abnormality is polychromatic cataracts which are present in the majority of patients. It may be the only manifestation of the disease (13, 16).

Mobius Syndrome

Mobius syndrome is characterized by bilateral horizontal eye movement abnormality, mask-like facies, a history of infantile feeding difficulties (ninth nerve), and atrophy of the distal part of the tongue (twelfth nerve). Hypoplastic limb anomalies and chest deformities have also been described. The etiology is felt to be aplasia of the cranial nerve nuclei. The motility disturbance can range from bilateral abduction deficits to bilateral horizontal gaze palsies. Convergence substitution is often used to compensate for the horizontal gaze defect. Rectus muscles may be fibrotic and the forced duction test may be abnormal. If seventh nerve function is severely impaired, exposure keratitis may occur as a result of inadequate lid closure. All patients have some degree of mental retardation. Most cases of Mobius syndrome are sporadic although dominant pedigrees have been reported.

Synergistic Divergence

Patients with this syndrome present with exotropia, monocular medial rectus palsy, and paradoxical abduction of the involved eye on gaze into the field of action of the paretic medial rectus muscle (on attempted abduction of the non involved eye, both eyes abduct). Electromyographic evidence suggests that there is anomalous innervation of the lateral rectus muscle by the nerve intended for the medial rectus. There is minimal or absent innervation of the lateral rectus by the sixth nerve. This is similar to the innervational abnormality seen in Duane's syndrome except that the major portion of the medial rectus nerve is now innervating the lateral rectus. Synergistic divergence has been seen in patients who have other innervation abnormalities such as Marcus Gunn jaw winking.

■ REFERENCES

1. Borchert MS, Sadun AA, Sommers JD, Wright KW, et al.: Congenital ocular motor apraxia in twins. Findings with MRI. J Clin Neuro Ophthalmol—1987:7:104.
2. Campbell IW and Wharty RH: Saccadic omission: why we do not see a grey out during saccadic eye movement. Vision Res—1978:18:1297–1303.
3. Fielder AR, Gresty MA, Dodd KL, et al.: Congenital ocular motor apraxia. Trans Ophthalmol Soc UK—1986:105:589.
4. Glaser JS, and Bachynski B: Infranuclear disorders of eye movement. In: Glaser JS (ed). Neuro-ophthalmology. Philadelphia—J.B. Lippincott Co., 1990:361–418.
5. Gutman I, Levartovski S, Goldhammer Y, Tadmor R, Findler G: Sixth nerve palsy and unilateral horner's syndrome. Ophthalmol, 1986:93:913–916.
6. Guy JR, and Day AL: Intracranial aneurysms with superior division paresis of the oculomotor nerve. Ophthalmol, 1989:96:1071–1076.
7. Hamed LM: Associated neurologic and ophthalmologic findings in congenital oculomotor nerve palsy. Ophthalmol, 1991:98:708–714.
8. Hanson MR, Hamid MA, Tomsak RL, et al.: Selective saccadic palsy caused by pontine lesions: clinical, physiological and pathological correlations. Ann Neurol—1986:20:209.
9. Harley RD: Paralytic strabismus in children. Etiologic incidence and management of the third, fourth and sixth nerve palsies. Ophthalmol, 1980:87:24–43.
10. Hoyt CS, Mousel DK, Weber AA: Transient supranuclear disturbances of gaze in healthy neonates. Am J Ophthalmol—1980:89:708–713.
11. Keane JR: Bilateral ocular motor signs after tentorial herniation in 25 patients. Arch Neurol—1986:43:806.
12. Keane JR: Ocular skew deviation. Arch Neurol—1975:32:185.
13. Kuhn E, Fiehn W: Adult form of myotonic dystrophy. In: Huber A, Klein D (eds). Neurogenetics and Neuro-ophthalmology. Amsterdam—Elsevier/North Holland, 1981:31.
14. Lees AJ: The Steele-Richardson-Olszewski syndrome (progressive supranuclear palsy). In: Marshen CD, Fahn S (eds). Movement Disorders. Boston—Butterworths, 1987:272.
15. Lepore FE, Glaser JS: Misdirection revisited. A critical appraisal of acquired oculomotor nerve synkinesis. Arch Ophthalmol—1980:98:2206–2209.
16. Lessel S, Coppeto J, Samet S: Ophthalmoplegia in myotonic dystrophy. Am J Ophthalmol—1971:71:1231.
17. Loewenfeld I, Thompson HS: Oculomotor paresis with cyclic spasms. A critical review of the literature and a new case. Surv Ophthalmol—1975:20:81.
18. Manning KA and Riggs LA: Vergence eye movements and visual suppression. Vision Res—1984:24:521–526.
19. Mansour AM, Reinecke RD: Central trochlear palsy. Surv Ophthalmol—1986:30:279–297.
20. McGettrick P, Eustace P: The WEBINO syndrome. Neuro-ophthalmology—1985:5:109.
21. Miller NR: Clinical Neuro-Ophthalmology. Baltimore—Williams and Wilkins, 1985:608–634.
22. Newman NJ: Mitochondrial disease and the eye. Ophthalmol Clin North Am—1992:5:405–424.
23. O'Conner PS, Tredici TJ, Green RP: Pupil-sparing third

nerve palsies caused by aneurysm. Am J Ophthalmol—1983:95:395.

24. Purvin V: Third cranial nerve palsy. In: Diagnostic Problems in Clinical Ophthalmology. Margo CE (ed). Philadelphia—W.B. Saunders, 1994:678–685.

25. Rucker CW: The causes of paralysis of the third, fourth and sixth cranial nerves. Am J Ophthalmol—1966:61:1293–1298.

26. Rush JA, Yong PR: Paralysis of cranial nerves III, IV, and VI: cause and prognosis in 1000 cases. Arch Ophthalmol—1981:99:76–79.

27. Savino PJ, Helliker JK, Gaskill GH, and Schatz NJ: Chronic sixth nerve palsies. Arch Ophthalmol—1982;100:1442.

28. Schatz NJ, Savino PJ, Corbett JJ: Primary aberrant oculomotor regeneration. Arch Neurol—1977:34:29–32.

29. Sergott RC, Felberg NT, Savino PJ, Bllzzard JJ, and Schatz NJ: The clinical immunology of Graves ophthalmology. Ophthalmol, 1981:88:484–487.

30. Sharpe JA, Rosenberg MA, Hoyt WF, et al.: Paralytic pontine exotropia. Neurology—1974;24:1076.

31. Simpron JA: Myasthenia gravis and myasthenia syndromes. In: Disorders of voluntary muscle. Walton J (ed). Edinburgh—Churchill Livingstone, 1981:585–624.

32. Sydnor CF, Seaber JH, Buckley EG: Traumatic superior oblique palsies. Ophthalmol, 1982:89:134–138.

33. Trobe JD: Isolated pupil-sparing third nerve palsy. Ophthalmol, 1985:92:58–61.

34. Troost BT, and Daroff RB: The ocular motor defects in progressive supranuclear palsy. Ann Neurol—1977:2:397.

35. Wall M, and Wray SH: The one and a half syndrome—a unilateral disorder of the pontine tegmentum: a study of 20 cases and review of the literature. Neurology—1983:33:971.

36. Werner DB, Savino PJ, and Schatz NJ: Benign recurrent sixth nerve palsies in childhood. Arch Ophthalmol—1983:101:601–608.

37. Zaret CR, Behrens MM, Eggers HM: Congenital ocular motor apraxia and brainstem tumor. Arch Ophthalmol—1980;98:328.

38. Zee DS, Hain TC, Carl JR: Abducting nystagmus in internuclear ophthalmoplegia. Ann Neurol—1987:21:383.

10 Nystagmus

Edward G. Buckley

Nystagmus is an involuntary, rhythmic, to and fro oscillation of the eyes. The movement can be pendular, jerk, rotary, elliptical or any combination. A pendular nystagmus has equal velocity in each direction. The term "jerk nystagmus" denotes a movement of unequal directional speed and by convention the nystagmus is named after the *fast* component. A left jerk nystagmus has a slow movement to the right and a fast movement to the left. Rotary nystagmus denotes a rotation (torsion) around the visual axis with no horizontal or vertical movement of the eye. Elliptical or circular nystagmus is a movement which involves a combination of vertical and horizontal displacements.

When describing a nystagmus, as much information about the movement as possible should be recorded including the type of movement, the frequency (the number of oscillations per unit of time; typically slow, medium or fast), the amplitude (the distance traveled during the movement; fine or course), and the direction which may be horizontal, vertical, rotary, oblique, or circular. A schemata is helpful in recording this information (Fig. 10–1). A complete description often aids in the diagnosis and follow up of the patient's subsequent course (2).

Nystagmus can result from dysfunction in the afferent visual system (Table 10–1), vestibular apparatus, or cerebellum and can be either congenital or acquired.

Congenital nystagmus is usually due to some type of identifiable disorder of the *anterior* visual pathway or is caused by a primary motor dysfunction. *Posterior* chiasmal lesions and cortical blindness do not cause nystagmus, although they may show slow roving eye movements. Acquired nystagmus is almost always a sign of a significant central nervous system abnormality.

Patients with nystagmus will often develop a head position to dampen the nystagmus and improve visual function (the "null point") (Fig. 10–2). The presence of a preferred head position is not helpful in deciding about etiology but may have some bearing on visual function and the type of nystagmus. Patients with a jerk nystagmus more often tend to develop a head position than patients with pendular nystagmus. This is because of a phenomena known as *Alexander's law,* which states that "a jerk nystagmus becomes worse when gazing in the direction of the fast component." Thus a right jerk nystagmus becomes much worse in right gaze and improves in left gaze (Fig. 10–3). A patient with a right jerk nystagmus will have a right face turn with a gaze left preference. *Spasmus nutans,* a benign form of acquired asymmetric or unilateral pendular nystagmus, will often have an associated head nod or bob. Adults with acquired nystagmus will also seek gage positions of decreased oscillation to improve visual function and decrease symptoms (with compensatory force turn).

■ NYSTAGMUS TYPES OF DIAGNOSTIC IMPORTANCE

Congenital Nystagmus

Congenital nystagmus is caused by either visual system abnormality involving the retina or optic nerve or a congenital motor abnormality—afferent pathy abnormalities is associated with poor vision and is termed sensory nystagmus, Primary motor nystagmus is congenital *motor nystagmus* (3) (Table 10–2). Characteristically congeni-

197

Nystagmus Notation

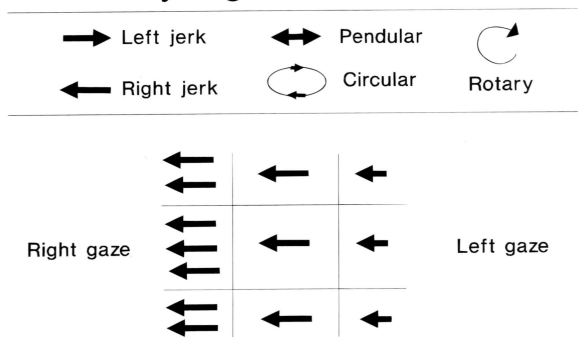

→ Left jerk   ↔ Pendular   ↻ Rotary

← Right jerk   Circular

Right gaze   Left gaze

Figure 10–1.

Nystagmus notation. The above schemata is useful in describing a patient's nystagmus. Directional arrows are used to indicate the direction of the nystagmus and its basic characteristics. Multiple arrows and the length of the arrow can be used to indicate frequency and amplitude respectively.

tal nystagmus is a conjugate horizontal nystagmus which remains horizontal on up and down gaze. It can take on any combination of wave forms including pendular, jerk or rotary. It is often associated with a compensatory head position and the frequency and amplitude may decrease with time. There may be periods where the nystagmus appears to worsen and these are usually associated with illness, fatigue, or stress. There is no oscillopsia and it is abolished during sleep. Congenital nystagmus is dampened by convergence and is often associated with an es-

Figure 10–2.
(LEFT) Patient with a left jerk nystagmus using a left head turn gaze right preference to obtain best visual acuity. (RIGHT) Same patient after a Kestenbaum surgical procedure to relocate the null point to the primary position.

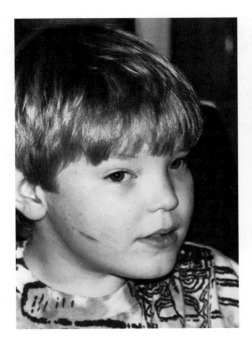
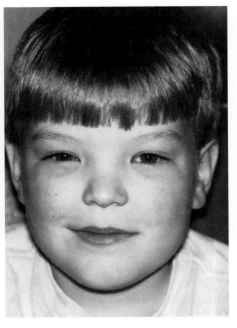

TABLE 10–1
Ocular Causes of Nystagmus

Achromatopsia
Aniridia
Cataracts
High myopia
Macular hypoplasia
Retinitis pigmentosa
Nystagmus associated with minimal fundus abnormalities
    Leber's congenital amaurosis
    Rod monochromacy
    Blue cone monochromacy
    Hereditary optic atrophy
    Optic nerve hypoplasia
    Ocular albinism
    Congenital stationary night blindness

TABLE 10–2
Clinical Characteristics of Congenital Nystagmus

Horizontal
Binocular
Symmetrical
Dampened by convergence
Associated esotropia
Optokinetic nystagmus inversion (two-third of patients)
Head oscillation
No oscillopsia
Abolished in sleep
Distinctive wave forms
Preferred gaze direction with improved visual function

otropia (Nystagmus Blockage Syndrome). In congenital jerk nystagmus, approximately two-thirds of the patients exhibit a paradoxical *inversion* of the optokinetic response (i.e., the direction of the quick recovery phase is the same as that of the drum rotation instead of in the opposite direction) (15). Some patients may have associated head nodding or shaking. The head nodding can be in a direction and amplitude different from the underlying nystagmus and provides no visual benefit (12).

Alexander's Law
Right Jerk Nystagmus

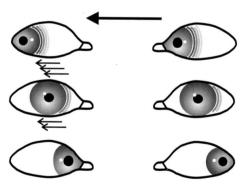

Figure 10–3.
Alexander's law. A jerk nystagmus usually becomes worse in amplitude and frequency in gaze directed toward the fast phase component. Therefore, a right jerk nystagmus becomes worse on right gaze and less in left gaze.

Some patients with congenital nystagmus will have a *paradoxical pupillary constriction* to darkness. As the room lights are turned off, the pupils instead of dilating, will momentarily constrict. After some time the pupils will undergo slow dilatation. This paradoxical pupillary constriction to darkness is indicative of optic nerve and/or retinal disease (congenital achromotopsia, congenital stationary night blindness, optic nerve hypoplasia).

Latent Nystagmus/Manifest Latent Nystagmus

Latent nystagmus is a special form of congenital nystagmus which is usually associated with congenital esotropia. It is a jerk nystagmus which is seen only under *monocular* conditions (9). When one eye is covered, both eyes develop a jerk nystagmus with the fast phase in the direction of the uncovered eye. Thus, when the right eye is covered, both eyes develop a left jerk nystagmus. If the left eye is covered then a bilateral right jerk nystagmus occurs. In some patients a latent nystagmus can become "manifest." This occurs most often in children who have markedly decreased vision in one eye, from either strabismic or organic amblyopia. In this situation the ocular system behaves as if one eye were covered (the amblyopic eye) and an obvious jerk nystagmus develops with the fast phase in the direction of the eye with the better vision. The diagnosis can be confirmed by covering the good eye and observing whether the jerk nystagmus changes direction. Only manifest latent nystagmus will exhibit this phenomena. Neither latent nor manifest latent nystagmus has ever been associated with central nervous system disease (2).

■ NYSTAGMUS OF LOCALIZING VALUE (TABLE 10–3)

Spasmus Nutans

Spasmus nutans is a high frequency, pendular, small amplitude, asymmetrical or unilateral nystagmus that begins anytime from 3–18 months of age. It is usually associated with head nodding and torticollis (24). The nystagmus is generally bilateral but it can be monocular, asymmetric and vary in different gaze positions. The

TABLE 10–3
Nystagmus of Localizing Value

Type	Location	Etiology
See-Saw	Suprachiasmal	Craniopharyngiomas
	Third ventricle	Arnold-Chiari
	Diencephalon	Retinitis pigmentosa
Periodic Alternating (PAN)	Cervicomedullary	Arnold-Chiari
	Cerebellum	Cerebellar disorders
	Fourth ventricle	MS, Posterior fossa
		tumors, encephalitis
Retraction	Dorsal Midbrain	Pinealoma
		Hydrocephalus
		Aqueductal stenosis
		Trauma, Tumor
		Infarction
Down-beat	Cerebellum	Cerebellar disease
	Medulla, cervical cord	Arnold-Chiari
		Multiple sclerosis
		High cervical tumors
		Syphilis
		Drug intoxication
		Paraneoplastic
		Metabolic disorders
		Hypomagnesmia
Up-beat	Anterior vermis cerebellum, cervicomedulla	Cerebellar disease
		Arnold-Chiari
		Drugs, Wernicke's
Gaze evoked	Cerebellar pontine angle	Tumor, infarction
Rebound	Cerebellum, Brainstem	Cerebellar disease
Oculopalatal myoclonus	Dentato-rubro-olivary (myoclonic triangle)	MS, Neurosyphilis infarction
Opsoclonus	Cerebellar-pontine pathway	Neuroblastomas
Ocular Flutter		Paraneoplastic
		Drugs, Encephalitis
		Chiasmal Tumor
Spasmus Nutans	Midbrain	Chiasmal Tumor
Dissociating abducting	Medial longitudinal fasciculus	MS, infarction

nystagmus is usually horizontal but may be vertical or torsional and often appears as a shimmering eye movement. On lateral gaze there is often greater nystagmus in the abducting eye (22). If head nodding is present, it is often not in the same direction as the nystagmus and may be more obvious when the patient is attempting to observe something at distance. The nystagmus tends to be abolished during head nodding, and this phenomena appears to be diagnostic for spasmus nutans. In most cases, spasmus nutans is a benign disorder that usually disappears by 3–4 years of age. There have been several cases of spasmus nutans that have been associated with chiasmal or supra-chiasmal tumors (3, 21). These children may or may not have other central nervous system findings, most typically optic atrophy. If the diagnosis is uncertain, the patient with presumed spasmus nutans should have a neuroradiologic investigation to rule out a central nervous system tumor. Spasmus nutans can occasionally be familial and has been present in monozygotic twins.

Periodic Alternating Nystagmus

Periodic alternating nystagmus (PAN) is a horizontal jerk nystagmus that periodically changes direction every 60–120 seconds (7). Typically, the patient has a jerk nystagmus in one direction that lasts for approximately 60–90 seconds, then the nystagmus slowly begins to decrease in amplitude and frequency. There is a period of no nystagmus which lasts from 10–20 seconds after which the nystagmus begins to jerk in the opposite direction. The nystagmus will continue in that direction with increasing amplitude and frequency for about 60–90 seconds and then the process repeats. Some patients will adopt an alternating head position to take advantage of the changing null position. The etiology of

See-Saw Nystagmus

congenital PAN is unknown. In patients who have acquired PAN there is most often an injury in the vestibulo-cerebellar pathway which carries visual information to the caudal brainstem and cerebellum. PAN is most commonly associated with an abnormality at the cranio-cervical junction—and in particular, the Arnold-Chiari malformation. It has also been associated with cerebellar disorders, demyelinating disease, vascular insufficiency, encephalitis, and posterior fossa tumors. Its association with vestibular hyper-responsiveness, downbeat nystagmus, and gaze evoked rebound nystagmus suggests failure of an ocular motor inhibitory system perhaps originating in the cerebellum (16). Evaluation of a patient with PAN should include magnetic resonance imaging with mid-sagittal sections. Treatment for this disorder is symptomatic and drugs such as Baclofen have been helpful in patients with the acquired form (16). Neurosurgical intervention has been beneficial in patients who have compression of the cerebellum from an Arnold-Chiari malformation.

See-saw Nystagmus

An unusual and quite dramatic type of nystagmus is "see-saw" nystagmus. See-saw nystagmus is a type of pendular nystagmus consisting of alternating and repetitive elevation and intorsion of one eye with simultaneous depression and extorsion of the other (17). The eye movement is similar to that of the eyes placed on either end of a child's see-saw (Fig. 10–4). Congenital variants of see-saw nystagmus exists but these either lack the torsional component or exhibit extorsion with elevation and intorsion with depression, a pattern opposite that of acquired see-saw nystagmus (4). Evidence suggests that a disturbance of the connections of the interstitial nucleus of Cajal may be responsible for the development of see-saw nystagmus (23).

See-saw nystagmus is often associated with a lesion in the rostral midbrain or suprasellar area (30). Large tumors such as a craniopharyngioma can present with see-saw nystagmus and a bitemporal hemianopia. See-saw nystagmus may also be seen in patients with head trauma, Arnold-Chiari malformations, septico-optic dysplasia, and retinitis pigmentosa. In patients with post-traumatic see-saw nystagmus, bitemporal hemianopia has been present in all cases, and some had endocrine abnormalities. An isolated chiasmal lesion does not suffice to produce see-saw nystagmus. Temporary see-saw nystagmus may occur after brainstem strokes without chiasmal or diencephalic like lesions. See-saw nystagmus has also been encountered as a congenital defect (12). Evaluation includes a computerized tomography (CT) or magnetic resonance imaging (MRI) scan to rule out an intracranial mass. The treatment for see-saw nystagmus is to remove the insighting etiology. If it per-

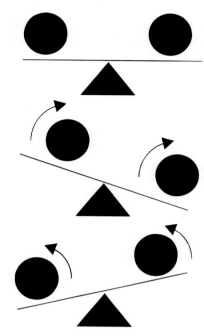

Figure 10–4.
See-saw nystagmus. Schematic representation of the eye movements seen in see-saw nystagmus. The eyes move as if placed on either end of a child's see-saw. The rising eye intorts and the falling eye extorts as if the eyes were rolling down the see-saw board. This pattern repeats itself.

sists after neurosurgical intervention, then Baclofen and Clonazepam have been helpful.

Convergence Retraction Nystagmus (Nystagmus Retractorius)

Convergence Retraction nystagmus is characterized by quick phases that converge and/or retract the eyes. It is best elicited on attempted fast upward gaze which is usually paralytic. A substitution eye movement occurs consisting of co-contraction of all the horizontal extraocular muscles and the eyes are pulled (retracted) into the orbit with convergence. It is easily seen by having the patient watch an optokinetic tape or drum rotating downward which causes the eyes to make a fast movement upward, thereby accentuating the retraction phenomena (28). Convergence retraction nystagmus is part of the dorsal midbrain syndrome (*Parinaud's syndrome*) and is associated with paralysis of upward gaze, light near dissociation of the pupils, eyelid retraction (Collier's sign), accommodative paralysis, defective convergence, and skew deviation. It is caused by lesions of the midbrain that disrupt the posterior commissure, and those located at or near the upper brainstem, posterior part of the third ventricle, and rostral part of the sylvian aqueduct. In the pediatric age group it is commonly secondary to congenital aqueductal stenosis, hydrocephalus, or pinealoma. In adults it is usually secondary to severe head trauma, tumor, hemorrhage, infarction, or inflammation. Treatment for convergence retraction nystagmus is mainly symptomatic.

Downbeat Nystagmus

Downbeat nystagmus is defined as a nystagmus in the primary position with the fast phase beating in a downward direction. It is associated with lesions at the caudal brainstem, upper cervical cord, or cerebellum. It usually is of maximal intensity when the eyes are deviated laterally and downward. The patient with down beating nystagmus can be asymptomatic or can present with vertical oscillopsia, blurred vision, or headache. When examining patients with downbeat nystagmus, one should be alert for associated signs of hereditary cerebellar degeneration such as gaze disturbances, ocular dysmetria, truncal ataxia, titubation, and optic atrophy. MRI scanning of the cervical medullary junction is often helpful in eliciting an etiology. The mechanism of downbeat nystagmus is postulated to be disruption of central vestibular pathways (8, 13). Downbeat nystagmus may co-exist with PAN, another type of nystagmus suggestive of an abnormality of the cranio-cervical junction (8, 20). A variety of miscellaneous conditions also have been reported to produce downbeat nystagmus (Table 10–3).

If downbeat nystagmus is associated with cervical medullary abnormalities, neurosurgical decompression may be curative. In patients with familial cerebellar ataxia, partial suppression of nystagmus has been reported after treatment with Clonazepam. In patients who are taking psychotropic drugs such as Dilantin, Lithium or Carbamazepine reducing the medication has significantly improved the nystagmus. Nystagmus surgery to shift the null point is also helpful and should be considered in any patient who has adopted a head position in order to relieve symptoms.

Upbeat Nystagmus

Upbeat nystagmus is a jerk nystagmus characterized by the fast component beating upward. While upbeat nystagmus may be congenital the phenomena most likely indicates an acquired pathologic lesion. Upbeat nystagmus may be seen after ingestion of drugs, particularly anti-epileptics and tranquilizers (5). Acquired upbeat nystagmus which is not drug induced may present in one of two patterns, each of which has a distinct localizing value. The first is a large amplitude upbeat nystagmus in the primary position increasing on upgaze and decreasing on downgaze. This is characteristically encountered with lesions involving the anterior vermis of the cerebellum. The second is a small amplitude up beat nystagmus in the primary position decreasing on up gaze and increasing on downgaze. This has been associated with cervicomedullary lesions (26). Primary position upbeat nystagmus is virtually always associated with significant brainstem pathology. Upbeat nystagmus may result from a defect in the vertical smooth pursuit system. Upbeat nystagmus has also been described as a complication of meningitis, and as a manifestation of Werincke's encephalopathy. The treatment for upbeat nystagmus is removal of inciting medications, treatment of the underlying anatomical defect, or vertical nystagmus surgery.

Gaze Evoked Nystagmus

Gaze evoked nystagmus which is large amplitude, low frequency in one gaze, and higher frequency smaller amplitude in the opposite gaze, is indicative of a mass compressing the brainstem located on the side of the slower nystagmus. The slow nystagmus has a frequency of less than two cycles per second. It represents a disturbance of the paramedian pontine reticular formation which is the reason for its gaze paretic nature. The faster jerk nystagmus results from destruction of the vestibular system. This combination of lesions occurs with compression of the brainstem at the cerebellar pontine angle. A type of gaze evoked nystagmus is seen in normal individuals and is often called "end point nystagmus." It usually occurs on looking far laterally or upward and is poorly sustained. It has lower amplitude, is equal on right and left gaze, and is unassociated with ocular abnormalities.

Bruns' nystagmus occurs with tumors of the cerebellar pontine angle such as acoustic neuromas and meningiomas. It is a low frequency large amplitude nystagmus, which occurs when the patient looks to the side of the lesion and a high-frequency small amplitude nystagmus which occurs when the patient looks toward the side opposite the lesion. Conjugate gaze evoked nystagmus worse in the direction of gaze may occur in patients with unilateral cerebellar disease when the eyes are directed toward the side of the lesion.

Rebound Nystagmus

Rebound nystagmus is characterized by either a decrease and change in direction of a gaze evoked horizontal nystagmus after prolonged ocular eccentric fixation, or a horizontal gaze evoked nystagmus that on refixation to primary position, temporarily beats in the opposite direction (18). Slow phases are in the direction of prior attempted eccentric gaze and the amplitude of the nystagmus rapidly diminishes until the eye is stable (23). Rebound nystagmus is observed most frequently in patients with chronic cerebellar diseases and in patients with brainstem lesions. It can also occur with diffuse neurologic disorders that include cerebellar degeneration. And can be seen in normal individuals in the dark.

Ocular Myoclonus

Ocular myoclonus is a vertical pendular nystagmus with a rate of 2–5 beats per second which is associated with movements of other structures such as the palate, facial muscles, tongue, pharynx, diaphragm, and extremities (14). It occurs with lesions in the myoclonic triangle which is made up of the ipsilateral red nucleus in the midbrain, the ipsilateral inferior olivary nucleus in the medulla, and the contralateral dentate nucleus in the cerebellum usually involving the connective pathways of the central tegmental tract and the inferior and superior cerebellar peduncle. Pathologic studies show a specific correlation with pseudohypertrophy of the inferior olivary nucleus which occurs months to years after brainstem or cerebellar infarction (mean interval ten months—range 0–4 years). It may also occur in patients with multiple sclerosis and neurosyphilis. The etiology is felt to be a disruption of the connections between the dentate nucleus and the contralateral inferior olivary nucleus that run via the red nucleus in the central tegmental tract (14). Ocular palatal myoclonus develops as a consequence of the olivary nucleus hypertrophy and is not a manifestation of the acute lesions. Once established, ocular myoclonus ordinarily persists even during sleep. A variety of medications have been used to treat the disorder including trihexyphenidyl, valproic acid, carbamazepine, and 1,5-hydroxytryptophan.

Opsoclonus/Ocular Flutter

Opsoclonus is an extremely rare and unusual form of eye movements. It is not truly a nystagmus, but rather a bizarre ocular oscillation. It is rapid, involuntary, and multi-vectorial. It can be present intermittently and often has a high frequency low amplitude movement. The movements are so vast and chaotic that they are not easily confused with other forms of nystagmus and have been termed "saccadomania" (11). Ocular flutter can be distinguished from opsoclonus since the oscillations in ocular flutter remain in the horizontal plane.

Both ocular flutter and Opsoclonus occur most commonly in adults and children as a consequence of nonspecific encephalitis (23). The eye movement disorder is usually preceded by viral symptoms and is often accompanied by cerebellar and long track signs. The illness usually resolves in a few weeks or months. When opsoclonus is associated with ataxia and myoclonus of the extremities, affected patients show "dancing eyes and dancing feet" (11). Opsoclonus/ocular flutter can be a sign of occult neuroblastoma and an otherwise normal child with opsoclonus/ocular flutter should have a complete systemic and neurologic evaluation including magnetic resonance imaging of the chest and abdomen and urinary levels of catecholamines (1, 29). Adults with opsoclonus should be evaluated for occult visceral carcinoma as a preneoplastic process (10). Substances including amitriptyline, chlordecon, haloperidol, and lithium may produce opsoclonus. When these substances are discontinued the abnormal eye movements improve or disappear.

■ OTHER FORMS OF NYSTAGMUS

Superior Oblique Myokymia

Superior oblique myokymia is an intermittent monocular torsional eye movement. The patient experiences oscillopsia, diplopia, or blurred vision. The oscillation is rapid, vertical or torsional and easiest seen with the aid of a slit lamp or ophthalmoscopy. The condition is usually benign and spontaneous remissions and re-elapses occur (19). It has been associated with multiple sclerosis, pontine tumors, lead intoxication, and adrenoleukodystrophy. The etiology of superior oblique myokymia is unknown but felt to be a spasm of the superior oblique muscle (25). Treatment consists of either carbamazepine which provides short term benefits, or strabismus surgery consisting of superior oblique tenectomy in combination with ipsilateral inferior oblique weakening for patients with persisting symptoms.

Heimann–Bielschowsky Phenomena

An unusual monocular course pendular vertical oscillation can occur in an eye which has experienced visual loss. The oscillations vary between one and five cycles per second and the amplitude is often large (up to 20 degrees) (27). Visual acuity in the eye is always extremely poor and a latent period of one to 20 years may elapse between loss of vision and onset of these movements (27). The etiology of this phenomena is unknown, however, the oscillation has been decreased or eliminated in several patients with improvement of vi-

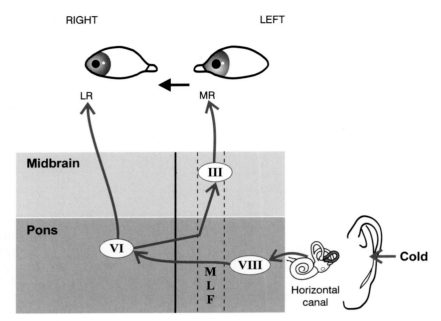

Caloric Stimulation (COWS)

RIGHT   LEFT

Figure 10–5.
Caloric stimulation. When cold water is placed in the ear, the semicircular canals are stimulated. This results in a signal which is conveyed to the contralateral horizontal gaze center (sixth nerve nucleus). This results in a fast phase movement (jerk nystagmus) to the opposite side. Therefore, cold water placed in the left external meatus will result in a right jerk nystagmus.

sual function (31), suggesting that this is caused by a visual sensory deficit. Muscle surgery has also been effective in reducing the oscillation.

Induced Nystagmus

Caloric

Stimulation of the vestibular system can be accomplished by caloric irrigation. Water irrigated into the external auditory canal will stimulate thermal convection of the endolymph in the semi-circular canals, resulting in a jerk nystagmus. The eye movements that occur during choleric irrigation are dependent upon the temperature of the water (warm- 44 degrees or cold- 30 degrees centigrade), visual fixation, alertness (awake or comatose), and unilateral or bilaterality of the stimulation. In the awake patient, a normal response consists of a jerk nystagmus with the slow phase toward the side of cold water irrigation and the fast phase away from the site of cold water irrigation (Fig. 10–5). A useful mnemonic which describes the fast phase component is COWS (Cold Opposite, Warm Same). A vertical nystagmus can be elicited by bilateral stimulation with bilateral cold water causing a slow phase downward movement and a fast phase upward (mnemonic CUWD- Cold Up, Warm Down). Visual fixation suppresses or abolishes caloric nystagmus in normal individuals (23). In the comatose patient, the normal response is a *tonic* conjugate ocular deviation toward the side of cold water irrigation and away from the side of warm water irrigation (Table 10–4). There is *no* fast phase component.

Optokinetic Nystagmus

Optokinetic nystagmus is a jerk nystagmus which is elicited by having the patient look at a repetitive moving target. Helmholtz noted the nystagmus in passengers on a train watching the passing scenery (6). The nystagmus occurs as the patient pursues the moving target and then makes a fast eye movement (saccade) in the opposite direction to pick up the next approaching object. Thus, if the objects are moving to the patient's left, the patient will pursue to the left and then make a fast eye movement to the right. The repetitive nature of this eye movement combination will appear to the observer to be a right jerk nystagmus. Both horizontal and vertical jerk nystagmus can be elicited with an OKN stimulus. The production of optokinetic nystagmus depends on intact visual and ocular motor pathways and is mainly a measure of pursuit ability (23) (Fig. 10–6). The final pathway appears to be through the vestibular neuronal

TABLE 10–4
Caloric Vestibular Stimulation
Eye Movement Direction Relative to Side Stimulated

	Awake (Jerk nystagmus-FAST phase)		Comatose (Tonic deviation-no nystagmus)	
	Unilateral	Bilateral	Unilateral	Bilateral
Cold Water	Opposite	Upward	Same	Downward
Warm Water	Same	Downward	Opposite	Upward

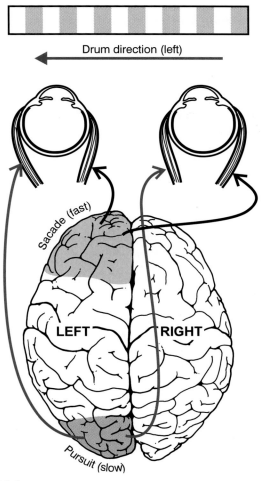

Figure 10–6.
Optokinetic nystagmus. An optokinetic target directed toward the patient's left tests the integrity of the left brain. The left occipital lobe pursues the target to the left and the left frontal lobe initiates a saccadic movement to pick up the anticipated coming targets. Therefore, the patient develops a right jerk nystagmus.

system. Inputs responsible for the optokinetic response originate in the visual cortex in the occipital lobe and travel in the efferent optomotor tract with a second pathway originating with a retinal signal which reaches the vestibular nuclei by an accessory optic pathway that includes pretectal nuclei such as the nucleus of the optic tract. The cortical pathway is felt to produce optokinetic nystagmus from small moving targets while the retinal pathway appears to be responsible when the entire peripheral visual field is moved. This second pathway would explain why animals can retain their optokinetic responses after cortical ablation including bilateral removal of the occipital poles.

Evaluating the optokinetic response can be helpful in confirming functional hysteria in "blind patients," identification of internuclear ophthalmoplegia, accentuating retraction nystagmus, confirming presence of congenital nystagmus, accessing gross visual acuity, and detecting loss of saccadic function in such disorders as supranuclear palsy and ocular motor apraxia.

Vestibular Nystagmus

Vestibular nystagmus is a horizontal-torsional primary position jerk nystagmus. Nystagmus due to peripheral vestibular disease beats in the same direction in all fields of gaze but has an increased amplitude on gaze in the direction of the fast component (Alexander's law) (Fig. 10–3). Visual fixation inhibits the nystagmus and its accompanying vertigo. The direction of the fast phase is away from the damaged end organ. Thus, a right jerk nystagmus would indicate a left peripheral vestibular abnormality. Marked vertigo can occur with the direction of spin toward the fast phase. If the disease involves the end organ then tinnitus and deafness may be present. Causes include infection (labyrinitis), Meniere's dis-

TABLE 10–5
Vestibular Nystagmus

Symptom or Sign	Peripheral (End-Organ)	Central (Nuclear)
Direction of nystagmus	Unidirectional, fast phase opposite lesion	Bidirectional or unidirectional
Purely horizontal nystagmus without rotary component	Uncommon	Common
Vertical or purely rotary nystagmus	Never present	May be present
Visual fixation	Inhibits nystagmus and vertigo	No inhibition
Severity of vertigo	Marked	Mild
Direction of environmental spin	Toward slow phase	Variable
Direction of past-pointing	Toward slow phase	Variable
Direction of Romberg fall	Toward slow phase	Variable
Effect of head turning	Changes Romberg fall	No effect
Duration of symptoms	Finite (minutes, days, weeks) but recurrent	May be chronic
Tinnitus and/or deafness	Often present	Usually absent
Common cause	Infectious (labyrinthitis) Meniere's disease, neuronitis, vascular, trauma, toxic	Vascular, demyelinating, neoplastic

Daroff RB, Troost BT, Dell'Osso LF: Nystagmus and related ocular oscillations. In *Neuro-Ophthalmology*, Glaser JS. Hagerstown: Harper & Row Pub. Inc., 1978, pp. 219–243.

ease, vascular disorders, trauma, and drug toxicity. A patient with unidirectional jerk nystagmus, vertigo in the direction of the fast phase component, past pointing, and a positive Romberg test in the direction of the slow component has acute dysfunction of the vestibular end organ on the side of the nystagmus slow phase (8). Nystagmus due to central vestibular disease (vestibular nuclei and pathways) may be unidirectional or bi-directional, and may be purely vertical or purely torsional (Table 10–5). A pure horizontal nystagmus without a torsional component is suggestive of central disease and visual fixation does not inhibit the nystagmus which may actually increase its intensity. The presence of a marked bi-directionality to the nystagmus (left beating on left gaze and a similar severe right beating nystagmus on right gaze) is almost always indication of a central origin. Central nystagmus is commonly caused by multiple sclerosis, central nervous system tumors, vascular disorders, and encephalitis (8).

■ REFERENCES

1. Atkin A and Bender M: Lightning eye movements (ocular myoclonus). J Neurol Soc—1976:27:71–78.
2. Buckley EG: Evaluation of the child with nystagmus. Seminar in Ophthalmol—1990:90:131–137.
3. Cogan DG: Congenital nystagmus. Can J Ophthalmol—1967:2:4.
4. Daroff RB: See-saw nystagmus. Neurology—1963:13:306.
5. Daroff RB, Troost BT: Upbeat nystagmus. JAMA—1973:225:312.
6. David NJ: Optokinetic nystagmus, a clinical review. J Clin Neuro-Ophthalmol—1989:9:258–266.
7. Davis DB, Smith JL: Periodic alternating nystagmus. Am J Ophthalmol—1971:72:757–762.
8. Dell'Osso LF, Daroff RB, Troost BT: Nystagmus and saccadic intrusions and oscillations. In: Glaser JL (ed): Clinical Neuro-Ophthalmology. Philadelphia: L. B. Lippincott, Co., 1990:325–356.
9. Dell'Osso LF, Schmidt D, Daroff RB: Latent, manifest latent, and congenital nystagmus. Arch Ophthalmol—1979:97:1877–1885.
10. Digre KB: Opsoclonus in adults-report of three cases and review of the literature. Arch Neurol—1986:43:1165–1175.
11. Ellenberger C, Netsley MG: Anatomic basis and diagnostic value of opsoclonus. Arch Ophthalmol—1970:83:307.
12. Felt RP, Biglan AW: Congenital see-saw nystagmus. J Pediatr Ophthalmol Strabismus—1981:22:13–16.
13. Gresty MA, Barratt H, Rudge P, Page N: Analysis of downbeat nystagmus. Arch Neurol—1986:43:52.
14. Guillain G: The syndrome of synchronous rhythmic palato-pharyngo-laryngo-oculo-diaphragmatic myoclonus. Proc R Soc Med—1988:31:1031–1038.
15. Halmagyi GM, Gresty MA, Leech J: Reversal of optokinetic nystagmus. Mechanism and clinical significance. Ann Neurol—1980:7:429–435.
16. Halmagyi GM, Ridge P, Gresty MA, Leigh JR, Zee DS: Treatment of periodic alternating nystagmus. Ann Neurol—1980:8:609–611.
17. Hamid LM: Nystagmus. In: Margo, CE (ed): Diagnostic problems in clinical ophthalmology. Philadelphia: W.B. Saunders—1994:704–710.
18. Hood JT, Kaylan A, Leech J: Rebound nystagmus. Brain—1973:96:507.
19. Hoyt WF, Keane JR: Superior oblique myokymia. Report and discussion on five cases of benign intermittent uniocular microtremor. Arch Ophthalmol—1970;84:461–467.
20. Keane JR: Periodic alternating nystagmus with downward beating nystagmus. Arch Neurol—1980:37:178.
21. Koenig SB, Nardich TP, Zaparackas Z: Optic glioma masquerading as spasmus nutans. J Pediatr Ophthalmol Strabismus—1982:19:20–24.
22. Leigh RJ, Zee DS: The neurology of eye movements. Philadelphia: F.A. Davis, 1983.
23. Miller NR (ed): Clinical neuro-ophthalmology. Baltimore: Williams & Wilkins, 1985.
24. Norton EWD, Cogan DG: Spasmus nutans: a clinical study of twenty cases followed two years or more since onset. Arch Ophthalmol—1954:52:442–446.
25. Rosenberg ML, Glaser JS: Superior oblique myokymia. A misnomer. J Clin Neuro Ophthalmol—1983:3:131.
26. Schatz NJ, Schlezinger NS, Berry RG: Vertical upbeat nystagmus on downward gaze: a clinical pathologic correlation. Neurology—1975:25:380.
27. Smith JL, Flynn JT, Spiro HJ: Monocular vertical oscillations of amblyopia. The Hermann-Bielschowsky Phenomena. J Clin Neuro-Ophthalmol—1982:2:85–91.
28. Smith JL, Zeepe I, Gary AJ, et al.: Nystagmus retractorius. Arch Ophthalmol—1959:62:864.
29. Solomon GE, Chutorias AM: Opsoclonus and occult neuroblastoma. N Engl J Med—1968:279:475.
30. Williams IM, Dickinson P, Ramsey RJ, Thomas L: See-saw nystagmus. Aust J Ophthalmol—1982:10:19–28.
31. Yee RD, Jelks GW, Baloh RW, Hourubia V: Uniocular nystagmus in monocular visual loss. Ophthalmology—1979;86:511–518.

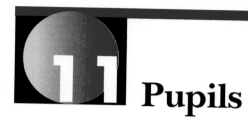

11 Pupils

Angela Scott, Edward G. Buckley

Examination of the pupils can provide valuable clues about the status of the visual and central nervous systems (20). Pupillary size is determined by the actions of the iris sphincter (parasympathetic innervation) and dilator (sympathetic innervation) muscles. It varies according to age, illumination, degree of mental stimulation or fatigue, and systemic conditions such as diabetes and infections. In general, the resting position of the pupil is small in infancy, becomes larger in the young and middle adult years, and then is smaller again in the elderly (9). Normal pupils should be isocoric. Lesions involving the efferent pathway or the iris substance will produce anisocoria. Physiologic anisocoria (defined as an inequality of greater than or equal to 0.4 mm) occurs in 19% of patients (8).

■ AFFERENT PUPILLARY PATHWAY

The afferent pupillary pathway begins when light stimulates the retinal photoreceptors generating an impulse to the small retinal ganglion cells (W-cells). Connections to these cells travel with the rest of the visual fibers, undergo hemidecussation at the optic chiasm exit the optic tract prior to reaching the lateral geniculate nucleus, and synapse within the pretectal nucleus in the midbrain (Fig. 11–1). Second order neurons leave the pretectal nucleus and project to the midline Edinger-Westphal subnucleus of both third nerves. Because of the hemidecussation of the *afferent* pupillary fibers at the optic chiasm, light directed into one eye results in identical innervation to the ipsilateral (direct response) and contralateral (consensual response) pupil (Fig. 11–1).

Since the pupillomotor fibers leave the afferent visual pathway just posterior to the optic chiasm, lesions involving the lateral geniculate nucleus and optic radiations can result in visual impairment with normal pupillary responses. Thus, patients can be completely blind from an occipital lobe lesion (cortical blindness) yet have completely normal pupillary responses to light.

■ PARASYMPATHETIC PATHWAY

The efferent parasympathetic pathway is responsible for constriction of the pupils to both light and near stimuli. These fibers travel from the Edinger-Westphal nucleus on the surface of the third nerve eventually joining the portion of the inferior division which innervates the inferior oblique muscle. Prior to reaching the inferior oblique muscle the parasympathetic neurons leave the inferior division of the third nerve and synapse in the ciliary ganglion. Neurons from the ciliary ganglion travel with the short ciliary nerves to the globe, passing through the suprachoroidal space to the iris sphincter muscle and ciliary body (Fig. 11–2).

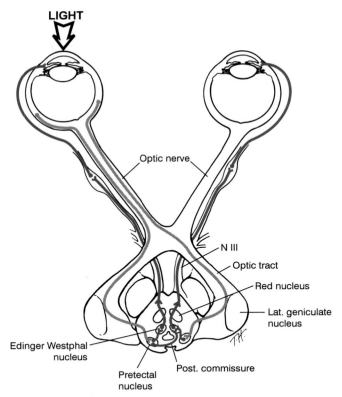

Figure 11–1.
Anatomy of a light reflex pathway with parasympathetic outflow to
the iris sphincter. Note light directed into one eye results in bilateral
pupillary constriction. Grey line equals afferent pathway, red line
equals efferent pathway.

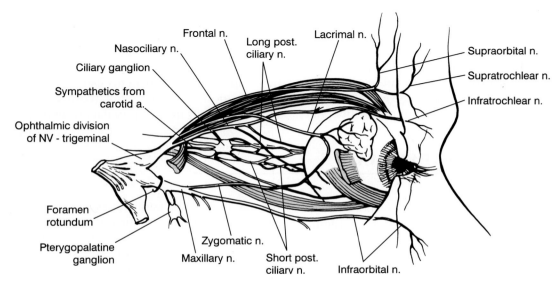

Figure 11–2.
Nerves of the orbit.

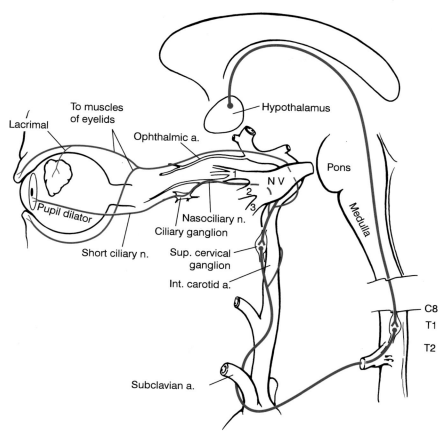

Figure 11–3.
The oculosympathetic pathway. The origin begins in the hypothalamus with connections down through the brainstem to synapse in the upper cervical cord (central or first neuronal pathway). Fibers then travel around the subclavian artery and over the base of the lung to join in the thoracic sympathetic trunk which then synapses in the superior cervical ganglion (pre-ganglionic or second neuronal pathway). The third order neuron travels with the first branch of the trigeminal nerve and passes through the ciliary ganglion to reach the pupillary dilator muscle.

■ SYMPATHETIC PATHWAY

The efferent sympathetic pathway produces pupillary dilation through its actions at the iris dilator muscle. This system originates in the posterior hypothalmus. Uncrossed fibers descend to synapse in the intermediolateral gray matter of the spinal cord at the level of C8 to T2 (the ciliary spinal center of Budge). Second order neurons ascend in the cervical sympathetic chain to synapse in the superior cervical ganglion in the neck. These neurons are in close proximity to the apex of the lung and can be affected by lesions in this area (Pancoast tumor). Post-ganglion fibers then travel with the internal carotid artery into the cavernous sinus, where they join the first division of the trigeminal nerve. Aneurysms of the internal carotid in the cavernous sinus can produce an ipsilateral Horner's syndrome with abducens, trochlear, or oculomotor nerve palsy and partial facial anesthesia. The fibers enter the orbit through the superior orbital fissure and travel to the eye by way of the nasociliary, long and short ciliary nerves (Fig. 11–3).

■ NEAR REFLEX

The near reflex is composed of the triad of pupillary constriction, convergence, and accommodation. The exact anatomic pathways are not known but appear to involve the cerebral cortex, with fibers projecting from the cortex to the Edinger-Westphal nucleus in the midbrain. These fibers travel ventral in the midbrain to the fibers serving the light response and thus can be spared from compression by more dorsally located midbrain lesions (light-near dissociation). Parasympathetic fibers for accommodation travel to the eye with the fibers serving pupillary constriction but end in the ciliary muscle.

■ AFFERENT PUPILLARY DEFECT

A relative "afferent" pupillary defect (RAPD), also known as a Marcus Gunn pupil, is a sign of asymmetric abnormality in the anterior "afferent" visual system (optic nerves, chiasm or tract) and is detected by comparing the pupillary responses to a light shown alternately into each eye. In effect, the pupils are being used as a "light meter" to measure quantitatively how well light is being conducted by the afferent visual system of the stimulated eye. If an asymmetric abnormality exists, less constriction of both pupils will be observed (i.e., more dilation) when light is shown into the involved eye "as compared to" the uninvolved eye (Fig. 11–4). This difference in light sensitivity is best appreciated by alternately shining a light source into the two eyes with a rhythmic motion (the swinging flashlight test) (Fig. 11–4). This test should be performed in a dimly lit room, with the patient fixing on a distant object to avoid the miosis seen with the near response. A bright light source is directed into one eye and both pupils are observed for their reaction. Light directed into a normal eye will produce equal brisk constriction of both pupils. After approximately one to two seconds the light is directed into the other eye. In the absence of pathology there usually is a small initial degree of pupillary constriction (due to the slight dilation that occurs as the light passes from one eye to another) followed by slight dilation to a steady state. If an abnormality is present in the afferent visual pathway, instead of constricting, both pupils will immediately dilate when the light is swung to the abnormal eye. This response (less constriction when the same light is directed into one eye as compared to the fellow eye) is designated as a "relative" afferent pupillary defect (because one optic nerve is being evaluated "relative to the other") and can be graded from trace to 4—depending on the degree of dilation. After one to two seconds the light source is returned to the first eye and the response is observed. The light is continually "swung" back and forth between the two eyes to confirm the accuracy of the observations (Fig. 11–4).

Since both pupils respond equally, only one functioning pupil is necessary to perform this test. In cases where the pupil is unable to react because of mechanical problems (i.e., posterior synechiae, third nerve palsy) or is not visible (i.e., hyphema, corneal opacity) one can still detect a relative afferent pupillary defect by performing the swinging flashlight test and observing the response of the "working" pupil (19). No afferent defect will be detected if both optic nerves are equally damaged since an imbalance in function is necessary for an afferent pupillary defect to be present.

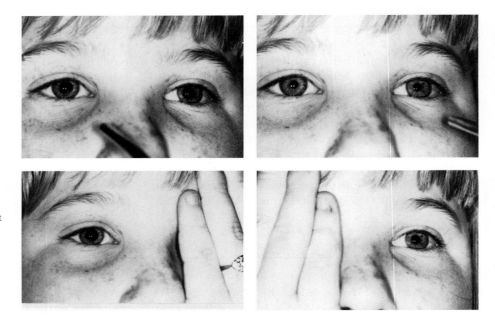

Figure 11–4.
Afferent pupillary defect. A patient with a right afferent pupillary defect. Light shown on the involved right eye results in minimal constriction of both pupils (top left). When redirected to the uninvolved left eye, both pupils constrict (top right). The same test can be performed with ordinary room light by measuring the pupillary diameter with the uninvolved eye covered (bottom left) and the involved eye covered (bottom right). Note that the pupil is larger on the involved right side.

The severity of the afferent pupillary defect correlates directly with the amount and location of the associated visual field loss (7). Central field loss has more impact than peripheral (21). Media opacities such as cataract and hyphema usually do not cause afferent pupillary defects (17). Amblyopia, even when profound, will only result in a very subtle defect, and organic disease should be suspected if one is present (14).

■ HORNER'S SYNDROME

Horner's syndrome is produced by a lesion of the sympathetic pathway (Fig. 11–3). This syndrome is classically associated with a triad of ptosis, miosis, and anhidrosis (Fig. 11–5). The pupillary abnormality is due to the interruption of sympathetic input to the iris dilator muscle—and is best manifest in darkness. When the lights are dimmed, the uninvolved pupil will dilate normally, while the Horner's pupil remains constricted, with only moderate dilation after 10–15 seconds. This phenomenon is known as the "dilation lag," and is specific for a Horner's pupil. The pupil constricts normally to both light and near.

The accompanying ptosis results from loss of sympathetic innervation to the Mueller's muscle of the ipsilateral upper eyelid (Fig. 11–3), producing 1–2 mm of ptosis. Another lid sign that may be useful is the apparent "upside down ptosis" due to lack of sympathetic innervation to the lower lid retractors, causing the lower lid to ride higher than usual. Since fibers for facial perspiration travel with the *external* carotid artery, anhidrosis will not be present in a *distal* lesion. Other signs are hyperemia of the conjunctiva and an apparent enophthalmos (not supported by exophthalmometry).

Horner's syndrome may be further localized to central (1st order), pre-ganglionic (2nd order), or post-ganglionic lesions (3rd order venous) (see Table 11–1). Central lesions include hypothalamic infarcts, tumors, or other intracranial abnormalities (6, 16). Symptoms and signs are usually not limited to the Horner's syndrome because of the proximity of other structures.

Pharmacologic testing is useful for identifying a Horner's syndrome as well as localizing the lesion to either pre- or post-ganglionic (5). Topical cocaine (4%–10%) blocks the re-uptake of norepinephrine from the synapse at the nerve terminal in the iris dilator muscle, thereby producing prolonged activity at the neuromuscular junction and dilation of a normal pupil. In Horner's syndrome, because of denervation, very little norepinephrine is released into the synapse, therefore, cocaine produces little dilation of the pupil. For localization of the insult, the hydroxyamphetamine 1% (Paredrine) test is useful (2, 5). Paredrine causes the release of norepinephrine from the nerve terminal into the synapse, producing dilation of the pupil. With lesions of the central or second-order neuron the pupil will dilate normally because the uninvolved third order neuron still produces norepinephrine. Pupils in post-ganglionic lesions (third order neuron) do not dilate because of impaired or absent production of norepinephrine by the damaged neuron.

Further workup of a pre-ganglionic Horner's syndrome includes chest x-ray and neurologic evaluation. Pre-ganglionic or second order Horner's are often produced by pathology at the lung apex or in the neck,

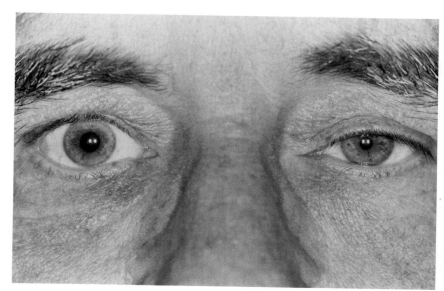

Figure 11–5.
Left Horner's syndrome. Note the characteristic ptosis and miosis. The miosis is greater with the room lights down. Note that the lower lid is also slightly ptotic and that the eye appears to be enophthalmic.

TABLE 11–1
Evaluation of Anisocoria

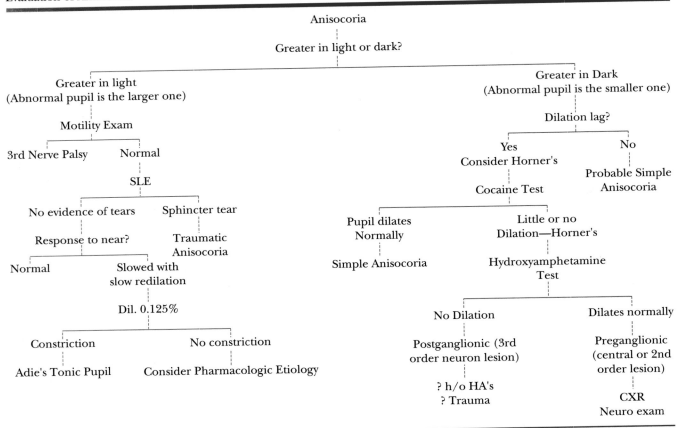

such as metastatic lung and breast tumors, radical neck surgery or injury. Post-ganglionic lesions, are usually believed to be benign and only rarely are due to more serious conditions. Etiologies include unilateral vascular headache, trauma, carotid disorders (aneurysms, dissections, or occlusion), inflammatory disorders, and local neoplasms (6, 12).

Congenital Horner's syndrome is relatively uncommon, accounting for only about five percent of all cases. In addition to the classic triad, patients demonstrate ipsilateral iris hypochromia. This finding is due to failure of normal iris melanocyte development because of impaired sympathetic innervation. Very rarely, ipsilateral hypochromia has been documented in cases of acquired Horner's syndrome in adults (3). Birth trauma to the brachial plexus is the most common etiology. Other causes include vascular occlusion, chest or neck tumors, pneumothorax and idiopathic maldevelopment (24). Acquired Horner's in childhood is suspicious for occult neuroblastoma. Appropriate workup should be performed.

■ ADIE'S SYNDROME

Adie's syndrome (tonic pupils), is characterized by a large pupil with little or no constriction to light and slowed constriction to a near stimulus (Fig. 11–6) (10). The anisocoria will be greater in light than dark. The involved pupil undergoes very slow redilation after discontinuation of near effort. The pathogenesis is believed to be an abnormality in the ciliary ganglion or short ciliary nerves (Figure 11–2).

Seventy percent of cases are in females, usually in the 20–40 age group. Eighty to ninety percent of cases are unilateral, however, studies show that the contralateral pupil will become involved at a rate of 4%

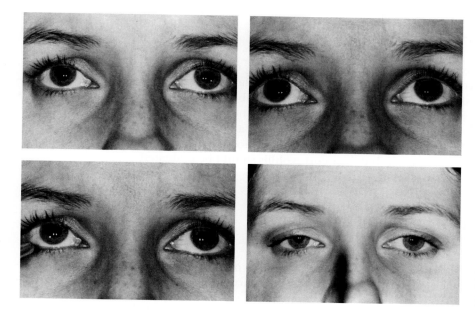

Figure 11–6.
Patient with a right Adie's pupil. Note that the pupils are larger under room light (top left) than with the lights off (top right). The pupil constricts purely to light (bottom left) and better to near (bottom right).

per year (18). Absent or decreased deep tendon reflexes are seen in approximately 50% of cases. The patient may be completely asymptomatic, with anisocoria noted only on routine examination. Others may complain of symptoms related to pupillary or ciliary muscle dysfunction, such as photophobia, blurred vision at near, or periocular discomfort.

On slit lamp examination, isolated segments of the pupil can be seen to constrict to the light (vermiform movements) and are due to segmental palsy. In long-standing cases, the involved pupil may actually become the smaller of the two pupils complicating the diagnosis.

Pharmacologic testing may be used to verify the diagnosis. An Adie's pupil will display denervation supersensitivity and will constrict easily to administration of dilute Pilocarpine (0.125%). Normal pupils generally will not constrict at this low concentration. It is impor-

tant that the tests be performed prior to instillation of any other eye drops or any manipulation of the cornea, as these measures may alter the epithelium and allow increased penetration of the drops.

Patients bothered by accommodative symptoms usually can be assured that this should decrease within one to two years. Some patients have received relief by treatment with pilocarpine 0.125% administered three times a day (4).

While tonic pupils are generally felt to be a benign condition, approximately 20% will be associated with other disorders. These conditions include herpes zoster, neurosyphilis, temporal arteritis, sarcoidosis, paraneoplastic syndromes, diabetes mellitus, and neuropathies such as Charcot Marie Tooth disease and Guillain Barré (10, 13). Further workup is warranted in atypical patients or patients with accompanying symptoms suspicious for inflammatory or neoplastic conditions.

■ LIGHT-NEAR DISSOCIATION

Loss of the pupillary response to light with preservation of the near reflex is termed light-near dissociation. The fibers serving the near reaction are believed to be located more ventrally within the pretectal midbrain, and therefore can be spared with more dorsally located lesions compressing the light response fibers.

Light-near dissociation has been described in a number of conditions, many involving a compressive or ischemic lesion in the midbrain. The dorsal midbrain syndrome, also known as Parinaud's syndrome, is often

produced by a pinealoma or other lesion compressing the pretectum (see Chapter 10, Nystagmus). Parinaud's pupils are typically large and may be slightly oval. Other associated findings are impaired upward gaze, convergence-retraction nystagmus on attempted up gaze, decreased convergence, lid retraction, hypoaccommodation, and skew deviation. Other causes of light-near dissociation include neurosyphillis, diabetes mellitus, myotonic dystrophy, familial amyloidosis, multiple sclerosis, temporal arteritis, and pituitary apoplexy (1, 11, 13, 15).

■ ARGYLL ROBERTSON PUPILS

One specific form of light-near dissociation is seen in neurosyphilis. The pupils, known as Argyll-Robertson pupils, are miotic, often irregular in shape, and unreactive to light but briskly reactive to near. This condition is usually bilateral and is associated with good vision. The response to mydriatics is reduced.

The precise location of the lesion is unknown, but believed to be near the Edinger-Westphal subnucleus of the third nerve, damaging fibers from both the ipsilateral and contralateral pretectal areas, sparing the corticotegmental fibers approaching the nucleus, thus preserving the near response. Histopathologic confirmation of such a lesion has not yet been documented. When the diagnosis of Argyll Robertson pupils, is made, neurosyphilis should be evaluated.

■ PHARMACOLOGICALLY DILATED PUPILS

Often pupillary dilatation can occur because of accidental or willful instillation of a mydriatic agent. This is commonly seen in healthcare personnel who work with "atropine-like" drugs, outdoors individuals who come in contact with plants (i.e., gardeners, hikers) which contain belladonna alkaloids, and in malingerers. This usually presents as an acute unilateral or bilateral pupillary dilation with no other third nerve abnormalities. The diagnosis is confirmed by the absence of pupillary constriction to 1% pilocarpine (22,23). These individuals will also have an impairment of accommodation resulting in near visual difficulties. The dilation and accommodative difficulties may persist for up to ten days.

■ REFERENCES

1. Bronster OJ, Rudolph SH, Shanzer S: Pupillary light-near dissociation in cranial arteritis. A case report. Neuro-ophthalmol—1983:3:65–70.
2. Cremer SA, Thompson HS, Digre KB, Kardon RH: Hydroxyamphetamine mydriasis in Horner's syndrome. Am J Ophthalmol—1990:110:71–76.
3. Diesenhouse MC, Palay DA, Newman NJ, To K, Albert DM: Acquired heterochromia with Horner's syndrome in two adults. Ophthalmol, 1992:99:1815–1817.
4. Flach AJ, Dolan BJ: Adie's Syndrome: a medical treatment for symptomatic patients. Ann Ophthalmol—1984: 1151–1154.
5. Grimson BS, Thompson HS: Drug testing in Horner's syndrome. In: Smith JL, Glaser JS (eds). Neuro-ophthalmology. St. Louis: C.V. Mosby, 1975:265–270.
6. Grimson BS, Thompson HS: Horner's syndrome: overall view of 120 cases. Topics in Neuro-ophthalmology. Baltimore—Williams & Wilkins, 1979:151
7. Johnson LN, Hill RA, Bartholomew MJ: Correlation of afferent pupillary defect with visual field loss on automated perimetry. Ophthalmol, 1988:95:1649–1655.
8. Lam BL, Thompson HS, Corbett JJ: The prevalence of simple anisocoria. Am J Ophthalmol—1987:104:69–73.
9. Loewenfeld, O and Lowenfeld, IE: The pupil in the eye, editor Dauson, H; New York, Academic Press, 1969.
10. Maitland CG, SCherokman BJ, Schiffman J, Harlan JW, Galdi AP: Paraneoplastic tonic pupils. J Clin Neuro-ophthalmol—1985:5:99–104.
11. Miller VR: Walsh and Hoyt's Clinical Neuro-Ophthalmology, 4th ed. Baltimore—Williams and Wilkins, 1985.
12. Monteiro MLR, Coppeto JR: Horner's syndrome associated with carotid artery atherosclerosis. Am J Ophthalmol—1988:105:93–94.
13. Nichols BP, Romanchuk KG: Pituitary apoplexy presenting with light-near dissociation of the pupils. J Clin Neuro-ophthalmol—1987:7:139–143.
14. Portnoy JZ, Thompson HS, Lennarson L, Corbett JJ: Pupillary defects in amblyopia. Am J Ophthalmol—1983: 96:609–614.
15. Seybold ME, Yoss RE, Hollenhorst RW, Moyer NJ: Pupillary abnormalities associated with tumors of the pineal region. Neurol, 1971:21:232–237.
16. Stone WM, de Toledo J, Romanul FCA: Horner's syndrome due to hypothalamic infarction. Clinical, radiologic, and pathologic correlations. Arch Neurol—1986: 43:199–200.
17. Striph GG, Halperin LS, Stevens JL, Chu FC: Afferent pupillary defect caused by hyphema. Am J. Ophthalmol. 1988:126:352–3.
18. Thompson HS: Adie's syndrome: some new observations. Trans Am Ophthalmol Soc—1977:75:587–626.
19. Thompson HS, Corbett JJ, Cox TA: How to measure the relative afferent pupillary defect. Surv Ophthalmol—1981:26:39–42.
20. Thompson HS, Franceschetti AT: Hippus semantic and historic considerations of the word. Am J Ophthalmol—1971:71:1116–1120.

21. Thompson HS, Montague P, Cox TA, Corbett JJ: The relationship between visual acuity, pupillary defect, and visual field loss. Am J Ophthalmol—1982:93:681–688.

22. Thompson HS, Pilley SF: Unequal pupils. A flow chart for sorting out the anisocorias. Surv Ophthalmol—1976:21: 45–48.

23. Weinstein JM, Zweifel TJ, Thompson HS: The clinical diagnosis of pupil disorders. Journal of Clinical Neuro 1979: 41:15–26.

24. Weinstein JM, Zweifel TJ, Thompson HS: Congenital Horner's syndrome. Arch Ophthalmol—1980:98: 1074–1078.

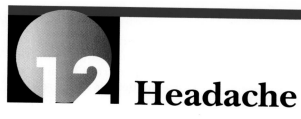

12 Headache

Saunders L. Hupp

Head, eye, or face pain with or without visual disturbance is a common complaint in an ophthalmic practice. The presence of a systemic disease and accompanying abnormalities on the physical examination may point to a source of the head pain, but often the complaints are not associated with any abnormalities on physical examination. Therefore, the physician must entertain a diagnosis on the basis of historical characteristics which may include syndromes of uncertain pathophysiology such as migraine, cluster, or tension headache (Table 12–1). Each of these common syndromes may cause a variety of pain and/or visual disturbances and must be differentiated from neurologic dysfunction due to ischemia, inflammation, seizure, and compression.

■ HEADACHE WITH NORMAL PHYSICAL EXAM

The following headache syndromes are characterized by normal physical examination accompanied by typical historical features.

Migraine

Migraine is a complex syndrome characterized by recurrent attacks of headache widely variable in intensity, frequency, and duration. Attacks are commonly unilateral and are usually associated with anorexia, nausea, and vomiting. In some cases they are preceded by, or associated with, neurological and mood disturbances. All the above characteristics, including headache, are not necessarily present in each attack or in each patient (1).

Recent evidence suggests that the prodromes of migraine may be of hypothalamic origin and the alterations in perception associated with spreading cortical neuronal changes. The pain of migraine and tension headache is probably not due to vasoconstriction, vasodilation, or muscle contraction, but more likely generated centrally with enhancement by inflammatory neuropeptides such as substance P (16).

The prevalence of migraine is related to both age and sex and probably markedly underestimated. Walsh and Hoyt estimate 10% of the general population experience migraine, but other studies suggest the prevalence in adults is much higher. Childhood migraine is less common than the adult form. Bille studied 8993 school children between the ages of 7 and 15 years and found 5–6% to have migraine (24, 27).

Common migraine (migraine without aura) is defined as headache accompanied by autonomic nervous system dysfunction such as nausea without other significant neurologic alterations (16). The head pain, which is often pounding or throbbing, can start anywhere on the cranium and usually spreads to involve one half or the whole head. Often the pain is retro-orbital, severe, and may be mistaken for eye or sinus disease. Although the headache is not heralded by dramatic visual or sensory phenomena, there may be a premonitory change in mood, frequent yawning, fluid retention, word finding trouble, or other nonspecific prodromal symptoms. The headache may last for hours—or less frequently, a day or more. The patient seeks a quiet dark environment or sleep for relief.

Classic migraine (migraine with aura) occurs when vi-

TABLE 12–1
Classification of Headache

I. Normal physical examination
   A. Characteristic historical features
      1. Migraine
      2. Tension/Muscle Contraction Headache
      3. Dietary headache
      4. Posttraumatic headache
      5. Altitude headache
      6. Asthenopia
   B. Non-distinctive history
      1. Conversion headache
      2. Atypical facial pain
II. Abnormal physical examination
   A. Giant cell arteritis
   B. Herpetic neuralgia
   C. Hypertension
   D. Central nervous system disease
      1. Variation of intracranial pressure
      2. Subdural hemorrhage
      3. Meningitis
      4. Raeder's syndrome
      5. Carotid dissection
      6. Tolosa-Hunt syndrome
   E. Cranial neuralgias
      1. Trigeminal neuralgia
      2. Glossopharyngeal neuralgia
      3. Greater occipital neuralgia
   F. Ocular inflammation
   G. Temporomandibular joint pain
   H. Sinus disease
   I. Dental disease
   J. Orbital disease

sual or sensory-motor disturbances precede or, more rarely, accompany the headache. Males and females are affected equally. Visual symptoms may include both positive and negative scotomata. The scintillating positive scotoma is the most frequent disturbance. They are usually of a hemianopic nature, drift or "march" toward the temporal periphery (Fig. 12–1), and last less than 1 hour (22). The positive scotoma may appear as sparkles, flashes of colors, or heat waves.

Negative scotoma unaccompanied by scintillations may take the character of homonymous, central, tunnel, or altitudinal visual field defects (20), including sudden and complete bilateral blindness. Vision may also be described as "blurred", or "looking through a film of water."

Cluster migraine (cluster headache) most often occurs in the third, fourth and fifth decades of life in patients with no previous headache history and with a striking male predominance of at least 5:1 (13, 16). The headache is unilateral in the oculo temporal region and is usually characterized as an excruciating, burning, sharp, deep ache. It begins and ends abruptly lasting

less than 2 hours. It may occur several times in a 24 hour period and is commonly nocturnal. Rather than lying down in a quiet dark room as preferred by most migraine sufferers, the cluster patient is often restless, paces about, holding on to his face. Frequently, the headache is accompanied by Horner's syndrome and other ipsilateral autonomic phenomena such as lacrimation, conjunctival injection, sweating, and rhinorrhea.

Complicated migraine is a broad category used to describe patients who develop otherwise unexplained paroxysmal neurologic dysfunction that rarely may be permanent. A history of classic or common migraine is variable. Headache need not be an important component of complicated migraine and if present it may be shorter and less severe than other forms of migraine. The neurologic disturbance may include positive or negative scotomas as well as ophthalmoplegia, hemiplegia, hemiparesis, hemisensory loss, or disturbances of higher cortical function (19, 20). The rarer symptoms of cortical dysfunction include disturbances of color vision (central achromatopsia), facial recognition (prosopagnosia), reading (alexia with or without agraphia) (2), transient global amnesia, and acute confusion or psychosis (9). An unusual prodrome encompassing alterations of time sense, body image, as well as distortion of vision such as illusions of enlargement, shrinking, and elongation, has been labeled the "Alice in Wonderland syndrome" (11, 23). Frequently disturbing and puzzling to both patient and doctor, these episodes are often recognized for what they really are only after the headache appears.

Acephalgic migraine or episodic migrainous neurologic dysfunction of the type associated with the "classical" form of migraine but *without headache* has been reported by several authors (12, 20, 25, 26). Alvarez reviewed 618 cases of classic migraine and found that 13% of patients, most frequently men, experienced acephalgic episodes (1). These acephalgic episodes usually affect patients over age 40 years of age and have been termed "migraine equivalents" or "migrainous accompaniments" (Table 12–2).

Ocular migraine (retinal migraine) (Table 12–3) is characteristically a transient monocular visual loss, usually occurring in young adults less than 40 years of age. There is often a history of common or classic migraine or, more rarely, cluster headache. After repeated attacks, or occasionally with single spells, the patient may be left with a permanent visual field defect. Duration of visual loss ranges from seconds to hours, with most cases lasting less than 30 minutes. It has been suggested that long-lasting amaurotic spells with recovery are most likely due to migraine, with one report of recovery of vision after 7½ hours of amaurosis (8). Headache is an inconstant accompaniment of ocular migraine and is usually located over or around the affected eye. In addition, the temporal relationship between headache and visual

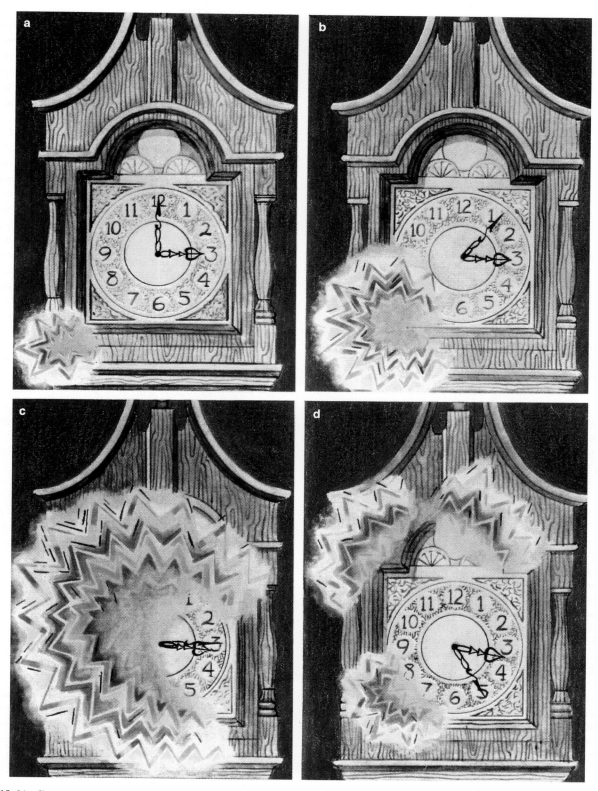

Figure 12–1(a–d).
Classical migrainous scintillating scotoma with march and expansion of fortification figures. (a) Initial small paracentral scotoma. (b) Enlarging scotoma 7 minutes later. (c) Scotoma obscuring much of central vision 15 minutes later. (d) Break-up of scotoma at 20 minutes.

TABLE 12–2
Accompaniments of Migraine

scintillating scotoma
paresthesia
dysarthria
hemiplegia
vertigo
blindness
blurred vision
hemianopia
transient monocular blindness
ophthalmoplegia
oculo-sympathetic palsy (Horner's syndrome)
mydriasis
confusion-stupor
cyclical vomiting
seizures
diplopia
deafness
recurrence of old stroke deficit
chorea

symptoms is variable, with visual loss occurring before, during, or after a headache.

Ophthalmoplegic migraine, a relatively uncommon condition, has been reported to occur in 2–17% of migraineurs (7). Males and females are equally affected. Typically, ophthalmoplegic migraine is more common in children. A migraine history in the child is often difficult to establish but a family history of migraine is frequent (5). Severe ipsilateral hemicranial headache is often a prominent feature of the syndrome and usually

TABLE 12–3
Causes of Transient Visual Disturbances of the Afferent Visual System

MONOCULAR
refractive error—myopia
vitreo-retinal traction
inflammation—vitritis/retinitis/optic neuritis
amaurosis fugax—retinal microembolism
papilledema
optic disc drusen
congenital dysplasia of the optic disc
coagulopathies
vasculitis
hypotension—arrhythmia/orthostatic
anemia
ocular migraine
BINOCULAR
migraine
seizure
occipital mass lesion (tumor or AVM)
occipital ischemia (embolic, vasculitis, hypoperfusion)

TABLE 12–4
Treatment of Migraine

1. General Measures to minimize conditions and agents that may precipitate migraine attacks
   Diet items
   Chocolate
   Alcohol
   Cheese
   Monosodium glutamate
   Nuts
   Hypoglycemia
   Stress
   Smoking
   Hypertension
   Birth control pills
2. Abortive Drugs
   Aspirin
   Acetaminophen
   Propoxyphene (Darvon)
   Fiorinal (aspirin, caffeine, butalbital)
   Midrin (isomethaptene mucate, acetaminophen, dichloral phenazone)
   Bellergal (phenobarbital, ergotamine tartrate, belladonna)
   Percodan (oxycodone, aspirin)
   Oxygen (100%, 3–5 liters/min)—cluster headache
   Esgic (acetaminophen, butalbital, caffeine)
   Empirin (aspirin, caffeine, phenacetin)
   Ergotamine tartrate
   Gynergen
   Ergostat
   Cafergot
   Wigraine
   DHE (dihydroergotamine mesylate)
   Non-steroidal anti-flammatory agents
   Naproxen
   Ibuprofen (Motrin)
   Sumatriptan
3. Prophylactic drugs
   Propranolol hydrochloride
   Methysergide
   Amitriptyline
   Calcium channel blockers
   Verapamil
   Nifedipine
   Lithium carbonate
   Cyprohepatadine
   Clonodine
   Indomethacin

precedes the attack although the headache may have significantly diminished or disappeared hours or days before the onset of the ophthalmoplegia. The third nerve is the most frequently involved ocular motor nerve followed in frequency by the sixth and the fourth nerves respectively (24). Usually the ophthalmoplegia resolves in a matter of three to four days without any permanent extraocular paralysis. The pupil is often involved and it is not uncommon to be left with slight mydriasis. Rarely, with repeated or prolonged episodes which may last as long as a month, the ophthalmoplegia may become partially or totally permanent. Aberrant regeneration is unusual but has been reported after this condition (21).

The *treatment* of migraine (Table 12–4) is often determined by the effect of symptoms on the patient's life style. If the attacks are not disabling or frequent, treatment may be nothing more than a thoughtful explanation of the frightening and uncomfortable symptoms coupled with reassurance that a more dangerous neurologic condition is not present. If specific treatment is to be initiated, it may be divided into three categories: general measures, abortive treatment of the acute attack, and prophylactic therapy aimed at preventing recurrence (Table 12–5).

Tension/Muscle Contraction Headache

Muscle tension headache is usually characterized by a tight pulling pain affecting both sides of the head. The pain is not intensified by body movement like the unilateral throbbing of migraine. Autonomic symptoms are uncommon as are photophobia or phonophobia. The patient is often able to continue normal activities rather than requiring rest and quiet. It is not uncommon for headache to begin with characteristics of tension and to evolve into a migraine syndrome.

Dietary Headache

The consumption or withdrawal of certain foods or beverages can result in head or facial pain. Nitrate or nitrite compounds, commonly used as preservatives, may act as vasal dilators and can induce a throbbing headache. Monosodium glutamate, a flavor enhancer often found in oriental foods, can be associated with headache and, in some instances, peripheral edema. Well-known is the headache of a "hangover" the day after ingestion of alcohol. Chronic cessation of the intake of caffeine after periods of chronic use can trigger a throbbing migrainous-like headache in susceptible persons.

Post Traumatic Headache

Head or neck pain may be just one symptom of a post traumatic condition which may include dizziness, insomnia, concentration difficulties, as well as mood and personality changes. The headache may be similar in character to that of a common migraine. The etiology of this head or neck pain is uncertain, and the physical examination is often entirely normal. The neck pain may be associated with a "whiplash" injury produced by sudden flexion and extension of the neck. Treatment of this condition is difficult and may include analgesics, sedatives, as well as tricyclic antidepressants.

Asthenopia

This retro-orbital, periocular, or brow pain is often associated with reading or other near vision tasks. As the visual effort is continued, the discomfort may be described as brow ache, lid heaviness, or some "tired" feeling about the eyes and is also referred to as eye strain. The localized discomfort about the eyes and orbits may also become generalized into a severe muscle contraction type headache. The key to recognition of this condition is its association with visual tasks. The clinician should search for uncorrected refracted errors, changes in power or axis of cylindric correction, or the presence of heterophorias.

■ HEADACHE SYNDROMES CHARACTERIZED BY AN ABNORMAL PHYSICAL EXAMINATION

Giant Cell Arteritis

Head pain in patients over the age of fifty that tends to localize over the branches of the temporal arteries should alert the clinician to the possibility of giant cell arteritis. Other accompanying features include scalp pain or tenderness, fever, proximal arthritis (polymyalgia rheumatica), and jaw claudication. Giant cell arteritis is characterized by arterial occlusion and may be accompanied by blindness from ischemic optic neuropathy or central retinal artery occlusion. The treatment is high dose corticosteroids and the diagnosis is confirmed by elevation of a sedimentation rate and biopsy of the superficial branches of the temporal artery.

Herpetic Neuralgia

Herpes zoster is often accompanied by severe pain of a burning and aching quality in the distribution of a cranial nerve, often a division of the 5th cranial nerve. More rarely, it can involve the 7th cranial nerve (Ramsay Hunt syndrome) and be associated with ipsilateral facial palsy (15). The diagnosis is usually apparent because of the accompanying vesicular rash, but in the pre-herpetic stage the head pain may precede the appearance of the typical rash by four to seven days. During this time, a diagnosis may be impossible. Involvement of the first division of the trigeminal nerve is frequently accompanied by a kerato-uveitis. The pain of the initial zoster infection usually resolves in 1 to 2 weeks, but it may persist for months or years, especially in the elderly. This post-herpetic phase of pain can be quite severe and triggered by simple touching of the involved area. Treatment of post-herpetic neuralgia is quite difficult and often requires a pain team approach.

Raeder's Syndrome

Severe ipsilateral head pain accompanied by a post-ganglionic Horner's syndrome and other cranial nerve abnormalities is defined as Raeder's syndrome (10). Cluster headache is a type of Raeder's syndrome and has been discussed in the section on migraines. If parasellar cranial nerves are involved, it is imperative to rule out inflammatory or mass lesions.

Carotid Dissection

Traumatic dissection of the internal carotid artery from the neck into the cavernous sinus region can produce ipsilateral head and neck pain accompanied by a post ganglionic Horner's syndrome and a bruit (6). The associated trauma need not be severe and may only be of a positional nature. Symptoms of multiple cranial nerve dysfunction or arterial occlusive disease may be present if the processes extends to the base of the brain or produces emboli. Arteriography, magnetic resonance imaging, or digital subtraction angiography may provide typical findings.

Tolosa-Hunt Syndrome

The combination of pain, ophthalmoplegia, and sensory loss (V1) involving cranial nerves III through VI, which pass through the superior orbital fissure is typical of the Tolosa-Hunt syndrome (17). This condition is often caused by an inflammatory process involving the anterior cavernous sinus and/or superior orbital fissure. The diagnosis is obtained by magnetic resonance imaging studies and the treatment is often corticosteroids.

Trigeminal Neuralgias

Trigeminal neuralgia or tic doloureux is characterized by excruciating pain in the distribution of one of the divisions of cranial nerve V. The third division of nerve V is the most commonly affected with the second and the first following in frequency. This paroxysmal pain usually only lasts 20 to 30 seconds and has a very characteristic triggering mechanism that may include such innocuous stimuli as a breeze or a light touch. The neurologic examination is otherwise normal until the triggering mechanism is initiated. Treatment includes oral agents such as phenytoin or carbamazipine, but often surgical intervention is necessary. Surgical procedures include radio frequency trigeminal gangliolysis or craniotomy with manipulation or direct destruction of the trigeminal nerve (4).

Greater Occipital Neuralgia

Periorbital pain that is associated with point tenderness in the occipital area is characteristic of greater occipital neuralgia (18). The pain is believed due to irritation of the greater occipital nerve as it pierces the tendinous insertion of the splenius capitis muscle at the base of the skull. The periocular pain is likely referred pain in the distribution of the trigeminal nerve. Often this condition is treated with injections of Xylocaine or corticosteroids to the area of point tenderness in the occiput.

Ocular Inflammation

Periorbital or retro-orbital pain may be secondary to ocular inflammation with irritation of branches of the first division of the trigeminal nerve. This pain is often associated with injection of the sclera and/or conjunctiva and intraocular signs should be present.

Temporomandibular Joint Pain

Inflammation or degenerative changes of the temporomandibular joint can produce irritation of the auriculotemporal and chorda tympani nerves producing an aching facial pain syndrome (14). This is more commonly seen in middle aged elderly adults and may be accompanied by head pain of the vertex, occiput, and supraorbital regions. It is very important to palpate the area of the temporomandibular joint for point tenderness and excessive mobility. Treatment of this condition includes non-specific analgesic medicines as well as the use of a bite plate at night to stabilize this joint.

Sinus Disease

Throbbing, dull head pain may be associated with sinus disease and at times difficult to differentiate from that of a common migraine or tension headache. The differentiating characteristic of sinus disease is the presence of tenderness over the affected sinus region accompanied by the appropriate sinus disease detected by radiologic investigation. The pain of frontal sinus disease is typically frontal, whereas the pain of ethmoid and sphenoid sinus disease may be retro-orbital. It is important to carefully look for other signs of orbital inflammation indicating spread into the adjacent orbital structures through the thin, bony walls.

Orbital Disease

Any orbital infection, inflammation, or mass lesion can incite a headache syndrome characterized by retro-orbital or periorbital pain. This pain is often of a dull, throbbing nature. Orbital signs are often present which will include proptosis, inflammation, swelling, or a palpable mass. Often, idiopathic or orbital inflammation or thyroid eye disease may produce pain with seemingly subtle clinical findings.

■ REFERENCES

1. Alvarez WC: The migrainous scotoma as studied in 618 persons. Am J Ophthalmol 49:489–504, 1960.
2. Bigley KG, Sharp FR: Reversible alexia without agraphia due to migraine. Arch Neurol 40:114–115, 1983.
3. Bille BS: Migraine in school children. A study of incidence and short term prognosis, and a clinical, psychological and electroencephalographic comparison between children with migraine and age matched controls. ACTA Paediat Scan. (Suppl 136) 51:1–151, 1962.
4. Dalessio DJ: Treatment of trigeminal neuralgia. JAMA 245:2519–2520, 1981.
5. Fenichel GM: Migraine in childhood: Brief review of this inherited disorder which strikes five percent of school-age children. Clin Pediatr 7:192, 1968.
6. Fisher CM: The headache and pain of spontaneous carotid dissection. Headache 22:60–65, 1981.
7. Friedman AP, Harter DH, Merritt HH: Ophthalmoplegic migraine. Arch Neurol 7:320–337, 1962.
8. Fujino T, Akiya S, Takagi S, et al: Amaurosis fugax for a long duration. J Clin Neuro-Ophthalmol 3:9–12, 1983.
9. Gascom G, Barlow C: Juvenile migraine presenting as an acute confusional state. Pediatrics 45:628–635, 1970.
10. Grimson BS, Thompson HS: Raeder's syndrome. A clinical review. Surv Ophthalmol 24:199, 1980.
11. Hachinski VC, Porchawka J, Steele JC: Visual symptoms in the migraine syndrome. Neurology 23:570–579, 1973.
12. Hedges TR Jr: Isolated ophthalmic migraine: its frequency, mechanisms, and differential diagnosis. In: Smith J.L. (ed). Neuro-ophthalmology. Symposium of the University of Miami and the Bascom Palmer Eye Institute. Vol 6, St. Louis: C.V. Mosby, pp.140–50, 1972.
13. Horton BT: Histiminic cephalgia: differential diagnosis and treatment. Proc Mayo Clin 31:325–333, 1956.
14. Howell FV: The teeth and jaws as sources of headache. In Dalessio DJ, editor: Wolff's headache and other head pain—New York—Oxford University Press, ed 4, p 385, 1980.
15. Hunt JF: Geniculate neuralgia. Arch Neurol Psychiatry. 37:253, 1937.
16. Hupp SL, Kline LB, Corbett JJ: Visual disturbance of migraine. Surv Ophthalmol 33:221–236, 1989.
17. Kline LB: The Tolosa-Hunt syndrome. Surv Ophthalmol. 27:79–95, 1982.
18. Knox DL, Mustonen E: Greater occipital neuralgia. An ocular pain syndrome with multiple etiologies. Trans Am Acad Ophthalmol Otolaryngol 79:513, 1975.
19. Kupersmith MJ, Warren FA, Hass WK: The non-benign aspects of migraine. Neuro-Ophthamol 7(1):1–10, 1987.
20. O'Connor PJ: Acephalgic migraine. Ophthalmology 88:999–1003, 1981.
21. O'Day J, Billson F, King J: Ophthalmoplegic migraine and aberrant regeneration of the oculomotor nerve. Br J Ophthalmol. 64(7):534–6, 1980.
22. Richards W: The fortification illusions of migraines. Sci Am 224:88–96, 1971.
23. Todd J: The syndrome of Alice in Wonderland. Canad. M.A.J. 73:701–704, 1955.
24. Walsh FB, Hoyt WF. Clinical Neuro-ophthalmology. 3rd ed. Williams and Wilkins, Baltimore, pp 1654–1689, 1969.
25. Whitty CWM: Migraine without headache. Lancet 2:283–5, 1967.
26. Wiley RG: The scintillating scotoma without headache. Ann Ophthalmol 11:581–5, 1979.
27. World Federation of Neurology Research Group on Migraine and Headache: Definition of Migraine: Third Migraine Symposium. London: Heiniman, London, 1970.

13 Cerebrovascular Abnormalities

Edward G. Buckley

■ ANEURYSMS

Cerebral aneurysms occur in approximately five percent of the population. There are two morphologic types termed saccular (berry aneurysm) and fusiforme. Saccular aneurysms are felt to be developmental defects in the wall of the artery due to an absent internal elastic lamina and tend to occur at arterial junctions in the carotid system involving the anterior communicating, middle cerebral, or in the region of the origins of the posterior communicating arteries (11) (Fig. 13–1). Fusiforme aneurysms most frequently affect the basilar artery, are characterized by tortuous dilatation with elongation of the artery, and are usually associated with atherosclerosis.

Clinical symptoms seen with cerebral aneurysms are due to progressive enlargement or rupture. Increased intracranial pressure associated with rapid enlargement can result in ophthalmic signs such as third nerve paresis, sixth nerve paresis, papilledema, subretinal or intraretinal hemorrhage, and vitreous hemorrhage (Terson's syndrome). Slow progressive enlargement of aneurysms can produce ocular symptomatology such as visual loss, visual field defects, or oculomotor nerve palsies depending on the location. Subarachnoid or intraventricular blood after rupture causes depression of consciousness, focal neurologic signs, and cerebral herniation.

Four types of cerebral aneurysms are of particular importance to ophthalmologists because of their frequent impact on the visual system. These are:

Intracavernous Carotid Aneurysm

Aneurysms of the cavernous portion of the carotid artery usually show slowly progressive enlargement with compression of the sixth, third, fifth, and fourth cranial nerves. An ipsilateral Horner's syndrome can occur from involvement of the sympathetics which are in close proximity to the carotid artery in the cavernous sinus. Ipsilateral visual loss can occur if enlargement extends superiorly. Ocular and forehead pain can often be a late symptom. Diagnosis can be confirmed by CT scan, MRI scan, or cerebral angiography (Figs. 13–2 and 13–3). Treatment with intravascular occlusion of the aneurysm by detachable balloons can be effective in relief of pain and improvement of the ophthalmoplegia.

Giant Aneurysms

Large (greater than 25 mm) intracranial carotid aneurysms tend to occur at the supraclinoid portion of the internal carotid artery and result in compression of the optic nerves and chiasm. Visual loss usually begins unilaterally with slow progression before enlargement is sufficient to compromise the contralateral nerve or chiasm. On visual field testing giant aneurysms have been associated with a characteristic ipsilateral nasal junctional scotoma. The majority of giant aneurysms occur in women in their 50's and 60's and rarely rupture. These large aneurysms can simulate a mass lesion such as a neoplasm or a pituitary tumor. Diagnosis is confirmed by CT, MRI, or cerebral angiography. The treatment consists of carotid ligation in the neck or detachable balloon catheterization.

Posterior Communicating Artery Aneurysm

Aneurysms of the posterior communicating artery arise at the junction of the carotid artery and tend to be asso-

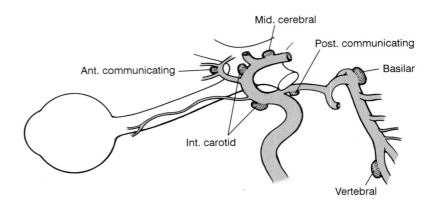

Figure 13–1.
A schematic illustrating the more common locations for intracranial aneurysms.

ciated with a painful complete third nerve palsy. The determination of pupillary involvement is important as pupillary sparing third nerve palsies are usually associated with microvascular disease while total pupillary paralysis occurs with ruptured or unruptured posterior communicating artery aneurysms. In the clinical setting of a sudden onset of painful third nerve palsy with severe headache and nuchal rigidity, angiography is indicated irrespective of pupil involvement. While the oculomotor palsy is usually complete, some preservation of function can occur, but it is quite uncommon for any single muscle to be entirely spared. The incidence of oculomotor palsy with posterior communicating artery aneurysm is approximately 50%. The diagnosis of posterior communicating artery aneurysms can be made ei-

ther with contrast enhanced CT, MRI angiography, or cerebral angiography. Treatment involves direct neurosurgical ligation of the aneurysm and should be performed promptly to try to preserve third nerve function.

Basilar Artery Aneurysm

Basilar artery aneurysms make up approximately 15% of all intracranial aneurysms. Frequent eye signs occur from compression of the brain stem, compromise of the oculomotor nerve, or pressure on the chiasm. *Saccular* basilar aneurysms tend to occur in middle-aged women and often present with subarachnoid hemorrhage without previous neurologic signs or symptoms (11). Neurologic signs when they do occur consist of episodic

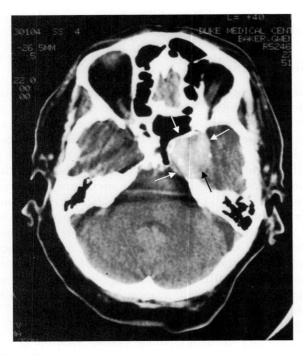

Figure 13–2.
CT scan of a patient with a left intercavernous carotid aneurysm. The patient presented with a progressive left sixth nerve palsy.

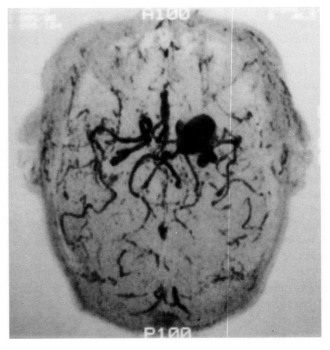

Figure 13–3.
MRI angiogram of patient shown in Figure 9.2. Note the large left carotid aneurysm.

diplopia, transient hemiplegia, nystagmus, visual field defects, skew deviation, up gaze palsy, and multiple cranial nerve defects. Isolated oculomotor paralysis has been reported. Patients with saccular aneurysms tended to die of rupture. *Fusiforme* basilar aneurysms tend to occur in older men and are commonly associated with hypertension, atherosclerotic cardiovascular disease, and abdominal aortic aneurysms. Neurologic signs are slowly progressive and consist of multiple cranial nerve palsies with long tract motor and sensory signs. Fusiforme basilar artery aneurysms do not tend to rupture and most patients succumb to their cardiovascular disease.

■ ARTERIAL VENOUS MALFORMATIONS

Arterial venous malformations (AVMs) are congenital abnormal communications between arteries and veins such that blood is shunted directly from the arterial to the venous circulation without an intervening capillary bed. Angiographically, AVMs can be classified depending on whether the arterial supply is dural or pial. Dural malformations are limited to the dura and receive only meningeal arterial blood. Pial malformations are intracranial lesions that are supplied only by cerebral or cerebellar arteries without meningeal contribution. Neurologic signs and symptoms which occur are secondary to the location of the AVM or complications of subarachnoid and intracerebral hemorrhage. Congenital AVMs often present with convulsions, headaches, progressive neurologic deficits and mental changes which are often due to hemorrhage or shunting of blood away from otherwise normal brain. In adults the most common presentation is a sudden onset of a headache, stiff neck, and decreased consciousness secondary to subarachnoid hemorrhage. Seizures are quite common occurring in 40% of patients. The initial symptoms of AVMs usually present between the ages of 10 and 30 years.

Dural AVMs are rare constituting 5–10% and occur predominantly in women over 40 years of age. They occur mainly in the posterior fossa and present with a variety of brainstem findings including abnormalities of the cranial nerves, long track signs, gaze palsies, ataxia, skew deviation, and nystagmus. In addition, hemifacial spasm in the young adult, hydrocephalus with signs of increased intracranial pressure, or reccurrent occipital or hemicranial headaches suggest the possibility of a posterior fossa AVM. Since most posterior fossa dural malformations occur near a major venous sinus, a pseudotumor-like picture (headaches, disc edema, cranial nerve palsies) can occur due to direct shunting of arterial blood into the venous system.

The more common (85%) pial arterial venous malformations are supplied primarily by the carotid circulation, affect men slightly more than women, and are associated with the triad of hemorrhage, seizures, and recurrent headaches. Clinical symptoms result from subarachnoid hemorrhage or intracerebral hemorrhage with hematoma formation. Ophthalmic signs occur when there is involvement of a portion of the visual radiations. Occipital lobe AVMs may be difficult to distinguish from migraines as they both include visual phenomena and headaches, but it is rare that "classic" migraine is mimicked by occipital AVM. Visual field testing will often reveal a homonymous hemianopia. Congenital AVMs can occupy the entire occipital pole for decades without producing visual field defects. Amaurosis fugax can be a presenting symptom of anteriorly located AVMs if blood is shunted to the meningeal circulation from the ophthalmic artery.

Diagnostic evaluation of AVMs consists of CT scanning, MRI scanning, or MRI angiography. The prognosis of symptomatic untreated vascular malformations is poor. Approximately 20% have intracranial hemorrhage and 40–80% of the patients become severely disabled or die of their disease. The combined morbidity/mortality of surgery is 25%. The mortality rate from hemorrhage is 30%. Asymptomatic patients with superficial AVMs fare better and often no intervention is required. A variety of intravascular techniques employing embolization with materials such as silastic and cyanoacrylate have been successful. Recently, stereotactic heavy–charged–particle Bragg-peak radiation has been used to treat inaccessible lesions which have high surgical or embolization risk. Ninety-two percent had complete obliteration after three years. The major disadvantage to this technique was a prolonged latency period before complete obliteration.

■ DURAL AND CAROTID CAVERNOUS SINUS FISTULAS

Carotid cavernous sinus fistulas are abnormal communications between a branch of the carotid artery and the cavernous sinus. Generally these shunts can be divided into two broad types depending on the origin of the arterial blood supply. The first is a direct high pressure shunt between the internal carotid artery and the cavernous sinus with 75% occurring as a result of head trauma. There is usually rapid onset of pulsatile exophthalmos, pain, conjunctival and episcleral injection, chemosis, ophthalmoplegia, and an orbital bruit (Figure 13–4). The ophthalmoplegia may be secondary to cranial nerve palsies from nerve compression in cavernous sinus (commonly the sixth) or mechanical limitation due to enlarged, engorged extraocular muscles. Ocular hypertension occurs due to increased episcleral venous pressure and some patients develop venous stasis retinopathy and central retinal vein occlusions (16). Since the two cavernous sinuses are connected, these signs and symptoms may be bilateral even in unilateral lesions. Sudden improvements suggest *thrombosis of the superior ophthalmic vein* which may also result in increased signs and symptomatology on the *opposite* side.

The second type are dural fistulas and result from a connection between the meningeal branches of the internal carotid or external carotid artery and the cavernous sinus and have much lower flow rates with less severe symptomatology. Typically, dural sinus fistulas are gradual in onset and frequently may be mistaken for conjunctivitis or thyroid ophthalmopathy. The episcleral and conjunctival vessels become dilated with arterial blood (arterialization) and have a corkscrew configuration (Figure 13–5, 13–6). There is either no or mild proptosis, minimal ophthalmoplegia, a small increase in intraocular pressure and often no bruit. They typically occur in post-menopausal women and are associated with atherosclerotic changes, hypertension, collagen vascular disease, or childbirth.

The diagnosis of carotid cavernous sinus fistulas can be confirmed by orbital ultrasound, CT or MRI scanning, MRI angiography, intravenous digital subtraction angiography, or arterial angiography. Findings useful in establishing a diagnosis include a dilated superior ophthalmic vein, mild *symmetric* enlargement of the ex-

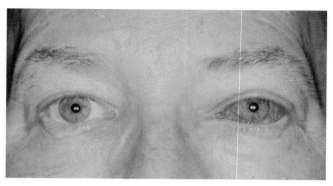

Figure 13–5.
Patient with a left dural sinus fistula. Note marked arterioralization of the episcleral vessels. There is no proptosis and no ophthalmoplegia.

traocular muscles, proptosis, and bulging of the outer wall of the cavernous sinus (Fig. 13–7). The best detailed information can be obtained with angiography but because of its risks this should only be performed if the information will alter the course of therapy. Dural fistulas have been known to disappear after angiography. Carotid cavernous sinus fistulas will close spontaneously in approximately 25–50% of patients with the higher frequency seen in the low flow dural shunts. The spontaneous closure is thought to be secondary to partial or complete thrombosis of the cavernous sinus. Acute worsening of symptoms may indicate that a spontaneous thrombosis has taken place and resolution of clinical symptoms may follow. Traumatic cavernous sinus fistulas are less likely to close spontaneously because of their higher flow rate. The indications for intervention include progressive loss of vision, persistent diplopia, corneal exposure due to proptosis, intractable glaucoma, or severe head pain. Most patients with dural

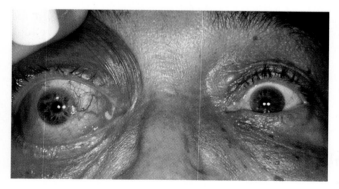

Figure 13–4.
Patient with a right carotid cavernous sinus fistula. Note marked proptosis, chemosis and episcleral injection. The patient also exhibited a total ophthalmoplegia.

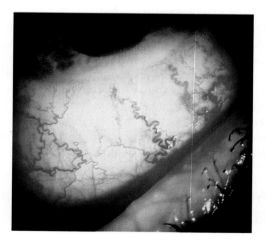

Figure 13–6.
Characteristic cork screw configuration of the conjunctival vessels in a patient with a dural sinus fistula.

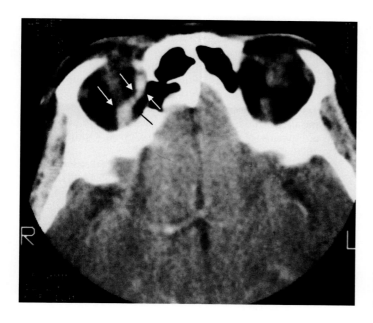

Figure 13–7.
CT scan of patient with right dural sinus fistula. Note dilated superior ophthalmic vein (arrows).

sinus fistulas do not need treatment. Glaucoma if it occurs can often be managed with medical or surgical interventions.

Treatment of carotid cavernous sinus fistulas is directed toward closure of the fistula or its feeding vessels. This can be accomplished with carotid ligation in the neck (no longer advocated), intravascular embolization with embolic materials such as glue (isobutyl-2-cyanoacrylate) and poly-vinyl alcohol particles. Intravascular balloons also have been used primarily for treating traumatic fistulas. Successful fistula closure occurs anywhere from 70–95%. Complications include carotid occlusion, neurologic deficits, sinus thrombosis, false or pseudo aneurysm, cranial nerve palsies, and visual field loss.

Glaucoma secondary to cavernous sinus fistulas has been successfully controlled with both medical and surgical interventions. Glaucoma filtering procedures have been successful as have laser trabeculoplasty. PANretinal photocoagulation has been shown to produce resolution of glaucoma as well as retinal neovascularization.

■ REFERENCES

1. Bogousslavsky J, Vinuela F, Barnett HJ, et al.: Amaurosis fugax as the presenting manifestation of dural arteriovenous malformation. Stroke—1985:16:891.
2. Bynke HG, Efsina HO: Carotid cavernous sinus fistula with contralateral exophthalmos. ACTA Ophthalmol—1970:48:971.
3. Farris BK, Smith JL, and David NJ: The nasal junction scotoma in giant aneurysms. Ophthalmol—1986:93:895.
4. Grayson WK, Soni SR, Spooner VA: Analysis of the recovery of third nerve function after direct surgical intervention for posterior communicating aneurysms. Br J Ophthalmol—1974:58:118.
5. Grove AS: The dural shunt syndrome. Pathophysiology and clinical course. Ophthalmol—1983:90:31–44.
6. Harris MJ, Fine SL, Miller NR: Photocoagulation treatment of proliferative retinopathy secondary to carotid-cavernous sinus fistula. Am J Ophthalmol—1980:90:515–518.
7. Hooke O, Norden G, Guzman J: Saccular aneurysms of the vertebral-basilar arterial system: a report of 28 cases. ACTA Neurol Scand—1963:39:271.
8. Kashii S, Solomon S, Moser F, Tostanowski J, and Burde R: Progressive visual field defects in patients with intracranial arteriovenous malformations. AJO 1990:109:556.
9. Keltner JL, Satterfield D, Dublin AB, and Lee B: Dural and carotid cavernous sinus fistulas. Ophthalmol 1987:94:1585–1600.
10. Kupersmith MJ, Berenstein A, Choi IS, et al: Percutaneous transvascular treatment of giant carotid aneurysms: Neuro-ophthalmic findings. Neurology—1984:34:328.
11. McCormick WF: Pathology and pathogenesis of intracranial saccular aneurysms. Semin Neurol—1984:4:291.
12. McKinna AJ: Eye signs in 611 cases of posterior fossa aneurysms: Their diagnostic and prognostic valve. Can J Ophthalmol—1983:18:3.
13. Newton TH and Cronquist S: Involvement of dural arteries in intracranial arteriovenous malformations. Radiology—1969:93:1071.
14. Nijensohn DE, Saiz RJ, Regan TJ: Clinical significance of basilar artery aneurysms. Neurology—1974:24:301.
15. Phelps CD, Thompson HS, Ossoining KC: The diagnosis and prognosis of atypical carotid-cavernous fistula (red-

eyed shunt syndrome). Am J Ophthalmol—1982:93: 423–36.

16. Sanders MD and Hoyt WF: Hydroxic ocular sequelae of carotid-cavernous fistulae. Study of the causes and failure before and after neuro-surgical treatment in a series of 25 cases. Br J Ophthalmol—1969:53:82–97.

17. Soni SR: Aneurysms of the posterior communicating artery and oculomotor paresis. J Neurol Neuro Surg. Psychiatry—1974:37:475.

18. Stein BM and Wolpert SM: Arteriovenous malformations of the brain. Arch Neurol—1980;37:1.

19. Steinberg GK, Fabrikant J, Marks M, Levy R, Frankel K, Phillips M, Shuer L, and Silverberg G: Stereotactic heavy-charged-particle Bragg-Peak radiation for intracranial arteriovenous malformations. N Eng J Med 1990:323:96–101.

20. Swearingen B, Heros RC: Common carotid occlusin for unclippable carotid aneurysms: an old but still effective operation. Neurosurgery—1987:21:288.

21. Trobe JD, Glaser JS, Quencer RC: Isolated oculomotor paralysis: The product of saccular and fusiforme aneurysms of the basilar artery. Arch Ophthalmol—1978:96:1236.

22. Wilkins RH: Natural history of intracranial vascular malformations: a review. Neurosurgery—1985;16:421.

V Strabismus and Pediatric Ophthalmology

Section Editor: Kenneth W. Wright

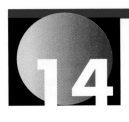

14 Motor Aspects of Strabismus

Kenneth W. Wright

■ EYE MOVEMENTS

Eye movements are clinically described in terms of monocular rotations called ductions and binocular movements called versions. *Ductions* are tested with one eye covered observing the extent of the movements of the uncovered eye.

Types of ductions include: *adduction*—nasal rotation; *abduction*—temporal rotation; *supraduction*—upward rotation; and *infraduction*—downward rotation. Clinically, a limitation of ductions may be recorded on a scale of −1, indicating slight limitation and almost full ductions, to a −4, indicating inability to move the eye past midline. Cycloduction or torsional movements are twisting eye movements, with excycloduction or *extorsion* representing a rotation of the 12-o'clock position temporally and incycloduction or *intorsion* representing a rotation of the 12-o'clock position nasally.

Versions are tested by observing how well the two eyes move together in synchrony, without covering an eye. Versions are defined as follows: *dextroversion*—right gaze; *levoversion*—left gaze; *supraversion*—upgaze; *infraversion*—downgaze. Version testing allows simultaneous comparison of eye movements, with one eye compared with the other. Versions are useful for identifying subtle muscle imbalances such as muscle underactions and overactions. This contrasts to ductions, which tests the ability of one eye to move, and identifies gross limitations of eye movements. Versions are graded on a scale of +1 to +4 for overaction and −1 to −4 for underaction. See Chapter 19 on oblique dysfunction for more on oblique muscle dysfunction.

■ EXTRAOCULAR MUSCLES

There are four rectus muscles and two oblique muscles, which act to move the eye around a fixed center of rotation (see Chapter 1 and Fig. 14–1). Horizontal rectus muscles have a single function: adduction for the medial rectus and abduction for the lateral rectus. The vertical rectus muscles (superior rectus and inferior rectus) and oblique muscles (superior oblique and inferior oblique), however, have three functions—one primary and two secondary (Table 14–1). Vertical rectus muscles are the major elevators and depressors of the eye, with the superior rectus primarily an elevator and the inferior rectus muscle primarily a depressor. Secondary functions include intorsion for the superior rectus, extorsion for the inferior rectus, and tertiary function of adduction for both vertical rectus muscles. Oblique muscle function is primarily torsional, the superior oblique producing intorsion and the inferior oblique producing extorsion. Torsional movements of the oblique muscles are secondary to their tangential (nasal to temporal) course. Secondary oblique functions include depression for the superior oblique, elevation for the inferior

233

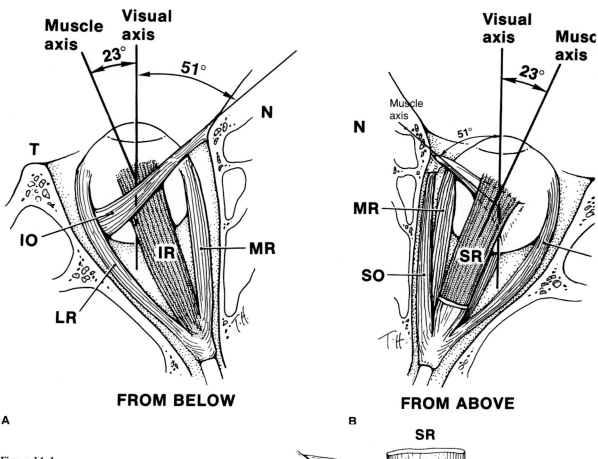

FROM BELOW

A

FROM ABOVE

B

Figure 14–1.
Drawing of extraocular muscles. Notice that the visual axis is 23° off the vertical muscle axis (inferior rectus and superior rectus) and 51° off oblique muscle axis (inferior oblique and superior oblique) (Fig. 14–1 A and B). **A,** The inferior oblique muscle view seen from below the eye. **B,** The superior oblique muscle view from above. Notice the superior oblique parallels and the inferior oblique with the functional origin being the trochlea. **C,** View behind the eye shows relationship of the extra ocular muscle. Notice that both oblique muscles lie below their corresponding rectus muscle (superior oblique is below the superior rectus and the inferior oblique is below the inferior rectus). (From Wright K: Color Atlas of Ophthalmic Surgery: Strabismus. Philadelphia: JB Lippincott, 1991.)

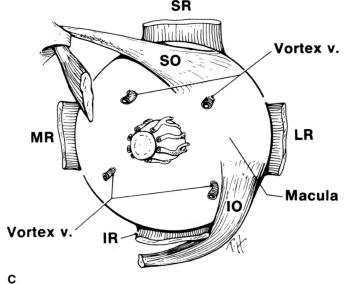

C

oblique, and tertiary function of abduction for both oblique muscles.

The multiple functions of the vertical rectus and oblique muscles occur because, unlike the horizontal rectus muscles, the pull of the vertical rectus muscles and oblique muscles is not parallel to the visual axis of the eye. With the eye in primary position, the axis of the vertical rectus muscles diverge 23° off the visual axis, while the oblique muscles course tangentially in a nasal to temporal direction 51° off the visual axis (Fig. 14–1). Thus, in addition to their vertical function, vertical rectus muscles pull in a nasal direction. Because the vertical rectus muscle insertions are anterior to the equator of the eye, this nasal pull produces the secondary functions of adduction for both vertical rectus muscles, intorsion for the superior rectus, and extorsion for the inferior rectus. The functional origin of the oblique muscles are at the anterior-nasal aspect of the orbit, with

TABLE 14–1
Extraocular Muscle Measurements

Muscle	Origin	Insertion: Distance from Limbus (mm)	Approximate Muscle Length (mm)	Tendon Length (mm)	Arc of Contact (mm)	Action from Primary Position
Medial rectus	Annulus of Zinn	5.5	40	4	6	Adduction
Lateral rectus	Annulus of Zinn	7.0	40	8	10	Abduction
Superior rectus	Annulus of Zinn	8.0	40	6	6.5	Elevation, intorsion, adduction
Inferior rectus	Annulus of Zinn	6.5	40	7	7	Depression, extorsion, adduction
Superior oblique	Orbit apex above annulus of Zinn	From temporal superior rectus insertion to 6.5 mm from optic nerve	32	26	12	Intorsion, depression, abduction
Inferior oblique	Lacrimal fossa	Macular area	37	1	10	Extorsion, elevation, abduction

the superior oblique above and inferior oblique below (Fig. 14–1). Note that the oblique and vertical rectus muscle functions are dependent on eye position. For example, with the eye rotated 51° into adduction, the inferior oblique muscle becomes almost a pure elevator and the superior oblique a pure depressor.

The anatomic origin of the superior oblique is the orbital apex, above the superior rectus muscle; however, its functional origin is at the trochlea (Fig. 14–1B). The superior oblique muscle has the longest tendon (25 mm) of the extraocular muscles. Starting a few millimeters posterior to the trochlea, the tendon passes through the trochlea then turns posterior-temporally to insert under the superior rectus muscle. The tendon insertion is broad and follows the temporal boarder of the superior rectus muscle, from the superior rectus insertion posteriorly to a point approximately 6.5 mm from the optic nerve (Fig. 14–1C). The posterior two thirds of the tendon insertion is responsible for the secondary functions of the superior oblique muscle: depression and abduction. These posterior tendon fibers pull the back of the eye up and in toward the trochlea, which moves the front of the front of the eye down and out, producing the secondary functions of depression and abduction.

The inferior oblique originates in the lacrimal fossa, which is located at the inferior-nasal aspect of the anterior orbit. It passes posterior-temporal, paralleling the course of the superior oblique tendon to pass under the inferior rectus muscle. After passing under the inferior rectus muscle, the inferior oblique inserts on the posterior lateral aspect of the globe along the inferior border of the lateral rectus muscle (Fig. 14–1). Inferior oblique muscle contracture pulls the back of the eye down and nasally, which moves the front of the eye up and out, producing the secondary functions of elevation and abduction. In contrast to the superior oblique, the inferior oblique muscle has the shortest tendon of the extraocular muscles, approximately 1 mm long.

■ PERIOCULAR FASCIA

A connective tissue fascia unites the superior rectus muscle to the overlying levator palprebal muscle. Recession of the superior rectus muscle can cause posterior displacement of the levator palprebral muscle and postoperative upper eye lid retraction. Careful dissection of these fascial attachments helps prevent upper lid retraction. The inferior rectus is between the inferior oblique muscle below and the sclera above. The inferior rectus and inferior oblique muscles are joined together by a connective tissue called Lockwood's ligament (Fig. 1–7B). Lockwood's ligament is continuous with the capsulopalprebral fascia and the lower lid retractors. These

ligaments are responsible for lower lid retraction after inferior rectus muscle recession. Removal of these connective tissue ligaments helps prevent postoperative lower lid retraction.

Tenon's capsule is a smooth connective tissue that lines the eye, separating the globe and muscles from surrounding orbital fat. The extraocular muscles penetrate Tenon's capsule as they approach the globe. At the point of muscle penetration, Tenon's capsule forms an elastic membrane called the *muscle sheath*. Together, Tenon's capsule and the muscle sheath provide a fascial barrier separating orbital fat from the extraocular muscles and globe. Tenon's capsule allows for free rotation of the globe with very little resistance. Traumatic violation of posterior Tenon's capsule or muscle sheath can result in scarring of orbital fat to the globe or extraocular muscle resulting in restriction of eye movements (Fig. 14–2). This specific type of scar is termed *fat adherence,* and can occur after accidental periocular trauma or as a complication of extraocular surgery including retinal, oculoplastic, or strabismus surgery (see p. 316, Fig. 20–4). A connective tissue of similar consistency to Tenon's capsule spans between the anterior aspect of the extraocular muscles and is termed the *intermuscular septum.* It is not involved with separating orbital fat from the globe but probably helps to hold the muscles in place. *Check ligaments* extend from the anterior aspect of the muscle to the overlying conjunctiva and more posteriorly to Tenon's capsule.

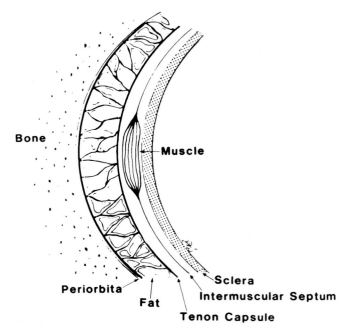

Figure 14–2.
Normal relationship of the orbital bone extraconal fat rectus muscle and sclera. Notice that Tenon's capsule separates extraconal fat from muscle and sclera. Intramuscle septum stretches from rectus muscle to rectus muscle and is between Tenon's capsule and sclera. (From Wright KW: The fat adherence syndrome and strabismus after retina surgery. Ophthalmology 1986;93:414.)

■ LAWS OF OCULAR MOTILITY

Axes of Fick and Listing's Law

All ocular movements represent a rotation of the eye around a fixed center. These rotations can be described as occurring around three axes (i.e., X, Y, and Z) that pass through the center of rotation of the eye and are termed the *Axes of Fick* (Fig. 14–3). The orientation of the axes of Fick are at right angles to the direction of ocular rotation (4). For example, the Z axis is vertically oriented and allows horizontal rotation, the X axis is horizontally oriented for vertical rotation, and the Y axis is oriented with the visual axis allowing for torsional rotations important during head tilting. Listing's plane consists of a plane that includes the Z and X axes (Fig. 14–3). *Listing's law* states that virtually all positions of gaze can be achieved by rotations around these two axes that lie on Listing's plane. Oblique eye movements are achieved by rotations around oblique axes on Listings plane, which are oriented between the X and Z axes (O axis in Fig. 14–3).

Sherrington's Law of Reciprocal Innervation

Monocular rotations require contraction of the acting muscle or *agonist* with simultaneous relaxation of the

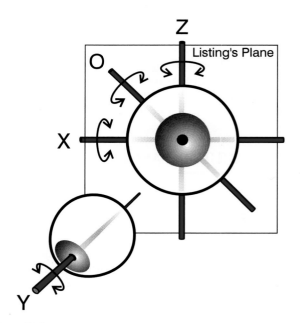

Figure 14–3.
Diagram of Listing's plane and XYZ axes of rotation (axis of Fick). X axis is responsible for vertical rotation, Z axis for horizontal rotation, and O axis for oblique rotation. Y axis is the center for torsional rotation.

TABLE 14–2
Monocular Movements

Agonist–Antagonist

Medial Rectus	—	Lateral Rectus
Superior Rectus	—	Inferior Rectus
Superior Oblique	—	Inferior Oblique

Synergists

Duction	Primary Mover	Secondary Mover
Supraduction	Superior rectus	Inferior oblique
Infraduction	Inferior rectus	Superior oblique
Adduction	Medial Rectus	Superior rectus/inferior rectus
Abduction	Lateral rectus	Superior oblique/Inferior oblique
Excyclo	Inferior oblique	Inferior rectus
Incyclo	Superior oblique	Superior rectus

opposing muscle or the *antagonist* (Table 14–2). For example, when the eye adducts, the medial rectus contracts (agonist) and the lateral rectus relaxes (antagonist) (Fig. 14–4). Other agonist/antagonist pairs include the superior rectus and inferior rectus for vertical rotations and the superior oblique and inferior oblique for torsional rotations. The oblique muscles

also are agonist/antagonist pairs for vertical rotations when the eye is in adduction. This relationship between agonist and antagonist muscles is referred to as *Sherrington's law of reciprocal innervation*. Remember, Sherrington's law refers strictly to monocular eye rotations, that is, ductions.

Synergist

In contrast to agonist and antagonist, the term *synergist* refers to muscles of the same eye that act to move the eye in the same direction. Thus, synergistic muscles have common functions and relate to monocular rotations. The inferior oblique and superior rectus muscles can both elevate the eye; therefore, they are synergists for supraduction. These muscles, however, are not synergists for horizontal or torsional rotations (Table 14–2).

Field of Action

The *field of action* of a muscle is that eccentric gaze position where a specific muscle contributes the most. For example, the superior oblique muscle is most active and contributes most when the eye moves down and nasally. Thus, the field of action of the superior oblique muscle is "down and in." One can evaluate the function of an extraocular muscle by having the patient look in the field of action of the muscle. To test superior oblique function, have the patient look down and nasally. If the superior oblique muscle is paretic, the eye will not fully rotate down and nasally. Figure 14–5 shows the field of action of the extraocular muscles of the right eye. Although the oblique muscles are major contributors to vertical eye movements in adduction, the superior and inferior recti also help to elevate and depress the eye in adduction. The oblique muscles, however, do not contribute significantly to vertical movements in abduction, as this is the sole responsibility of the superior and inferior recti.

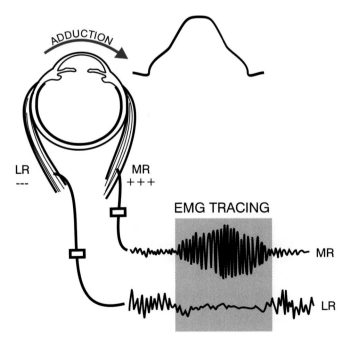

Figure 14–4.
Sherrington's law of reciprocal innervation (agonist/antagonist). Diagram shows left eye moving in adduction with the left medial rectus muscle the agonist and firing on EMG recordings while the left lateral rectus is the antagonist and relaxes shown by EMG recording.

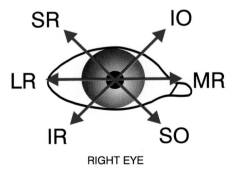

Figure 14–5.
Field of action of the extraocular muscles. Diagram shows right eye, and the arrows point to the direction of gaze where a specific muscle is the major mover. To test a specific muscle, have the patient look in the direction of the arrow.

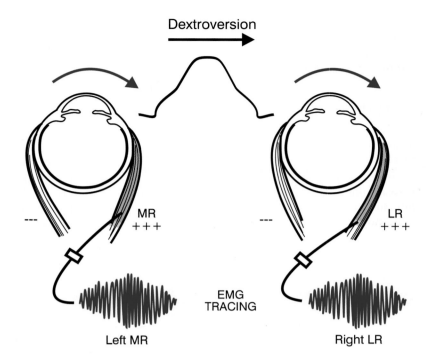

Figure 14–6.
Hering's law of yoke muscles, patient looking to the right (dextroversion with yoke left medial rectus muscle and right lateral rectus muscle firing as evidence by EMG recordings seen in red). The left lateral rectus and right medial rectus muscles are yoke antagonists, and they relax during dextroversion. Hering's law relates to binocular coordinated eye movements.

Hering's Law of Yoke Muscles

Our eyes do not move independently but move together in concert. Even if one eye is blind, the eyes move together. A horizontal version movement to the right requires contraction of the left medial rectus and right lateral rectus muscles, along with simultaneous relaxation of their agonists, the left lateral rectus and right medial rectus muscles (Fig. 14–6). The paired agonist and antagonist muscles from each eye are referred to as *yoke muscles*. In the example above, the left medial and the right lateral rectus muscles are yoke agonist muscles. *Hering's law* states that yoke agonist and yoke antagonist muscles must receive equal innervation. Hering's law refers to binocular eye movements (versions) in contrast to Sherrington's law, which describes monocular rotations (ductions).

Binocular Fusion

Binocular fusion is the process of merging the images from each eye and maintaining binocular eye alignment on the visual target. There are two aspects of binocular fusion: sensory fusion and motor fusion. *Sensory fusion* is the cortical process of blending the images from each eye into a single binocular stereoscopic image. Sensory fusion only occurs when the eyes are well aligned except for the abnormal state of anomalous retinal correspondence (i.e., ARC) (see Chapter 16). Sensory fusion and ARC will be discussed in more detail in Chapter 16. *Motor fusion* is the mechanism that allows fine tuning of eye position to maintain eye alignment so that the foveas of each eye are aligned with the same object of regard. It

acts as a locking mechanism that keeps the eyes aligned on visual targets as they move throughout our visual space and controls innate tendencies for the eyes to drift off target. These correctional eye movements provided by motor fusion are termed *fusional vergence* movements. There is an important distinction between motor fusion and sensory fusion. Motor fusion is the mechanism of motor realignment of the eyes to keep each fovea on target, whereas sensory fusion is the brain integrating the images from each eye.

There are three types of vergence movements: convergence, divergence, and vertical vergence. *Convergence* is the strongest vergence movement. It is used to follow objects moving from distance to near and to correct tendencies for the eyes to drift out (exodeviations). With convergence, both eyes move toward each other or inward. One can demonstrate convergence by looking at the tip of a pencil, then slowly bringing the pencil toward one's nose. The eyes will converge to hold eye alignment on the pencil as the pencil approaches the nose. In contrast to version movements where both eyes move in the same direction, vergence movements are disconjugate as the eyes move in opposite directions. Convergence, for example, results in the left eye moving to the right and the right eye moving to the left. *Divergence* is the opposite of convergence and is an outward or temporal movement of both eyes that occurs when an object moves from near to distance. Divergence also corrects the tendency for the eyes to drift in (esodeviations). *Vertical vergence* keeps our eyes vertically aligned and consists of elevation of one eye with depression of the fellow eye. Vertical vergence corrects tendencies for the eyes to vertically separate (hyperdeviation). Divergence is a much weaker mechanism than convergence but is significantly stronger than vertical vergence. The strength of vergence movements can be measured in prism diopters and are called *fusional vergence amplitudes*. See below for a discussion of how to measure fusional vergence amplitudes.

■ STRABISMUS

Strabismus is the term for ocular misalignment or an underlying tendency toward misalignment. When the eyes are misaligned, one eye will fixate with the fovea and the fellow eye deviates, so the image falls on a peripheral retinal point (Fig. 14–7). This is termed *heterotropia* or just *tropia*, and refers to the presence of a manifest strabismus. Another form of strabismus is a tendency for the eyes to drift, but that tendency is controlled by fusional vergence or motor fusion. This latent deviation that is held in check by motor fusion is called a *heterophoria* or simply *phoria*.

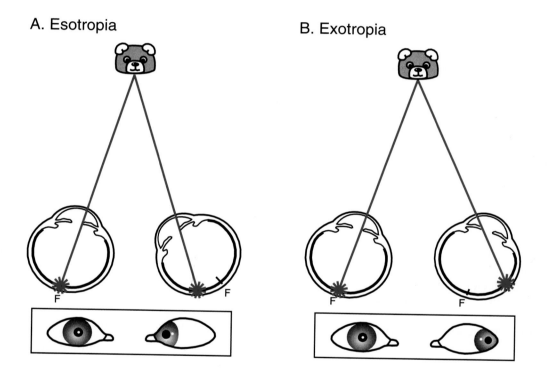

A. Esotropia   B. Exotropia

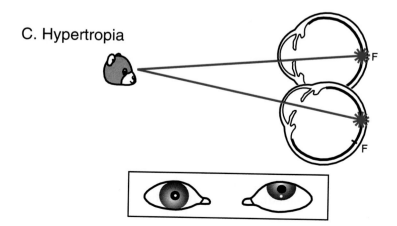

C. Hypertropia

Figure 14–7.
Diagram shows both retinal orientation and eye position for esotropia, exotropia, and hypertropia. **A,** Esotropia with the retinal image falling on the fovea of the fixing eye and nasal to the fovea in the deviated eye. **B,** Exotropia with the retinal image falling on the fovea of the fixing eye and temporal to the fovea in the nonfixing eye. **C,** Hypertropia with the retinal image falling on the fovea of the fixing eye and above the fovea in the hypertropic eye.

Heterotropia

A heterotropia can be horizontal, vertical, torsional, or a combination of the three. *Orthotropia* means the eyes are aligned, and there is no tropia. *Esotropia* (ET) refers to an inturning strabismus with the image in the deviated eye falling nasal to the fovea (Fig. 14–7A). *Exotropia* (XT) is an outward deviation with the image falling temporal to the fovea in the deviated eye (Fig. 14–7B). *Hypertropia* (HT) is a vertical strabismus with one eye deviated above or below the other eye. With a hypertropia, the image in the hypertropic eye is above the fovea (Fig. 14–7C). The term hypotropia also can be used to describe vertical strabismus, but by convention the term hypertropia is usually used. A left hypertropia is the same as a right hypotropia. Cyclotropia refers to a torsional misalignment of the eyes. *Incyclotropia* (intorsion) is a rotational deviation where the 12-o'clock position of the eye is rotated nasally. *Excyclotropia* (extorsion) is a temporal rotation of the 12-o'clock position of the eye. Normally the fovea should be aligned between the middle and the lower pole of the optic disc by indirect ophthalmoscopy (Fig. 14–8). If the fovea is below the lower pole of the optic disc (above the disc in the indirect ophthalmoscopic view), this indicates objective extorsion (Fig. 14–9A). The fovea oriented above the middle of the optic disc (below the middle in the indirect ophthalmoscopic view) indicates intorsion (Fig. 14–9A).

Heterophoria

In contrast to a tropia where there is a manifest strabismus, a heterophoria or phoria is a tendency toward ocular misalignment, but motor fusion maintains appropriate eye alignment. The presence of a phoria is a sign that motor fusion is present. A phoria will become manifest and break down into a tropia if fusion is broken. This occurs by occluding one eye or severely blurring

the vision of one eye (Fig. 14–10). A large phoria may break down spontaneously into a tropia when the patient is tired or has taken a central nervous system depressant, as under these conditions motor fusion is compromised. The breakdown of a phoria into a tropia is why some adult patients experience double vision when very fatigued or after taking a sedative or imbibing alcohol. A phoria that is so difficult to fuse that it spontaneously breaks down into a manifest tropia is termed an *intermittent tropia.*

Phorias are described by the same prefixes as tropias but with the suffix phoria: *esophoria* an inturning, *exophoria* an out-turning, and *hyperphoria* a vertical tendency to deviate. Torsional motor fusion is weak to nonexistent; therefore, a tendency to torsional misalignment is manifest as a tropia, and, for practical purposes, torsional phorias do not exists. Torsional misalignment is, however, tolerated surprisingly well. The brain will accept and sensorily fuse up to 5° of torsional misalignment.

Tropia-Phoria (Monofixation Syndrome)

Patients with a tropia of less than 10 prism diopters will often have peripheral fusion and have a phoria coexisting with a small tropia. This is called the *monofixation syndrome* and is associated with peripheral binocular fusion, *gross stereopsis,* central fixation of the preferred eye, and central suppression of the foveal area in the fellow eye (see Chapter 2). Tropias greater than 10 prism diopters preclude fusion as the disparity of the images is too great to allow for even peripheral fusion. Patients with a tropia greater than 10 prism diopters will not have motor fusion and will not have a coexisting phoria (see Chapter 16 for further discussion).

Comitant Versus Incomitant Strabismus

Strabismus can be classified as either comitant or incomitant. *Comitant strabismus* is when the ocular rotations are full, and the deviation is the same in all fields of gaze. Most types of congenital and childhood onset strabismus are comitant. If a strabismus is comitant, this indicates that the ductions are normal, and there is no significant restriction or paresis. *Incomitant strabismus,* however, is a deviation that is significantly different in different fields of gaze. It is almost always associated with abnormal ocular rotations caused by muscle paresis, muscle overaction, or ocular restriction. Causes of muscle *paresis* include third, sixth, or fourth cranial nerve paresis, lost or slipped muscle, or neuralmuscular disease such as myasthenia gravis or chronic progressive external ophthalmoplegia (CPEO). *Restrictive* causes of incomitant strabismus include periocular scarring, orbital fat adherence to the globe or extraocular muscle, orbital floor fracture with entrapment of a rectus mus-

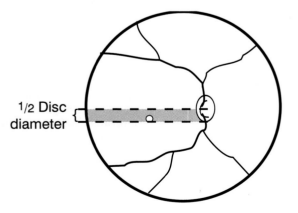

Figure 14–8.
Diagram of the fundus shows the normal fovea disc relationship. The fovea should be located between the center and lower pole of the disc (Direct view).

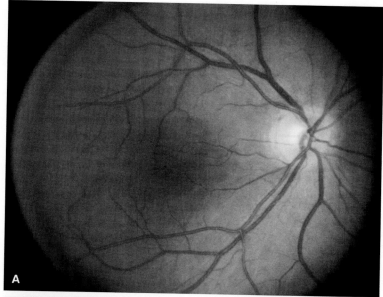

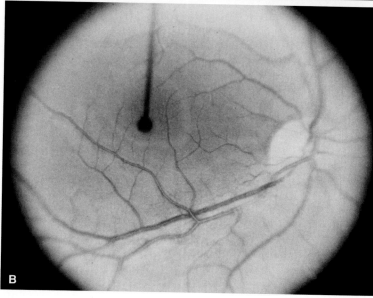

Figure 14–9.
A, Fundus photograph of a patient with an acute fourth nerve palsy and excyclotorsion. Notice that the fovea falls below the lower pole of the optic disc. **B,** Fundus photograph of a patient with superior oblique overaction and intorsion. Notice that the fovea falls above the upper half of the optic disc (Direct view).

cle or orbital fat, a tight contracted muscle, and muscle fibrosis. Clinically, a combination of muscle weakness and restriction often coexist. The antagonist of a paretic muscle will secondarily contract, hence adding a component of restriction.

Tests for Eye Alignment

Eye alignment can be determined objectively without verbal responses from the patient by light reflex testing, red reflex testing, and the cover tests (see Chap. 3). Tests such as the Maddox rod, red cover, Lancaster red/green, and amblyoscope require subjective responses and will be covered in the sensory chapter.

Light reflex testing is based on the first Purkinje image,

which is a vertical image located just behind the pupil; it is not a true corneal reflex. If the light reflexes are centered symmetrically (slightly nasal to the pupil center because of physiologic positive angle Kappa), the eyes are aligned. The two light reflex tests are the Hirschberg and Krimsky tests. The *Hirschberg* test evaluates the location of the light reflex in relation to the pupil without prisms (Fig. 14–11). Each millimeter of deviation off center corresponds to 15PD of misalignment. The Krimsky test is used in strabismic patients to quantitate the amount of deviation with prisms. The *Krimsky* test is performed by progressively adding prisms until the light reflexes are centered in each eye. The amount of prism required to center the reflexes is the size of the deviation. The Krimsky test can be performed

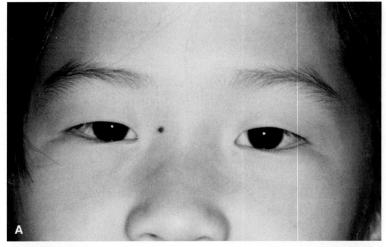

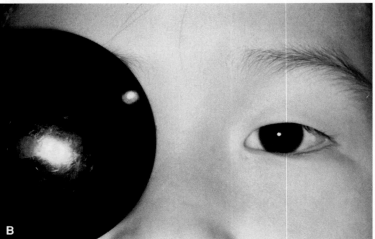

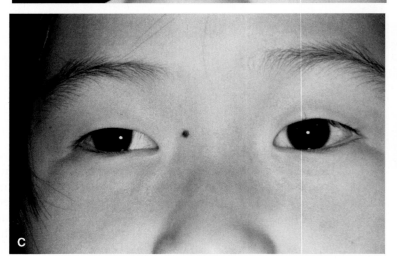

Figure 14–10.
A, Patient with a large exophoria. The eyes are straight during binocular viewing (no tropia), however, there is an underlying tendency for the eyes to drift out (exophoria). This tendency is held intact by binocular motor fusion. **B,** One eye is covered to dissociate the eyes and to break fusion. You cannot see it, but the right eye behind the cover is turned out. **C,** When the cover is removed, one can see that the right eye has drifted out as fusion was disrupted by the cover. Within a few seconds after this photograph was taken, the patient blinked, and regained straight eyes and binocular fusion.

by placing the prism in front of either eye if the deviation is comitant. If there is limitation of ocular rotation (i.e., incomitant deviation), however, measure the primary deviation by placing the prism in front of the eye with limited rotations and the secondary deviation by placing the prism in front of the normal eye.

Red reflex testing can be used to assess eye alignment. This is done by using a direct ophthalmoscope to illuminate each eye to obtain a binocular red reflex (stand approximately 1 meter from the patient). If the simultaneous red reflexes are equal, the eyes are straight. Patients with strabismus will show a brighter reflex from

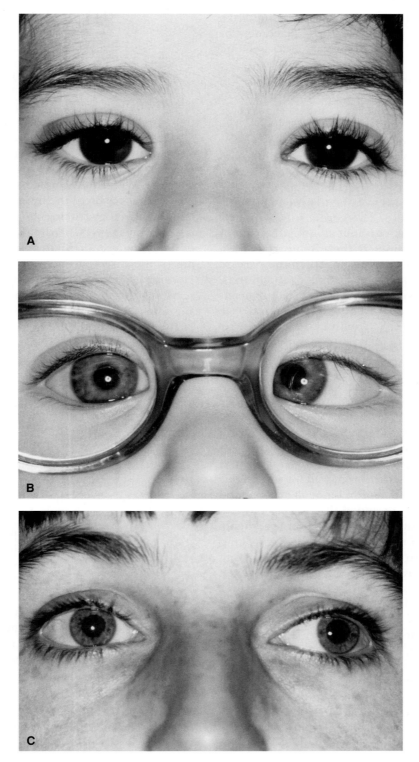

Figure 14–11.
Krimsky light reflex test. **A,** Patient with straight eyes-orthotropia. Notice that the light reflexes are centered. **B,** Esotropia. The light reflex is centered in the fixing eye, and displaced temporally left eye. **C,** Exotropia. The light reflex is centered in the fixing eye, however, it is displaced nasally in the left eye.

the deviated eye. This test is known as the *Brueckner test*. The Brueckner test also identifies large amounts of anisometropia, media opacities (e.g., cataracts), and gross retinal pathology (e.g., posterior retinal detachment or a large retinoblastoma), and is a useful infant screening test.

Cover tests are the most accurate way of identifying and measuring strabismus. There are two basic types of cover tests. The cover/uncover test and alternate cover test. The *alternate cover test* is used to dissociate fusion and measure the full deviation, tropia, plus any underlying phoria. Alternate cover testing does not differentiate a phoria from a tropia, it measures the full dissociated deviation. The test is performed by covering the fixing eye for a few seconds to suspend fusion and force fixation to the fellow eye. The cover is then quickly moved to the opposite eye without allowing the patient to obtain binocular vision. If there is no refixation movement on alternate cover testing, then the eyes are aligned, and there is no phoria or tropia (orthophoria). Refixation movements on alternate cover testing means there is a tropia, a phoria, or both (tropiaphoria) (see monofixation in Chap. 16). If shifting the occluder results in the uncovered eye to move out temporally to refixate, that means that eye was turned in under the cover and identifies an esodeviation. With an exodeviation, the eye is out under the occluder and alternate cover testing produces a nasalward or an inward refixation movement.

The *cover/uncover test* identifies the presence of a tropia. The test is performed by briefly covering one eye while the fellow eye is observed for a refixation shift. If no shift occurs, the occluder is removed for several seconds to allow re-establishment of binocular vision, and the fellow eye is briefly occluded. If covering one eye causes a refixation movement of the fellow eye, then a tropia is present. No shift on cover/uncover testing means the eyes are straight during binocular viewing (orthotropia), but there may be a phoria. The cover test is most useful in conjunction with the alternate cover test in patients with relatively straight eyes. No shift on cover/uncover testing and a shift on alternate cover testing indicates a phoria, no tropia. A small shift on cover/uncover testing, with a larger shift on alternate cover testing means there is a small tropia and a larger phoria (monofixation syndrome). If the shift on cover/uncover testing is the same as the shift on alternate testing, there is a pure tropia with no phoria. Identifying a phoria is important, as the presence of a phoria indicates motor fusion. Remember, if there is a question of a small deviation, always perform a cover/uncover test first to identify a tropia shift. A shift on alternate cover testing only indicates that either a phoria or a tropia is present, but it does not distinguish between these entities.

Prisms to Measure Strabismus

Prisms are used to quantitate the amount of deviation and to optically align the eyes (Fig. 14–12). A prism bends light toward the base of the prism, and the power of a prism is measured in prism diopters. One prism diopter will shift an image 1 cm at a distance of 1 meter, or a displacement that equals approximately 0.5°. If a patient has an exotropia of 30 prism diopters, this equals an angle of approximately 15° (see Chapter 3). One can optically neutralize strabismus by placing a prism in front of the deviated eye, with the apex pointed in the direction of the deviated eye (Fig. 14–12B). With this orientation, the image in the deviated eye moves on to the fovea. The deviation also can be neutralized by placing the prism in front of the fixing eye (Fig. 14–12C). When a prism is placed in front of the fixing eye, the fixing eye has to refixate by moving in the direction of the prism's apex. Because of Hering's, law the fellow eye also moves in the same direction, thus rotating the deviated eye into proper alignment. Notice that when a prism is placed in front of the fixing eye, the retinal image moves toward the base of the prism, but the patient sees an image jump in the direction the prism's apex is pointing. One can neutralize a strabismus by placing the prism over the deviated eye, the fixing eye, or split the prism over both eyes. Remember the prisms are oriented so the apex points in the same direction as the deviation; base out—apex nasal for esotropia, base in—apex temporal for exotropia, and base down—apex up for hypertropia.

To measure the size of a deviation, use the alternate cover test in conjunction with prism neutralization. Place a prism in front of one eye (either eye if the deviation is comitant) oriented appropriately to neutralize the deviation. Then perform alternate cover testing and look for a refixation movement. Change the prism (more or less prism) until there is no refixation movement. The prism that neutralizes the deviation such that there is no shift by alternate cover testing represents the size of the deviation in prism diopters. Strabismus surgery is usually based on the prism-alternate cover test measurement, as surgery is aimed to correct the full deviation, phoria, and tropia.

Simultaneous Prism Cover Test. The *simultaneous prism cover test* is a modification of the cover/uncover test. With this test, a prism is added to the cover/uncover test. Use this test to measure the size of a small tropia in patients with a coexisting phoria (i.e. the monofixation syndrome). The test is performed by covering the fixing eye while a prism is simultaneously placed in front of the deviated eye. If the appropriate prism is placed in front

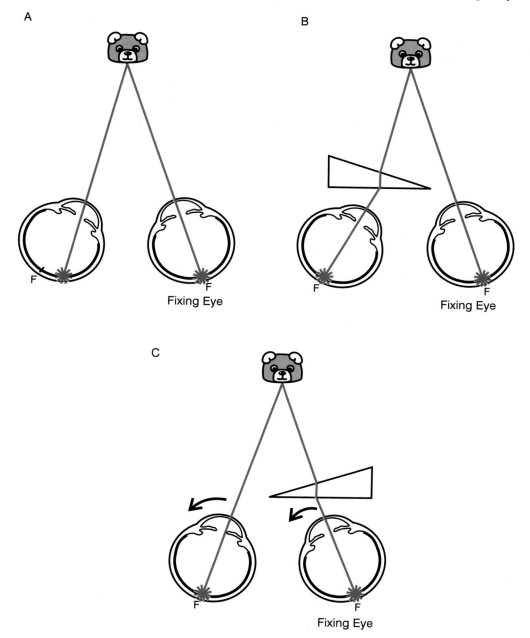

Figure 14–12.
Diagram shows the use of a prism to neutralize esotropia. **A,** A left esotropia patient fixing right eye. Notice that the image falls nasal to the fovea. **B,** A base out prism is placed in front of the deviated eye. Since a prism deflects light toward its base, the retinal image moves temporally onto the fovea, thus neutralizing the deviation. You can see that in Figure 14–12B, the image now falls on each fovea. **C,** Prism is placed in front of the fixing right eye. This initially displaces the retinal image temporally off the fovea. The fixing eye then has to rotate nasally to refixate the image on to the fovea. Because of Hering's law, both eyes move when the fixing eye moves to refixate (right eye nasally and left eye temporally). Temporal movement of the left eye shifts the fovea nasally to align with the target (compare Figure 14–12A with Figure 14–12B). Thus, one can correct or neutralize a deviation by placing the prism in front of either the fixing eye or the deviated eye.

of the deviated eye, there is no refixation shift of the deviated eye. The process of covering the fixing eye and simultaneously placing a prism in front of the deviated eye is repeated until there is no shift from the deviated eye. The prism that neutralizes the tropia shift represents the size of the tropia in prism diopters.

Measurement of Primary Versus Secondary Deviations. Patients with incomitant strabismus and limited ductions will have a smaller deviation when the sound eye is fixing (*primary deviation*) and a larger deviation when the eye with limited ductions fixates (*secondary deviation*) (Fig. 14–13). The secondary deviation is always larger

A. Primary deviation—ET 25$^\Delta$

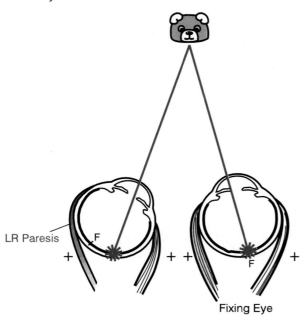

LR Paresis

Fixing Eye

B. Secondary deviation—ET 40$^\Delta$

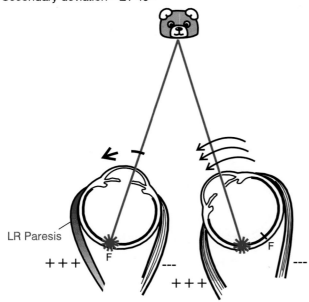

LR Paresis

Figure 14–13.
Diagram shows a patient with a left lateral rectus paresis. The primary deviation is when the patient fixates with the nonparetic eye (A) and the secondary deviation is when the patient fixates with the paretic eye (B). **A,** Primary deviation measures 25 prism diopters (nonparetic eye fixing). Because the nonparetic eye (right eye) can easily come to primary position, little inervational input is necessary, and the deviation is relatively small. **B,** Secondary deviation measures 40 prism diopters. Patient fixates with the left paretic eye. Because the left lateral rectus is paretic, it requires a large amount of innervational input to bring the eye to primary position (dotted arrow). Thus, the left lateral rectus receives +3 innervation. Because of Hering's law, the right medial rectus, its yoke muscle also receives +3 innervation. Because there is no paresis or restriction in the right eye, the right eye over-rotates, producing a large secondary deviation.

than the primary deviation, whether the strabismus is caused by restriction, paresis, or both. This difference between the primary and secondary deviation occurs because when the eye with limited rotations fixates more innervational activity is required to bring the eye to primary position than when the sound eye fixates. Because of Hering's law, when the agonist muscle of the eye with limited movement receives increased innervational activity to fixate in primary position, its yoke muscle on the fellow sound eye receives an equal amount of increased innervation causing a large over-shoot. Because the sound eye moves freely, the increased innervational muscle force causes it to overshoot, resulting in a larger deviation (Fig. 14–13B).

In patients with restriction or paresis, measure the primary deviation by placing the prism over the eye with limited rotations, and measure the secondary deviation by placing the prism over the good eye. Placing the prism over the eye with limited rotations allows this eye to stay in its position of rest, resulting in a relatively small deviation. Placing the prism in front of the eye with normal ocular rotations forces the eye with limited rotations to come to primary position to fixate, thus bringing out the larger secondary deviation.

Angle Kappa. In some patients, the fovea is not located at the center of the posterior pole of the eye. If the fovea is displaced temporally, then the eye must turn out temporally to fixate. This is not eccentric fixation because the patient fixates with the true fovea. This is called a *positive angle kappa*, and the eye will appear turned out and look exotropic, yet there is no shift on cover testing (Fig. 14–14). Retinopathy of prematurity is the most common cause of a positive angle kappa associated with temporal dragging of the macula, followed by a temporal retinal scar secondary to toxocara. Patients with an esotropia and a positive angle kappa may falsely appear to have straight eyes. Most nondiseased eyes have a slight physiologic positive angle kappa usually less than 5%. A *negative angle kappa* occurs when the fovea is displaced nasally so the eye turns in to fixate, giving the appearence of esotropia. This is much less common than a positive angle kappa, and again the cover test shows no shift.

One can clinically access the angle kappa by performing a monocular Hirschberg light reflex test. A positive angle kappa has a nasally decentered reflex, while a negative angle kappa shows a temporally deviated light reflex. Notice that the angle kappa relates to the eye position during monocular viewing and is associated with central foveal fixation (albeit a displaced fovea). In contrast, eccentric fixation represents peripheral, nonfoveal fixation, and is associated with poor vision (see Chapter 15, for a description of eccentric fixation).

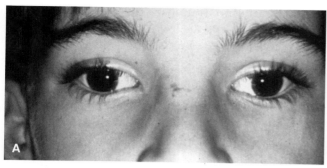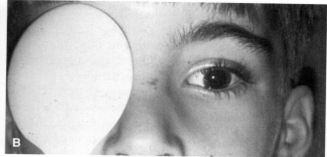

Figure 14–14.
A, Positive angle kappa with both eyes appearing exotropic secondary to temporal dragging of the macula associated with retinopathy of prematurity. **B,** Cover test shows no shift, as the left eye remains in the abducted position even when monocularly fixating with the right eye covered.

Prism-Induced Strabismus. Strabismus can be induced in a subject with straight eyes by placing a prism in front of one eye. To create a certain type of strabismus, orient the prism opposite to how you would neutralize a deviation. A base out prism induces exotropia, a base in prism induces esotropia, and a base up prism over the right eye induces right hypertropia.

Measuring Fusional Vergence Amplitudes. *(also see Chap. 3).* Fusional vergence amplitudes are measured by inducing a deviation (eso, exo, or hyper) and seeing if motorfusional vergence will realign the eyes. A deviation can be induced by placing a variable prism (usually a prism bar or Risley Prism) over one eye. Start with a small prism that can easily be fused and increase the prism until fusion breaks. Before the fusion breakpoint, patients usually will observe blurred vision; this is called the blur point. Record both the blur point and the breakpoint. Measure convergence with a base out prism, divergence with a base in prism, and vertical vergence with a vertically oriented prism. Because our normal vertical vergence amplitudes are small, even small vertical misalignments are difficult to control by motor fusion. A tendency for the eyes to diverge, however, is easier to control because of innate large fusional convergence amplitudes. Table 14–3 shows normal fusion vergence amplitudes.

Thus, from Table 14–3, the maximum base out prism that can be fused is approximately 35 prism diopters (convergence), the maximum base in prism that can be fused is 6 to 10 prism diopters (divergence), and the maximum vertical prism that can be fused is usually 2 to 3 prism diopters (vertical vergence). Prisms

larger than these maximums will break fusion and induce a tropia. In clinical situations where there is a long-standing strabismus with fusion, fusional vergence amplitudes can build to be quite large. Patients with congenital superior oblique palsy, for example, can have vertical fusion vergence amplitudes up to 25 to 30 prism diopters.

Types of Convergence

There are at least five mechanisms that can invoke convergence: (1) fusional convergence, (2) tonic convergence, (3) voluntary convergence, (4) proximal or instrument convergence, and (5) accommodative convergence (5).

Fusional convergence requires binocular vision and is stimulated when an approaching object causes the retinal images to shift temporal to the fovea. Fusional convergence repositions this image shift with a binasal movement (convergence) to keep the images on each fovea to maintain binocular vision. Occluding one eye suspends fusional convergence.

Voluntary convergence is the voluntary act of converging and is associated with accommodation.

Proximal or *instrument convergence* is convergence that is stimulated by the feeling that an object is near. When using a microscope, one may over converge because of the sense that something is close.

Accommodative convergence is a neurologic reflex that is stimulated by a blurred retinal image and links accommodation (focusing) with convergence. As an object approaches from the distance, one must accommodate to keep the image clearly in focus. As accommodation occurs, a reflex convergence also occurs to keep the eyes on the approaching target. The *near reflex* includes accommodation, convergence, and pupillary miosis. This synkinetic reflex of accommodation and convergence is not dependent on binocular vision and occurs when one eye is occluded or in patients who are blind in one eye.

TABLE 14–3
Normal Fusion Vergence Amplitudes

	Distance (6 meters)	Near (⅓ meter)
Convergence	20–25 PD	30–35 PD
Divergence	6–8 PD	8–10 PD
Vertical vergence	2–3 PD	2–3 PD

Accommodative Convergence : Accommodation Ratio (AC/A ratio)

The relationship between the amount of accommodative convergence (in prism diopters) associated with a given amount of accommodation (in diopters) is referred to as the accommodative convergence/accommodation ratio (AC/A ratio). The normal AC/A ratio is between 4 and 6 prism diopters of convergence for every diopter of accommodation. Patients with a high AC/A ratio will overconverge at near, while a low AC/A ratio results in lack of convergence, or relative divergence at near. The normal AC/A ratio is between 4 and 6 PD/D.

Methods for measuring the AC/A ratio include the heterophoria method, clinical distance-near relationship, and the lens gradient method. All of these methods are based on changing the patient's accommodation, then measuring the associated change in convergence. Accommodation is changed by moving the fixation target from distance to near (heterophoria method, clinical distance-near relationship) or by changing the amount of accommodation needed for a specific fixation distance by introducing various amount of plus or minus spherical lenses (lens gradient method).

For AC/A ratio calculations, use 6 meters (20 feet) for distance, and one-third meter (14 inches) for near. Esodeviations are represented as positive numbers and exodeviations as negative numbers. Notice that the number of diopters of accommodation needed to focus at a specific point is the reciprocal of the fixation distance in meters. Focusing at a distance of 6 meters requires 0.166 (1/6) diopters of accommodation, while focusing at near requires 3 (3/1) diopters. For practical purposes, there is insignificant accommodation at 6 meters, so 6 meters is considered optical infinity, and accommodation is considered 0 in the distance.

The clinical distance-near relationship and the lens gradient method are the most clinically useful. The clinical distance-near relationship provides information about the overall change in convergence when one looks from distance to near, including the effects of proximal convergence. The lens gradient method measures the pure AC/A ratio. It is important when measuring the AC/A ratio to use accommodative targets and to have the patient wear their full optical correction.

Heterophoria Method

The heterophoria method uses the difference between the distance and near deviation and the interpupilary distance to determine the AC/A ratio. Notice that the larger the interpupilary distance, the greater the AC/A

ratio. A wide interpupillary distance requires a high AC/A ratio to keep the eyes adequately converged on a near target.

$$AC/A = IPD + \frac{N - D}{DA}$$

IPD = interpupillary distance (cm), D = distance deviation (PD), N = near deviation (PD), and DA = diopters of accommodation for near fixation (1/3 m = 3 diopters).

Example:

Distance = ET 30
Near = ET 42
Interpupillary distance = 50 mm
Diopters of accommodation at near = 3 D

$$AC/A = 5 + \frac{(42 - 30)}{3} = +9$$

high AC/A ratio

Clinical Distance-Near Relationship

The clinical distance-near relationship is a simple comparison of the distance and near deviation. Calculate the clinical distance near relationship by subtracting the distance deviation from the near deviation. If the distance-near difference is within 10 prism diopters, it is considered normal. A near deviation that is 10 prism diopters greater at near than distance is considered high. The clinical distance near relationship is a simple and useful method for identifying a high AC/A ratio.

N − D = Clinical distance near relationship
    D = distance deviation viewing target at 6 meters (20 feet)
    N = near deviation viewing target at 1/3 meter

Example 1: D = ET 15   AC/A relationship 35 − 15 = **20**
            N = ET 35   High AC/A ratio

Example 2: D = XT 15   AC/A relationship 20 − (−15) = **35**
            N = ET 20   High AC/A ratio

Lens Gradient Method

With the lens gradient method, accommodation is changed by having the patient view an accommodative target through supplemental plus or minus spherical lens at a fixed distance. A plus lens relaxes accommodation, and a minus lens increases accommodation. The AC/A ratio is calculated by dividing the difference between measurements with and without a supplemental lens by the power of the supplemental lens. Measurements are usually made with and without a −3.00 supplemental lens in the distance, as distance measurements minimize proximal convergence.

$$AC/A = \frac{\text{Deviation without lens} - \text{Deviation with lens}}{\text{lens in diopters}}$$

Example 1:

Deviation without lens = ET 45

Deviation with +3.00 lens = ET 15 AC/A = $\dfrac{45 - 15}{3} = 10$

Example 2:

Deviation without lens = XT 5

Deviation with −3.00 lens = ET 10 AC/A = $\dfrac{-5 - 10}{-3} = 5$

The lens gradient formula can be used to calculate the effect of a spectacle lens on a strabismic deviation given an estimated AC/A ratio. A −2.00 myope has a normal AC/A ratio of 5 and an exophoria of 10 prism diopters without glasses. What is the effect of giving the myopic correction on the strabismus? The minus 2.00 lens increases accommodation by 2.00 diopters, and since the AC:A ratio is 5 to 1, 10 prism diopters of convergence occurs, which neutralizes the exophoria resulting in orthophoria.

A child with 30 prism diopters esotropia has a +5.00 cycloplegic refraction. Assuming the AC/A ratio is normal (5), what will be the effect of prescribing the full hypermetropic correction? With an AC/A ratio of 5, a +5.00 diopter lens will reduce the esotropia by 25 prism diopters, leaving a small residual esotropia of 5 prism diopters. Thus, prescribing the hypermetropic glasses would have a good chance of correcting the esotropia, with only a small residual deviation.

Smooth Pursuit and Saccadic Eye Movements

Smooth pursuit eye movements are slow movements used to follow objects at velocities up to 30° per seconds. Saccadic eye movements are rapid eye movements used for quick refixation. Rapid eye movements have velocities up to 250° per second. Saccadic eye movements are so fast, there is no time for visual feedback to adjust the amount of movement, and they cannot be controlled voluntarily. This is why they are referred to as ballistic, as it is theorized that the amplitude of a saccadic movement is preprogrammed based on the amount of retinal eccentricity of the target. Vision during a saccadic eye movement is suppressed. This process of eliminating vision during a saccade is termed saccadic omission. The presence of a saccadic eye movement is an important clinical sign, as a saccadic eye movement requires intact muscle function, so the presence of a normal saccadic eye movement indicates good muscle function. When evaluating a patient with limited ductions, the absence of a saccadic eye movement indicates muscle weakness, whereas a good saccadic movement that stops abruptly indicates good muscle function in the presence of an ocular restriction. This abrupt stopping of a fast eye movement is analogous to the restrictive movement of a dog on a leash who runs rapidly, only to be tethered at the end of the leash. A good way to test for saccadic eye movements is to stimulate optokinetic nystagmus (OKN) by using a rotating drum. OKN testing is especially helpful for examining saccades in young children who do not voluntarily follow a rapidly moving target (also see Chap. 9).

Principles of Strabismus Surgery

The goal of strabismus surgery is to correct ocular misalignment by altering the muscle function or muscle mechanics. Indications for strabismus surgery include establishment or enhancement of binocular fusion, elimination of diplopia, correction of a face turn associated with incomitant strabismus or nystagmus, and to improve cosmetic appearance. Strabismus surgery can be divided into three general categories including: (1) recession, (2) resection, and (3) transposition. In addition, a more recently developed treatment is chemodenervation or botulinum injection.

Muscle Recession

The torque or rotational force that is created by an extraocular muscle contraction is proportional to the length of the moment arm (mechanical lever) and the muscle force (muscle strength).

where

$$m \times F = T$$

m = moment arm F = muscle force T = torque

Figure 14–15 is a diagram of the horizontal rectus muscles showing the relationship of the moment arm to the muscle axis and center of rotation. Notice that the moment arm intersects the center of rotation and is perpendicular to the muscle axis. A muscle recession is a procedure that moves the muscle insertion to a new location closer to the muscle's origin, thus creating slack in the muscle. Notice that in Figure 14–15B, the medial rectus muscle insertion has been moved posteriorly 7 mm from its original insertion. This represents a 7 mm recession (maximal recession for MR). Even with this large recession, the moment arm remains unchanged. This is because the rectus muscles have a long arc of contact anterior to the perpendicular of the moment arm. A rectus muscle recession therefore changes the rotational force or torque by producing muscle slack rather than changing the moment arm. Slackening a muscle reduces its muscle strength as per the muscle length tension curve or "Starling's" curve. Figure 14–16 is a generalization of the length tension curve for extraocular muscles. Note that the curve is exponential, and, toward the end of the curve, a small degree of slackening produces a large degree of weakening.

Thus, a standard rectus muscle recession does not

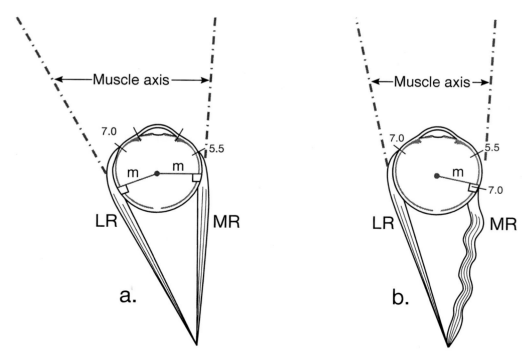

Figure 14–15.
A, Diagram of medial and lateral rectus muscle. Notice that this is the left eye and that the medial rectus muscle has a straight course to the eye and a short arc of contact, whereas the lateral rectus muscle courses temporally to wrap around the globe and it has a longer arc of contact. The moment arm (m) is a line perpendicular to the muscle axis that intersects the center of rotation of the eye. The muscle insertion distance from limbus is 7.0 for lateral rectus muscle (LR), and 5.5 for medial rectus muscle (MR). **B,** A 7-mm recession of the medial rectus muscle (usually considered the maximum recession for the medial rectus) places the muscle near the equator of the eye. Despite this posterior location, the moment arm remains unchanged with the eye in primary position. The muscle, however, is slackened. The major effect of a recession is muscle slackening rather than a reduction in the moment arm.

LENGTH TENSION CURVE

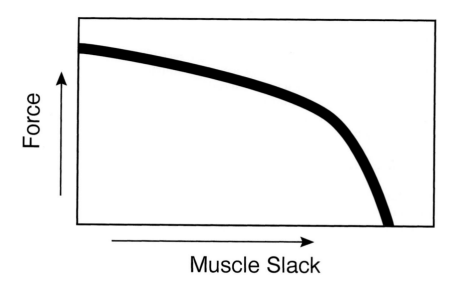

Figure 14–16.
Diagram of the length tension curve with force plotted vertically and muscle slack or tension plotted horizontally. Notice that the more the muscle is slackened, the less force that a muscle can produce. This is an exponential curve with a small amount of slackening causing a large amount of force reduction toward the end of the curv

change the moment arm significantly, but its effect is proportional to the slack created. Clinically, this is important as large recessions deal with the end of the length tension curve. This means that small errors on large recessions will produce large effects. For example, on the medial rectus muscle, each 0.5 mm of recession will give approximately 5 prism diopters of esotropia correction up to a recession of 6 mm (Table 14–4). After 6 mm of recession, each 0.5 mm of recession produces 10 prism diopters of correction. Thus, an over-recession of only 1 mm on bilateral 6-mm recessions would result in a 20 prism diopters of overcorrection!

Rectus muscle recessions have more of an effect in the field of action of the muscle. That is, a right medial rectus recession will produce an exoshift in primary position and more of an exoshift in left gaze, with very little exoshift in right gaze. As the eye rotates toward the recessed medial rectus muscle, the slack that is created by the recession is increased, and the moment arm is shortened slightly. As the eye looks away from the recessed muscle, the muscle is tightened by the rotation, thus lessening the effect. This is why a bilateral medial rectus recession has a greater effect at near. One can use

this induced incomitance of a muscle recession to correct incomitant strabismus. If a patient has a small esotropia in primary position and a large esotropia in left gaze, one would consider a right medial rectus recession. Recession procedures can be performed on rectus or oblique muscles. Recession of the inferior oblique is a popular procedure for weakening the inferior oblique muscle and is described in more detail in Chapter 19, Oblique Dysfunction and A and V Patterns. Recession of the superior oblique provides less consistent results, as moving this broad insertion results in a change of the complex vector forces.

Resection

A muscle resection consists of removing part of the muscle and replacing the shortened muscle at its original insertion site. This procedure tightens the muscle. Rectus resections have a relatively small effect on the length tension curve, as most of the effect relates to creating a tether or leash. This can be verified clinically by assessing the incomitance induced by a rectus resection. A right medial rectus resection limits abduction of the

TABLE 14–4
Strabismus Surgery Numbers

A. BILATERAL SURGERY

Esotropia

Deviation (prism diopters)	MR OU Recession (mm)	LR OU Resection* (mm)
15	3.0	3.5
20	3.5	4.5
25	4.0	5.5
30	4.5	6.0
35	5.0	6.5
40	5.5	7.0
50	6.0	8.0
60	6.5	
70	7.0	

* When lateral rectus resection is performed for residual esotropia after a large medial rectus recession (>6.0 mm,), these resection numbers should be lowered.

Exotropia

Deviation (prism diopters)	LR OU Recession (mm)	MR OU Resection (mm)
15	4.0	3.0
20	5.0	4.0
25	6.0	5.0
30	7.0	5.5
35	7.5	6.0
40	8.0	6.5
50	9.0	

B. UNILATERAL SURGERY

Esotropia

Deviation (prism diopters)	MR Recession (mm)	LR Recection (mm)
15	3.0	3.5
20	3.5	4.5
25	4.0	5.5
30	4.5	6.0
35	5.0	6.5
40	5.5	7.0
50	6.0	7.5
60	6.5	8.0

Exotropia

Deviation (prism diopters)	LR Recession (mm)	MR Resection (mm)
15	4.0	3.0
20	5.0	4.0
25	6.0	5.0
30	7.0	5.5
35	7.5	6.0
40	8.0	6.5
50	9.0	7.0

right eye, thus creating an esotropia shift in right gaze. A right medial rectus resection could correct exotropia in primary position, which increases in right gaze. It should be noted that tightening both medial rectus muscles creates an esoshift, which is greater in the distance than near, because tightening the medial rectus muscles limits the normal distance divergence.

Another technique to tighten a muscle is to perform a *tuck*. This procedure consists of folding the muscle onto itself, thus shortening the muscle. The author described a technique for tucking a rectus muscle, which preserves the anterior ciliary blood flow.[6] The muscle is secured posteriorly and then sutured to the scleral anteriorly. The redundant tucked muscle disappears over time, and reoperating on a tucked muscle shows no residual mass effect on the muscle tuck for tucks of 5.5 mm or less.

Resections can be teamed with recessions in the same eye, and this procedure is called a *recession-resection* or "R and R." A recession-resection procedure produces significant incomitance, which can persist over months and even years. The effect of the procedure is additive as a recession limits ocular rotation toward the recessed muscle and a resection away from the resected muscle. A recession of the right medial rectus muscle and resection of the right lateral rectus produces an exoshift in primary position, which increases in left gaze. The right eye does not adduct as well since the medial rectus is weak and the lateral rectus is tight. For the most part, resections are limited to rectus muscles.

The four rectus muscles provide a constant posterior pull. Rectus muscle recessions tend to weaken this posterior pull, inducing a relative proptosis and secondary lid fissure widening. Rectus resections, however, pull the eye back posteriorly and can cause enophthalmus and lid fissure narrowing. Clinically significant postoperative proptosis or enophthalmus occurs only when multiple muscles of one eye receive the same procedure—either a recession or a resection, very asymmetric surgery is performed, or a large amount of recession or resection is performed on tight muscles such as in Graves disease.

Faden

The faden procedure is a suture that is placed though a rectus muscle to secure the muscle to the sclera posterior to the equator, usually 12 to 14 mm posterior to the muscle insertion. This procedure reduces the moment arm when the eye rotates toward the fadened muscle. It therefore weakens the rotational force when the eye rotates to the operated muscle. It is most useful on the medial rectus muscle as it has the shortest arch of contact, so the faden effect occurs earlier in the rotation. The faden does not have a significant effect in primary posi-

tion and has only a slight effect for correcting incomitance. When used, it is usually performed with a recession of the same muscle.

Transposition

Transposition surgery is based on changing the location of the muscle insertion so the muscle pulls the eye in a different direction (i.e., changes the vector of forces). Transposition surgeries can be used to treat a rectus muscle paresis or a lost muscle. A right lateral rectus palsy would result in limited abduction and an esotropia that increases in right gaze. This can be treated by transposing the part or all of the superior rectus and inferior rectus laterally (see Fig. 20–1). Because the vertical muscles do not fire on attempted abduction, the amount of abduction would relate to the elasticity of the transposed muscles, not to active contraction of the muscles.

Another use of transposition surgery is to correct for a small vertical deviation. One can vertically off set the horizontal rectus muscles in combination with horizontal rectus surgery to correct small vertical deviations. A patient with an esotropia and a small right hypertropia, for example, can be corrected by a recession-resection procedure right eye with infraplacement of the horizontal rectus muscles inferiorly. By transposing the horizontal rectus muscles inferiorly, they act to pull the eye down, thus correcting the hypertropia.

Transpositions also can be used to correct vertical incomitance or A and V patterns (see Chap. 19 Oblique Dysfunction and A and V Patterns, Fig. 19–11).

Chemodenervation (Botulinum Injection)

Eye position can be altered by injecting botulinum toxin into a rectus muscle, as botilinum toxin produces a temporary muscle paralysis. The paralysis stretches the injected muscle and causes a contracture of its antagonists. The stretching of the injected muscle and tightening of its antagonists produces a long-lasting change in eye position. One could correct an esotropia by injecting the medial rectus muscle with botulinum. This would cause a temporary paralysis of the medial rectus muscle, inducing a consecutive exotropia. The exotropia would last for approximately 2 to 3 months, until the medial rectus muscle regains its strength. During that paralytic period, the medial rectus would stretch, and the lateral rectus would contract, thus producing the lasting effect. An injection of botulinum into the ipsilateral medial rectus muscle of patients with a six nerve palsy has been advocated to prevent muscle contraction (3). In general, multiple injections are often required to maintain the alignment, and strabismus surgery remains the treatment of choice for both comitant and paralytic strabismus (1, 2).

■ REFERENCES

1. Biglan AW, et al.: Management of strabismus with botulinum A toxin. Ophthalmology 1989;96:935–943.
2. Ing MR: Botulinum alignment for congenital esotropia. Ophthalmology 1993;100:318–322.
3. Rosenbaum A, Kushner BJ, Kirschen D: Vertical rectus muscle transposition and botulinum toxin (oculinum) to medial rectus for abducens palsy. Arch Ophthamol 1989;107:820.
4. Von Noorden G: Binocular Vision and Ocular Motility. St. Louis: Mosby, 1990.
5. Wright KW: Pediatric Ophthalmology and Strabismus. St. Louis: Mosby, 1995.
6. Wright KW, Lanier AB: Effect of a modified rectus tuck on anterior segment circulation in monkeys. J Pediat Ophthalmol Strab 1991;28.

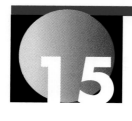

Visual Development and Amblyopia

Kenneth W. Wright

■ VISUAL DEVELOPMENT

At birth, our visual acuity is quite poor, probably in the range of counting fingers, because of the immaturity of visual centers in the brain. Visual acuity rapidly improves during the first 3 to 4 months of life because of dramatic functional and structural development of visual centers such as the lateral geniculate nucleus and the striate cortex (Fig. 15–1). Normal visual development is stimulated by signals generated from clear in-focus retinal images. A blurred or distorted retinal image provides abnormal stimulation and stimulates abnormal neurodevelopment of visual centers in the brain, which results in poor vision or *"amblyopia"*. Visual development is most critical during the first 3 to 4 months of life; this is termed the *critical period of visual development.*. A key developmental milestone is central fixation and accurate smooth pursuit, which should be present by 2 to 3 months of age in most visually normal infants. Visually normal infants may occasionally show delayed visual maturation, however, poor fixation past 6 months of age is usually pathologic and should be fully investigated.

In concert with monocular visual development is the development of binocular vision. Animal studies by Weisel and Hubel (33) and Rakic (20) have shown that binocular cortical connections are present from birth. Although binocular anatomy is present at birth, refinement of these connections is necessary to obtain binocular visual function. Requirements for normal binocular visual development include equal retinal stimulation with clearly formed images and proper eye alignment.

The presence of strabismus or a unilateral blurred retinal image will disrupt normal binocular development.

At birth, eye alignment is variable, with approximately 70% of infants showing a small variable exodeviation, 30% having essentially straight eyes, and <0.5% having a variable esodeviation (26). By 2 months of age, the majority of infants will have established proper alignment, but a small intermittent exodeviation may persist for up to 6 months. The persistence of an esotropia after 2 months of age, however, is in most cases pathologic. Binocular vision begins to develop in early infancy. Human studies have documented binocular interaction at 2 to 3 months of age (3, 16), whereas stereopsis develops later, between 3 and 6 months of age (2, 12).

Smooth Pursuit Asymmetry

Another aspect of binocular visual development is the development of smooth pursuit symmetry. For the first few months of life, healthy infants demonstrate better smooth pursuit for temporal to nasal directed eye movements than nasal to temporal eye movements during monocular viewing (1). This bias for temporal to nasal moving objects and the poor smooth pursuit for nasal to temporal moving objects is termed smooth pursuit asymmetry and is only seen when one eye is covered. Smooth pursuit asymmetry can be detected clinically by using an optokinetic (OKN) stimulus. If OKN asymmetry is present, there will be a diminished response when

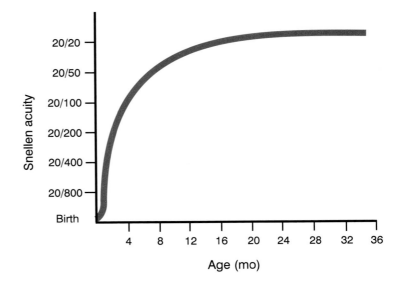

Figure 15–1.
Curve represents visual acuity development with age on the horizontal axis and Snellen acuity on the vertical axis. Note the exponential increase in visual acuity during the first few months of life.

the drum rotates nasal to temporal compared with temporal to nasal rotation. By approximately 5 to 6 months of age, smooth pursuit and OKN responses become symmetrical (17). Disruption of normal binocular development, however, will result in persistent smooth pursuit asymmetry throughout life. Clinical disorders that disrupt early binocular visual development such as congenital esotropia, unilateral cataracts, and anisometropic amblyopia, all have been associated with persistent smooth pursuit asymmetry (9, 28, 32).

■ BINOCULAR VISION AND STEREOPSIS

Normal binocular vision is a process of integrating retinal images from two eyes into a single three-dimensional perception. This process of binocular vision requires binocular fusion, which is the process of merging the images from each eye. Two forms of binocular fusion include sensory fusion and motor fusion. *Sensory fusion* is the cortical integration of the two images, while *motor fusion* represents the corrective movements of the eyes required to maintain eye alignment on a target of regard (see Binocular Fusion, in Chap. 14). To obtain binocular vision, the eyes must be in proper alignment so that the images of the two eyes fall on *corresponding retinal points*: i.e. retinal areas from each eye that are physiologically linked to the same cortical area. By geometric theory, when an observer fixates on a specific point, objects to the side of this point automatically will fall on corresponding retinal points if these objects lie on a circle that crosses through the optical centers of each eye (Fig. 15–2). This circle is termed *Vieth-Mueller's circle.* Physiologic experiments have shown that Vieth-Mueller's circle is not accurate, and that the circle of corresponding points is actually an ellipse, which is termed the empirical horopter. Objects that are in front of or behind the empirical horopter will stimulate noncorresponding retinal points (Fig. 15–2, points A and B). Objects in front of the horopter will stimulate bitemporal retina, and objects distal to the horopter will stimulate binasal retina. The empirical horopter is actually a theoretical line and is infinitely thin. Three-dimensional objects have components that fall in front of and behind the horopter; thus, all three-dimensional objects stimulate noncorresponding retinal points. The brain has the ability, however, to fuse or merge images that fall on slightly noncorresponding retinal points. This finite area off the horopter where fusion is possible is called *Panum's fusional area* (Fig. 15–2). Objects within Panum's fusional area produce single binocular vision with *stereoscopic vision.* The brain's ability to identify that images are falling on slightly noncorresponding points produces the perception of stereoscopic vision. Points that fall outside Panum's fusional area fall on retinal points that are so noncorresponding (too disparate) that they cannot be fused, and this will cause *physiologic diplopia.* In everyday life, we are constantly experiencing physiologic diplopia, however, it is almost always ignored. You can experience physiologic diplopia by fixating on a distance target such as a light-switch at approximately 10 feet, and then place a pencil vertically straight up a few inches in front of your nose. While you are fixating on the light-switch in the distance, notice that the pencil is double. In this example, the light switch represents the central fixation point of the empirical horopter. Since the pencil is in front of the horopter, the pencil stimulates noncorresponding

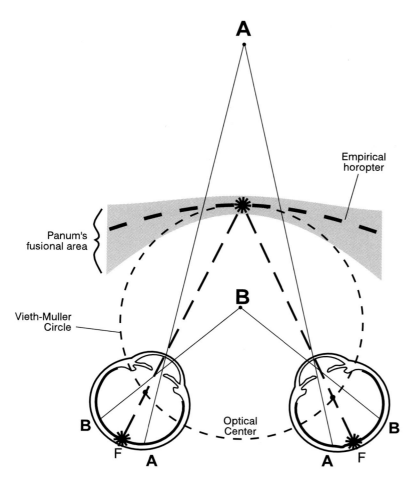

Figure 15–2.
Schematic drawing of Panum's fusional area, empirical horopter, and Vieth-Müller's circle. Panum's fusional area is marked in pink. Objects that lie on the empirical horopter will stimulate corresponding retinal points. Three-dimensional objects that fall within Panum's fusional area stimulate slightly disparate retinal points (noncorresponding), which are fused into a single stereoscopic image. Objects that fall in front of or behind Panum's fusional area will cause physiologic diplopia. Point A represents a point distal to Panum's fusional area that stimulates noncorresponding binasal retinal points, which project to the temporal visual field producing uncrossed diplopia. Point B is proximal to Panum's fusional area and stimulates noncorresponding bitemporal retinal points, which project to the nasal visual field causing crossed diplopia.

bitemporal retinal points (Fig. 15–2, letter B). The temporal retina projects to the contralateral hemifield and causes crossed diplopia. Notice that if you close the left eye, the right pencil disappears. Now fixate on the pencil at near and notice that there will be two light switches in the distance. The horopter is now located at the pencil, and the light switch is distal to the horopter (Fig. 15–2, letter A). Points distal to the horopter produce uncrossed diplopia because they stimulate binasal retina that project to the ipsilateral hemifield. Panum's fusional area is narrow in the center and widens in the periphery. This is consistent with the high resolution small receptive fields of the central macular area, whereas the peripheral retina has larger receptive fields, lower resolution, and are more tolerant of deviations off the horopter.

Bifoveal Fusion

The term bifoveal fusion relates to the normal state of binocular vision consisting of excellent motor fusion and high-grade stereo acuity of 40 to 50 seconds arc. Absence of stereo acuity does not mean there will be a complete absence of depth perception. Patients with monocular vision can perceive depth by way of monocular clues. Motion parallax (patient moves head side side and sees near objects move more than distance objects), object overlap, shadows and the relative size of objects provide monocular clues for depth. Monocular clues are so powerful that patients with monocular vision can do well in most professions, including ophthalmic microsurgery (5).

■ ADAPTATIONS TO ABNORMAL VISUAL STIMULATION

As stated above, normal visual development requires stimulation by equally clear retinal images and proper eye alignment. Normally, around 70% of striate cortex neurons are binocular and respond to visual stimulation of both eyes. The minority of striate cortical cells are monocular responding to only one eye. A unilateral blurred retinal image or strabismus during the period of visual development changes this architecture, decreasing the number of binocular cortical cells and increasing the percentage of monocular cortical cells (6, 7, 15). Animal studies by Crawford and von Noorden (6, 7) have shown that even 2 weeks of strabismus during early visual development will cause irreversible loss of binocular vision. Human studies verify the fragility of binocular visual development, as a unilateral cataract or strabismus during early infancy uniformly results in loss of binocularity unless early and effective treatment is provided (35, 39). In addition to loss of binocularity, loss of visual acuity also may result because of abnormal early visual experience (amblyopia).

Suppression is an adaptive mechanism that eliminates the confusion caused by unequal visual stimulation in children. A unilateral blurred retinal image or an ocular deviation in children under 8 to 9 years of age will provoke suppression to block out information from the eye with the blurred image or the deviated eye. This unconscious inhibition of information from one eye, because it cannot be fused with information from the fellow eye, occurs at the level of the striate cortex and is termed *cortical suppression* (37). Cortical suppression is probably the predominant mechanism that reduces binocular cortical cells resulting in a loss of binocular vision; it is a contributing factor to most types of amblyopia. For a discussion of clinical sensory adaptations, see Chapter 16, Sensory Adaptations and Sensory Examination.

■ AMBLYOPIA

The term amblyopia is derived from Greek and means dull vision (amblys = dull, ops = eye). Poor vision is caused by abnormal development in visual areas of the brain, which is in turn caused by abnormal visual stimulation during early visual development. The pathology associated with amblyopia is not specific to the eye, rather it is located in the visual areas of the brain including the lateral geniculate nucleus and the striate cortex (13, 30). This abnormal development is caused by three mechanisms: (1) blurred retinal image called *pattern distortion*; (2) *cortical suppression*, or (3) both *cortical suppression plus pattern distortion*. Strabismic patients who show strong fixation preference constantly suppress cortical activity from the nonpreferred eye, and strabismic amblyopia develops secondary to cortical suppression. Patients with strabismus who alternate fixation, alternate suppression, and do not have amblyopia. These patients, however, do not develop binocular vision. Monocular pattern distortion (e.g., anisometropia or unilateral cataract) causes amblyopia by two mechanisms: cortical suppression (because of the unequal images) and pattern distortion. Bilateral pattern distortion (bilateral congenital cataracts or bilateral high hypermetropia) will result in bilateral amblyopia. If the images are symmetrically blurred, no suppression occurs, but bilateral pattern distortion causes abnormal neurodevelopment and bilateral amblyopia. Virtually all clinical types of amblyopia can be classified into one of three mechanistic categories: (1) strabismic (pure suppression); (2) monocular pattern distortion (suppression plus pattern distortion), or (3) bilateral pattern distortion (pure pattern distortion) (Table 15–1).

Amblyogenic Period

The severity amblyopia is dependent on several factors, including when the abnormal stimulus began, the length of exposure to abnormal stimulation, and the severity of the image blur. The more severe the image blur, the earlier the onset, and the longer the duration of a malapropos stimulus, the more severe the impact on neurodevelopment and the more severe the impact on visual acuity. Children are most susceptible to amblyopia during the critical period of visual development, which is the first 3 to 4 months of age. Stimulation with a severely blurred retinal image during this time results in dense, often irreversible amblyopia. This is why visually significant congenital cataracts must be operated on and visually rehabilitated within the first few weeks of life. Amblyopia can occur, however, in older children. Acquired strabismus or an acquired media opacity, such as a cataract, can cause amblyopia up to 7 or 8 years of age, albeit of lesser severity.

The earlier the intervention, the better the prognosis for amblyopia. Even so, patients who present late with amblyopia can show significant improvement (11, 29, 34). Even children who present after 8 years of age may benefit from amblyopia therapy (4, 18). Patients who present after the critical period with presumed congenital cataracts also may show significant visual improvement with aggressive amblyopia management (24). Faced with the older child with amblyopia, it is often difficult to decide whether to proceed with amblyopia therapy. In children younger than 10 years of age, it is a good idea to perform a limited patching trial. If, after a 2 to 3 month trial of aggressive amblyopia therapy no improvement occurs, one can document that amblyopia therapy was tried and failed.

Strabismic Amblyopia

Infantile esotropia has the highest incidence of strabismic amblyopia, with amblyopia developing in approximately 50% of patients. Strabismic amblyopia is uncom-

TABLE 15–1
Classification of Amblyopia

A. Strabismis Amblyopia
   (Pure Suppression)
   1. Congenital esotropia (strong fixation preference)
   2. Congenital exotropia (strong fixation preference)
   3. Accommodative esotropia (strong fixation preference)
B. Monocular Pattern Distortion Amblyopia
   (suppression plus pattern distortion)
   1. Anisometropic amblyopia
      a. Hypermetropic
      b. Myopic
      c. Astigmatic (meridional amblyopia)
   2. Media Opacity (Monocular pattern deprivation amblyopia)
      a. Unilateral cataract
      b. Unilateral corneal opacity (eg, Peter's anomaly)
      c. Unilateral vitreous hemorrhage or vitreous opacity
C. Bilateral Pattern Distortion Amblyopia
   (pure pattern distortion)
   1. Ametropic amblyopia
      a. Bilateral high hypermetropia
      b. Astigmatic (meridional amblyopic)
   2. Media opacity (Binocular pattern deprivation amblyopia)
      a. Bilateral congenital cataracts
      b. Bilateral corneal opacities (eg. Peter's anomaly)
      c. Bilateral vitreous hemorrhages

mon in patients with intermittent strabismus such as intermittent exotropia or patients with incomitant strabismus and fusion such as Duane's syndrome or Brown's syndrome.

Monocular Pattern Distortion Amblyopia

Unilateral pattern distortion (i.e., blurred retinal image) in the visually immature produces suppression in addition to pattern distortion, both of which disrupt normal visual development and contribute to amblyopia. Two types include anisometropic amblyopia and unilateral media opacity.

Anisometropic Amblyopia

Anisometropic amblyopia is caused by a difference in refractive errors. Children with anisometropic amblyopia often go undetected because there are no overt signs of the amblyopia such as strabismus. These patients with straight eyes have peripheral fusion and usually develop some stereopsis between 3000 and 70 seconds arc (monofixation syndrome). Even as little as 1 diopter of hypermetropic anisometropia can cause significant amblyopia, and moderate hypermetropia of +3.00 can cause severe amblyopia with visual acuity of approximately 20/200. Myopic anisometropia, how-

ever, must be at least 4.00 to 6.00 diopters difference in order to cause amblyopia. This is because children with myopic anisometropia use the less myopic eye for distance and the more myopic eye for near. Myopic anisometropic amblyopia is usually mild. If an astigmatism is asymmetric (differences of +1.50 or more), this also can result in anisometropic amblyopia.

Unilateral Media Opacity

A monocular media opacity such as a cataract occurring in the amblyogenic period (up to 7 or 8 years of age) can cause amblyopia and loss of binocularity. The earlier the onset, the more severe the amblyopia. Congenital opacities occurring during the critical period can be devastating to visual development and should be treated immediately for best visual results. A visually significant congenital cataract, for example, is a surgical urgency and must be removed in the first few weeks of life to prevent dense irreversible amblyopia. Rehabilitation after 2 to 6 months usually results in extremely poor visual acuity (20/400 or worse).

Bilateral Pattern Distortion Amblyopia

Bilateral symmetrical pattern deprivation is not associated with suppression, and the resulting amblyopia is usually less severe than unilateral pattern deprivation. Conversely, it can be more devastating to the overall visual function of the patient because it is a bilateral process.

Ammetropic Amblyopia (Bilateral Hypermetropic Amblyopia)

High hypermetropia (usually more than +5.00) can result in decreased vision and amblyopia if not treated in early childhood (19). These children are often undetected until school age, because their eyes are well aligned and young children do not usually complain of poor vision. When these children first get their optical correction, visual acuity does not improve dramatically. Improvement occurs slowly over several months to years. Their final visual acuity is usually in the range of 20/30 to 20/25. Bilateral amblyopes do not fully accommodate, so it is important to give the full hypermetropic correction. Even young infants should be given spectacle correction if their refractive error is +5.00 or more.

Meridional Amblyopia

Bilateral symmetrical astigmatisms of +3.00 or more also can result in bilateral amblyopia. Amblyopia secondary to a large astigmatism is called meridional amblyopia. To avoid meridional amblyopia, it is suggested to prescribe astigmatic correction if the astigmatism is +2.00 or more in preschool children, and astigmatisms over +3.00 should be treated in virtually any child, even infants, even if astigmatisms are bilateral.

Bilateral Media Opacity

Bilateral congenital opacities such as Peter's anomaly and congenital cataracts can result in severe bilateral amblyopia with nystagmus, depending on the severity of the induced image blur. Nystagmus associated with bilateral congenital or neonatal blindness is termed sensory nystagmus. Dense bilateral congenital cataracts cause severe amblyopia and sensory nystagmus in more than 80% of patients if not treated by 2 months of age (22). The presence of sensory nystagmus in a patient with bilateral media opacities suggests a poor prognosis and dense amblyopia with visual acuity of 20/200 or worse. Even older patients with sensory nystagmus, however, can show significant visual acuity improvement, with dampening of the nystagmus (in some patients) if the opacity is removed and a clear image is established (34).

Amblyopic Vision

The most distinctive characteristic about amblyopic vision is that visual acuity is poor and there is decreased two point discrimination. Amblyopia is usually defined as a difference of at least two Snellen lines of visual acuity. Amblyopia however can range from missing just a few letters on the 20/20 line to dense amblyopia of hand motion vision. Contrast sensitivity also is affected; however, the most significant loss of visual function is spatial resolution. Another characteristic of amblyopic vision is the *crowding phenomenon*. Patients with amblyopia will have better visual acuity to single optotype presentation than reading a line of multiple optotypes. Another phenomenon associated with amblyopic vision is the visual acuity difference between the two eyes diminishes as the overall luminance of the room diminishes. This phenomenon can be demonstrated by using neutral density filters to create scotopic conditions.

Eccentric fixation is a characteristic of severe amblyopia. Patients with eccentric fixation do not use their fovea but view instead with a perifoveal area. When the sound eye is covered, the amblyopic eye does not look directly at a target, but fixates off center. Monocular fixation is not steady and there is a drifting of fixation. The visual acuity in patients with eccentric fixation is usually 20/200 or worse. Note that eccentric fixation is different than anomalous retinal correspondence (ARC). ARC is a binocular sensory adaptation present only during binocular viewing, and is not an indication of dense amblyopia (see Chapter 16 for a description of ARC). Eccentric fixation is present under monocular or binocular conditions, and is a sign of severe, often irreversible amblyopia.

■ DETECTION OF AMBLYOPIA IN PREVERBAL CHILDREN

Amblyopia can be diagnosed in children who are too young to cooperate with optotype acuity tests such as Allen cards, E game, and Snellen acuity. Clinically the most useful test is fixation testing.

Fixation Testing

Basically there are two types of fixation testing, monocular fixation, and binocular fixation preference. *Monocular fixation testing* assesses whether the patient fixes with the fovea (centrally) and the quality of fixation. Each eye should be occluded in turn, and fixation should be assessed for three separate factors: *quality* and accuracy (good, fair, poor), *location* (central versus eccentric), and *duration* (maintained versus sporadic). Abbreviations often used to describe fixation include GCM for good, central, and maintained; CSM for central, steady, and maintained; and FF for fix and follow. Eccentric fixation is an important sign to note as it indicates severe amblyopia. When testing monocular fixation, the fixation target should be slowly moved through the visual field to assess the quality of fixation. The target and its size should be documented in the chart. It is important to be aware of the normal timetable for visual maturation, although this may vary widely in individuals. The newborn has only sporadic saccadic eye movements with very poor fix and follow; by 6 weeks, most infants will show some smooth pursuit and central fixation, and by 8 weeks the vast majority of infants will have central fixation with accurate smooth pursuit and easily demonstrable optokinetic drum responses. Smooth pursuit is asymmetric until age 6 months, with monocular temporal to nasal pursuit being better than nasal to temporal pursuit (9) (see Chap. 14).

Binocular fixation preference testing detects unilateral amblyopia and compares the vision of one eye with the other. This test is based on the fact that strong fixation preference in patients with strabismus indicates amblyopia or decreased vision in the nonpreferred eye (36, 43). Binocular fixation preference testing is more sensitive than monocular fixation testing, as significant amblyopia can be present (20/100 to 20/200), yet the patient may show normal central monocular fixation. Binocular fixation preference testing, however, will identify even mild amblyopia (two to three lines Snellen acuity difference) (36, 40, 43). Remember to assess monocular fixation before fixation preference testing to rule out the possibility of bilateral symmetric visual loss in preverbal children.

Standard Fixation Preference Testing

This is a reliable method for diagnosing amblyopia in patients with large angle strabismus (36, 43). If a patient with strabismus spontaneously *alternates fixation*, using one eye then the other, this indicates equal fixation preference and no amblyopia (Fig. 15–3). In contrast, *strong fixation preference* for one eye indicates amblyopia. The stronger the fixation preference, the worse the amblyopia. The degree of fixation preference can be estimated by briefly covering the preferred eye to force fixation to the nonpreferred eye. Remove the cover from the preferred eye then observe how well and how long the patient will maintain fixation with the nonpreferred eye before refixating back with the preferred eye (Fig. 15–4). If fixation immediately goes back to the preferred eye after the cover is removed, this indicates strong fixation preference for the preferred eye and amblyopia of the deviated eye. If the patient maintains fixation with the nonpreferred eye through smooth pursuit, through a blink or for at least 5 seconds, this shows the nonpreferred eye holds fixation well, and indicates no significant amblyopia is present (vision within two to three Snellen lines difference). The ability to maintain fixation with the nonpreferred eye while following a moving target is a very reliable indicator of equal vision and no significant amblyopia.

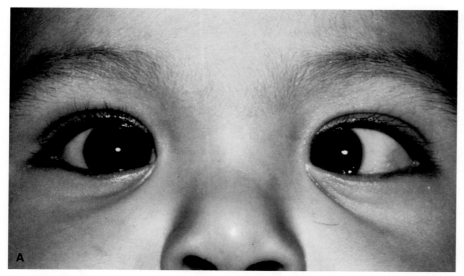

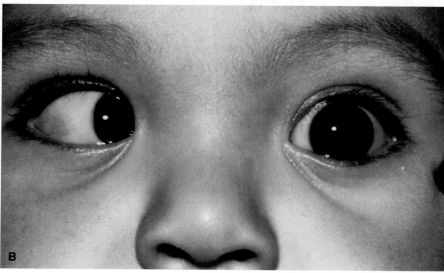

Figure 15–3.
Infant with congenital esotropia and alternating fixation. In Figure A, patient is fixing right eye. In Figure B, patient has switched fixation to the left eye. Alternating fixation indicates equal visual preference, no amblyopia.

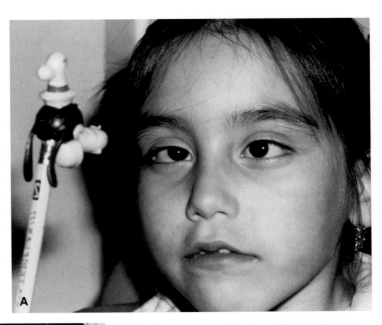

Figure 15–4.
Patient with esotropia and fixation preference for the left eye. In Figure A, patient is fixing left eye. In Figure B, left eye is covered forcing fixation to the nonpreferred right eye. The cover is then removed to see if patient will hold fixation with the right eye under binocular viewing conditions. In C, the cover has been removed, and patient maintains fixation with the right eye under binocular viewing conditions. Because the patient is able to hold fixation well with the right eye (through smooth pursuit or through a blink), this indicates no amblyopia even though there is a preference for the left eye.

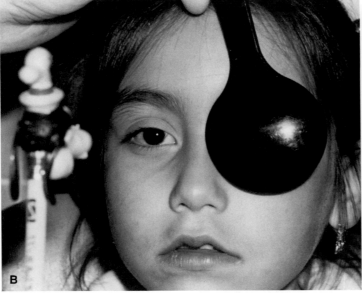

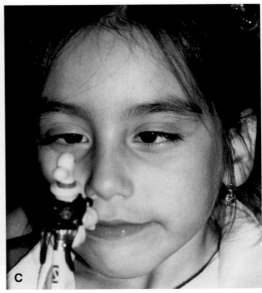

Vertical Prism Test (Induced Tropia Test)

Standard fixation testing is not useful in children with small angle strabismus (less than 10 prism diopters) and in patients with straight eyes. Patients with deviations less than 10 prism diopters often have the monofixation syndrome (see Chap. 16). These patients show strong fixation preference even though the vision may be equal. Thus many nonamblyopic patients with small angle strabismus will falsely appear to have amblyopia by standard fixation preference testing. Additionally, standard fixation preference testing cannot be performed on patients with straight eyes because one does not know which eye is fixing. The vertical prism test, or 10 diopter prism test developed by Wright and coworkers, allows fixation preference testing to accurately diagnose amblyopia in patients with straight eyes or small angle strabismus (36,40).

The vertical prism test is performed by placing a 10 to 15 prism diopter prism base up or base down in front of one eye, thereby inducing a vertical strabismus. If the eye behind the prism is fixating, then both eyes will move up as the fixing eye views through the prism. If the eye without the prism fixes then the eyes view straight ahead in primary position (Fig. 15–5). Thus, with the induced vertical strabismus, it is possi-

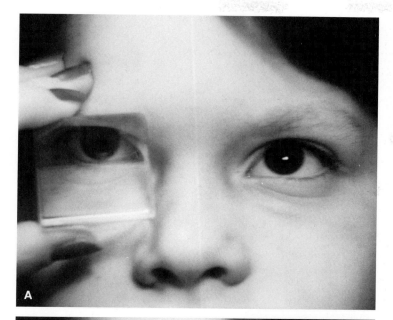

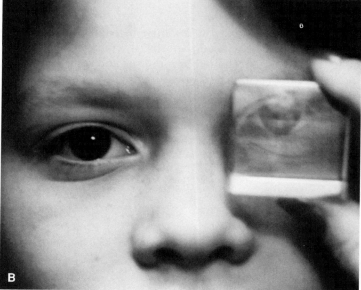

Figure 15–5.
Patient with straight eyes being tested with the vertical prism test using a base down prism. One can determine which eye is fixing by observing the eye position. If the patient views through the eye with the prism, both eyes move up. Fixation with the eye without the prism causes no refixation movement and the eyes remain straight ahead in primary position. **A,** A base down prism is placed in front of the right eye. Can you tell which eye is fixing? The right eye is fixing through the prism because both eyes are in upgaze. **B,** The base down prism is placed in front of the left eye. Again, which eye is fixing? The right eye is fixing, because the eyes are in primary position looking straight ahead. The vertical prism test induces a vertical deviation, and allows assessment of fixation preference. This patient showed strong fixation preference for the right eye.

ble to determine which eye is fixing in patients with straight eyes or small angle tropias. Patients with equal vision will be able to hold fixation with either eye, but patients with amblyopia show strong preference for the dominant eye. If the monofixation syndrome is present, the vertical prism will dissociate the eyes, which eliminates their facultative suppression scotoma and breaks peripheral fusion, allowing correct assessment of amblyopia by fixation testing. This eliminates the overdiagnosis of amblyopia associated with standard fixation testing in patients with small angle strabismus. The vertical prism test is useful in clinical conditions such as anisometropic amblyopia, unilateral ptosis, postoperative congenital esotropia, microstra-

bismus, and other conditions that are associated with unilateral amblyopia.

Special Tests

Teller acuity cards and the pattern visual-evoked potential are useful for estimating visual acuity in situations that require verification of results by fixation testing (10, 27). Teller acuity cards are gray rectangular cards with stripes (technically termed gratings) on one end (Fig. 15–6). Infants and children inherently prefer to look at formed images; so if the infant has the ability to see the stripes, the infant will demonstrate an eye movement toward the stripes. The infant is presented a card with the

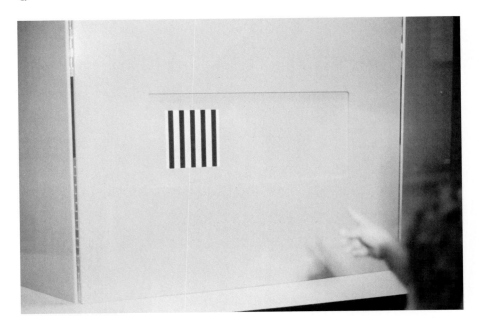

Figure 15–6.
Photograph of Teller acuity card presented behind a gray screen. Note the vertical black and white grid pattern. The patient is pointing to the grid.

stripes oriented either on the left or right side. The examiner is behind the card and observers the infants eye movements through a peep hole in the center of the card. Varying widths of stripes are used to determine the thinnest stripes that provoke the appropriate eye movements. One problem with stripes or grating acuity tests is their tendency to underestimate the severity of amblyopia.

The *pattern visual-evoked potential* (PVEP) measures brain wave activity in response to pattern stimulation. Luminance balanced patterns (usually black and white checks) are presented by monitors and scalp electrodes over the occipital area measure potential changes in the brain. The patterns reverse and the occipital brain activity is recorded and analyzed by computer. The pattern stimulus can be changed to measure a variety of acuity levels; however this test only gives a visual acuity estimate (24, 25, 42).

■ TREATMENT OF AMBLYOPIA

Critical to the treatment of amblyopia is early detection and early intervention. The strategy for treating amblyopia is to (1) provide a clear retinal image and (2) correct ocular dominance if present.

Clear Retinal Image

The first step to treating amblyopia is to make sure that there is a clear retinal image. Correct significant refractive errors and remove visually significant opacities within the visual axis. Remember that amblyopic eyes do not fully accommodate, and it is important to prescribe full hypermetropic correction. In patients with anisometropic amblyopia and peripheral fusion, it is often possible to fully correct the amblyopia just by providing the appropriate optical correction. Patients with strabismic amblyopia may or may not require optical correction but virtually all require occlusion therapy to correct ocular dominance.

Correct Ocular Dominance
Occlusion Therapy

Occluding or patching the sound eye interrupts suppression and forces the amblyopic eye to fixate. In patients with peripheral fusion, full-time occlusion may break down the peripheral fusion and induce strabismus. Consider part occlusion in patients with fusion to allow some binocular visual fusion. If part-time occlusion therapy fails, then full-time patching therapy may be necessary. In children who have large-angle manifest strabismus or in children with no fusion because of dense amblyopia, full-time occlusion therapy can be used. The follow-up interval for full-time occlusion is 1 week per the child's age in years. A 3-year-old child receiving full-time occlusion should be seen back at least every 3 weeks to check the vision in the good eye. Overpatching the good eye in young children can result in reverse amblyopia (i.e. decreased vision of previously good eye), although this is rare in children older than 3 years of age. In infants, reverse amblyopia can be severe, and, for this reason, it is often suggested that children younger than 1 year of age receive part-time occlusion.

Penalization Therapy

Penalization therapy is based on blurring the vision in the sound eye to force fixation to the amblyopic eye. Penalization therapy is effective only when fixation switches to the amblyopic eye. Atropine penalization in patients with significant hypermetropia (usually more than +3.00) of the sound eye is an excellent way to treat amblyopia (21). Atropine penalization consists of placing atropine 0.5% or 1% in the sound eye each day and removing optical correction from the sound eye. An in-office test to predict if penalization will work consists of using cyclopentolate to cycloplege the good eye, then remove the optical correction from the good eye and give the amblyopic eye full optical correction. Under these conditions, if fixation switches to the amblyopic eye, then penalization will improve vision. If the patient continues to fixate with the sound eye for distance and near, then it is unlikely that penalization will work (38). Atropine penalization in young children and infants can cause reverse amblyopia and vision should be carefully monitored (31, 38).

Bilateral Light Occlusion

Bilateral light occlusion or bilateral patching can prolong the critical period of visual development. Dark-rearing studies in animals have shown that prolonged dark-rearing causes very little adverse effect and can significantly prolong visual central nervous system plasticity (8). In humans, bilateral light occlusion for up to 2.5 weeks has no significant detrimental effect on visual development (14, 41).

Other Methods

Pleoptics is a method of treating dense amblyopia with eccentric fixation. It is based on flashing an extremely bright ring of light around the fovea of the amblyopic eye to temporarily "blind" the eccentric fixation area forcing fixation to the fovea. This method has not been shown to be more effective than occlusion therapy, and for the most part it has been abandoned. Another method for treating amblyopia is active foveal stimulation. *CAM* treatment consists of the patient viewing a rotating spiral of high contrast pattern. The CAM stimulator also has been abandoned by most clinicians.

■ REFERENCES

1. Atkinson J: Development of optokinetic nystagmus in the human infant and monkey infant: an analogue to development in kittens. In: Freeman RD (ed): Developmental Neurobiology of Vision. New York: Plenum Press, 1979.
2. Birch EE, Gwiazda J, Held R: Stereoacuity development of crossed and uncrossed disparities in human infants. Vision Res 1982;22:507.
3. Braddick O, et al.: Cortical binocularity in infants. Nature 1980;288:363–365.
4. Brown MH, Edelman PM: Conventional occlusion in the older amblyope. Am Orthop J 1976;26:54–56.
5. Burden: The Stigma of Strabismus, Arch Ophthal 1994;112:302.
6. Crawford MLJ, von Noorden GK: Optically induced concomitant strabismus in monkeys. Invest Ophthalmol Vis Sci 1980;19:1105.
7. Crawford MLJ, von Noorden GK: The effects of short-term experimental strabismus on the visual system in macaca mulatta. Invest Ophthalmol Vis Sci 1979;18:496–505.
8. Cynader M: Prolonged sensitivity to monocular deprivation in dark-reared cats: effects of age and visual exposure. Dev Brain Res 1983;8:155–164.
9. Demer JL, von Noorden GK: Optokinetic asymmetry in esotropia. J Pediatr Ophthalmol Strabismus 1988;25:286.
10. Dobson V, Teller DA: Visual acuity in human infants: a review and comparison of behavioral and electrophysiological studies. Vision Res 1978;18:1469.
11. Ellis FD, Schlaegel TF: Unexpected visual recovery: organic amblyopia? Am Orthoptic J 1991;31:7.
12. Fox R, Aslin RN, Shea SL, Dumais ST: Stereopsis in human infants. Science 1980;207:323.
13. Hendrickson AE, Movshon JA, Eggers HM, Gizzi MS, Boothe RG, Kiorpes L: Effects of early unilateral blur on the macaque's visual system, II: anatomical observations. J Neurosci 1987;7:1327–1339.
14. Hoyt CS: The long-term visual effects of short-term binocular occlusion of at-risk neonates. Arch Ophthalmol 1980;98:1970.
15. Ikeda H, Tremain K: Amblyopia and cortical binocularity. Transactions Ophthalmological Society U.K., 1980. Vol 100, pg 452.
16. Leguire LE, Rogers GL, Bremer DL: Visual-evoked response binocular summation in normal and strabismic infants. Invest Ophthalmol Vis Sci 1991;32:126–133.
17. Naegele JR, Held R: The postnatal development of monocular optokinetic nystagmus in infants. Vis Res 1982;22:341.
18. Oliver M, et al: Compliance and results of treatment for

amblyopia in children more than 8 years old. Am J Ophthalmol 1986;102:340–345.

19. Raab E: Refractive amblyopia. Intl Ophthalmol Clin 1971; 11:155.

20. Rakic P: Prenatal genesis of connections subserving ocular dominance in rhesus monkey. Nature 1976;261:467.

21. Repka MX, Ray JM: The efficacy of optical and pharmacological penalization. Ophthalmology 1993;100: 769–775.

22. Rogers GL, Tishler CL, Tsou BH, Hertle RW, Fellows RR: Visual acuities in infants with congenital cataracts operated on prior to 6 months of age. Arch Ophthalmol 1981:99:999.

23. Romano PE, Noorden GK von: Atypical responses to the four-diopter prism test. Am J Ophthalmol 1969;67:935.

24. Sokol S, Hansen VC, Moskowitz A, Greenfield P, Towle VL: Evoked potential and preferential looking estimates of visual acuity in pediatric patients. Ophthalmology 1983;90:552.

25. Sokol S: Visually evoked potentials: theory, techniques and clinical applications. Surv Ophthalmol 1976;21:18.

26. Sondhi N, Archer SM, Helveston EM: Development of normal ocular alignment. J Ped Ophthalmol Strab 1988;25:210–211.

27. Teller DY, Morse R, Borton R, Regan D: Visual acuity for vertical and diagonal gratings in human infants. Vision Res 1974;14:1433.

28. Tychen L, Lisberger SG: Maldevelopment of visual motion procession in humans who had strabismus with onset in infancy. J Neurosci 1986;6:2495–2508.

29. Vereecken EP, Brabant P: Prognosis for vision in amblyopia after the loss of the good eye. Arch Ophthalmol 1984;102:220.

30. von Noorden GK, Crawford MLJ, Levacy RA: The lateral geniculate nucleus in human anisometropic amblyopia. Invest Ophthalmol Vis Sci 1983;24:788–790.

31. von Noorden GK: Amblyopia caused by unilateral atropinization. Ophthalmology 1981;88:131–133.

32. Westall Carol A, Woodhouse JM, Brown VA: OKN asymmetries and binocular function in amblyopia. Ophthal Physiol Opt 1989;9:269–276.

33. Wiesel TN, Hubel DH: Ordered arrangement of orientation columns in monkeys lacking visual experience. J Comp Neuro 158:307,1974.

34. Wright KW, Christensen LE, Noguchi BA: Results of late surgery for presumed congenital cataracts. Am J Ophthalmol 1992;114:409–415.

35. Wright KW, Edelman PM, McVey JH, Terry A, Lin M: High grade stereo acuity after early surgery for congenital esotropia. Arch Ophthalmol 1994;112:913–919.

36. Wright KW, Edelman PM, Walonker F, Yiu S: Reliability of fixation preference testing in diagnosing amblyopia. Arch Ophthalmol 1986;104:549.

37. Wright KW, Fox BES, Erikson KJ: PVEP evidence of true suppression in adult onset strabismus. J Pediatric Ophthal Strab 1990;27:196–201.

38. Wright KW, Guyton DL: A test for predicting the effectiveness of penalization on amblyopia. In: Henkind P, ed. Acta: XXIV International Congress of Ophthalmology. Philadelphia: JB Lippincott, 1983;896–901.

39. Wright KW, Matsumoto E, Edelman PM: Binocular fusion and stereopsis associated with early surgery for monocular congenital cataracts. Arch Ophthalmol 1992;110: 1607–1609.

40. Wright KW, Walonker F, Edelman P: 10-diopter fixation test for amblyopia. Arch Ophthalmol 1981;99: 1242–1246.

41. Wright KW, Wehrle MJ, Urrea PT: Bilateral total occlusion during the critical period of visual development. Arch Ophthalmol 1987;105:321.

42. Wright KW, Eriksen J, Shors TJ: Detection of amblyopia with P-VEP during chloral hydrate sedation. J Pediatr Ophthalmol Strabismus 1987;24:170–175.

43. Zipf RF: Binocular fixation pattern. Arch Ophthalmol 1976;94:401–405.

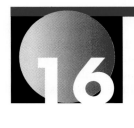

16 Sensory Adaptations and Sensory Examination

Kenneth W. Wright

■ SENSORY ADAPTATIONS TO STRABISMUS

Proper eye alignment and clear retinal images during infancy stimulate the development of *bifoveal fusion,* with motor fusion and high grade stereoscopic vision. As discussed in Chapter 15, a blurred image or strabismus interferes with binocular vision and provokes suppression. A variety of sensory adaptations can occur in response to abnormal visual stimuli and suppression. The specific type of sensory adaptation that develops depends on when the sensory insult occurs and its severity (3). Below are specific clinical sensory adaptations divided into two broad categories based on the onset of the abnormal stimulus. This classification is probably an over simplification as there may be congenital abnormalities of central fusion that contribute to the sensory status, but it aids in understanding this often complicated field.

1. Visually mature (after 7–10 years of age)
2. Visually immature (early childhood, before 7 years of age)

■ SENSORY ADAPTATIONS OF THE VISUALLY MATURE

Generally speaking, the visual system is mature by 9 to 10 years of age. Beyond this age, there is insufficient cortical plasticity to invoke cortical suppression. There are, however, some exceptions to this rule, which are stated below under Prolonged Plasticity.

Diplopia

In visually mature patients (older than 7 to 10 years of age), acquired strabismus causes diplopia (double vision). Diplopia occurs when an image falls on the fovea of the fixing eye and an eccentric retinal point of the deviated eye. The red filter test can be useful for examining patients with diplopia. The red filter test consists of placing a red filter in front of one eye and having the patient view a fixation target or a fixation light (Fig. 16–1). In a patient with acquired esotropia, one image falls on the fovea of the fixing eye, while the image in the deviated eye falls nasal to the fovea. Because nasal retina projects to the temporal hemifield, the patient sees the diplopic image on the same side as the deviated eye. This is called *uncrossed diplopia,* that is, with the red filter over the right eye, the red light is seen to the right of the white light (Fig. 16–2). Patients with acquired exotropia will have *crossed diplopia* as the retinal image in the exo-deviated eye falls on the temporal retina, which projects to the nasal hemifield, contralateral to the deviated eye (Fig. 16–3). With exotropia, the red light is seen on the opposite side of the red filter. If the red filter is over the right eye, the red light will be to the left of the white

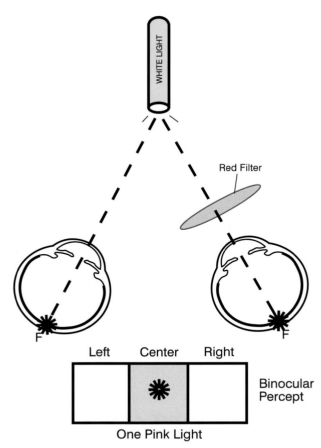

Figure 16–1.
Diagram of the red filter test being performed on a normal patient with orthotropia and normal retinal correspondence. The red filter is over the right eye, and patient sees one pink light.

umented that patients with acquired strabismus and tunnel vision from unilateral glaucoma often experience confusion. This is because the peripheral field of the deviated eye is eliminated and the patient is forced to use the fovea of both eyes.

Rivalry

Rivalry is a phenomenon of normal binocular vision that prevents the simultaneous perception of different images on corresponding retinal points. More simply put, rivalry prevents confusion. If a series of parallel lines are presented to each eye with the lines in one eye rotated 90° to the fellow eye, the observer will perceive that the lines disappear where they cross, causing a

light. A trick used to remember this is, the S in esotropia means the same side for uncrossed diplopia, and the X in exotropia stands for a cross for crossed diplopia. In patients with vertical strabismus, the image in the hyperdeviated eye falls above the fovea and projects to the inferior field so the hypertropic eye sees the image below.

Visual Confusion

Some patients with acquired strabismus will fixate with both foveas even though there is a manifest deviation. These patients will spontaneously perceive two different images that are superimposed. For example, a patient with exotropia, with one eye fixing on a lampshade and the fellow eye fixing on a window, will perceive the lampshade superimposed on the window. Confusion is very rare, as patients with acquired strabismus almost always experience diplopia, because they suppress foveal information from the deviated eye. The author has doc-

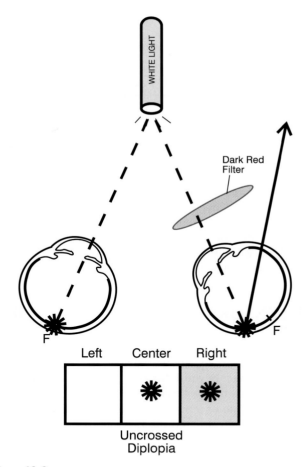

Figure 16–2.
Red filter test performed on a patient with esotropia and uncrossed diplopia. Note that the image in the right eye is falling on nasal retina which projects to the temporal visual field. The patient sees a white light from the fovea of the left eye in the center of the visual field and a red light from the right eye is on the right side or on the same side as the red filter (i.e., uncrossed diplopia).

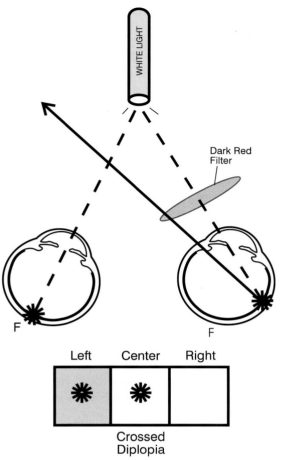

Figure 16–3.
Red filter test on a patient with exotropia and crossed diplopia. With exotropia, the image in the deviated eye falls on temporal retina, which projects to the opposite visual field. The white light is seen in the center of the visual field from the fixing left eye and sees the red light from the right exotropic eye to the left or on the opposite side of the red filter (i.e., crossed diplopia).

patchy drop out of some of the lines. You can experience rivalry by placing a pencil vertically oriented in front of one eye and a horizontally oriented pencil in front of the fellow eye. Put the pencils approximately 2 inches in front of each eye. Note that there is a patchy drop out of one of the images where the two pencils overlap. The term retinal rivalry is a misnomer as it probably involves inhibition or suppression of visual processing in the occipital cortex.

Prolonged Plasticity

Classically, visual plasticity is believed to end by 7 to 10 years of age. This would mean that older patients with acquired strabismus could not develop suppression. Occasionally, however, adult patients with acquired strabismus learn to ignore or suppress diplopia. Some have called this ignoring, which is a voluntary process. Visual-evoked potential studies have shown that adult patients can eliminate diplopia through cortical suppression (4). Another clinical example of prolonged visual plasticity relates to adult patients with amblyopia who lose vision in their good eye. Even though these patients are well beyond the usual period of visual plasticity, significant visual acuity improvement can occur in the amblyopic eye.

■ SENSORY ADAPTATIONS OF THE VISUALLY IMMATURE

Strabismus that occurs during the first few years of life, and specifically before 8 to 10 years of age, disrupts normal binocular development, causing specific functional adaptations of binocular vision. The type of sensory adaptation is dependent on when the strabismus occurred, the size of the strabismus, and whether the strabismus was intermittent or constant. Once a binocular adaptation is established in childhood, it usually persists throughout adult life.

Monofixation Syndrome

Marshall Parks (1) described the monofixation syndrome. This is an adaptation to a small angle strabismus (less than 10 prism diopters) or a moderately blurred unilateral retinal image that occurs in infancy or early childhood. The patient adapts to the small angle strabismus or unilateral image blur by suppressing the central visual field (i.e., central suppression scotoma) of the

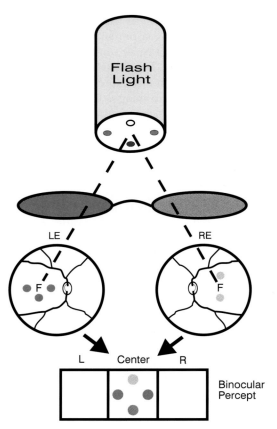

Figure 16–4.
Worth four dot on a normal patient with orthotropia. The subject is fusing so the white light, which is seen through both filters, combines resulting in a total of four lights seen two red and two green. One of the red lights is often seen as being slightly lighter than the other red light and it may flicker to green. This is the white light which appears red to one eye and green to the other eye but is fused.

nonpreferred eye but maintains binocular fusion in peripheral fields and fixes centrally with the preferred eye. Central suppression is dependent on fixation with the preferred eye, as occluding the preferred eye eliminates suppression of the deviated eye. The suppression is localized to the central visual field, because the central retina is organized with high spatial resolution and small receptive fields, so even small differences in image clarity or retinal image position will be recognized. The peripheral fields, however, have relatively low spatial resolution and large receptive fields. Small differences in image clarity and small image displacements are not appreciated by the peripheral retina, so the peripheral images are sensorily fused. The size of the suppression scotoma is proportional to the amount of image disparity (i.e., size of the deviation) in strabismic patients, and the amount of image blur in patients with anisometropia. If the suppression scotoma is larger than 10 prism diopters, peripheral fusion will be disrupted, and monofixation syndrome will not occur. Patients with

more than 10 prism diopters of strabismus or severe unilateral image blur will not develop peripheral fusion or allow the monofixation syndrome.

Characteristics of the monofixation syndrome include motor fusion with fusional vergence amplitudes, and a central suppression scotoma measuring up to 5° (10 prism diopters). The *Worth four dot test* is an excellent way to diagnose the monofixation syndrome. The test is performed by having the patient wear red/green glasses, by convention placing the red filter over the right eye and the green filter over the left eye. A flashlight with four illuminated dots (two green, one red and one white) is presented to the patient (Fig. 16–4). The eye with the red filter sees two red lights; the red light and the white light which appears red through the red filter. The eye with the green filter sees three green lights; two green lights and one white light which appears green through the green filter. The white light is the only light that is seen by both eyes. The normal response to the Worth four dot test is to see four dots, two red and two green. The white light that is seen by both eyes appears as single light, usually red but it may flicker to slightly green. The Worth four dot test stimulates peripheral retina when used at near, and central retina when the flash light is placed in the distance (Table 16–1). Patients with the monofixation syndrome fuse the near Worth four dot (subtending 6°) as the dots fall outside the central suppression scotoma. The distance Worth four dot (6 meter box) subtends 1.25°, so the dots of the distance Worth four dot fall within the monofixation suppression scotoma, and only the dots from the preferred eye are seen (either two red or three green). This response is pathognomonic for the monofixation syndrome (Fig. 16–5).

Most patients with monofixation syndrome show some stereo acuity in the range of 3000 to 70 seconds arc and motorfusion with near normal vergence amplitude. Despite the presence of stereopsis, many patients also have amblyopia ranging from one or two Snellen lines difference, to severe amblyopia, up to 20/200 visual acuity. Typically, the monofixation syndrome is associated with a small angle tropia seen on simultaneous prism cover test and a larger phoria seen on alternate cover testing. Thus, a good way to identify a monofixation syndrome in young children unable to cooperate

TABLE 16–1
Worth-Four-Dot Flashlight

Distance from Patient	Angle
⅙ meter	12 °
⅓ meter (14 inches)	6° (Standard Worth-four-dot)
½ meter	4 °
1 meter	2 °

A. Near Worth Four Dot (Esotropia 8△)

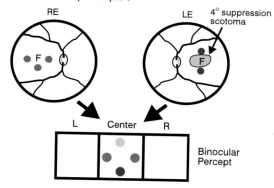

B. Distance Worth Four Dot (Esotropia 8△)

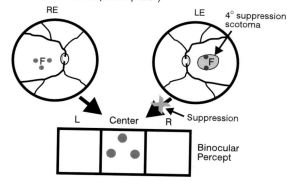

C. Distance Worth Four Dot - Preferred Eye Covered

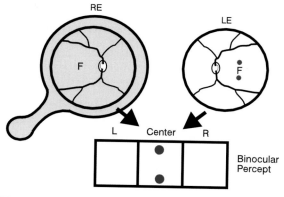

Figure 16–5.
Diagram showing the monofixation syndrome examined with the Worth four dot test. Patient has a small angle esotropia of 8 prism diopters and a suppression scotoma left eye of 8 prism diopters (4°). **A,** Near Worth four dot subtends 6° (12 prism diopters), so the dots fall outside the central suppression scotoma. The patient has peripheral fusion and reports the normal fusion response and sees four dots. **B,** The distance Worth four dot subtends 1.25° and therefore falls within the central suppression scotoma. Since the red dots falling within the suppression scotoma left eye are not perceived, patient reports seeing three green dots from the right eye, and none of the dots from the left eye. **C,** The distance Worth four dot test performed with the preferred eye (RE) covered. By covering the preferred eye, the suppression scotoma disappears. With the right eye covered, the patient now sees the two red lights from the left eye.

with sensory testing is to identify a tropia less than 8 to 10 prism diopters in the presence of a larger phoria. Causes of the monofixation syndrome include anisometropic amblyopia, unilateral partial cataract, and small angle strabismus.

Anomalous Retinal Correspondence (ARC)

Normally, both foveas are physiologically linked through lateral geniculate-occipital cortical connections, and the foveas are the centers of reference for the eye. This is called normal retinal correspondence. *Anomalous retinal correspondence (ARC)* is a sensory adaptation to strabismus. To avoid diplopia, the immature visual system reorganizes to accept an eccentric retinal point of the deviated eye as the center of reference. This anomalous center of reference is called the *pseudofovea* (Fig. 16–6). Note that the ARC adaptation is only pre-

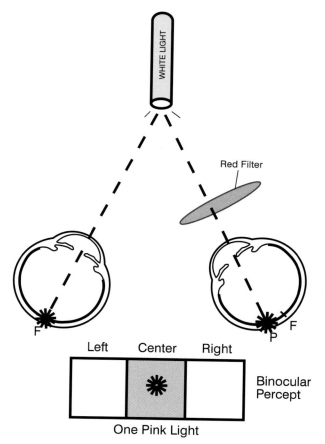

Figure 16–6.
Diagram of the red filter test in a patient with esotropia and anomalous retinal correspondence (ARC). Patient fixing left eye and the right eye is esotropic. The red filter in front of the deviated eye produces a red retinal image which falls nasal to the true fovea but directly on the pseudofovea. Because during binocular viewing, patients with ARC use their pseudofovea as the center of reference, this patient sees one pink light, no diplopia. If the dominant eye was to be covered, the pseudofovea would disappear and the patient would fixate with the true fovea.

sent under binocular viewing conditions, as occluding the fixing eye results in refixation of the deviated eye to the true fovea and elimination of the pseudofovea.

Figure 16–6 shows the red filter test on a patient with ARC and a right esotropia. The right retinal image is nasal to the true fovea, but the patient does not see double as the image falls on the pseudofovea. Neutralizing the esotropia with a base out prism in front of the right eye moves the image onto the true fovea (Fig. 16–7). The patient, however, experiences crossed diplopia as the image is now temporal to the pseudofovea, and temporal retina projects to the contralateral hemifield. This type of diplopia is termed *paradoxical diplopia*. Remember, that under binocular viewing, patients with ARC perceive the pseudofovea to be the central reference point of the retina, not the true fovea.

Even though patients with ARC are able to superimpose images via the pseudofovea, true motor fusion does not occur. Patients with ARC do not have fusional vergence amplitudes and do not have stereopsis. ARC is seen in patients with early childhood onset strabismus and deviations greater than 15 prism diopters. ARC is clinically important because adult patients with strabismus and ARC may have paradoxical diplopia after corrective strabismus surgery. All adult patients should be checked for ARC by neutralizing the deviation preoperatively with prisms to see if the patient has double vision. If double vision occurs, then there is a risk of persistent postoperative diplopia. The majority of patients with ARC and postoperative diplopia will be able to ignore or suppress the double vision; however, patients should be warned that in rare instances diplopia may persist.

Large Regional Suppression

Large regional suppression occurs in patients with large angle strabismus or severe unilateral retinal image blur. Patients with congenital esotropia or intermittent exotropia often show large regional suppression. These patients may alternate suppression or show strong fixation preference. Patients with intermittent strabismus may switch their adaptation between bifoveal fusion and large regional suppression. This occurs in patients with intermittent strabismus, such as patients with intermittent exotropia or patients with congenital incomitant

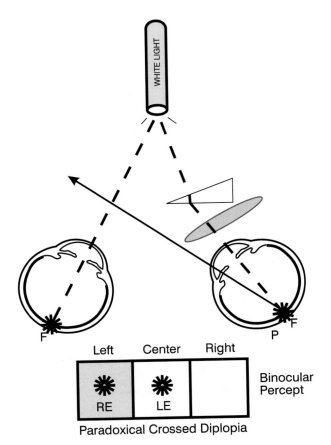

Figure 16–7.
Red filter test on an esotropic patient with ARC. A base out prism is placed in front of the deviated eye to neutralize the esotropia. Note that the retinal image now falls on the true fovea but temporal to the pseudofovea. Since temporal retina projects to the opposite field the patient experiences crossed diplopia even though the image in the deviated eye is placed on the true fovea. Remember, the pseudofovea is the center of reference during binocular viewing in patients with ARC, and a retinal image that is displaced off the pseudofovea is perceived to be off center.

strabismus such as Duane's syndrome, congenital superior oblique paresis, or Brown's syndrome. Interestingly, these patients show excellent bifoveal fusion with good stereopsis when their eyes are aligned, yet during the tropia phase they show large regional suppression. During the large regional suppression phase, there is no stereopsis and no motor fusion.

■ SENSORY TESTING

Sensory tests are useful for identifying normal binocular vision and sensory adaptations to abnormal stimuli. Sensory tests can be divided into two broad categories: (1) diplopia tests and (2) haploscopic tests.

Diplopia Tests

Diplopia tests are based on stimulating both eyes by a single fixation target and placing a colored filter over

TABLE 16–2
Diplopia Tests

1. Maddox rod	Most dissociating
3. Worth four dot test (room lights off)	
2. Red filter test	
3. Worth four dot test (room lights on)	
4. Bagolini lenses	Least dissociating

one or both eyes. The color filter distinctly tints the retinal images so the examiner can tell which image corresponds to which eye. If the eyes are in alignment, the target will fall on each fovea, and the patient will see a single target. Patients with strabismus will see two targets unless they suppress (Fig. 16–1). Table 16–2 lists diplopia tests according to their ability to dissociate fusion. Tinted filters in front of the eyes can disrupt fusion and thus some diplopia tests are dissociating. Diplopia tests produce uncrossed diplopia with esotropia, crossed diplopia with exotropia and an inferiorly displaced image from the hypertropic eye, in patients with normal retinal coresponder.

Maddox Rod Test

This test can be used for identifying horizontal, vertical, and especially torsional deviations. The single Maddox rod is totally dissociating as there are no common targets seen by both eyes (no binocular fusion clues). The Maddox rod is made up of multiple cylindrical high plus lenses stacked on top of each other, giving it a washboard appearance (also see Chap. 3 and Fig. 3–50). When the patient views a light through the Maddox rod a linear streak of light is seen which is oriented 90° to the cylindrical ribs of the Maddox rod.

Single Maddox Rod for Horizontal and Vertical Deviations

The single Maddox rod test is performed by placing the Maddox rod over one eye, nothing over the fellow eye as the patient views a point light source (penlight or muscle light). If the patient sees the streak of light passing through the penlight, the patient is orthophoric. If the streak of light is displaced isilateral to the Maddox rod (uncrossed diplopia), this indicates either an esophoria or an esotropia is present. A streak that is displaced to the opposite side to the Maddox rod (crossed diplopia) indicates either an exophoria or an exotropia. Because the Maddox rod presents different images to each eye the test is completely dissociating (breaks up fusion). A phoria therefore will become a tropia when tested with the Maddox rod. Thus, the Maddox rod test, and other dissociating tests for that matter, do not distinguish between phorias and tropias. To make the distinction between a phoria and a tropia, assess the eye alignment objectively (cover uncover test) before administering the dissociating diplopia test.

Double Maddox Rod for Torsional Deviations

The double Maddox rod determines subjective torsion. The patient is asked to align the two streaks of light so they are parallel. In orthophoric patients, the streaks will overlap so that only one line is seen. In these patients a prism can be used to induce a deviation and separate the lines. Patients without torsion will see parallel lines and will not adjust the lenses. Those with intorsion rotate the 12-o'clock position nasally, and those with extorsion rotate the lens temporally (Fig. 16–8). The double Maddox rod test measures subjective torsion and does not localize which eye is torted. To find the total

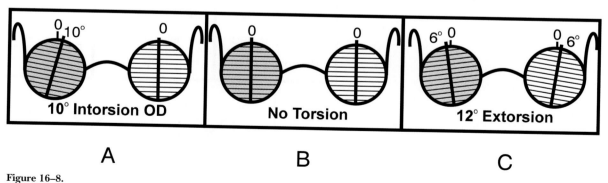

Figure 16–8.
Double Maddox rod with the red lens on the right eye and the clear lens on the left eye. **A** shows 10° of intorsion right eye, **B** shows no torsion, and **C** shows 12° of intorsion. Note that torsion is additive as seen in **C** with 6° of right intorsion and 6° left intorsion.

torsion between the two eyes with the double Maddox rod, sum the monocular torsion of each eye. Note that a patient with intorsion views the world as being extorted, and likewise extorsion causes objects to be perceived as being intorted.

Red Filter Test

This test is described above under diplopia. The red filter test is one of the simplest sensory tests and is performed by placing a red filter over one eye while having the patient observe a fixation target or fixation light (Fig. 16–1). If the eyes are aligned so the image of the object of regard falls on both foveas the patient will see one pink light. Esotropia produces uncrossed diplopia (Fig. 16–2), and exotropia produces crossed diplopia (Fig. 16–3).

Worth Four Dot

This test is described above under monofixation syndrome. During testing, leave the ambient lights on so that the patient also can see peripheral objects, thus preserving peripheral fusion. If the lights are turned off, the only object seen by both eyes would be the white dot, which provides a relatively weak binocular fusion stimulus. Thus, Worth four dot with lights out is a very dissociating test (Table 16–2). Patients with normal fusion will report seeing four lights, two red and two green (Fig. 16–4). By moving the flashlight away from the pa-

tients, the dots subtend a smaller visual angle and stimulate a smaller area of central retina (Fig. 16–5). Table 16–1 lists the stimulus angle for the Worth four dot flashlight at various distances from the patient. The standard near Worth four dot flashlight at one third of a meter subtends an angle of 6° while the standard distance Worth four dot box (not the flashlight) at 20 feet subtends 1.25°.

Bagolini Striated Lenses

With this test, the patient wears clear glasses that have linear scratches that create a streak of light when the patient fixates on a single light source. These striations are oriented obliquely, one eye at 45° and the fellow eye at 135°. Patients with normal binocular vision will see an intact cross. Since the lenses are clear glass, this test almost provides normal view and is the least dissociating of the diplopia tests. Patients with large areas of suppression will see only one line, while central suppression associated with monofixation results in a cross with the center of one line missing. Figure 16–9 shows responses to various sensory adaptations. Note that patients with ARC see an intact cross.

Haploscopic Fovea to Fovea Tests

With haploscopic fovea to fovea tests, there are two movable fixation targets, one for each eye. These targets can be moved separately to be placed in alignment with

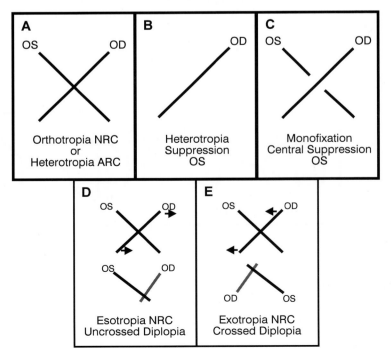

Bagolini Lens

Figure 16–9.
Diagram showing responses to Bagolini lens testing for various sensory adaptations. Bagolini lenses are an excellent way to test for sensory adaptations as they provide almost normal free view and they are the least dissociating of the sensory tests.

each fovea. Haploscopic fovea-to-fovea tests include the Lancaster red/green test, the amblyoscope, and the after-image test. The after-image test does not use a haploscopic device, but each eye is stimulated separately, marking each fovea separately.

Lancaster Red/Green Test

This test is useful for measuring deviations in various fields of gaze in adult patients with acquired strabismus and diplopia. Figure 16–10 shows the Lancaster red/green test in a patient with an exotropia and small left hypotropia. A red lens is in front of the right eye and the green lens is in front of the left eye. The examiner holds a red light projector and the patient holds a green light projector. These projectors project a streak of colored light on a grid screen. The examiner places the red light in the center of the screen and asks the patient to place the green light on top of the red light. The patient directs the green light to the left and slightly down to align the green light with the fovea of the left eye. In contrast to diplopia tests where crossed eyes (esotropia) give uncrossed diplopia, with the Lancaster red/green test the direction of the light separation is in the same direction as the eye separation. In Figure 16–10 there is a left exotropia and a small left hypotropia, and note that the darker streak is to the left (ipsilateral) and below the red streak. If the patient is orthophoric, the patient will align the light directly on top of the examiner's light so that the two lights will be superimposed. The examiner s streak controls the location of the fixing eye, so when the examiner holds the red light, the right eye (behind the red filter) is the fixing eye and if the examiner holds the green light then the left eye (behind the green filter) becomes the fixing eye. By changing the light the

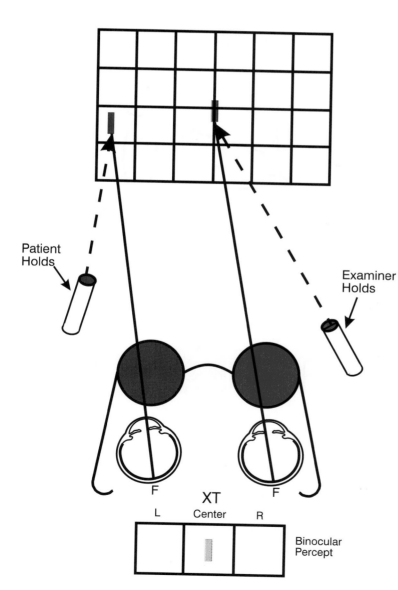

Figure 16–10.
Diagram of Lancaster red green test. The examiner holds the red projection light, which projects a streak onto the screen grid. Patient holds the green light (seen as black in this diagram). Red green glasses with the red filter over the right eye and green filter over the left eye are placed on the patient. The examiner's red projected streak controls the position of the eye behind the red filter (right eye). The patient who is holding the green light is told to place the green streak on top of the red streak. By doing this, the patient lines up each streak with each fovea. The examiner can change the position of the eye behind the red filter by moving the red streak and in this diagram the right eye is the fixing eye. Lancaster red green test is used on adult patients with diplopia and NRC (normal retinal correspondence).

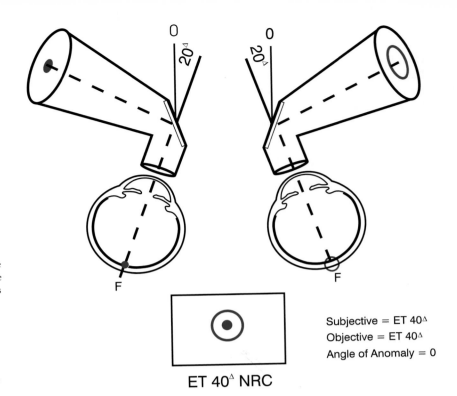

Figure 16–11.
Diagram of the amblyoscope in a patient with an esotropia of 40 prism diopters and NRC. The arms of the amblyoscope are angled until the patient sees the red dot inside the red ring. This requires 20 prism diopters of angulation each eye to place each target on the fovea of each eye. The subjective angle is the angle of amblyoscope arms after the patient sees the red dot centered within the red ring (40 prism diopters). The objective angle is the angle measured by alternate cover testing by alternately occluding the arms of the amblyoscope (40 prism diopters). The angle of anomaly is the difference between the objective and subjective angle (0). With NRC the objective angle equals the subjective angle.

ET 40$^\Delta$ NRC

Subjective = ET 40$^\Delta$
Objective = ET 40$^\Delta$
Angle of Anomaly = 0

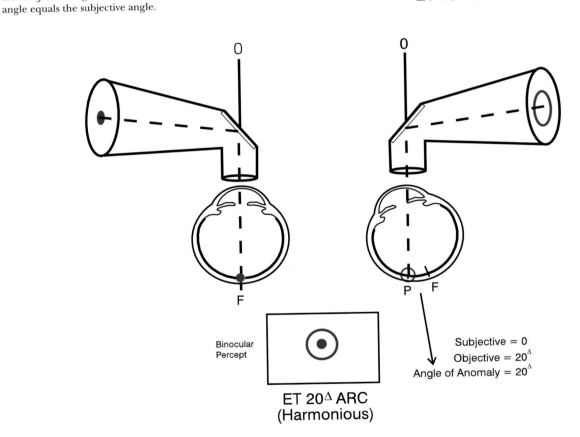

Binocular Percept

ET 20$^\Delta$ ARC
(Harmonious)

Subjective = 0
Objective = 20$^\Delta$
Angle of Anomaly = 20$^\Delta$

Figure 16–12.
Diagram of the amblyoscope examining a patient with a 20 prism diopters esotropia and ARC. The patient directs the examiner to keep the arms of the amblyoscope parallel as this aligns the targets with the true fovea of the left eye and the pseudofovea of the right eye. The subjective angle is therefore 0 as the arms of the amblyoscope are parallel. The objective angle (actual amount of deviation reference to the true foveas) is 20°. The objective angle is measured by alternate cover testing because during monocular viewing the true fovea is used. The angle of anomaly is the difference between the subjective and objective angles. In this case, the angle of anomaly is 20 prism diopters, which equals the objective angle. If the angle of anomaly equals the objective deviation, then the location of the pseudofovea matches the deviation, and this is termed harmonious ARC.

examiner holds, the primary and secondary deviation can be measured.

Amblyoscope

The amblyoscope consists of two arms, one for each eye (Fig. 16–11). The arms of the amblyoscope can be moved to measure either the subjective or objective angle. The subjective angle is measured by moving the amblyoscope until the two pictures in each arm are superimposed. The objective angle is measured by alternating target presentation from right eye to left eye, then moving the arms until there is no shift. This is analogous to alternate cover testing. In patients with normal retinal correspondence, the subjective angle will equal the objective angle because patients with normal retinal correspondence use their true foveas under monocular or binocular conditions. Patients with anomalous retinal correspondence, however, will show a small or no subjective angle and a larger objective angle (Fig. 16–12). The angle of anomaly is the difference between the subjective and objective angle, and this represents the displacement of the pseudofovea from the fovea. In Figure 16–12, the subjective angle is 0 because the location of the pseudofovea matches the angle of deviation (objective angle). Thus, the objective angle is equal to the angle of anomaly (i.e., 20 prism diopters). This is called *harmonious ARC.* If the location of the pseudofovea does not correct for the angle of deviation, then the angle of anomaly does not equal the objective angle, and the subjective angle is not 0. This is called *unharmonious ARC.*

After Image Test

This test consists of a linear strobe light that bleaches the central retina under monocular conditions with the patient fixating at the center of the strobe light. The middle of the strobe light is masked to spare the fovea. The strobe light produces an after image line which tags the location of each fovea, a horizontal line to one eye and a vertical line to the fellow eye (Fig. 16–13). After the foveas are tagged both eyes are opened to allow binocular viewing. Patients with normal retinal correspondence (NRC) will perceive a cross to the after image test, whether the eyes are aligned or if there is strabismus. This is because tagging is performed under monocular conditions each fovea is marked even if strabismus is present. With NRC, the foveas are the center of reference; so the patient sees both after images aligned as a cross. Patients with anomalous retinal correspondence (ARC), however, will see the after images separated, and they do not see a cross (Fig. 16–14). In ARC, fixation reverts to the true fovea during monocular viewing. Since the after image is stimulated under monocular conditions, it tags the fovea of patients with

ARC. After the after image is established, binocular vision is allowed. Now, under binocular viewing, patients with ARC use the pseudofovea as their center of reference. The true foveas are tagged however; so the after image on the true fovea is perceived as being eccentric to the pseudofovea.

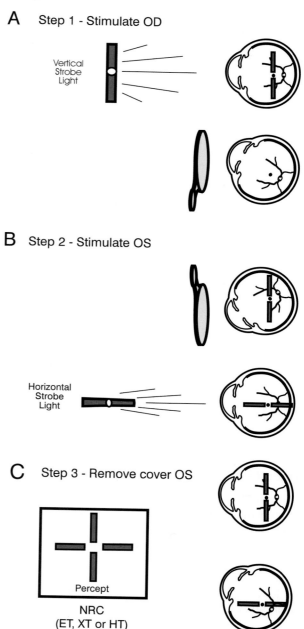

Figure 16–13.
Diagram demonstrating the after-image test. **A,** The vertical strobe light is flashed on the right eye while the left is flashed to desaturate the right eye while the left eye is covered. **B,** The right eye is covered and the left eye is stimulated with a horizontally oriented strobe light. **C,** The occluders are removed and the patient describes the location of the after-images. If the patient has NRC, they will see a cross whether or not they have strabismus. This is because each fovea was tagged during monocular conditions, and in NRC the fovea is the center of reference.

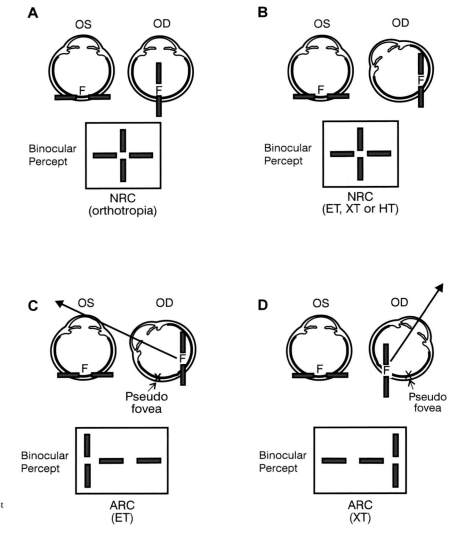

Figure 16–14.
Diagram showing results of the after image test in patient with various sensory adaptations.

Other Tests

Other tests for suppression include the vectographic test and the four prism diopter base out test. The *vectographic test* uses polarized glasses and a polarized projector to stimulate each eye individually. Some letters are seen by both eyes and some are seen only by one eye, right or left. Patients who suppress one eye will only see the letters projected to the fixing eye and will not see the letters of the suppressed eye, so some letters will be skipped. The *four base out test* is performed by introducing a four prism diopter base out prism in front of one eye and observing for a convergence eye movement. If there is no convergence, then the patient is suppressing that eye. A convergence eye movement indicates fusion. A version eye movement in the direction of the apex of the prism indicates lack of fusion and suppression of the contralateral eye. Unfortunately, there are many atypical responses associated with the four base out test (2).

◼ REFERENCES

1. Parks MM: The monofixational syndrome. Trans Am Ophthalmol Soc 1969;67:609–657.
2. Romano PE, Noorden GK von: Atypical responses to the four-diopter prism test. Am J Ophthalmol 1969;67: 935.
3. Wright KW: Pediatric ophthalmology and strabismus. St. Louis, Mosby, 1995:119–138.
4. Wright KW, Fox BS, Erikson KJ: PVEP Evidence of true suppression in adult onset strabismus. J Pediatric Ophthal Strab 1990;27:196–201.

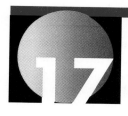

17 Esodeviations

Kenneth W. Wright

In contrast to exodeviations, which are typically intermittent and associated with high-grade stereopsis, esodeviations usually present as a constant tropia, often with amblyopia, and often poor potential for binocular fusion and stereopsis. These differences may relate, at least in part, to differences between our innate convergence and divergence fusional amplitudes. Strong innate fusional convergence provides control of exodeviations, thus allowing development of binocular fusion and stereopsis (intermittent exotropia for example). Conversely, fusional divergence amplitudes are weak, so esodeviations are poorly controlled. This leads to a constant tropia at an early age, constant suppression, loss of binocular fusion potential, and amblyopia in patients with strong fixation preference. Not all esotropic patients have such a poor prognosis. Patients with late onset acquired esotropia may have intermittent esotropia and large fusional divergence amplitudes; these patients have an excellent prognosis for binocular fusion. Esodeviations can be classified into several categories, as outlined in Table 17–1.

■ INFANTILE ESOTROPIA (CONGENITAL ESOTROPIA)

Infantile or, as it is often termed, congenital esotropia, is classically defined as an esotropia which is present before 6 months of age. The esotropia may present at birth; however, in many cases the esotropia is acquired during the first 6 months of life. Small transient exodeviations are common in normal neonates, but esodeviations in newborns are rare (2). A constant esotropia that is present after 2 months is probably pathologic and usually does not resolve spontaneously.

No consistent inheritance pattern for infantile esotropia has been established, but it is clear that it tends to run in families. Some pedigrees appear to be autosomal-recessive, others dominant, and in many cases there is no family history of strabismus. The variability of inheritance patterns suggests heterogeneity for the phenotype of infantile esotropia. Thus, it is not surprising that the pathogenesis of infantile esotropia is probably multifactorial. In some cases, hypermetropia and accommodative convergence play a major role (see infantile accommodative esotropia below), while in others the cause of the infantile esotropia is unclear. Various etiologies have been suggested, including increased accommodative convergence, primary motor abnormality, and genetic cortical fusion deficit (7, 26). This author prefers a motor etiology over a primary fusion deficit as high grade stereopsis has been achieved after very early surgical alignment. The sixth and fourth cranial nerves are the longest nerves, and myelinization occurs from the brain stem distally towards the muscles. Perhaps a delay in the functional maturation of the sixth nerve relative to the third nerve produces a mild bilateral lateral rectus muscle paresis, which results in an infantile esotropia. In some cases, infantile esotropia is associated with developmental delay, cerebral palsy, or other diseases such as Down's syndrome. Perhaps in these cases, there are other factors that contribute to the esotropia. Suffice it to say that the cause of infantile esotropia remains unknown.

TABLE 17-1
Esotropia

1. Infantile esotropia (common)
2. Accommodative esotropia (common)
3. Acquired non-accommodative esotropia (uncommon)
4. Nystagmus Compensation Syndromes (uncommon)
5. Cyclic esotropia (rare)
6. Esophoria (common)
7. Divergence insufficiency (rare)
8. Sensory esotropia (common)

Clinical Manifestations

Infantile esotropia is characterized by large-angle constant esotropia usually presenting in the first few weeks to 6 months of life (Fig. 17–1). There may be a history that the angle of deviation increased during the first few months of life, with the deviation usually measuring between 40 to 70 prism diopters at the time of presentation. Patients may alternate fixation or show strong fixation preference for one eye which indicates amblyopia. Amblyopia occurs in approximately 50% of children with infantile esotropia (12). There is often some limitation of abduction to voluntary version testing, however doll's head maneuver and abduction saccades reveals normal lateral rectus function. Patients with infantile esotropia often have mild to moderate hypermetropia in the range of +2.00 to +3.00. If the angle of deviation is relatively small (less 40 prism diopters), or variable in size, prescribe the full hypermetropic correction. Consider the possibility of infantile accommodative esotropia if the hypermetropia is +3.00 or more in these patients.

Associated motor anomalies frequently associated with infantile esotropia include inferior oblique overaction in approximately 70% of cases, dissociated vertical deviation (DVD) in 75% of cases, and latent nystagmus in approximately 50% of cases. Dissociated vertical deviation, latent nystagmus, and inferior oblique overaction usually are seen at age 1 or 2 years, often several months to years after the esotropia has been corrected.

Another motor anomaly associated with infantile esotropia is monocular OKN asymmetry (see Chapter 15). Under monocular conditions, there is a bias for objects moving in a temporal to nasal direction. This results in a poor OKN response for the drom rotating in a nasal to temporal direction versus a temperal to nasal direction (22). OKN asymmetry is normally seen in all infants younger than 4 months of age but should become symmetrical by 6 months. OKN asymmetry persists throughout life in patients who have early disruption of binocular visual development. This includes patients with monocular congenital cataracts, severe anisometropic amblyopia, and infantile esotropia (1, 3, 22, 25). For more on smooth pursuit asymmetry, see Chapter 15.

Systemic diseases such as Down's syndrome, albinism, and cerebral palsy are frequently associated with infantile esotropia. Most investigative studies on infantile esotropia, however, exclude patients with these systemic diseases and consider pure infantile esotropia as being an entity without associated systemic disease or a neurologic condition.

Infantile Esotropia and Face Turn

Cross-Fixation

Patients with large-angle esodeviations (50 to 70 prism diopters) often fixate with the adducted eye and *cross-fixate*. When the fixing eye is in adduction, there will be a face turn to the side of the adducted eye (Fig. 17–2). Objects on the patients left are viewed with the right eye, and objects to the right are seen by the left eye.

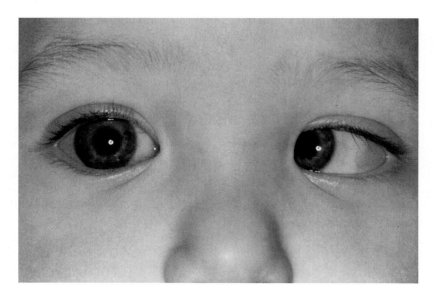

Figure 17–1.
Eight-month-old with infantile esotropia. Note the large-angle deviation which is typical of infantile esotropia.

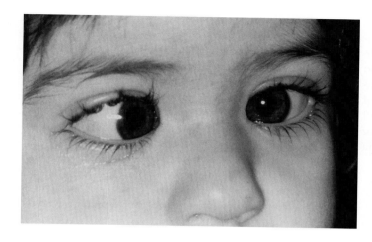

Figure 17–2.
Two-year-old with infantile esotropia and cross fixation. Patient is fixing left eye with a face turn to the right. Note that the fixing eye is in adduction. Ciancia's syndrome is similar to cross fixation except it is a more severe form. Patients with nystagmus compensation syndrome and manifest latent nystagmus and face turn also fix with their adduction eye, but the deviation is usually much smaller (less than 30 prism diopters).

Cross-fixation indicates that the patient will use either eye, however, even with cross-fixation there may be mild amblyopia (11). If patients are able to follow with smooth pursuit with either eye, then no significant amblyopia exists (27).

Ciancia's Syndrome

Ciancia's syndrome probably represents a severe form of infantile esotropia with cross-fixation and tight medial rectus muscles. Findings include large-angle esotropia, limited abduction (good abduction saccades), face turn with the fixing eye in adduction, and early end point type jerk nystagmus on attempted abduction (6). In Ciancia's syndrome, the reason for the face turn is probably tight medial rectus muscles, whereas in nystagmus compensation syndrome the nystagmus is primary, and the face turn is a compensatory mechanism to damp the nystagmus (see Nystagmus Compensation Syndrome below). The treatment of Ciancia's syndrome is maximal (7.0 mm) bilateral medial rectus recessions (20).

Nystagmus Compensation Syndrome

Esotropia associated with nystagmus, fixing eye in adduction, and a face turn toward the fixing eye was, at one time, classified as *nystagmus blockage syndrome* or *nystagmus compensation syndrome* (23). The theory was that patients with nystagmus, esotropia, and a face turn have congenital nystagmus and use accommodative convergence to block or damp the nystagmus to improve near vision. The accommodation stimulates overconvergence, which results in an esotropia. Recent studies however have shown that nystagmus compensation syndrome associated with congenital nystagmus, and overaccommodative convergence is extremely rare (24). The vast majority of patients with nystagmus, esotropia, and face turn actually have manifest latent nystagmus (see below) (10). The true nystagmus compensation syndrome is a small, variable, and intermittent esotropia, which is present only at near and is associated with pupillary miosis.

Manifest Latent Nystagmus

Manifest latent nystagmus (MLN) is a jerk nystagmus associated with infantile esotropia. The nystagmus increases when one eye is occluded or when fusion is disrupted by the presence of strabismus. The fast phase is toward the side of the fixing eye, and the null point is in adduction.

Patients with MLN with intermittent face turn have a small intermittent esotropia partially controlled with weak peripheral fusion. When fusion breaks, the esotropia becomes manifest, the nystagmus increases, and the patient adopts a face turn to place the fixing eye in adduction to reduce or damp the nystagmus. The treatment of esotropia, MLN with face turn is directed to promoting binocular fusion to reduce the MLN, thereby eliminating the need for a null point. Fusion is improved by correcting the underlying esodeviation, either with hypermetropic spectacles or strabismus surgery (31).

Differential Diagnosis

The differential diagnosis of infantile esotropia includes Duane's syndrome, congenital fibrosis syndrome, congenital sixth nerve palsy (Mobius' syndrome, see Chapter 9) and infantile myasthenia gravis. These disorders are associated with limited abduction and therefore can be differentiated from infantile esotropia in which the ductions should be full. This differentiation may be difficult in patients with large-angle infantile esotropia and tight medial rectus muscles. Even in these patients, however, vestibular stimulation by doll's head maneuver reveals near full ductions and good abduction saccades in patients with primary infantile esotropia.

Other diagnoses in the differential include pseudoesotropia secondary to large epicanthal folds and infantile accommodative esotropia (see below). Infantile accommodative esotropia may be difficult to distinguish from infantile esotropia. The key to the diagnosis of infantile accommodative esotropia is the presence of straight eyes for several months, then a variable small angle esodeviation associated with hypermetropia of +3.00 or more (see infantile accommodative esotropia below).

Pseudoesotropia

Pseudoesotropia is a common condition that needs to be distinguished from infantile esotropia. With pseudoesotropia, the infant has a wide nasal bridge and wide prominent epicanthal folds, which give the appearance of esotropia, but the eyes are orthotropic (Fig. 17–3). It can be difficult to convince parents that the eyes are truly straight, so it may be helpful to instruct the parents on how to perform the Hirschberg light reflex test. Follow-up is important in patients with pseudoesotropia because a true esotropia will develop in a small percentage.

Treatment of Infantile Esotropia

In most cases, the treatment of infantile esotropia is surgical, usually bilateral medial rectus recessions. In patients with small-angle esotropia (under 35 prism diopters), even mild hypermetropia of +2.00 to +3.00 should be prescribed since glasses alone may correct the deviation. Patients with large angle esotropia (40 prism diopters or more) usually do not respond to mild hypermetropic spectacle correction. If the hypermetropia is +3.00 or more, however, spectacles should be given a trial even if the deviation is large. Amblyopia should be treated before surgery. This is important because after

surgery, parents often feel the problem is solved and may not return for follow-up visits. In addition, if the eyes are straightened, it is more difficult to assess fixation preference, since the vertical prism test is required. One rare exception to treating the amblyopia first rule is in patients with a large-angle esotropia and an amblyopic eye, which is fixed in adduction (strabismus fixus). In these cases, unilateral strabismus surgery on the amblyopic eye may be required to bring the eye into primary position so a clear retinal image is provided. Older children or adults with irreversible amblyopia should have monocular surgery on the amblyopic eye (recession-medial rectus and resection lateral rectus), to avoid the risk of surgery on the good eye.

Timing of Surgery

The standard approach has been to operate between 6 months and 2 years of age. This is based primarily on a study by Ing (14), which showed that peripheral fusion (monofixation syndrome) can be achieved if the eyes are aligned by 2 years of age. More recently, the author has shown in a few patients that excellent fusion with high-grade stereopsis can be obtained when surgery is performed before 6 months of age (earliest 13 weeks) (28). The author suggests that very early surgery should be considered only if the following criteria are met: large angle esotropia (40 prism diopters or more), constant or increasing deviation documented by two visits 2 weeks apart, and the infant is a good anesthesia risk. Patients with small angle (less than 30 PD), variable angle, or intermittent esodeviations should be treated with hypermetropic spectacles when appropriate, or if not hypermetropic they should be followed closely until approximately 6 months of age and operated on if still esotropic. It is important to note that even brief periods of strabismus during the early period of visual development results in permanent loss of binocularity. Craw-

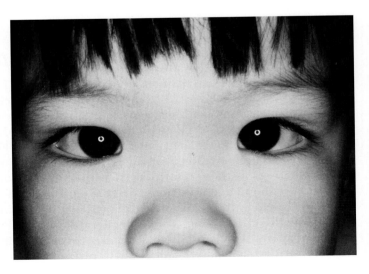

Figure 17–3.
Three-year-old with pseudoesotropia. Patient was referred with a question of right esotropia.

ford and von Noorden (8, 9) showed that even 2 to 3 weeks of prism-induced esotropia in infant monkeys resulted in irreversible loss of binocular cortical cells.

Treatment Goal

The goal of treating congenital esotropia is to achieve at least some binocularity and fusion. In all but a few rare cases, the best sensory result is monofixation syndrome with peripheral fusion and subnormal stereopsis (7, 14, 18, 28). In a small group of patients, high-grade stereopsis has been shown to be obtainable if alignment is established between 3 and 4 months of age (28). Perhaps one day our goal will be high-grade strereoacuity with central bifoveal fusion, but for now the goal is monofixation. To achieve the monofixation syndrome, the eyes must be aligned within 8 to 10 prism diopters of orthotropia before 2 years of age. Patients older than 2 years of age with infantile esotropia have a very poor prognosis for fusion (14).

Postoperative Care

Close follow-up is important because amblyopia will develop in approximately 20% of patients after surgery. Patients also should be followed for the development of DVD and inferior oblique overaction.

Residual Esotropia

If, after surgery, there is a significant esotropia of 10 to 15 prism diopters or more, further treatment is indicated. First, consider prescribing hypermetropic correction, especially if the cycloplegic refraction shows +2.00 or more. If the residual esotropia persists after 6 to 8

weeks, additional surgery should be considered. If the initial bimedial rectus recessions were 5.0 mm or less, consider re-recessing the medial rectus muscles. A bilateral re-recession of 2.0 mm roughly corrects 25 prism diopters of residual esotropia. If the initial recession of the medial rectus muscles were greater than 5.0 mm, then perform a resection or the Wright modified tuck (30) of the lateral rectus muscles. Be careful about performing large lateral rectus tightening procedures against previously recessed medial rectus muscles, as overcorrections are frequent.

Consecutive Exotropia

If a large consecutive exotropia occurs, be sure to check for an adduction deficit, as poor adduction may indicate a slipped medial rectus muscle. A slipped medial rectus muscle requires exploration and advancement of the slipped medial rectus muscle. Small exotropias under 20 prism diopters should be followed for at least 6 to 8 weeks before considering further surgery.

Botulinum

The use of botulinum for infantile esotropia remains under investigation (17). Botulinum injections to the medial rectus muscle might have a theoretic advantage, as they would produce an incomitant result so the patient could adopt a face turn to obtain fusion. There are, however, some practical problems involved with the use of botulinum, including postinjection ptosis leading to amblyopia, induced vertical deviations, and the temporary nature of botulinum, resulting in the need for multiple injections to sustain a long-term effect (3A, 14A).

■ ACCOMMODATIVE ESOTROPIA

Accommodative esotropia is caused by overconvergence associated with accommodation. Hypermetropia of +2.00 diopters or more is the most common cause of accommodative esotropia, and this is termed hypermetropic accommodative esotropia or refractive esotropia. A high AC/A ratio and weak divergence fusional amplitudes can also cause esotropia in patients with relatively low amounts of hypermetropia (high AC/A accommodative esotropia). Many patients show a combination of accommodative esotropia and a basic esotropia, and they are termed *partially accommodative esotropia*. These patients improve with hypermetropic spectacle correction but require surgery for the residual esotropia (Fig. 17–4).

Clinical Features

Accommodative esotropia is acquired and can present any time between early infancy to late childhood, but most frequently starts between 18 months and 4 years of age. Initially the deviation is small and intermittent with the esotropia seen mostly during near fixation, or when the child is tired. Over time (sometimes only a few weeks) the deviation may increase to become constant, and amblyopia may develop. The diagnosis of accommodative esotropia is based on a significant reduction or elimination of the esotropia after prescribing full hypermetropic correction or bifocals. In contrast to congenital esotropia, the deviation in accommodative es-

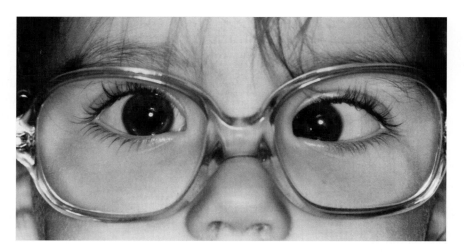

Figure 17–4.
A 3-year-old with partially accommodative esotropia. Patient is wearing full hypermetropia correction of +3.00 in both eyes, however, a residual esotropia persists.

otropia is acquired, and fusion has already occurred during early visual development; thus, these patients have relatively good fusion potential. The earlier the eyes are straightened the better the chances for re-establishing fusion. Motor sequelae such as dissociated vertical deviation, latent nystagmus, inferior oblique overaction, and OKN asymmetry are not usually associated with accommodative esotropia.

Infantile Accommodative Esotropia

Accommodative esotropia may occur in early infancy as young as 2 to 3 months of age (4). Often, these cases are diagnosed as congenital esotropia (19). Infantile accommodative esotropia, however, is associated with hypermetropia of +3.00 or more, the deviation is variable, usually intermittent, and relatively small (less than 40 prism diopters). Infants with esotropia, and +3.00 or more refractive error should be given full hypermetropic correction in an attempt to correct the esodeviation. Approximately 50% of children with infantile accommodative esotropia will require surgery in addition to glasses. In general, accommodative esotropia has a better prognosis than infantile esotropia if treated early, because the eyes are straight during the critical period of visual development, allowing development of binocular vision.

Treatment of Hypermetropic Accommodative Esotropia

Key to the management of hypermetropic accommodative esotropia is the immediate dispensing of full hypermetropic spectacle correction. Glasses should be worn full time and prescribed even in infants as young as 2 months of age.

Cyclopegic Refraction

A good cycloplegic refraction is critical. The standard cycloplegic agent is cyclopentolate 1% in children older than 2 years and 0.5% in infants. The refraction should be performed 30 to 40 minutes after the last cylopentolate drop. The mydriatic effect lasts for 6 to 24 hours, but the cycloplegia is only present for 20 minutes to 1 hour. Patients with very dark irides, high refractive errors, with variable readings on retinoscopy should be considered for an atropine refraction. Atropine, 1% (0.5% in infants) is given twice a day for 3 days before and including the day of the visit. With atropine, mydriasis lasts 7 to 14 *days,* and cyloplgia approximately 24 hours (peak 1 to 3 hours). See Table 17–2 for a summary of commonly used cycloplegic/mydriatic agents in children.

Use of Spectacles

Spectacles are the treatment of choice in most cases, but extended-wear contact lenses can be prescribed as a substitute for spectacles. Placing the corrective lens on the corneal plane with contact lenses reduces accommodative effort, and in fact has a slight advantage over spectacles. Some children will have trouble relaxing into their full hypermetropic correction. In these cases, short course (1 week) with topical atropine to both eyes once a day will relax accommodation and will improve compliance.

If after prescribing full hypermetropic correction a residual esotropia of 10 prism diopters or more persists, and there is no evidence of binocular fusion, one should consider further treatment. If there is a residual esotropia for near but straight eyes with fusion in the distance try bifocals (see below). If there is a residual esotropia for distance with full hypermetropic correction, then surgery is necessary. Remember, most patients with accommodative esotropia have fusion potential. The treatment goal is to re-establish binocular fusion, not just to align the eyes for cosmesis.

Bifocal Add

As stated above, patients who are straight in the distance with fusion (esotropia less than 10 prism diopters), but

TABLE 17–2
Cycloplegic/Mydriatic Agents in Children

Agent	Strength (%)	Mydriasis		Cycloplegia		Side Effects
		Maximum (minutes)	Recovery time	Maximum (minutes)	Recovery time	
Phenylephrine	2.5 only	20	2 hrs	none		Tachycardia, hypertension
Tropicamide	0.5, 1	20–40	2–6 hrs	30	2–6 hrs	
Cyclopentolate	0.5,1,2	30–60	6–24 hrs	20–60	6–24	Psychosis, seizure
Homatropine	2,5	40–90	1–3 days	30–70	1–3 days	Ataxia
Atropine	0.5,1	40 days	7–14 days	60–180	6–12 days	Flushing, tachycardia, fever, delirium

have a residual esotropia greater than 10 prism diopters at near are candidates for a bifocal add in addition to their hypermetropic correction. If after prescribing full hypermetropic correction a residual esotropia greater than 10 PD persists in the distance which precludes fusion, then bifocals are not indicated because bifocals will not help establish fusion in the distance. This is termed partially accommodative esotropia and patients require surgery plus hypermetropic spectacles (see below).

The near add relaxes accommodative convergence, thus reducing the near esotropia to allow for binocular fusion (Fig. 17–5). When prescribing bifocals, usually start with +3.00 or +2.50 add using the least amount that allows fusion. Make sure the bifocal segment is high and bisects the pupil. Executive flat-top bifocals are usually the best for children, however, blended-add bifocals may be useful in some patients where the appearance of the bifocal line is a problem. In many cases, bifocals can be weaned over time, slowly reducing the bifocal add, thus encouraging fusional divergence (16).

Surgery for Partially Accommodative Esotropia

If the hypermetropic spectacle correction improves the esodeviation but does not fully correct it, the entity is termed partially accommodative esotropia. Strabismus surgery is indicated in these patients to re-establish proper eye alignment and binocular fusion. The standard surgery for partially accommodative esotropia is bilateral medial rectus recessions. Some advocate surgery based on the residual esotropia with correction. With this approach there is an approximately 25% undercorrection (21, 29). Because of the high incidence of undercorrection, others recommend that patients have *augmented surgery*, prism adaptation, or *enhanced* surgery (15, 29). This author found excellent results (approximately 90% success) by operating on a target angle that was midway between the near deviation without correction and the near deviation with correction (29). However, in patients with a high AC/A relationship, this aug-

mented formula will overcorrect some patients for distance. In these patients with a large distance/near disparity, an alternative formula would be to average the near deviation without correction (larger deviation) and the distance deviation with correction (smallest angle). After surgery, patients uniformly require hypermetropic correction. If a small consecutive exotropia is present, one can reduce the amount of hypermetropia to invoke accommodative convergence. If a residual esotropia of 10 prism diopters or more is present, and the patient is not fusing, then further surgery is required.

Prism Adaptation

Another method for reducing undercorrections is prism adaptation.[21] This is based on neutralizing the residual esotropia with press-on prisms to disclose the full latent deviation. Base out press-on prisms are placed on the full hypermetropic correction to neutralize the residual esotropia. The patient is seen again in 2 weeks, and additional prism power is added if the deviation increases. The prism is increased until the angle is stable. Surgery is then performed, based on the full prism adapted angle.

Miotic Agents

Miotic drops such as phospholine iodide (echothiophate iodide) can help correct hypermetropic accommodative esotropia and are helpful in patients with a high AC/A ratio. Phospholine Iodide acts to block cholinesterase, thus acetylcholine is more active and there is a parasympathomimetic effect. As a result, the iris sphincter and ciliary muscles contract, producing miosis and increased accommodation for a given accommodative effort. Thus, a smaller amount of accommodation is needed to focus the image at near, hence, there is less convergence. It does not significantly affect the extraocular muscles. By reducing the accommodative effort, accommodative convergence also diminishes, thus correcting the esotropia. Miotic agents can

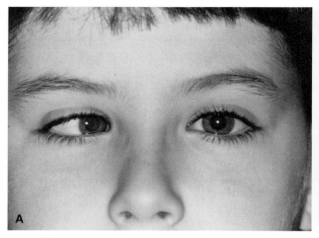

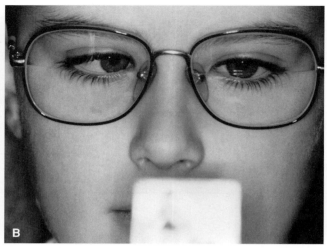

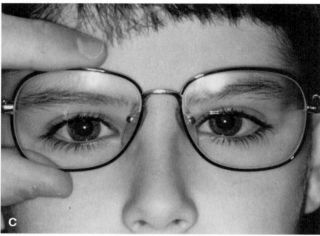

Figure 17–5.
An 8-year-old with a high AC/A ratio and esotropia for near while wearing her full cycloplegic hypermetropic correction of +2.00. Note that the eyes were straight when viewing in the distance, through the upper segment (not shown). **B,** A large angle esotropia persists when viewing through the upper segments of her glasses. **C,** When patient views through the bifocal add of +3.00, the eyes are straightened providing binocular fusion.

occasionally be successful in treating patients with relatively small angle accommodative esotropia, but hypermetropic spectacle correction is the treatment of choice. In children who absolutely refuse to wear glasses, or cannot wear contact lenses, miotic agents may be tried. They also may be useful for short periods of time when glasses are an inconvenience, for example, during the summer months when children are swimming. When prescribing miotics, start with a low dose of phospholine iodide 0.03%, 1 drop every morning. If this is not sufficient, increase the dose to phospholine iodide 0.125%, once or even twice a day.

Miotics do have side effects. Ocular side effects include iris cysts in 20% to 50% of cases, which may occur anytime from several weeks to several months after starting treatment (5). Iris cysts tend to regress after discontinuing phospholine iodide; however, the author has seen persistent large iris cysts several years after the discontinuation of treatment. Cotreatment with phenylephrine may help prevent iris cysts. Rare ocular complications include lens opacities, retinal detachments, and angle closure glaucoma in adults. Topical phospholine iodide has a systemic effect, and it lowers cholinesterase

activity in the blood for several weeks. Miotics such as phospholine iodine prolong the effect of succinylcholine, which may result in prolonged respiratory paralysis postoperatively. Patients receiving miotics who are undergoing general anesthesia should avoid succinylcholine, or cease miotic use for at least 6 weeks before having succinylcholine anesthesia.

High AC/A Ratio Esotropia

Some patients with accommodative esotropia have minimal or no hypermetropia, and their esodeviation is small or nonexistent in the distance and quite large at near. These patients have a high AC/A ratio and are best treated with bifocal spectacle correction even though the upper segment is a plano sphere. As discussed above, miotics also can be used in high AC/A ratio esotropia. If bifocal glasses fail to correct the esotropia, then strabismus surgery may be indicated. Since the eyes are straight in the distance, it is difficult to know how much surgery to perform. In these unusual cases, prism adaptation may be helpful because it brings out any latent distance deviation.

ACQUIRED NONACCOMMODATIVE ESOTROPIA

Most cases of acquired accommodative esotropia have significant hypermetropia of at least +2.00 or more diopters. Occasionally, however, a patient will present with primary acquired esotropia without significant hypermetropia. In patients with acquired esotropia, it is important to rule out the possibility of a neurologic process such as myasthenia gravis, chronic progressive external ophthalmoplegia, or a mild sixth nerve paresis associated with an intracranial mass, especially if the esotropia is greater in the distance (see divergence pare-

sis below). If the neurological work-up is negative, the cause of acquired nonaccommodative esotropia is usually a decompensated congenital esophoria. These patients tend to have strong tonic fusional divergence, and they may have a latent deviation much larger than is seen by alternate cover testing. Undercorrections are frequent in patients with acquired nonaccommodative esotropia and therefore prism adaptation can be helpful in disclosing the full latent deviation. Surgery should be based on the prism adapted angle.

CYCLIC ESOTROPIA

This is a rare form of esotropia, and most ophthalmologists may only see one case in an entire career. Patients with cyclic esotropia will have straight eyes most of the time, however, periodically, every 24 to 48 hours, a manifest esotropia develops. Cyclic esotropia usually occurs between 2 to 6 years of age and is often progressive, eventually becoming a constant esotropia. If cyclic esotropia is suspected, have the parents mark the calendar

with straight days versus esotropia days to document the cyclic pattern. A complete ocular examination is indicated in these patients with a good cycloplegic refraction to rule out latent hypermetropia. Strabismus surgery may be indicated in patients with cyclic esotropia. In these cases, perform surgery based on the full esodeviation during the tropia phase (13).

ESOPHORIA

Small esophorias, between 4 to 8 prism diopters, are relatively common. Even small esophorias can cause asthenopic symptoms such as headaches and reading fatigue. The first line of treatment is to prescribe a reading add to relax accommodative convergence. Base-out prisms also can help in these patients, however,

prescribe less than the full deviation to stimulate fusional divergence. Patients with large esophorias will have difficulty fusing and may break down into an acquired nonaccommodative esotropia, which may require surgery.

DIVERGENCE PARESIS

Divergence insufficiency or "divergence paresis" is an esodeviation that is greater in the distance than near. Clinically, most esodeviations are greater at near than distance, however, in some cases, primary esotropia without a specific neurological etiology will present with the deviation greater in the distance than near. Patients

with divergence insufficiency, however, must be carefully evaluated as divergence insufficiency can be a sign of central nervous system disease or a mild bilateral sixth nerve paresis. Neuroimaging studies are indicated in patients with acquired divergence paresis.

■ SENSORY ESOTROPIA

Sensory esotropia is an esodeviation caused by unilateral blindness. The general teaching has been that if the visual loss occurs before 2 years of age, then patients will develop esotropia; however, if the vision loss occurs after 2 years of age, exotropia develops. This is only a general rule, with many exceptions; the presence of an esotropia is not a good marker for the onset of blindness. The treatment of sensory esotropia is a recession/resection procedure of the blind eye, avoiding surgery on the better seeing eye.

■ REFERENCES

1. Aiello A, Borchert MS, Wright KW: Independence of optokinetic nystagmus asymmetry and binocularity in infantile esotropia. Arch Ophthalmol 1994;112:1580–1583.

2. Archer SM, Sondhi N, Helveston EM: Strabismus in infancy. Ophthalmology 1989;96:133–137.

3. Atkinson J: Development of optokinetic nystagmus on the human infant and monkey infant. In: Freeman RD (ed): Developmental neurobiology of Vision, New York: Plenum Publishing Corp, 1979, p 277.

3A. Biglan AW, et al.: Management of strabismus with botulinum A toxin. Ophthalmology 1989;96:935–943.

4. Baker JD, Parks MM: Early onset accommodative esotropia. Am J Ophthalmol 1980;90:11.

5. Chin NV, Gold AA, Breinin GM: Iris cysts and miotics. Arch Ophthalmol 1964;71:611.

6. Ciancia A: La esotropia en el lactante, diagnostico y tratamiento. Arch Chil Oftalmol 1962;9:117.

7. Costenbader FD: Infantile esotropia. Trans Am Ophthalmol Soc 1961;59:397.

8. Crawford MLJ, von Noorden GK: The effects of short-term experimental strabismus on the visual system in macaca mulatta. Invest Ophthalmol Vis Sci 1979;18:496–505.

9. Crawford MLJ, von Noorden GK: Optically induced concomitant strabismus in monkeys. Invest Ophthalmol Vis Sci 1980;19:1105.

10. Dell'Osso LF, Ellenberger Jr C, Abel LA, Flynn JT: The nystagmus blockage syndrome. Investigative Ophthalmol Vis Sci 1983;24:1580.

11. Dickey CF, Metz HS, Stewart SA: The diagnosis of amblyopia in cross-fixation. J Pediatr Ophthalmol Strabismus 1991;28:171–175.

12. Dickey CF, Scott WE: Amblyopia—the prevalence in congenital esotropia versus partially accommodative esotropia. In: Lenk-Schager M (ed): Orthoptic Horizons—Transactions of the Sixth International Orthoptic Congress. Harrogate, Great Britain 1987:106.

13. Helveston EM: Cyclic strabismus. Am Orthoptic J 1971;23:4851.

14. Ing MR: Early surgical alignment for congenital esotropia. Ophthalmology 1983;90:132–135.

14A. Ing MR: Botulinum alignment for congenital esotropia. Ophthalmology 1993;100:318–322.

15. Jotterand VH, Isenberg SJ: Enhacing surgery for accommodative esotropia. Ophthalmic Surg 1988;19:263–266.

16. Ludwig IH, Parks MM, Getson PR: Long-term results of bifocal therapy for accommodative esotropia. J Pediatr Ophthalmol Strabismus 1989;26:264–270.

17. Magoon E: Chemodenervation of strabismic children. Ophthalmology 1989;96:931–934.

18. Parks MM: Congenital esotropia with a bifixation result, report of a case. Documenta Ophthalmologica 1984;58:109–114.

19. Pollard ZF: Accommodative esotropia during the first year of life. Arch Ophthalmol 1976;94:1912.

20. Prieto-Diaz J: Large bilateral medial rectus recession in early esotropia with bilateral limitation of abduction. J Pediatr Ophthalmol Strabismus 1980;17:101–105.

21. Prism Adaptation Research Group: Efficacy of prism adaptation in the surgical management of acquired esotropia. Arch Ophthalmol 1990;108:1248–1256.

22. Tychen L, Lisberger SG: Maldevelopment of visual motion processing in humans who had strabismus with onset in infancy. J Neurosci 1986;6:2495–2508.

23. von Noorden GK: The nystagmus compensation (blockage syndrome). Am J Ophthalmol 1976;82:283.

24. von Noorden GK, Munoz M, Wong SY: Compensatory mechanisms in congenital nystagmus. Am J Ophthalmol 1987;104:387–397.

25. Westall CA, Schor CM: Asymmetries of optokinetic nystagmus in amblyopia: the effect of selected retinal stimulation. Vision Res 1985; 25: 1431–1438.

26. Worth C: Squint, its causes, pathology and treatment. Ed 6, London: Bailliere, Tindall and Cox, 1929.

27. Wright KW, Edelman PM, Walonker F, Yiu S: Reliability of fixation preference testing in diagnosing amblyopia. Arch Ophthalmol 1986;104:549.

28. Wright KW, Edelman PM, Terry A, McVey J, Lin M: High grade stereo acuity after early surgery for congenital esotropia. Archiv Ophthalmol 1994;112:913–919.

29. Wright KW, Bruce-Lyle L: Augmented surgery for esotropia associated with high hypermetropia. J Pediatr Ophthalmol Strabismus 1993;30:167–170.

30. Wright KW, Lanier, AB: Effect of a modified rectus tuck on anterior segment circulation in monkeys. J Pediatr Ophthalmol Strab 1991;28:77–81.

31. Zubcov AA, et al.: Treatment of latent nystagmus. Am J Ophthalmol 1990;110:160–167.

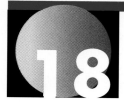

18 Exodeviations

Kenneth W. Wright

Exodeviations can be classified as shown in Table 18–1, with intermittent exotropia being the most common form. In contrast to esotropia, intermittent exotropia is associated with high-grade stereopsis and bifoveal fusion. This may be because of our innate strong fusional convergence amplitudes, which allow for at least partial control of exodeviations, whereas our divergence is weak so esodeviations cannot be fused, and the deviations tend to be constant. Most newborn infants, in fact, have a small transient exodeviation, which resolves by 4 months of age.[1] Small exophorias, usually less than 10 prism diopters, are common in the general population and should be considered normal. An exception to the general rule that exodeviations are associated with good fusion is the rare condition, congenital exotropia. These patients have a large deviation, poor fusion potential, and often an underling systemic disease.

■ INTERMITTENT EXOTROPIA

Intermittent exotropia is an exodeviation that is controlled part of the time by fusional convergence. Think of intermittent exotropia as a large exophoria that intermittently breaks down into a manifest exotropia (Fig. 18–1). This is by far the most common type of exodeviation. The pathogenesis of intermittent exotropia is unknown.

Clinical Manifestations

Intermittent exodeviation usually occurs between 2 and 6 years of age but may present any time between infancy and adulthood. Initially, an exotropia may only be seen when the patient is fatigued or ill. Symptoms include blurred vision, asthenopia, visual fatigue, and photophobia with squinting. The photophobia and squinting are believed to be mechanisms for eliminating diplopia or confusion; however, this theory has come into question by Wiggins and von Noorden (25). The natural history of intermittent exotropia is variable. Approximately 70% will show an increasing frequency of the exotropia state and progressive loss of fusion, 20% will stay the same, and a very small percentage will improve over time (24).

During the exophoric phase, patients have bifoveal fusion with excellent stereo acuity ranging between 40 and 50 seconds arc. When tropic, most patients demonstrate hemiretinal suppression, but some have anomalous retinal correspondence (ARC). Occasionally, patients with late onset intermittent exotropia (after age 5 or 6) will have normal retinal correspondence (NRC) and diplopia; however, this is unusual. Significant amblyopia is rare in patients with intermittent exotropia. Oblique dysfunction such as superior oblique or inferior oblique overaction can coexist with intermittent exotropia. Small hyperdeviations (less than 5 to 8 prism diopters) are fairly common, and they spontaneously resolve with correction of the exotropia.

Classification of Intermittent Exotropia

Intermittent exotropia can be classified by the difference between the distance and near deviation (3). The classification below is clinically useful as it helps deter-

TABLE 18–1
Exodeviations

1. Intermittent exotropia (most common)
   a. Basic
   b. Pseudodivergence excess (increased tonic fusional convergence)
   c. True divergence excess
      1. High AC/A ratio
      2. Normal AC/A ratio, increased proximal convergence
2. Convergence insufficiency (common)
3. Sensory exotropia (common)
4. Congenital exotropia (extremely rare)

mine the target angle when considering the surgical plan.

Basic Intermittent Exotropia

The distance and near deviation is similar, within 10 prism diopters.

Example:	Distance	XT 35 PD
	Near	XT 30 PD
	Operate for	XT 35 PD

Pseudo Divergence Excess

The exodeviation appears to be more than 10 prism diopters greater at distance than at near, but after prolonged monocular occlusion (30-minute patch test, see below), the near deviation increases to within 10 prism diopters of the distance deviation.

Example:	Distance	XT 35 PD
	Near	XT 15 PD
Near after patch test		XT 30 PD
	Operate for	XT 30 to 35 PD

Patch Test (Monocular Occlusion)

The patch test suspends tonic fusional near convergence and discloses the full latent deviation. Approxi-

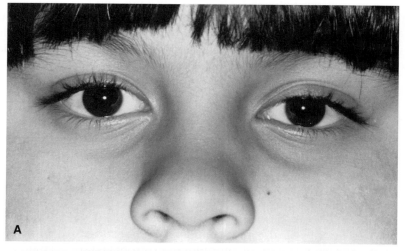

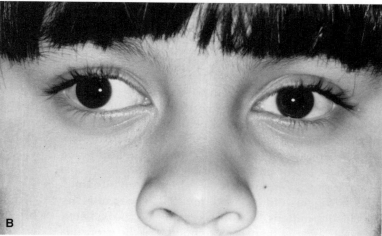

Figure 18–1.
Six-year-old with intermittent exotropia. **A,** Patient in the phoric phase with straight eyes and high grade stereopsis. **B,** Shows patient in tropic phase with large right exotropia. Patient is suppressing right eye and does not have diplopia.

mately 80% of patients with apparent divergence excess actually have pseudodivergence excess (4, 13, 23).

If the distance measurement is more than 10 prism diopters greater than the near measurement (divergence excess pattern), the patch test is indicated to differentiate pseudo divergence excess from true divergence excess. This is important as the patch test can help identify the surgical target angle. The patch test is performed by placing a patch over one eye for 30 to 60 minutes to suspend tonic fusional convergence. The deviation is then measured by alternate cover testing for distance and near without allowing the patient to regain fusion.

True Divergence Excess

True divergence excess is when the exotropia is more than 10 prism diopters greater in the distance than near, even after prolonged monocular occlusion. The term divergence excess does not indicate the etiology of the distance-near disparity, as it can be caused by either a high AC/A ratio, an increased proximal convergence, or both (13).

Divergence Excess Types

High AC/A Ratio. Patients with a high AC/A ratio will show less of an exodeviation at near than distance. The diagnosis of high AC/A ratio is made by completely dissociating the eyes with prolonged monocular occlusion, then measuring the deviation with and without a +3.00 near add. Patients with high AC/A ratio true divergence excess are prone to overcorrection at near if the distance measurement is used as the target angle for surgical correction. In this group of patients, reduce the amount of surgery and use a target angle halfway between the distance and near measurements done after the patch test.

Example: Distance   XT 38 PD
                 Near   XT 10 PD
Near after patch test   XT 15 PD
Near after patch test with +3.00   XT 36 PD

$$\text{Operate for} \quad \text{XT 25 PD} = \frac{(15 + 36)}{2}$$

$$\text{High AC/A} = \left(\frac{36 - 15}{3.00}\right) = 7 \text{ PD/D}$$

Increased Proximal Convergence (Normal AC/A Ratio). Rarely, a patient will show a true divergence excess pattern, but the AC/A ratio is normal. Increased proximal convergence is probably the cause of the distance near-disparity in these cases. In contrast to the high AC/A ra-

tio group, these patients show better results when surgery is based on an angle close to the distance measurement (13).

Measuring Intermittent Exotropia

It is important to determine the full exodeviation in patients with intermittent exotropia. Patients may show variable angles of deviations depending on the time of day and the mental status of the patient. The patch test helps dissociate the eyes to bring out the full deviation for both distance and near. Another technique is to perform the far distance test and have the patient look out of the window at a distant target, well past 20 feet. This helps relax proximal convergence and will disclose the full distance deviation. It is a good idea to obtain more than one measurement before performing surgery to get an idea of the true deviation.

Indications for Surgery

The most important indication for therapeutic intervention is an increasing tropia phase with diminished fusion control. Patients who show very infrequent breakdown of fusion, perhaps only once or twice a week and who show no increase in the tropia phase, can be monitored conservatively. Patients who show poor fusion recovery and an increasing tropia phase (>50%) should be treated. A good test for fusional recovery is to have the patient fixate on a distance target and temporarily occlude one eye. After removing the occluder, note how long it takes for the patient to recover fusion. Immediate recovery of fusion shows good fusional control. Another point to note when considering surgery is the age of the patient. Patients who have surgery at younger than 4 years of age have a higher incidence of developing amblyopia and loss of stereopsis postoperatively than when surgery is performed in older children (8). It is best to postpone surgery in children with intermittent exotropia until 4 to 5 years of age unless the patient demonstrates progressive loss of fusion control. In these cases, nonsurgical treatments as described below can be tried. If fusion continues to decompensate, however, early surgery is indicated.

Nonsurgical Treatment

In general, nonsurgical treatment is not very effective and is usually used as a temporizing measure or as a postoperative treatment for a small residual exotropia. One frequently used method to control intermittent exotropia in patients with myopia is to prescribe more minus power than is found on cycloplegic refraction (i.e., over-minus). Increasing the myopic correction increases accommodative convergence thus helping to control the intermittent exotropia. Over-minus by approximately 1.50 to 3.00 diopters (5).

Part-time monocular occlusion also can improve fusional control of intermittent exotropia (9,11). With this treatment, the dominant eye is occluded 3 to 4 hours a day to stimulate the nonpreferred eye. Some have suggested that this provides a type of antisuppression therapy. In cases where there is equal ocular preference, alternate eye patching is indicated. In general, I have found part-time occlusion therapy to be of minimal value in most patients. For young patients (younger than 4 years of age), occlusion therapy may be considered as a way of temporizing until the child is old enough for surgery. Patch the dominant eye 3 to 4 hours per day, or alternate the patching if there is equal visual preference.

Orthoptic therapy such as antisuppression orthoptic therapy and diplopia awareness therapy is usually not indicated as this can lead to intractable diplopia in later life.

Surgical Treatment

The procedure of choice for intermittent exotropia is bilateral lateral rectus recessions. Symmetrical surgery (bilateral lateral rectus recessions) is usually preferred over a monocular surgery (recession lateral and ipsilateral medial rectus resection) because bilateral surgery produces a comitant result. A large monocular recession/resection procedure can cause an esotropia and uncrossed diplopia on side gaze ipsilateral to the recession/resection. Adults who have had large recession/resections for intermittent exotropia often complain of diplopia in sidegaze for several months or longer. An important question is how much surgery to perform and should surgery be based on the distance or near deviation? Examples under the classification of intermittent exotropia above provide a guide to determining the surgical target angle. Some advocate reducing the amount of surgery if the exotropia diminishes by approximately 50% in side gaze (16), but this author has rarely reduced the amount of surgery because of lateral incomitance.

■ OBLIQUE DYSFUNCTION AND A- AND V-PATTERNS

(Also see Chapter 19 Oblique Dysfunction and A and V Patterns)

If significant oblique dysfunction is present, the oblique muscles should be operated on at the same time as the horizontal muscles. Patients with significant A- and V-patterns without oblique dysfunction should have the horizontal rectus supra- or infraplaced as appropriate. V-pattern intermittent exotropia undergoing bilateral lateral rectus recessions require supraplacement one half tendon width, whereas A-patterns require infraplacement. Intermittent exotropia associated with superior oblique overaction and A-pattern is a difficult situation, because superior oblique weakening procedures can lead to superior oblique palsy. Patients with intermittent exotropia have excellent fusion and a superior oblique palsy in these patients results in diplopia. Two strategies to avoid superior oblique paresis would be to use horizontal muscle supra- or infraplacement instead of superior oblique weakening or use a controlled superior oblique weakening procedure such as the superior oblique tendon silicone expander (26).

Another pattern often associated with intermittent exotropia is X-pattern with increasing exodeviation in upgaze and downgaze relative to primary position. X-pattern is often associated with an upshoot and downshoot in adduction that resembles oblique dysfunction. In most cases, there is no true oblique muscle dysfunction, and the X-pattern along with the up and down shoot disappears after bilateral lateral rectus recessions. Tight lateral rectus muscles are probably the cause of the up shoot and the X-pattern. As the eye adducts against the tight lateral rectus muscle, the muscle can slip up or down when the eye moves up or down, pulling the eye up and out, or down and out. This vertical leash effect of a tight or co-contracting lateral rectus muscle is one cause for up and down shoots associated with Duane's co-contraction syndrome (see Chap. 20).

Postoperative Management

The immediate postoperative goal is to achieve a small consecutive esodeviation approximately 8 to 15 prism diopters (18, 20). Patients should be informed that a transient postoperative esotropia with diplopia may occur. In most patients, the consecutive esodeviation will resolve within 1 to 2 weeks; however, some patients may require a month or longer. Even large consecutive esodeviations can resolve spontaneously. In children younger than 4 years of age, a consecutive esotropia even for a relatively brief period can lead to suppression, amblyopia, and loss of binocularity (8). Some authorities have advocated part-time alternate eye occlusion therapy for younger patients with consecutive esotropia to help prevent unilateral suppression and amblyopia until the esodeviation spontaneously resolves. Hardesty et al. (10) have suggested prescribing prism glasses to neutralize the esodeviation during the early postoperative period. Press-on prisms can be given to patients of all ages to provide fusion until the esotropia resolves. Hardesty et al. recommend slightly undercorrecting the esodeviation to stimulate divergence (10). Because there is a danger of losing binocular fusion, I try to delay surgery on children younger than 4 years of age (8). If the exotropia is poorly controlled and getting worse, early surgery may be necessary.

A persistent overcorrection of more than 2 weeks' duration should be corrected. Conservative treatment includes prism glasses, bifocals, and miotics. Persistent consecutive esodeviations at near are frequent in patients with true divergence excess and a high AC/A ratio. These patients often require long-term bifocal therapy. It is prudent to warn patients with a high AC/A ratio that these bifocal glasses may be needed postoperatively. A persistent esodeviation after 6 weeks, not controlled by conservative measures, should be considered for reoperation. In most cases, bilateral medial rectus recessions are indicated, especially if the esotropia is greater at near.

Residual exodeviations usually occur late, anywhere from weeks to years after surgery. If a significant residual exotropia occurs, consider re-recessing both lateral rectus muscles if the primary recessions were less than 6.0 mm. For primary recessions greater than 6.0 mm, consider bilateral medial rectus resections or tucks. Be conservative about the amount of medial rectus tightening as you are tightening against previously recessed laterals.

Prognosis

Short-term success for intermittent exotropia is relatively good, with approximately 80% of patients achieving straight eyes at 6 months to 1 year. Long-term follow-up results are not as good, as Richard and Parks (19) reported a 56% success rate with one surgery at 2 to 8 years (mean, 4 years) follow-up. Thirty-eight percent of these patients were undercorrected, whereas only 6% were overcorrected. These authors noted that an additional

surgery improved their success rate to approximately 80%. Using postoperative prism therapy, Hardesty et al. reported an 80% success rate after no more than two surgeries with a 10-year follow-up period (10). A clinical observation is that intermittent exotropia tends to recur, and late residual exodeviations are common.

Convergence Insufficiency

Convergence insufficiency is the inability to converge, which results in an exodeviation at near (Fig. 18–2). Clinical symptoms include asthenopia, reading fatigue, blurred vision at near, and diplopia at near (15). Key ocular signs include remote near point of convergence (greater than 8 to 10 cm from nose), decreased near fusional convergence amplitudes, and a large exophoria at near. The exophoria at near intermittently breaks down into a manifest exotropia. Reduced fusional convergence amplitudes as measured by base-out prism is an important sign. Normal fusion convergence amplitudes are between 30 and 35 prism diopters. Patients with convergence insufficiency often show fusional convergence amplitudes of less than 20 prism diopters.

Treatment

Convergence insufficiency is the one type of strabismus that is best treated with orthoptic exercises. Convergence exercise is the treatment of choice and is successful in the majority of patients. The two most useful convergence exercises are near point exercises (pencil push-ups) and base-out prism convergence exercises. These exercises are dependent on the patient recognizing diplopia and the fusion breakpoint. Patients who do not recognize diplopia can be aided by a red filter over the dominant eye using a light as a fixation target. Rarely, surgery is necessary. If surgery is deemed necessary, small unilateral or bilateral medial rectus resec-

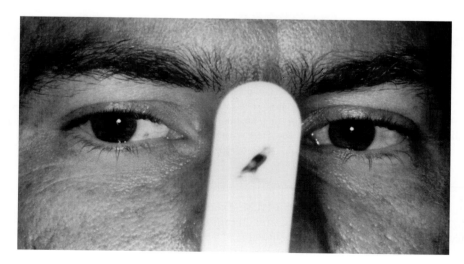

Figure 18–2.
Adult patient with convergence insufficiency. Note the left eye is fixing on the fixation target and the right eye is exotropic. The patient had no significant deviation for distance fixation. Convergence insufficiency is best treated by convergence exercises.

tions have been advocated (12, 22). In my experience, medial rectus resections are not very effective for managing convergence insufficiency. Creating tight medial rectus muscles will limit divergence in the distance but does not significantly increase convergence at near (17).

Accommodative Insufficiency

Primary accommodative insufficiency is rare; however, it can be a cause of reading fatigue and asthenopia (7). It is a lack of appropriate accommodation for near. Hypoaccommodation can be diagnosed by dynamic retinoscopy, the Costenbader accommodometer or near vision card held at close working distance. Unlike convergence insufficiency where the symptoms are relieved by occluding one eye, accommodative insufficiency is present under monocular or binocular conditions. If patching one eye relieves asthenopic symptoms, then consider convergence insufficiency or another disorder of binocular interaction (phoria or aniseikonia). If monocular occlusion does not improve symptoms, then the asthenopia is not caused by an abnormality of binocular interaction and consider accommodative insufficiency.

Convergence insufficiency can be associated with accommodative insufficiency (14, 21). Accommodative insufficiency can be acquired secondary to systemic disorders such as Parkinson's disease, oral lithium, or local ciliary body dysfunction with Adie's pupil (2). Accommodative exercises are a treatment for primary accommodative insufficiency, however, exercises result in only modest improvement (14). Patients with true primary accommodative insufficiency usually require a reading add. Prescribe the lowest power necessary to relieve symptoms to continue stimulation of accommodation. Other causes for asthenopia include latent hypermetropia and presbyopia in older patients.

■ CONGENITAL EXOTROPIA

This is a very rare entity, as most ophthalmologists will only see one or two cases in their career. Congenital exotropia may occur primarily without other systemic abnormalities, however, congenital exotropia is more commonly associated with systemic disorders such as ocular albinism, craniofacial abnormalities, and cerebral palsy. It is important to remember that more than 70% of healthy newborns will have a small intermittent exodeviation that resolves by 2 to 6 months of age (1). In contrast, congenital exotropia is a large, constant deviation that persists. The differential diagnosis of congenital exotropia includes congenital third nerve palsy (Fig. 18–3). Congenital third nerve palsy is usually unilateral and is often a partial third nerve palsy. Neuroimaging is indicated if the cause of the third nerve paresis is unknown. Treatment is bilateral lateral rectus recessions performed in early infancy usually after 6 months of age. The prognosis for fusion is poor (similar to infantile esotropia), and patients often require more than one surgery.

Sensory Exotropia

Unilateral vision loss can result in an exodeviation, which is termed sensory exotropia. Historically, it has been taught that vision loss before 4 years of age results in a sensory esotropia whereas vision loss after 4 years of age results in a sensory exotropia. Clinical experience, however, shows that blindness can result in either an esotropia or an exotropia regardless of age of onset. In a study by Cheng et al. (6), patients with unilateral congenital cataracts developed essentially equal distribution between sensory esotropia and sensory exotropia. The management of sensory exotropia is usually surgery with a recession/resection procedure on the blind eye.

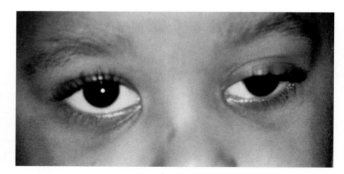

Figure 18–3.
Child with congenital third nerve palsy. Note the left eye is "down and out" and there is a left ptosis. Pupils may or may not be involved.

■ REFERENCES

1. Archer SM, Sondhi N, Helveston EM: Strabismus in infancy. Ophthalmology 1989;96:133–137.
2. Brown B: The convergence insufficiency masquerade. Am Orthoptic J 1990:40:94–97.
3. Burian HLM: Exodeviations: Their classification, diagnosis and treatment. Am J Ophthalmol 1966;62: 1161–1166.
4. Burian HM, Franceschetti AT: Evaluation of diagnostic

methods for the classification of exodeviations. Trans Am Ophthalmol Soc 1970;68:56.

5. Caltrider N, Jampolsky A: Overcorrecting minus lens therapy for treatment of intermittent exotropia. Ophthalmology 1983;90:1160.

6. Cheng KP, Hiles DA, Biglan AW, Pettapiece MC: Visual results after early surgical treatment of unilateral congenital cataract. Ophthalmology 1991;98:903–910.

7. Chrousos GA, O'Neill JF, et al.: Accommodative deficiency in healthy young adults. J Pediatr Ophthalmol Strabismus 1988;25:176–179.

8. Edelman PM, Murphree AL, Brown MH, Wright KW: Consecutive esodeviation... then what? Am Orthoptic J 1988;38:111–116.

9. Freeman RS, Isenberg SJ: The use of part-time occlusion for early onset unilateral exotropia: J Pediatr Ophthalmol Strabismus 1989;26:94.

10. Hardesty HH, Boynton JR, Keenan P: Treatment of intermittent exotropia. Arch Ophthalmology 1978;96:268.

11. Henderson JW, Iacobucci I: Occlusion in the preoperative treatment of exodeviations. Am Orthopt J 1965;15:42.

12. Hermann JS: Surgical therapy for convergence insufficiency. J Pediatr Ophthalmol Strabismus 1981;18:28.

13. Kushner BJ: Exotropic deviations: a functional classification and approach to treatment. Am Orthoptic J 1988;38:81–93.

14. Mazow ML, Musgrove K, Finkelman S: Acute accommodative and convergence insufficiency. Am Orthoptic J 1991;41:102–109.

15. Mazow ML: The convergence insufficiency syndrome. J Pediatr Ophthalmol Strabismus 1971;8:243–244.

16. Moore S: The prognostic value of lateral gaze measurements in intermittent exotropia. Am Orthop J 1969;19:69.

17. Nardi M, et al.: Divergence pseudoparalysis: a case report. Graefe's Arch Clin Exp Ophthalmol 1986;224:371–373.

18. Raab EL, Parks MM: Recession of the lateral recti: Early and late postoperative alignments. Arch Ophthalmol 1969;82:203.

19. Richard JM, Parks MM: Intermittent exotropia. Surgical results in different age groups. Ophthalmology 1983;90:172.

20. Scott WE, Keech R, Mash J: The postoperative results and stability of exodeviations. Arch Ophthalmol 1981;99:1814.

21. von Noorden GK, Brown DJ, Parks M: Associated convergence and accommodative insufficiency. Doc Ophthalmol 1973;34:393–403.

22. von Noorden GK: Resection of both medial rectus muscles in organic convergence insufficiency. Am J Ophthalmol 1976;81:223.

23. von Noorden GK: Divergence excess and simulated divergence excess: diagnosis and surgical management. Ophthalmologica 1969;26:719.

24. von Noorden GK: Binocular vision and ocular motility, theory and management of strabismus. CV Mosby, St. Louis. 1985. p 310.

25. Wiggins RE, von Noorden GK: Monocular eye closure in sunlight. J Pediatr Ophthalmol Strabismus 1990;27:16.

26. Wright KW, Min BM, Park C: Comparison of superior oblique tendon expander to superior oblique tenotomy for the management of superior oblique overaction and brown syndrome. J Pediatr Ophthalmol Strabismus 1992;29:92–97.

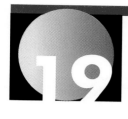

Oblique Dysfunction and A and V Patterns

Kenneth W. Wright, Jyoti Raina

■ A AND V PATTERNS

A significant difference in the horizontal deviation from upgaze to downgaze is described as an A or V pattern. An A pattern is more divergence in downgaze versus upgaze of at least 10 prism diopters, while a V pattern is increasing divergence in upgaze versus downgaze by 15 prism diopters. An example of an A pattern is upgaze ET 20, downgaze XT 5, and a V pattern is upgaze XT 15, downgaze ET 10. A and V patterns are caused by oblique muscle overaction, oblique muscle paresis, or unknown cause.

■ EVALUATING OBLIQUE DYSFUNCTION

When an oblique muscle over- or underacts, all three functions of the muscle will be involved: vertical, horizontal, and torsional. Clinical quantification of oblique dysfunction, however, is based for the most part on the vertical hyper- or hypofunction seen on version testing. To assess oblique function, the eye under examination is moved into the field of action of the muscle, which is elevation in adduction for the inferior oblique, and depression in adduction for the superior oblique. The amount of overaction or underaction of the adducted eye is graded on a scale of +1 to +4 for overaction and −1 to −4 for underaction.[16] When evaluating oblique dysfunction, the abducting eye should be fixing so that the adducting eye is free to manifest oblique dysfunction. For example, if the right inferior oblique is being

evaluated, a version movement to the left is directed, the right eye is partially covered and the right eye observed behind the cover for an up-shoot. Figure 19–1 shows degrees of inferior oblique overaction on version testing. For the characteristics of individual oblique muscle dysfunction see below.

The amount of A or V pattern associated with oblique dysfunction is an additional parameter to quantitate the amount of oblique dysfunction. In general, large patterns of more than 20 prism diopters are indicative of at least +2 over- or underaction. The amount of abnormal fundus torsion seen on indirect ophthalmosopy also can be used to help quantitate the amount of oblique dysfunction (see Chapter 14, Motor Aspects of Strabismus, Figs. 14–8 and 14–9).

■ OBLIQUE OVERACTION

Overaction of an oblique muscle can be primary, of unknown cause, or secondary to a muscle paresis. Primary oblique overaction is commonly found in association with horizontal strabismus and is the most frequent

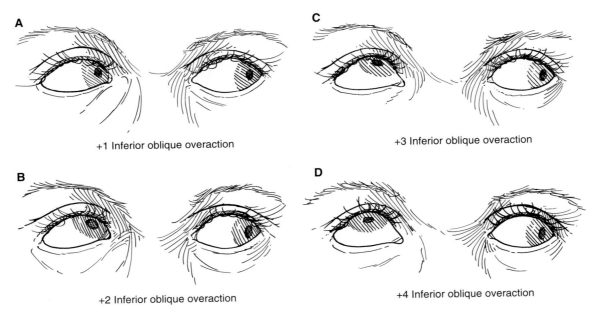

A

+1 Inferior oblique overaction

B

+2 Inferior oblique overaction

C

+3 Inferior oblique overaction

D

+4 Inferior oblique overaction

Figure 19–1.
Quantification of degree of inferior oblique overaction, +1 to +4. Note the abducting eye is fixing, and it is directed straight across horizontally, not elevated.

cause of A- and V-pattern strabismus. An oblique muscle paresis will cause an overaction of its antagonist (Sherrington's law of agonist-antagonist muscles). A superior oblique paresis, for example, produces ipsilateral inferior oblique overaction. Oblique overaction also can be caused by paresis of its yoke muscle in the contralateral eye (Hering's law of yoke muscles). A left inferior rectus paresis, for example, causes apparent overaction of the right superior oblique muscle if the patient fixes with the paretic left eye.

In general, recently acquired oblique muscle paresis is usually associated with significant underaction of the paretic agonist and with relatively mild overaction of the antagonist oblique muscle. Long-standing oblique muscle paresis, however, is usually associated with significant overaction of the antagonist oblique muscle. In some cases, there may be more overaction of the antagonist muscle than underaction of the paretic muscle. The head tilt test and Parks three-step test described below is useful for diagnosing the paresis of a vertical rectus muscle or oblique muscle.

Head Tilt Test

In patients with a vertical deviation, the head tilt test should be performed to distinguish primary oblique dysfunction from oblique dysfunction secondary to a vertical or oblique muscle paresis. A positive head tilt test is a strong indication there is a paresis, whereas a negative head tilt usually indicates a primary oblique dysfunction. If the vertical deviation changes by more than 5 prism diopters on right tilt versus left tilt, then the head tilt test is positive. The head tilt test is also a

critical part of the Parks three-step test, which is used to diagnose which oblique or vertical rectus muscle is paretic.

Tilting the head normally invokes torsional eye movements to correct and maintain the appropriate retinal orientation. A tilt right for example invokes intorsion of the right eye and extorsion of the left eye. The intortors are the superior oblique and the superior rectus muscles, while the extortors are the inferior oblique and the inferior rectus muscles. Note that for each pair of torsional muscles there is one elevator and one depressor. For intorsion the superior oblique is the depressor, the superior rectus is the elevator, and for extorsion the inferior oblique is the elevator, the inferior rectus is the depressor. This arrangement keeps vertical forces balanced during the head tilt. If one of the torsional muscles are paretic however, then there will be an imbalance of vertical forces and a vertical deviation on head tilt testing. Figure 19–2 shows this concept for a right superior oblique paresis. As the head tilts to the right, the right superior oblique and right superior rectus contract to intort the right eye. Since the superior oblique is paretic the superior rectus is unopposed and elevates the eye creating an increasing right hyperdeviation on head tilt to the right.

Parks Three-Step Test

The Parks three-step test incorporates the head tilt test with the pattern of incomitance to determine which muscle is paretic. When a patient presents with a vertical deviation, first perform the head tilt test to see if a paretic muscle is present. If the head tilt test is positive

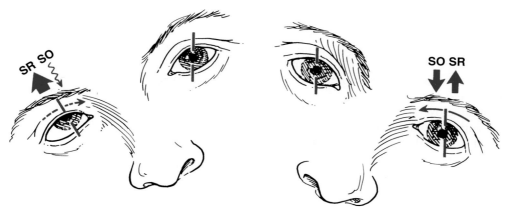

Figure 19–2.

Diagram of a right superior oblique paresis with a positive head tilt to the tilt right. As the head tilts to the right, the left eye extorts and the right eye intorts. The extorters of the left eye are the inferior rectus and the inferior oblique. Their vertical functions cancel each other and there is no vertical over shoot. The intorters of the right eye are the superior rectus and superior oblique muscles. Since the right superior oblique is paretic, the elevation effect of the superior rectus is unopposed and a right hypertropia occurs on tilt to the right.

(more than 5 prism diopters difference right tilt versus left tilt), then perform the Parks three-step test to determine which oblique or vertical rectus muscle is paretic. The three steps are first, determine the hyperdeviation in primary position, second, where is the hypertropia greatest, right or left gaze, and third, on head tilt to which side is the hypertropia greatest, tilt right or tilt left.

TABLE 19–1

First Step Hyper in Primary		Second Step Hyper Increases in which Gaze		Third Step Increased Hyper with Head Tilt	
RHT	RSO	**R**	RIR	**R =**	LIO
	RIR		LIO	**L =**	RIR
	VS				
	LSR	**L**	RSO	**R =**	RSO
	LIO		LSR	**L =**	LSR
LHT	RSR	**R**	RSR	**R =**	RSR
	RIO		LSO	**L =**	LSO
	VS				
	LSO	**L**	RIO	**R =**	LIR
	LIR		LIR	**L =**	RIO

Example: WHICH MUSCLE IS PARETIC?

STEP 1: RIGHT HYPERTROPIA
Right IR or SO   vs   Left SR or IO
(underacting muscles in right versus left eye).

STEP 2: RHT INCREASES IN LEFT GAZE
Left SR   or   Right SO
(the muscles with field of action in left gaze).

STEP 3: RHT INCREASES HEAD TILT TO THE RIGHT
Right tilt induces intorsion of right eye and extorsion of left eye. Both of the muscles in contention (RSO and LSR) are intorters, but only the RSO produces right intorsion, so the answer is RSO palsy.

ANSWER = RSO palsy

Table 19–1 lists the responses to Parks three-step test for all vertical and oblique muscle palsies.

Problems with the Head Tilt Test

A positive head tilt test and the Parks three-step test are not infallible for diagnosing vertical muscle paresis. Patients with dissociated vertical deviations will show a positive head tilt, as will some patients with restrictive causes for vertical strabismus. In addition, the head tilt test is designed to diagnose a single paretic muscle, and it may not be reliable when multiple muscles are involved with restriction or paresis.

■ SUPERIOR OBLIQUE PALSY

A superior oblique palsy or paresis is the most common cause for an isolated vertical deviation (also see Neuro-ophthalmology section IV). The typical findings of a *unilateral superior oblique paresis* include an ipsilateral hyper-

tropia which increases on contralateral side gaze and a positive head tilt test with the hyperdeviation increasing on head tilt to the ipsilateral shoulder. For example, a right superior oblique paresis shows a right hypertropia, which increases in left lateral gaze and increases on head tilt to the right (Fig. 19–3 and example above). Typically, there is associated ipsilateral superior oblique underaction and ipsilateral inferior oblique overaction. In some cases (e.g., congenital superior oblique paresis), there may be relatively little superior oblique underaction and mostly inferior oblique overaction (Fig. 19–3). Patients with a unilateral superior oblique paresis adopt a compensatory head tilt to the side opposite to the paresis to reduce the hypertropia and fuse. Congenital superior oblique palsy is the most likely diagnosis in patients presenting with a hyperdeviation in primary position and a compensatory head tilt.

Bilateral superior oblique paresis is associated with bilateral inferior oblique overaction and bilateral superior oblique underaction and produces a right hypertropia in left gaze and a left hypertropia in right gaze. Other signs include V pattern, extorsion greater than 10°, and a reversing head tilt test, with a right hypertropia tilt right, and a left hypertropia tilt left (Fig. 19–4). In downgaze, the superior oblique muscle functions of ab-

duction and intorsion counteract the adduction and extorsion of the inferior rectus muscles. If the superior oblique muscles are weak, however, the inferior rectus muscles are unopposed, which causes an esotropia shift and extorsion in downgaze. This type of V pattern with little change from upgaze to primary position but a significant esotropia shift from primary position to downgaze has been termed *arrow pattern* by the author (Fig. 19–4). The presence of an arrow pattern with extorsion increasing in downgaze is diagnostic for an acute bilateral superior oblique palsy and is often seen with traumatic superior oblique palsies.

A *bilateral asymmetric superior oblique paresis* can look like a unilateral superior oblique paresis and this is termed *masked bilateral* superior oblique palsy. Suspect a masked bilateral paresis if the hypertropia precipitously diminishes in lateral gaze toward the side of the obviously paretic superior oblique muscle. For example, a right superior oblique palsy with a RHT 15 in primary position that diminishes to RHT 2 in right gaze indicates a possible masked bilateral paresis with a mild

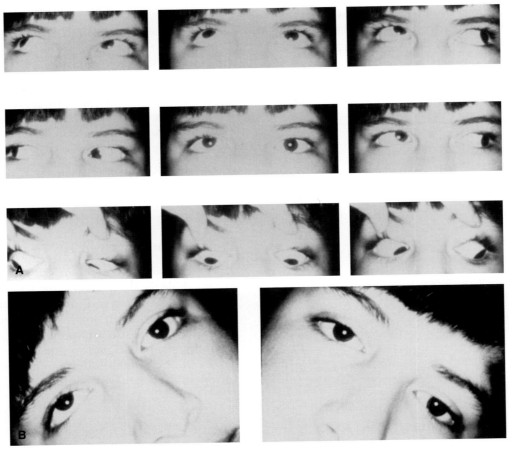

Figure 19–3.
A, Composite 9 gaze photograph of a patient with a congenital right superior oblique palsy. Note the large RHT in primary position that increases in left gaze. There is right inferior oblique overaction +3, and superior oblique underaction −2. In straight right gaze it looks like the left superior oblique is overacting, but the right superior oblique is slightly tight because of secondary contracture. **B,** Positive head tilt test with large RHT on tilt right.

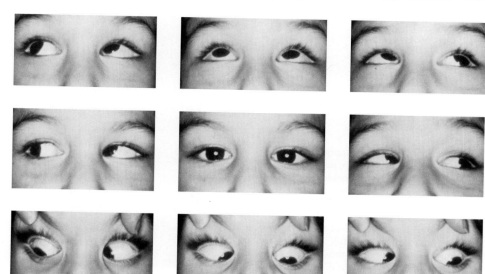

Figure 19–4.
Bilateral congenital superior oblique paresis with V pattern (arrow pattern sub-type with ET increasing from primary position to downgaze. Note a RHT in left gaze and a LHT in rght gaze. There is bilateral inferior oblique overaction (right eye, +1; left eye, +2), and bilateral superior oblique underaction (both eyes, −2). Head tilt (not shown) would have shown a RHT tilting right, and LHT tilting left.

paresis of the left superior oblique muscle. The left inferior oblique should be examined closely for trace overaction. The presence of a V pattern and bilateral extorsion on fundus examination also suggest bilateral involvement in patients with a presumed unilateral palsy. If surgery is performed on only one side of a masked bilateral superior oblique paresis, the contralateral superior oblique paresis will become evident postoperatively. Thus, unilateral surgery can unmask a masked bilateral superior oblique paresis. Clinical signs of unilateral versus bilateral superior oblique paresis are shown in Table 19–2.

Falling Eye

Significant underaction of the superior oblique muscle and fixation with the paretic eye will produce the classic finding called the *falling eye*. When a patient with a superior oblique palsy fixes with the paretic eye and tries

to look down and nasally into the field of action of the paretic superior oblique muscle, the weak superior oblique requires a large amount of innervation to make the eye movement. Because of Hering's law, the yoke muscle (contralateral inferior rectus muscle) receives an equally large amount of innervation. Since the contralateral inferior rectus has normal function, this increased innervation produces a large secondary contralateral hypotropia or falling eye (Fig. 19–5).

Traumatic Superior Oblique Paresis

Traumatic superior oblique paresis is usually associated with severe closed head trauma, loss of consciousness, and cerebral concussion, but even very mild head trauma, without loss of consciousness can cause a superior oblique paresis. It is caused by the tentorium contusion near the posteriorly exiting trochlear nerves.

Trochlear nerve damage occurs when the tentorium

TABLE 19–2
Unilateral vs. Bilateral Superior Oblique Paresis

Clinical Sign	Unilateral	Bilateral
Superior oblique underaction	Ipsilateral underaction	Bilateral underaction
Inferior oblique Overaction	Ipsilateral overaction	Bilateral overaction
V-pattern	Less than 10 prism diopters	Greater than 10 prism diopters with arrow pattern (convergence in down-gaze)
Hypertropia	Greater than 5 prism diopters	Less than 5 prism diopters (except asymmetric paresis)
Head tilt test	Increasing hyper on ipsilateral head tilt (Rt. SOP = RH tilt right)	Positive head tilt to both sides (RHT on tilt to right and LHT on tilt to left)
Extorsion	Less than 10°	Greater than 10°

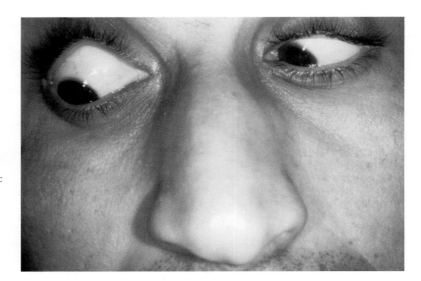

Figure 19–5.
Photograph of a traumatic superior oblique palsy in the left eye showing the falling eye in the right. The paretic eye (left eye) is fixing in the field of action of the paretic superior oblique muscle requiring a great deal of innervation. Because of Hering's law of equal innervation of yoke muscles, the right inferior rectus muscle also receives a great deal of innervation. Since the right inferior rectus is at full strength, it overacts and pulls the right eye down thus causing the appearance of falling eye right eye.

shifts inferiorly and traumatizes the trochlear nerves as they exit the midbrain. Since the two trochlear nerves exit the midbrain together only a few millimeters apart, the nerve trauma is almost always bilateral. Thus, most cases of traumatic superior oblique paresis are bilateral, although the paresis may be asymmetric. The pattern of strabismus is extremely variable. Classically there is a small hypertropia in primary position, a left hypertropia in right gaze and a right hypertropia in left gaze, a V-arrow pattern with an esotropia in downgaze, and extorsion worse in downgaze. Because the strabismus is acquired, patients older than 6 years of age will experience torsional, vertical, and horizontal diplopia that increases in downgaze. The management of traumatic superior oblique paresis is to watch the patient conservatively for at least 6 months. During this time, serial measurements of the deviation should be taken to establish a pattern of possible recovery. Alternate patch-

ing will eliminate the diplopia and may help to reduce secondary contracture of the ipsilateral superior rectus muscle. After 6 months of observation, if the superior oblique paresis persists, surgery can be considered (see Treatment below).

Congenital Superior Oblique Palsy

The cause of congenital superior oblique palsy is unknown. In some cases, the superior oblique paresis is associated with a lax tendon and rarely an absent superior oblique tendon (7, 12). Plager suggests performing exaggerated forced duction test of the superior oblique tendon at the begining of surgery to see if the tendon is lax or absent (12). These authors advocate tightening the superior oblique tendon (SO tuck) if forced ductions indicate a lax superior oblique tendon (7, 12).

Patients with congenital superior oblique palsy often

TABLE 19–3
Unilateral Superior Oblique Paresis

Clinical Manifestation	Procedure
Inferior oblique overaction. Hyperdeviation in primary position <10PD. Deviation is greatest in up-gaze.	Inferior oblique weakening
Superior oblique underaction with mininal inferior oblique overaction Hyperdeviation in primary position <10PD. Deviation greatest in down gaze.	Small superior oblique tuck or Inferior oblique weakening
Inferior oblique overaction with superior oblique underaction Hyperdeviation in primary position >10 prism diopters	Ipsilateral inferior oblique weakening with contralateral inferior rectus recession or Ipsilateral superior oblique tuck with contralateral inferior rectus recession

TABLE 19–4
Treatment of Bilateral Superior Oblique Palsy

Clinical Manifestation	Procedure
Pure Excyclodiplopia >8 Minimal hypertropia, <8PD, small V pattern, and minimal inferior oblique overaction and superior oblique underaction	Bilateral Harada-Ito
Bilateral superior oblique underaction Big arrow pattern (>15PD increase in esotropia from primary to down gaze), >10° extorsion in primary position increasing in downgaze, and reversing hypertropias in side-gaze	Bilateral full superior oblique tendon tuck with bilateral medial rectus inferior transposition ½ tendon width
Asymmetric bilateral superior oblique palsy (masked bilateral) Hyperdeviation in primary position >10 prism diopters, asymmetric inferior oblique overaction	Unilateral superior oblique tuck plus inferior oblique weakening procedure or superior oblique strengthening procedure on the less paretic side (masked side)

show a pattern of a unilateral paresis or an asymmetric bilateral paresis. There is usually a large hypertropia in primary position and significant inferior oblique overaction usually with relatively less superior oblique underaction (Fig. 19–3). Even though the paresis is present at birth, the first clinical sign of congenital superior oblique paresis often presents in late childhood or even adulthood. Normal vertical fusional amplitudes are weak and even small hyperdeviations of 3 to 5 prism diopters cannot be fused. Patients with congenital superior oblique paresis, however, develop large vertical fusional amplitudes, and fuse large hypertropias up to 35 prism diopters. The presence of large vertical fusion amplitudes is an important clinical sign that the hyperdeviation is long-standing, rather than acutely acquired and is suggestive of a congenital superior oblique palsy. Over time the fusional control weakens resulting in a deviation that becomes manifest in later life.

In addition to large fusional vergence amplitudes, patients with congenital superior oblique paresis adopt a compensatory head tilt opposite to the palsy to minimize the deviation and establish binocular fusion. Patients with congenital superior oblique paresis typically have good stereopsis and show the hyperdeviation intermittently when they are fatigued. Even though patients with congenital superior oblique paresis have high grade stereopsis, most also have the ability to suppress, so most do not experience diplopia.

Other Causes of Superior Oblique Paresis

The majority of superior oblique pareses are either congenital or traumatic, but other causes include vascular disease with brain stem lacunar infarcts, multiple sclerosis, intracranial neoplasm, herpes zoster ophthalmi-cus, diabetes and associated mononeuropathy, and iatrogenic after superior oblique tenotomy. If no specific cause of an acquired superior oblique paresis can be found, a neurologic work-up including neuroimaging should be performed (see Eye Movement Disorders, Chapter 9, Table 9–2).

Treatment of Superior Oblique Paresis

The treatment of superior oblique paresis (SOP) depends on the pattern of the strabismus. Preoperative evaluation for inferior oblique overaction and superior oblique underaction is critical. Cardinal position of gaze measurements are also important to determine the pattern of strabismus and where the deviation is greatest. Most treatment strategies identify where the deviation is greatest, then design a surgery to correct the deviation in primary position while the reducing incomitance (8). For example, a right unilateral superior oblique palsy with a hypertropia less than 10 prism diopters, and inferior oblique overaction, minimal superior oblique underaction can be treated with a simple ipsilateral inferior oblique weakening procedure (e.g., inferior oblique recession or partial anteriorization). If the hypertropia in primary position is greater than 10 to 12 prism diopters, then an isolated inferior oblique recession will not be enough to correct the hypertropia. In this case, one should add a contralateral inferior rectus recession in addition to an ipsilateral inferior oblique recession. Late overcorrections after inferior rectus recessions have been known to occur, so be conservative in regard to recessing the contralateral inferior rectus muscle.

Patients who have a bilateral superior oblique paresis with extorsion and a large arrow pattern with an esotropia greater than 10 prism diopters in downgaze should be considered for bilateral superior oblique tucks and bilateral medial rectus recessions with infraplacement. Patients with bilateral traumatic superior oblique paresis after closed head trauma may have partial recovery, and may be left with extorsional diplopia, without significant oblique dysfunction, V pattern or hypertropia. In these cases, extorsion can be corrected by the Harada-Ito procedure, which consists of selectively tightening the anterior 25% to 33% of the superior oblique tendon fibers (Fig. 19–6).

Tightening the entire width of the superior oblique tendon (i.e., SO tuck), has theoretical utility for improving superior oblique function. A SO tuck however, usually results in some improvement of superior oblique function, but the tight tendon also creates restrictive leash to elevation in adduction (i.e., *iatrogenic Brown's syndrome*). Perhaps the best indication for an SO tuck is a mild superior oblique paresis associated with a small hypertropia, −1 superior oblique underaction and a deviation that is greatest in downgaze. The tuck also has been suggested in patients with congenital su-

perior oblique paresis secondary to a congenitally lax superior oblique tendon (7, 12).

Table 19–3 lists the treatment for three common presentations of unilateral superior oblique paresis and Table 19–4 lists treatment strategies for bilateral superior oblique paresis.

Primary Inferior Oblique Overaction

Primary inferior oblique overaction is most commonly associated with a horizontal strabismus such as congenital esotropia or intermittent exotropia. Isolated primary inferior oblique overaction also can occur without associated horizontal strabismus. Although primary inferior oblique overaction is bilateral in most cases, it can be quite asymmetric, with the lesser overacting inferior oblique difficult to detect (11). When inferior oblique overaction is identified, it is important to differentiate primary inferior oblique overaction from a secondary inferior oblique overaction (i.e., superior oblique paresis). It can be difficult to differentiate primary inferior oblique overaction from secondary overaction, as patients with marked inferior oblique overaction may have significant superior oblique underaction secondary to the tight inferior oblique muscle. Conversely, patients with a superior oblique paresis often have inferior oblique overaction. In addition, indirect ophthalmoscopy will show significant objective extorsion in both primary and secondary inferior oblique overaction. The key to distinguishing primary from secondary inferior oblique overaction is the head tilt test. The head tilt test is negative in primary inferior oblique overaction, and positive with secondary overaction (see SOP above). In both groups, there is the typical upshoot of the adducting eye and both types usually manifest a significant V-pattern, especially if there is bilateral inferior oblique overaction. The type of V-pattern, however, can help differentiate primary vs. secondary inferior oblique overaction. Patients with primary inferior oblique overaction have a *Y-pattern* with a significant exotropia shift occurring from primary position to upgaze, but relatively little change between primary position and downgaze. The Y pattern occurs because the inferior oblique muscles act as abductors in upgaze. In counter distinction, a V pattern associated with superior oblique paresis (especially bilateral) shows an arrow pattern with an esotropia shift which occurs from primary position to downgaze. Table 19–5 compares the clinical signs of primary inferior oblique overaction with secondary inferior oblique overaction caused by superior oblique paresis.

Since the inferior oblique muscle is an elevator, abductor and intortor, these elements are exaggerated in direct proportion to overaction. When quantitating inferior oblique overaction look at the entire function of the muscle, including the upshoot, amount of V-pattern

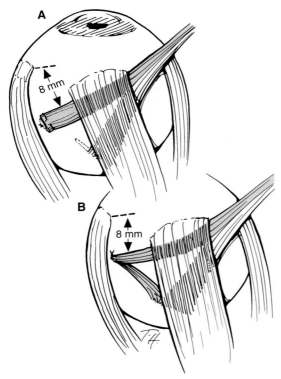

Figure 19–6.
Harada Ito procedure. **A,** Disinsertion technique: where anterior fibers of superior oblique tendon are disinserted and moved temporally to a spot close to the superior border of the lateral rectus muscle and 8 mm posterior to the lateral rectus insertion. **B,** Pullover technique. The anterior superior oblique tendon fibers are isolated and pulled terminally as with the disinsertion technique, but they are displaced without disinsertion.

TABLE 19–5
Primary Inferior Oblique Overaction vs. Superior Oblique Palsy

Clinical Sign	Primary Overaction	Secondary Overaction
Inferior oblique overaction	Yes	Yes
V-pattern	Yes, Y-pattern	Yes, "arrow" pattern
Head tilt test	Negative	Positive
Subjective torsion	No	Yes (except in congenital superior oblique palsies)
Objective extorsion (fundus examination)	Yes	Yes
Underaction of ipsilateral superior oblique muscle	No (minimal if any)	Yes

(Y-pattern subtype) and fundus extorsion (5, 16). Figure 19–1 shows various degrees of inferior oblique muscle overaction on a scale of one to four.

Mimickers of Inferior Oblique Overaction

Inferior oblique overaction is the most common, but by no means the only cause of an ocular upshoot in adduction. Dissociated vertical deviation (DVD) can look just like inferior oblique overaction, because DVD will become manifest in sidegaze as the adducted eye is occluded by the nasal bridge. This results in a hyperdeviation in sidegaze, which mimics inferior oblique overaction. DVD is differentiated from inferior oblique overaction by occluding the affected eye in abduction as well as adduction and evaluating for a change in the vertical deviation. If the elevation is the same in adduction and abduction, then this is DVD. An increasing hyperdeviation in adduction suggests inferior oblique overaction. DVD commonly coexists with inferior oblique overaction in patients with infantile esotropia. In these cases the distinction can be extremely difficult. The presence of a V-pattern (Y subtype), a true hyperdeviation in lateral gaze with a hypotropia of the contralateral eye, and objective extorsion on indirect ophthalmoscopy indicate inferior oblique overaction and not DVD.

An upshoot in adduction can also be caused by a tight lateral rectus muscle associated with a large exotropia or lateral rectus co-contraction in Duane's syndrome. As the eye adducts and slightly elevates the tight lateral rectus pulls the eye up causing pseudo-overaction of inferior oblique. Aberrant innervation of the inferior oblique or superior rectus muscle also has been documented as another cause of an upshoot associated with Duane's syndrome.

Treatment of Inferior Oblique Overaction

Surgery is indicated when the inferior oblique overaction and V-pattern interfere with fusion or are a cosmetic problem. In general, +2 or more inferior oblique overaction should be considered surgically significant while +1 or less overaction usually does not require treatment. There are, however, two important exceptions to this rule. The first exception is in patients with bilateral asymmetric inferior oblique overaction in whom one eye shows minimal overaction. In these cases, both inferior oblique muscles should be weakened, even if one only shows trace overaction. Unilateral inferior oblique weakening surgery in an asymmetric bilateral case unmasks the inferior oblique overaction of the unoperated eye. The other exception where inferior oblique surgery should be considered despite minimal upshoot on sidegaze is bilateral overaction associated with a significant V-pattern, Y-subtype. Patients who have a significant divergence from primary position to upgaze should have inferior oblique weakening even when minimal overaction seen on versions.

In most cases, inferior oblique overaction is bilateral, and bilateral surgery should be performed. Patients with amblyopia of two lines or greater difference, however, should have monocular surgery limited to the amblyopic eye in order to avoid the risk (although slight) of surgical complications to the nonamblyopic eye. When inferior oblique overaction coexists with horizontal strabismus, both should be corrected at the same operation. Staged planning of two separate operations does not improve surgical results and requires a second anaesthesia. When planning simultaneous horizontal and inferior oblique surgery, the horizontal surgical numbers are not altered. While the inferior oblique muscles have an abduction function, weakening the inferior obliques does not significantly alter the horizontal alignment.

Surgical Techniques for Weakening the Inferior Oblique Muscles

Surgical techniques for correcting inferior oblique overaction include myectomy, recession and anteriorization (Fig. 19–7) (1, 4, 9). Note that in Figure 19–7C, the anteriorized inferior oblique muscle now is no

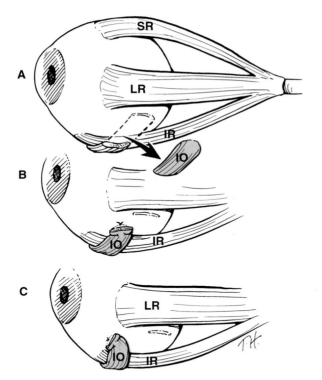

TABLE 19–6
Surgical Techniques for Inferior Oblique Overaction

Degrees of Overaction	Possible Techiques
+1	• Recession (small)
+2	• Recession (large) • Myectomy
+3	• Recession with partial anteriorization • Myectomy
+4	• Full anteriorization (bilateral surgery only) • Extirpation/denervation • Myectomy

Figure 19–7.
Inferior oblique weakening procedures **A,** Myectomy. Hatch marks show the temporal portion of the muscle removed in the procedure. **B,** Recession-slight anteriorization. The muscle is recessed towards the inferior rectus muscle so the new insertion is closer to the origin. The new insertion is slightly anterior to the natural arch of contact of the muscle. **C,** Full anteriorization with J deformity. The muscle is recessed and transposed anteriorly to inferior rectus insertion. The posterior border of the muscle anteriorized thus creating the J deformity. This proceedure can induce a hypotropia. It is performed for severe inferior oblique overaction, and performed bilaterally to avoid the induced hypotropia.

longer an elevator and abductor, but is now anterior to the equator and pulls the front of the eye down and is actually a depressor. This is why full anteriorization procedures can lead to an ipsilateral hypodeviation (3, 14), and should only be performed bilaterally for severe inferior oblique overaction. The authors prefer the graded—anterior transposition procedure. The advantage over myectomy is that it is reversible and that the inferior oblique muscle is left intact for reoperation. Surgical options for various degrees of inferior oblique overaction are listed on Table 19–6. Figure 19–8 shows a graded anteriorization for a specific degree of inferior oblique overaction.

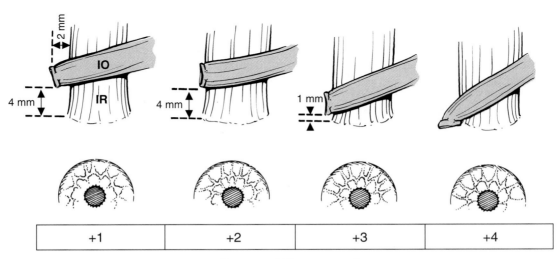

Degree of IO overreaction

Figure 19–8.
Surgeon's view of author's graded technique for inferior oblique weakening based the degree of inferior oblique overaction. The more anterior the new insertion the greater the effect of the surgery. Surgery A is for +1 inferior oblique overaction and D is for +4 and should only be performed bilaterally.

■ SUPERIOR OBLIQUE OVERACTION

The cause of superior oblique overaction (SOOA) is unknown. It may be related to an associated paresis of the contralateral inferior rectus muscle, thus producing a secondary overaction of the yoke superior oblique muscle. The author has noted several patients with superior oblique overaction who also have an underacting contralateral inferior rectus muscle.

Clinical Features of SOOA

Superior oblique overaction is an exaggeration of the normal function of the superior oblique muscle including depression, abduction, and incyclotorsion. Patients with SOOA show a downshoot of the adducting eye in lateral gaze, abduction in downgaze causing an A-pattern and objective incyclotorsion which is seen on indirect ophthalmoscopy. The A-pattern is not symmetrical, but shows more divergence from primary position to downgaze, than from upgaze to primary position. This type of A-pattern is termed a lambda pattern (λ) (Fig. 19–9).

Superior oblique overaction often occurs in association with horizontal strabismus such as intermittent ex-

otropia. Most patients with superior oblique overaction do not show subjective incyclotorsion by Maddox rod testing, even though indirect ophthalmoscopy reveals intorsion. This is because of sensory adaptation as the superior oblique overaction has been present since early infancy. Like inferior oblique overaction, superior oblique overaction is usually bilateral.

Another characteristic of superior oblique overaction is limited elevation in adduction. This is secondary to a contracted tight superior oblique muscle.

Differential Diagnosis of SOOA

The differential diagnosis of limited elevation in adduction includes, superior oblique overaction, Brown's syndrome, and inferior oblique paresis (Table 19–7). *Brown's syndrome* is caused by a tight superior oblique muscle tendon complex (see Chapter 20). In Brown's syndrome there is no superior oblique overaction and forced ductions are positive to elevation in adduction. In addition, the syndrome is often associated with an exodeviation when the eyes move from primary position to upgaze (Y-pattern) whereas supe-

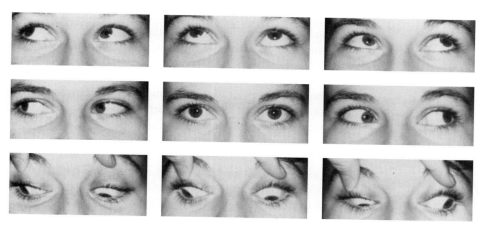

Figure 19–9.
Bilateral superior oblique overaction (+3 in both eyes) with typical A pattern lambda subtype, with increasing divergence in downgaze.

TABLE 19–7

	Brown's Syndrome	Primary Superior Oblique Overaction	Inferior Oblique Paresis
Bilateral Involvement	Unusual	Common	Unusual
Pattern	"Y" (divergence in up gaze)	Lambda (divergence in down gaze)	"A" (convergence in up gaze)
Superior Oblique Overaction	No	Yes	Yes
Inferior Oblique Underaction	Yes	Minimal or Moderate	Yes
Standard Forced Ductions	Positive	Negative	Negative
Head Tilt Test	Negative	Negative	Positive
Torsion	None to slight intorsion in up gaze	Intorsion (increasing in down gaze)	Intorsion increasing in up gaze
Greatest vertical deviation	Up gaze	Down gaze	Up gaze

rior oblique overaction is associated with a lambda A-pattern.

Inferior oblique paresis also can be confused with superior oblique overaction because there is overaction of the ipsilateral superior oblique in this condition. In fact, cases of primary superior oblique overaction may represent a mild inferior oblique paresis. Unlike primary superior oblique overaction, inferior oblique paresis is associated with a positive head tilt test and the largest hyperdeviation occurs when the patient looks up and in. Congenital inferior oblique paresis is rare. It is often unilateral and associated with a large hypotropia in primary position. Acquired inferior oblique paresis can be secondary to a lacunar midbrain infarct or rarely, head trauma. Patients with acquired inferior oblique paresis experience cyclovertical diplopia. The surgical treatment of unilateral inferior oblique paresis is an ipsilateral superior oblique weakening procedure such as the silicone expander. A contralateral superior rectus recession is added if the hypotropia is 10 prism diopters or more, as is usually the case.

■ TREATMENT OF SOOA

The ideal superior oblique weakening procedure produces a measured slackening of the muscle-tendon complex without disrupting the functional mechanics of the insertion. Many surgical approaches to weaken the superior oblique have been tried (2, 13). Presently the two most commonly used procedures are the superior oblique tenotomy and the Wright silicone tendon expander (17, 18). The tenotomy technique involves cutting the tendon in two, while the silicone tendon expander consists of inserting a segment of a 240 retinal silicone band between the cut ends of a nasal tenotomy to elongate the tendon (Fig. 19–10). Table 19–8 lists the length of the silicone for a specific amount of superior oblique overaction (15, 17).

Other superior oblique weakening procedures include tenectomy, recession, posterior tenotomy, and split tendon elongation (2, 13). In a comparative study, the author found the silicone tendon expander to be superior to tenotomy especially in patients with preoperative fusion (15). Superior oblique tenotomy on patients with high-grade stereopsis and fusion carries a significant risk for creating a secondary superior oblique paresis and causing postoperative diplopia (10). In these cases, the silicone tendon expander is preferred. Another situation where superior oblique weakening procedures can cause problems is in patients with pre-existing DVD. Weakening the superior obliques will exacerbate DVD. In these cases, options are to treat the A pattern with horizontal rectus muscle transpositions rather than weakening the superior obliques, or to plan an undercorrection of the superior oblique overaction with the silicone tendon expander. The advantage of the superior oblique silicone tendon expander is that it lengthens the superior oblique tendon in a controlled manner and holds the cut tendon ends apart at a fixed distance. This reduces postoperative superior oblique paresis, allows for controlled weaken-

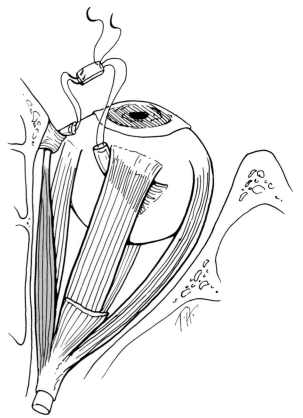

Figure 19–10.
Wright's superior oblique silicone expander: A segment of a retinal 240 band is sewn between the cut ends of the superior oblique tendon. This procedure lenghtens the tendon in a graded fashion, separating the tendon end a specific amount. The silicone keeps the ends from growing back together.

TABLE 19–8
Silicone Expander Length Chart

Superior Oblique Overaction	Length of Silicone
+1	4 mm
+2	5 mm
+3	6 mm
+4	7 mm

ing, and makes it possible to find cut tendon ends if re-operation is necessary.

Treatment of A and V Patterns

Patients with A and V patterns who have minimal or no inferior oblique overaction can be managed by offsetting or transposing the horizontal rectus muscles superiorly or inferiorly. In cases with a significant oblique dysfunction, it is appropriate to operate on the obliques rather than perform a transposition. For large A and V patterns that are disproportionate to the amount of oblique dysfunction, combining horizontal rectus muscle offsets with oblique surgery should be considered.

The horizontal offset procedure changes vector forces, so if the medial rectus muscle is infraplaced, the medial rectus muscles will have increased function when the eyes rotate up, thus collapsing the V pattern. Conversely, when the eye rotates down, the infraplaced medial rectus muscles slacken, resulting in divergence of the apex of the V. The direction for moving a horizontal rectus muscle for an A and V pattern is shown in Figure 19–11. For example, a patient with A-pattern exotropia can be managed by bilateral lateral rectus recessions and infraplacement of the lateral rectus muscles. One-half tendon width of vertical displacement results in approximately 15 prism diopters of pattern correction. A full tendon width vertical displacement results in approximately 25 prism diopters of correction

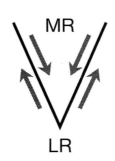 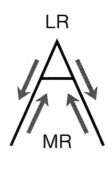

Figure 19–11.
Vertical transposition of horizontal muscles for A and V patterns. The red arrows indicate the direction of movement with the lateral rectus (LR) moved up for a V pattern and down for an A pattern. The medial rectus are moved down for a V pattern and up for an A patern. Thus, medial rectus is moved toward the apex of the A or V, and the lateral rectus moved away from the apex of the A or V. This transposition holds true whether the muscles are recessed, or resected.

and is reserved for extremely large A or V patterns. Vertical transposition of horizontal rectus muscle by one full tendon width reduces the vector forces at the horizontal plane. A full tendon width infraplacement of the lateral rectus muscles would predispose to an overcorrection (esotropia) postoperatively. In these cases, the amount of recession is slightly reduced in anticipation of a overcorrection.

■ REFERENCES

1. Apt L, Call NB: Inferior oblique muscle recession. Am J Ophthalmol 1978;95:95.
2. Berke RN: Tenotomy of the superior oblique for hypertropia. Trans Am Ophthalmol Soc 1946;44:304–342.
3. Bremer DL, Rogers GL, Quick LD: Primary position hypotropia after anterior transposition of the inferior oblique. Arch Ophthalmol 1986;104:229–232.
4. Elliot L, Nankin J: Anterior transposition of the inferior oblique. J Pediatr Ophthalmol Strabismus 1981;18:35.
5. Guyton DL: Clinical assessment of ocular torsion. Am Orthopt J 1983;33:7.
6. Harada M, Ito Y: Visual correction of cyclotropia. Japanese J Oph 1964;8:88
7. Helveston EM: Classification of superior oblique muscle palsy. Ophthalmology 1992;99:1609–1615.
8. Knapp RP: Classification and treatment of superior oblique palsy. Am Orthop J 1974;24:18–22.
9. Mims JL, Wood RC: Bilateral anterior transposition of the inferior obliques. Arch Ophthalmol 1989;107:41.
10. Parks MM: Bilateral superior oblique tenotomy for A-pattern strabismus in patients with fusion (commentary). Binocular Vision 1988;3:39.
11. Parks MM: The overacting inferior oblique muscle. Am J Ophthalmol 1974;77:787.
12. Plager DA: Traction testing and superior oblique palsy. J Pediatr Ophthalmol Strabismus 1990;27:136–140.
13. Romano P, Roholt P: Measured graduated recession of the superior oblique muscle. J Pediatr Ophthalmol Strabismus 1983;20:134–140.
14. Stager DR, Weakley DR, Stager D: Anterior transposition of the inferior oblique: anatomic assessment of the neurovascular bundle. Arch Ophthalmol 1992;110:360.
15. Wright KW, Min BM, Park C: Comparison of superior oblique tendon expander to superior oblique tenotomy for the management of superior oblique overaction and Brown syndrome. J Pediatr Ophthalmol Strabismus 1992;29:92–99.
16. Wright KW: Current approaches to inferior oblique muscle surgery. In: Hoyt CS (ed). Focal points 1986: clinical modules for ophthalmologists. Am Acad Ophthalmol, 1986;1.
17. Wright KW: Superior oblique silicone expander for Brown's syndrome and superior oblique overaction. J Pediatr Ophthalmol Strabismus 1991;28:101–107.
18. Wright KW: Surgical procedure for lengthening the superior oblique tendon. Invest Ophthalmol Vis Sci 1989; 30(suppl):377.

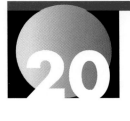

20 Complex Strabismus: Paralytic and Restrictive Strabismus, Ocular Torticollis, and Dissociated Vertical Deviation

Kenneth W. Wright, Jyoti Raina

The types of strabismus described in the previous chapters (e.g., congenital esotropia, accommodative esotropia, and intermittent exotropia) are associated with full ocular ductions. In this chapter, we review the evaluation and management of incomitant strabismus, caused by limited ocular rotations associated with paralysis and restriction. In addition a discussion of ocular torticollis and dissociated vertical deviation (DVD) is presented.

■ PARALYTIC AND RESTRICTIVE STRABISMUS

The first step in the evaluation of strabismus associated with limited ocular rotations is to determine the diagnosis of paresis or restriction or both (1). Causes of paresis include cranial nerve palsy, congenital agenisis of an extraocular muscle, or a traumatically ruptured or disinserted muscle (e.g., poststrabismus surgery slipped). Ocular restriction is caused by a tight extraocular muscle (e.g., thyroid disease, congenital fibrosis syndrome, Brown's syndrome), periocular scarring to the eye or eye muscles (e.g., fat adherence), or an orbital fracture with orbital fat and or muscle entrapment. In some cases, restriction and paresis can coexist. Examples include an extra ocular muscle palsy, which produces a large deviation, which causes secondary contracture of the antagonist muscle, or a traumatically disinserted or damaged muscle with associated periocular scarring.

Diagnostic tests that differentiate paresis from restriction include forced ductions, force generation test, saccadic velocity measurements, intraocular pressure changes in various fields of gaze, and lid fissure changes in sidegaze.

Forced ductions are performed by grasping the eye with a forceps, then passively moving the eye into the field of limited ocular rotation. If the eye shows a resistance to rotation with the forceps (positive forced ductions), then there is a restriction. If forced duction testing shows full ocular rotations (negative forced ductions), yet on duction testing there is limited movement, then a muscle weakness is the cause of limited rotations, not a restriction.

Force generation test directly measures muscle force. The eye is grasped with a forceps, and the patient is asked to look into the field of limited rotation. The examiner feels the pull of the muscle against the forceps, and compares this with the fellow eye or the antagonist muscle. If there is diminished pull from the muscle into the field of limited rotation, then a paresis is present. Forced ductions can be used in conjunction with forced generation testing. If forced ductions are positive, and the forced generation test shows poor muscle function, then the diagnosis is a combination of restriction and paresis.

Saccadic velocity measurements can help differentiate restriction versus paresis by observation without touching the eye, so this method can be used on young children as well as adults. The test is based on the fact that normal muscle function is required to generate a saccadic eye movement, therefore the presence of a saccade indicates the normal muscle function. Saccadic eye movements can be stimulated by a rotating optokinetic drum, and can be measured by electroculargram (EOG) recordings, or by clinical estimation. A restriction is associated with a normal saccadic velocities, but the eye stops abruptly when the restriction is met. This is termed the dog on a leash sign, as ocular velocity pattern is an analogy to a dog running until it abruptly stops at the end of the leash. In contrast, a paretic muscle does not have the power to generate a saccadic eye movement, and the eye shows slow eye movement that does not generate a saccad.

Another sign of restriction is increased intraocular pressure (IOP) on attempted duction into the field of restriction. Lid fissure narrowing occurs on ductions away from a tight muscle, and lid fissure widening occurs on ductions toward a paretic muscle (also see Duane's syndrome, Fig. 20–2).

■ PARALYTIC STRABISMUS

This section discusses the management of third and sixth nerve paralysis. For the management of fourth nerve palsies, see Chapter 19, on Oblique Muscle Dysfunction. The evaluation and differential diagnosis of cranial nerve palsies is covered in the chapter entitled Neuro-ophthalmology.

Acquired Third and Sixth Cranial Nerve Paresis

After the appropriate neurologic evaluation, the initial management of an acquired third or sixth nerve paresis is observation for at least 6 months before considering strabismus surgery. An observation period is important because the majority of patients will show at least some recovery, and some will even regain complete function. During the observation period, secondary contracture of the antagonist muscle may occur, especially if the deviation is large. Muscle contraction occurs, as the antagonist muscle is slackened by the ocular deviation. Over several months, the antagonist takes up the muscle slack and becomes contracted and tight. Part-time occlusion of the nonparetic eye forces fixation to the paretic eye and may reduce secondary contracture. In the case of acute sixth nerve palsy, some advocate injecting botulinum into the ipsilateral medial rectus muscle to create a temporary medial rectus paresis, thus preventing medial rectus muscle contracture. The effects of botulinum slowly wears off after 3 to 8 months. The use of botulinum is controversial. Drawbacks include limited abduction and adduction of the paretic eye, which can be annoying to the patient, diffusion to other extraocular muscles, causing a vertical deviation or more frequently ptosis, and persistent medial rectus paresis that lasts past the 6-month observation period (9, 12). If the deviation is relatively small, press-on prisms can be tried to neutralize the deviation in primary position and stimulate fusion.

Surgical Management of Sixth Nerve Palsy

The management of sixth nerve paresis is based on the amount of lateral rectus function present (Table 20–1). If the lateral rectus function is less than 50% of normal, then an ipsilateral medial rectus muscle recession and a vertical muscle transposition procedure are indicated.

There are two basic transposition procedures: the full-tendon transfer (Knapp procedure) and the split tendon transfer (Hummelsheim and Jensen procedures) (Fig. 20–1). The Knapp procedure is described

TABLE 20–1
Surgical Management of Sixth Nerve Paresis

A. Good lateral rectus function	• Recess ipsilateral medial rectus muscle, (adjustable suture), resection of ipsilateral lateral rectus muscle, and small contralateral medial rectus recession with or without faden.
B. Poor lateral rectus function	• Ipsilateral medial rectus recession, (adjustable suture) and transfer of superior and inferior rectus muscle temporally (Hummelsheim split tendon transfer preferred by author)
	• Botulinum to ipsilateral medial rectus muscle and lateral transposition of vertical rectus mucles.

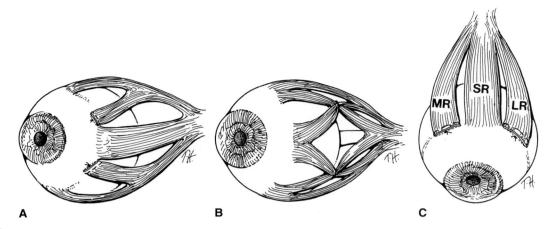

Figure 20–1.
Transposition procedures for muscle palsies. (From Wright, K: Color Atlas of Ophthalmic Surgery: Strabismus. Philadelphia: J. B. Lippincott, 1991.) **A,** Diagram of the *Hummelsheim* procedure, which is a split tendon transfer of half the superior and inferior rectus muscles laterally. This procedure can be performed either vertically or horizontally. The split-tendon transfer has an advantage over a full-tendon transfer as some of the anterior ciliary vessels are left intact, thus reducing the chances for a postoperative anterior segment ischemia. **B,** *Jensen* procedure is a split-tendon transfer procedure where the muscle is not disinserted but there is a muscle union between adjacent muscles. Note in the diagram that half the superior rectus is joined with half of the lateral rectus and half the inferior rectus is joined with half the lateral rectus. This increases lateral forces and is used for sixth nerve palsy. **C,** Diagram shows full muscle transfer or *Knapp* procedure of the medial and lateral rectus muscles superiorly. This is used for double elevator palsy, but a full-tendon transfer can be used on the superior and inferior recti for the management of sixth nerve palsies.

below for the treatment of double elevator palsy, but can be modified by transposing the superior and inferior rectus muscles laterally, to treat sixth nerve palsies. A full-tendon transfer disrupts major contributors to the anterior segment circulation and therefore carries a significant risk of anterior segment ischemia. Split-tendon transfer procedures have the advantage of preserving half of the vertical rectus anterior cilliary vessels, reducing the incidence of postoperative anterior segment ischemia. A possible disadvantage of the split tendon transfer procedure is its lesser effect. Split-tendon procedures, however, can produce strong abduction forces if the muscle being transposed is fully mobilized, by splitting the muscle at least 14 mm posterior to the muscle insertion. For nonresolving sixth nerve palsies, botulinum toxin injection to the ipsilateral medial rectus muscle in combination with strabismus surgery has been recommended (3, 15).

If lateral rectus function is good, then recess the ipsilateral medial rectus (with or without adjustable suture), and reset the ipsilateral lateral rectus muscle. Also consider weakening contralateral medial rectus muscle (yoke to the paretic lateral rectus muscle) with a recession or a recession plus a faden. Weakening the contralateral medial rectus muscle helps to match yoke function, thus improving lateral incomitance.

Surgical Management of Third Nerve Palsy

There is no good procedure for a complete third nerve palsy, however, a large ipsilateral recession of the lateral

rectus and resection of the medial rectus with superior oblique tenotomy can improve the condition. Often there is a ptosis, and one may consider a silicone frontalis sling to raise the lid (see Chapter 27). If there is poor superior rectus function and no Bell's phenomenon, then the patient is at risk for corneal exposure development after lid sling procedure. In these patients, it is wise to undercorrect the ptosis to avoid exposure. Silicone material is preferred because it can be easily removed if corneal exposure occurs. Superior oblique tendon transfer to medial rectus insertion has been described to correct the exotropia, but this procedure has resulted in inadequate horizontal alignment and postoperative limitation of depression (16).

Slipped and Lost Muscle

An important complication of strabismus surgery is a slipped or lost muscle. Orbital trauma also can result in a lost or damaged muscle. The medial rectus is most commonly lost or slipped muscle after strabismus surgery. A slipped muscle after strabismus surgery is caused by suturing the muscle capsule or anterior Tenon's capsule instead of true muscle tendon. Anterior Tenon's capsule and muscle capsule are then secured to sclera, so the muscle slips posteriorly while a pseudo tendon of connective tissue is attached to sclera.

A lost muscle is when the muscle retracts posteriorly there is no connection of the muscle to sclera. The medial rectus muscle is the most difficult to retrieve, as there are no fascial connections to oblique muscles, which keep the muscle from retracting posteriorly. In contrast, the inferior, superior, and the lateral recti have check ligaments that connect to adjacent oblique muscles.

Typical signs of a slipped or lost muscle include decreased muscle function with limited ductions and lid fissure widening on attempted duction into the field of the lost muscle. On occasion, the presentation may be subtle with slight limitation of duction as the only finding. The key observation is an incomitant deviation with underaction of the slipped muscle.

The management of slipped or lost muscle is to find and advance the muscle to anterior sclera if possible. Full-thickness locking bites through muscle fibers must be obtained. If a lost muscle cannot be retrieved, then a transposition procedure such as the Hummelsheim should be performed.

Congenital Absence of Extraocular Muscles

Although virtually all extraocular muscles have been described as being absent, the inferior rectus is most commonly so affected (10). The condition is often associated with craniofacial dysostosis, anencephaly (2) or other congenital anomalies. An absent rectus is managed by a Hummelsheim-type procedure to substitute for the absent muscle.

Duane's Syndrome

Duane's retraction syndrome (DRS) is caused by a congenital hypoplasia of the sixth nerve nucleus with misdirection of the medial rectus nerve, splitting to innervate both the medial rectus and the lateral rectus muscles and is usually unilateral and rarely bilateral (6, 13). Because both the medial and lateral rectus muscles are innervated by the nerve to the medial rectus muscle, both muscles fire and contract simultaneously on attempted adduction. This co-contraction of the medial and lateral rectus muscles on adduction gives rise to the term Duane's co-contraction syndrome. This co-contraction causes globe retraction with lid fissure narrowing on attempted adduction. On attempted abduction, however, the lid fissure widens because the lateral rectus muscle is paretic, and the medial rectus muscle tone is inhibited per Sherrington's law (7) (Fig. 20–2). Duane's syndrome is associated with a variety of systemic disease, including Goldenhars' syndrome and prenatal use of the teratogen thalidomide.

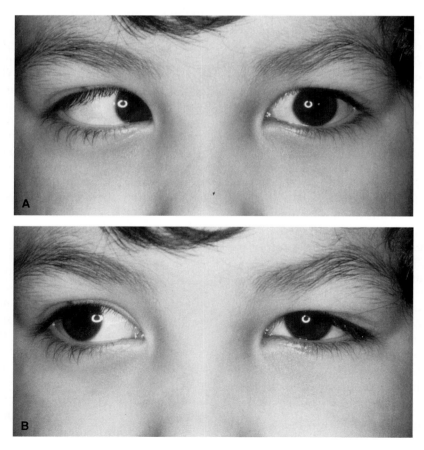

Figure 20–2.
Duane's retraction syndrome in the left eye. **A,** Widening of palpebral fissures on attempted abduction. **B,** Narrowing of palpebral fissures on adduction.

Duane's syndrome can be classified into three categories plus synergistic divergence: type I, poor abduction; type II, poor adduction; and type III, poor adduction and abduction (14, 17, 18). These clinical types of Duane's syndrome represent different innervational abnormalities. In type I, the medial rectus muscle receives most of the medial rectus nerve innervation and the lateral rectus minimal innervation from the medial rectus nerve (Fig. 20–3A). This is the most common type of Duane's syndrome (14). It is usually associated with the Duane's eye fixed in an adducted position, an esotropia in primary position, and a compensatory face turn in the direction of the Duane's eye (i.e., left face turn for a left Duane's type I syndrome) (14). Duane's type III is the second most common and is caused by equal innervation of the medial and lateral rectus muscles by the medial rectus nerve (Fig. 20–3C). Because the medial and lateral forces are similar, the eye will rest in approximately primary position, and there will be no significant face turn. In some cases of Duane's type III, an exotropia is present in primary position because the lateral rectus receives slightly more innervation than the medial rectus muscle. This causes a face turn away from the Duane's eye. Type II Duane's is rare and is associated with poor adduction but good abduction (Fig. 20–3B). Electromyography (EMG) recordings on type II Duane's patients show the lateral rectus muscle to contract appropriately on abduction, but it also contracts paradoxically on adduction (17). This probably represents a partial innervation of the lateral by the sixth nerve nucleus as purposeful abduction is present, in addition to aberrant sixth nerve innervation of the medial rectus muscle. Another rare form of Duane's syndrome is *synergistic divergence* (19). In this case, the nerve to the medial rectus muscle aberrantly innervates the lateral rectus muscle with significantly more fibers than go to the medial rectus muscle, so the Duane's eye

paradoxically abducts on attempted adduction (Fig. 20–3D). A patient with right synergistic divergence will diverge on left gaze.

Duane's syndrome may be associated with an upshoot and or a downshoot on attempted adduction, which looks similar to inferior oblique and superior oblique overaction. EMG studies have identified a variety of aberrant innervation patterns, which explain the vertical movements on adduction (17, 18). In some cases, the upshoot and downshoot are caused by strong inappropriate firing of the lateral rectus muscle on adduction. This leash effect pulls the eye up or down as the eye rotates slightly up or down past the horizontal plane. In other cases, the vertical recti are aberrantly innervated by part of the medial rectus nerve, so the vertical muscle fires on adduction.

Management of Duane's Syndrome

Strabismus surgery may be indicated to correct a face turn or reduce an upshoot or downshoot associated with Duane's syndrome. Type I Duane's syndrome with an esotropia in primary position and a face turn toward the Duane's eye requires an ipsilateral medial rectus recession usually about 6.0 to 6.5 mm. This moves the Duane's eye to primary position, thus correcting the face turn. If the patient has an exotropia Duane's with the Duane's eye in abduction and a face turn away from the Duane's eye (usually Type III), then a lateral rectus recession should be performed. These patients have significant innervation of the lateral rectus muscle, and therefore frequently show upshoots and downshoots. If an upshoot and downshoot coexist, then a Y-splitting of the lateral rectus in addition to a recession should be performed. The Y-splitting procedure involves dividing the lateral rectus muscle into two halves, and placing

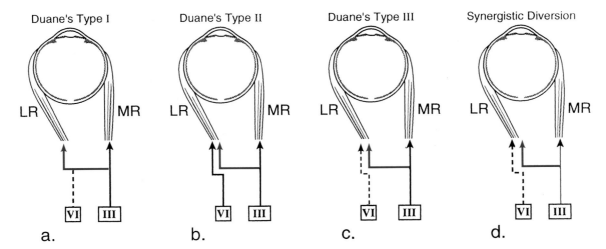

Figure 20–3.
Diagrammatic representation of misdirection of nerve fibers in Duane's syndrome. The aberrant nerve pathway is shown in red, and the dotted lines represent hypoplasia or agenesis. (Modified from Wilcox et al., in Am J Ophthalmol 1981;91:1–7.)

one half above and one half below the scleral insertion of the lateral rectus muscle.[22] The Y-split of the lateral rectus muscle inhibits upshoots and downshoots by placing some of the muscle above and below the horizontal plane of the eye. Retroequatorial fixation (faden) of lateral rectus also has been performed in these patients with aberrant vertical movements.

Mobius Syndrome

Mobius syndrome is characterized by a combination of facial palsy, sixth nerve palsy often a with partial third nerve palsy, and distal limb abnormalities such as syndactylism or even amputation defects. Craniofacial anomalies can occur and include micrognathia, tongue abnormalities, and facial or oral clefts. Ocular motility abnormalities include failure to abduct and retraction on adduction, typical of Duane's syndrome in some patients. The facial palsy usually spares the lower face, however, orbicularis function is weak. Skeletal abnormalities also include pectoralis muscle deficits. The inheritance pattern is variable and may be familial, however, most are sporadic.

■ RESTRICTIVE STRABISMUS

Fat Adherence Syndrome

Fat adherence syndrome occurs after traumatic violation of Tenon's capsule causes extraconal fat to adhere to the sclera and or rectus muscle. Extraconal fat septi connect to the periorbitum, so fibrosis associated with the fat adherence syndrome can extend from the sclera to the orbital bone thus creating a restrictive strabismus (Fig. 20–4). Fat adherence is difficult to treat because after Tenon's capsule is violated and fat adherence is established, it is almost impossible to re-establish the fascial barrier that separates orbital fat from the globe. Teflon or silicone sheaths have been tried, but they eventually become encapsulated in scar. The best treatment of fat adherence syndrome is to avoid penetrating posterior Tenon's capsule during strabismus or retinal surgery. Fat adherence syndrome has been described after various periocular surgeries including strabismus surgery, retinal surgery, orbital surgery, and surgery such as glaucoma implant surgery.

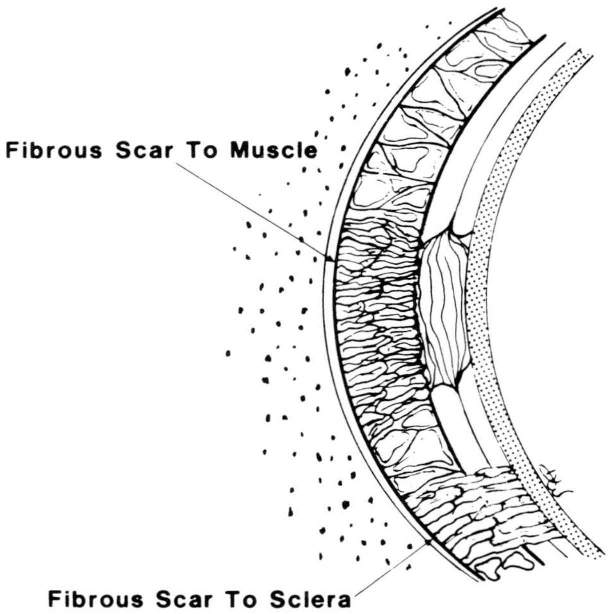

Grave's Ophthalmopathy

Grave's ophthalmopathy is related to thyroid dysfunction, however thyroid function studies may be normal. Initially, there is an acute phase during which there is an inflammatory lymphocytic infiltration of the extraocular muscles resulting in extraocular muscle enlargement and proptosis. This active phase usually lasts several months to 1 year. Orbital imaging studies show thickened extraocular muscles, especially posteriorly. The second phase is a cicatricial phase with quiescence of inflammation and secondary contracture of the muscles. All muscles are usually involved, but the inferior rectus and medial rectus are most severely involved. Strabismus develops in the cicatricial phase, with a restrictive esotropia and hypotropia being most common. The management of Grave's ophthalmopathy is careful observation during the acute inflammatory phase. Treatment with systemic steroids and even external beam radiation may be indicated for severe disease with signs of optic nerve compression by inflamed extraocular muscles. Orbital decompression also is useful if vision is compromised or if there is severe proptosis. After the inflammatory phase has subsided and strabismus measurements have stabilized, strabismus surgery may be considered. Surgery should be limited to recession procedures to release the tight muscles. A right hypotropia with tight right inferior rectus muscle can be managed by a right inferior rectus recession (less than

Fibrous Scar To Muscle

Fibrous Scar To Sclera

Figure 20–4.
Diagram showing fat adherence after violation of Tenon's capsule overlying the rectus muscle and in an area away from the rectus muscle. Note that a fibrous scar throughout the fat septae can attach periosteum to the muscle and/or sclera. This scar causes a restrictive leash, which limits eye movements. (Published courtesy of Ophthalmology 1986;93:411–415.)

15 prism diopters) using an adjustable suture technique, with a left superior rectus recession if the deviation is large (more than 15 to 20 prism diopters). As late overcorrections after inferior rectus recessions have been described, it is advisable to adjust to a slight initial undercorrection.[8]

Congenital Fibrosis Syndrome

Congenital fibrosis syndrome of the extraocular muscles is usually inherited as an autosomal-dominant trait. The cause is unknown, but the syndrome is associated with fibrotic replacement of extraocular muscle tissue.

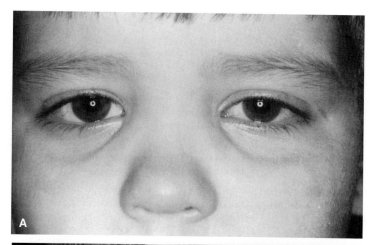

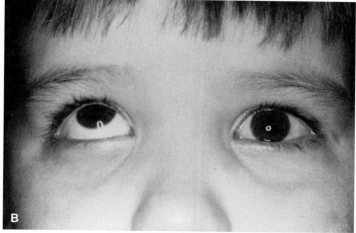

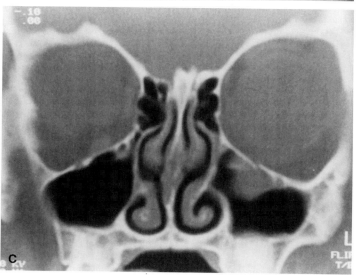

Figure 20–5.
Orbital floor fracture in the left eye. **A,** In primary gaze, there is no significant deviation. **B,** Restricted elevation in the left eye in upgaze. **C,** Computed tomography scan shows herniation and entrapment of inferior orbital fat into the maxillary antrum. Note the inferior rectus is not entrapped and is within the orbit.

The clinical features may be classified into five groups: (1) generalized fibrosis syndrome; (2) fibrosis of inferior rectus with blepharophimosis; (3) strabismus fixus; (4) vertical retraction syndrome; and (5) unilateral fibrosis blepharoptosis and enophthalmos (5). Forced ductions are positive. The medial rectus muscle is most commonly affected, although the fibrosis can be generalized and effect virtually all of the rectus muscles. Treatment is recession of the fibrotic muscle. These cases can be technically difficult because exposure of the muscle is limited, especially in cases with fibrotic medial rectus muscle.

Orbital Floor Fracture

Restrictive strabismus in orbital floor fractures is due to entrapment of fat and possibly muscle. This causes inferior rectus muscle fibrosis and scarring to the damaged floor, causing restriction of elevation and positive forced ductions (Fig. 20–5). Often there also will be limited depression, which can persist even after the floor fracture has been repaired. The cause of the limited depression is probably the inferior rectus being tethered by inferior scarring, so the inferior rectus muscle cannot transmit its full pull to the globe. Signs of a blowout fracture includes diplopia due to restricted vertical eye movement, enophthalmos, and numbness of face below the traumatized orbit and along the upper teeth. Strabismus surgery is indicated if diplopia persists 6 to 8 weeks after repair of the floor fracture. For more details on the management of orbital fractures see Chapter 26 on Ocular Plastics.

Brown's Syndrome

Brown's syndrome consists of an inability to elevate an eye when the eye is in adduction (Figs. 20-6A and 20-6B). The most common cause is a congenitally tight superior oblique muscle tendon complex, termed *true congenital Brown's syndrome.* Clinical findings include limited elevation in adduction, an exodeviation in attempted upgaze, and an ipsilateral hypotropia that increases in upgaze (4). Most patients with Brown's syndrome have good binocular vision with a compensatory

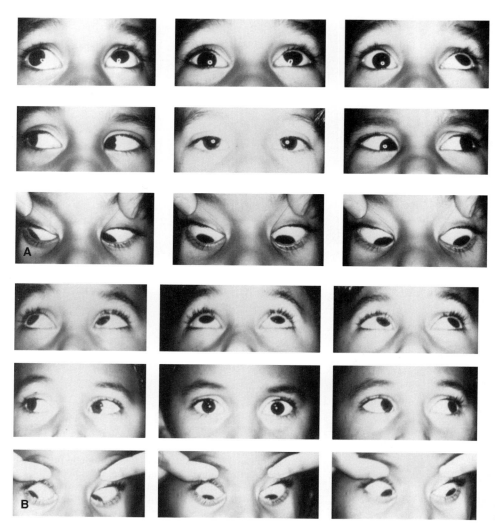

Figure 20–6.
Patient with Brown's syndrome in the right eye. **A,** Preoperative picture shows defective elevation in adduction. **B,** Postoperative pictures show improvement of elevation in adduction after silicone expander.

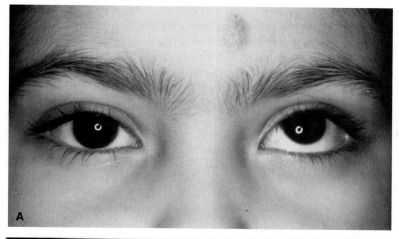

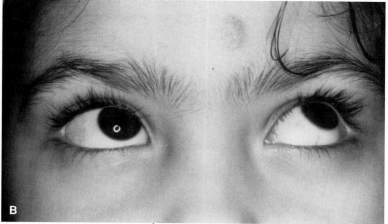

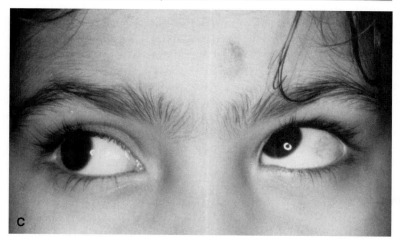

Figure 20–7.
Double elevator palsy in the right eye. **A,** Right eye does not elevate in upgaze. **B,** Poor elevation in adduction. **C,** Poor elevation in abduction.

chin elevation and slight face turn away from the Brown's eye.

The management of true congenital Brown's syndrome is conservative unless there is a significant vertical deviation in primary position. In most cases, it is better to wait until the child is visually mature before performing surgery, because an induced strabismus after surgery is not uncommon and can lead to the loss of binocular vision. If surgery is indicated, the procedure of choice is superior oblique tenotomy with silicone expander (23) (See Fig. 19–10.) Other treatment modalities include superior oblique tenotomy with ipsilateral inferior oblique recession.

Other causes of Brown's syndrome or pseudo-Brown's syndrome include congenital fibrotic band to the globe, floor fracture, peritrochlear scarring or superior oblique tendon sheath syndrome, trochlear inflammation (rheumatoid arthritis), glaucoma implant under superior oblique tendon in the superior nasal quadrant, or fat adherence syndrome. Virtually any periocular condition that results in limited elevation in adduction can mimic Brown's syndrome. Superior oblique overaction or inferior oblique palsy also can be misdiagnosed as Brown's syndrome. With superior oblique overaction, the vertical deviation is greatest in downgaze, and in both superior oblique overaction and inferior oblique paresis there is an A pattern rather than an exodeviation in upgaze.

Double Elevator Palsy

Double elevator palsy is a limited elevation of one eye across the board in adduction and abduction (Fig. 20–7). The term double elevator implies paresis of superior rectus and inferior oblique muscle; this is, however, a misnomer as in 70% of cases the deficient eleva-

tion is due to restriction, secondary to a tight inferior rectus.[11] Double elevator palsy may be mistaken for Brown's syndrome, although the limited elevation is worse in adduction than in abduction in the latter. The condition presents clinically as a hypotropia; often a chin elevation and ptosis are present. True ptosis because of levator weakness is present in 50% to 60% of cases whereas pseudoptosis may occur in almost all patients with a large hypotropia. Other associated findings include jaw winking, Duane's syndrome, and other misdirection syndromes (21). Surgery is indicated if vertical strabismus is present in primary gaze. If supraduction forced ductions are positive, indicating a tight inferior rectus, the tight muscle should be recessed. If forced ductions are negative, indicating a superior rectus paresis, then a Knapp transposition or vertical Hummelsheim or vertical Jensen transposition procedure should be used (Fig. 20–1).

■ OCULAR TORTICOLLIS

Patients with a face turn may have an ocular problem, or the face turn may be secondary to a skeletal abnormality of the neck (Fig. 20–8). A simple way to differentiate ocular torticollis from skeletal torticollis is to have the patient close their eyes and move their head from side to side. Skeletal torticollis will have restricted neck movement, whereas ocular torticollis should show a relatively free range of motion of the neck. Ocular torticollis can have three components: face turn (horizontal head posturing), chin elevation or depression, and head tilt (tilting to the left or right). The two most common causes of ocular torticollis are incomitant strabismus and nystagmus. Another face turn syndrome is esotropia associated with abduction nystagmus; this is covered in the esotropia chapter (Chapter 17). When examining a patient for ocular torticollis, the first step is to passively move the head opposite to the face posturing and look for evidence of nystagmus or strabismus.

Ocular Torticollis Associated with Incomitant Strabismus

A variety of incomitant strabismus can cause ocular torticollis, including Duane's syndrome, Brown's syndrome, double elevator palsy, cranial palsies, A and V patterns, and restrictive strabismus. In patients with restrictive or paralytic strabismus, the face turn can be corrected by surgically moving the eye with limited ductions into primary position. For example, in right sixth nerve palsy, there is a face turn to the right with the right eye stuck in adduction. The face turn can be corrected by moving the paretic right eye to primary position by recessing the medial rectus muscle, and per-

forming a vertical muscle transposition (see management of sixth nerve palsy above). A chin elevation associated with a double elevator palsy would be corrected by elevating the double elevator palsy eye.

Ocular Torticollis Associated with Nystagmus

Patients with congenital nystagmus may have less nystagmus in an eccentric position of gaze. This position of gaze where the nystagmus is least is called the null point. Patients with an eccentric null point will adapt a compensatory face posturing to place the eyes at the null point to dampen the nystagmus and improve vision (Fig. 20–8). The compensatory face posturing may be a face turn, head tilt, chin elevation or depression, or a combination. A patient with a null point to left and downgaze, for example, will adapt a right face turn and a chin elevation, thus placing the eyes at the null point.

The treatment of nystagmus related head posturing is based on using eye muscle surgery to move the null point from an eccentric position to primary position. Move the null point by moving the eyes. For example, if a patient has a null point to the right, the eyes would be shifted to right gaze and a compensatory face turn to the left (Fig. 20–8). The face turn can be corrected by moving both eyes to the left into primary position (left eye, recess medial—reset lateral; and right eye, reset medial—recess lateral). This procedure is termed the *Kestenbaum* or *Parks–Kestenbaum* procedure. A chin depression is treated by large bilateral superior rectus recessions (or inferior rectus resections), and a chin elevation by bilateral inferior rectus recessions (or superior rectus resections). Table 20–2 quantitates the Kesten-

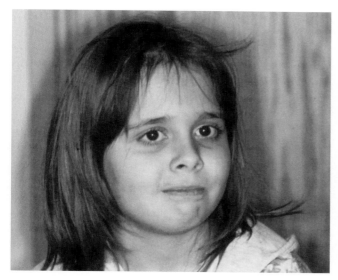

Figure 20–8.
Face turn to left in a patient with nystagmus. Note the eyes are in right gaze. Correct the face turn by moving the eyes to the left.

baum procedure for various degrees of face turn. An initial over correction is desirable as the face turn tends to recur.

Dissociated Vertical Deviation and Dissociated Horizontal Deviation

Dissociated vertical deviation (DVD) describes the tendency for an eye to elevate, abduct, and extort when the binocularity is suspended or the patient spontaneously dissociates (often when fatigued) (Fig. 20–9). Note that with a true hypertropia, there is a corresponding hypotropia of the nonfixing eye. In contrast, with DVD there is no hypotropia of the nonfixing eye; in fact occluding one eye results in a hypertropia of the covered nonfixing eye. Alternate cover testing results in a downward refixation movement of each eye. DVD, therefore, violates Hering's law of yoke muscles because one eye moves without a similar movement in the same direc-

tion from the fellow eye. DVD is often associated with congenital esotropia, and it may occur in virtually any condition that disrupts binocular vision (i.e., monocular congenital cataract, unilateral optic nerve hypoplasia, etc.). On version testing, DVD can look like inferior oblique overaction because vision of the adducting eye is blocked by the bridge of the nose. This disociates the eyes, causing the DVD of the adducting eye to be manifest. The two can be distinguished as DVD has no true hypotropia of the opposite eye and the hyperdeviation is the same in abduction and adduction. In inferior oblique overaction, there is a hypotropia of the opposite eye, and the deviation increases in as the eye moves into adduction. DVD and inferior oblique overaction often coexist with congenital esotropia (20).

The cause of dissociated vertical deviation is unknown, but it is associated with abnormal binocular visual development. Certain brain stem nuclei such as the interstitial nucleus of Cajal regulate vertical/vestibular torsional movements and receive inhibitory input from binocular cells in the occipital cortex. Perhaps lack of binocular inhibitory input to this or related nuclei results in disinhibition and overactivity of a vertical movements giving rise to what we clinically see as DVD.

The treatment of DVD is surgical if it manifests greater than approximately 50% of the time and or is a cosmetic problem. DVD is almost always bilateral and surgery is usually performed bilaterally. Large recessions of the superior rectus muscles or inferior rectus resections are the procedures most commonly performed. Strabismus surgery rarely, if ever, cures DVD. Unilateral surgery of the amblyopic eye is indicated if there is amblyopia of three lines or more. If DVD and inferior oblique overaction coexist, then an anterior transposition of the inferior oblique is indicated, as this will address both problems with one procedure.

Dissociated horizontal deviation (DHD), which may be unilateral or bilateral, is a subtype of DVD and is often seen in patients with corrected congenital esotropia.[20] This is a dissociated condition like DVD, but the exo-component of DVD is exaggerated. Cover-uncover testing may show no shift or often a small esotropia, but pro-

TABLE 20–2
Kestenbaum Face Turn to Left (the Eyes Shifted to a Right Null Point)

Face Turn (degrees)	Right Eye		Left Eye	
	Recess Lateral Rectus (mm)	Reset Medial Rectus (mm)	Recess Medial Rectus (mm)	Reset Lateral Rectus (mm)
<20	7	6	5	8
30	9	8	6.5	10
45	10	8.5	7	11
>50	11	9.5	8	12.5

(Table modified from Archer 1993 (1) and Wright 1991 (22))

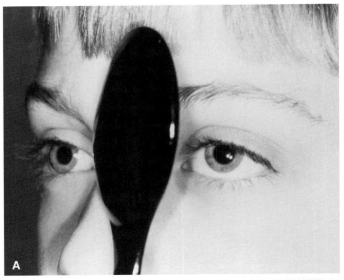

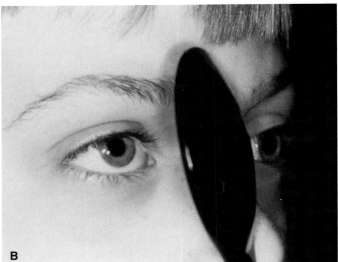

Figure 20–9.
Dissociated vertical deviation (DVD) in both eyes. **A,** With the left eye covered, there is a left hyper, and **B,** with the right eye covered there is a right hyper. Note that the eye behind the cover is not only elevated but is also slightly exodeviated. In some patients, the horizontal component is predominant, with little or no hyperdeviation, and this is termed dissociated horizontal deviation (DHD).

longed occlusion produces an exodeviation. Think of DHD in patients with a small residual esotropia, who also have a dissociated exodeviation. The treatment of DHD is recession of the ipsilateral lateral rectus muscle.

■ REFERENCES

1. Archer SM: Strabismus surgery planning. In: Del Monte MA, Archer SM (eds): Atlas of Pediatric Ophthalmology and Strabismus Surgery, New York: Churchill Livingstone, 1993, p. 14.
2. Barnes RJ: Anencephaly with absence of superior oblique tendon. Survey Ophthalmol 1972;16:371–374.
3. Biglan AW, et al.: Management of strabismus with botulinum A toxin. Ophthalmology 1989;96:935–943.
4. Brown HM: True and simulated superior oblique tendon sheath syndrome. Doc Ophthalmol 1973;34:123.
5. Hertel RW, Katowitz JA, Young PL, et al.: Congenital unilateral fibrosis, blepharoptosis, and enophthalmos syndrome. Ophthalmology 1992;99:347–355.
6. Hotchkiss MG, Miller NR, Clark AW, et al.: Bilateral Duane's retraction syndrome, a clinical-pathologic case report. Arch Ophthalmol 1980;98:870–874.
7. Huber A: Electrophysiology of the retraction syndromes. Br J Ophthalmol 1974;58:293–300.
8. Hudson HL, Feldon SE: Late overcorrection of hypotropia in Grave's ophthalmopathy. Ophthalmology 1992;99:356–360.
9. Lee J, et al.: Resuts of a prospective randomized trial of

botulinum toxin therapy in acute unilateral sixth nerve palsy. J Pediatr Ophthalmol Strabismus 1994;31:283–286.

10. Mets MB, Parks MM, Freeley DA, Cornell FM: Congenital absence of inferior rectus muscle. Report of three cases and their management. Binocular Vision 1987;2:77–86.

11. Metz HS: Double elevator palsy. Archi Ophthalmol 1979;97:901.

12. Metz HS, Dickey CF: Treatment of unilateral acute sixth nerve palsy with botulinum toxin. Am J Ophthalmol 1991;112:381–384.

13. Miller NR, Kiel SM, Green WR, Clark AW: Unilateral Duane's retraction syndrome. Arch Ophthalmol 1982; 100:1468–1472.

14. Raab EL: Clinical features of Duane's syndrome. J Pediatr Ophthalmol Strabismus 1986;23:64–68.

15. Rosenbaum A, Kushner BJ, Kirschen D: Vertical rectus muscle transposition and botulinum toxin (oculinum) to medial rectus for abducens palsy. Arch Ophthamol 1989; 107:820.

16. Saunders RA, Rogers CT: Superior oblique transposition for third nerve palsy. Ophthalmology 1982;89:310.

17. Scott AB, Wong GY: Duane's syndrome: an electromyographic study. Arch Ophthalmol 1972;87:142–147.

18. Strachan IM, Brown BH: Electromyography of extraocular muscles in Duane's syndrome. Br J Ophthalmol 1972;56:594–599.

19. Wilcox LM, Gittinger JW, Breinen GM: Congenital adduction palsy and synergistic divergence. Am J Ophthalmol 1981;91:1–7.

20. Wilson ME, Parks MM: Primary inferior oblique overaction in congenital esotropia. Accommodative esotropia and intermittent exotropia. Ophthalmology 1989;96: 952–957.

21. Wright KW, Liu GY, Murphree AL, et al.: Double elevator palsy, ptosis and jaw-winking. Am Orthoptic J 1989;39: 143–150.

22. Wright KW: Color Atlas of Ophthalmic Surgery: Strabismus. Philadelphia: J. B. Lippincott; 1991, p. 136.

23. Wright KW: Superior oblique silicone expander for Brown's syndrome and superior oblique overaction. J Pediatr Ophthalmol Strabismus 1991;28:101–107.

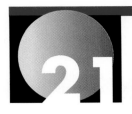

21 Pediatric Lens Abnormalities

Kenneth W. Wright

■ PEDIATRIC CATARACTS

Cataracts in children present a special challenge, because early visual rehabilitation is critical to prevent irreversible amblyopia. Congenital cataracts occur in approximately 1:250 live births, and pose the most difficult challenge. Up until the 1980s, many ophthalmologists would not even attempt surgery on unilateral congenital cataracts because of the poor prognosis. Now, with early intervention, operating as early as the first week of life, the prognosis is much improved. For the differential diagnosis of pediatric leukokoria, see Table 22–4, Chapter 22.

Morphology of Infantile Cataracts

Infantile cataracts can be classified by the location of the lens opacity. The nucleus is demarcated by the Y sutures (Fig. 21–1). Opacities involving or central to the Y sutures are nuclear cataracts and usually indicate that the cataract was present since birth. Sutural cataracts are cataracts which follow the Y sutures (Fig. 21–2). These cataracts involve the peripheral aspect of the nucleus and may be progressive and expand into the cortex and central nuclear areas.[3] Cataracts that are located peripheral to the Y sutures are cortical cataracts. Cortical cataracts that are layered in an onion skin-like layer pattern, with clear zones between the opacities are termed lamellar cataracts or zonular cataracts (Fig. 21–3). The visual prognosis for lamellar cataracts is relatively good because they are acquired, with the lens being relatively clear during the early period of visual development. Lamellar cataracts can be inherited or can indicate a metabolic disease such as hypoglycemia or galactosemia.

Anterior Cataracts

Anterior polar cataracts involve the anterior capsule and anterior cortex at the center or pole of the lens. Typically, anterior polar cataracts are small, nonprogressive, and usually do not interfere with visual acuity. These patients must be followed up closely, however, because there are cases where the cataract does progress (19, 27). One type of anterior polar cataract is the anterior pyramidal cataract. This anterior polar cataract takes the shape of a pyramid or cone (Fig. 21–4). The cone is made of fibrous tissue and probably represents an abnormality of surface ectoderm separation during lens development.

Anterior subcapsular cataracts are opacities immediately under the anterior capsule in the anterior lens cortex. *Alport's syndrome* is classically described as associated with *anterior lenticonus* (anterior bowing of the anterior capsule), with or without an anterior polar subcapsular cataract. Systemic findings include neurosensory hearing loss and hemorrhagic nephritis with late renal failure and renal hypertension (32, 33). Alport's syndrome is fairly common and accounts for approximately one sixth of familial glomerular nephritis. Only 15% of patients, however, have ocular abnormalities. Various modes of inheritance have been described, including X-linked dominant (most common), autosomal-recessive, and autosomal-dominant. There is no specific treat-

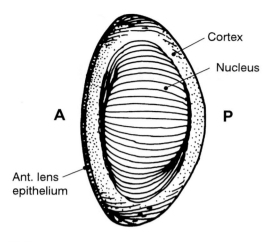

Figure 21–1.
Diagram of neonatal lens showing anterior lens epithelium lens nucleus located between the Y sutures and the cortex peripheral to the Y sutures. A: anterior, P: posterior.

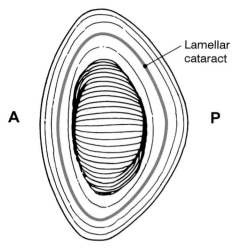

Figure 21–3.
Drawing of a lamellar cataract with the opacity (identified in red) occurring in the cortex just peripheral to the lens nucleus.

ment, and management is directed toward the renal failure.

Posterior Cataracts

Of the posterior lenticular opacities, posterior lenticonus and persistent hyperplastic primary vitreous (PHPV) are the most common unilateral posterior cataracts in childhood.

Posterior lenticonus is a congenital thinning and posterior bowing of the posterior capsule (Fig. 21–5). Early in infancy, the cortex is relatively clear; however, over time the area of cortex surrounding the abnormal pos-

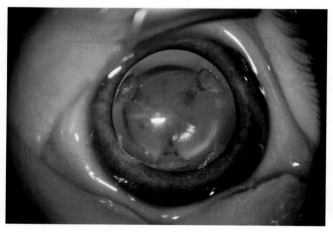

Figure 21–2.
Photograph of a 4-week-old infant with a congenital sutural nuclear cataract. Note the anterior Y suture is oriented upright. The peripheral clear red reflex represents clear lens cortex, whereas the central opacity involves the sutures and nucleus.

terior capsule opacifies, and the cataract progresses. Even when the opacification is minimal, lenticular astigmatism can be a cause of amblyopia. The visual prognosis for posterior lenticonus is relatively good since the opacity is progressive, and the visual axis is usually relatively clear during the early visual developmental period (37).

Persistent hyperplastic primary vitreous (PHPV) represents abnormal regression of the primitive hyaloid vascular system. This produces a fibrovascular tissue that emanates from the optic disc as a stalk, and courses to the back of the lens where it forms a retrolental membrane (Fig. 21–6). This membrane may extend to the ciliary processes, and, over time, the fibrovascular membrane can contract, pulling the ciliary processes centrally (Figs. 21-6A and 21-6B). If left untreated, severe forms of PHPV can lead to shallowing of anterior chamber, angle-closure glaucoma, and eventual loss of the eye in late childhood. PHPV varies in severity with the mildest form represented by a Mittendorf's dot with a fine vessel extending from the disc to a dot of fibrosis on the posterior capsule, usually measuring less than 2 mm. The most common form is an optic nerve stalk that inserts on the posterior capsule and causes a posterior central opacity (Fig. 21-6C). On rare occasions, PHPV can be associated with fibrosis and traction on the macula, resulting in poor visual potential. Overall, the prognosis with PHPV is relatively good if the retina is normal. PHPV tends to be a progressive problem, and the opacity may be relatively mild at birth, so in many cases the amblyopia is less severe than what would be expected with a large congenital opacity. Even when surgery is performed relatively late in infancy, good visual results have been reported (21, 37).

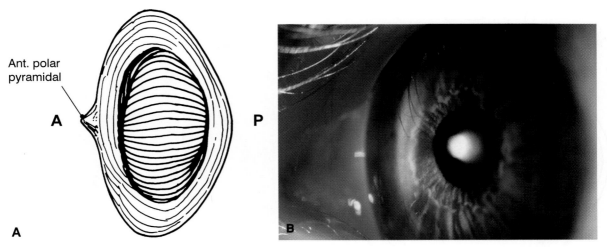

Figure 21–4.
Anterior polar cataract. **A,** Drawing of a pyramidal anterior polar cataract with an anterior conical opacity consisting of fibrous tissue. **B,** Companion photograph showing white conical area of fibrosis coming off the anterior capsule, through the pupil, and protruding into the anterior chamber. Over time, progressive cortical changes occurred, and this patient required cataract surgery. At the time of surgery, the fibrotic conical opacity was difficult to fragment, and required removal with intraocular forceps.

Posterior subcapsular cataracts involving the posterior lens cortex may be idiopathic or they may be associated with Down's syndrome, chronic steroid use, or blunt trauma.

The oil drop cataract is the term typically given to a faint opacity in the central aspect of the posterior cortex, which is seen on retroillumination and is associated with *galactosemia.* Galactosemia, if diagnosed early, can result in reversal of the cataract through dietary restric-tion as long as dietary restriction is instituted before lenticular cortical scarring (7).

Other Forms

Christmas Tree Cataract

Christmas tree cataracts consist of multiple small flecks of various colors that reflect light and give the appear-

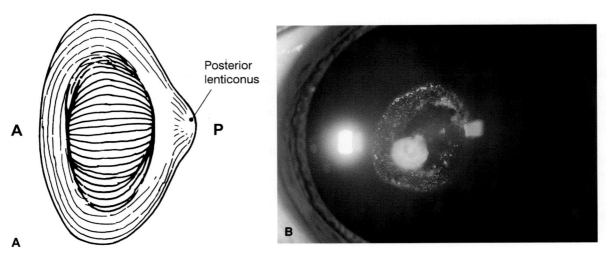

Figure 21–5.
Posterior lenticonus is a posterior bowing of the posterior capsule with capsular thinning. This capsular ectasia produces a progressive posterior capsular opacity. **A,** shows a diagram of posterior lenticonus with the posterior ectasia seen in red. **B,** is a slit lamp photograph of posterior lenticonus. The circular opacity represents the area of thinning and posterior bowing of the posterior capsule.

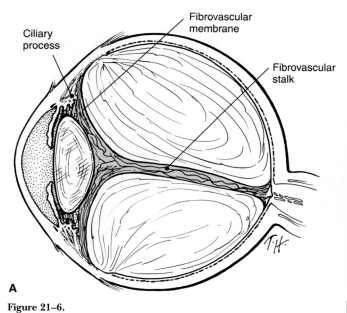

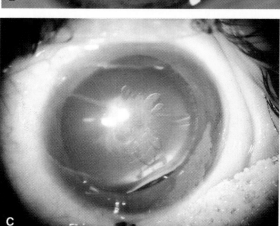

Figure 21–6.
Persistent hyperplastic primary vitreous (PHPV). **A,** Diagram of
PHPV showing a fibrovascular stalk, which emanates from the optic
nerve and extends to the posterior capsule of the lens to form a
retrolental fibrovascular membrane. In severe forms of PHPV, the
fibrovascular membrane contracts with time pulling the ciliary body
centrally, shallowing the anterior chamber, thus causing angle
closure glaucoma. **B,** is a clinical photograph of severe PHPV with
the fibrovascular membrane pulling the ciliary processes centrally.
The dark black tissue with the scalloped border is the ciliary body
being pulled to the center of the pupil by the fibrovascular
membrane. The pink appearance of the membrane is secondary to
vascularization of the membrane. **C,** is a mild form of PHPV without
significant traction on the ciliary body. The central opacity is located
at the contact point of the fibrovascular stalk. The stalk is not seen in
this photograph, but extends from the optic nerve to the posterior
capsule of the lens.

ance of a lighted Christmas tree. These cataracts can be
associated with myotonic dystrophy, pseudohypoparathyroidism, and hypoparathyroidism.

Cerulean Cataract

Cerulean or blue-dot cataracts consist of multiple small
opacities scattered throughout the cortex, which are
bluish-white in color. The cerulean cataract can be associated with Down's syndrome or may be idiopathic,
occurring during early puberty. These cataracts are usually bilateral and generally cause minimal visual loss.

Membranous Cataract

A membranous cataract is a cataract in which the cortex
has been absorbed, and the anterior and posterior capsule come into close proximity. Often, there is calcification within the lens capsule bag. Membranous cataracts
can be associated with trauma, intrauterine infections,

or anomalous lens development associated with anterior chamber dysgenesis syndromes.

Systemic Evaluation

The causes and evaluation for unilateral versus bilateral congenital cataracts are listed in Tables 21–1 and
21–2, and 21–3.

Unilateral Cataract

In general, unilateral infantile cataracts are caused by a
systemic disease (Table 21–1). Exceptions to this rule include intrauterine infections such as rubella. Approximately 20% of rubella cataracts are, in fact, unilateral.
Thus, the presence of a unilateral cataract does not totally exclude the possibility of an associated systemic disease such as congenital rubella, but it is highly suggestive that the cataract is caused by local dysgenesis. Two
common types of unilateral cataracts are posterior lenti-

TABLE 21–1
Etiology of Unilateral Cataracts

1. Idiopathic (50%)
2. Posterior lenticonus (10%)
3. Persistent hyperplastic primary vitreous (PHPV) (10%)
4. Anterior polar (10%)
5. Other (9%)
   a. Anterior segment dysgenesis
   b. Posterior pole tumors (RARE)
6. Traumatic (10%)
   (rule out child abuse)
5. Intrauterine infection (rubella) (1%)

Note: Asymmetric bilateral lens opacity may be misinterpreted as an unilateral cataract.

TABLE 21–2
Etiology of Bilateral Cataracts

1. Idiopathic (60%)
2. Hereditary cataracts (30%), without systemic disease
   a. Autosomal dominant (most common pattern)
   b. Autosomal recessive
   c. X-linked
3. Systemic diseases (5%)
   a. Hallermann-Streiff syndrome (midfacial hypoplasia, dwarfism)
   b. Lowe's syndrome (oculo-cerebro-renal syndrome)
   c. Smith Lemli Optiz
   d. Galactosemia
   e. Hypoglycemia
   f. Trisomy
      1) Down syndrome (21)
      2) Edward syndrome (28)
      3) Patau syndrome (13)
   g. Alport syndrome
   h. Myotonic dystrophy
   i. Fabry's disease (ceramide trihexosidase deficiency)
   j. Hypoparathyroidism
   k. Marfan's syndrome
   l. Pseudohypoparathyroidism
   m. Conradi syndrome
   n. Diabetes mellitus
   o. Peroxismals biogenesis disorder
   p. Wilson's disease
4. Intrauterine infection (3%)
   a. Rubella
   b. Cytomegalovirus
   c. Varicella
   d. Syphilis
   e. Toxoplasmosis
   f. Herpes simplex
5. Ocular abnormalities (2%)
   a. Aniridia
   b. Anterior segment dysgenesis

TABLE 21–3
Systemic Evaluation of Pediatric Cataracts

I. History:
   A. Family history is critical.
   B. Age of onset of cataract.
   C. Developmental milestones.
   D. Trauma (battered child syndrome?)
III. Pediatric physical examination:
   Consult geneticist or dysmorphologist.
VI. Ocular physical exam:
   Diagnose specific morphological features of the cataract: i.e., PHPV, posterior lenticonus, anterior polar cataract.
V. Laboratory: for
   A. Unilateral cataracts
      TORCH Titer and VDRL
   B. Bilateral cataracts
      1. Routine
         a. TORCH Titer and VDRL
         b. Urine for reducing substance (after milk feeding)
      2. Optional:
         a. Red cell galactokinase (developmental cataracts).
         b. Urine for amino acids (developmental delay and glaucoma).
         c. Calcium and phosphorus (cataracts and metabolic disorders).

conus and persistent hyperplastic primary vitreous (PHPV). The work-up for a unilateral congenital or infantile cataract should include a full ophthalmic examination, and, if the examination does not clearly reveal a specific diagnosis, serum TORCH titers should be obtained to rule out intrauterine infection (Table 21–3). If a titer is positive, IGM assays should be performed because IGM does not cross the placenta and IGM indicates fetal immunoglobin and fetal infection.

Bilateral Cataract

Bilateral cataracts are often inherited; autosomal-dominant being the most common inheritance pattern. Systemic disease can cause bilateral cataracts, and approximately 5% to 10% of bilateral cataracts are associated with a systemic disorder (11). Systemic diseases that cause bilateral cataracts are listed in Table 21–2. The work-up for bilateral congenital or infantile cataracts should include a careful medical examination by a pediatrician who has been alerted to the fact that the child has cataracts or by a geneticist or dysmorphologist. Laboratory work-up should include a urine for reducing substance after a milk feeding and TORCH titer (Table 21–3). The laboratory work-up is not necessary if the cataracts can be definitely defined as hereditary without other systemic abnormalities.

Cataracts and Infantile Glaucoma

Cataracts associated with glaucoma are a difficult problem. The differential diagnosis of congenital cataracts with glaucoma include Lowe's syndrome, congenital rubella syndrome, anterior segment dysgenesis syndromes, and aniridia with cataract. The management should include making the specific diagnosis of glaucoma and cataracts, then controlling the glaucoma with topical and oral medication before surgery. If the glaucoma is severe, one should consider a combined surgical approach, performing the glaucoma surgery and cataract surgery at the same operation.

Lowe's Syndrome (Oculocerebrorenal Syndrome). This is an X-linked disorder seen as bilateral congenital cataracts, often with bilateral congenital glaucoma. Infants have severe developmental delay, hypotonia, and renal failure, with aminoaciduria (13). The prognosis is poor as there is progressive neurologic and renal deterioration, with death often occurring in late childhood. A dilated slit-lamp examination of the patient's mother shows multiple punctate white snow flake opacities of the lens (check the lens periphery).

Rubella Syndrome. Systemic findings include congenital heart defects, hearing loss, and mental retardation. Ocular finding include cataracts (15%), salt and pepper retinopathy (25%), strabismus (20%), microphthalmus (15%), optic atrophy (10%), corneal haze (10%), glaucoma (10%), and phthsis bulbi (2%). The retinopathy does not usually effect vision and is stable, not progressive. Cataracts are caused by the invasion of the lens by the rubella virus (31). Rubella cataracts are usually bilateral (80%), but they are unilateral in 20% of cases. Rubella cataracts may present with a hazy cornea caused by either congenital glaucoma or keratitis. Treatment of the cataract involves removing all the lens cortex because these patients are prone to postoperative inflammation, especially if residual cortex is left after surgery. Live virus has been recovered from lens material.

■ TREATMENT OF PEDIATRIC CATARACTS

Timing of Surgery and Amblyopia

The strategy for treating congenital or infantile cataracts is to provide a clear retinal image as soon as possible to avoid irreversible amblyopia. The most common cause for poor vision after pediatric cataract surgery is amblyopia, which can be unilateral or bilateral (2). Because of this, a unilateral or bilateral congenital cataract, which is visually significant, must be visually rehabilitated as soon as possible, even during the first week of life (2). The urgency of treatment is very important, especially for bilateral cataracts. Bilateral congenital cataracts that obscure the visual axis will result in sensory nystagmus and a bilateral poor visual outcome if not treated by 2 months of age (30).

Bilateral Light Occlusion

Bilateral total light deprivation has been shown to prolong visual plasticity in animals (9). Studies in humans show that bilateral light occlusion for up to 2 weeks in human neonates is safe and does not adversely affect final visual acuity (18, 38). I equate it to leaving the baby in the womb for a little longer, where there is no light stimulation so visual development is put on hold. In neonates with congenital cataracts or media opacities from other causes, bilateral occlusion has been used to prevent amblyopia and extend the critical period of visual development (15, 36, 38). Bilateral occlusion is used in neonates younger than 4 months of age and is initiated as soon as a visually significant unilateral or bilateral cataract is identified. Occlusion of both eyes is continued until a clear retinal image is established in both eyes (surgery and fitting of contact lens), a process that should take no longer than 2 weeks. Bilateral occlusion is not recommended if the infant is older than 4 months or if the visual potential is extremely poor.

Is the Opacity Visually Significant?

One of the important questions in an infant with a partial cataract is whether the cataract should be removed. Determining if an infantile cataract is visually significant can be difficult. As a rule of thumb, Parks suggests that central nuclear or posterior lens opacities 3 mm or larger are usually visually significant (28). Anterior polar opacities are less likely to cause amblyopia unless the opacity extends into the cortex and blocks the entrance pupil. The clinical evaluation should include an evaluation of fixation and following eye movements. Preferential looking and the pattern visual-evoked potential also can be helpful for determining amblyopia. These tests, however, provide estimates of vision and are best used as supplemental data. Direct ophthalmoscopy and the red reflex test are probably the most useful test in newborn infants. A central opacity that blocks visualization of fundus details with the direct ophthalmoscope is indicative of a visually significant cataract. In children who are old enough to cooperate with optotype acuity, a visual acuity of 20/70 or worse usually indicates a need for surgery. A progressive loss of stereoacuity in a patient with unilateral cataract is also an important finding.

Surgical Technique

Pediatric cataracts and cataracts in young adults (younger than 30 years of age) can be removed by vitrectomy instrumentation using suction and suction cutting modalities. With pediatric cataracts, there is no need for nuclear expression or phacoemulsification, which is needed in senile cataracts because of the mineralized hard nucleus. Intracapsular cataract extraction is definitely contraindicated in pediatric cataracts as the vitreous has an adhesion to the posterior capsule in children (Wieger's capsulohyaloid ligament). Removal of the entire lens via an intracapsular technique results in a high incidence of vitreous loss and vitreoretinal traction.

The technique for removing pediatric cataracts consists of performing an anterior capsulectomy using the suction and cutting mode of a vitrectomy instrument such as the Ocutome. Once the anterior capsule is removed, the suction mode is used to aspirate cortex and nucleus. Some cutting may be necessary to break up firm cortex or nucleus. Minimal cutting should be used during cortex removal to avoid inadvertent rupture of the posterior capsule. After the cortex has been thoroughly removed, aspirate anterior capsule lens epithelial cells from the undersurface of the anterior capsule. This helps reduce the incidence of secondary cortex growth and cortex pearls. In children older than 2 to 3 years of age, consider intraocular lens placement, especially for patients with a unilateral cataract. In infants, perform a posterior capsulectomy and small anterior vitrectomy, using low suction and high cutting rate, as the posterior capsule inevitably will become opacfied.[25] A peripheral skirt of posterior capsule can be left so that secondary posterior chamber intraocular lens implantation can be performed when the child is older. In older children who can cooperate with a postoperative YAG laser capsulotomy (usually older than 3 years), leave the posterior capsule intact anticipating a YAG capsulotomy after surgery.

Complications of cataract surgery are unusual (28) but can include retinal detachment (rare), immediate or late glaucoma (5%), retinal hemorrhages (6) (if the eye is soft at the end of surgery), secondary cortex growth (Elschnig pearls), and endophthalmitis. Aphakicystoid macular edema is very unusual (29).

Management of Aphakia

Contact Lenses

The standard of care for pediatric aphakia has been extended wear or flexible wear contact lenses. Silicone lenses and gas-permeable hard lenses are the lenses of choice in children. Fit the silicone lens relatively flat, based on the flat K, as a steep lens can result in the suck-on syndrome where the lens attaches onto the cornea like a suction cup, causing corneal edema. During the first year of life, an extended wear lens regime is preferred to ensure a constant clear retinal image. For the first year of life, prescribe +2.00 to +3.00 diopters over the refraction to induce myopia, providing a clear image at near. In older infants and toddlers, reduce the overcorrection to a +1.00 to +1.50 to induce mild myopia. In general, bifocals are prescribed for bilateral aphakes, and monocular aphakes are corrected for near at one meter by over plusing by one diopter. Omnivision does allow for some fusion and even stereopsis.

Intraocular Lenses

Intraocular lenses have now become an accepted method for treating aphakia in children (12, 17, 22). One must be selective, however, when considering lens implantation in the pediatric age group. During the first year of life, there is a dramatic increase in the axial length and a change in the lens power (approximately 10 to 14 diopters) (14). Because of this, implanting intraocular lenses with full lens power for emmetropia in an infant is contraindicated, as the patient will be severely myopic in late childhood. By 2 years of age, however, the eye is almost adult size. On average there is only 1 mm of axial elongation or 3.00 diopters of myopic shift from 2 years of age until the eye reaches adult size at age 10 years. Therefore, for the most part, intraocular lenses are limited to children older than 2 years of age with acquired or progressive cataracts. The intraocular lens power used in children older than 2 years of age is calculated for emmetropia. Since the posterior capsule invariably opacifies (25), a secondary YAG capsulotomy is usually necessary. In children who may not cooperate with postoperative YAG capsulotomy, consider performing a posterior capsulectomy and small anterior vitrectomy during the primary surgery after intraocular lens insertion.

Epikeratophakia

Epikeratophakia has a limited role in the management of pediatric aphakia. There are patients, however, who are late contact lens failures and are not candidates for intraocular lens implantation (26). I have used epikeratophakia in a patient with Marfan's syndrome who had lensectomy to restore vision but who had become contact lens intolerant. Unfortunately, epikeratophakic grafts are no longer commercially available.

Aphakic Spectacles

Aphakic spectacles are not a great option in children. They are unsightly, they are easily lost, and they do not provide constant correction of the aphakia, as infants in bed do not wear glasses well. Contact lenses are the treatment of choice for both unilateral and bilateral

TABLE 21–4
Patching Regime for Unilateral Congenital Cataracts (If
vision rehabilitated before two to three weeks of age)

Age (months)	Occlusion Therapy
0–1 month	No patching
0–2 months	2 hours per day
2–4 months	3 hours per day
4–6 months	50% of waking hours as indicated
6–12 months	Up to 80% of waking hours as indicated

aphakia in children. Aphakic spectacles can be used as
a back-up for contact lenses in bilaterally aphakic children. Aphakic spectacles also can be used in patients
with unilateral cataracts who have strabismus and no
binocular fusion potential. In this case, the spectacles
are only worn when the good eye is patched.

Occlusion Therapy

There is some controversy regarding to the amount of
patching for patients with monocular cataracts. The
amount of patching should be determined based on the
severity of amblyopia and how soon the retinal image
was cleared. If the cataract was operated during the first
week of life and contact lens immediately placed without complication, then minimum patching is required
for the first month of life. In general, do not patch more
than 50% waking hours during the first 6 months of life
if early visual rehabilitation has been achieved. The advantage of part-time occlusion is that is allows for the
possibility of binocular vision development (15, 36).
Table 21–4 provides a suggested patching regime if the
cataract is operated early, and the contact lens fit by 4
weeks of age. If a patient with congenital cataract is seen
later (after 1 to 2 months of age), then more aggressive
patching is indicated. Retrospective studies using full-
time occlusion therapy uniformly show an absence of
binocular vision and 100% strabismus, whereas part-
time occlusion allows for some binocular development,
even in patients with monocular cataracts (15, 36). Patients with unilateral congenital cataracts require long-
term occlusion therapy, usually until 7 to 9 years of age.
Critical to the management of monocular congenital
cataracts is educating the parents about amblyopia and
the importance of a clear retinal image and occlusion
therapy.

Visual Prognosis

Monocular Cataracts. If surgery and optical correction is
provided early, by 2 months of age, visual acuity outcomes are relatively good, even for monocular congenital cataracts (4, 15, 30, 36). Birch and Stager (4) reported that a mean visual acuity of 20/60 (range,
20/800 to 20/30) was achieved if surgery was performed

before 2 months of age, whereas surgery after 2 months
of age resulted in poor visual acuity, ranging from hand
motions to 20/160. Cheng et al. (5) found that similar
results were achieved if surgery was performed before
17 weeks of age (6), however, all patients received full-
time occlusion therapy and all patients had the complication of postoperative strabismus.

Historically, patients with monocular cataracts have
a very poor prognosis for obtaining fusion, and virtually
all studies report that strabismus will develop in almost
100% of patients. Wright, (36) and Gregg and Parks
(15) reported that good visual acuity and binocularity
with stereopsis is possible in patients with monocular
cataracts. The key points in these cases were binocular
occlusion until visual rehabilitation, very early surgery
with immediate contact lens fitting, and part-time
monocular occlusion (less than 50%) for amblyopia
during the first few months of life.

Children with cataracts are not always seen during
the first few months of life. When faced with a child who
has a unilateral or bilateral cataract, the clinician must
determine whether to perform surgery on the cataract
or whether there is irreversible amblyopia. Reports by
Kushner (23) and Wright (37) indicate that many older
children with presumed congenital cataracts can show
significant visual acuity improvement. There is a relatively good prognosis for PHPV, posterior lenticonus,
and lamellar cataracts, even when the patient is seen after the critical period of visual development. Lack of
strabismus (straight eyes) is also a good prognostic sign
in patients with unilateral cataracts (37).

Binocular Cataracts. It is sometimes said that binocular
cataracts are less amblyogenic than monocular
cataracts. This is misleading, because even though a
monocular cataract causes a very dense amblyopia,
binocular cataracts also can cause significant amblyopia,
even legal blindness. It is very important that binocular
cataracts be treated with the utmost urgency, with
surgery during the first few weeks of life. If a visually significant bilateral congenital cataract is not cleared by 2
months of age, the majority of patients will develop sensory nystagmus and very poor visual acuity (30). Patients
with unoperated bilateral cataracts and sensory nystagmus can show visual acuity improvement and improvement of the nystagmus, even if surgery is performed
late, after the critical period of visual development. I
have reported that visual acuity as good as 20/50 to
20/70 can be achieved, even when surgery is performed
late (37). Surgery by 2 months of age is definitely the
treatment of choice. However, older children who are
seen later should be considered for cataract surgery,
even though they have bilateral cataracts and nystagmus. The exception to this is in patients with an abnormality of the retina or optic nerve such as aniridia. In patients with aniridia, cataract surgery usually does not
improve vision, because macular hypoplasia limits the
visual acuity potential.

■ ECTOPIA LENTIS (SUBLUXED LENS)

Displacement of the crystalline lens from its normal position is termed ectopia lentis or subluxed lens. The most common cause of bilateral subluxed lens is Marfan's syndrome, whereas the most common cause of a unilateral subluxed lens is probably trauma. The various causes of lens subluxation are listed in Table 21–5.

The laboratory assessments of a patient with ectopia lentis depends on the history and physical examination. If a clearly identifiable cause for the subluxation is found, a full laboratory work-up is not needed. Table 21–6 lists the clinical evaluation of subluxed lens.

Marfan's Syndrome

Marfan's syndrome the most common cause of subluxed lenses. It is a connective tissue disorder that is autosomal-dominant. Recent research has shown that Marfan's syndrome is caused by an incorrect expression of a gene product for the 350 kD glycoprotein called fibrillin, which makes up the extracellular microfibrol network (10).

Ocular manifestations of Marfan's syndrome include lens subluxation in approximately 80% of patients (24). The lens is usually displaced up and out; however, it may occur in any direction, but complete dislocation rarely occurs (Fig. 21–7). Other ocular findings include hypoplastic iris with pupillary miosis (difficult to dilate), lenticular myopia (axial length usually normal), flat corneal curvature, and possibly a increased incidence of spontaneous retinal detachment.

Systemic findings are consistent with the abnormal microfibrillar network and include aortic arch dilatation, dissecting aortic aneurysms, femoral hernias, and arachnodactyly (long thin fingers). Patients tend to be very tall, and their upper body segment is much shorter by comparison to their legs and arms. Scoliosis may occur and this may be quite deforming. Pectus excavatum and joint laxity are also present.

TABLE 21–5
Causes of Subluxed Lens

    A. Systemic Associations (Bilateral subluxation)
       1. Marfan's syndrome (by far, most common)
       2. Weill-Marchesani
       3. Homocystinuria
       4. Hyperlysinemia
       5. Sulfite oxidase deficiency
    B. Isolated Ocular Causes
       1. Trauma (unilateral)
       2. Aniridia (may be unilateral)
       3. Ectopia lentis et pupillae (bilateral)
       4. Autosomal dominant (bilateral)
       5. Anterior uveal coloboma (usually unilateral)
       6. Idiopathic (unilateral or bilateral)

TABLE 21–6
Clinical Evaluation of Subluxed Lens

A. History
   1. History of trauma, systemic illness, mental retardation seizures, etc.
   2. Family history, history of cardiovascular disease, sudden death in adolescence or early adulthood, skeletal abnormalities.
B. Complete Eye Exam
   1. Anterior segment, corneal diameter, anterior chamber depth, lens position, area of subluxation, iris, zonule attachments to the lens, phakodonesis.
   2. Refraction, rule out myopia and astigmatism.
   3. Keratometry
   4. Ultrasound
   5. Retinal exam
C. General Appearance
   1. Height
   2. Length of arms vs. Torso
   3. Length of fingers
   4. Joint flexibility
D. Laboratory Tests
   1. Cardiologist and cardiac ultrasound to rule out Marfan's
   2. Urine for amino acid
   3. Hand X-rays for possible brachiodactyly associated with Weill-Marchesani.
   4. Urine for sodium-nitroprusside (rule out homocystinuria)

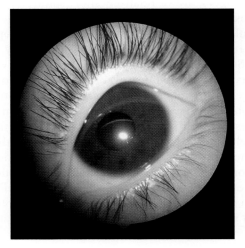

Figure 21–7.
Photograph of a subluxed lens associated with Marfan's syndrome. Classically, the lens is displaced up and out (superior-temporally), but in this case the lens is down and in (inferior-nasally).

Homocystinuria

Homocystinuria is caused by a deficiency of the enzyme cystathionine synthetase which results in abnormal methionine metabolism. Laboratory screening tests for homocystinuria include urine for amino acids (homocystine) and blood levels, which shows elevated homocystine and methionine. Sodium nitroprusside urine test screens for homocystinuria. Homocystinuria is rare, occurring in approximately 1:200,000 births.

Ocular manifestations include ectopia lentis, myopia, rarely secondary glaucoma, and possible retinal detachment. The zonules are weak and abnormal and lens accommodation is poor. In contrast to Marfan's syndrome, approximately one third of homocystinuria patients eventually develop complete lens dislocation either into the vitreous or anterior chamber. Subluxation in homocystinuria is symmetrical and occurs in almost all patients. Systemic findings include cerebral vascular thrombosis, myocardial infarction, pulmonary embolism, and intermittent claudication, all of which contribute to death at an early age. Homocystinuria patients are at increased anesthesia risk because of the possibility of thromboembolic disease.

Skeletal abnormalities are very mild in comparison to Marfan's syndrome, however, pectus excavatum, joint laxity, hernias, and scoliosis can occur. Some infants with homocystinuria will show developmental delay.

Weill-Marchesani Syndrome (Spherophakia-Brachymorphia)

Weill-Marchesani is usually inherited as an autosomal-recessive trait and consists of both ocular and skeletal abnormalities. The skeletal abnormalities are the reverse of Marfan's syndrome, as patients with Weill-Marchesani syndrome show brachymorphia, short stubby fingers, are of relatively short stature, and have hypoflexibility of the joints.

Ocular manifestations include microspherophakia (small round lens) and subluxation in virtually all patients. Subluxation is progressive with the lens eventually becoming completely dislocated. Dislocation into the anterior chamber is common. Secondary pupillary block glaucoma is an important consideration in Weill-Marchesani syndrome (20, 34, 35). Because of the risk of developing pupillary block glaucoma and the fact that once pupillary block occurs it is very difficult to treat, some authors have suggested a prophylactic laser peripheral iridotomy in all patients with Weill-Marchesani syndrome. In addition, patients should be prescribed miotic agents to prevent anterior dislocation of the lens. The risk of glaucoma is extremely high, with approximately 80% of patients developing angle-closure glaucoma.

Sulfite Oxidase Deficiency

This is an extremely rare disorder associated with increased sulfite in the urine. Systemic findings include hemiplegia, progressive choreoathetoid movements, seizures, and decreased mentation. There is cortical atrophy, most prominent in the parietal and frontal lobes. Over time, there is progressive subluxation and dislocation of the lens.

Ectopia Lentis et Pupillae

This is an ocular anomaly, which consists of lens subluxation and corectopia (displaced pupil). The pupil is often misshapen, either oval or slit-like, and the pupil is difficult to dilate. Persistent pupillary membranes with or without lenticular adhesions may occur. Ectopia lentis et pupillae is frequently bilateral and is often associated with myopia, glaucoma, and retinal detachment (8).

Treatment of Ectopia Lentis

A mild subluxation with most of the pupil covered by the lens is compatible with excellent visual acuity and does not necessarily need treatment. If the edge of the lens bisects the visual axis, this often results in image distortion and amblyopia. In these cases, a trial of pupillary dilation should be initiated. Phakic and aphakic correction should be attempted to find the best vision. Part-time occlusion therapy along with pupillary dilation may be enough to improve visual acuity. My experience, however, is that a subluxed lens that bisects the pupil often results in significant image distortion, even when the pupil is dilated. In these cases, surgical removal of the lens is indicated to clear the visual axis. Removal of the lens should be performed using a closed eye vitrectomy technique (1). One can approach the subluxed lens from an anterior (corneal) or posterior (pars plana) approach. The efficacy and safety of the anterior limbal versus posterior pars plana approach has been found to be approximately the same, perhaps with a slightly increased risk for retinal detachment using pars plana approach (16). Recent results have shown that lensectomy for subluxed lens can be performed safely and visual outcomes are good (1, 16). Marfan's lenses should not be removed by intracapsular techniques as zonules remain firm and removing the lens en bloc can result in retinal detachment.

■ REFERENCES

1. Behki R, Noel LP, Clarke WN: Limbal lensectomy in the management of ectopia lentis in children. Arch Ophthalmol 1990;108:809–811.
2. Beller R, Hoyt CS, Marg E, Odom JV: Good visual function after neonatal surgery for congenital monocular cataracts. Am J Ophthalmol 1981;91:559.
3. Bercovitch L, Donaldson DD: The natural history of congenital sutural cataracts: case report with long-term follow-up. Am J Pediatr Ophthalmol Strabismus 1982;19:108.
4. Birch EE, Stager DR: Prevalence of good visual acuity following surgery for congenital unilateral cataract. Arch Ophthalmol 1988;106:40.
5. Cheng KP, Hiles DA, Biglan AW, Pettapiece MC: Visual results after early surgical treatment of unilateral congenital cataract. Ophthalmology 1991;98:903–910.
6. Christiansen SP, Munoz M, Capo H: Retinal hemorrhage following lensectomy and anterior vitrectomy in children. J Pediatr Ophthalmol Strabismus 1993;30:24–27.
7. Cordes FC: Galactosemia cataract: a review. Am J Ophthalmol 1960;50:1151–1158.
8. Cross HE: Ectopia lentis et pupillae. Am J Ophthalmol 1979;88:381–384.
9. Cynader M, Derman N, Hein A: Recovery of function in cat visual cortex following prolonged deprivation. Exp Brain Res 1976;25:139–156.
10. Dietz HC, et al.: Science 1993;259:681.
11. Francois J: Syndromes with congenital cataract. 16th Jackson Memorial Lecture. Am J Ophthalmol 1961;52:207.
12. Gimbel HV, et al.: Implantation in children. J Pediatric Ophthalmol Strabismus 1993;30:69–79.
13. Ginsberg J, Bove KE, Fogelson MH: Pathological features of the eye in the oculocerebrorenal (Lowe) syndrome. J Pediatr Ophthalmol Strabismus 1981;18:16–24.
14. Gordon RA, Dunzs PB: Refractive development of the human eye. Arch Ophthalmol 1985;103:785–789.
15. Gregg FM, Parks MM: Stereopsis after congenital monocular cataract extraction. Am J Ophthalmol 1992;114:314–317.
16. Hakin KN, et al.: Management of the subluxed crystalline lens. Ophthalmology 1992;99:542–545.
17. Hiles DA: Intraocular lens implantation in children with monocular cataracts. Ophthalmology 1984;91:1231–1237.
18. Hoyt CS: The long-term visual effects of short-term binocular occlusion of at-risk neonates. Arch Ophthalmol 1980;98:1967–1970.
19. Jaafar MS, Robb RM: Congenital anterior polar cataract: a review of 63 cases. Ophthalmology 1984;91:249–254.
20. Jensen AD, Cross HE, Paton D: Ocular complications in the Weill-Marchesani syndrome. Am J Ophthalmol 1974;77:261–269.
21. Karr, DJ, Scott WE: Visual acuity results following treatment of persistent hyperplastic primary vitreous. Arch Ophthalmol 1986;104:662.
22. Koenig SB, et al.: Pseudophakia for traumatic cataracts in children. Ophthalmology 1993;100:1218–1223.
23. Kushner BJ: Visual results after surgery for monocluar juvenile cataracts of undetermined onset. Am J Ophthalmol 1986;102:468.
24. Maumenee IH: The eye in the Marfan syndrome. Trans Am Ophthalmol Soc 1981;69:685.
25. Morgan KS, Karciolglu Z: Secondary cataracts in infants after lensectomies. J Pediatr Ophthalmol Strabismus 1987;24:45–48.
26. Morgan KS, McDonald MB, Hiles DA, et al.: The nationwide study of epikeratophakia for aphakia in older children. Ophthalmology 1988;95:526.
27. Nelson LB, Calhoun JH, Simon JW, Harley RD: Progression of congenital anterior polar cataracts in childhood. Arch Ophthalmol 1985;103:1842.
28. Parks MM: Management of cataracts in infants. Pediatric Ophthalmology and Strabismus: Transactions of the New Orleans Academy of Ophthalmology. New York: Raven Press, 1986, pp. 119–139.
29. Pinchoff BS, Ellis FD, Helveston EM, Sato SE: Cystoid macular edema in pediatric aphakia. J Pediatr Ophthalmol Strabismus 1988;25:240.
30. Rogers GL, Tishler CL, Tsou BH, Hertle RW, Fellows RR: Visual acuities in infants with congenital cataracts operated on prior to 6 months of age. Arch Ophthalmol 1981;99:999.
31. Scheie HG, Schaffer DB, Plotkin SA, Kertesz ED: Congenital rubella cataracts: surgical results and virus recovery from intraocular tissue. Arch Ophthalmol 1967;77:440–444.
32. Streeten BW, Robinson MR, Wallace R, Jones DB: Lens capsule abnormalities in Alport's syndrome. Arch Ophthalmol 1987;105:1693–1697.
33. Thompson SM, Deady JP, WIllshaw HE, White RH: Ocular signs in Alport's syndrome. Eye 1987;0:146–153.
34. Willi M, Kut L, Cotlier E: Pupillary-block glaucoma in the Marchesani syndrome. Arch Ophthalmol 1973;90:504–508.
35. Wright KW, Chrousos GA: Weill-Marchesani syndrome with bilateral angle-closure glaucoma. J Pediatr Ophthalmol Strabismus 1985;22:129–132.
36. Wright KW, Matusmoto E, Edelman PM: Binocular fusion and stereopsis associated with early surgery for monocular congenital cataracts. Arch Ophthalmol 1992;110:1607.
37. Wright KW, Christensen LE, Noguchi BA: Results of late surgery for presumed congenital cataracts. Am J Ophthalmol 1992;114:409–415.
38. Wright KW, Wehrle MJ, Urrea PT: Bilateral total occlusion during the critical period of visual development. Arch Ophthalmol 1987;105:321.

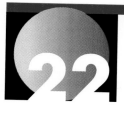

22 Retinopathy of Prematurity and Pediatric Retinal Tumors

Kenneth W. Wright

■ RETINOPATHY OF PREMATURITY

In the late 1940s and early 1950s, retinopathy of prematurity (ROP), or as it was then called retrolental fibroplasia (RLF), was the most common cause of blindness in children (Fig. 22–1). Premature infants born during this period were placed in incubators and treated with almost 100% oxygen. Dr. Arnold Patz was one of the pioneers who, in the mid 1950s, showed that hyperoxia was a critical factor that caused the development of ROP in premature infants (39). After oxygen was curtailed, a dramatic decrease in the incidence of severe ROP occurred. Unfortunately, morbidity and mortality rates also increased because of hypoxic brain damage. The use of oxygen monitoring by arterial blood gas and pulse oximeters has greatly improved survival rate and reduced morbidity in premature infants. The survival rate for a 26-week-old gestation, 700 g premature neonate is now approximately 50%, whereas almost none of these infants survived in the early 1960s. Because of the increased survival of low birth-weight infants, the incidence of ROP is again increasing. The ophthalmologist plays a critical role in the management of ROP, since the window for treatment is narrow. It is the ophthalmologist who is responsible for identifying and treating high-risk infants.

Etiology

The exact cause of ROP remains controversial; however, it is clear that oxygen plays a major role in the development of ROP. One of the most widely accepted theories on the pathogenesis of ROP is that increased oxygen causes vasoconstriction of immature retinal vessels (5, 39). Premature infants do not have a fully vascularized retina, and the retinal vasculature is immature. Figure 22–2 shows the extent of retinal vascularization emanating from the optic nerve relative to gestational age in weeks. Note that the vessels start at the optic nerve and progressively grow toward the ora serrata. The nasal retina is vascularized first, and then the temporal retina later. A small skirt of avascular temporal retina is present even in full-term infants. This is why ROP is most commonly seen at the temporal retina and has been reported in full-term infants (30). There also are a few scattered reports of ROP occurring in full-term infants without exposure to oxygen, but some may represent a misdiagnosis.

Vasoconstriction of the immature vessels produces secondary ischemia of the peripheral retina (5). This hypoxia leads to the stimulation of local vasoproliferative factors, resulting in the development of abnormal vessels and arteriolar-venous shunts at the border of vascular and avascular retina. These shunt vessels can progress to form neovascularization. Shunt vessels and neovascular vessels leak protein and invoke retinal fibrosis. Scarring and retinal fibrosis cause retinal traction, which can result in retinal detachment. Almost all cases of ROP are associated with hyperoxia. Providing a stable, controlled, low oxygen environment, while maintaining adequate oxygen saturation for the premature infant is one of the most important challenges in the neonatal intensive care unit.

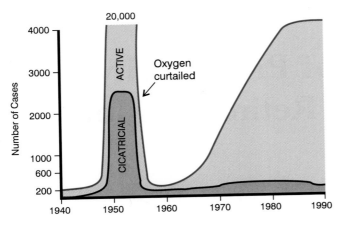

Figure 22–1.
Graph showing incidence of ROP over time from the 1940s to the 1990s. Note that around 1955 the incidence of cicatricial and active ROP dropped significantly as this is the point in time when oxygen was curtailed. In the late 1960s through the 1990s, survival of very low birth weight infants increased along with the incidence of active ROP (red area). Note that the incidence of severe cicatricial ROP has remained relatively low during this period.

Risk Factors

The most significant risk factor for developing ROP is the degree of prematurity as measured by birth weight (21, 38). Table 22–1 shows the incidence of ROP compared with birth weight. In infants weighing between 1000 and 1250 g, almost 50% will show some sign of ROP; however, only 2% will reach threshold.[38] Vision-threatening ROP almost never develops in children weighing more than 1250 g, and, therefore, screening mostly begins in infants weighing less than 1250 to 1500 g (14–16, 38). This rule however applies to children receiving curtailed oxygen. On a project Orbis mission to an underdeveloped country, I examined several children with bilateral stage 5 cicatricial ROP (total retinal detachment), with birth weight more than 1800 g. These infants were not monitored and received uncurtailed oxygen for prolonged periods of time.

As stated above, hyperoxia is also an important risk factor, as transcutaneous oxygen tensions over 80% correlated significantly with increased incidence and severity of ROP (22). Other risk factors include gestational age, respiratory distress syndrome, infections, intracranial hemorrhage, and blood transfusions. Blood transfusions supply the neonate with adult hemoglobin, which dissociates oxygen more freely, thus providing increased tissue oxygen dose.

Classification of ROP

The Committee for the Classification of Retinopathy Of Prematurity has published an international classification of ROP. (45, 46) This classification uses three parameters: (1) zone of the disease (posterior to anterior location); (2) clock hours of involvement (circum-

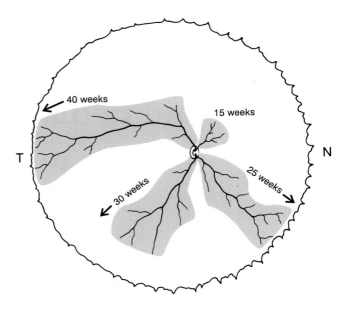

Figure 22–2.
Diagram showing the vascularization pattern of the fetal retina. Retina vessels grow out of the optic nerve towards the peripheral retina. Since the distance from the optic nerve to the nasal retina is shortest, the nasal retina becomes vascularized first. Even a full-term infant will have a narrow skirt of avascular retina in the temporal periphery (T: temporal retina; N: nasal retina).

ferential extent of ROP); and (3) stage (degree of abnormal vasculature). Figure 22–3 shows the various zones with zone 1 being the most posterior zone, demarcated by a circle centered on the optic nerve, the radius of which extends twice the distance from the disc to the fovea. Zone 2 is a circle centered on the optic nerve with the radius being the distance from the optic nerve to the nasal ora serrata. Zone 3 is the temporal crescent of peripheral retina not included in zones 1 and 2. If ROP is present nasally, it must be in zone 1 or 2.

Stages of ROP

The stages of ROP denote the severity of the disease and include normal immature retina, active ROP, and regressed ROP. Consult Table 22–2 and Figures 22–4 and 22–5 for an overview of the stages of ROP.

TABLE 22–1
Incidence of ROP Versus Birth Weight

Birth Weight grams	Any ROP %	Stage 3 %	Pre-threshold %	Threshold %
<750	90	37	39	15
750–999	78	22	21	7
1000–1250	47	8	7	2
Total Group	66	18	18	6

Modified from Palmer et al, 1991 (38)

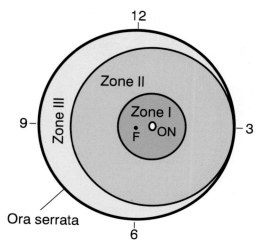

Figure 22–3.
International classification of ROP "zones." Zone 1 is the circumferential area around the optic nerve with a radius twice the distance from the optic nerve to the fovea (dark red area). Zone 2 has a diameter from the optic nerve to the nasal retina (pink zone). Zone 3 is the temporal crescent of retina not covered by zone 1 or zone 2 (light pink area).

Normal Immature Retina

This is not truly ROP but normal immature retina with a peripheral avascular zone (Fig. 22–4). Normal immature retina can be distinguished from stage 1 ROP by the transition between vascular and avascular retina. Normal retinal vessels have a pattern of arborization (tree branching) that provides uniform vascular coverage, and there is no sharp demarcation line at the junction of vascular and avascular retina as there is on ROP.

TABLE 22–2
Stages of Retinopathy of Prematurity

Stage	Retinal Findings
Normal	Normal vascularized retina with arborization of vessels, no demarcation line between the peripheral avascular zone
1.	Demarcation line with straightening of the peripheral vessels as they connect to the demarcation line.
2.	Elevated ridge with volume straightened peripheral vessels inserted into ridge
3.	Ridge with neovascularization extending off the retina into the vitreous.
4.	Subtotal retinal detachment A. Extrafoveal B. Retinal detachment including fovea
5.	Total retinal detachment—Funnel configuration open, narrow or closed, anterior or posterior.

Active ROP

In stage 1 ROP, there is a sharp demarcation line between the vascular and avascular zone, which represents an arteriolar–venous shunt. The peripheral vessels line up in a straight parallel configuration and feed into the shunt (Fig. 22–4). These abnormal vessels take on a pattern reminiscent of the bristles of a broom. The shunt is flat at stage 1, seen only as a demarcation line delineating vascular from avascular retina. This is the mildest form of ROP and has a very good prognosis.

Stage 2 ROP is a progression of the demarcation line in stage 1 to an elevated ridge (Fig. 22–4). This occurs

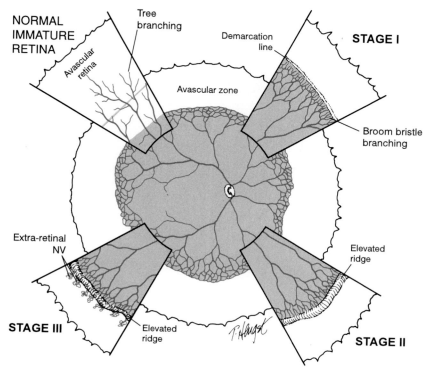

Figure 22–4.
Diagram of the vascular pattern associated with normal immature retina, and stage I to stage III ROP. The upper left is a diagram of normal immature retina showing the typical tree branching vascular pattern. Upper right shows stage I ROP with straightening of the peripheral vessels to insert at the shunt-demarcation line. There is the distinctive broom bristle branching pattern with the vessels ends lining up along the shunt. Lower right stage II ROP showing an elevated ridge, which represents an enlarged shunt. Lower left stage III ROP with extraretinal extension of neovascularization (NV), in addition to a shunt.

as the vascular shunt enlarges. Studies using fluorescein angiography have documented that the abnormal shunt vessels leak. Normal immature retina and stage 1 or 2 ROP in zone 3, without plus disease, has an excellent prognosis.

Stage 3 ROP is the presence of a ridge with extraretinal extension of neovascular tissue into the vitreous (Fig. 22–4). There is a ragged appearance to the ridge, and there may be local hemorrhage because of the fragile neovascular tissue. Stage 3 is an indication of severe disease and must be followed closely with at least weekly examinations.

Plus disease is the presence of dilated and tortuous retinal vessels in the posterior pole. It is a sign of severe disease and may coexist with stage 2 or stage 3 ROP (Fig. 22–5). Stage 3 ROP and plus disease indicates significant risk of vision loss and may require laser or cryotherapy (Table 22–3).

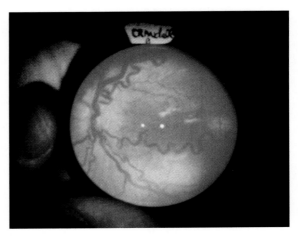

Figure 22–5.
Photograph of plus disease showing tortuous and dilated retinal arcades emanating from the optic nerve.

Regression vs Cicatricial ROP

After the active stage of ROP, the disease regresses. This can take the form of a benign normal regression pattern or a cicatricial pattern.

Normal Regression

Normal regression of ROP occurs when retinal vessels grow past the shunt–demarcation line to vascularize the peripheral retina, without significant fibrosis or scarring. Clinically, normal regression is diagnosed by identifying vessels that grow past the shunt into the avascular retina in a normal branching pattern, along with the involution of the shunt and or neovascularization.

Cicatricial ROP

Cicatricial ROP is retinal scarring as a result of severe active ROP, usually stage 3. The degree and severity of cicatricial ROP depends on the severity of the active disease and is quite variable. The hallmark of cicatricial ROP is retinal fibrosis and secondary retinal traction. In the mild form, cicatricial ROP produces peripheral traction that pulls the vascular arcades temporally, straightening the vessels. More severe temporal traction will drag the macula temporally, which may or may not interfere with vision, but will produce a positive angle kappa. A positive angle kappa occurs because the eye must abduct to fixate with the temporally displaced macula. This gives the false appearance of an exotropia (see Fig. 14–14).

Stages 4 and 5

Severe fibrosis and traction can lead to retinal detachment, which may be partial (stage 4) or total (stage 5)

(see Table 22–2). Epiretinal traction can roll the retina into a scroll detachment. Circumferential traction causes a funnel detachment as seen in Figure 22–6. In addition to tractional retinal detachment, serous detachments without traction also can occur.

Management of ROP

The most important aspect of the management of ROP is early detection. The multicenter trial of Cryotherapy

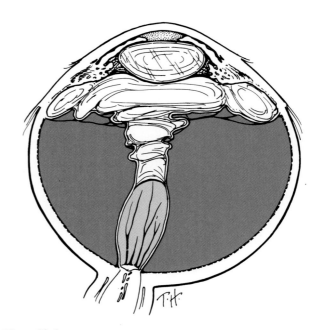

Figure 22–6.
Stage V ROP with total retinal detachment. The red area in the cutaway of the closed funnel detachment showing retinal vessels inside the funnel. Note that the retrolental membrane is pushing the lens and iris diaphragm anteriorly. There is a high incidence of angle closure glaucoma in these patients.

TABLE 22–3
Protocol for Premature Infants

A.	Screen all premature infants under 1500 gr.	Initial fundus exam at four weeks after birth.
B.	No ROP Immature retina:	Repeat exam in one month. If one month follow up shows normal regression pattern see back in six months for full exam and cycloplegic refraction.
C.	Mild ROP:	(Stage 1 or 2): Repeat exam every two weeks to monitor for progression.
D.	Pre-threshold	(Zone 1 any ROP, Zone 2 stage 2 with *Plus disease*, or Zone 2 stage 3): Note that pre-threshold is extremely important and repeat exams should be performed every week until either threshold is reached or regression is unequivocally seen.
E.	Threshold	(Zone 1 or 2 with five contiguous clock hours or 8 accumulative clock hours of stage 3 in the presence of *Plus disease*): Once threshold is reached, cryotherapy or laser therapy must be performed within 72 hours.
F.	Stage 4	Scleral buckle may be indicated. If it is a serous detachment follow, no surgery (23, 36).
G.	Stage 5	Consider vitreoretinal surgery; but universally poor visual outcome (27, 49).

for Retinopathy of Prematurity (CROP) has shown a 50% reduction in vision-threatening sequelae to ROP when cryotherapy is applied in the active stage before development of retinal detachment (14–16). The initial neonatal nursery examination should be performed during the first months of life for all infants weighing less than 1500 g (14–16). Patients in the neonatal intensive care unit are dilated before examination (e.g. *cyclomydril*). Drops should be instilled twice at 5-minute intervals. Scleral depression is required to visualize the peripheral retina. It is important to remember to inform the patients' family members and nurses of the ocular status and the proposed follow-up after the examination.

Table 22–3 summarizes the protocol for examining and treating immature infants. If immature retina is found in zone 3 on initial screening, but no ROP, then repeat the examination every month until a normal regression pattern is established. Once normal regression is complete, plan a long-term follow up in 6 months for a ocular examination including cycloplegic refraction. If stage 1 or stage 2 ROP is found, a repeat examination should be performed approximately every 2 weeks depending on the severity and zone, to monitor for progression. Once a normal regression pattern is identified, follow-up examinations can be spaced to approximately every month. Patients with stage 3 ROP or stage 2 ROP in zone 2 with plus disease must be monitored very closely, as this represents prethreshold disease. In these cases, the examination should be performed at least every week, as these patients are at significant risk for progressing to threshhold disease. Patients who develop stage 3 ROP over 5 contiguous clock hours or 8 accumulative clock hours with plus disease have reached *threshold ROP,* and require cryotherapy or laser therapy. Treatment should be given within 72 hours of identifying threshold disease. Table 22–3 lists the protocol for following premature infants.

Cryotherapy and Laser Therapy

Cryotherapy and laser therapy ablate the peripheral hypoxic avascular retina (8). Ablation therapy is given to the avascular retina, not directly to the shunt or the neovascularization. If left untreated, threshold disease is associated with an unfavorable outcome in approximately 50% of cases, whereas cryotherapy or laser therapy reduces this to approximately 20% to 25% (14–16). Argon, xenon, and the diode laser have been shown to be effective, with results similar to cryotherapy (11, 25, 32, 33, 47). Laser therapy has become a popular form of treatment.

Vitreoretinal Surgery

The surgical management of stage 4 or 5 ROP is controversial. Scleral buckling procedure may be indicated for some stage 4 cases (23, 36). Stage 5 has an extremely poor prognosis even with modern vitreoretinal techniques. The retina can be at least partially anatomically reattached in approximately 25% to 48% of cases, however postoperative visual function is universally poor (27, 49). The heroic vitreoretinal surgery required to repair a stage 5 retinal detachment should be performed only after a full discussion of realistic expectations with the parents regarding the poor prognosis (17, 23, 49).

Medical Treatments

The most important medical treatment, also the most difficult, is to keep a low stable tissue dose of oxygen during the infants stay in the neonatal intensive care unit. Other treatment modalities include the administration of *surfactant,* which reduces respiratory distress syndrome (41). High-dose vitamin E supplementation has been advocated in the past. The use of high-dose vitamin E is decreasing as there are significant side effects (e.g., *necrotising entercolitis*), the efficacy is questionable. Now most centers give only low dose physiologic vitamin E supplementation (18, 26).

Differential Diagnosis

The *differential diagnosis* of ROP includes PHPV, FEVR, Norrie's disease, and the causes of leukokoria (Table 22–4). The diagnosis of ROP is usually straightforward based on the history of prematurity, oxygen exposure, and characteristic fundus findings. Nonetheless, these are rare diseases that can be confused with ROP.

Familial Exudative Vitreo Retinopathy (FEVR). This is an autosomal-dominant inherited peripheral retinopathy that, in the early stage, looks very similar to ROP (37). Findings include peripheral neovascularization, avascular retina, and retinal exudates. The disease may evolve to produce retinal traction, macular dragging, retinal folds, retinal breaks, and retinal detachment.

Norrie's Disease: This is a rare x-linked recessive disease that includes retinal dysplasia that is usually bilateral, deafness (33%), and mental retardation (25%). The retina may be detached at birth, may mimic PHPV, or mimic retinoblastoma consisting of retinal psuedotumors.

TABLE 22–4
Differential Diagnosis of Leukokoria

Cataract
Coats Disease
Coloboma of Choroid and optic nerve
Corneal Opacity
Familial Exudative Vitreoretinopathy (FEVR)
High Myopia/Anisometropia
Medulloepithelioma and Other Posterior Pole Tumors
Myelinated Nerve Fibers
Norrie's Disease
Persistent Hyperplastic Primary Vitreous (PHPV)
Retinal Detachment (trisomy 13, Meckel syndrome, Warburg syndrome, Norrie's disease, and incontinentia pigmenti)
Retinal Dysplasia
Retinoblastoma
Retinopathy of Prematurity
Toxocariasis
Uveitis (posterior)
Vitreous Hemorrhage

Late Complications of ROP

ROP holds an increased incidence for myopia, astigmatism, anisometropia, amblyopia, and strabismus (31, 40). Patients with severe stage 5 ROP can have glaucoma as a late complication. Late retinal detachment also is a complication, especially in patients with high myopia.

■ PEDIATRIC POSTERIOR SEGMENT TUMORS

Retinoblastoma

Retinoblastoma is a malignant tumor of the sensory retina and is the most common ocular malignancy in childhood. Critical to the treatment of retinoblastoma is early identification, because cure rates are greater than 90% if the tumor is localized within the eye. A white reflex within the pupil is called *leukokoria* and is a serious sign that deserves immediate evaluation (Fig. 22–7). The differential diagnosis of leukokoria in children is listed in Table 22–4 with retinoblastoma in bold letters to emphasize its importance, since it is a potentially lethal disease.

Clinical Signs

The most common presenting signs of retinoblastoma are leukocoria and strabismus. Retinoblastoma may present with findings that mimic other ophthalmic disorders, such as primary angle-closure glaucoma, vitreous hemorrhage, retina detachment, hyphema, hypopion, and preseptal cellulitis. Usually retinoblastoma presents with a quiet eye; however, tumor necrosis can lead to in-

traocular hemorrhage, inflammation, and a red and painful eye. Angle-closure glaucoma occurs when the posterior pole fills with tumor, thus pushing the lens–iris diaphragm anteriorly. Although retinoblastoma is rare (estimated at 1:20,000 live births), the ophthalmologist must hold high suspicion for this disease in any child younger than 5 years of age with an unexplained posterior pole lesion.

Retinoblastoma can grow subretinally (exophytic) into the vitreous (endophytic) (Fig. 22–8), or rarely occurs as a diffuse infiltrating mass that grows along the retina, and into the vitreous looking much like a posterior uveitis (9). Retinoblastoma tumors have a yellow or slightly pink gelatinous appearance (Fig. 22–8). There may be white areas within the tumor that represent calcification (Fig. 22–7B). Calcification is a hallmark of retinoblastoma and is best detected by computed tomography scan (Fig. 22–7B) or ocular ultrasound. Calcification is associated with tumor necrosis, which occurs as the tumor outgrows its blood supply. The presence of calcium in a retinal mass is highly suggestive of retinoblastoma; however, other diseases that have tissue necrosis (e.g., Coats' disease) can show calcifica-

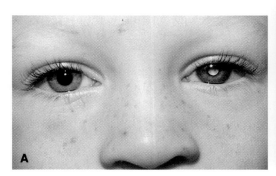 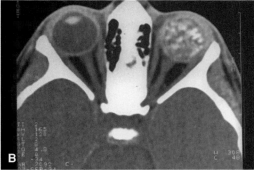

Figure 22–7.
A, Photograph of a 19-month-old with left leukokoria secondary to retinoblastoma. **B,** Computed tomography scan showing extensive intraocular calcification associated with retinoblastoma. Calcification represents area of tumor necrosis.

tions, and rarely retinoblastoma tumors will not be calcified.

Genetics

Retinoblastoma is caused by a mutation in a growth suppressor gene. The site of the gene for retinoblastoma is chromosome 13q14, and the gene has been sequenced (13, 19, 20). Both alleles must be affected for the development of retinoblastoma tumor, as one intact suppressor gene is all that is necessary to regulate retinal cell growth. Knudson was the first to suggest this two hit hypothesis (32). Although retinoblastoma is often cited as an autosomal-dominant disorder, it is a predisposition that is autosomal-dominant. Retinoblastoma is actually an autosomal-recessive trait, since both alleles must be affected to express the disease. There are two recognized mechanisms that cause a mutation of both alleles, thus causing retinoblatoma: *hereditary retinoblastoma* and *sporadic retinoblastoma.*

Hereditary Retinoblastoma

In the hereditary form of retinoblastoma, a mutation of both retinoblastoma genes occurs by inheriting one abnormal gene from one parent (germinal mutation) and then acquiring a spontaneous mutation of the other allelic gene at the retinal cell level later in development (somatic mutation). Patients with hereditary retinoblastoma have one defective retinoblastoma gene in virtually all cells in their body. Because of this, patients with the hereditary retinoblastoma are predisposed to acquiring secondary nonocular tumors such as osteosarcoma in late childhood and adulthood.

Since all the retinal cells in the inherited form have one abnormal gene (one hit) and a predisposition to develop retinoblastoma, most inherited retinoblastomas are bilateral with only 15% being unilateral. Hereditary retinoblastoma is often multifocal with mul-

tiple tumors developing in each eye. Patients with the hereditary form present early, on the average by around 12 months of age. The inherited form can come from a parent with known retinoblastoma, from a germinal mutation in the egg or sperm, or a mutation at the time of conception. In these latter cases, the family history is negative for retinoblastoma. In fact, the majority of new cases of bilateral hereditary retinoblastoma are due to a new germinal mutation, as only 10% have a positive family history. If a parent has retinoblastoma, there is a 50% chance of passing the predisposition (one retinoblatoma gene) to a child. Because not all children with one mutated allele develop a mutation in the second allele, the chances of the child developing retinoblastoma is 40%. If there is no family history of retinoblastoma and a child is born with bilateral retinoblastoma, the chances that another sibling will develop retinoblastoma is approximately 8%. Remember that most germinal mutations are not present in the germinal stem cells of the parents, so subsequent children are at low risk. With DNA testing, in most cases, carriers of a germinal mutation of the retinoblastoma gene can be identified.

A large deletion in the area of the retinoblastoma gene may involve other local genes and cause an identifiable defect in the karyotype at chromosome 13q14. These patients may have the clinical characteristics of facial dysmorphism, developmental delay, mental retardation, and low-set ears. This phenotype only occurs in 3% of retinoblastoma cases where there are multiple genes that are deleted in addition to the retinoblastoma gene.

Sporadic Retinoblastoma

The sporadic form of retinoblastoma is caused by a spontaneous mutation of both alleles at the retinal cell level (two somatic mutations). This requires two independent mutational events that are not inherited. Sporadic retinoblastoma presents as a unilateral–unifocal

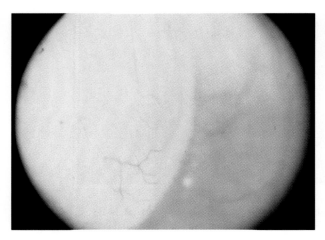

Figure 22–8.
Fundus photograph of endophytic retinoblastoma. Notice the yellow-white appearance of the domed mass. Normal attached retina is seen in the background to the left.

tumor. It must be noted however that 15% of hereditary retinoblastoma occurs as a unilateral tumor albeit usually multifocal. Approximately 60% of all retinoblastoma cases are the nonhereditary form.

Staging of Retinoblastoma

Retinoblastoma has been classified by Reese Ellsworth as to the prognosis of the eye (Table 22–5). This classification has been mistakenly extrapolated to estimate the prognosis for survival. It states that multiple or solitary tumors less than 10 disc diameters in size located posterior to the equator have an outcome that is very favorable (less than 4 disc diameters) or favorable (less than 10 disc diameters). Any tumor at or anterior to the equator, a tumor larger than 10 disc diameters, or a tumor extending to the ora serrata has a doubtful to unfavorable prognosis. Massive tumors involving over half the retina or the presence of vitreous seeding indicates a very unfavorable prognosis for salvaging the eye.

The classic histologic findings of retinoblastoma are *Flexner-Wintersteiner rosettes* and less commonly seen are *fleurettes*. Pathologic signs of poor systemic prognosis include extrascleral extension, extension of the tumor into the optic nerve posterior to the lamina cribrosa, and possibly choroidal involvement. Local extension into the orbit and metastasis through the subarachnoid space into the brain are the most common routes of tumor spread. Bone marrow, liver, and lungs also are distant sites for metastasis.

Pinealoblastoma (Trilateral Retinoblastoma)

Pinealoma associated with bilateral retinoblastoma has been termed trilateral retinoblastoma. This is a rare occurrence and has an extremely poor prognosis (6, 35,

44). The pineal body is considered a third eye and has an embryologic link to the retinal tissue.

Examination and Workup of Retinoblastoma

When a patient presents with a presumed retinoblastoma, it is important to perform a careful retinal examination with scleral depression of both eyes and obtain a computed tomography scan. Ocular ultrasound may be useful to help differentiate the tissue type. In general, the diagnosis of retinoblastoma is based on the clinical appearance and the presence of calcification on computed tomography scan or ocular ultrasound. Elevated aqueous LDH levels are suggestive of retinoblastoma but are not diagnostic.

Careful detailed drawings should be made of the lesions. Magnetic resonance imaging is helpful for determining if there is extrascleral extension; however, MRI will not identify calcification. Computed tomography scan is indicated to identify calcium, but lack of calcium does not rule out retinoblastoma. At one time, bone marrow aspiration and biopsy and lumbar puncture were routinely ordered in all patients with retinoblastoma. Recently, most experts have suggested limiting these tests to cases where extrascleral extension is suspected.

Treatment

Large tumors involving the macula are associated with poor visual prognosis and are generally treated by enucleation. Smaller unilateral tumors can be treated with external beam radiation (approximately 4000 rad). If the tumor is bilateral, then every attempt should be made to save at least one eye (2, 3). External beam radiation is most useful for posteriorly located tumors.

TABLE 22–5
Reese-Ellsworth Eye Prognosis Classification

Group 1: Very favorable
- Solitary tumor less than 4 DD in size, at or behind equator
- Multiple tumors, none over 4 DD in size, all at or behind equator

Group 2: Favorable
- Solitary tumor, 4 to 10 DD in size, at or behind equator
- Multiple tumors, 4 to 10 DD in size, behind equator

Group 3: Doubtful
- Any tumor anterior to equator
- Solitary tumor, larger than 10 DD, behind equator

Group 4: Unfavorable
- Multiple tumors, some larger than 10 DD in size
- Any lesion extending anteriorly to the ora serrata

Group 5: Very unfavorable
- Massive tumors involving over half the retina
- Vitreous seeding

Radioactive plaque treatment also has been used and has the advantage of minimizing radiation to normal tissue. External beam radiation may have the disadvantage of inducing or speeding up the development of secondary tumors in patients with the hereditary form of retinoblastoma and causes facial asymmetry (4, 34). Some have advocated the use of chemotherapy to decrease the size of the tumor followed by laser or cryotherapy. Small peripheral tumors can be treated with cryotherapy or laser photocoagulation. If tumor extends past the lamina cribora even if the cut end of the optic nerve is clear of tumor, systemic chemotherapy is usually indicated.

A child with unilateral retinoblastoma must be followed closely because in 20% of these patients, a new tumor will develop in the good eye. This risk diminishes greatly after 2 years of age. In cases of hereditary retinoblastoma, siblings are at risk for developing the tumor and should be followed with serial scleral depression retinal examinations, unless DNA analysis demonstrates the sibling does not carry a retinoblastoma gene.

Tumor Regression

After treatment, tumors will undergo regression and tumor necrosis. Type I regression is associated with a persistent calcific mass, which is white and has the appearance of cottage cheese. Type II regression consists of translucent grayish tissue, which has the appearance of uncooked fish flesh. The type II regression pattern may be difficult to differentiate from viable tumor. The regression patterns are sometimes seen in otherwise normal patients and are believed to be caused by spontaneous regression of retinoblastoma. These cases of spontaneous regression are very rare, and all retinoblastoma cases should be treated aggressively.

Prognosis

When a unilateral retinoblastoma, without extrascleral extension and without extension past the lamina cribrosa, is treated with enucleation, it is associated with long-term survival greater than 90%. If the tumor cells extend posterior to the lamina cribrosa, the survival rate is approximately 60%, even if the cut end of the optic nerve is free of tumor. Extrascleral extension of tumor cells beyond the surgical transection site of the optic nerve is associated with a long-term survival rate of less than 20%. External beam radiation in patients without extrascleral extension results in a cure in approximately 85% of patients. Successfully treated patients with retinoblastoma have a risk period for extraocular spread of tumor between 12 and 18 months.

If the patient has hereditary retinoblastoma, there is a risk for secondary malignant tumors developing in later life. These tumors often are in the area of external beam radiation but also can occur in remote sites. Secondary tumors include malignant melanoma, fibrosarcoma, leiomyosarcoma, osteosarcoma, and renal cell carcinoma. In patients who receive radiation therapy, secondary tumors develop earlier than in patients who have not had radiation. The incidence for development of a secondary tumor in patients with hereditary retinoblastoma is probably more than 50% follow-up of more than 30 years.

Medulloepithelioma

Medulloepithelioma is a tumor that arises from the ciliary body or iris (12). It occurs sporadically and can occur virtually any time during life but most commonly is seen in children between 4 to 8 years of age. The tumor probably stems from nonpigmented ciliary epithelium.

The tumor is slow growing and tends to stay localized within the eye. Survival rates are excellent if the tumor is localized to the eye (10). The tumor usually arises from the ciliary body; however, rare reports of optic nerve and retinal involvment have been described. Since the tumors arise from the ciliary body, they are usually not detected until they are quite large. Often, patients have angle-closure glaucoma, pain, poor vision, or an anterior chamber cyst or mass. Cataract, rubeosis, and PHPV have been associated with medulloepitheliomas.

The treatment is usually enucleation; however, iridocyclectomy can be curative if the entire lesion is removed.

Uveal Melanoma

Although they are extremely rare in children, uveal melanomas may still occur. Tumors may involve the iris, cilliary body, or choroid (42, 43). The diagnosis of melanoma should be entertained in patients with an enlarging pigmented mass. Other causes of a pigmented intraocular mass in children include melanocytoma, choroidal nevus, pigmented neurofibroma, juvenile xanthogranuloma, and a retinal pigment epithelial hamartoma. Uveal melanomas may arise from ocular and oculodermal melanocytosis (48). Ocular ultrasound is an important tool for establishing the proper diagnoses as it is in adults.

The prognosis of uveal melanomas in children parallels that of adults. A review of choroidal and ciliary body tumors in children by Barr, McLean, and Zimmermann showed that, of 42 patients, 13 died of metastatic disease, an incident similar to the adult population (7). Poor prognostic features include extraocular extension, large basal diameter (greater than 10 mm), aggressive cell type, and red painful eye with tumor necrosis at the time of presentation. The treatment is usually enucleation.

Leukemia

Leukemia can involve all ocular structures, however, the retina is the most commonly involved site. Acute lymphoblastic leukemia (ALL) is the most common leukemic cell type. Retinal involvement includes cotton–wool spots, exudates, dilated veins, and most commonly retinal hemorrhages (24). Hemorrhages may take on the appearance of a Roth spot with white centers and surrounding hemorrhage. Other ocular manifestations include retinal infiltrates, vitreous involvement, exudative retinal detachment, optic nerve involvement, iris infiltrate, hypopyon (1), ring corneal ulcers, and conjunctiva and perilimbal infiltrates (28). Treatment, for the most part, is directed toward the systemic disease by the hematology team. However, local radiation to anterior lesions (conjunctiva, anterior chamber, or iris) with low-dose external beam radiation has been found to be effective.

■ REFERENCES

1. Abramson DH, et al.: Treatment of bilateral groups I-III: Retinoblastoma with bilateral radiation. Arch Ophthalmol 1981;99:1761–1762.

2. Abramson DH, et al.: Simultaneous bilateral radiation for advanced bilateral retinoblastoma. Arch Ophthalmol 1981;99:1763–1766.

3. Abramson DH, et al.: Second non-ocular tumors in retinoblastoma survivors: Are they radiation induced? Ophthalmology 1984;91:1351–1355.

4. Ashton N: Oxygen and the growth and development of retinal vessels. In vivo and in vitro studies. Am J Ophthalmol 1966;62:412–435.

5. Bader, et al.: Bilateral reintoblastoma with ectopic intracranial retinoblastoma: Trilateral retinoblastoma. Cancer Genet Cytogenet 1982;5:203–213.

6. Barr CC, McLean IW, Zimmerman LE: Uveal melanoma in children and adolescents. Arch Ophthalmol 1981;99:2133.

7. Ben-Sira I, Nissenkorn I, Grunwald E, et al.: Treatment of acute retrolental fibroplasia cryotherapy. Br J Ophthalmol 1980;64:748–762.

8. Bhatnagar R, Vine AK: diffuse infiltrating retinoblastoma. Ophthalmology 1991;98:1657–1661.

9. Broughton WL, Zimmerman LE: A clinicopathologic study of 56 cases of intraocular medulloepitheliomas. Am J Ophthalmol 1987;85:407–418.

10. Capone A Jr, Diaz-Rohena R, Sternberg P Jr, Mandell B, Lambert HM, Lopez PF. Diode-laser photocoagulation for zone 1 threshold retinopathy of prematurity. Am J Ophthalmol 1993;116:444–450.

11. Canning CR, McCartney AC, Hungerford J: Medulloepithelioma (diktyoma). Br J Ophthalmol 1988;72:764–767.

12. Cavenee WK, Dryja TP, Phillips RA, et al.: Expression of recessive alleles by chromosomal mechanisms in retinoblastoma. Nature 1983;305:779–784.

13. Cryotherapy for Retinopathy of Prematurity Cooperative Group: Multicenter trial of cryotherapy for retinopathy of prematurity: preliminary results. Arch Ophthalmol 1988;106:471–479.

14. Cryotherapy for Retinopathy of Prematurity Cooperative Group: Multicenter trial of cryotherapy for retinopathy of prematurity: one year outcome, structure and function. Arch Ophthalmol 1990;108:1408–1416.

15. Cryotherapy for Retinopathy of Prematurity Cooperative Group: Multicenter trial of cryotherapy for retinopathy of prematurity: 3½-year outcome, structure and function. Arch Ophthalmol 1993;111:339–344.

16. DeJuan E, Shields S, Machemer R: The role of ultrasound in the management of retinopathy of prematurity. Ophthalmology 1988;95:884–888.

17. Ehrenkranz RA: Vitamin E and retinopathy of prematurity: still controversial. J Pediatr 1989;114:801–803.

18. Friend SH, Bernards R, Rogeli S, et al.: A human DNA segment with properties of the gene that predisposes to retinoblastoma and osteosarcoma. Nature 1986;323:643–646.

19. Fung YKT, Murphree AL, Zhang FH, et al.: In vitro growth suppresion of normal and tumor cells by the human Rb gene. 1987.

20. Flynn JT, Bancalari E, Bachynsk BN, et al.: Retinopathy of prematurity: diagnosis, severity and natural history. Ophthalmology 1987;94:620–629.

21. Flynn JT, Bancalari E, et al.: A cohort study of transcutaneous oxygen tension and the incidence and severity of retinopathy of prematurity. N Engl J Med 1992;326:1078–1080.

22. Greven C, Tasman W: Scleral buckling in stages 4B and 5 retinopathy of prematurity. Arch Ophthalmol 1990;97:817–820.

23. Guyer DR, Schachat AP, Vitale S, et al.: Leukemic retinopathy. Relationship between fundus lesions and hematologic parameters at diagnosis. Ophthalmology 1989;96:860–864.

24. Hunter DG, Repka MX: Diode laser photocoagulation for threshold retinopathy of prematurity. A randomized study. Ophthalmology 1993;100:238–244.

25. Johnson L, Bowen FW, Abassi S, et al.: Relationship of prolonged pharmacological serum levels of vitamin E to incidence of sepsis and necrotizing enterocolitis in infants with birth weights 1,500 grams or less. Pediatrics 1985;15:619–638.

26. Kalina RE: Treatment of retinal detachment due to

retinopathy of prematurity. Documented disappointment (editorial). Ophthalmology 1991;98:3–4.

27. Kincaid MC, Green WR: Ocular and orbital involvement in leukemia. Surv Ophthalmol 1983;27:211–232.

28. Abramson DH, Wachtel A, Watson CW, et al.: Leukemic hypopyon. J Pediatr Ophthalmol Strabismus 1981;18:42.

29. Knudson AG Jr: Hereditary cancer, oncogenes, antioncogenes. Cancer Res 1985;45:1437–1443.

30. Kushner BJ, Gloeckner E: Retrolental fibroplasia in full-term infants without exposure to supplemental oxygen. Am J Ophthalmol 1984;97:148–157.

31. Kushner BJ: Strabismus and amblyopia associated with regressed retinopathy of prematurity. Arch Ophthalmol 1982;100:256–261.

32. Landers MB III, Toth CA, Semple HC, Morse LS. Treatment of retinopathy of prematurity with argon laser photocoagulation. Arch Ophthalmol 1992;110:44–47.

33. McNamara JA, Tasman W, Vander JF, Brown GC: Diode laser photocoagulation for retinopathy of prematurity: Preliminary results. Arch Ophthalmol 1992;110:1714–1716.

34. Messmer EP, Fritze H, Mohr C, et al.: Long-term treatment effects inpatients with bilateral retinoblastoma: Ocular and mid-facial findings. Graefes Arch Clin Exp Ophthalmol 1991;229:309.

35. Nelson SC, et al.: Successful therapy for trilateral retinoblastoma. Am J Ophthalmol 1992;114:23–29.

36. Noorily SW, Small K, deJuan E, Machemer R: Scleral buckling for stage 4B retinopathy of prematurity. Ophthalmology 1992;99:263–268.

37. Ober RR, Bird AC, Hamilton AM, Sehmi K: Autosomal dominant exudative vitreoretinopathy. Br J Ophthalmol 1980;64:112–120.

38. Palmer EA, Flynn JT, Hardy RH, on behalf of the cryotherapy for retinopathy of prematurity cooperative group: In-cidence and early course of retinopathy of prematurity. Ophthalmology 1991;98:1628–1640.

39. Patz A, Hoeck LE, DeLaCruz E: Studies on the effect of high oxygen administration in retrolental fibroplasia. Nursery observations. Am J Ophthalmol 1952;27:1248–1253.

40. Quinn GE, et al.: Development of myopia in infants with birth weights less than 1251 grams. Ophthalmology 1992;99:329–340.

41. Repka MX, Hardy RJ, Phelps DL, Summers CG: Surfactant prophylaxis and retinopathy of prematurity. Arch Ophthalmol 1993;111:618–620.

42. Rosenbaum PS, Boniuk M, Font RL: Diffuse uveal melanoma in a five year old child. Am J Ophthalmol 1988;106:601–606.

43. Shields CL, Shields JA, Milite J, et al.: Uveal melanoma in teenagers and children. A report of 40 cases. Ophthalmology 1991;98:1662–1666.

44. Shields JA, Pesin SR: Seven cases of trilateral retinoblastoma. Am J Ophthalmol 1989;107:121–126.

45. The Committee for the Classification of Retinopathy of Prematurity: An international classification of retinopathy of prematurity. Arch Ophthalmol 1984;102:1130–1134.

46. The Committee for the Classification of Retinopathy of Prematurity: An international classification of retinopathy of prematurity. The classification of retinal detachment. Arch Ophthalmol 1987;105:906–913.

47. The Laser ROP Study Group: Laser therapy for retinopathy of prematurity. Arch Ophthalmol 1994;112:154–156.

48. Velazquez N, Jones IS: Ocular and oculodermal melanocytosis associated with uvea melanoma. Ophthalmology 1983;90:1472–1476.

49. Zillis JD, de Juan E, Machemer R: Advanced retinopathy of prematurity: the anatomic and visual results of vitreous surgery. Ophthalmology 1990;97:821–826.

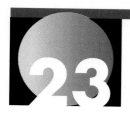

23 Pediatric Ophthalmology Syndromes

Kenneth W. Wright, Jyoti Raina

■ PHAKOMATOSES

The phakomatoses involve the formation of hamartomas that typically involve the skin and nervous system. The term phakos is Greek for birthmark or mole. There are many diseases that fall in the phakomatoses group of disorders; however, we will cover the six conditions commonly associated with ocular manifestations.

Neurofibromatosis (Von Recklinghausen's Disease)

Neurofibromatosis is an autosomal-dominant disease and has two forms, neurofibromatosis I (von Recklinghausen's disease) and neurofibromatosis II (bilateral acoustic neurofibromatosis). Prenatal diagnosis is possible by chromosome analysis.

Neurofibromatosis I

Neurofibromatosis I (NF-1) is the classic form of neurofibromatosis described by von Recklinghausen. It is the most common form of the phakomatosis, occurring in approximately 1 in 3000 of the general population. The most outstanding clinical features include cutaneous nevi called cafe au lait spots, plexiform neurofibromas of the lids pigmented freckling around the axillary or inguinal areas, optic nerve glioma, Lisch iris nodules, and bony lesions including sphenoid dysplasia or thinning of the long bone cortex. The primary embryologic defect involves primitive neural crest cells and neuroectoderm. The clinical diagnostic criterion for NF-1 is the presence of two or more of the characteristics listed in Table 23–1.

Ophthalmic and Facial Findings. One of the most consistent findings of NF-1 is the presence of Lisch nodules of the iris. These are iris hamartomas composed of melanocytes. They appear as well-circumscribed small nodules in the iris that are slightly raised and have a brownish appearance (Fig. 23–1). They are present in approximately 30% of affected children younger than 6 years of age and in more than 90% of patients in late childhood and adulthood. Plexiform neuromas can occur in the eyelid and often cause an "S"-shaped deformity of the lid margin. Facial asymmetry and hemihypertrophy also can be associated with NF-1. Neurofibromas of the conjunctiva, corneal nerve thickening, and glaucoma secondary to trabecular meshwork outflow obstruction also may occur. Retinal findings include small glial tumors or optic nerve pallor secondary to an optic nerve glioma.

Optic nerve gliomas occur in approximately 15% of patients with NF-1; however, almost 70% of children with optic nerve gliomas have NF-1. These tumors tend to be slow growing and are usually managed conservatively by observation. Computed tomography and magnetic resonance imaging findings show the characteristic fusiform shape of the optic nerve glioma.

Gliomas of the chiasm have a worse prognosis and should be suspected in a patient with NF-1 and optic nerve pallor and no proptosis.

Systemic Findings. Patients with NF-1 can develop intracranial tumors at any time, including gliomas, meningiomas, and ependymomas. Benign tumors can undergo malignant transformation into neurofibrosarcoma and malignant schwannomas. Other malignant

TABLE 23–1
Criteria for Diagnosing Neurofibromatosis I

Must have two or more of the following criteria
1. Café-au-lait maculas, 6 or more, at least 5 mm in diameter
   for prepubertal children
   Greater than 15 mm in diameter for postpubertal individuals.
2. Freckling of the axillary or inguinal skin areas
3. One plexiform neuroma or two or more neurofibromas, any type
4. Optic nerve glioma
5. Lisch nodules (iris hamartomas)
6. Osseous lesions (sphenoid dysplasia or thinning of long bone cortex)
7. Family history, first degree relative with NF I

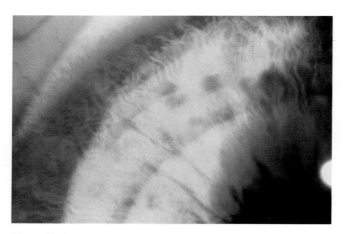

Figure 23–1.
Lisch nodules on iris in neurofibromatosis Type I. They are brownish raised nodules.

transformations include pheochromocytoma, medullary carcinoma, and chronic myelogenous leukemia. Other systemic findings include cystic lesions of the lung, cardiac rhabdomyoma, and neurofibromas of virtually any organ. Mapping studies identify that the proximal portion of the long arm of chromosome 17 (chromosome band 17q11.2) is the location of the mutation.

Neurofibromatosis II

Neurofibromatosis II (NF-2) consists of bilateral acoustic neuromas and posterior subcapsular cataracts. The acoustic neuromas or schwannomas develop during the second to third decade of life. Other tumors associated with NF-2 include brain or spinal cord tumors, meningiomas, schwannomas, astrocytomas, and neurofibromas. Unlike NF-1, where there is usually cutaneous involvement, NF-2 usually does not involve the skin. NF-2 is inherited as an autosomal-dominant trait and has been mapped to chromosome 22 (22q11.21-q13.1).

NF-2 is an extremely rare disorder, affecting approximately 1 of 50,000. Clinical presentation relates to auditory symptoms such as hearing loss, tinnitus, dizziness, or headache. The diagnostic criteria for NF-2 are described in Table 23–2.

Von Hippel-Lindau Disease

Von Hippel-Lindau disease consists of a vascular lesion (hemangioblastoma) that classically affects the retina (angiomatosis retinae) and the cerebellum. Patients can show signs of cerebellar dysfunction or vision loss. Other organ systems can become involved, including angiomas of the kidney, pancreas, liver, and spleen. Renal cell carcinoma occurs in approximately one third of patients. Cutaneous involvement is unusual; however, pigmented macular lesions of the skin may develop in some patients in the third or fourth decades of life. Patients most commonly die of either cerebellar hemangioblastomas or renal cell carcinomas. Fortunately, this is a rare disorder, occurring in less than 1 in 40,000 patients. The inheritance is autosomal-dominant with incomplete penetrance. The chromosomal abnormality has been mapped to 3p25-p26 and is a tumor suppressor gene abnormality.

Ocular findings are mainly hemangioblastomas of the retina. (Fig. 23–2). The retinal vascular tumors can be found between the ages of 10 and 40 years, which is earlier than the cerebellar presentation. Initially, the tumor is extremely small and looks like no more than a slight aneurysmal dilatation of peripheral retinal vessels. Over time, the vascular tumor increases in size to form a smooth domed tumor, which is fed by a tortuous dilated tumor vessel emanating from the optic nerve. This creates a arterial venous shunt. Tumors may be present anywhere in the retina but are most commonly seen in the midperiphery or may involve the optic disc. Leakage from the tumor can cause lipid exudate of the retina and may take on the appearance of Coats' disease. Involvement may be bilateral or multifocal in one eye. Almost 100% of patients with von Hippel-Lindau disease will have retinal involvement.

TABLE 23–2
Criteria for Diagnosing Neurofibromatosis II

1. Bilateral acoustic neuromas or eighth nerve mass on CT or MRI scan.
   OR
2. Family history of NF-2 (first degree relative) and patient with unilateral acoustic neuroma
   OR
Two of the following
Juvenile posterior subcapsular cataract
Neurofibroma
Meningioma
Schwannoma

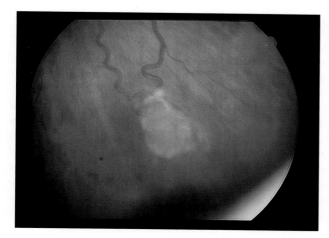

Figure 23–2.
Retinal hemangioblastoma in von Hippel Lindau. Note the two feeder vessels that connect with the yellowish vascularized retinal mass.

Tuberous Sclerosis (Bourneville's Disease)

Tuberous sclerosis is a disease of tumors such as astrocytic hamartomas and angiofibromas, which involve multiple organs. The classic presentation includes the triad of seizures, mental retardation, and facial angiomas. These features have variable expressivity; however, seizures are the most common manifestation, occurring in almost 20% of patients. Virtually all patients will have an abnormal electroencephalograph.

Ocular findings include astrocytic hamartomas of the retina or optic disc and retinal pigment epithelial defects. The astrocytic hamartomas classically appear as a smooth white or gray mass with a mulberry or tapioca texture (Fig. 23–3). Lid involvement with angiofibromas also can occur. Retinal lesions do not require treatment.

Systemic findings of tuberous sclerosis include angiofibromas over the nose and cheeks, which often are termed adenoma sebaceum. Depigmented macules or ash-leaf spots and cafe au lait spots also can be seen. Ash-leaf spots are best identified by illumination with a blue light or fluorescent lamp. Cerebral lesions include white matter abnormalities, subependymal nodules, cortical tubers, and subependymal giant cell astrocytoma. These lesions may be present in up to 50% of affected individuals. Table 23–3 lists associated findings of tuberous sclerosis.

Tuberous sclerosis is a rare disorder and is inherited as an autosomal-dominant trait with variable penetrance. The majority of patients are seen, however, as a new mutation without a family history of tuberous sclerosis. Tuberous sclerosis has been found in two types, type 1, involving chromosome 9q33-q34 and type 2, linked to chromosome 11q23. Patients with tuberous sclerosis should be followed with neuroimaging, renal ultrasound, and cardiac work-up (see Table 23–3). Genetic counseling is important because patients may have

mental retardation, and accurate communication to the family is important.

Sturge-Weber Syndrome

Sturge-Weber syndrome is an angiomatosis including a facial cutaneous hemangioma (port-wine stain), which may be unilateral or bilateral and involves the first and second division of the trigeminal nerve (see Fig. 45–7). Leptomeningeal (pia and arachnoid) angiomatosis, childhood seizures (contralateral side), and mental retardation also may occur. Expressivity of the disease is variable, and most patients do not manifest the entire syndrome.

Ocular findings include eyelid hemangiomas (nevus flammaeus or port-wine stain), tortuous conjunctival vessels with episcleral vascular plexi, and choroidal hemangiomas. The choroidal hemangiomas are diffuse and have a tomato catsup appearance. It is often diffi-

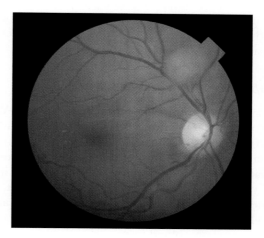

Figure 23–3.
Retinal astrocytic hamartoma in a patient with tuberous sclerosis. The lesion is seen just superior to the superior temporal arcades.

TABLE 23–3
Associated Findings of Tuberous Sclerosis

Ocular findings
1. Ocular astrocytic hamartomas of the retina
2. Retinal pigmentary abnormalities
3. Sector iris hypopigmentations
4. Angiomas of the lid

Systemic findings
1. Seizures
2. Facial cutaneous angiofibromas (butterfly distribution)
3. Fingernails and toenails with subungual fibromas
4. Ash-leaf spots
5. Forehead and scalp fibrous plaques
6. Dental enamel pits
7. Renal cysts or tumors
8. Pulmonary involvement, cardiac rhabdomyoma

cult to see the choroidal hemangioma because of its diffuse nature, and comparison of eye to eye is helpful in making the diagnosis. Choroidal hemangiomas can be found in approximately 40% of patients. Heterochromia of the iris can be noted in patients with unilateral cutaneous hemangiomatosis. Glaucoma occurs in approximately 30% of patients with Sturge-Weber syndrome. Upper and lower eyelid involvement is believed to be an indicator of glaucoma development. Glaucoma is probably secondary to increased episcleral venous pressure. Glaucoma is difficult to manage medically, and surgery has important potential risks, most importantly intraoperative or postoperative choroidal effusion or choroidal hemorrhage. Systemic findings include focal or generalized motor seizures in approximately 80% of affected individuals, hemangiomatous involvement of the mouth and lips, and the classic radiologic finding of railroad track calcifications in the leptomeninges.

Unlike most other forms of phakomatosis such as neurofibromatosis, Sturge-Weber syndrome is not associated with a recognized Mendelian inheritance pattern, and a positive family history is unusual.

Klippel-Trenaunay-Weber Syndrome

This syndrome appears to be related to Sturge-Weber syndrome in that it is not inherited by classic Mendelian patterns and is associated with cutaneous hemangiomas. The syndrome includes cutaneous hemangiomata, hypertrophy of bones and soft tissue, ipsilateral varicosities, and arterial venous fistula. The cutaneous hemangiomas can be quite large and are extremely difficult to remove surgically because of the danger of massive blood loss.

Louis-Bar Syndrome (Ataxia-Telangiectasia)

Louis-Bar syndrome is characterized by cerebellar ataxia and ocular and cutaneous telangiectasia. The ocular telangiectasias involve the conjunctiva and appear between 4 and 7 years of age. Diffuse cerebellar atrophy occurs, and oculomotor apraxia develops with deficient saccadic generation, cerebellar nystagmus, and strabismus. Systemic manifestations include signs of cerebellar atrophy with choreoathetosis, dysarthria, hypotonia, and ataxia. Immunologic compromise occurs, which may be secondary to thymus gland hypoplasia; pulmonary infections are common. Hematologic cancer, such as leukemia, lymphoma, lymphosarcoma, and Hodgkin's disease, is associated with Louis-Bar syndrome.

Louis-Bar syndrome is inherited as an autosomal-recessive trait and is due to a gene that functions to repair DNA. Patients with Louis-Bar syndrome are, therefore, susceptible to radiation.

Wyburn-Mason Syndrome (Racemose Angiomatosis)

Wyburn-Mason syndrome is sporatic and consists of arteriovenous malformations that involve the retina, midbrain, and thalamus. Ocular characteristics include dilated tortuous retinal vessels often occurring in the inferior temporal quadrant of the retina. The tortuous vessels represent a large arteriovenous shunt. Angioma also can involve the orbit and cause proptosis. Systemic findings include cavernous sinus angiomata or angiomata along the basilar or posterior cerebellar artery. Intracranial hemorrhage or compression of surrounding structures can cause headaches and neurologic symptoms.

■ CRANIOFACIAL ABNORMALITIES

Hypertelorism

Hypertelorism is an increased distance between the orbits. Clinical estimate of hypertelorism can be determined by measuring interpupillary distance; however, radiologic measurements are most accurate.

Telecanthus

A wide intercanthal distance and normal interpupillary distance is termed telecanthus. This is a condition of soft tissue that often improves over time as the nose develops and the nasal bridge skin is pulled forward.

Craniosynostosis

Craniosynostosis results from premature closure of the cranial sutures. This results in inhibited skull growth perpendicular to the closed suture. Increased growth occurs at the opened sutures. Since the pattern of premature closure is quite variable, there is a large spectrum of presentations with varying skull shapes. Craniosynostosis is often associated with strabismus and can be associated with missing or congenitally displaced extraocular muscles. The most common craniosynostosis are inherited as an autosomal-dominant trait including Crouzon's, Apert's, and Pfeiffer's syndromes. In addition to cranial and facial abnormalities, patients with Apert's and Pfeiffer's syndrome have syndactyly.

Apert's Syndrome

Apert's syndrome is caused by a synostosis of the coronal suture. Associated findings include midfacial hypoplasia, protrusion of the lower jaw, high arched

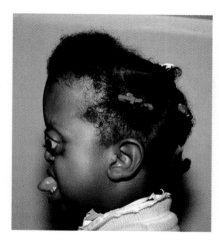

Figure 23–4.
Facial features showing severe proptosis and flattening of forehead and micrognathia in Crouzon's disease.

Pfeiffer's Syndrome

Pfeiffer's syndrome is similar to Apert's syndrome, although in Pfeiffer's syndrome there are characteristic broad, short thumbs and great toes. The orbits are extremely shallow, there is severe proptosis, often with corneal exposure, and strabismus is common.

Crouzon's Syndrome

Crouzon's syndrome is similar to Apert's and other types of craniosynostoses with the coronal suture being most frequently involved, however, other combinations of suture synostosis are common (Fig. 23–4). With Crouzon's syndrome, there are no anomalies of the hands or feet as there are in Apert's and Pfeiffer's syndromes. Proptosis can be severe and vision-threatening because of optic nerve compression or corneal exposure secondary to proptosis. Abnormal extraocular muscles and the absence of extraocular muscles are frequently reported in Crouzon's and in Apert's syndromes. There is maxillary hypoplasia, a hook-shaped nose, and a flat forehead. Other associated abnormalities include deafness and delayed development.

palate, and syndactyly of the fingers and toes. Other features include proptosis, antimongoloid slant of the palpebral fissures, strabismus, and hypertelorism. The strabismus is often characterized by esotropia with a V pattern. Shallow orbits can cause severe proptosis, optic nerve atrophy, and subluxation of the globes.

■ MANDIBULOFACIAL DYSOSTOSES

The mandibulofacial dysostoses represents abnormal differentiation of the first branchial arch and include Goldenhar's syndrome and Treacher-Collins syndrome.

Goldenhar's Syndrome

Goldenhar's syndrome or oculoauricular dysostosis is a form of hemifacial microsomia. It most commonly presents as a sporadic occurrence. Two to three percent of future siblings are at risk for development of Goldenhar's syndrome. Typical findings include unilateral facial asymmetry with mandibular hypoplasia, usually involving the right side of the face. Preauricular appendages or ear tags, malformation of the ear, hearing loss due to external ear lesions, or middle or inner ear malformations also are present. Vertebral abnormalities include fusional defects, scoliosis, and spina bifida. Microsomia is common and associated with mandibular malformations. Ocular findings include epibulbar or conjunctival lipodermoids often associated with vertebral abnormalities, limbal dermoids, eyelid colobomas, and subcutaneous dermoids of the lids (Fig. 23–5). Other systemic findings are unusual but may include heart, lung, and kidney malformations.

Treacher-Collins Syndrome

Treacher-Collins syndrome is inherited as an autosomal-dominant trait with incomplete penetrance and variable expressivity. Features include coloboma or notching of the lower lid, hypoplasia of the malar and mandibular bones, malformations of the external ear, atypical hair line with projections toward the cheek, absence of the zygomatic arch antimongoloid slant of the palpebral fissures, hypoplasia of the lower jaw, and a blind fistula between the angles of the mouth and ears. Unlike Goldenhar's syndrome, which is usually unilateral, Treacher-Collins syndrome is bilateral. Lacrimal punctum may be absent, and other, less frequently encountered anomalies include upper lid coloboma and ptosis.

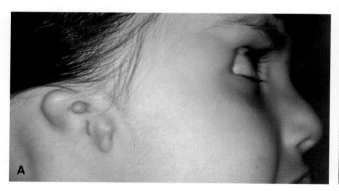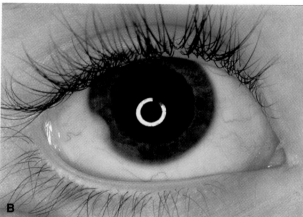

Figure 23–5.
A, Microtia with preauricular tags in Goldenhar's syndrome. **B,** Limbal dermoid.

■ OTHER CRANIOFACIAL DISORDERS

Stickler's Syndrome

Stickler's syndrome is an autosomal-dominant trait with high penetrance associated with facial and skeletal abnormalities, high myopia, and a high incidence of retinal detachment. The classic facial appearance includes malar hypoplasia with flattened midface, flattened nasal bridge, micrognathia, and cleft or high-arched palate. These facial signs represent the *Pierre-Robin sequence.* Mitral valve prolapse occurs in approximately 50% of cases, and a progressive arthropathy is present in almost all patients but it may be subtle and only show as flattening of the epiphyseal centers on radiographs. Ocular features of Stickler's syndrome include high myopia and vitreoretinal degeneration, causing a high incidence of retinal detachment. The vitreous is liquified with optically empty areas with vitreous veils and condensations. Other ocular findings include glaucoma and cataracts.

Cockayne Syndrome

This is a syndrome of premature aging, dwarfism, birdlike facies, and retinal degeneration. Mental retardation, seizures, cerebellar ataxia, nystagmus, muscle rigidity, and neurosensory deafness are part of the neurologic sequelae. The disease is progressive, usually becoming evident by 2 years of age, with deafness often occurring during late adolescence.

Retinal findings include a retinitis pigmentosa picture with a "salt and pepper" retinal pigment epithelial degeneration, waxy optic disc pallor, and attenuated retinal vessels. Other ocular findings include corneal opacification, band keratopathy, cataracts, nystagmus, and poor pupillary response with hypoplastic irides. There is no specific treatment.

Rubenstein-Taybi Syndrome

Mental retardation, broad toes and thumbs, short stature, and an antimongoloid slant of the palpebral fissures are characteristics of this syndrome. In addition, more than 90% of patients will have a high-arched palate and a beaked or straight nose, which gives an elfin facial appearance. Rubenstein-Taybi syndrome is sporadic, and laboratory studies of muscle biopsies show a pattern consistent with denervation atrophy of the muscle. There is no specific treatment for the syndrome.

Hallerman-Streiff Syndrome

This is a sporadic, midfacial hypoplasia that is associated with congenital cataracts in 100% of cases. Characteristics include micromandibular hypoplasia, beaked nose, and dwarfism. Microcornea makes aphakic contact lens fitting difficult.

Fetal Alcohol Syndrome

Fetal alcohol syndrome is associated with maternal ingestion of large amounts of alcohol during the first trimester of pregnancy. The most obvious findings of fetal alcohol syndrome are facial abnormalities including flat philtrum, thin vermilion border of the upper lid, flat facies, and large epicanthal folds. Newborns are usually low birth weight, show developmental delay, and are often associated with mild to moderate mental retardation. Telecanthus, ptosis, strabismus, optic nerve hy-poplasia, and anomalies of the anterior segment including anterior chamber dysgenesis syndromes have been described.

■ ALBINISM

Albinism is a lack of melanin pigment, which can occur primarily involving the eye (ocular albinism) or can occur systemically (oculocutaneous albinism).

Oculocutaneous Albinism

Oculocutaneous albinism can be divided into tyrosi-nase-positive and tyrosinase-negative types. With ty-rosinase-positive oculocutaneous albinism, hair root studies show positive tyrosinase activity. Advances in molecular genetics have shown that there are many possible genetic defects which will cause a specific al-bino phenotype. For example, tyrosinase positive ocu-locutaneous albinism has been found to be secondary to abnormalities involving at least three separate genes, (tyrosinase gene mutations, P gene mutations, and tyrosinase related protein type I (TRP-1)). In addition, a variety of mutations on a specific albinism gene may result in different phenotypic expression with the same gene causing both tyrosinase-positive and tyrosinase-negative oculocutaneous albinism. Molecular genetics is the basis for a new classificaiton of albinism, however, most clinicians still use the clinical classification of tyrosinase positive and tyrosinase negative oculocutaneous albinism. Patients with tyrosi-nase positive oculocutaneous albinism show progressively increased pigmentation, as they are able to produce melanin. Tyrosinase-negative oculocutaneous albinism is a severe hypopigmentation disorder that tends to be static and is associated with very poor visual acuity. The eye findings associated with albinism include nystagmus, hypopigmentation of the iris, transil-lumination defects of the iris, and hypopigmented fundus. Both tyrosinase-positive and tyrosinase-negative oculocutaneous albinism are inherited as an autosomal-recessive trait. Transillumination defects of the iris are important to differentiate true albinism from otherwise normal patients with hypopigmentation (Fig. 23–6).

Ocular Albinism

Ocular albinism is hypopigmentation that is localized to the eye. Patients with ocular albinism may have brown or dark hair and will not look like the typical albino patient. Ocular albinism is usually inherited as x-linked, or autosomal-recessive trait. Typical findings of ocular albinism are transillumination defects of the iris, nystagmus, and hypopigmented fundus. Macular hypoplasia also can be associated with ocular albinism. Strabismus is commonly seen with both oculocutaneous and ocular albinism. Hemifield VEP studies show excess of decussation at the chiasm, and patients with albinism show decreased binocularity. Decreased vision associated with albinism is related to macular hypoplasia. Vision tends to improve over time as pigmentation increases, especially in patients with tyrosinase-positive albinism.

Hermansky-Pudlak Syndrome

This is a tyrosinase-positive albinisim associated with prolonged bleeding time secondary to abnormal platelet aggregation. Lung disease and ulcerative colitis develop at approximately 30 to 40 years of age. Because

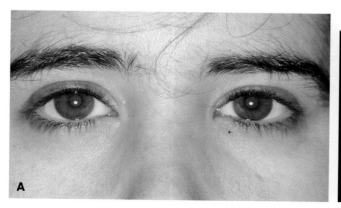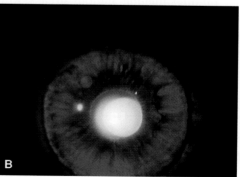

Figure 23–6.
A, Hermansky-Pudlak syndrome with ocular albinism but iris are brown. **B,** Despite brown eyes, the iris transilluminates on slit-lamp examination.

of the platelet abnormalities, patients show bruisability, increased nosebleeds, and increased bleeding after minor surgical procedures (Table 23–6).

Chédiak-Higashi Syndrome

This is a tyrosinase-positive oculocutaneous albinism and is associated with decreased lymphocytic effectiveness to prevent infections secondary to defective micro-tubule assembly. Bacterial infections are dangerous in these patients and in childhood can be fatal.

Waardenberg Syndrome

This is not obviously a pigment dilution disease but is associated with white forelocks, hypopigmented fundus, and heterochromia secondary to hypopigmentation of all or part of the iris. Other findings include telecanthus, confluent eyebrows, and sensorineural deafness.

■ CONNECTIVE TISSUE DISORDERS

Marfan's Syndrome

Marfan's syndrome is a connective tissue disorder that is inherited as an autosomal-dominant and is the most common cause of bilateral subluxed lenses. See Chapter 29, for further discussion.

Ehlers-Danlos Syndrome

There are various forms of Ehlers-Danlos syndrome with the ocular form or form VI consisting of blue, fragile sclera with spontaneous perforation of the globe, keratoconus and *angioid streaks* (Bruchs membrane breaks). Patients with Ehlers-Danlos syndrome have thin extensible skin, hyperextensibility of joints, and skin that easily scars.

Pseudoxanthoma Elasticum

This is an autosomal-dominant or autosomal-recessive disease that effects the elastic component of connective tissue. There is calcification of the elastic component of vessels and of Bruch's membrane. Because of the vasculopathy, multiple systems become affected including coronary heart disease, renal failure and hypertension, neurologic disease, and gastrointestinal hemorrhages. Mitral valve prolapse occurs in more than 70% of cases. Skin is elastic and hyperextensible.

Ocular findings include angioid streaks, which are breaks in Bruch's membrane and which radiate from the optic disc peripherally. The elastic layer of Bruch's membrane is replaced by calcific changes. Subretinal neovascularization occurs as vessels grow through breaks in Bruch's membrane. There is no specific treatment except for support treatment for complications of the vasculopathy and retinal neovascularization.

Osteogenesis Imperfecta

Osteogenesis imperfecta has at least five clinical subtypes. This is a disease of alpha type I collagen and affects connective tissue. Ocular signs include blue sclera, which results from visualization of the choroid through thin sclera. The scleral thickness is approximately half that of normal. Other ocular findings include keratoconus, megalocornea, and posterior embryotoxon. Rarely, patients will have cataracts, glaucoma, and spontaneous rupture of the globe. Patients are prone to longbone fractures of the extremities and spine.

Blue Sclera

Blue sclera is due to visibility of uveal tissue through thin sclera. The common ocular and systemic conditions associated with blue sclera are listed below.

1. Myopia
2. Buphthalmos
3. Scleral staphyloma
4. Congenital ocular melanosis
5. Aniridia
6. Ehlers-Danlos syndrome
7. Marfan's syndrome
8. Osteogenesis imperfecta
9. Paget's stndrome
10. Pierre Robin syndrome

■ METABOLIC STORAGE DISEASE

Mucopolysaccharadosis

Mucopolysaccharadosis (MPS) are a group of storage diseases caused by an error of carbohydrate metabolism. At present, there are six types of MPS syndromes, five recessively inherited, and Hunter's syndrome, which is x-linked. The classification of MPS into groups I to VII is based on the type of enzyme deficiency. Type V is presently vacant, as it recently has been identified as a subtype of type I. Type I is subdivided into

TABLE 23–4
Features of MPS

| Type | Ocular Features | | | Systemic Features | | | Prognosis |
	Corneal Clouding	Retinal Degeneration	Optic Nerve Atrophy	Coarse Facial Features	Mental Retardation	Skeletal Dysplasia	
I-H (Hurler)	+, by 6 mos	+	+,	+	+	+	death by 10 yrs
I-S (Scheie)	+, by 12-24 mos	+	+	+	variable	+	may live to middle age
I-HS (Hurler-Scheie)	+	+	−	+	variable	+'	better than I-H
II (Hunter)	rare	+	+	+	+	+	death by 15 years
III (Sanfilippo's)	−	+	+	+	variable	+	death by 2nd or 3rd decade
IV (Morquio's)	by age 10	rare	−	+	mild	+	may survive to 6th decade
VI (Maroteaux Lamy Synd)	after age 5	−	+	+	−	+	death in 2nd decade
VII (Sly Synd)	mild	−	−	variable	+	+	may live to middle age

three categories based on the severity of the disease; Type 1-H (Hurler syndrome), Type 1-S (Scheie syndrome), and Type 1-HS (Hurler-Scheie syndrome).

Table 23–4 summarizes the clinical features of the MPS syndromes. Systemic and ocular features are variable and subtype-specific. Typically, systemic abnormalities include coarse facial features, short stature, and mental retardation (Fig. 23–7). Various types of mucopolysaccharides are found in the urine, depending on the enzyme deficiency. Common ocular findings include corneal stromal clouding, pigmentary retinal degeneration, and optic nerve atrophy. Corneal clouding usually coexists with skeletal abnormalities and is present in all types, except type III and most Hunter's syndrome. Pigmentary retinopathy is associated with the presence of mental retardation.

MPS are progressive diseases with variable prognosis depending on the type. Usually patients live well into middle age; however, patients with type I and type VI tend to have respiratory infection and heart failure. There is no specific systemic treatment. Patients with visually significant corneal opacities may benefit from corneal transplantation. There may in fact be clearing of the surrounding recipient corneal bed 1 or 2 years after transplantation. Table 23–5 lists the differential diagnosis for a pediatric cloudy cornea.

Tyrosinemia

An error in tyrosine metabolism leads to high serum levels and increased urinary excretion of tyrosine and parahydroxyphenylpyruvate.

Tyrosinemia type I and neonatal tyrosinemia have no characteristic skin or eye lesions.

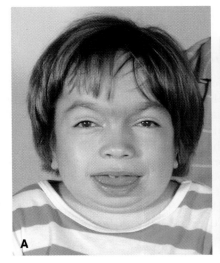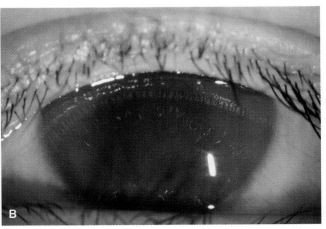

Figure 23–7.
A, Typical Hurler's facies. **B,** Slit-lamp photograph of cloudy cornea in mucopolysaccharidosis.

TABLE 23–5
Differential Diagnosis of Cloudy Cornea

In Infancy

1.	Birth trauma (forceps injury)	Unilateral, central, stromal and/or epithelial opacity due to breaks in DM. Usually resolves though amblyopia may result from slow resolution.
2.	Congenital glaucoma	Unilateral or bilateral epithelial and stromal opacity later. Increased corneal diameter with high IOP.
3.	Mucopolysaccharidosis (Hurler's, Scheie's)	Bilateral, diffuse opacities by 6–12 months. Progressive, do well with PK.
4.	Mucolipidoses Type IV	Bilateral corneal clouding in first year of life. Conjunctival biopsy shows typical inclusion cells (I-cells).
5.	Congenital hereditary endothelial dystrophy (CHED)	Bilateral, diffuse corneal thickening. AR form is stationary, while AD form is progressive.
6.	Congenital hereditary stromal dystrophy (CHSD)	Bilateral, central, flaky, corneal clouding: AD non progressive.
7.	Sclerocornea	Bilateral or unilateral peripheral opacity. Associated with other abnormalities (Goldenhar syndrome).
8.	Peter's anomaly	Central corneal opacity with defects in posterior stroma, DM and endothelium. 80% are bilateral.
9.	Limbal dermoid	Unilateral, temporal opacity. Increasing size or post-excision scarring may cause astigmatism and amblyopia.

In Childhood

1.	Mucopolysaccharidosis	Bilateral, diffuse opacities. Type I and VI present early in childhood.
2.	Cystinosis	Bilateral cystine corneal deposits. Widespread systemic crystal deposition. Renal involvement in infantile form (Fanconi's syndrome).
3.	Corneal blood staining	Unilateral diffuse brown staining following hyphema. Slow resolution can result in amblyopia.
4.	Interstitial keratitis	Bilateral with corneal edema and vascularization in acute stage (salmon patch). In quiescent stage "ghost vessels" in stroma.
5.	Rubella keratopathy	Microcornea, central epithelial and stromal opacities and cataract. The infantile glaucoma type is associated with raised IOP and megalocornea.
6.	Familial dysautonomia (Riley Day syndrome)	AR, opacity and keratopathy secondary to reduced lacrimation or decreased corneal sensation.
7.	Tyrosinemea	Corneal erosions, culture negative ulcers, epithelial pseudodendrites.

Tyrosinemia type II or Richner Hanhart syndrome has a clinical triad of skin lesions, ocular manifestations, and mental retardation. The ocular features are typically seen as corneal lesions and appear early in childhood. Painful, erosive, or hyperkeratotic skin lesions over palms and soles coexist with or precede ocular lesions. Pseudodendritic corneal erosions, culture-negative ulcers, and intraepithelial linear or stellate opacities have been described.

Estimation of serum tyrosine levels are imperative in a child with bilateral photophobia and pseudodendritic corneal lesions. Early detection and dietary restriction of phenylalanine and tyrosine lead to reversal of ocular and skin changes and even prevention of mental retardation.

Mucolipidosis

Some of the clinical features of this condition overlap those found in mucopolysaccharidoses and sphingolipidoses. Mucolipidosis is characterized by the presence of peculiar inclusion cells (I-cells) in cultured fibroblasts. A conjunctival biopsy is diagnostic. Table 23–6 lists the clinical features of the subtypes.

Gangliosidosis

This rare group of storage disorders represents errors of sphingolipid metabolism. These are characterized by intracellular storage of phospholipids and glycolipids in the ganglion cell layer of retina besides other tissues of the body. The fovea being devoid of ganglion cells presents a characteristic "cherry red" appearance against a white background of lipid laden ganglion cells, in the initial stages of disease. Table 23–7 lists the differential diagnosis of a cherry red spot. Table 23–8 shows the salient features of the different subtypes of gangliosidoses.

Niemann Pick Disease

This condition is due to a disorder of sphingomyelin metabolism. It is characterised by presence of foam cells

TABLE 23–6
Clinical Features of Mucolipidoses

Type	Enzyme def	Ocular features	Systemic features	Prognosis
I	α-N acetylneuraminidase	corneal clouding, cherry red spot, optic atrophy	mental retardation, dysostosis multiplex	uncertain, no known treatment
II	multiple lysosomal enzymes	late corneal clouding, correlating with survival, no cherry red spot	Hurler-like facies, dysostosis multiplex, mental retardation	early death
III	multiple lysosomal enzymes	ground glass corneal clouding, hyperopic astigmatism	Hurler-like facies, skeletal dysplasias, aortic valve disease	progressive joint stiffness, hyperopia should be corrected
IV	ganglioside neuraminidase	corneal clouding, retinal degeneration, optic nerve atrophy	progressive psychomotor retardation, no skeletal dysplasia or facial dysmorphism	poor visual prognosis due to retinal degeneration

(intracellular deposits of sphingomyelin) in bone marrow, peripheral blood smear, liver spleen and brain. These are classified into types A–E on biochemical and clinical bases. They all present with a cherry red spot.

Type A is most common (85%), and 80% are Ashkenazi Jews. They have early and severe central nervous system (CNS) involvement.

Type B is visceral involvement with apparently normal CNS involvement.

Type C is moderate CNS involvement. Ocular features also include supranuclear paralysis of extraocular muscles.

Type D has later onset but severe involvement of CNS.

Type E has mild, chronic adult onset, with no CNS involvement.

Sialodosis

In this condition enzyme neuraminidase is deficient and it exists as two types, and is the typical "cherry red spot, myoclonus" syndrome.

Type I Myoclonus syndrome begins in the second decade in these patients of normal appearance and intelligence. Type II patients have a more severe and progressive systemic involvement. Corneal clouding besides cherry red spots have also been reported in this subtype.

Farber's Disease

Deficiency of ceramidase has been demonstrated in some of these patients. They are known to also present with cherry red spots, besides the systemic features of lumps on wrists, ankles, and joints. In the infantile form of the disease, death occurs due to pulmonary compli-

cations. The adult-onset group develop progressive neurologic disease.

Metachromatic Leukodystrophy

This is an autosomal-recessive condition with deficiency of arylsulfatase leading to widespread demyelination of brain and spinal cord. A classic cherry red spot has been described in addition to optic atrophy in these patients. Depending on the age at onset, infantile, juvenile, adolescent, and adult forms have been described. The infantile form is most common and has the worst prognosis.

Wilson's Disease

This rare condition is characterized by widespread deposition of copper due to deficiency of alpha 2 ceruloplasmin. The genetic defect has been mapped to chromosome 13q near esterase D locus and is named gene for Wilson's disease. *Kayser Fleisher ring* is the most specific ocular finding. This is present in all cases, although its appearance may be delayed in some children. This is a golden brown ring of copper deposits at the level of

TABLE 23–7
Differential Diagnosis of a Cherry Red Spot

Gangliosidosis
Niemann Pick disease
Farber's disease
Sialodosis
Mucolipidosis
Ocular trauma
Central retinal artery occlusion

TABLE 23–8
Gangliosidoses

Types	Deficient Enzyme	Ocular Features	Systemic Features	Prognosis
GM I Type I (Landing disease)	A, B and C-Beta galactosidase	Cherry red spot in 50% of cases. Tortuous conjunctival vessels, cloudy, cornea, optic atrophy, myopia	Psychomotor retardation, Hurler-like facial features, hepatosplenomegaly and congestive heart failure	Death by two years
GM I Type II (Derry disease)	B and C galactosidase	No cherry red spot, nystagmus, esotropia, pigmentary retinopathy	Ataxia, psychomotor retardation	Death by third to tenth year of life
GM II Type I (Tay Sachs Disease)	Isoenzyme hexaminidase A (autosomal recessive typically affecting European Jews)	Cherry red spot in 90% by six months, nystagmus, optic atrophy, attenuation of retinal vasculature	Hypotony, abnormal sensitivity to sound, seizures	Death by two to two and a half years
GM II Type II (Sandhoff disease)	Hexaminidase A & B	Cherry red spot, strabismus, minimal corneal clouding, normal optic nerve	Progressive psychomotor retardation	Death by two to twelve years
GM II Type II Burnheimer Seitelberger disease	Partial deficiency of hexasaminose A	No cherry red spot	Psychomotor retardation	Death by 15 years

Descemet's membrane. Typically it develops superiorly, then inferiorly, and finally in the horizontal meridian. It recedes in an identical manner after penicillamine therapy or liver transplantation.

Some patients also present with a green "sunflower" cataract. This is actually an anterior subcapsular deposit of granular pigment rather than a cataract.

Copper deposition in the liver, spleen, and CNS can cause a wide spectrum of clinical presentations as jaundice, hepatosplenomegaly, cerebral degeneration, and mental instability.

Fabry Disease

This is inherited in an x-linked recessive fashion and is due to deficiency of enzyme galactosidase. Typically, patients present with episodes of excruciating pain involving fingers and toes and angiokeratomas of skin. The most common ocular features are corneal verticillata or whorl dystrophy of cornea and a "Fabry cataract." Corneal verticillata are bilateral, brownish deposits at the level of Bowman's membrane located inferiorly on the cornea. Corneal verticillata also have been described in patients on the antiarrythmic drugs indomethacin, chloroquine, and meperidine.

Fabry cataract is unique with spoke-like granular lens opacities. Aneurysmal dilatation of inferior bulbar conjunctival vessels also have been reported in 78% of cases as well as retinal tortuosity. Common systemic features include angiokeratomas and cardiac and renal lesions.

Cystinosis

Widespread systemic and ocular cystine crystal deposition occurs in this autosomal-recessive disease without known biochemical defects. The common sites include the kidney, leucocytes, and bone marrow. The ocular tissues affected are the conjunctiva, cornea, iris, lens, and retina. Photophobia and pain may result from corneal deposits. These initially appear in the periphery and then progress to involve full thickness of the central cornea. Pigmentary retinopathy also has been reported in some cases. Depending on the age at onset, three forms have been described.

1. The infantile form, also known as Fanconi's syndrome, presents with progressive renal failure growth retardation and renal rickets.
2. The adult form is asymptomatic with normal renal function and life expectancy.
3. In the adolescent form, the symptoms of renal failure are variable and generally appear in the second decade. Retinopathy is typically absent in this group.

While treatment with oral cystaemine prevents additional deposits in ocular tissue and the kidney, it does not reverse pre-existing damage. Children with renal transplantation do well but survive only to the second or third decade of life. Topical cystaemine and corneal grafts have been used with some success.

Alkaptonuria (Ochronosis)

This AR disease is due to deficiency of the enzyme homogentisic acid oxidase. The characteristic features are the presence of homogentisic acid in the urine, widespread cartilage, and connective tissue pigmentation, cardiac valvular sclerosis, premature arterial sclerosis, and degenerative arthritis involving large peripheral joints. Tissue pigmentation is due to benzoquinoacetic acid and its polymers, which are indistinguishable from melanin.

Ocular involvement in the form of ochronic pigment deposition in the conjunctiva limbus or cornea is seen in 80% of patients. Typically, the scleral patches are triangular and anterior to the insertion of the horizontal recti. The treatment is purely symptomatic as dietary restriction is not helpful.

Alagille Syndrome (Arteriohepatic Dysplasia)

The diagnosis of this condition is made clinically in an infant with cholestatic jaundice and posterior embryotoxon. The typical facial features of deep-set hyperteloric eyes, broad forehead, long nose, and pointed chin become more obvious with age. At present, the most commonly reported ocular finding is a prominent Schwalbe's line (15%) with or without iris strands. Pigmentary chorioretinal atrophy and myopia also have been described. Variable systemic features of liver impairment, pulmonary valve stenosis, vertebral deformities, endocrine system and kidney involvement are well known. Cholestasis improves with age.

TABLE 23–9
Features of Chromosomal Anomalies

	Ocular Features	Systemic Features
	TRISOMY SYNDROMES	
Trisomy 13 or Patau Syndrome	Microphthalmia, coloboma, cataract, PHPV, intraocular cartilage, retinal	Cleft lid/palate, polydactyly, CVS and, CNS malformation
Trisomy 18 or Edwards syndrome	Corneal opacities, coloboma, microophthalmia	Characteristic facies, rocker bottom feet, renal abnormality, apneic spells
Trisomy 21 or Down syndrome	Epicanthus, upward slanting of palpebral fissures (mongoloid slant), myopia, strabismus, keratoconus	Characteristic mongoloid facies, protruding tongue, Simian palmar crease, hypotonia, cardiac
	DELETION SYNDROMES	
4 p deletion	Coloboma, coarse iris, exophthalmos	Midline scalp defects, cleft or high arched palate, deformed nose
5 p deletion (cri du chat syndrome)	Cataract, glaucoma, foveal hypoplasia, optic atrophy, coloboma,	"Cat-like cry" (abnormality in larynx), hypotonia, microcephaly
11 p deletion WAGR Syndrome (Wilm's tumor aniridia,	Aniridia (band p 13) cataract, glaucoma, corneal dystrophy, macula hypoplasia, strabismus	Mental retardation, pre-disposition to Wilms's tumor, genito-urinary abnormalities
13 q deletion	Retinoblastoma (band q 14) Cataract	Dysmorphic features, microcephaly
	DUPLICATION SYNDROMES	
Duplicated 22 q "Cat eye syndrome"	Coloboma of uveal tract, microphthalmia	Imperforate anus/anal atresia with rectovesical or rectovaginal fistula
	ANEUPLOIDY SYNDROMES	
Turner Syndrome 45XO	Ptosis, cataract, refractive errors, corneal scar, blue sclera, color blindness (incidence as in normal males)	Sexual infantilism, short stature, webbed neck, broad shield chest, multiple pigmented nevi, coarctation
Klinefelter Syndrome	Brushfield spots, myopia, choroidal atrophy, coloboma, micro-ophthalmia	Mental retardation increasing with number of X chromosomes, radio-

Chromosomal Anomalies

The common ocular manifestations exhibited by many of the identifiable chromosomal anomalies include hypertelorism, epicanthus, blepharoptosis, up and down slanting of palpebral fissures, strabismus, and microphthalmia. Nearly all patients with chromosomal defects present with some degree of mental retardation. The more specific and common ocular and systemic features of well-known chromosomal anomalies are described in Table 23–9.

Aicardi Syndrome

Aicardi syndrome is caused by an x-linked dominant gene that is lethal in males. Virtually all reported cases have occurred in females. The syndrome consists of infantile spasms or seizures, absence of the corpus callosum, progressive mental retardation, and characteristic chorioretinal lacunae. Initial neurologic evaluations may show normal examination during early infancy, however, progressive mental retardation, hypotonia, and seizures occur usually within 4 to 6 months after birth. The disease is generally fatal, with death occurring during childhood. Multiple skeletal anomalies have been described including scoliosis, spina bifida, vertebral abnormalities, cleft lip and palate, and fused ribs. Ocular abnormalities include chorioretinal lacunae of the fundus, micro-ophthalmus, colobomas of the choroid and optic nerve, optic nerve hypoplasia, peripapillary glial tissue, and the morning glory syndrome. The fundus appearance is characteristic of Aicardi syndrome and consists of bilateral circumscribed chorioretinal lesions with pigmented borders. The central aspect of these lesions are hypopigmented. Strabismus, nystagmus, and ptosis occur along with deterioration of the neurologic status. There is no specific treatment for this disorder except for supportive measures.

Prader-Willi Syndrome

Prader-Willi syndrome is characterized by hypotonia, obesity, small hands and feet, mental retardation, strabismus, and occasionally hypopigmentation or albinism. These patients have an insatiable appetite and will eat virtually anything. Their appetite increases with age, and parents often are forced to lock their refrigerator to prevent malignant obesity. Partial deletion of long arm chromosome 15 is responsible.

■ DYSLEXIA AND LEARNING DISABILITIES

Dyslexia is a very difficult problem for children, parents, and teachers alike. Because dyslexia usually occurs in children with otherwise normal intellectual capabilities, teachers and parents often look to a visual defect as the cause for poor reading. In fact, there has been no definite evidence of any relationship between peripheral visual abilities and reading problems (1–4, 6). Studies have consistently shown that normal readers and patients with dyslexia have similar incidence of peripheral visual defects. This concurs with my clinical experience since I have had a number of patients with very poor visual acuity, nystagmus, and limited ocular rotations (Duane's syndrome); yet these patients have excellent reading skills. On the other hand, I have examined many children with dyslexia who have absolutely normal visual acuity, binocularity, and ocular motility. Although the vast majority of dyslexic children will have normal ophthalmologic examinations, they should have a complete ophthalmic examination including cycloplegic refraction. Convergence insufficiency and latent hypermetropia are conditions that may interfere with reading and lead to near fatigue and asthenopia. Mild hypermetropia of +1.50 or less rarely causes asthenopia and does not interfere with reading.

Many optometric practitioners claim that dyslexic children have an oculomotor deficit that disrupts the normal reading pattern. They go on to rationalize that eye exercises improve ocular coordination, and thus can improve reading skills. Much of this thinking has come from early publications of the American Optical Company, Bureau of Visual Science, 1950. Studies by Goldberg and Schiffman at Johns Hopkins University using electronystagmography clearly demonstrated that ocular coordination and motility is normal in dyslexic children (2). Additionally, they showed that the degree of comprehension produces the pattern of ocular movement and not the innate ocular motility potential that determines the degree of comprehension. That is to say, children that have difficulty comprehending and reading will show abnormal fixation and refixation movements as they read, however, their ocular motility will be normal. A patient who can read French fluently will show normal eye motility when reading French, however, they will show abnormal eye movements when reading English. These and other studies have shown that reading and learning disabilities are not caused by a lack of ocular coordination or any form of ocular motor problems in the vast majority of children.

Vision therapy, perceptual training, and motor training have no role in the treatment of the dyslexia. Dyslexic children require reading tutoring and one-on-one education, not eye exercises or balance beam training. A joint organizational statement has been issued from the executive committees and councils of the American Academy of Pediatrics and the American Academy of Ophthalmology. It emphatically states that children with learning disabilities have the same incidence of ocular abnormalities as children who are normal achievers and are reading at grade level. Visual training, eye muscle exercises, and reading with tinted glasses frequently result in unwarranted expense and often misplace resources where they could be used for tutoring (5).

■ REFERENCES

1. Goldberg HK: Role in patching in learning. Am J Ophthalmol 1969;6:123.
2. Goldberg HK, Arnott W: Ocular motility in learning disabilities. J Learn Disabil 1970;3:160.
3. Goldberg HK: Dyslexia/Learning Disabilities. Second ed. Vol II. Philadelphia: W.B. Saunders, 1983, pp 1305–1318.
4. Helveston EM, et al.: Visual funtion and academic performance. Am J Ophthalmol 1985:99:346–355.
5. Metzger RL, Werner DB: Use of visual training for reading disabilties: a review. Pediatrics 1984;73:824–829.
6. Vellutino FR: Dyslexia. Scientific American 1987;256:34–41.

VI Oculoplastic

Section Editor: David T. Tse

24 The Lacrimal System

David T. Tse, Kevin R. Scott

■ ANATOMY AND PHYSIOLOGY

The lacrimal system is comprised of three integral components responsible for the production, distribution, and drainage of tears. The main and accessory lacrimal glands secrete a tear film that protects the ocular surface and helps maintain optimal vision. The eyelids and their blinking action help distribute tears across the cornea and transport tears to the puncta. The lacrimal excretory system drains tears from the lacus lacrimalis (Lid tear lake) into the inferior meatus. Conditions altering the complex interplay of anatomy and physiology of these components will result in symptomatic epiphora (tearing). Proper clinical distinction between anatomic and physiologic dysfunction and accurate localization of the anatomic defect are essential for treatment.

■ SECRETORY SYSTEM

The main lacrimal gland is located in the superior lateral portion of the anterior orbit. Directly posterior to the orbital rim is a concavity within the orbital plate of the frontal bone that forms the fossa glandular lacrimalis. The *lacrimal gland* is supported within the fossa by various attachments. The suspensory ligament of Soemmering fixes the superior surface of the gland to the periorbita of the frontal bone. The main structural support to the gland is provided by the lateral horn of the levator aponeurosis and the Whitnall's ligament. The lateral horn of the levator aponeurosis divides the lacrimal gland into an orbital and palpebral lobe, with the palpebral lobe laying beneath the levator aponeurosis. The orbital lobe contains approximately two thirds of the volume of the lacrimal gland, and the palpebral lobe constitutes the remainder.

The secretory ducts of the lacrimal gland coalesce and pass through the palpebral lobe to the conjunctiva. The 12 to 14 lacrimal excretory ducts open to the palpebral conjunctiva, 4 to 5 mm above the lateral aspect of the upper tarsal margin. They are seen as fine dots when the upper lid is everted. All the excretory ducts pass through the palpebral lobe of the lacrimal gland; consequently, inadvertent excision of this portion of the gland will compromise main lacrimal gland secretions.

The accessory lacrimal glands consist of the glands of Wolfring, located at the superior tarsal border, and the glands of Krause, situated in the conjunctival fornix. These structures contain small nests of lacrimal glands that drain directly to the conjunctiva. The glands of Krause number approximately 20 to 40 in the upper fornix and only 6 to 8 in the lower fornix. The glands of Wolfring are less common, numbering approximately 3 at the superior tarsal border and only 1 at the inferior tarsal border. The role of the accessory lacrimal glands is primarily for the maintenance of basal tear secretion.

The lacrimal nerve provides sensory innervation of the lacrimal gland. The lacrimal gland secretion is produced by stimulation of a reflex arc as well as central stimulation. The afferent limb of the reflex pathway is supplied by the fifth cranial nerve. The efferent limb is through the facial (seventh) cranial nerve that originates in the pons above the superior salivatory nucleus. Interruption of the reflex arc results in the loss of reflex tear production.

Stimulation of any of the branches of the trigeminal nerve may result in reflex tearing. Stimulation of the ophthalmic division of the trigeminal nerve from defects in the corneal epithelium, or spasm of the ciliary body (iritis) is a frequent source.

■ TEAR DISTRIBUTION SYSTEM

The *tear film* distribution system consists of the eyelids and the tear meniscus along the eyelid margin. Blinking spreads the tear film, resurfaces areas of dryness, adds fresh components to the tears, and removes debris. Blinking produces a vertical distribution of tears, while horizontal tear flow occurs in the tear meniscus at the eyelid margin. The lacrimal puncta conduct the tear fluid from the tear meniscus and lacrimal lake into the ampulla and canaliculi (Fig. 24–1). This is effected by a *lacrimal pump* mechanism that actively pumps tear into the sac with each blink. The two most popular theories are those of Jones (1–3) and Doane (4).

Jones suggested that the "lacrimal pump" has three major components: the pretarsal orbicularis muscle, preseptal orbicularis muscle, and the lacrimal diaphragm. Each muscle has two heads, superficial and deep. The deep head of the pretarsal orbicularis muscle (Horner's muscle) originates around the ampulla of the canaliculus and inserts on the posterior lacrimal crest. The superficial head of the pretarsal orbicularis and preseptal orbicularis fibers insert in a dense conjoined medial canthal tendon anterior to the fundus of the lacrimal sac. The deep head of the preseptal muscle (Jones' muscle) inserts on the fascia overlying the sac and the posterior lacrimal crest. The lacrimal diaphragm is an extension of the periorbita and forms the lateral wall of the lacrimal sac.

The pumping sequence begins with the lids in the open position, in which capillary action siphons the tears into the ampulla of the canaliculus. The sac is collapsed when the lids are opened. Eyelid closure initiates compression of the lacrimal ampulla, accompanied by shortening of the canaliculus via contraction of the deep heads of the pretarsal orbicularis (Horner's muscle). Continued orbicularis muscle contraction shortens the canaliculus, propelling tears medially toward the sac. The deep heads of the preseptal muscles simultaneously pull the lacrimal diaphragm laterally, creating a negative pressure gradient within the tear sac. As the lids open, the sac collapses, and tears are discharged into the nasolacrimal duct. The ampulla and canaliculus expand synchronously to draw in more tears, initiating a new cycle. Reflux from the lacrimal sac into the canaliculus system is prevented by the valve of Rosen-müller at the junction of the upper and lower canaliculis (Fig. 21–1).

Using high-speed cinematography to assess the dynamics of the blinking pattern and tear drainage, Doane documented the following sequence of events:

1. With the lids open, the lacrimal excretory system is fully expanded.
2. With the lids one third closed, the puncta are occluded by contact of lid margins.
3. As lid closure progresses to two thirds closed, the canaliculi and sac are squeezed.
4. With complete lid closure, compression of the entire lacrimal system is produced. Partial vacuum is formed within the excretory system as the lids begin to open.
5. With the lids one third open, there is a release of pressure on the canaliculi. The puncta remain occluded.
6. With the lids two thirds open, puncta "pop" open, followed by a rapid flow of tear fluid into the punctal opening lasting as long as several seconds.
7. The eyelid blinking cycle is repeated.

Doane also observed that tears flow over the cornea only with blinking, and that the punctum and marginal

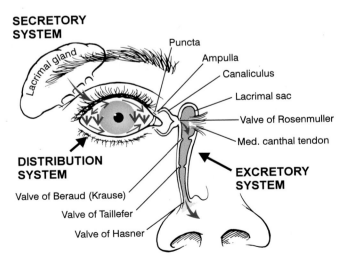

Figure 24–1.
Three integral components of the lacrimal system.

tear strip both move 2 to 5 mm nasally with each blink. Doane's theory of lacrimal pump function postulated a complete collapse of the lacrimal excretory system on eyelid closure. In contrast, Jones suggested that eyelid closure compressed the ampulla and canaliculi but expanded the lacrimal sac. Both theories proposed that the chief propulsive force lies with the compression and nasal movement of the canaliculi. They further agreed that there is a valve effect within the canaliculi in preventing reflux from the sac. Jones stressed the ingress of tears at the punctum as due to capillary action, while Doane's theory suggested a negative pressure effect in siphoning tears into the canaliculi.

In patients with physiologic dysfunction, symptomatic *epiphora* results from a failure of functional mechanisms involving the tear distribution system. This may be caused by anatomic abnormalities, such as eyelid malpositions, lid imbrication, kissing puncti, and conjunctivochalasis. Eyelid malpositions include ectropion, entropion, and lid retraction. Abnormal lid margin apposition to the globe, as in punctal eversion and tarsal ectropion, may prevent tears from reaching the canaliculi with each blink. Entropion and secondary trichiasis can cause ocular irritation and reflex tearing that overwhelms the drainage system. Superimposed on eyelid malposition is the element of palpebral conjunctival injection and keratinization induced by chronic exposure. Frequently, this leads to a vicious cycle of reflex tearing and rubbing of the eye by the patient. Lid retraction associated with Graves' ophthalmopathy or anterior lamella shortage can lead to incomplete blink and reflexive tearing. The retracted position of the eyelid creates an abnormal gradient for normal tear migration toward the puncta.

The lacrimal pump mechanism relies on the frequent contracture of the pretarsal and preseptal orbicularis muscle during blinking for proper functioning. Patients with generalized facial akinesia, such as Parkinson's disease or progressive supranuclear palsy, may manifest epiphora on the basis of an ineffective lacrimal pump. In seventh nerve palsies, paralytic lower lid ectropion, along with poor orbicularis tone, contribute to the symptom of epiphora. Patients with an inflexible eyelid secondary to a burn, scar tissue, or scleroderma may have inadequate tear drainage due to deficiency in lacrimal pump function. Proper recognition of the underlying anatomical defect will enable the surgeon to select the appropriate treatment to relieve patient's tearing symptom. Specific surgical procedures for correction of various eyelid malpositions are described in the preceding section.

Lid Imbrication Syndrome

Lid imbrication syndrome (5) is an abnormality of lid apposition in which the upper lid overrides the lower

lid. This syndrome classically presents as an unrecognized cause of chronic ocular irritation. Patients often complain of foreign body sensation, irritation, burning, and tearing. This condition is best evaluated by having the patient tilt his head backward and shining a flashlight toward the upper lid. The physical finding of the upper lid overriding the lower lid is pathognomonic for the disease (Fig. 24–2). Rose bengal staining of the superior lid margin tarsal conjunctiva is a reliable aid for diagnosing lid imbrication syndrome. The pathogenesis of lid imbrication is due to laxity of the upper lid. Treatment ranges from tear substitutes to horizontal lid shortening of the upper lid.

Kissing Puncti

Kissing puncti is a condition in which the upper punctum is in apposition with the lower punctum on primary gaze (Fig. 24–3). The normal medial canthal fissure, caruncle, and lacrimal papillae are not visible (Fig. 24–3A). The punctal openings are effectively occluded, precluding ingress of tears into the canalicular system with each blink. The etiology of this eyelid malposition problem is unclear, but horizontal lid laxity, with medial displacement of the punctum and blepharoptosis (6) may be contributory. One simple method to assess the importance of this anatomic problem as a contributing factor in epiphora is to pull the lower punctum laterally with a piece of tape (Fig. 24–3B). When the puncta are no longer in apposition, or "kissing," the dye clearance test is repeated. If there is an improvement in the rate of dye clearance while the punctum is moved laterally, then one can predict that a horizontal tightening procedure should improve the patient's tearing symptom.

Conjunctivochalasis

Conjunctivochalasis is an isolated bilateral condition in which redundant bulbar conjunctival tissue billows over

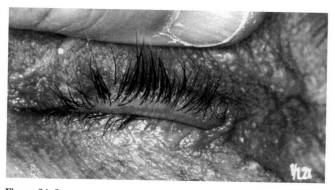

Figure 24–2.
Eyelid imbrication viewed from below; upper lid is overriding the lower lid.

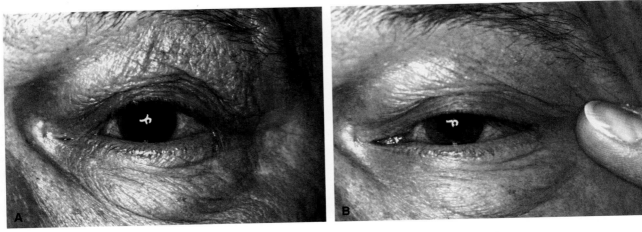

Figure 24–3.
A, Apposition of puncti on primary gaze. **B,** Widening of the medial canthal fissure when the lower lid is pulled laterally.

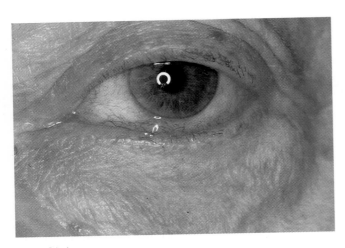

Figure 24–4.
Conjunctivochalasis.

the eyelid margin or covers the lower punctum (7). The redundancy is usually located centrally, a few millimeters below the inferior limbus (Fig. 24–4). The redundant tissue causes tearing by mechanically disrupting the normal meniscus and impeding tear flow. Conjunctivochalasis can be corrected by an elliptical resection of the redundant conjunctival tissue.

■ EXCRETORY SYSTEM

The *lacrimal excretory system* consists of the punctum, canaliculus, common canaliculus, lacrimal sac, and the nasolacrimal duct (Fig. 24–1). The tears enter the lacrimal excretory system at the punctum in the posterior eyelid margin. The punctum has a diameter of approximately 0.3 mm, but this may vary with the tone of the surrounding fibroelastic ring. The initial 2 mm of the canaliculus is vertically oriented. The lumen of the ampulla may be up to 2 to 3 mm wide. The canaliculus then courses horizontally for approximately 8 to 10 mm to the lacrimal sac. Before entering the lacrimal sac, the upper and lower canaliculis fuse, forming the common canaliculus. A dilation of the internal common punctum may be present and is called the sinus of Maier. The common canaliculus enters the lacrimal sac at the level of the medial canthal tendon. Nearly 90% of all canali-

culi merge to a common duct, while in 10% of the eyes each canaliculus opens independently into the sac. The lacrimal sac lies in a bony fossa, formed by the lacrimal bone and the nasal process of the maxilla. The nasolacrimal duct runs within the osseous canal, which is formed by the lacrimal, maxillary, and ethmoid bones. The nasolacrimal duct gains entrance into the inferior meatus, approximately 1.5 cm behind the anterior border of the inferior turbinate.

Multiple valves have been identified in the nasolacrimal system; however, most "valves" generally represent mucosal folds and are of no functional significance. One valve of importance is the valve of Rosenmüller at the entrance of the common canaliculus into the lacrimal sac (Fig. 24–1). This mucosal fold prevents reflux of lacrimal sac content back through the canaliculi.

Repeated probings may compromise the integrity of this valve. As a result, blowing of the nose will occasionally result in air being regurgitated through the nasolacrimal system onto the globe. The other nasolacrimal valve of significance is the *valve of Hasner*, which is implicated in congenital *nasolacrimal duct obstruction* (Fig. 24–1). This structure prevents retrograde reflux of air, nasal secretions, and nasal flora into the nasolacrimal duct.

■ CONGENITAL DISORDERS AND MANAGEMENT

Embryologically, the nasolacrimal drainage system develops from an invagination of surface ectoderm, which originates in the naso-optic fissure. Canalization occurs first in the central portion of the nasolacrimal passageways and then proceeds segmentally in both directions. Normally, the process of canalization is completed by the end of the 9-month gestational period. This system may fail to open anywhere throughout its course; however, the distal end of the *nasolacrimal duct (NLD)* is the most common site of obstruction. The blockage of tear drainage results from a thin membrane, at the level of the valve of Hasner, failing to perforate at birth. Additionally, there are a multitude of other less common anatomic variations within this system that can cause obstruction, including impaction of the inferior turbinate or a complete bony obstruction of the nasolacrimal duct.

The incidence of symptomatic congenital nasolacrimal duct obstruction ranges from 1% to 5%, of which one fourth to one third are bilateral. The incidence of obstruction in premature infants is much higher. Since the ability to produce tears is present at birth, stagnation of tears within the nasolacrimal sac frequently results in tearing and mattering of the lashes within the first few weeks of life.

Pediatric Epiphora

The proper work-up of a child with *epiphora* should begin with a careful history. It is important to establish the onset, duration, and severity of tearing, as well as a history of ocular infection or facial trauma. It also is incumbent on the ophthalmologist to rule out the more visually threatening causes for tearing, before concluding it is related to an obstruction of the nasolacrimal duct. For instance, congenital glaucoma may have tearing as the initial presenting symptom. A detailed history and examination may reveal additional symptoms and signs of glaucoma: photophobia, blepharospasm, breaks in Descemet's membrane, an increased corneal diameter, or clouding of the cornea. Additionally, a careful examination can help to eliminate the following: entropion, ectropion, trichiasis, distichiasis, epiblepharon, punctal atresia, conjunctivitis, foreign bodies, and rare disorders such as crocodile tears in association with Duane's retraction syndrome.

For an adequate evaluation of a tearing newborn or young child, either loupes, or in a cooperative child, a slit lamp is required. A systematic approach to the examination will aid in eliminating these additional causes of tearing. The key components of the ocular examination include determination of eyelid and lash position and documenting punctal patency, corneal clarity, and corneal diameter.

In cases of *nasolacrimal duct obstruction*, inspection alone may reveal an increased tear lake, epiphora, mattering of the lashes, or a distended lacrimal sac. Gentle pressure over the lacrimal sac will frequently result in regurgitation of the stagnant material from within the sac. When possible, document if the discharge refluxes from the upper, lower, or both puncta. This is an indirect verification of the patency of the canalicular system.

A thorough evaluation of the lacrimal drainage system in newborns and young children is often limited. Therefore, the ophthalmologist must rely primarily on the history and external examination. The modified fluorescein dye disappearance test, as described by Katowitz and Welsh (8), is a simple and useful method in assessing the integrity of the outflow system. In this test, a drop of 0.5% proparacaine is first instilled into the fornix, followed by 1 to 2 drops of 2% fluorescein solution. In a patent outflow system, the fluorescein is normally cleared from the tear lake within 10 minutes. The qualitative comparison of the rate of fluorescein egress from both sides is determined by directing a slit-lamp cobalt blue light at the eyes of the patient from several feet away. This should be done in a partially darkened room. From this distance, the light should illuminate the entire face of the child and is generally nonthreatening. Since a crying child precludes proper interpretation of this test, the parent should remain with the child throughout the test. A delay in fluorescein clearance is suggestive of an outflow obstruction. One should also examine the nose and pharynx with a blue light. The presence of fluorescein indicates at least some flow of dye through the NLD system.

Medical Management of NLD Obstruction

There is general agreement that the best initial management of an NLD obstruction is a combination of nasolacrimal sac massage and topical antibiotics to reduce the amount of mucopurulent discharge. Massage of the nasolacrimal sac has been shown to be effective in increasing the rate of spontaneous resolution of the distal membranous nasolacrimal duct obstruction.

Proper massage technique involves the parent placing his or her index finger over the medial canthal tendon and applying pressure in a nasal and downward direction to increase the hydrostatic pressure within the lacrimal sac. The parents are instructed to keep their fingernail trimmed to avoid trauma to eyelid skin. Massage should be performed four times a day with 5 to 10 repetitions each time. Following digital massage, topical sulfacetamide, 10% solution, may be instilled four times daily.

Timing of Initial NLD Probing

Controversy exists about the optimal timing for initial probing in a patient with congenital nasolacrimal duct obstruction. This controversy results primarily because a high percentage will spontaneously resolve with conservative medical management alone.

Katowitz and Welsh (8) reported 54% of congenital nasolacrimal duct obstructions resolved spontaneously by 6 months, and only an additional 17% resolved by 13 months. Peterson and Robb (9) reported similar results, with 54% resolving within 6 months, and only an additional 14% spontaneously resolving by 13 months. Katowitz and Welsh also reported that delaying initial probing beyond 13 months of age resulted in decreasing success as well as increasing complexity of therapy required to achieve success.

In patients with persistent symptoms of NLD obstruction despite an optimal course of medical therapy, consideration for probing should be given. We recommend that the initial probing be performed between 6 months and 1 year of age. This will allow most patients to resolve spontaneously, yet maintain the maximum response to a first probing.

Nasolacrimal Duct Probing

Additional controversy exists over whether to perform the initial probing in the office with a papoose restraint or under general anesthesia. Our individual preference is to perform probing under general anesthesia because it permits a more controlled, gentle, and complete evaluation of the nasolacrimal system. Additionally, this approach to NLD probing allows a comprehensive examination under anesthesia, as well as a controlled infracturing of the inferior turbinate, if needed.

Since there is no consensus on timing and location of probing, the parents need to be fully informed of the possibility for spontaneous resolution, balanced against the ocular discomfort for the child and inconvenience for them with continued medical management. They also should be informed of the reduced success rate if probing is performed after 13 months of age. Exceptions to the 6- to 12-month rule arise in cases of acute purulent dacryocystitis or a dacryocystocele (amniotocele). Treatment of these cases will be outlined later.

Surgical Technique

The instruments needed for probing include cotton gauze, nasal speculum, bayonet forceps, Freer periosteal elevator, assorted Bowman probes, punctal dilator, clear suction catheter, 2% fluorescein dye, irrigation cannula, 3-mm syringe, nasal atomizer, and 4% cocaine solution. The nose is then sprayed with 4% cocaine solution on the involved side. With use of a fiberoptic headlight, loupes, nasal speculum, and bayonet forceps, the nose is packed under and around the inferior turbinate with a strip of cotton gauze moistened with 4% cocaine. The solution should be squeezed out of the gauze before packing the nose to avoid toxicity. One to two percent cocaine solution can be used in very young or frail children. The anesthesiologist should be informed of the use of cocaine, and a dose of 3 mg/kg must not be exceeded.

After 5 minutes, the packing is removed and the nasal cavity inspected. If the inferior turbinate is hypertrophic and impacted against the lateral wall, the blunt end of a Freer periosteal elevator is used to gently infracture the turbinate toward the septum. The tip of the periosteal elevator is inserted under the inferior turbinate, and gentle pressure is applied to the turbinate until a slight crack is felt. This maneuver is performed using both hands to allow a slow, steady movement, which guards against inadvertent injury to the nasal septum.

The superior punctum is dilated with a punctal dilator. A size 0 Bowman probe is bent slightly to create a smooth curvature, which facilitates passage down the nasolacrimal duct. The probe is introduced into the punctum for approximately 1.5 to 2 mm in a vertical direction and rotated laterally to parallel the lid margin. As the probe is advanced toward the lacrimal sac, lateral traction on the upper lid is applied. This traction avoids the formation of accordion folds in the canaliculus (Fig. 24–5). A soft stop encountered while advancing the probe may represent a stricture or membranous blockage within the canaliculus or the common internal punctum. After reaching the nasolacrimal sac, a "hard" stop is felt against the bony lacrimal sac fossa. If there is any question whether the sac has been reached, relax the traction on the lid and attempt to advance the probe medially. If this results in movement of the eyelid toward the nose, then the tip of the probe is still in the canaliculus.

The tip of the probe should remain in contact with the bone while the probe is pivoted 90° superiorly and advanced inferiorly in a slightly posterolateral direction. The direction of the probe is in vertical alignment with the second incisor tooth. The probe is gently pushed downward until the membranous obstruction is reached. A slight inferior pressure will result in a "give,"

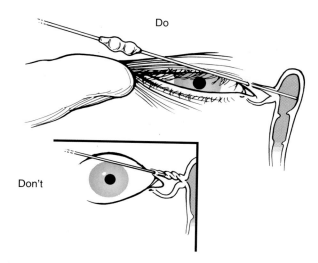

Do

Don't

Figure 24–5.
Nasolacrimal duct probe. Top diagram shows proper technique. Bottom diagram shows improper technique without lateral lid traction so the punctum is folded, increasing the possibility for a false passage.

allowing the probe to enter the inferior meatus. A nasal speculum is inserted into the external naris in an attempt to directly visualize the probe. The nasal speculum should be inserted so the blades separate vertically to avoid damaging the septum.

If the probe cannot be visualized, a size 3 Bowman probe can be used to make a metal-on-metal contact with it. Not advancing the probe far enough or false passage of the probe in a submucosal plane are common causes for not being able to make contact with the probe. Following confirmation, the probe is removed, and an irrigation cannula on a 3-ml syringe is inserted through the superior canaliculus into the lacrimal sac. Two percent fluorescein solution is gently irrigated through the system. Yellow-green tinged fluid should easily be retrieved with a clear suction cannula positioned under the inferior turbinate. If the fluorescein solution regurgitates out of the opposite canaliculus and no fluorescein is recovered from the nasopharynx, then stenosis of the NLD should be suspected. Additionally, a scraping sensation felt while passing the probe may signify a marked stenosis of the duct. These findings should be reviewed with the parents and are helpful in explaining why additional procedures may be necessary in the future, should probing fail.

When a bilateral obstruction exists, the same procedure is repeated on the contralateral side. To avoid confusion when irrigating the second side, all residual fluorescein from the first side must be suctioned from the nasopharynx.

Postoperative Management

After the nasolacrimal system has been probed and patency established, the patient is started on a regimen of sulfacetamide, 10% solution, 4 times daily for 1 week. The patient is seen in 3 weeks, and the fluorescein dye disappearance test is repeated. If the patient is still symptomatic, and the dye disappearance test is delayed, a trial of massage and antibiotics is initiated for 4 to 6 weeks. After this period, persistent epiphora and mattering should be treated with a repeat probing, along with silicone intubation.

Nasolacrimal Intubation

Silicone intubation is indicated for patients who have had a seemingly adequate initial probing but who remain symptomatic. Frequently, it has been noted that the patients who required silicone intubation were those with a tight probe passage through the nasolacrimal duct on initial probing, or those for whom difficulty on irrigation into the nose was encountered, despite confirmation of the probe in the proper location.

Katowitz and Welsh (8) reported 63 patients with congenital nasolacrimal duct obstruction who had an initial NLD probing at or after 24 months of age. One third of these patients responded to a first probing. In 71% of those patients who had failed the initial probing, symptoms resolved following nasolacrimal intubation. Therefore, if during the initial probing of a child older than 24 months in which the NLD appears to be tight, we convert to a primary nasolacrimal duct intubation with silicone stent.

Endotracheal anesthesia is used in all silicone intubation procedures. The technique and precautions are the same as those outlined previously for the nasolacrimal probing. After several minutes, the nasal packing is removed, and the nasal cavity is inspected. The inferior turbinate is then infractured, as previously described. The Crawford silicone stent, with a stainless steel probe and an olive tip, is our preferred intubation set. The newest modification of the original Crawford silicone stent has the added advantage of a suture within the tubing. Before using the stent, the stainless steel probe is bent slightly or curved for easier advancement into the nose.

The superior punctum is gently enlarged with a punctal dilator.

The Crawford probe is introduced into the superior punctum and advanced through the nasolacrimal system in the same fashion as that outlined for the nasolacrimal probing. Once the probe is in the nasal cavity, metal-on-metal verification of its proper placement is made with a modified groove director inserted into the inferior meatus.

Once contact is made, the probe is pulled superiorly several millimeters to allow the groove director to be advanced underneath the inferior turbinate and against the lateral nasal wall (10). The probe is advanced into the groove, and the olive tip is engaged by the keyhole groove at the end of the director (Fig. 24–6). The groove director is then withdrawn from the nose, while the probe is pulled in the opposite direction to avoid disengagement. The second stainless steel probe is similarly passed through the inferior canaliculus and retrieved from the inferior meatus. The advantages of this retrieval method are as follows: (1) it avoids the use of a hook to fish for the probe, thereby minimizing trauma to the nasal mucosa; (2) the groove director protects the floor of the nose because the tip of the lacrimal probe does not come in contact with the nasal mucosa during the entire procedure, thereby further reducing trauma to tissues; (3) the groove director traps the lacrimal probe if it directs itself posteriorly; and (4) retrieval is easy because the groove director guides the olive tip into the keyhole, ensuring capture.

The two ends of the Crawford silicone stent are pulled from the nose until the tubing forms a small loop between the two punctum. A muscle hook is used to engage the tubing between the two punctum, while the silicone tubing is pulled from the nose inferiorly under slight tension. A Castroviejo locking needle holder is used to grasp the tubing just at the level of the external naris. The Crawford tube is cut at the attachment site to the stainless steel probes.

When using the Crawford silicone stent with a suture within the tubing, a Crawford stripper is used to remove the silicone from both ends, without cutting the suture inside. The suture is then tied in four single square knots and cut close to the knots (Fig. 24–7). Before releasing the nasal end of the tubing, the tension of the silicone tubing between the punctum should be checked and approximately 3 to 4 mm of temporal slack is needed to avoid "cheese-wiring" of the punctum. After this is confirmed, the muscle hook is removed first before releasing the knots from the needle holder.

The tubing is then released to hang loosely under the inferior turbinate. If desired, a 5-0 Prolene suture can be placed just within the nasal vestibule on the lateral wall to fixate the stent, thereby reducing the chance for displacement into the nasolacrimal sac. If the intubation is performed using a silicone stent without an internal suture, then the silicone tubing is tied to itself in a similar fashion with four knots. The use of four single throws will keep the total knot size small, which allows for easy passage out of the canalicular system should the knots become inadvertently pulled into the lacrimal sac. In an attempt to avoid displacement of the silicone stent into the nasolacrimal sac, a 5-0 Prolene suture can be placed just within the nasal vestibule on the lateral wall to fixate the silicone stent.

Postoperative Management

Following silicone stent intubation, the patient is prescribed a steroid-antibiotic solution 4 times a day for 1 week. The patient is re-evaluated at 1 week following silicone stent placement. If the patient is without any stent-related problems or evidence of persistent dacryocystitis, the stent is kept in place for 6 months to 1 year.

Complications of Silicone Intubation

Silicone tubing within the nasolacrimal system is generally well tolerated. Problems can occur, however, if the tubing is tied too tightly with "cheese-wiring" through the punctum and canaliculus. Because of this possibility, the punctum needs to be checked on each postoperative visit and the tubing removed if cheese-wiring is noted. A slight enlargement of the punctum is common and does not necessitate removal. A pyogenic granuloma can form near the punctum and should be excised with light cautery applied to the base. If the tubing has already been in place for several months and the patient is asymptomatic, the tubing, along with the pyogenic granuloma, should be removed.

Occasionally, the tubing may cause conjunctival and corneal irritation secondary to persistent contact during adduction of the eye. If the keratoconjunctivitis is not relieved by topical lubricant at bedtime, then the tubing should be removed.

Prolapse of the stent, with the knots dislodged into the lacrimal sac is a common problem associated with silicone intubation. To avoid this problem, fixation

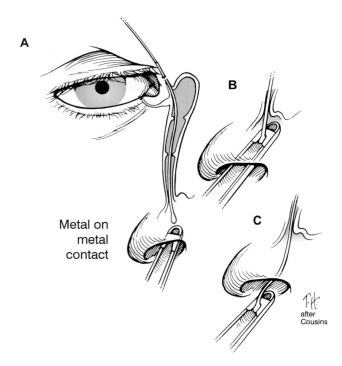

A

B

C

Metal on metal contact

after Cousins

Figure 24–6.
Silicone tube intubation.

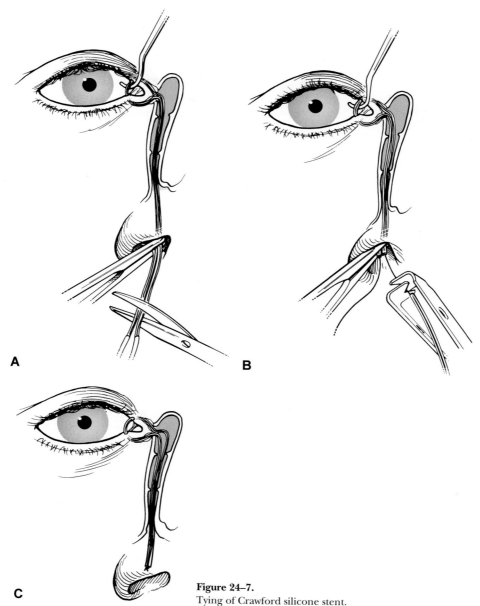

Figure 24–7.
Tying of Crawford silicone stent.

within the naris may be considered. Additionally, various authors have described the use of a silicone button, retinal sponge material, and ventricular shunt tubing attached to the intranasal portion of the silicone to guard against retraction of the knots into the lacrimal sac. Should the knots prolapse into the nasolacrimal sac, the silicone tubing can be removed through the superior canaliculus, provided not too many knots were placed originally. Avoid cutting the silicone stent until the knots are externalized.

On rare occasions, dacryocystitis may persist or recur with the silicone stent in proper position, which necessitates removal of the stent and subsequent dacryocystorhinostomy (DCR).

Silicone Stent Removal

In general, the silicone stent can be removed in the office, without the need for general anesthesia. In a small and uncooperative child, a papoose restraint may be necessary. With the head stabilized, the silicone tubing is visualized under the inferior turbinate or at its fixation point within the naris. The tubing is then grasped with an alligator forceps and pulled from the nose, after cutting the loop at the medial canthus. If unable to locate the stent within the nose, the loop at the medial canthus is grasped with a forceps and the knots are pulled into the sac. The knots are then rotated out of the superior canaliculus and the stent cut with scissors.

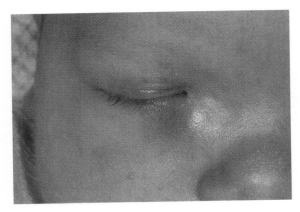

Figure 24–8.
Amniocele: the blueish bulge in the area of the nasolacrimal sac.

ical management alone, an in-office nasolacrimal probing can be performed to the level of the lacrimal sac to prevent the development of dacryocystitis. Typically, this is all that is needed to decompress the sac, and the child can then be treated for a typical nasolacrimal duct obstruction with massage and topical antibiotics. Occasionally, a full probing may be needed to effectively decompress the sac.

This condition must be differentiated from a capillary hemangioma and a meningoencephalocele. Capillary hemangiomas tend to have a more reddish and solid appearance, with moderate to high internal reflectivity by ultrasound. Additionally, capillary hemangiomas can develop above or below the medial canthal tendon. A meningoencephalocele tends to be pulsatile, occurring mainly above the medial canthal tendon and has a cystic appearance by ultrasound.

Acute dacryocystitis during the neonatal period usually is caused by an amniotocele and presents with distention of the lacrimal sac, purulent discharge, and surrounding erythema. Since this condition may rapidly progress to periocular cellulitis, intravenous antibiotics and an urgent nasolacrimal probing is indicated. If the distended sac begins to point on the skin surface, drainage with a small-gauge needle is indicated to decompress the sac. The aspirate is sent for cultures and Gram stain to guide the initial antibiotic therapy.

Chronic infection involving the lacrimal sac, as a complication of congenital lacrimal obstruction, is far more common than the acute form. It may be present with little or no apparent discomfort, variable enlargement of the tear sac, and little or no mucoid secretion. In some instances, pressure over the lacrimal sac will produce almost no reflux through the canaliculi. In other instances, the chronic dacryocystitis may take a suppurative form, presenting with a large ectatic sac which drains readily on digital compression of the sac. The secretion is purulent and thick. In either case, whether the chronic dacryocystitis is accompanied by gross purulent discharge or not, an appropriate initial step should be to perform therapeutic probing.

In a very uncooperative child, inhalation anesthesia, using a face mask, may be necessary for the removal of a silicone stent.

The patient is seen 3 weeks after stent removal, and a modified fluorescein dye disappearance test is repeated to document the patency of the system. If tearing symptom persists and the fluorescein dye disappearance is delayed, a DCR procedure along with silicone stent placement should be considered.

Dacryocystocele (Amniotocele)

A dacryocystocele (amniotocele) is a distention of the nasolacrimal sac in the neonate. This condition presents as a cystic-appearing bluish mass in the area of the nasolacrimal sac below the medial canthal tendon (Fig. 24–8). The lesion typically enlarges secondary to a ball-valve effect at the level of the common internal punctum, in conjunction with an NLD obstruction. Amniotic fluid, mucus, or tears accumulate within the sac and may become secondarily infected. Our preference is to initially treat a dacryocystocele conservatively with massage and topical sulfacetamide, 10% solution, 4 times a day. If there is no improvement after a few days of med-

■ ACQUIRED EPIPHORA

Acquired epiphora is a common complaint that requires a logical clinical and anatomical approach to both its understanding and management. Tearing is due to either excessive tear production or inadequate tear drainage. The patient with symptomatic epiphora may have either a normal anatomic system overwhelmed by overproduction of tears, or a drainage system that is anatomically compromised and unable to handle normal tear production (Table 24–1). Abnormal tear distribution can also result in epiphora. The

surgeon must determine which of these two situations exists before intervention can be initiated.

Hypersecretion

Acquired hypersecretion of tears leads to epiphora by overwhelming an anatomically normal lacrimal drainage system. This occurs most frequently in persons past puberty and particularly in the elderly. The most common causes of increased tear production include environ-

TABLE 24–1
Major Causes of Epiphora Associated With Each Component of the Lacrimal System

Hypersecretion	Distribution	Excretory Obstruction
V_1 branch of the trigeminal nerve	**Abnormal blink**	**Cong. anomalies**
foreign body	facial akinesia	atresia of puncta
pollutants	Parkinson's disease	atresia of canaliculus
allergy	Progressive supranuclear palsy	atresia of NLD
glaucoma	facial burn	amniotocele
exposure keratopathy	scleroderma	facial anomalies
aberrant lashes	**Eyelid malposition**	Conjunctival shrinkage disease
lacrimal gland tumor	ectropion	**Acquired Lacrimal Drainage**
Posterior fossa brain tumor	entropion	Canaliculitis
	retraction	Dacryocystitis
	Lid imbrication	Dacryolith
V_2 branch of the trigeminal nerve	Punctal apposition	Acquired punctal/canalicular stenosis
nasal lesions	Conjunctivochalasis	**Primary acquired NLD obstruction**
V_3 branch of the trigeminal nerve		**Secondary acquired NLD obstruction**
dental problem		1^0 neoplasms
Miscellaneous		2^0 to sinus neoplasms
Graves' disease		infections
Refractive errors		inflammation
amentropia, tropia, phoria		trauma
Raeder's syndrome		radiation
Crocodile tears		drugs
drugs		
dry eyes—meibomian gland disease		
blepharitis—evaporative dry eyes		

mental irritants, allergens, chronic conjunctivitis, marginal blepharitis, and other ocular inflammations such as keratitis and iritis. Among other irritants are foreign particles, upper respiratory infection, bright light, and accommodative strain. Allergic phenomena may include contact reactions to medications such as local anesthetics, mydriatics, antibiotics, sulfonamides, mercurials and idoxuridine, as well as to secondary ingredients such as naphazoline, phenylephrine preservatives, and lanolin bases. In older patients, irritation and resultant epiphora may be paradoxically caused by xerophthalmia (dry eye) and tear film abnormalities. A dry eye stimulates hypersecreation and causes reflex epiphea. For a description of dry eye syndrome, see Chapter 49.

Reflex irritation stemming from teeth, nasal sinuses, or nose also may cause lacrimation. When persistent tearing has no apparent ocular cause, consideration must be given to the possibility of a decayed tooth, nasal polyps, inflammation of the nasopharyngeal area, the maxillary antrum or the sphenoidal and posterior ethmoidal air cells, and chronic sinusitis with atrophic rhinitis.

Excessive lacrimation may often accompany the initial stages of lacrimal cyst and tumor involvement, or Mikulicz's syndrome. In fact, in the presence of swelling in the lacrimal gland fossa, tearing is a significant clue to lacrimal gland involvement. Lacrimation also may be produced by drugs that stimulate the lacrimal gland,

such as strong parasympathomimetic agents. A syndrome of tearing photophobia and torticollis in young children between 1 month and 2 years caused by a posterior fossa brain tumor has been described (12).

Stimulation of the trigeminal nerve, most particularly the V_1, which innervates the eye, will result in tearing. Neuropathic disorders that produce anomalous lacrimation include trigeminal neuralgia and the "crocodile tears" syndrome. The latter phenomenon, also known as the gustolacrimal reflex, is characterized by profuse lacrimation during the act of eating—particularly salty, spicy, or hot food. Although not well understood and reported rarely, the acquired form of this condition has been observed to develop generally some 6 months after the onset of facial palsy—either of Bell's type or as a result of herpes zoster, trauma, or intracranial surgery. It is postulated that the degeneration of the greater superficial petrosal nerve excites collateral growth from the lesser superficial petrosal nerve, which is involved in salivary secretion. These collateral sprouts "cross" and make functional connection with the lacrimal gland, thus establishing a reflex arc that provokes lacrimation on chewing. The condition also may be congenital. Since dry eye can cause epiphera, evaluation for dry eye should be part of the evaluation of epiphera including the Schirmer test.

Schirmer's Test

Schirmer I Test (Hyposecretion). This test measures the aqueous component of the tear film and does not differentiate between basic and reflex tear production. It yields only a gross estimate of tear production. The examination room should be dimly lit, and the patient is asked to maintain a straight gaze. Both eyes are tested simultaneously. The Schirmer I test is performed without topical anesthesia. It is important to gently blot the inferior fornix with a cotton tipped applicator before inserting the filter paper. A piece of 41 Whatman filter paper 5 × 35 mm in dimension, is folded on one side 5 mm from the end. The folded end is inserted into the inferior fornix at the temporal third of the lower lid. A normal range of wetting is between 10 and 30 mm after 5 minutes. A wetting of more than 30 mm does not have any differential diagnostic value. If less than 8 mm of wetting, a hyposecretion condition can be assumed.

Jones' Test (Basal Secretion). If the Schirmer I test is abnormal, a basic secretion test can be performed. This test differentiates basal secretion from reflex secretion. The aqueous component of the tear film is comprised of a basic, nonreflex secretion from the accessory glands (Krause and Wolfring), and a reflex secretion from the main lacrimal gland. A drop of topical anesthetic is instilled onto the eye and the tear film in the inferior fornix is cautiously removed with a cotton applicator. The topical anesthetic eliminates reflex lacrimation and provides a better gauge of basic tear production. The filter paper is inserted into the inferior fornix similar to the Schirmer I test. Wetting of less than 10 mm in 5 minutes indicates a decreased basal secretion.

Schirmer II Test (Reflex Secretion). If the results of the Schirmer I and Jones' tests are below normal, the Schirmer II test will yield information on reflex tearing capability. The conjunctiva is again anesthetized, and the filter paper is placed into the temporal third of the inferior fornix. The nasal mucosa of the middle turbinate is stimulated with a cotton applicator without anesthetizing the mucosal membrane. After 2 minutes, the amount of wetting of the filter paper is measured. The amount by which the Schirmer II test exceeds basic production represents reflex secretion. If there is no wetting at all, this finding indicates a failure of reflex secretors.

Lacrimal Drainage System Obstruction

Once tear overproduction has been eliminated as a causative factor, the surgeon is effectively left with diagnosing and managing an anatomic disorder causing a relative or absolute outflow obstruction. The evaluation of the lacrimal drainage system begins with the external and slit-lamp examinations seeking to answer the following questions: Is the patient's blink adequate? Is there eyelid malposition, lid imbrication, or conjunctivochalasis? Are the puncta positioned properly? Are the puncta open or closed? Is the lacrimal sac palpable or can material be expressed from the puncta with digital pressure over the sac? In answering these questions, one can begin to determine whether the obstruction lies in the upper or lower lacrimal system.

Upper Lacrimal System Obstruction

Normal lid contour, with proper anatomic positioning of the puncta within the tear meniscus, is required for adequate tear drainage. Displacement of the punctum from its normal position is most frequently the result of lower eyelid ectropion. Evaluation and appropriate surgical correction of eyelid malpositions should be completed before undertaking any lacrimal drainage system repair. When punctal stenosis is a secondary phenomenon, caused by chronic punctal eversion, simple correction of the underlying eyelid malposition along with punctal dilation may be sufficient to reestablish drainage. Swelling and redness around the punctum and canaliculus may indicate canaliculitis.

In addition to external and slit-lamp examinations, the likely site of obstruction within the lacrimal drainage system can be identified by the following series of functional tests.

Lower Lacrimal System Obstruction

If the puncta and canaliculi have been evaluated and considered normal, attention is turned to the lacrimal sac and nasolacrimal duct. In the normal individual, the lacrimal sac is never palpable. Should the initial examination of a patient complaining of epiphora demonstrate a distended lacrimal sac, a nasolacrimal duct obstruction is almost certainly present. Likewise, expression of purulent discharge with gentle pressure over the lacrimal sac is all but pathognomonic for nasolacrimal duct obstruction. If neither punctal stenosis nor distension of the sac is present, then Jones I and II dye tests are needed to further localize the site of obstruction (see below).

Intranasal Examination. A nasal speculum examination should be performed to assess the position of normal nasal structures. Nasal septal deviation may cause crowding of the internal nose with turbinate impaction. Rhinitis-induced turbinate swelling, tumors, or polyps can obstruct the nasolacrimal ostium. Children with dacryocystitis occasionally may have foreign bodies impacted under the inferior turbinate. Destruction or inflammation of the turbinates secondary to Wegener's granulomatosis or inhalation cocaine abuse can sometimes be identified. Such findings during nasal inspection will direct the clinician toward further diagnostic tests. Position of the anterior end of the middle turbinate should be appraised to determine if adequate space is available for a planned dacryocystorhinostomy or conjunctivodacryocystorhinostomy procedure.

Fluorescein Dye Disappearance Test

The fluorescein dye disappearance test is a rapid, semiquantitative screening method for the presence of lacrimal drainage system obstruction. The test is best performed by simultaneously instilling a single drop of concentrated 2% fluorescein solution into each inferior fornix. Ten to fifteen minutes after instillation, the degree of fluorescein clearance is grossly quantified. Observing the patient at a distance with the cobalt blue light of the slit lamp may be of aid in detecting subtle differences. Any asymmetry between eyes or an obvious delay in the clearance of dye from both eyes can be easily appreciated. Symmetric delays are more difficult to diagnose and require detailed study with the primary and secondary Jones dye tests.

If the fluorescein dye disappearance test documents a functional delay in the presence of a stenotic punctum, a review of possible etiologic factors should first be conducted. Punctal stenosis may be caused by trauma, such as that induced by repeated canalicular probings; chronic use of topical cholinesterase inhibitors or antiviral agents; ocular pemphigoid; infections, such as herpes zoster; and the presence of a congenital punctal membrane.

With the elimination of the etiologic factors and verification of the functional block, punctal stenosis is managed by means of a punctoplasty procedure. Attempts to repeatedly dilate the punctum will lead to restenosis and risk possible iatrogenic trauma and creation of false passage. The technique of punctoplasty will be discussed later.

Jones I Test—Primary Dye Test

The primary Jones test is a second method of establishing the overall patency of the lacrimal drainage system and corroborates the results of the dye disappearance test. First, the nasal mucosa is anesthetized with aerosolized 4% cocaine or another similar anesthetic agent. The fluorescein solution previously instilled into the fornix for the dye disappearance test will be searched for under the inferior turbinate. While spreading the external naris vertically with a nasal speculum, a calcium alginate swab is inserted under the inferior turbinate. The applicator tip is examined for evidence of fluorescein dye.

The presence of dye is described as a positive test, which indicates a patent drainage system and obviates the need for further testing. The absence of dye, or a negative test, is suggestive of two possibilities. First, fluorescein dye failed to enter the sac due to an upper system (i.e., punctum, canaliculus, or common punctum) obstruc-

tion. In this situation, a delay in dye clearance during the dye disappearance test should corroborate this finding. Second, fluorescein dye was able to enter into the sac, but could not be recovered under the inferior turbinate due to either a partial or complete nasolacrimal duct obstruction. In both circumstances, dye clearance also could be delayed. To further localize the site of obstruction, or to differentiate a partial from a complete nasolacrimal duct obstruction, a Jones II test is performed.

Jones II Test—Secondary Dye Test

Following a negative Jones I test, the fornices are irrigated free of residual fluorescein. A lacrimal irrigation cannula (23 to 27 gauge) on a saline-filled 3-ml syringe is inserted through the lower punctum and into the canaliculus. It is important not to advance the tip into the lacrimal sac. While the patient's head is tilted forward and the nose positioned over a metal basin, saline is gently irrigated into the sac. There are three potential outcomes:

1. Recovery of dye-tinged fluid from the nose indicates a patent canalicular system, but a partial nasolacrimal duct obstruction. The dye is able to enter into the sac, but does not passively enter into the nose; hence, a negative Jones I test, because of resistance at the level of nasolacrimal duct. However, in this instance, the resistance is overcome by the pressure of the irrigating fluid.
2. Recovery of only clear fluid from the nose indicates a relative stenosis of the upper canalicular system, usually at the level of punctum or common canaliculus. In this situation, dye is not able to enter the sac; hence, no dye is recovered in the nose with active irrigation of fluid into the sac. A delay in dye clearance (on dye disappearance test), coupled with the detection of canalicular stricture on probing should be confirmatory.
3. No fluid recovered from the nose, with fluid reflux out of the canaliculi. Three possible scenarios may occur in this particular circumstance:
   - Reflux of clear fluid around the irrigation cannula, without distension of the lacrimal sac. This is indicative of a severe canalicular stricture, involving the canaliculus intubated with the irrigation cannula.
   - Reflux of clear fluid out of the nonintubated canaliculus, without distension of the lacrimal sac. Occasionally, a jet stream of fluid may be seen refluxing out of the upper canaliculus upon irrigation. This is indicative of a complete stricture at the level of common canaliculus.
   - Reflux of clear or dye-tinged fluid, with distension of the lacrimal sac. This is suggestive of a complete nasolacrimal duct obstruction. The pres-

TABLE 24–2
Interpretation of Excretory Test Results in the Evaluation of Epiphora

Disappearance Test	Jones I Test	Jones II Test	Diagnosis/Site of Obstruction	Needs to Reassess
Rapid	+	No need to perform	Patent drainage system; probable hypersecretion	Reflexive tearing
Normal	+	+, dye recovery in nose	Patent system; functional	Reflexive tearing; tear distribution component
Normal	−	+, dye recovery in nose	Partial nasolacrimal duct obstruction	Palpate sac; nasal speculum exam
Delayed	−	+, Clear fluid in nose	Punctal/canalicular stenosis; partial NLD obstruction	Punctum/canaliculus; tear distribution component
Delayed	−	−, Reflux of dye-tinged fluid from opposite punctum, with sac distension	Complete nasolacrimal duct obstruction	Palpate sac, nasal speculum exam
Delayed	−	−, Reflux of clear fluid from opposite punctum	Complete common canaliculus obstruction	Probe canaliculus with a double-0 Bowman probe
Delayed	−	−, Reflux of clear fluid around irrigation cannula	Severe canalicular stricture	Probe canaliculus

+ = recovery of dye in nose
− = no recovery of dye in nose
NLD = nasolacrimal duct

ence of dye in the fluid refluxing out indicates that the dye was able to enter into the sac through a patent upper system, but became stagnant within the sac because of an outlet obstruction (Table 24–2).

Diagnostic Intracanalicular Probing

When the secondary Jones test indicates canalicular obstruction, the involved canaliculus should be probed to localized the point of stenosis. A probing instrument (00 Bowman probe) is passed through the anesthetized lower and upper canaliculi into the sac, feeling for stricture along their course. Upon reaching an obstruction, the examiner grasps the probe with a forceps where it enters the punctum and measures the distance to the impeded end of the probe with a millimeter ruler. The distance measured indicates the site of obstruction (Table 24–3).

Diagnostic Imaging Techniques

Radiographic studies are mandatory when sinus disease, neoplasm, mucoceles, or fractures in the area of the lacrimal fossa region are suspected. Dacryocystography may be helpful in evaluating a patient with suspected lacrimal sac tumor in which other studies are inconclusive. Characteristically this study reveals a distended sac with a mottled density or a filling defect. Based on the

outcome of these functional tests, one can identify a likely point of obstruction and initiate appropriate treatment.

Diseases of the Upper Lacrimal Drainage System

Punctal Stenosis

For patients with isolated punctal stenosis, punctoplasty is a simple and effective first step to relieve the tearing symptom. Several punctoplasty procedures have been described in the past. In the one-snip procedure, a single vertical incision into the ampulla is made through the posterior wall of the punctum with a sharp Westcott scissors. In most instances, a Jones two-snip punctoplasty is performed by creating a 2-mm high, V-shaped opening posteriorly. Even with excision of a wedge of punctal tissue, appositional closure of the punctum can oc-

TABLE 24–3
Interpretation of Probing

Measured Distance	Site of Obstruction
1–9 mm	Prior to common canaliculus
10–11 mm	At common canaliculus
12–15 mm	In sac

cur. To reduce the incidence of postoperative closure, we have had the most success with a three-snip puncto-plasty followed by placement of a circular silicone stent within the canalicular system. The rationale for the placement of a silicone stent here is analogous to stent placement to ensure patency of the internal ostium following a dacryocystorhinostomy (DCR). The silicone stent not only prevents appositional closure secondary to the healing process, but also mechanically dilates the stenotic canaliculi, if this is also present.

Three-Snip Punctoplasty Procedure

After application of topical anesthetic, peripunctal infiltration of the inferior punctum is carried out with 2% lidocaine with epinephrine. The punctum is dilated with a punctal dilator. The posterior rim of the punctum is grasped with a 0.12-mm forceps and one blade of a sharp Westcott scissors is inserted into the ampulla. A vertical snip incision is made at the lateral aspect of the posterior rim. A second vertical snip incision is made at the medial aspect of the punctum while grasping the posterior edge of the punctum with 0.12-mm forceps. The posterior flap of tissue is excised by a horizontal third snip joining the inferior margins of the first two cuts. The wedge of tissue excised is made within the ampulla and not in the horizontal portion of the canaliculus, as has been previously described in another variation of the three-snip punctoplasty. It is important to visualize the epithelial lining of the ampulla.

The newly formed opening is a defect in the posterior wall of the ampulla, properly positioned to serve as an opening for tear drainage. Light bipolar cautery may be applied to control bleeding. A circular "doughnut" silicone stent is then placed in the upper system to ensure patency.

Circular Doughnut Silicone Stent Placement
(Pigtail Probing)

Doughnut silicone intubation describes the shape of the stent once it is intubated into the upper lacrimal system and encircles it for 360°. The stent passes from one punctum through its corresponding canaliculus, into the opposite canaliculus and exits the other punctum, forming a complete circle. The Worst round eyed pigtail probe is used. It is important to avoid the use of the crocheted probe as iatrogenic canalicular damage is common. The use of the Worst *pigtail probe* requires a thorough knowledge of the anatomy of the upper lacrimal drainage system. In most patients (90%), the canaliculi join to form the common canaliculus before entering the lacrimal sac. In the remaining 10%, the canaliculi gain entrance into the lacrimal sac independently and, thus, the smooth, continuous drainage system that facilitates introduction of the probe is not present. This latter group can be difficult, or impossible to intubate using the pigtail probe.

The eyed pigtail probe is introduced into the upper punctum and gently rotated through the canalicular system after peripunctal anesthetic infiltration (see Fig. 26–1). Excessive force is not necessary, and difficulty intubating the system may indicate stenosis or obstruction of the canaliculi. If resistance is encountered, it is worthwhile to attempt to intubate the system from the inferior canaliculus. One should never try to force the probe into the canalicular system. Once the tip of the pigtail probe enters the canaliculus, the shaft is digitally rotated to advance the tip toward the sac. The spiral portion of the probe should be kept in the same plane as the canaliculi. It is important to recall that the common canaliculus lies immediately posterior to the medial canthal tendon. A slight posteriorly directed probe rotation should facilitate its passage. If the probe cannot be retrieved after multiple attempts, one trick is to pass a size O Bowman probe into the sac through the opposite canaliculus. Metal-on-metal contact with the tip of the pigtail probe and the Bowman probe should be felt in the sac. While constantly maintaining metal-on-metal contact, the tip of the pigtail probe is guided through the opposite canaliculus as the Bowman probe is slowly withdrawn. If this maneuver again fails to pass the pigtail probe through, then the procedure should be aborted to minimize further trauma to the canalicular system.

Continued rotation of the probe allows the tip to exit the opposite punctum. A 5-0 Prolene suture is threaded through the eyehole. The pigtail probe is then gently rotated in a retrograde fashion, pulling the Prolene suture through the canalicular system (see Fig. 26–2). Sterile ophthalmic antibiotic ointment is applied to one end of the Prolene suture as lubricant and a 23-mm piece of silicone tubing (0.6-mm outside diameter) is threaded onto the Prolene suture. For an adult, a tubing longer than 25-mm will make the ring too large. To prevent inadvertent removal of the suture, the two ends of the Prolene suture are secured with a hemostat (see Fig. 26–3).

A gentle continuous pull of the Prolene suture exiting one punctum, while advancing the stent through the opposite punctum, leads to rotation of the silicone stent into the canalicular system (see Fig. 26–4). After intubation of the system, approximately 2.0 mm of stent should protrude from each punctum. Excess may be removed by cutting partially through the tubing (without cutting the suture within), then grasping the surplus with toothed forceps and avulsing it from the remainder of the stent. The hemostat is then momentarily released and the excess tubing removed. Care should be taken not to inadvertently pull the suture out.

The Prolene suture is then tied with four single throws, thus uniting the ends of the stent to form a circular configuration (see Fig. 26–5). The suture is cut close to the knot. The knot retracts partially into the lumen of the tubing. The doughnut stent is then rotated 180° to position the anastomosis in the region of the common canaliculus. This rotation prevents erosion of the punctum and irritation of the conjunctiva should the ends of the sutures become exposed.

The silicone stent is removed in 8 to 12 weeks. On removal, the stent is rotated to expose the knot and the ends of the tubing. The suture is then cut, allowing the suture and the tubing to be pulled out as a single unit.

Finally, the silicone stent intubation technique detailed earlier is also useful in repairing traumatic canalicular lacerations. The pigtail probe allows rapid identification and intubation of the transected proximal canaliculus. The silicone stent is intended to reduce constriction at the site of the canalicular anastomosis.

Canaliculitis

Patients presenting with persistent symptoms of chronic or recurrent unilateral conjunctivitis, mucoid discharge, epiphora, ocular surface irritation, and localized tenderness in the peripunctal region should prompt an evaluation for signs of canaliculitis. Clinical clues include medial eyelid thickening or erythema, "pouting" of the punctum, and expressible mucopurulent canalicular debris. Diagnosis is made on expressing yellowish cheesy concretions from the involved canaliculus with two cotton-tipped applicators (Fig. 24–9). Cytologic examination of the concretions usually will show Gram-positive branching filaments. The etiologic agents responsible for the vast majority of cases of canaliculitis are *Actinomyces israeli*, *Streptomyces*, and *Arachnia propionica*. Fungal organisms such as *Candida albicans*, *Aspergillus niger*, *Fusarium*, and *Nocardia* have been reported. Treatment consists of emptying the canaliculus either by simple curettage through a dilated punctum or by canaliculotomy. Marsupialization of the

canaliculus is performed by horizontally incising the canaliculus on the posterior surface, and using a fine chalazion curette to evacuate the concretion from the dilated canaliculus and its diverticuli. The lacrimal drainage system is then lavaged with penicillin G 100,000 U/ml solution or a 1% tincture of iodine. The initial postoperative treatment should include oral penicillin and topical polymyxin. The antibiotic regimen can be modified depending on the culture and sensitivity results.

Diseases of the Lacrimal Sac and Nasolacrimal Duct

Dacryocystitis

Dacryocystitis is an inflammation of the lacrimal sac that occurs primarily because of nasolacrimal duct obstruction that is either present at birth or acquired. The etiology of dacryocystitis is not clearly understood. However, it is believed that there may be an underlying anatomic abnormality present, predisposing to stasis of tear flow. Congenital impatency, midfacial fracture, dacryolith, lacrimal sac tumor, sinus infection, allergic rhinitis, and systemic disease all have been implicated in dacryocystitis. Stagnation of tears and mucus within the lacrimal sac results in local inflammation and subsequent infection. The most common organisms encountered are pneumococci, streptococci, staphylococci, and diphtheroids. Other organisms isolated included *Klebsiella pneumoniae*, *Hemophilus influenza*, *Pseudomonas aeruginosa*, and *Actinomyces*.

Infection of the lacrimal sac may manifest clinically as either acute or chronic dacryocystitis. In the acute condition, the patient presents with a painful swollen mass below the medial canthal tendon. Conjunctival injection, tearing, and mattering are typically seen. The cellulitis is usually confined anterior to the orbital sep-

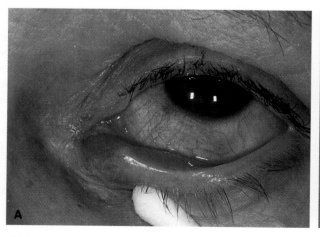
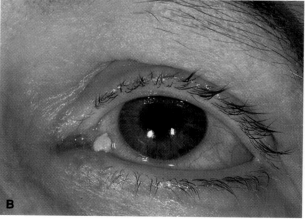

Figure 24–9.
A, Pouting of the inferior punctum as a characteristic feature of canaliculitis. **B,** Sulfur granule expressed from punctum.

tum and may extend across the entire lower lid and cheek. The lacrimal sac region is exquisitely painful to palpation, and pressure on the sac will often fail to result in regurgitation of mucopurulent material. Occasionally, the swollen sac may decompress externally to form a dacryocutaneous fistula.

Initial treatment should include systemic antibiotic and frequent hot compresses applied over the lacrimal sac region. Systemic therapy in the form of cephalexin 250 mg 4 times a day for 7 to 10 days is given. A dacryocystorhinostomy procedure is indicated, after resolution of the acute phase of infection.

Chronic dacryocystitis may present with little or no apparent discomfort, variable enlargement of the tear sac, and little or no mucoid secretion. In some instances, pressure over the lacrimal sac will produce almost no secretion reflux through the puncta. In other instances, the chronic dacryocystitis may take a suppurative form, presenting with a large nontender ectatic sac below the medial canthal tendon, which drains readily when the sac is decompressed by digital manipulation (Fig. 24–10). The secretion is purulent and thick in these cases. The patient may complain of chronic red eye, tearing, mattering along lid margin, and a thick discharge upon awakening. The definitive treatment is a DCR procedure to create a new drainage conduit for the lacrimal sac.

Dacryocystorhinostomy (DCR)

Dacryocystorhinostomy (DCR) is a drainage procedure designed to bypass the site of nasolacrimal duct obstruction by forming a fistula between the lacrimal sac and the nasal cavity. This procedure is performed in adults who have chronic epiphora or dacryocystitis secondary to complete or partial obstruction of the nasolacrimal duct, and in children who have recurrent dacryocystitis or have failed previous probings and sili-

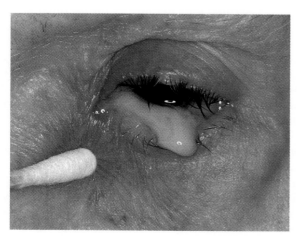

Figure 24–10.
Chronic dacryocystitis.

cone intubations. This procedure is indicated for these conditions when the upper and lower canaliculus are patent. A DCR procedure is contraindicated when malignancy of the lacrimal sac is suspected. Additionally, a DCR should not be performed on a patient with acute dacryocystitis. One should wait until the infection has been cleared with systemic antibiotics and for an opportunity to reassess the patient's symptoms and patency for the lacrimal drainage system by appropriate diagnostic tests.

Preoperative Evaluation. Before surgery, a thorough nasal speculum examination of the nostrils should be performed. The surgeon needs to rule out any nasal abnormalities, such as deviated nasal septum, polyps, or tumors, which could compromise the success of the procedure. It also is necessary to assure that there is adequate space adjacent to the planned internal ostium.

To avoid bleeding, the patient is advised to refrain from taking aspirin, aspirin-containing products such as Alka-Seltzer, and anti-inflammatory agents for at least 2 weeks before surgery. In patients with systemic hypertension, good blood pressure control before surgery is mandatory since cocaine and epinephrine are used during this procedure. Patients with discharge from the sac are instructed to massage the sac and to use topical antibiotics for several days before surgery.

Surgical Technique

Anesthesia and Skin Marking. A DCR procedure can be performed under either general or local anesthesia. However, local anesthesia combined with mild sedation is preferred because it has the advantages of superior hemostasis, fewer postoperative side effects, and wider patient acceptance. Even when using general anesthesia, nasal packing with cocaine-moistened cotton strips, coupled with external subcutaneous injection of a lidocaine solution that contains epinephrine, should be given to facilitate hemostasis. Improved visualization of anatomy from meticulous control of hemostasis is the key to the success of this procedure.

Upon arrival in the operating room, the patient's nasal cavity on the involved side is sprayed with 4% cocaine solution. The cocaine solution will vasoconstrict the vascular mucosa and provide mucosal anesthesia to minimize discomfort during subsequent packing. The maximum recommended dosage of cocaine is 3 mg/kg. Five minutes later, the anterosuperior nasal cavity adjacent to the lacrimal fossa is packed with a strip of cotton gauze moistened with 4% cocaine solution. Nasal packing should be performed with the aid of a fiberoptic headlight, nasal speculum, and bayonet forceps.

The bayonet forceps should be directed toward the medial canthus, placing the packing in the middle meatus, between the head of the middle turbinate and inferior turbinate. Proper placement of the packing within the nasal cavity is important since it serves not only to vasoconstrict and anesthetize the mucosa, but it also acts as a barrier to prevent inadvertent laceration of the nasal septum when the mucosa is incised during the procedure. It must also be emphasized that excessive upward packing force be avoided to prevent perforation of the cribriform plate. Another strip of cotton gauze is inserted into the posterior nasal cavity to catch any oozing that may run toward the oropharynx. This is especially useful while operating on an awake patient.

After the nostril has been packed with the cotton gauze, a marking pen is used to mark the proposed incision site. The proposed linear skin incision is located midway between the medial canthal angle and the dorsum of the nose (Fig. 24–11). A line is drawn 10 to 12 mm medial to the medial canthal angle, beginning at the level of the inferior edge of the medial canthal tendon, extending downward and laterally in a straight line toward the nasal alar fold for a distance of 1.5 cm. This incision is parallel to the angular vessels and lies within the thicker nasal skin. Do not curve the incision to involve the thinner eyelid skin because postoperative cicatricial contracture will result in a bowstring scar.

Local anesthesia is obtained by subcutaneous infiltration of lidocaine 2% with 1:100,000 dilution of epinephrine into the operative site and in the region of the infratrochlear nerve above the medial canthal tendon. Subcutaneous injections along the anterior lacrimal crest and into the lacrimal fossa are also given. A 30-gauge needle with a 5-ml syringe is used, and no more than 3 to 4 ml of anesthetic is needed. Anterior ethmoidal nerve block is frequently unnecessary. Subcutaneous injection along with nasal packing should be completed 10 to 15 minutes before surgery, so that adequate vasoconstriction and anesthesia will have been achieved before incision.

Skin incision over the preplaced marking is made with a 15 Bard-Parker blade. The incision should be no deeper than the subcutaneous fascia. If the area has been infiltrated 10 minutes before the operation with the lidocaine–epinephrine mixture, bleeding is minimal. With the skin edges tented up by forceps, the remaining strands of superficial fascia are cut with Stevens scissors. All bleeding points and subcutaneous vessels are cauterized with a wet-field bipolar cautery. Frequently, the angular vessels can be readily identified and retracted away with a rake retractor. If the angular vessels are severed inadvertently, it is best managed by ligating or cauterizing each end of the cut vessel. Curved Stevens scissors penetrate the orbicularis muscle fibers just nasal to the anterior lacrimal crest, and the blades are spread vertically to expose the periosteum of the frontal process of the maxilla. With the blunt rake retractors spreading the incision, the periosteum is incised 3 to 4 mm anterior and parallel to the crest with the sharp end of a Freer elevator. The periosteal incision extends from just below the medial canthal tendon to the inferior orbital rim.

As the periosteum is reflected toward the anterior lacrimal crests, bone bleeding from the sutura notha is frequently encountered. Sutura notha, a small vascular groove situated 1 to 2 mm from the anterior lacrimal crest, is often mistaken by surgeons for the edge of the crest, and they will incorrectly begin rounding for the lacrimal fossa. Bone bleeding from this indentation can be stopped with bone wax. Once the anterior lacrimal crest is reached, the surgeon should be cautious in rounding the edge. One should be gentle not to push the elevator against the sac too hard or without control. The tip can lacerate the sac, causing bleeding and making flap anastomosis difficult later in the procedure. The periosteum posterior to the crest is loosely adherent and the blunt end of the Freer elevator is used to reflect the lacrimal sac laterally. As the lacrimal sac and proximal nasolacrimal duct are reflected laterally to expose the full dimension of the lacrimal fossa, the suture line between the lacrimal bone and maxillary bone in the middle of the fossa can be identified. The periosteum anterior to its line of incision is also elevated for a few millimeters so that it will not be excised during bone removal.

Osteotomy. The tip of a small, curved hemostat is placed over the suture line and the thin bone is ruptured with a gentle push (Fig. 24–12). One has to be careful not to push the tip of the hemostat too deeply to perforate the mucosa, thereby causing bleeding to obscure the surgical site. The bony opening can be enlarged by spreading the hemostat blades. A 90° Hardy-Sella punch is then introduced through the bony

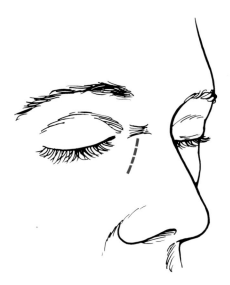

Figure 24–11.
Linear skin incision for a standard DCR.

opening to begin bone removal. The heel of the Hardy-Sella punch is used to push away the mucosa while engaging the bony edge. This is to ensure that the nasal mucosa will not be damaged with each bite of the instrument. The bone removed includes the anterior lacrimal crest down to the nasolacrimal duct, and the superior nasal wall of the nasolacrimal canal.

The nasal (medial) wall of the bony nasolacrimal canal is the most difficult, yet the most important piece of bone to remove. A flat-tipped, front-biting rongeur is used to break the thick anterior attachment of the canal from the maxilla. Removal of this osseous ridge facilitates communication of the nasal cavity with the membranous nasolacrimal duct and lacrimal sac. When removing bone from the superoposterior aspect of the nasal window, rotation or rocking of the rongeur while engaging the bone should be avoided. This is to prevent an inadvertent bony fracture extending into the adjacent cribriform plate, resulting in cerebrospinal fluid leakage. The area of bone removal will vary widely in adults, depending on the anatomy of the lacrimal drainage system and nose. In general, the osteotomy opening is about 15 × 15 mm, with the boundaries extending anteriorly to about 5 mm anterior to the anterior lacrimal crest, posteriorly to the posterior lacrimal crest, superiorly to the medial canthal tendon, and inferiorly to the inferior orbital rim. Once osteotomy has been completed, bleeding from bone can be stopped by

sealing the edges with bone wax. If mucosal bleeding is encountered, a small amount of lidocaine 2% with epinephrine (1:100,000) can be injected into the mucosa with a 30-gauge needle to provide hemostasis. A cotton pledget soaked in 4% cocaine can also be placed against the mucosal surface for hemostasis.

Incision into the Sac. Complete hemostasis should be obtained before opening the lacrimal sac. A 00 Bowman probe is inserted through the superior canaliculus into the lacrimal sac, tenting up the medial wall of the sac. A size 6600 Beaver blade is used to cut over the probe until the tip of the probe protrudes from the sac, thus verifying a full-thickness incision through both the periosteal and mucosal layers of the lacrimal sac (Fig. 24–13). One blade of a Westcott scissors is then inserted through the lacrimal sac opening, and the incision is enlarged in a superoinferior direction, extending from the top of the fundus to the nasolacrimal duct. Following sac opening, the interior of the sac is carefully examined for tumor or dacryolith. A probe also should be inserted into the sac and the tissue surrounding the internal ostium inspected. If there is evidence of common canalicular stenosis or scarring in preventing smooth passage of the probe, the internal ostium can be resected with a Westcott scissors. A silicone stent must then be inserted to prevent stricture or complete closure.

Incision of Nasal Mucosa. An H-shaped incision is designed, and the mucosa is incised with a size 6600 Beaver blade at the point where the Bowman probe protrudes from the lacrimal sac and hits the nasal mucosa. The horizontal incision should be made along a line di-

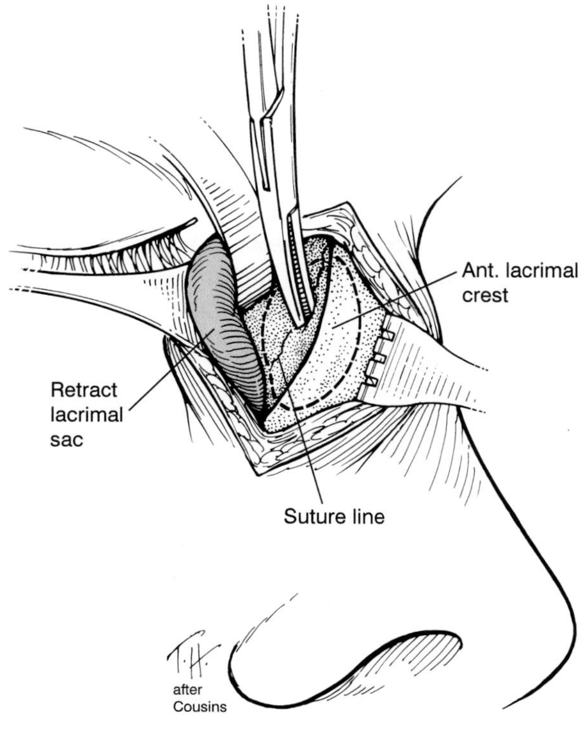

Figure 24–12.
Exposure of the anterior lacrimal crest and lacrimal sac fossa. Puncture through the thin bone with a curved hemostat.

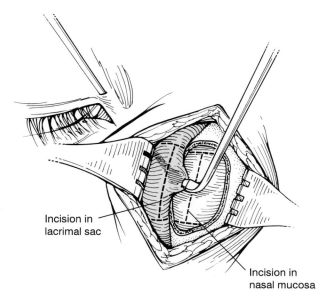

Figure 24–13.
Incising the medial wall of the lacrimal sac.

rectly opposite the lacrimal sac incision. Westcott scissors can extend the mucosal incision superiorly and inferiorly to provide anterior and posterior flaps with dimension similar to those of the lacrimal sac flaps. Through the mucosal incision, the preplaced nasal packing can be seen, thus verifying the proper positioning of the mucosal incision (Fig. 24–14). The nasal packing helps to insulate the nasal septum and middle turbinate from injury while the mucosa is being incised. Additionally, the packing in the nostril would prevent mucosal bleeding from running toward the oropharynx. Mucosal bleeding from the edges of the incision is then cauterized. Once hemostasis has been assured, the packing is removed from the nostril with a bayonet forceps. To avoid wound contamination, never pull the packing out through the osteotomy site; it should always be removed through the external naris.

Anastomosis of Posterior Flaps. The posterior flaps of the lacrimal sac and nasal mucosa are joined with two interrupted 4-0 Vicryl sutures on a semicircular needle. A short half-circle needle facilitates the passage of the suture in a tight, deep space (Fig. 24–15). Union of the posterior flaps should overlap the posterior osteotomy edge. Lumen of the lacrimal sac and middle meatus should be inspected. Extreme care should be taken to avoid cheese-wiring of the flaps while passing the needle or tying the sutures. Occasionally, tying these preplaced sutures in a confined space can be difficult.

One simple way of tying the sutures is the slipknot technique. The suture knots are tied external to the incision and slide into position without undue tension on the flaps. After passing the suture through the edges of the flaps, the suture is cut long. It does not matter which suture one starts with, as long as the proper sequence is followed while tying. The suture end A is looped over suture end B as the first step. Suture A is looped under suture B and then over suture A. This creates the first loop in the knot. As one continues with the slipknot forma-

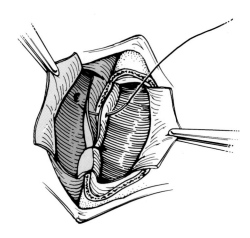

Figure 24–15.
Closure of the posterior flaps.

tion, a second loop identical with the first is created with the same sequence: A going over B, A under B, and then A over A. The final knot is tightened and should be firmly secured before sliding it down into the area of flap anastomosis. The sutures are then cut a few millimeters above the knot (Fig. 24–16).

Silicone Stent Placement. After uniting the posterior flaps, both upper and lower puncta are dilated with a punctal dilator. One end of a Crawford silicone tube is inserted into the upper canaliculus, through the newly created ostium, and into the middle meatus. The olive tip of the probe is guided out of the nasal cavity by a groove director. The probe is withdrawn from the external naris with the silicone tubing trailing. The procedure is then repeated through the lower canaliculus so that both ends of the tubing are delivered out of the nose (Fig. 24–17).

Anastomosis of Anterior Flaps. After placement of the silicone stent, the anterior lacrimal sac flap is united with the anterior nasal mucosal flap with two 4-0 Vicryl sutures (Fig. 24–18). The anterior flap should be tied with sufficient tension to prevent sagging of the flaps and to obstruct the internal ostium or scarring to the posterior flap anastomosis.

Skin Closure. Upon completion of the mucosal anastomosis and intubation with silicone stents, the cut edges of the periosteum are united with two 5-0 chromic sutures. The orbicularis muscle layer is also reapproximated with 5-0 chromic sutures. The skin incision is closed with 6-0 nylon sutures in a vertical mattress fashion.

Tying of Silicone Stent. The tubing is tied tightly with four square knots under moderate tension over a metal probe placed across the external naris, while the por-

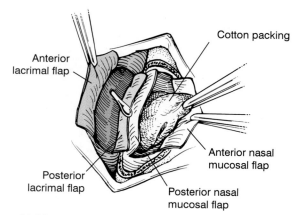

Anterior lacrimal flap

Cotton packing

Anterior nasal mucosal flap

Posterior lacrimal flap

Posterior nasal mucosal flap

Figure 24–14.
Exposure of the nasal packing after incising the nasal mucosa.

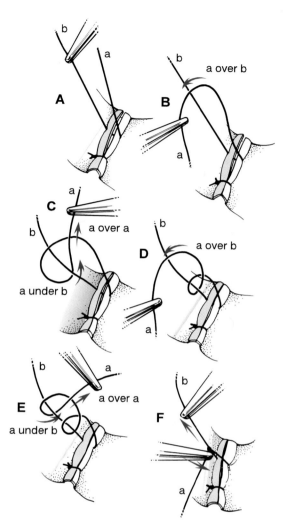

Figure 24–16.
Tying of the suture with a slipknot.

tion of the tube at the medial canthal angle is held with a muscle hook. The ends of the silicone tube are cut close to the knots. The metal probe is removed, and the knots retract into the nostril and hang loosely in the middle meatus.

Postoperative Management. Bacitracin ophthalmic ointment is placed on the incision site and instilled into the inferior fornix 3 times a day for 1 week. A 1-week course of oral cephalexin 250 mg 4 times a day.

The patient's postoperative activity is unrestricted, except for avoidance of nose blowing. A nasal decongestant spray is given twice daily for 1 week. Skin sutures are removed in 5 to 7 days, and the silicone stents are usually left in place for 3 to 6 months. The patient is instructed to wipe the eyelids in a unidirectional fashion toward the bridge of the nose, rather than outward toward the lateral canthus. This will minimize the chance of catching the loop at the medial canthal region and pulling the stent out.

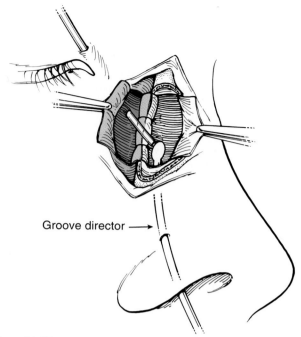

Figure 24–17.
Passing of the silicone stent over the posterior flaps. Retrieval of the stent with a groove director.

Conjunctivodacryocystorhinostomy (CDCR)

Conjunctivodacryocystorhinostomy (CDCR) is a lacrimal bypass procedure designed to circumvent stenosis or obstruction of the canalicular system by establishing a drainage conduit between the lacrimal lake and the nasal cavity. Common causes of canalicular obstruction include unsuccessful repair of a lacerated canaliculus, damage to the canaliculi from repeated probings, viral or chlamydia infections of the conjunctiva and lacrimal sac, chronic use of miotics or antiherpetic drugs, partial or total loss of the canalicular system secondary to tu-

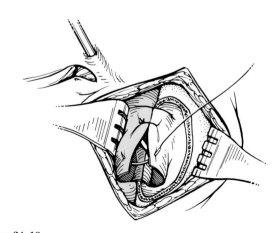

Figure 24–18.
Closure of the anterior flaps.

mor removal, congenital malformation of the lacrimal drainage system, inflammatory conditions such as sarcoidosis, iatrogenic thermal punctal closure, and idiopathy. Dacryocystorhinostomy (DCR) with Jones tube placement also may be indicated for failed DCR revisions in which the canaliculi are patent but nonfunctional.

Preoperative Evaluation. Preoperative examination of the nasal cavity is imperative to rule out a deviated septum, enlarged middle turbinate, or any nasal abnormalities. A severely deviated nasal septum toward the operative side will invariably compromise proper placement and function of the Jones tube; hence, correction of this problem before CDCR surgery may be advisable. Preoperative recognition of an enlarged middle turbinate will alert the surgeon of a possible intraoperative need for partial turbinectomy to improve visualization and positioning of the tube.

Patients should be advised that the glass tubes will remain with them for the rest of their lives, and that direct trauma to the medial canthal region can cause breakage.

Surgical Technique. A standard DCR is performed, as described in the preceding section, up to the step of uniting the posterior flaps of the nasal mucosa and lacrimal sac. After anastomosis of the posterior flaps, the position of the middle turbinate is inspected. If the anteroinferior tip is situated above the plane of the posterior flaps and will likely affect the orientation of the Jones tube, it is then resected with a front-biting Takahashi forceps or angled scissors. Brisk bleeding will be encountered, but can be minimized by injecting lidocaine with epinephrine 15 to 20 minutes before resection. The use of a sheet of Surgicel (or Gelfoam soaked in thrombin) over the cut surface and packing with cocaine-moistened cottonoid will greatly enhance hemostasis.

The caruncle is infiltrated with a small amount of 2% lidocaine with 1:100,000 dilution of epinephrine on a 30-gauge needle. The needle then penetrates the conjunctiva medial to the caruncle and is aimed toward the internal ostium in a 30° to 40° inferonasal direction. As the needle is advanced forward, anesthetic is infiltrated along this path. Instead of excising the caruncle, as is frequently recommended, a horizontal snip incision is made on the caruncle with a Westcott scissors. Preservation of the caruncle permits it to serve as a collar for a snug fit on the canthal flange and prevents nasal migration of the tube.

A von Graefe knife is inserted through the incision on the caruncle and pushed along the needle track toward the posterior flap junction. The direction of the stab incision should be such that the tube will rest in a dependent drainage position once placed. Advance-

ment of the knife blade through a dense fibrous tissue should be under firm digital control, as sudden "give" in tissue resistance may occur, thereby thrusting the knife forward. Once the tip of the knife is visualized within the internal ostium, the knife is moved up and down in small sawing movements to enlarge the track. Care should be taken not to inadvertently incise the lid margin with the sharp edges of the blade or to puncture the nasal septum with the knife tip. The von Graefe knife is withdrawn and a small-diameter Weiss gold dilator is introduced into the track to widen the aperture from the medial canthus to the nasal cavity. The use of a trephine to core out any tissue along the track to facilitate tube insertion is discouraged, since fibrous tissue is needed to envelop the tube and hold it into position. A Bowman probe is passed into the newly created tissue track, through the internal ostium until it makes contact with the nasal septum. A hemostat grasps the probe at the medial canthus, flush with the caruncle, and the length of the internal tract is estimated. The distance from the probe end to the hemostat is measured, and a Jones Pyrex tube, 3 to 4 mm shorter than the recorded length, is selected from the tube kit. A 4-mm diameter flange is preferred, since it lessens the chance of inward tube migration; however, if it crowds the medial canthal region, it should be exchanged for a smaller-diameter flange.

A Bowman probe is passed into the lumen of the selected Jones tube; the probe is then inserted into the tissue tunnel until the tip is visualized in the osteotomy site. While using the Bowman probe as a guide, the Jones tube is pushed into the tunnel with the finger tip. One should not use excessive force to advance the tube into the ostium. If resistance is encountered, a larger-size gold dilator should be used to progressively enlarge the aperture. Once the tube is embedded within the tract, the flange should be partially hidden within the lacrimal recess at the medial canthus. Internally, the shaft of the tube should be resting over the posterior flap anastomosis, and its distal end at least 2 to 3 mm away from the nasal septum. If the tube abuts the nasal septum, or its distal end does not extend into the nasal cavity by about 2 mm, the tube should be removed and an appropriately sized tube reintroduced. Once satisfied with its placement, the position of the tube is again verified through a nasal speculum inspection with the aid of a headlight. One must be certain that the end of the tube is not in contact with the septum and that it is not hidden from view by the middle turbinate.

The anterior flaps are anastomosed with two 4-0 Vicryl sutures. The periosteal edges are reapproximated with several 5-0 Chromic sutures. The orbicularis muscle and skin are closed in separate layers. A 6-0 nylon suture is tied around the collar of the Pyrex tube, with both arms going beneath the orbicularis, exiting the skin, and tied in the medial canthal area. This is an elective step that ensures tube position and prevents accidental displacement in the perioperative period. The skin sutures are removed in 7 days. The suture anchoring the tube may be removed in 3 weeks.

Postoperative Care. In addition to the routine postoperative care for a DCR procedure, Jones tubes require frequent cleaning and intermittent replacement. Four weeks after surgery, a nasal speculum examination is performed, without vasoconstricting the nasal mucosa. This assures a true topographic survey of the tube position relative to the nasal septum under normal conditions. The tube should be replaced if it is too long or too short. Similarly, the tube should be replaced if the flange is too large and is irritating the globe.

For the tube replacement or cleaning process, topical anesthetic drops are instilled onto the eye. The tube collar is grasped with a 0.3-mm forceps and pulled out of the CDCR ostium. Immediately, a dilator is inserted into the fistulous track as a temporary stent. The external surface of the tube is cleaned with soap and water. The inner lumen is cleaned by forcing a small wad of cotton through with a Bowman probe. After cleaning, the Jones tube is ready for reinsertion. The dilator is removed from the CDCR ostium. The clean Jones tube is slid onto the Bowman probe, and the probe is inserted into the ostium. The tube is returned to its well-healed fistulous track by gently pushing on the flange. After the tube exchange, the patient is instructed to irrigate the Pyrex tube with sterile normal saline on a regular basis. The solution is instilled into the medial canthal region and the patient quickly sniffs in the fluid, flushing out the lumen. Ideally, the tube is removed, cleaned, inspected, and possibly exchanged once a year.

Tumors of the Lacrimal Excretory System

Primary tumors of the lacrimal sac are relatively rare (11). The clinical triad of a painless irreducible mass extending above the medial canthal tendon, chronic dacryocystitis that irrigates freely, and bloody reflux either spontaneously or on irrigation should alert the clinician to the possibility of a primary lacrimal sac tumor. The presence of a mass within the sac contributes to mechanical obstruction of the nasolacrimal duct, and epiphora is frequently the earliest and most constant symptom. In the early stages, it may be possible to irrigate through the lacrimal sac containing a tumor before tumor growth occludes the drainage system. Later, there is swelling in the area of the sac, accompanied by a purulent discharge. Extension of the tumor outside the lacrimal sac and fossa may cause nasal pain and epistaxis.

Tumors of epithelial cell origin are the most common. Benign lacrimal sac masses include granuloma, polyp, papilloma, and hemangioma. Malignant lesions include squamous cell carcinoma, transitional cell carcinoma, anaplastic carcinoma, and adenocarcinoma. Malignant melanoma, malignant lymphoma, undifferentiated sarcoma, neurilemmoma, hemangiopericytoma, and fibrous histiocytoma also have been reported.

Confirmation is achieved by radiographic studies and dacryocystography. Because clinical features of intrinsic lacrimal sac tumors are alike, specific diagnosis depends on tissue studies following tumor removal. For malignant tumors, radical surgical excision followed by radiation therapy are the mainstay of therapy. Most often, dacryocystectomy is required, and growth beyond the lacrimal sac necessitates more extensive surgery.

■ REFERENCES

1. Jones LT: An anatomic approach to problems of the eyelids and lacrimal apparatus. Arch Ophthalmol 1961; 66: 137.
2. Jones LT: Epiphora. II. Its relation to the anatomic structures and surgery of the medial canthal region. Am J Ophthalmol 1957; 43; 203–212.
3. Jones LT: Anatomy of the tear system. Int Ophthalmol Clin 1973;13:3–22.
4. Doane MG: Blinking and the mechanics of the lacrimal drainage system. Ophthalmology 1981;88:844.
5. Karesh JW, Nirankari VS, Hameroff SB: Eyelid imbrication: an unrecognized cause of chronic ocular irritation. Ophthalmology 1993;100:883–889.
6. Glatt HJ: Epiphora caused by blepharoptosis. Am J Ophthalmol 1991;111:649–650.
7. Liu D: Conjunctivochalasis. Ophth Plast Reconstruct Surg 1986;2:25–28.
8. Katowitz JA, Welsh MG: Timing of initial probing and irrigation in congenital nasolacrimal duct obstruction. Ophthalmology 1987;94:698.
9. Peterson RA, Robb RM: The natural course of congenital obstruction of the nasolacrimal duct. J Pediatr Ophthalmol Strabismus 1978;15:246.
10. Tse DT, Anderson RL: A new modification of the standard lacrimal groove director for nasolacrimal intubation. Arch Ophthalmol 1983;101:1938.
11. Ryan SJ, Font RL: Primary epithelial neoplasms of the lacrimal sac. Am J Ophthalmol 1973;76:73–88.
12. Marmor MA, Beauchamp GR, Maddox SF: Photophobia, Epiphera, and Torticollis: A Masquerade Syndrome. J Ped Ophthal Strab 1990;27:202–204.

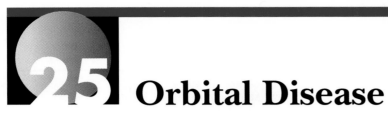

25 Orbital Disease

Thomas E. Johnson

Evaluation of the patient with an orbital space-occupying mass or inflammatory process requires a careful history and physical examination performed by a physician with a good knowledge of orbital anatomy and physiology. Orbital disorders can be life- or vision-threatening, so the rapid arrival at an accurate diagnosis is essential.

Ancillary studies, such as computed tomography (CT), magnetic resonance imaging (MRI), and ultrasound often are needed in the evaluation of orbital diseases, and their selective use adds invaluable information.

■ HISTORY

A careful history of the present illness is essential. The age of the patient is important, since children and adults tend to suffer from different orbital disease processes. For example, infantile hemangiomas are common in children, whereas lymphomas are seen almost exclusively in adults. A history of the onset and progression of symptoms should be elicited. Orbital disease processes may be acute, subacute, or chronic in their presentation and progression, and this information is very helpful in arriving at a differential diagnosis. For example, inflammatory lesions tend to occur acutely, whereas benign neoplasms such as benign

mixed tumors of the lacrimal gland usually present with a slow, indolent course. Also, the presence of symptoms such as pain, visual changes, and diplopia are helpful in differentiating different orbital processes. The past medical history may reveal a systemic disease associated with the orbital disorder, such as a primary malignancy that has metastasized, or a history of sinus disease that predisposed the patient to develop orbital cellulitis. A thorough review of symptoms may reveal other clues, such as fever and weight loss, that help to arrive at the diagnosis.

■ EXAMINATION

A thorough examination, including a complete ocular examination, should be performed. Best-corrected visual acuity is measured, and refractive changes should be noted. Orbital tumors that indent the posterior globe may produce a hyperopic shift in refraction. Intraocular pressure is recorded, as well as ocular motility. Pupillary examination for detection of an afferent de-

fect should be performed. A dilated fundus examination may reveal choroidal and retinal striae due to the mass effect of a neoplasm, and optic nerve changes, such as edema or pallor, may be observed.

An orbital examination includes observation of the periorbital tissues. Lid changes, such as edema, ecchymosis, and inflammation are noted. Tumors, which may

TABLE 25–1
Causes of Pseudoproptosis

1) Ipsilateral large eye (buphthalmos)
2) Contralateral small eye (microphthalmos)
3) Contralateral enophthalmos
4) Contralateral ptosis
5) Ipsilateral eyelid retraction
6) Facial asymmetry
7) Iatrogenic (oversized prosthesis)

TABLE 25–2
Causes of Unilateral Enophthalmos

1) Orbital fractures
2) Metastatic scirrhous carcinoma (breast)
3) Anophthalmic socket
4) Ipsilateral sinus disease

produce characteristic lid abnormalities include capillary hemangiomas, with frequently noted "strawberry" birthmarks, and metastatic neuroblastoma, which may cause lid ecchymosis in affected children. Inflammatory lesions often result in marked lid erythema and edema.

Next, ocular displacement is recorded. Many tumors produce a straight "axial" proptosis, where the eye is pushed directly outward. An example is the cavernous hemangioma in adults, which often is localized within the muscle cone of the orbit. Other lesions displace the globe depending upon their location within the orbit. Lacrimal gland tumors tend to push the globe downward and inward, whereas frontal-ethmoid sinus mucoceles push the globe downward and out. The amount of globe displacement from the midposition should be recorded as accurately as possible using a millimeter ruler. The amount of outward displacement, or proptosis, is measured, and the Hertel exophthalmometer is a widely used instrument for this purpose. When making serial measurements, it is important to always use the same base. Certain orbital processes, such as dysthyroid

orbitopathy and bilateral lymphoid tumors, may result in bilateral proptosis.

Pseudoproptosis refers to an apparent proptosis of one eye, which is not actually protruding abnormally (123). Conditions that simulate proptosis include eyelid retraction, contralateral enophthalmos, enlargement of one eye, and orbital asymmetry (Tables 25–1 and 25–2).

A neurologic examination should be performed to detect any sensory or motor deficits that may have resulted from the orbital disorder. Corneal sensation must be checked to rule out trigeminal nerve involvement.

A physical examination of the head and neck area is also performed. One should examine for preauricular and cervical lymphadenopathy, which may be present in either infectious or neoplastic disorders. Oral examination may be helpful, especially for patients with lymphangiomas of the orbit, who may also exhibit oral lesions. In addition, if orbital mucormycosis is suspected, palatal eschar may be evident and helpful in making this urgent diagnosis. If metastatic disease is suspected, a complete general physical is needed, usually in conjunction with an internist, to detect the primary malignancy.

■ ANCILLARY STUDIES

Ancillary studies are often always needed for a complete orbital evaluation. Ultrasound is a noninvasive, reliable technique that provides helpful information regarding the size, shape, location, internal reflectivity, vascularity, and mobility of different lesions. Also, the technique is sensitive in detecting mild extraocular muscle thickening, for example in Graves' disease. Additionally, this technique is used to detect optic nerve sheath distension due to either neoplasia or increased subarachnoid fluid, as in benign intracranial hypertension. Standardized echography consists of combined standardized A-scan, contact B-scan, and Doppler ultrasound (15). The standardized A-scan provides a one-dimensional view of the lesion, and reflectivity patterns are reported to closely correlate with histologic diagnosis when performed by a well-trained examiner. B-scan echoes represent a two-dimensional cross-section, and are used to

delineate a lesion's shape and proximity to normal anatomical structures. Doppler is used to investigate the vascularity of different lesions. Since ultrasound is a noninvasive procedure that does not use ionizing radiation, it can be used as often as necessary when following different orbital tumors and disease processes. Computed tomography (CT) scans are extremely useful in orbital evaluation and provide information on the size, extent, location of the tumor, as well as the condition of the globe and other orbital structures. The presence of bony excavation and erosion is well demonstrated with CT. In addition, contrast enhancement demonstrates the vascularity of certain lesions. A complete study should include both axial and coronal views. Computed tomography scanning provides an excellent display of orbital tumors and serves as a road map for the orbital surgeon. Magnetic resonance imaging (MRI) scanning also is very helpful and has the advantages of displaying soft tissue planes near the apex, as well as providing sagittal views. Also, radiation exposure is not encountered with this technique (18). However, bone changes are not as well demonstrated as with CT scanning. Additionally, intraocular ferrous foreign bodies may be dislodged with MRI, resulting in possible blindness (64, 127). Of course, consultation with a radiologist is of definite benefit in evaluating these imaging studies. It should be noted that echography, CT, and MRI are complementary techniques, and their combined use often provides valuable information that cannot be obtained by any single technique alone.

Other selective, less commonly used, ancillary studies in orbital evaluations include venography and arteri-

ography. Venography may be used in the evaluation of suspected vasculogenic lesions such as orbital varices, and arteriography may aid in the diagnosis of carotid cavernous fistulas and arteriovenous malformations. Digital subtraction angiography is performed using intravenous injection, and is therefore safer than conventional arteriography.

An exciting new technique for evaluating orbital disease processes is color Doppler imaging (CDI). It combines B-scan echography with color encoded vascular information and is most useful in evaluating vascular lesions, arteriovenous malformations, carotid-cavernous fistulas, and varices. It also is used to assess flow in normal vessels within the orbit. It is noninvasive and carries little risk for patients (26).

■ ORBITAL INFECTIONS
(Orbital and Preseptal Cellulitis)

Orbital infections may be vision- and life-threatening, and prompt evaluation and treatment of patients with these infections is essential. *Preseptal cellulitis (periorbital cellulitis)* is an infectious inflammation of the tissues anterior to the orbital septum, more often encountered in children with upper respiratory infections. Orbital cellulitis is an infectious inflammatory process involving the orbital tissues posterior to the orbital septum (61). Orbital cellulitis is a condition requiring urgent treatment. If untreated, vision- and life-threatening complications can develop, such as meningitis, brain abscess, cavernous sinus thrombosis, and death. Orbital cellulitis can occur at any age, but occurs most frequently in children and young adults. More than 50% of cases are secondary to a contiguous spread from an adjacent sinusitis, with the ethmoid sinus being the most common (96). Orbital cellulitis also can occur after trauma, orbital fracture repair, strabismus surgery (121), dacryocystorhinostomy, or glaucoma valve implant placement. Infections of the face, lacrimal sac, and lacrimal gland can extend into the orbit.

Patients with orbital cellulitis characteristically present with pain, proptosis, fever, decreased ocular motility, and decreased visual acuity. Patients with preseptal cellulitis exhibit external inflammatory signs, but have normal ocular motility, pupillary responses, and visual acuity.

The work-up of the suspected orbital cellulitis patient requires a careful history, complete ophthalmic evaluation, physical examination, and CT scanning of the orbital tissues. Blood cultures are often helpful, and bacteremia is more common in very young patients. Also, conjunctival and nasopharyngeal cultures may help identify the bacterial cause of the infection. A lumbar puncture should be obtained if there are meningeal

or other signs of central nervous system involvement. Other orbital inflammations, such as inflammatory pseudotumor, ruptured dermoid cyst, and orbital neoplasms, are included in the differential diagnosis.

The most common *bacterial pathogens* in preseptal cellulitis include *Haemophilus influenza, Staphylococcus aureus,* and *Streptococcus pneumonia.* Children younger than 4 years of age are especially susceptible to infection with *H. influenza* because of their lack of antibodies to the capsular antigen of *H. influenza.* The incidence of infection with this bacteria has decreased in recent years because vaccination against *H. influenza* is available. The same organisms encountered in preseptal cellulitis are commonly found in orbital cellulitis, and polymicrobial infection is the rule. Additionally, anaerobes and Gram-negative organisms are causative agents.

Infants with preseptal cellulitis are usually admitted for intravenous therapy, whereas older children and adults with preseptal infections can usually be treated with oral antibiotics on an outpatient basis, depending on the severity of disease. All patients with orbital cellulitis are admitted for intravenous antibiotics. Cefuroxime is an excellent choice for children, as it is effective against *H. influenza* that is ampicillin-resistant, as well as *S. aureus,* streptococci, and anaerobes (96). In adults, Cefuroxime alone, a combination of penicillin and a penicillinase-resistant penicillin such as nafcillin, or chloramphenicol with nafcillin can be used (72). For patients with penicillin allergy, a cephalosporin or vancomycin may be substituted. Antibiotic selection is tailored to the individual patient, taking into account the cause of the infection, the patient's drug sensitivities, and age. Usually a 7- to 10-day course of intravenous therapy is required, followed by a course of oral antibiotics for 10 to 14 days. Nasal decongestants are added

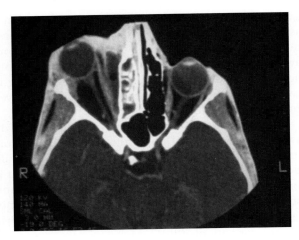

Figure 25–1.
Axial CT displays right ethmoid sinusitis, orbital cellulitis, and subperiosteal abscess.

is no visual loss, afferent pupillary defect, or worsening proptosis (16). Abscesses not responding promptly to antibiotics or causing worsening of vision need to be drained promptly. Concomitant sinus drainage should be considered but is not needed in every case.

Fungal infections also may cause orbital disease. Aspergillus is a fungus ubiquitous in the environment and is usually considered a harmless saprophyte. Paranasal sinus and orbital infections may occur in immunocompromised hosts, as well as in healthy, immunocompetent individuals, in which Aspergillus produces a chronic, fibrosing, granulomatous inflammation (32). Treatment includes surgical debridement of involved tissues, and use of Amphotericin B.

Mucormycosis is a fulminant opportunistic fungal infection caused by fungi of the class Zygomycetes. This devastating infection occurs in debilitated individuals, such as those in diabetic ketoacidosis or immunocompromised hosts (25, 31). Infection begins in the paranasal sinuses and secondarily spreads to the orbit. The large, nonseptate hyphae cause vascular occlusion, leading to infarction and necrosis of tissue (31). This disease is often fatal. Management includes prompt normalization of the underlying metabolic abnormality and debridement of all involved infected tissue (71). Orbital and sinus exenteration, coupled with both systemic and local treatment with Amphotericin B, is needed. In addition, hyperbaric oxygen therapy may be beneficial (87). Early intervention may be vision- as well as life-saving, and limited rhino-orbital mucormycosis occasionally may be managed without orbital exenteration (71).

for those patients with sinusitis-related orbital cellulitis. An otolaryngology consultation is imperative in managing orbital cellulitis related to sinus disease.

Complications of orbital cellulitis include subperiosteal abscess formation (36) (Fig. 25–1), orbital abscess (42), loss of vision, meningitis, cavernous sinus thrombosis, brain abscess (41), and even death. Subperiosteal abscess formation should be suspected if patients fail to improve or deteriorate on intravenous antibiotics. In most cases, prompt surgical drainage is needed to prevent visual complications. Small abscesses may be closely observed on antibiotic treatment if there

■ INFLAMMATORY ORBITAL DISEASE

Dysthyroid Orbitopathy (Graves' Disease)

Thyroid-related orbitopathy is the most common cause of unilateral and bilateral proptosis in adults (17). It is most often associated with hyperthyroidism, but may occur in the setting of hypothyroidism or euthyroid status. Children may be affected, but it most commonly affects adults, with women being affected about four times more often than men.

The cause of this inflammatory orbitopathy is unknown, but it is believed to be immune-related, with the extraocular muscles the inflammatory target. Clinically, patients present with unilateral or more commonly bilateral proptosis, usually of slow onset (Fig. 25–2). Initial complaints consist of mild ocular discomfort, usually due to exposure keratopathy. Signs include retraction of the upper and lower eyelids, lid lag on downgaze (von Graefe's sign), restriction of downward traction of the upper eyelid (Grove's sign), conjunctival chemosis, and motility disturbance. Vision may be affected by

corneal exposure changes or optic nerve compression from enlarged extraocular muscles. Compression of the optic nerve at the tight orbital apex is the most serious complication encountered in this condition.

Early in the course of the disease, the extraocular muscles and the retrobulbar fat are infiltrated with lymphocytes and plasma cells. Later, fibrotic changes usually occur, resulting in a restrictive myopathy and strabismus. All muscles are usually involved, with inferior and medial recti being most frequently affected. Motility disturbance with symptomatic diplopia is a common presentation. The acute inflammatory phase is usually self-limited and resolves within a few months to a year. In the chronic phases, the patient may have residual exophthalmos, strabismus due to restrictive myopathy, lid retraction, and exposure keratopathy.

Computed tomography usually displays fusiform enlargement of the extraocular muscles in which the muscle insertions are characteristically spared (Figs. 25–3 and 25–4). This feature is in contrast to inflammatory

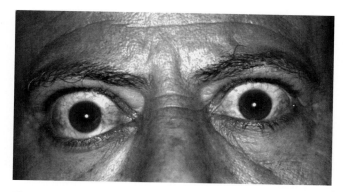

Figure 25–2.
Bilateral exophthalmos, lid retraction, and injection over rectus muscle insertions in man with dysthyroid orbitopathy.

pseudotumor, in which the inflammatory process characteristically involves the muscle as well as the muscle tendon (118). Proptosis is evident on CT, and occasionally there is an apparent increase in volume of the orbital fat. In more severe cases with compressive optic neuropathy, there is crowding of the optic nerve at the orbital apex by massively enlarged extraocular muscles. In their initial evaluation, patients with thyroid-related orbitopathy should have their thyroid status evaluated with appropriate serum thyroid function tests. Ultrasound examination is a valuable tool to confirm the echographic characteristics of enlarged extraocular muscles and to serially follow the muscles throughout the course of the disease (15). Other causes of enlarged extraocular muscles, such as metastatic carcinoma, pseudotumor, and carotid-cavernous fistula, should be considered in the differential diagnosis. In patients with concomitant ptosis, one also should consider the diagnosis of myasthenia gravis.

Management of dysthyroid orbitopathy varies, depending on the stage of the disease and the potential threat to the cornea and optic nerve. During the early stages, conservative treatment with ocular lubricants may be the only treatment needed. When inflammatory signs are severe or optic nerve compression is evident, systemic corticosteroids may be used. In addition, radiation therapy may be used for compressive optic neuropathy when corticosteroids fail or if a patient develops unacceptable side effects to steroids (8). Surgical orbital decompression, in which the floor, medial wall, and occasionally the lateral wall are removed, is an effective way to relieve optic nerve compression and severe exposure keratopathy (4). Strabismus is the most common complication associated with orbital decompression.

Eyelid retraction is another common manifestation of Graves' ophthalmopathy, generating both functional and cosmetic problems. The cause of lid retraction is poorly understood, but several factors may be contributory. These factors include: Mueller's muscle overaction from sympathetic stimulation, levator contraction, and overaction of the levator-superior rectus complex in response to a hypophoria induced by fibrosis and retraction of the inferior rectus. Upper lid muellerectomy along with recession of the levator aponeurosis is effective in minimizing retraction (120). For the lower lid, recession of the retractors, with or without an interpositional graft (hard palate or sclera) is also effective in rendering protection to the corneal surface (69).

Idiopathic Orbital Inflammatory Disease (Orbital Pseudotumor)

Idiopathic orbital inflammatory disease or "pseudotumor" is a nonspecific inflammation involving the orbital tissues. There is no recognizable cause (infection, rup-

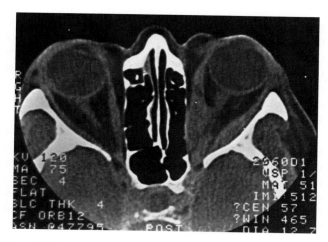

Figure 25–3.
Axial CT of patient with dysthyroid orbitopathy and enlarged extraocular muscles. Note the characteristic sparing of the muscle insertions.

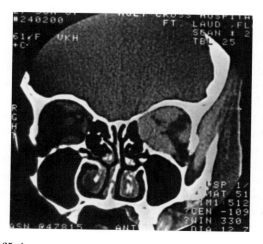

Figure 25–4.
Coronal CT of patient in Fig. 25–3 reveals marked enlargement of left medial, inferior, and superior rectus muscles, with relative sparing of the lateral rectus.

tured dermoid cyst, foreign body, hemorrhagic lymphangioma), or underlying systemic disease (Wegener's granulomatous, polyarteritis nodosa, sarcoidosis) (7). Lymphoid tumors, including benign and atypical lymphoid hyperplasia, as well as lymphoma, are also not included in the definition of pseudotumor. Lymphoid tumors differ enough clinically, radiographically, and histologically to be excluded from the group of idiopathic orbital inflammations.

Orbital pseudotumors may involve any site, tissue, or group of tissues within the orbit. They may be localized or diffuse, and can present acutely, subacutely, or chronically (94). Males and females are equally affected, and there is no racial predilection. Pseudotumors occur most frequently in middle-aged adults, but can affect young children as well as elderly patients (7). The disease tends to be unilateral, although it may occur bilaterally, especially in children. One study reported 45% of children had or subsequently developed bilateral orbital involvement (79). Pseudotumor also may be recurrent or alternate from one side to the other. Pseudotumor is probably the most frequent cause of proptosis in adults after thyroid-related orbitopathy. In biopsied orbital lesions, Henderson (40) reported an incidence of inflammatory pseudotumor of 4.2%, and Rootman (94) reported an incidence of 23/484 (4.7%). The incidence is probably much higher, because in most cases the diagnosis can be made clinically, and a biopsy is not performed.

The clinical presentation is dominated by inflammatory signs and may be variable. The acute form of the disease is the most striking, with an abrupt onset from days to weeks of any combination of periocular pain and discomfort, proptosis, chemosis, pain on eye movement, diplopia, ptosis, eyelid edema and erythema, decreased vision, and constitutional symptoms. Not all of these signs and symptoms are usually present in a given patient. Intraocular findings may include retinal and choroidal striae, optic nerve hyperemia and swelling, uveitis, and exudative retinal detachment (96).

Rootman and Nugent (94) classified acute orbital pseudotumors according to their orbital location, and described five patterns: anterior, diffuse, apical, myositic, and lacrimal. Patients with anterior pseudotumors usually present with manifestations of inflammation involving the globe and anterior orbit with pain, lid swelling, ptosis, diplopia, uveitis, papillitis, optic neuropathy, and exudative retinal detachment. On CT scanning, there is diffuse anterior orbital inflammation in close relation with the globe and associated scleral and choroidal thickening. On echography, sclerotenonitis with accentuation of Tenon's space may be noted. In diffuse orbital pseudotumor, the clinical manifestations are similar to anterior pseudotumor but are usually more severe, with increased papillitis, choroiditis, and optic neuropathy. Computed tomography reveals involvement of the entire orbit, with a soft tissue infiltrate from the apex to the posterior margin of the globe. Patients with posterior pseudotumors present with less proptosis, pain, and visible inflammation, but with a tendency toward the early development of optic neuropathy. Computed tomography reveals the inflammatory mass confined to the orbital apex, although often there is anterior extension along the course of the extraocular muscles or optic nerve. Patients with lacrimal gland pseudotumors present with pain, tenderness, and injection of the temporal upper eyelid and conjunctival fornix, and with a palpable lacrimal gland, and an S-shaped deformity of the upper lid. The globe is displaced downward and inward, and there is usually minimal proptosis. Pouting of the lacrimal ducts may be observed, and CT demonstrates inflammation confined to the superolateral orbit. Patients with myositic pseudotumors have one or more inflamed extraocular muscles and usually present with the sudden onset of retrobulbar pain, exacerbated by ocular movement. In addition, there is be reduced motility, diplopia, and injection over the insertion of the affected rectus muscles. Computed tomography reveals diffuse enlargement of the extraocular muscle, including the insertion. This is in contrast to dysthyroid orbitopathy, where the muscle insertion is characteristically spared from the inflammatory process, as visualized on CT scanning (118).

In cases of orbital pseudotumor, bone destruction is uncommon, although three patients were reported with surgically proven orbital pseudotumor with bone destruction and intracranial extension (30).

Orbital pseudotumors do not always have an acute, fulminant presentation. Chronic pseudotumors may occur as the sequelae of acute, recurrent orbital inflammations, but more commonly present without a history of acute inflammation. Chronic pseudotumors have signs and symptoms that develop gradually over months to years, and patients present with symptomatic proptosis, diplopia, or decreased vision, with few cutaneous or inflammatory signs. If the sclerosing pseudotumor is localized anteriorly in the orbit, it may be palpable as a rock-hard mass. This chronic, sclerosing variety is often complicated by permanent motility dysfunction and visual loss and may eventually result in a firm, fixed orbit with a blind, immobile eye.

Tolosa Hunt syndrome is considered a variant of pseudotumor that affects the superior orbital fissure and cavernous sinus. It has been described as painful external ophthalmoplegia, and patients usually present with a steady boring pain behind the eye, as well as motility dysfunction due to impairment of cranial nerves III, IV, and VI. In addition, there may be hypesthesia of the periorbital skin due to involvement of the trigeminal nerve and decreased vision when the optic nerve is involved. Proptosis may result from orbital venous congestion. Treatment with oral corticosteroids is usually effective (49).

Trochleitis is an unusual variant of pseudotumor, combined with superior oblique myositis (119). Tychsen and co-workers studied 13 patients presenting with aching pain and point tenderness over the trochlea. Ultrasound and CT were consistent with peritrochlear inflammation and myositis, and pathologic results revealed peritrochlear inflammation in two patients. Locally injected corticosteroids is an effective treatment.

Sinus involvement is usually absent in pseudotumor. However, Eshaghian and Anderson reported two cases of orbital pseudotumor that involved the paranasal sinus with bony irregularities. Both were initially believed to be malignant sinus neoplasms with orbital extension (24).

The histopathologic findings in pseudotumor are variable, depending on where the biopsy was taken and when in the course of the disease it was sampled. Classically, there is a nonspecific polymorphic infiltrate of inflammatory cells including lymphocytes, plasma cells, macrophages, eosinophils, and rarely neutrophils. Varying amounts of fibrous tissue are seen. In children, biopsies may exhibit a heavy eosinophilic infiltrate (80). As the disease progresses, more fibrous tissue is noted, and inflammatory cells become more widely separated by tracts of collagen. Jakobiec has noted frequent perivascular lymphocytic cuffing but not a true vasculitis with destruction of the muscularis (49). Necrosis of orbital fat may be observed with a resultant granulomatous response. In chronic, sclerosing pseudotumor there is a paucicellular inflammatory infiltrate, with dense fibrous connective tissue.

Orbital pseudotumors may also affect children. Blodi and Gass described 140 pseudotumor patients and found that 16% were in patients younger than 20 years (7). Mottow and Jakobiec found 6.6% of their 227 patients were younger than 20 years (79), and Rootman and Nugent reported that 30% of their acute pseudotumor patients were younger than 20 years (94). Shields et al. reviewed 250 consecutive cases of orbital biopsies in children and found 16.4% were inflammatory lesions (111).

Mottow and Jakobiec described 29 childhood pseudotumors and stated they differ from adult pseudotumors in three ways: (1) bilaterality is more common in children, and was seen in 45% of cases, (2) iritis is commonly seen in childhood pseudotumor, and is unusual in adults, and (3) trauma was related in 8 of 29 childhood cases. Children often present with constitutional symptoms such as headache, fever, vomiting, pharyngitis, anorexia, abdominal pain, and lethargy (79). Biopsies performed on 16 of 29 children revealed tissue eosinophilia in nine biopsies. Also, six of the patients had peripheral blood eosinophilia (80).

The differential diagnosis of orbital pseudotumor includes orbital cellulitis, ruptured dermoid cyst, lymphangioma, lymphoid tumor, and, in children, rhabdomyosarcoma, metastatic neuroblastoma, and Ewing's sarcoma. In the myositic subtype, the differential also includes thyroid-related orbitopathy. However, in dysthyroid orbitopathy, the onset is usually slower, and the disorder is usually bilateral, although often asymmetrical. Also included in the differential diagnosis of patients with enlarged extraocular muscles are metastatic carcinoma, direct carotid cavernous fistula, and spontaneous dural cavernous fistula (118). Systemic disorders with vasculitis may be confused with orbital pseudotumor. Wegener's granulomatous may involve the orbit. However, the inflammation in Wegener's is usually bilateral, with concomitant sinus disease, as well as renal and bronchopulmonary disease. Systemic lupus erythematosus also has been associated with acute orbital inflammation caused by a markedly enlarged extraocular muscle (33).

The etiology of idiopathic orbital inflammation is unknown. It is believed to be an orbital immune reaction, although no local autoantigens in the orbit have been identified. Possibilities include a blood-borne antigen or antibody localizing in the orbit, which has a rich vasculature. The agent may be a bacterial or viral product that is no longer replicative (49).

In many cases, treatment of orbital pseudotumor may be initiated without a preceding orbital biopsy. Some authors believe that performing a biopsy in an acutely inflamed orbit may exacerbate the inflammation, leading to a worse ultimate outcome. Mottow and Jakobiec reported that permanent functional impairments were seen more commonly in patients who underwent surgical exploration. In the patients who had orbital biopsy, they noted a greater degree of visual loss, a higher percentage of permanent exophthalmos, and a greater degree of residual proptosis. Also, motility disturbances were more profound in these patients (79). Other authors also have cautioned against orbital biopsies when the diagnosis is securely made using clinical, ultrasonographic, and CT findings. Rootman states that biopsies of extraocular muscles or within the confines of the orbital apex might prove detrimental but suggests biopsy of lacrimal gland inflammations, since biopsies in this area appear to be safe, and there is a relatively high incidence of neoplasia at this site (94).

The mainstay of treatment in acute orbital pseudotumors is oral corticosteroids. There is often a rapid and pathognomonic dramatic response within 48 to 72 hours of initial dosage (77).

High doses are usually needed, such as 80 to 100 mg of prednisone each day in adults. These high doses need to be maintained for 2 to 3 weeks to prevent a relapse. Then a slow, steady taper is carried out over an additional 3 weeks. Kennerdell recommends an initial dosage of 1.0 to 1.5 mg/kg/day of oral prednisone (66). Mottow and Jakobiec also noted a dramatic response in children treated with oral prednisone (79).

There is a less dramatic response in subacute and chronic cases.

Radiotherapy also is used in the treatment of pseudotumor. The indications for its use are: (1) steroids fail or systemic complications are unacceptable; (2) signs and symptoms recur during decreasing steroid dosage; (3) systemic corticosteroids are contraindicated. Low-dose supervoltage radiation in the range of 1000 to 2000 rad is given in divided doses over a 10- to 15-day course, using a lateral port and shielding the eye. Sergott and Glaser reported that 15 of 21 orbits responded favorably to radiotherapy without recurrence with a follow-up period of 25 months (101).

Immunosuppressive agents such as cyclophosphamide and chlorambucil have been used in recalcitrant cases, refractory to both corticosteroid therapy and radiotherapy.

Treatment of idiopathic sclerosing inflammation of the orbit is especially difficult. Rootman et al. recently reported 16 patients with sclerosing pseudotumor, and treatment resulted in complete resolution in only 2 of 16 patients. Blindness resulted in 3 of 16, and restricted movement in 10 of 16. They suggested earlier administration of aggressive therapy with immunosuppressive agents. Corticosteroid treatment combined with azathioprine, cyclosporine, or cyclophosphamide was suggested, combined with monitoring by experienced individuals in a multidisciplinary team (93).

Vasculitis

Multisystem diseases characterized by vasculitis can involve the orbit. These include Wegener's granulomatosis, polyarteritis nodosa, lupus erythematosus, hypersensitivity angiitis, giant cell arteritis, lethal midline granuloma, and others. Lupus is a multiorgan autoimmune disease that may rarely cause proptosis secondary to a severe myositis of the extraocular muscles (33). Polyarteritis nodosa is an idiopathic, nongranulomatous inflammatory disease that causes vasculitis of small- and medium-sized arteries. Wegener's granulomatosis is a multisystem disease that involves the upper and lower respiratory tract, as well as the kidneys. It is characterized by the classic triad of necrotizing granulomas and vasculitis of the upper and lower respiratory tract, focal necrotizing glomerulonephritis, and varied degrees of small-vessel vasculitis. A limited form, which does not include renal involvement, has been described (9). Ocular complications of this disease include conjunctivitis, episcleritis, scleritis, corneal ulceration, uveitis, retinal vasculitis, optic neuropathy, nasolacrimal duct obstruction, orbital cellulitis, and orbital masses. Orbital involvement may result in optic nerve compression with visual loss. The disease is rapidly fatal untreated. The treatment of choice is a combination of cyclophosphamide and corticosteroids. Orbital decompression also may be needed in the setting of compressive optic neuropathy (117).

Orbital Tumors

Children and adults tend to develop different types of orbital neoplasms. For example, infantile hemangiomas are common in children, and cavernous hemangiomas are seen almost exclusively in adults. There is some overlap, and some lesions, such as orbital meningiomas and dermoid cysts, affect both groups. In this chapter, we have attempted to classify different orbital neoplasms according to which age group they are most commonly encountered.

■ PEDIATRIC ORBITAL TUMORS

Most large series of orbital tumors in children report that about 90% of lesions are benign, and benign cystic lesions and vasculogenic lesions make up the majority of these tumors (12, 111, 133). In developing countries, there is a higher incidence of malignant orbital tumors, many of which result from secondary orbital invasion by neglected intraocular retinoblastomas (59, 81).

Dermoid Cysts

Dermoid cysts are benign cystic lesions that are choristomas, tumors composed of tissues not usually found at the involved site. They arise from tissue being pinched off at bony suture sites during embryogenesis, and are usually noted in early childhood. Dermoid cysts are characteristically painless, slow-growing tumors, and

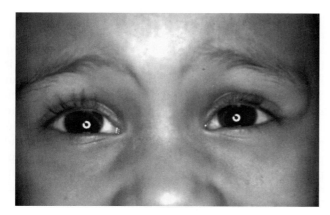

Figure 25–5.
Typical superior temporal superficial dermoid cyst OS in a young child.

may occur in the anterolateral orbit (the most common site) (Fig. 25–5), the superomedial orbit, or the deep orbit (Fig. 25–6). The lesions are well-encapsulated, and surgical excision is the treatment of choice. Trauma with leakage of the cystic contents may result in acute inflammation, producing a picture similar to orbital cellulitis. With complete excision, the prognosis is excellent. On histopathologic examination, the cysts are lined with stratified squamous epithelium, filled with keratin, and contain adnexal structures within the cyst wall (hair shafts, sweat glands, and meibomian glands). Epidermoid cysts are very similar but do not contain adnexal structures within the cyst walls. Dermoid cysts can also be diagnosed in adults, but are more likely to involve the deep orbital tissues and grow to a very large size (Fig. 25–7).

Dermolipomas are common congenital choristomatous growths, usually located in the temporal aspect of the conjunctiva near the lateral canthus. They contain fatty tissue and dermal appendages, appear pink-white to pink-yellow in color, and are not freely movable. Surgical excision may be difficult since they are infiltrative, and there is a significant risk of damage to

the lacrimal gland ductules or the extraocular muscles. A conservative approach to management is best in most cases.

Vascular Lesions

Infantile Hemangioma (Capillary Hemangioma)

The most common periocular vascular tumor of childhood is the infantile (capillary) hemangioma (35). This lesion is a hamartoma, composed of tissue normally found at the involved site. The lesions present at birth or during the first few months of life, progress rapidly during the first year, and usually spontaneously regress by the time the child reaches 4 to 7 years of age. Superficial tumors often have a characteristic reddish "strawberry" appearance and may swell in size when the child is crying (Fig. 25–8). Deeper lesions may appear bluish in color. The tumors may involve the eyelids, deep orbit, or a combination of these two locations (Figs. 25–9 and 25–10). If the lesion is deep, everting the eyelid is useful to identify the bright red vessels of the hemangioma. Other superficial hemangiomas may be noted in the head and neck region (Fig. 25–8). These benign tumors may induce amblyopia by occlusion of the visual axis, induction of astigmatism causing an anisometropia (90), and production of strabismus. Haik et al. described 101 patients with infantile hemangiomas and found an 80% complication rate in 50 patients, with a follow-up of more than 5 years; 60% of the complications were due to amblyopia (35). When the hemangiomas produce or threaten to cause amblyopia, treatment is needed. Treatments have included surgical excision, systemic corticosteroids, radiation, sclerosing agents, and other methods. The current treatment of choice consists of injection of intralesional steroid injections directly into

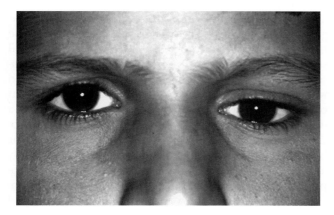

Figure 25–6.
13-year-old boy with downward displacement of the left eye due to deep orbital dermoid. (See Figure 25–7.)

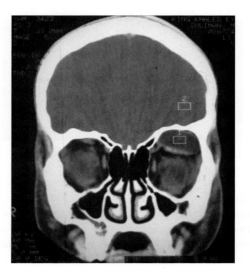

Figure 25–7.
Coronal CT scan displays superior deep left orbital dermoid cyst with expansion of the left orbit.

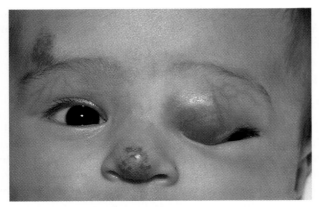

Figure 25–8.
Young child with large infantile hemangioma involving the left upper lid and orbit, occluding the visual axis and predisposing to amblyopia. Note other smaller facial hemangiomas.

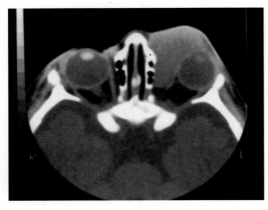

Figure 25–9.
Nonenhanced CT scan of child in Figure 25–8. Note the orbital extension of the lesion, and the marked contrast enhancement.

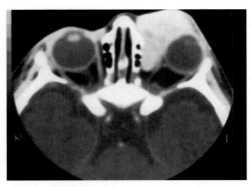

Figure 25–10.
Contrast enhanced CT scan of child in Figure 25–8.

the tumor (73, 74). The mechanism of action of corticosteroids is believed to be an increased vascular sensitivity to circulating catecholamines, rather than an anti-inflammatory action (74). This modality is considered safe and effective. Local complications have included depigmentation, subcutaneous fat atrophy, crystalline deposits, and eyelid necrosis. Systemic complications include adrenal suppression with growth retardation, usu-

ally after multiple injections (21). Visual loss due to retrograde embolization and central retinal artery occlusion has been reported (98, 113). This complication is believed to be volume- and pressure-dependent, and it has been recommended that one not inject more than 2.0 ml of volume, or exceed a dose of 40 mg of triamcinolone acetate combined with 6 mg of betamethasone (75). Deans and co-workers described a renewed interest in surgical excision of selected tumors (21). In the past, ophthalmologists have avoided the surgical approach due to risks of significant bleeding, unacceptable scarring, and inadequate results. Surgical excision is often difficult because of the infiltrative nature of the tumors and the risk of bleeding in these young patients. In carefully selected patients, a surgical approach involving dissection on the tumor's surface without entering its substance may prove successful. Patients with lesions extending into the dermis, or those with tumors that are bright red and do not allow movement of the overlying skin, are not good candidates for this surgical approach (21).

Lymphangiomas

Lymphangiomas are benign vascular tumors that usually appear in childhood, although at a later age than infantile hemangiomas (44). These lesions have been described as hemodynamically isolated vascular hamartomas, with no established connection to the arterial or venous circulation (92). The etiology of these lesions is obscure, since the orbit is not believed to have a lymphatic drainage system. The tumors may be superficial (involving the conjunctiva only), deep orbital, or combined, with both superficial and deep components. Not uncommonly, the first sign of the tumor is the rapid onset of proptosis due to an acute bleed within the tumor (chocolate cyst). The ensuing proptosis may be massive, and compression of the optic nerve may necessitate urgent surgical decompression. The lesions may increase in size during a viral upper respiratory infection.

Treatment of these tumors is quite difficult. They are not radiosensitive or corticosteroid responsive. Surgical excision of these lesions is also difficult, because they are infiltrative and may involve normal orbital structures. In addition, intraoperative and postoperative hemorrhage may occur, occasionally associated with permanent visual loss. Conservative management of acute proptosis secondary to hemorrhage within a diffusely infiltrating lymphangioma has been advocated. This management consists of activity limitation or bedrest, cold compresses, monitoring of visual acuity and pupillary light reaction, and maintenance of appetite (129). On histopathology, the lesions are nonencapsulated and contain endothelial-lined spaces and channels, some containing serous fluid and others containing blood (38). Blood breakdown products and lymphoid aggregates are also seen.

Neural Tumors

Neurofibromas can also involve the orbit. Localized neurofibromas may be occasionally encountered, but plexiform neurofibromas are much more common. Plexiform neurofibromas are peripheral nerve tumors composed of proliferating Schwann cells, endoneural fibroblasts, and axons. These infiltrative, vascular lesions are usually found in the lateral upper eyelid and orbit and are pathognomonic for neurofibromatosis type 1 (Fig. 25–11). The onset is usually in the first decade of life, and the lesions characteristically feel like a "bag of worms" on palpation (95). Plexiform neurofibromas may be associated with pulsatile exophthalmos, due to transmitted cranial pulsations caused by dysplasia of the orbital bones, and absence of the greater wing of sphenoid bone in Von Recklinghausen's disease (Fig. 25–12). Management of the tumors is quite difficult, due to the infiltrative and vascular nature of the lesions, and is mainly surgical. Recently, the carbon dioxide laser has been introduced in the management of these lesions (67). Proptosis in neurofibromatosis type 1 also

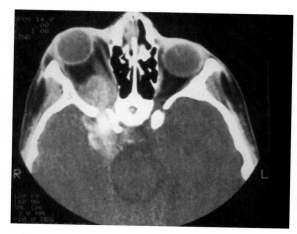

Figure 25–13.
Axial CT scan exhibits orbital invasion by intracranial meningioma. Note the hyperostosis of the apical orbital bones.

can be caused by diffuse uveal neurofibroma, producing an enlarged, thickened eye (Fig. 25–13).

Optic Nerve Tumors

Optic nerve gliomas, or juvenile pilocytic astrocytomas, are relatively rare primary neoplasms of glial cells of the optic nerve, which occur primarily in young children, usually apparent during the first decade of life. Children present with painless, progressive proptosis, associated with variable amounts of visual loss. The incidence of neurofibromatosis type 1 in patients with optic nerve gliomas has been reported between 10% and 70% in published series (22). Wright and co-workers found a high incidence of *neurofibromatosis* in those patients having a stable clinical course (11 of 16), but a lower incidence in patients demonstrating progressive enlargement of the tumor (4 of 15) (131). Most cases are unilateral, and bilateral tumors are believed to be pathognomonic of neurofibromatosis. Mucinous degeneration or bleeding into the tumor may result in abrupt worsening of proptosis and visual loss. Gliomas may occur anywhere in the course of the optic nerve and may extend to the chiasm and intracranially (22).

Treatment is controversial. Lesions confined to the optic nerve and not threatening the chiasm, especially when good vision is maintained, may be observed. Surgical resection of gliomas is reserved for blindness, severe pain, or disfiguring proptosis. When the tumor grows rapidly and when the chiasm is involved or threatened, a neurosurgical procedure may be required. Radiation therapy also has been used for nonresectable tumors and in some chiasmal and optic tract lesions (43).

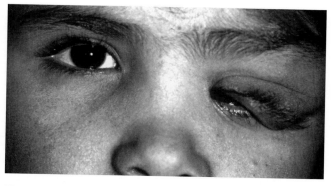

Figure 25–11.
Large, disfiguring plexiform neurofibroma involving left upper lid and orbit in a young girl with neurofibromatosis type 1.

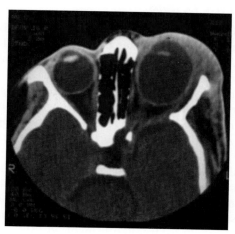

Figure 25–12.
Axial CT of patient in Fig. 25–11 reveals left lid and orbital plexiform neurofibroma, buphthalmic left eye due to diffuse uveal neurofibroma, and absence of the greater wing of sphenoid.

Meningiomas

Meningiomas are neural tumors that are uncommonly encountered in children. They most commonly arise from meningothelial cap cells found in the arachnoid layer of the meninges (128). These tumors may arise from the orbital portion of the optic nerve or secondarily invade the orbit from the intracranial cavity (Fig. 25–13). Sphenoid wing meningiomas cause hyperostosis of adjacent bone. A third, rare group of meningiomas arise within the orbital cavity but are not connected to the optic nerve and do not extend into the intracranial cavity. These tumors are referred to as ectopic (extradural) meningiomas (60).

Meningiomas are much more common in adults than in children, and women are affected more often than men (114). In children, meningiomas tend to behave aggressively and often are associated with neurofibromatosis type 1 (Fig. 25–13). Treatment of these tumors is difficult and may involve observation alone when the lesion is confined to the optic nerve and good visual acuity is maintained. Surgical resection or debulking may be needed if the eye is blind or if progression is noted. Adjunctive radiation therapy can be used (68).

■ FIBRO-OSSEOUS TUMORS

Fibrous Dysplasia

Tumors involving fibrous connective tissue, bone, and cartilage can involve the orbit. One of the more common lesions is fibrous dysplasia, which usually presents within the first two decades of life. These lesions are hamartomas, and are believed to be secondary to an idiopathic arrest of the maturation of bone at the woven stage. Lesions may involve one bone or contiguous bones (monostotic) or multiple bones (polyostotic) (78, 125). Children present with facial asymmetry, proptosis, and globe displacement. The frontal bone is most commonly affected, resulting in downward ocular displacement. Involvement of the sphenoid bone may result in optic nerve compression. Malignant transformation, although uncommon, has been reported. Computed tomography reveals characteristic translucent zones within the bone, as well as large sclerotic areas. There may be a ground glass appearance (Fig. 25–14). Management includes observation in lesions without optic nerve compression and surgery in more advanced cases, often involving a neurosurgical approach (125).

Aneurysmal Bone Cyst

Aneurysmal bone cysts are benign solitary lesions that can be observed in every part of the skeleton and un-

commonly involve the orbit bones in children and young adults. These lesions may represent a local reaction to injury, a primary vascular disturbance, or a secondary manifestation of a primary bone lesion (56). Clinically, patients with orbital involvement present with painless proptosis, ptosis, frontal headaches, diplopia, and gradual loss of vision. Computed tomography shows an intraosseous mass with bony erosion, often with a multicystic appearance.

Histologically, the lesions exhibit a multicystic appearance with nonendothelial-lines spaces that can be blood-filled or empty. In addition, they show solid areas composed of spindle cells, histiocytes, hemosiderin, and multinucleated giant cells. Osteoid formation is common. Surgical excision and curettage has been the treatment of choice with a favorable prognosis.

Giant-cell formation is a nonspecific response seen in many tumors that affect the orbit, including giant cell tumors (osteoclastomas), giant-cell (reparative) granulomas, brown tumors of hyperparathyroidism, and the "cholesterol granulomas" (85).

Histiocytic Lesions

The group of disorders characterized by an abnormal proliferation of histiocytes has been termed Histiocytosis X. The three related conditions are eosinophilic granuloma, Hand-Schüller-Christian disease, and Letterer-Siwe disease. The newer term for this group of disorders is Langerhans cell histiocytosis, since the proliferating cell has been found to be the Langerhans cell, a specialized histiocyte found in the epidermis (105).

Eosinophilic granuloma is the most common variant and results in a solitary osseous lesion in the orbit, most often in children. The lesions exhibit bony erosion and soft tissue expansion, and the frontal or zygomatic bones are the most frequently involved (5).

Hand-Schüller-Christian disease has the classic triad of diabetes insipidus, bilateral proptosis, and bony punched-out lesions in the cranial bones. This variety almost always affects infants and young children. Cuta-

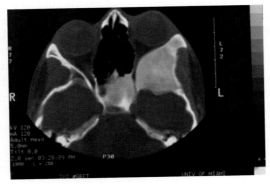

Figure 25–14.
Axial CT scan of young boy with monostotic fibrous dysplasia with characteristic "ground glass" appearance of bone.

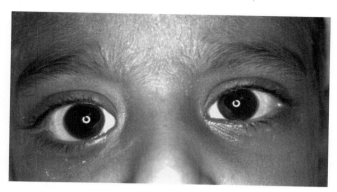

Figure 25–15.
4-year-old boy with Hand-Schüller-Christian disease and proptosis OD (57). From Johnson T et al: Clincopathological correlation. Saudi Bull Ophthalmol 1988;3:31.

neous involvement also may be apparent (57) (Figs. 25–15, 25–16, and 25–17).

Letterer-Siwe disease carries the worst prognosis, and patients can have widespread visceral involvement with hepatosplenomegaly, lymphadenopathy, jaundice, anemia, respiratory insufficiency, and osseous defects, as well as thrombocytopenia. Orbital involvement with this variety is uncommon. The mortality rate is high.

Computed tomography of orbital lesions usually demonstrates osteolytic lesions in the superior or superotemporal orbit. Histopathologic examination shows a combination of histiocytes, eosinophils, and multinucleated giant cells. The characteristic Langerhans cells can be demonstrated to contain Birbeck granules in the cytoplasm of the histiocytes on electron microscopy (105).

Management of localized orbital lesions includes local curettage, at times combined with low-dose radiation therapy. Children with systemic disease are treated with a combination of radiation therapy, chemotherapy, and corticosteroids, coordinated by a pediatric oncologist (97).

Metastatic Orbital Tumors of Children

Metastatic tumors may involve the orbital tissues in children, and neuroblastoma is the most common (2). Musarella and co-workers described 405 children with neuroblastoma from the Children's Hospital in Toronto, and found that 20% of patients had ophthalmic involvement (82). Neuroblastomas arise from primitive neuroblasts that may metastasize to one or both orbits from a primary lesion, usually within the abdomen (Fig. 25–18). Other primary sites include sympathetic and parasympathetic tissue within the mediastinal, cervical, and pelvic areas. The average age of onset is 2 years. Patients usually present with the rapid onset of painless proptosis, and often eyelid ecchymosis is noted secondary to the rapid growth of the tumor with resultant necrosis and hemorrhage (Fig. 25–19). Orbital lesions may produce lytic bony lesions and bone erosion, and metastases are bilateral in 40% of cases (82) (Fig. 25–20). Other ocular findings can include Horner's syndrome and opsoclonus-myoclonus (dancing eyes and dancing feet). Urine vanillylmandelic acid (VMA) may be elevated in (82) children with metastatic neuroblastoma. Histologic examination shows an undifferentiated small round cell neoplasm, and Wright rosettes are rarely found in the metastatic lesions. Electron microscopy may be needed to make the diagnosis and may show neurosecretory dense core vesicles, neu-

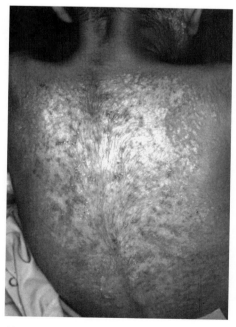

Figure 25–16.
Diffuse skin changes in patient in Fig. 25–15 are due to cutaneous involvement of Histiocytosis X. From Johnson T et al: Clincopathological correlation. Saudi Bull Ophthalmol 1988;3:31.

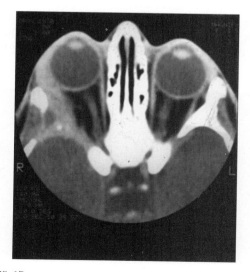

Figure 25–17.
Axial CT of patient in Fig. 25–15 demonstrates right lateral orbital lesion, with destruction of lateral orbital wall. From Johnson T et al: Clincopathological correlation. Saudi Bull Ophthalmol 1988;3:31.

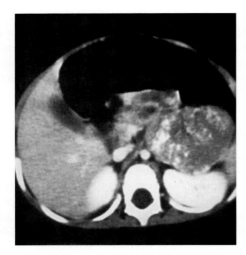

Figure 25–18.
Abdominal CT demonstrates primary abdominal neuroblastoma, originating in adrenal gland (arrows).

rotubules, and abortive axon formation (49). Treatment usually consists of a combination of chemotherapy and radiation therapy for bony metastases. The overall prognosis of the patient with orbital metastasis is poor, and one series reported a survival rate of only 11% at 3 years (82).

Other less common metastatic orbital tumors of childhood include Ewing's sarcoma of bone and Wilms' tumor.

Primary Malignant Orbital Tumors

Rhabdomyosarcoma

Rhabdomyosarcoma is the most common primary malignant neoplasm of the orbit in children (49, 95). These tumors arise from undifferentiated mesenchymal tissues that normally differentiate into striated muscle within the orbit. Patients usually present with a rapidly progressive, painless proptosis, and the usual age of onset is between 7 and 8 years (Fig. 25–21). This

diagnosis must be entertained in any child with acquired proptosis. Immediate biopsy is indicated if the diagnosis of rhabdomyosarcoma cannot be ruled out. Congenital lesions have been reported (23), as have cases during adulthood. Lesions are divided into embryonal, alveolar, and pleomorphic forms. Embryonal tumors are the most common within the orbit. Histopathology of the embryonal subtype reveals fascicles of spindle cells with small hyperchromatic nuclei, and a loose, myxoid stroma (49). Often, the cytoplasm will show cross striations suggestive of striated muscle differentiation. In the past, treatment consisted of orbital exenteration, with a poor survival rate. Now, treatment consists of a combination of radiation therapy combined with chemotherapy to treat any micrometastases (1, 126). This treatment is performed in coordination with a pediatric oncologist and radiation therapist. If the tumor is found to be confined to the orbit at presentation, the survival rate has been found to be greater than 90% at 3 years using this combination of radiation and chemotherapy (126). Therefore, an urgent evaluation and orbital tumor biopsy is recommended for any patient suspected of having an orbital rhabdomyosarcoma. Treatment side effects include cataracts, corneal and retinal changes, enophthalmos, lacrimal duct stenosis, facial asymmetry, bony hypoplasia, and defects in dentition (126).

Leukemia and Lymphoid Tumors

Children with leukemia can develop orbital masses as a result of their disease. Granulocytic sarcoma, or

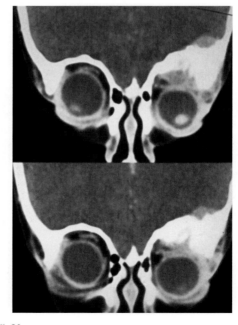

Figure 25–20.
Coronal CT of patient in Fig. 25–19 exhibits destructive left orbital mass with intracranial extension.

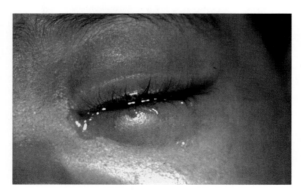

Figure 25–19.
Lid ecchymosis in 15-month boy with neuroblastoma metastatic to left orbit.

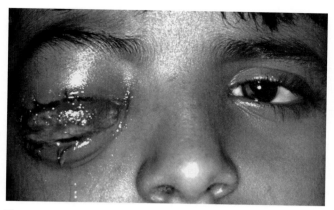

Figure 25–21.
9-year-old boy presented with 45-day history of painless proptosis OD, due to an embryonal rhabdomyosarcoma.

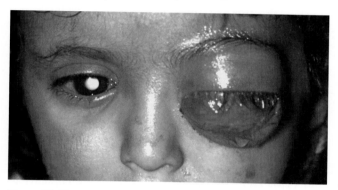

Figure 25–22.
Unfortunate young girl with bilateral *retinoblastoma* and secondary orbital extension on the left. Note leukocoria OD (59). From Johnson TE et al: Pediatric orbital tumors in Saudi Arabia orbit 1990; p. 211. From Orbit, The International Journal on Orbital Disorders, Oculoplastic and Lacrimal Surgery. Copyright by AEolus Press.

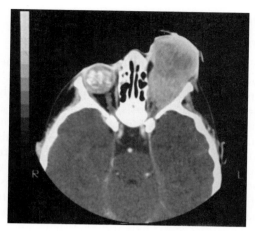

Figure 25–23.
Axial CT of patient in Fig. 25–22 demonstrates left orbital RB and intraocular calcifications OD (59). From Johnson TE et al: Pediatric orbital tumors in Saudi Arabia orbit 1990; p. 211. From Orbit, The International Journal on Orbital Disorders, Oculoplastic and Lacrimal Surgery. Copyright by AEolus Press.

chloroma, is a malignant orbital tumor that occurs in conjunction with acute myeloblastic leukemia (20, 135). The orbital mass may arise during the course of myeloblastic leukemia, or precede the blood and bone marrow findings. These lesions are often initially misdiagnosed. In a series of 33 patients from the Armed Forces Institute of Pathology, Zimmerman and Font reported that granulocytic sarcoma was most frequently misdiagnosed as lymphoma, a very unusual tumor in childhood (135). Histopathology shows a large cell or undifferentiated round cell neoplasm, and the Leder stain for esterase may be helpful in discerning the granulocytic origin of the cells (49). Treatment involves chemotherapy and possible localized radiotherapy, coordinated by a pediatric oncologist (49).

Retinoblastoma with Orbital Extension

Secondary orbital tumors are uncommon in children, and the most common lesion is orbital extension of retinoblastoma (RB). Shields et al. (111), in their series of 250 consecutive orbital biopsies in children, found 9 cases, all of which demonstrated only small areas of involvement discovered on microscopic examination after enucleation. However, series of childhood orbital tumors from developing countries have found a much larger percentage of orbital retinoblastomas, and two series reported orbital retinoblastomas as their most common tumor in the pediatric age group (59, 81). Secondary RB appears to be much more common in developing countries (Figs. 25–22 and 25–23). The most likely causes are genetic factors, consanguineous marriages, and delays in presentation (99). Once frank orbital disease occurs, the survival rate is very low, with a mortality rate approaching 90% (99).

■ ADULT ORBITAL TUMORS

Orbital Dermoid Cyst

Orbital dermoid cysts are benign cystic lesions usually seen in children, (see above) but they can also be found in older patients. Occasionally, superficial dermoids are observed, but deep orbital dermoids are more often encountered in adults. These tumors are usually located in the superior orbit, and may grow to a large size with relatively few symptoms. Expansion, thinning, and excavation of the orbital bones can occur, and the tumor may come in contact with the dura or even extend intracranially. Management is surgical, often requiring a lateral orbitotomy approach.

Vascular Orbital Tumors in Adults

Cavernous Hemangioma

Cavernous hemangioma has been described as the most common primary orbital tumor in adults (37). These benign vascular lesions generally produce slowly progressive, painless proptosis. They are usually found within the muscle cone, but can have an extraconal location. Larger tumors can induce a hyperopic shift and retinal striae, as well as increased intraocular pressure and optic nerve compression. Most patients have unilateral solitary lesions, although multiple lesions have been found to involve the same orbit (58). Unilaterality is usually the rule, although patients with bilateral simultaneous cavernous hemangiomas have been documented (29).

On echographic evaluation, there is found a firm, round to oval mass, usually within the muscle cone, which has a regular structure and medium to high reflectivity (83). Computed tomography and MRI reveal a round to oval, well-circumscribed mass with little contrast enhancement due to the tumor's relative lack of feeding and draining vessels (Fig. 25–24). On histopathologic examination, cavernous hemangiomas are well-encapsulated lesions containing large vascular spaces lined by endothelial cells and separated by thick fibrous septae. Small tumors may be observed, but larger lesions are treated by surgical excision, often using a lateral orbitotomy approach. With complete excision, the prognosis for vision is excellent.

Hemangiopericytoma

Hemangiopericytomas are uncommon vascular tumors that are more commonly encountered in the lower ex-

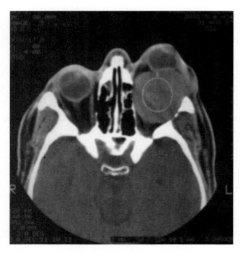

Figure 25–24.
Axial CT reveals a large left intraconal cavernous hemangioma causing proptosis and indentation of the globe, without bony erosion. This is the typical location of orbital cavernous hemangioma.

tremities and retroperitoneum, but also can involve the orbit. These tumors are composed of an abnormal proliferation of pericytes (91, 108). They usually occur in middle-aged adults, with a mean age of 42 in the large series from the Armed Forces Institute of Pathology (19). Men appear to be affected more often than women, and the tumors also have been reported in children (63).

Patients present with progressive proptosis, a palpable mass, diplopia, decreased vision, and varying amounts of pain. Patients usually present with a more rapid onset and progression than patients with cavernous hemangioma (108), and there is a predilection for the superior orbit (91).

Computed tomography shows a round to oval, well-circumscribed tumor that enhances with contrast. At surgery, the tumor is pink to violaceous, well-circumscribed, with large feeding vessels. On microscopic examination, there is a prominent vascular pattern, with sinusoidal spaces forming branching channels, giving a "staghorn" appearance. In addition, there are solid areas of ovoid to spindle-shaped cells (49). Tumors are classified as benign, borderline, or malignant, depending on histopathologic features including nuclear atypia and number of mitotic figures. One study demonstrated over 50% of lesions were benign, 15% were borderline, and 33% were malignant on histopathologic examination (19). Hemangiopericytomas have the capacity to metastasize, and 15% of patients in the series from the Armed Forces Institute of Pathology died with widespread metastases 6 to 32 years after the diagnosis was made (19).

Management includes complete surgical excision with the pseudocapsule to prevent recurrences and metastases. Patients should have extended follow-up due to the unpredictable pattern of behavior, and because metastatic disease can occur after many years.

Orbital Varix

An orbital varix consists of a dilatation of a pre-existing venous channel, usually within the superior orbit. Patients experience fullness of the orbit and proptosis, which increases with the Valsalva maneuver, or with placing the head in a dependent position. Management is usually conservative. Observation alone is advisable if the varix is not causing significant problems. Patients with severe pain, diplopia, and poor cosmesis may benefit from careful surgical excision. Complete excision may be difficult due to involvement with normal orbital structures and the risk of significant bleeding (6).

Arteriovenous Shunts

The orbital vessels can be involved in arteriovenous shunting, with the most common shunts being post-

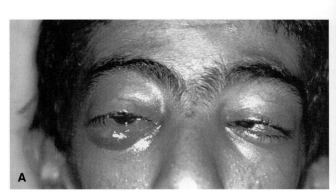
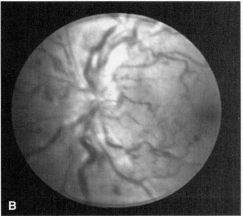

Figure 25–25.
A, Bilateral proptosis and chemosis due to bilateral traumatic carotid cavernous fistula. **B.** Fundus photo demonstrates disc edema and hyperemia, as well as congestion and tortuosity of retinal veins due to reversal of flow.

traumatic carotid-cavernous fistulas and low flow dural cavernous fistulas. Post-traumatic fistulas result when there is a tear in the intracavernous sinus portion of the internal carotid artery, with retrograde blood flow into the orbital veins (91). This results in proptosis, chemosis, a pulsatile bruit, arterialization of conjunctival veins, increased intraocular pressure due to decreased venous outflow, and lid swelling. Glaucoma can occur and may be refractory to medical management. Signs and symptoms are usually unilateral, but may be bilateral (Fig. 25–25). Computed tomography shows marked enlargement of the superior ophthalmic vein and symmetric enlargement of the extraocular muscles (Fig. 25–26). Color Doppler imaging is a new, noninvasive technique to diagnose and monitor these fistulas (26). Treatment is almost always needed in high-flow fistulas, and the

treatment of choice is embolization using detachable balloons or tissue adhesive (65).

Dural carotid cavernous fistulas are usually low-flow fistulas that occur spontaneously, usually in postmenopausal women, and can be associated with minor trauma, hypertension, or straining (34). The symptoms are milder than seen in high flow fistulas. Patients present with a red, chemotic eye, mild proptosis, and prominent conjunctival and episcleral vessels, which may have a "corkscrew" appearance (Fig. 25–27). There is often no bruit, but intraocular pressure can be increased. Acute angle-closure glaucoma has been described as the presenting sign of a spontaneous carotid cavernous fistula (14). The etiology is obscure, but it is believed that the fistulas begin with thrombosis of the cavernous sinus, followed by recanalization. Micro-

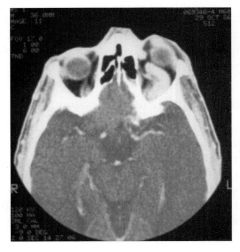

Figure 25–26.
Axial CT displays markedly dilated left superior ophthalmic vein secondary to traumatic carotid cavernous fistula.

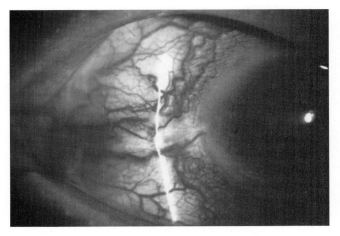

Figure 25–27.
Arterialization of conjunctival and episcleral veins in patient with carotid-cavernous fistula. Note that the dilated vessels extend to the corneal limbus, in contrast to dysthyroid orbitopathy, where they extend only to the rectus muscle insertions.

scopic meningeal branches of the internal and external carotid arteries become sufficiently enlarged to cause a significant shunt (91). Grove theorized that the dural shunts were congenital, and patients became symptomatic when thrombosis of the venous drainage posterior to the cavernous sinus occurred, shunting blood anteriorly into the orbital veins (34). Often these fistulas need no treatment. Many will spontaneously close or may close during diagnostic angiography (65).

Neural Tumors of Adults

Schwannoma (Neurilemoma)

The Schwannoma, or neurilemoma, is a peripheral nerve tumor composed of Schwann cells, which usually occurs in adults. Most tumors arise from peripheral nerves within the orbit, the most common being the supraorbital and supratrochlear nerves (107). Most are unilateral and solitary, and result in slowly progressive, painless proptosis. Diplopia can occur due to involvement of the orbital portion of cranial nerves III, IV, or VI, and apical involvement can result in optic neuritis. Most are benign, although malignant Schwannomas, as well as malignant transformation of benign lesions, can occur (102). Computed tomography and MRI scans reveal a well-circumscribed solid mass, oval in shape, with its long axis in the anteroposterior direction, due to its origin from a peripheral nerve. Histopathologic examination shows two cellular configurations, the Antoni A and Antoni B patterns. The Antoni A pattern shows solid cellular areas with spindle cells containing round to oval nuclei in a palisading pattern. The Antoni B pattern shows a looser, myxoid tissue with cells suspended in a mucinous background (49). The cytoplasmic S-100 protein stain is usually positive. Treatment is surgical, and most tumors are not radiosensitive. The prognosis for vision and life is generally good in benign lesions, but poor in malignant tumors (107).

Meningiomas

Orbital meningiomas were discussed under pediatric orbital tumors, but are found much more frequently in adults. Meningiomas involving the orbit can be primary, secondary, or rarely ectopic (extradural). Primary orbital meningiomas arise from the arachnoid layer of the intraorbital optic nerve. These slow-growing neoplasms are more common in middle-aged females (3), and usually present in the third to sixth decades of life (114). They usually produce a slowly progressive painless axial proptosis, associated with slowly progressive vision loss and transient visual obscurations (114). Visual field changes include enlargement of the blind spot, peripheral constriction, and central or cecocentral scotomas (128). Lesions located near or in the orbital apex pro-

duce an earlier, more profound visual loss than those located more anteriorly. High resolution CT scanning shows the following patterns: tubular thickening of the optic nerve, fusiform enlargement involving the middle and posterior segments of the nerve, anterior and posterior perioptic globular masses, and occasionally focal calcifications (114). A linear negative optic nerve shadow within the lesion (railroad tracking) indicates an intrasheath meningioma that has not yet erupted through the dura (47). Fundus examination shows optic disc edema and refractile bodies. Later, optociliary shunt vessels and optic atrophy are noted (114). The shunt vessels are believed to be collateral vessels that shunt venous blood away from the congested veins at the lamina cribrosa (128). The main histologic subtypes include meningotheliomatous (syncytial), transitional, psammomatous, fibroblastic, and angioblastic (106). Management is difficult because of the location of the tumors and their unpredictable biologic behavior. Patients with good vision and in whom the tumor is not threatening to spread intracranially may be managed with observation alone. Treatment is reserved for those tumors exhibiting aggressive growth, causing decreased visual acuity, or threatening intracranial spread. Treatment options include radiation or surgical excision, with subtotal or complete removal of the tumor, followed by radiation therapy (68).

Secondary orbital meningiomas are those that originate intracranially, usually within the arachnoid of the sphenoid bone, and invade the orbit. About one third of patients with intracranial meningiomas have ophthalmologic symptoms, such as visual loss, field defects, and diplopia (3). The amount of visual loss is related to the location of the original tumor. Lateral sphenoid lesions produce fewer symptoms than medial lesions near the sella, which tend to affect the optic nerve early (106). Plain radiographs often reveal hyperostosis in the region of the sphenoid bone, and CT scanning reveals a soft tissue mass and hyperostosis of the sphenoid and orbital bones. The management is mainly surgical, usually involving a neurosurgical approach, and the role of radiotherapy remains controversial.

Lacrimal Gland (Fossa) Lesions

Adult orbital tumors often originate in the lacrimal gland. Inflammatory and lymphoid tumors of the gland are seen about five times more often than epithelial tumors in clinical practice (49). Benign mixed tumors comprise about half of all epithelial lesions of the lacrimal gland (39). The nonepithelial tumors are comprised of lymphoid tumors and inflammatory pseudotumors. Bacterial or viral infections can cause an acute dacryoadenitis. Affected patients may have similar signs and symptoms to those with acute inflammatory pseudotumor of the lacrimal gland. Other specific inflammations, including sarcoidosis and Wegener's granulomatosis, can localize in the lacrimal gland. Sarcoidosis is a multisystem granulomatous disease of unknown cause that can cause bilateral lacrimal gland enlargement.

Benign Lacrimal Gland Tumors

Dacryops

A benign epithelial cyst of the palpebral lobe of the lacrimal gland is referred to as a dacryops. This is a ductal cyst of the palpebral lobe of the lacrimal gland. Small, asymptomatic lesions may be observed, while larger dacryops are usually excised, taking care not to damage the lacrimal ductules (11). Weatherhead described cysts arising from the ductal epithelium of the accessory lacrimal glands of Wolfring (Wolfring dacryops) near the superior tarsal border, most commonly in patients with a previous history of trachoma (124).

Herniated Orbital Fat

An abnormality that may be confused with a lacrimal gland neoplasm is herniated orbital fat, which can become visible in the superotemporal conjunctiva. The herniated fat has a similar appearance to a dermolipoma. This abnormality appears spontaneously in older patients, and is believed to be due to dehiscences in Tenon's capsule, allowing orbital fat to herniate forward. Herniated fat also can appear after trauma or surgery. Clinically, it appears as a yellow, soft, indentable mass, with a smooth, convex border, which moves forward and appears larger on retropulsion of the globe. Dermolipomas, in contrast, are usually pink-white to pink-yellow in color and are flat and diffuse. Additionally, they not mobile or indentable, and have smooth, straight, or slightly concave borders, and do not change in size with retropulsion. Surgical removal of herniated fat is only required if the tissue is cosmetically unacceptable and annoying to the patient (62).

Benign Mixed Tumor (Pleomorphic Adenoma)

Pleomorphic adenoma (benign mixed tumor) is the most common benign epithelial tumor of the lacrimal gland. These tumors usually occur in adults in their late 20s to early 60s (132). Patients present with a slowly progressive, painless proptosis, with displacement of the globe downward and inward (Fig. 25–28). A firm, lobular, nontender mass may be palpable in the anterior portion of the orbit. Symptoms are often reported for more than 1 year, whereas patients with malignant lacrimal gland neoplasms usually present with symptoms of less than 1 years' duration, with associated pain (132). Echographic evaluation reveals a regular to slightly irregularly structured round to oval mass within

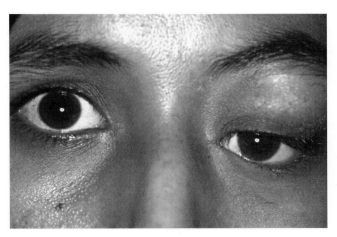

Figure 25–28.
26-year-old woman with painless proptosis and displacement of OS downward and inward of long duration.

the orbital lobe of the lacrimal gland, with medium to high reflectivity. Computed tomography shows a round to oval, well-circumscribed mass in the lacrimal fossa (Fig. 25–29). There may be bony expansion and excavation, but bony erosion is uncommon (53). Pleomorphic adenoma also has been reported to involve the palpebral lobe of the lacrimal gland (86). Management includes complete surgical excision of the tumor without rupturing its pseudocapsule. An incisional biopsy should not be performed if the tumor appears benign clinically and radiologically (115). There are often small tumor excrescences that extend through the pseudocapsule, so it is advisable to remove a small amount of normal tissue surrounding the neoplasm. Rupture of the capsule increases the risk of recurrence and the risk of malignant transformation. Recurrent tumors tend to be infiltrative and difficult to excise surgically. Rootman recommends a modified lateral orbitotomy and exci-

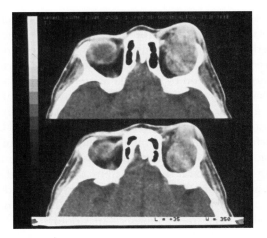

Figure 25–29.
Axial CT of patient in Fig. 25–28 reveals globular, well-circumscribed lacrimal gland mass with bony excavation. Complete surgical excision revealed a pleomorphic adenoma (benign mixed tumor).

sion using an extraperiosteal approach on the lateral portion, excision of a margin of orbital fat medially, and careful dissection of the palpebral lobe (95). With complete excision, the prognosis is excellent. Gross examination shows the lesions are gray-white, lobular, and contain a pseudocapsule. On microscopic examination, one sees two morphologic cell components: benign epithelial cells arranged in a double layer forming ducts and stellate spindle cells contained in a loose stroma. The stromal component contains epithelial cells that have undergone metaplasia and have pseudocartilage, osteoid, or myxoid characteristics (49).

Malignant Lacrimal Gland Tumors

Adenoid Cystic Carcinoma

Adenoid cystic carcinoma (cylindroma) is the most common malignant epithelial tumor of the lacrimal gland (76). The peak incidence is in the fourth decade of life, and there is no apparent sex predilection. Wright has noted a bimodal distribution, with a peak incidence in the second and fourth decades of life (130). Patients present with proptosis, with medial and downward displacement of the globe. Pain is a frequent symptom due to perineural invasion of the tumor. Symptoms typically have been present for less than 1 year when the patient is treated. Ultrasound evaluation reveals a hard mass usually within the orbital lobe of the lacrimal gland, which has a slightly irregular structure and medium to high reflectivity. Computed tomography shows a round to oval mass in the lacrimal fossa, and advanced lesions can show bone destruction (53). Histopathologic examination shows solid areas and cords of small, hyperchromatic cells with scant cytoplasm and large, atypical nuclei. Five histopathologic subtypes have been identified: Swiss cheese (cribriform), sclerosing, basaloid, comedocarcinoma, and tubular (ductal) (103). Lower tumor grades are associated with a predominantly Swiss cheese pattern, and patients with this subtype have been reported to have a longer survival (76). Management usually requires an initial incisional biopsy to confirm the diagnosis, followed by a complete metastatic work-up. If the diagnosis is confirmed on permanent histologic sections and the tumor is confined to the orbit, orbital exenteration, combined with removal of all involved bone, is performed (115). Rootman recommends an en bloc excision of the orbit using a multidisciplinary team consisting of an orbital surgeon, neurosurgeon, and craniofacial surgeon. Radiation therapy may be added postsurgically in large, advanced lesions (95). Even with radical surgery, the prognosis is very poor.

Other malignant epithelial tumors of the lacrimal gland include pleomorphic adenocarcinomas, mucoepidermoid carcinomas, adenocarcinomas, and other miscellaneous carcinomas.

Lymphoid Tumors of the Orbit

Lymphoproliferative tumors commonly involve the orbit and range from benign lymphoid hyperplasias to malignant lymphomas. The main difficulty with these neoplasms is in determining which will remain confined to the orbital tissues and which will have concurrent or eventually develop systemic lymphoma. Approximately 60% of orbital lymphomas present as localized lesions, and systemic dissemination subsequently develops in approximately 15% of patients with localized disease (97). Lymphoid tumors are composed mainly of lymphocytes, with varying populations of plasma cells, eosinophils, and fibrous tissue.

Clinically, orbital lymphoid tumors occur almost exclusively in adults and are very uncommon in children. If orbital lymphoma is diagnosed in a child, one should suspect a granulocytic sarcoma, as the orbital mass may precede blood or bone marrow findings in myelogenous leukemia, and the tumors may appear similar histologically (20). Patients usually present with the gradual onset of painless proptosis, combined with motility disturbances, displacement of the globe, and often lacrimal gland enlargement. Any of the orbital tissues may be involved, but there is a predilection for the lacrimal gland, and, in the majority of cases, there is a prominent extraconal component to the lesion. Often a firm, well-defined orbital mass is palpable beneath the skin in the anterior orbit. Most orbital lymphoid tumors are unilateral, but about 25% of patients demonstrate bilateral involvement (97). The anterior orbit and conjunctiva may be involved without deep orbital involvement, and the conjunctival component appears as a smooth, pink, "salmon patch." Benign and malignant lymphoid lesions cannot be distinguished by clinical, ultrasonographic, or radiographic examinations. A biopsy is always needed.

Lymphomas and orbital pseudotumors have similar echographic characteristics. They are regular to slightly irregular in structure, with low to medium reflectivity and low sound attenuation. Computed tomography usually shows a well-defined, homogeneous, oblong, oval orbital mass that molds to the eye and orbital bones without causing bony erosion or excavation, and appears isodense to the extraocular muscles (Figs. 25–30 and 25–31).

An incisional biopsy is needed to differentiate benign from malignant lesions. In most cases, an anterior transseptal biopsy can be performed. Fresh tissue should be sent for cell-marker studies and molecular genetic studies, if available.

Benign lymphoid hyperplasia tends to exhibit small mature-appearing lymphocytes, often with germinal centers, and sometimes plasma cells and histiocytes. These lesions are polyclonal, with an admixture of T and B lymphocytes. They have a 15% to 25% incidence

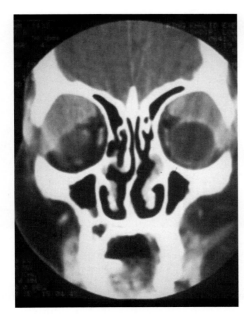

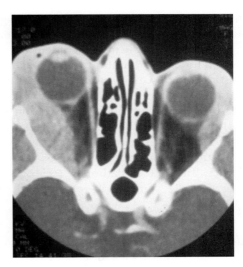

Figure 25–31.

Figure 25–30.
Here, and in figure 25–31, axial and coronal CTs exhibit bilateral orbital lymphoid lesions involving the lacrimal glands. Biopsy revealed malignant lymphoma. Note that the lesions mold to the globes and surrounding bone, and do not cause bony excavation or erosion.

of associated systemic disease at 5 years (49, 51). Malignant lesions tend to exhibit atypical, immature lymphocytes with nuclear pleomorphism, nuclear cleavage, and the absence of follicle formation, and are monoclonal B cell proliferations. Lesions diagnosed as malignant lymphoma have about a 60% chance of being associated with systemic disease (51). Atypical lymphoid hyperplasia, which is a "gray zone," displays cells of intermediate differentiation, with benign as well as malignant features. These tumors have a 40% chance of associated systemic disease at 5 years (49, 51). Immunohistochemical methods are used to study surface immunoglobulin on the B lymphocytes and determine if the lesion is polyclonal or monoclonal. Molecular genetic studies, examining gene rearrangements using DNA hybridization, are considered even more sensitive than immunohistochemical techniques. They are able to detect monoclonality in as few as 2% to 5% of cells, populations that may escape detection using immunohistochemical techniques (52). Further studies will show if these newer techniques are helpful in determining which patients with orbital lymphoid tumors will ultimately develop systemic lymphoma.

Management of these patients requires a multidisciplinary approach involving the ophthalmologist, oncologist, and radiation therapist. Patients found to have benign reactive lesions usually respond well to low-dose radiation therapy (97). All patients found to have an orbital lymphoma should undergo a complete metastatic work-up including a general physical examination,

chest x-ray, bone marrow aspiration/biopsy, serum protein electrophoresis, computed tomography scanning of the abdomen, pelvis, and chest, and other appropriate investigations for systemic disease (50). If systemic lymphoma is found, chemotherapy is usually initiated. Additionally, radiation therapy can be applied to the orbit, shielding the globe, for any residual tumor. If the tumor is found to be confined to the orbit without evidence of systemic lymphoma, radiation therapy alone is given (50). Close follow-up is essential, since systemic disease may develop even years after treatment of the primary orbital lymphoid tumor.

Mesenchymal Tumors (Fibrous histiocytoma)

Fibrous histiocytoma is the most common adult mesenchymal orbital neoplasm (49). This tumor can present in any age group, but most commonly occurs in middle adult life. It is usually unilateral, and the most frequent location is the upper nasal orbital quadrant. Lesions are classified as benign, locally aggressive, or malignant, with the majority being benign. Font and Hidayat described 150 cases from the Armed Forces Institute of Pathology, and found an age range of 4 to 85 years, with a median age of 43 years. Males and females were equally affected, and the superior orbit was involved in 41% of cases. In this series, 94 tumors were classified as benign, 39 locally aggressive, and 17 malignant (28). Besides the deep orbital tissues, these neoplasms may involve the eyelids, tarsus, and the epibulbar surface (46, 48, 54). Computed tomography shows the tumors usually are well-circumscribed, round or irregular masses, and are often difficult to differentiate from other neoplasms. Bony erosion is rare (104). The differential diagnosis includes such neoplasms as cavernous hemangioma, hemangiopericytoma, peripheral nerve sheath tumors, rhabdomyosarcoma, and metastatic carcinoma, among others. The management is surgical, as the lesions are not radiosensitive. Occasionally, exenteration of the orbital contents is required when there is widespread infiltration by a malignant fibrous histiocytoma. Gross pathologic examination shows the tumors are rubbery, firm, gray-white or yellow-tan lesions. Histopathologic examination shows a mixture of spindle-shaped fibroblast-like cells and ovoid histiocytic cells, often in a storiform pattern (49). There is a high recurrence rate after surgical excision. In the Armed Forces Institute of Pathology series, the recurrence rate was 42%, and the 10-year survival rate was 89% (28).

Secondary Orbital Tumors

Secondary orbital tumors are those that extend into the orbit from adjacent structures such as the eyelids, conjunctiva, globe, paranasal sinuses, nasal cavity, lacrimal sac, nasopharynx, and intracranial cavity. Secondary tumors invade the orbit by spread through perineural or perivascular spaces, bony foramina, or direct extension through bony erosion. These tumors occur most commonly in adults. The most frequent childhood secondary orbital tumor is retinoblastoma, and orbital involvement is now uncommon in developed countries but is seen frequently in developing countries. Secondary tumors make up a large percentage of lesions in series' of orbital tumors. The Wills Hospital series reported that 70 of 645 orbital biopsies (11%) were secondary tumors (110), and the Mayo Clinic series reported 107 of 764 (14%) of orbital tumors were secondary epithelial tumors (39).

Eyelid tumors that may secondarily invade the orbit include basal cell carcinoma, sebaceous gland carcinoma, squamous cell carcinoma, malignant melanoma, and sweat gland tumors. These neoplasms usually occur in adults, and orbital invasion results from neglected or incompletely excised tumors. Once orbital invasion has occurred, exenteration of the orbital contents, as well as removal of all involved bone is usually needed.

Of conjunctival tumors that may secondarily invade the orbit, **squamous cell carcinoma** is the most important (109). This malignant epithelial neoplasm usually arises from the bulbar conjunctiva near the limbus. It initially appears as a white or pink vascular lesion located either nasally or temporally within the palpebral aperture (Fig. 25–32). It may become elevated and exhibit leukoplakia (134). Orbital invasion can occur months to years after initial resection of the conjunctival lesion or due to neglected tumors (10, 45). Patients with orbital invasion present with diplopia, restricted motility, and globe displacement (Fig. 25–33). This disease is more common in underdeveloped tropical countries, where squamous cell carcinoma occurs in younger patients, and is more aggressive (116). **Mucoepider-**

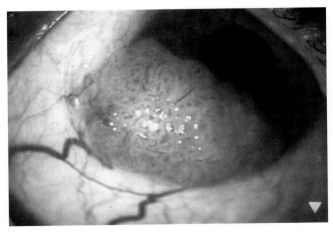

Figure 25–32.
Conjunctival squamous cell carcinoma originating at the corneoscleral limbus, with two large feeder vessels.

moid carcinoma is a variant of squamous cell carcinoma in which the tumor is composed of an admixture of mucus-producing cells and epidermoid elements and tends to behave more aggressively than conventional squamous cell carcinoma, with frequent orbital invasion (88). Again, once orbital invasion has occurred, orbital exenteration and removal of any involved bone usually is required.

The two most common intraocular tumors that may secondarily invade the orbit are uveal melanoma and retinoblastoma. **Malignant melanomas** of the uvea arise from melanocytes of the uveal tract and have the capacity to metastasize. It has been estimated that 10% to 15% of patients have extrascleral extension at the time of enucleation for uveal melanoma (70). The tumor cells reach the orbital tissues by invasion through scleral emissaria. Orbital extension of uveal melanoma usually necessitates a total or modified orbital exenteration, and the 5-year mortality rate is at least 80% (70). A study by Kersten et al. (70) indicated that orbital exenteration

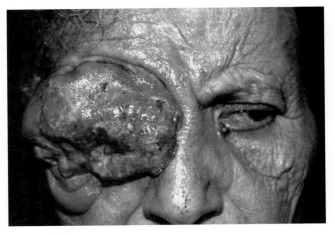

Figure 25–33.
Elderly Saudi Arabian woman with massive orbital squamous cell carcinoma which originated in the conjunctiva.

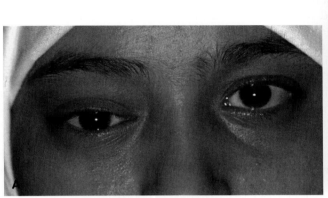

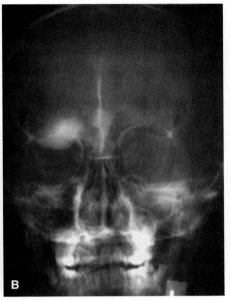

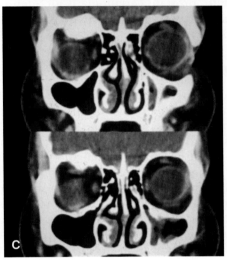

Figure 25–34 (A).
15-year-old girl with proptosis and downward displacement OD for one year duration. **Figure 25–34 (B).** Plain X-ray shows sinus osteoma extending from right frontal sinus into orbit. **Figure 25–34 (C).** Coronal CT scans reveal frontal sinus osteoma with secondary orbital extension.

of patients with secondary orbital melanoma may not improve long-term survival rates.

Tumors also may invade the orbit from the paranasal sinuses. Squamous cell carcinoma is the most common sinus carcinoma, and it may invade the orbit by direct erosion through bone, through osseous fissures, and through foramina. These tumors usually occur in adults and often are relatively asymptomatic in their early stages. In a study by Johnson and Krohel, 47 of 79 patients with sinus and nasal tumors had secondary orbital involvement, and the maxillary sinus was the most frequently involved (55). Treatment usually involves a combination of surgery, irradiation, and chemotherapy, and the prognosis is usually poor. Osteomas are benign tumors of bone, which can secondarily involve the orbit from extension from the paranasal sinuses. Frontal bone involvement most com-

monly produces symptoms, with proptosis and displacement of the globe (Fig. 25–34). Most occur in adults, and computed tomography readily identifies the well-defined, densely sclerotic, round to oval masses arising from the sinuses and projecting into the orbit. Three microscopic subtypes include ivory, mature, and fibrous. Treatment involves surgical excision. There is an association of sinus osteomas with Gardner's syndrome, in which patients develop multiple osteomas, soft tissue tumors, intestinal polyposis, and occasionally colonic carcinoma. Sinus mucoceles arising from the ethmoid and frontal sinuses can secondarily involve the orbit and produce orbital manifestations.

Tumors of nasal and pharyngeal origin may secondarily invade the orbit. **Nasopharyngeal carcinoma** is an important epithelial neoplasm that occurs in adults and may extend into the sinuses and orbit. Many are not resectable at the time of discovery, and treatment usually involves radiotherapy. Esthesioneuroblastoma is a malignant neurogenic neoplasm that arises from the olfactory sensory epithelium in the nasal fossa and may secondarily involve the orbit, usually in adults (89).

Meningioma is the most important intracranial neoplasm that may secondarily invade the orbit. Most begin in the region of the sphenoid bone (sphenoid wing meningioma). Medially located tumors enter the orbit through the superior and inferior orbital fissures and the optic canal. These tumors produce hyperostosis of the bones at the orbital apex and may result in a profound visual loss. Meningiomas are cytologically benign and do not metastasize. Therefore, radical surgery is usually not required. Removal or debulking of the tumor may be needed if visual structures are threatened, and this requires a neurosurgical procedure.

Lacrimal sac tumors, both benign and malignant, also can secondarily invade the orbit. The majority of malignant tumors are squamous cell carcinomas. Other lacrimal sac tumors that may secondarily invade the orbit include transitional cell carcinomas, adenocarcinomas, mucoepidermoid carcinomas, oncocytic adenomas, adenoid cystic carcinomas, angiosarcomas, lymphomas, malignant melanomas, fibrous histiocytomas, neurilemomas, and hemangiopericytomas (49). Presenting features may include epiphora, a mass in the sac region above the level of the medial canthal tendon, bloody tears, and pain. Management involves complete surgical excision of the tumor and involved bone, usually followed by radiation therapy. Orbital invasion may require exenteration.

Metastatic Orbital Tumors in Adults

Metastatic orbital tumors are uncommon and are less common than intraocular metastases by a ratio of up to 8:1 (112). Breast cancer is the most frequent primary source of orbital metastases, followed by lung cancer (39, 112). Other tumors more likely to metastasize to the orbit include prostate, gastrointestinal, renal cell, carcinoid tumors, and skin melanomas. Metastases usually occur in the setting of known malignancies but also may occur as the presenting symptom in 20% to 30% of patients (39).

Patients may present with sudden proptosis, pain, inflammatory signs, decreased motility, bony destruction, ptosis, visual loss, and paresthesias (39). One variant of breast carcinoma, **scirrhous carcinoma,** may result in enophthalmos due to cicatrization. This phenomenon has been observed less commonly with gastrointestinal, lung, and prostate carcinomas. An undiagnosed orbital tumor biopsy in a woman should be submitted for estrogen receptor assay (ERA) to aid in the diagnosis of breast cancer, as well as to help in the selection of treatment (95). The treatment of orbital metastases is usually palliative, using radiation therapy and/or chemotherapy. One study found the average time until death after diagnosis of orbital metastases was 13 months (112). Metastatic prostate carcinoma is an adenocarcinoma that may respond favorably to radiation therapy and to hormonal manipulation (95).

Exenteration

Orbital exenteration is the removal of all the orbital contents, including the globe, extraocular muscles, orbital soft tissues, periorbita, and part or all of the eyelids. This procedure is most commonly performed in the treatment of malignant orbital and eyelid tumors with orbital invasion, as well as other secondary malignancies invading the orbit from the nose, paranasal sinuses, and intracranial cavity (13). Certain neoplasms, such as rhabdomyosarcoma, at one time were managed with exenteration but are now more effectively treated with a combination of radiation and chemotherapy. Other less common indications for orbital exenteration include the treatment of nonmalignant conditions such as sclerosing pseudotumor with blindness and chronic pain, and mucormycosis.

■ REFERENCES

1. Abrahamson DH, Ellsworth RM, Tretter P, Wolff VA, Kitcher FD: The treatment of orbital rhabdomyosarcoma with irradiation and chemotherapy. Ophthalmology 1979;86:1330–1335.
2. Albert DM, Rubenstein RA, Scheie HG: Tumor metastases to the eye. Part II. Clinical study in infants and children. Am J Ophthalmol 1967;63:727–732.
3. Anderson D, Khalil M: Meningioma and the ophthalmologist. A review of 80 cases. Ophthalmology 1981;88:1004–1009.
4. Anderson RL, Linberg JW: Transorbital approach to decompression in Graves' disease. Arch Ophthalmol 1981;99:120–124.
5. Baghdassarian SA, Shammas HF: Eosinophilic granuloma of the orbit. Ann Ophthalmol 1977;9:1247–1251.
6. Beyer R, Levine MR, Sternberg I: Orbital varices: A surgical approach. Ophthalmic Plast Reconstr Surg 1985;1:205–210.
7. Blodi FC, Gass JDM: Inflammatory pseudotumor of the orbit. Br J Ophthalmol 1968;52:79–93.
8. Brennan MW, Leone CR, Janaki L: Radiation therapy for Graves Disease. Am J Ophthalmol 1983;96:195–199.

9. Bullen CL, Liesegang TJ, McDonald TJ, DeRemee RA: Ocular complications of Wegener's granulomatosis. Ophthalmology 1983;90:279–290.

10. Bullock JD, Augsburger J: Squamous cell carcinoma of the orbit. Ann Ophthalmol 1980;2:255–258.

11. Bullock JD, Fleishman JA, Rosset JS: Lacrimal ductal cysts. Ophthalmology 1986;93:1355–1360.

12. Bullock JD, Goldberg SH, Rakes SM: Orbital tumors in children. Ophthalmic Plast Reconstr Surg 1989;5:13–16.

13. Buus DB, Tse DT: Exenteration. In: Tse DT, Wright KW (eds). Oculoplastic Surgery. Philadelphia, JB Lippincott, 1992 p. 373.

14. Buus DR, Tse DT, Parrish RK: Spontaneous carotid cavernous fistula presenting with acute angle closure glaucoma. Arch Ophthalmol 1989;107:596–597.

15. Byrne SF, Glaser JS: Orbital tissue differentiation with standardized echography. Ophthalmology 1983;90:1071–1090.

16. Catalano RA, Smoot CN: Subperiosteal orbital masses in children with orbital cellulitis: Time for a reevaluation? J Pediatr Ophthalmol Strabismus 1990;27:141–142.

17. Char DH: Thyroid Eye Disease (2nd Edition) New York, Churchill Livingstone, 1990.

18. Char DH, Sobel D, Kelly Wm, Kjos BO, Norman D: Magnetic resonance scanning in orbital tumor diagnosis. Ophthalmology 1985;92:1305–1310.

19. Croxotto JO, Font RL: Hemangiopericytoma of the orbit. A clinicopathologic study of 30 cases. Hum Pathol 1982;13:210–218.

20. Davis JL, Parke DW, Font RL: Granulocytic sarcoma of the orbit. A clinicopathologic study. Ophthalmology 1985;92:1758–1762.

21. Deans RM, Harris GJ, Kivlin JD: Surgical dissection of capillary hemangioma. An alternative to intralesional corticosteroid. Arch Ophthalmol 1992;110:1743–1747.

22. Dutton JJ: Gliomas of the anterior visual pathway. Surv Ophthalmol 1994;38:427–452.

23. Ellenbogen E, Lasky MA: Rhabdomyosarcoma of the orbit in the newborn. Am J Ophthalmol 1975;80:1024–1027.

24. Eshaghian J, Anderson R: Sinus involvement in inflammatory orbital pseudotumor. Arch Ophthalmol 1981;99:627–630.

25. Ferry AP, Abedi S: Diagnosis and management of rhino-orbitocerebral mucormycosis (phycomycosis). A report of 16 personally observed cases. Ophthalmology 1983;90:1096–1104.

26. Flaharty PM, Lieb WE, Sergott RC, Bosley TM, Savino PJ: Color doppler imaging. A new noninvasive technique to diagnose and monitor carotid cavernous sinus fistulas. Arch Ophthalmol 1991;109:522–526.

27. Font RL, Gamel JW: Epithelial tumors of the lacrimal gland: An analysis of 265 cases. In: Jakobiec FA (ed). Ocular and Adnexal Tumors. Birmingham, AL, Aseculapius, 1978.

28. Font RL, Hidayat AA: Fibrous histiocytoma of the orbit. A clinicopathologic study of 150 cases. Hum Pathol 1982;13:199.

29. Fries PD, Char DH: Bilateral orbital cavernous hemangioma. Br J Ophthalmol 1988;72:871.

30. Frohman LP, Kupersmith MJ, Lang J, et al.: Intracranial extension and bone destruction in orbital pseudotumor. Arch Ophthalmol 1986;104:380–384.

31. Gass JDM: Ocular manifestations of acute mucormycosis. Arch Ophthalmol 1961;65:226–237.

32. Green WR, Font RL, Zimmerman LE: Aspergillosis of the orbit. Report of ten cases and review of the literature. Arch Ophthalmol 1969;82:302–313.

33. Grimson BS, Simons KB: Orbital inflammation, myositis, and systemic lupus erythematosus. Arch Ophthalmol 1983;101:736–738.

34. Grove AS: The dural shunt syndrome. Pathophysiology and clinical course. Ophthalmology 1984;91:31–44.

35. Haik BG, Jakobiec FA, Ellsworth RM, Jones IS: Capillary hemangioma of the lids and orbit: An analysis of the clinical features and therapeutic results in 101 cases. Ophthalmology 1979;86:760–789.

36. Harris GJ: Subperiosteal abscess of the orbit. Arch Ophthalmol 1983;101:751–757.

37. Harris GJ, Jakobiec FA: Cavernous hemangioma of the orbit. A clinicopathologic analysis of 66 cases. In: Jakobiec FA (ed). Ocular and Adnexal Tumors. Birmingham, Aesculapius, 1978.

38. Harris GJ, Sakol PJ, Bonavolonta G, Conciliis CD: An analysis of thirty cases of orbital lymphangioma. Pathophysiologic considerations and management recommendations. Ophthalmology 1990;97:1583–1592.

39. Henderson JW, Farrow GM: Orbital Tumors (2nd ed.). New York, Brian C. Decker (Thieme-Stratton), 1980.

40. Henderson JH: Orbital Tumors (3rd ed.), New York, Raven Press, 1994, p. 394.

41. Hodges E, Tabbara KF: Orbital cellulitis: review of 23 cases from Saudi Arabia. Br J Ophthalmol 1989;73:205–208.

42. Hornblass A, Herschorn BJ, Stern K, Grimes C: Orbital abscess. Surv Ophthalmol 1984;29:169–178.

43. Hoyt WF, Baghdassarian SA: Optic gliomas of childhood: natural history and rationale for conservative management. Br J Ophthalmol 1969;53:793–798.

44. Iliff WJ, Green WR: Orbital lymphangiomas. Ophthalmology 1979;86:914–929.

45. Illif WJ, Marback R, Green WR: Invasive squamous cell carcinoma of the conjunctiva. Arch Ophthalmol 1975;93:119–122.

46. Iwamoto T, Jakobiec FA, Darrell RW: Fibrous histiocytoma of the corneoscleral limbus. The ultrastructure of a distinctive inclusion. Ophthalmology 1981;88:1260–1268.

47. Jakobiec FA, Depot MJ, Kennerdell JS, Shults WT, Anderson RL, et al.: Combined clinical and computed tomographic diagnosis of orbital glioma and meningioma. Ophthalmology 1984;91:137–155.

48. Jakobiec FA, DeVoe AG: Fibrous histiocytoma of the tarsus. Am J Ophthalmol 1977;84:794.

49. Jakobiec FA, Font RL: Orbit. In: Spencer WH (ed). Ophthalmic Pathology. An Atlas and Textbook. Philadelphia, WB Saunders, 1986, pp. 2459–2860.

50. Jakobiec FA, Knowles DM: An overview of ocular adnexal lymphoid tumors. Tr Am Ophth Soc vol. LXXXVII: 420–444, 1989.

51. Jakobiec FA, McLean I, Font R: Clinicopathologic characteristics of orbital lymphoid hyperlasia. Ophthalmology 1979;86:948–966.

52. Jakobiec FA, Neri A, Knowles DM: Genotypic monoclonality in immunophenotypically polyclonal orbital lymphoid tumors. A model for tumor progression in the lymphoid system. The 1986 Wendell Hughes Lecture. Ophthalmology 1987;94:980–994.

53. Jakobiec FA, Yeo JH, Trokel SL, et al.: Combined clinical and computed tomographic diagnosis of primary lacrimal fossa lesions. Am J Ophthalmol 1982;94: 785–807.

54. John T, Yanoff M, Scheie HG: Eyelid fibrous histiocytoma. Ophthalmology 1981;88:1193–1195.

55. Johnson LN, Krohel GB, Yeon EB, Parnes SM: Sinus tumors invading the orbit. Ophthalmology 1984;91: 209–217.

56. Johnson TE, Bergin DJ, McCord CD: Aneurysmal bone cysts of the orbit. Ophthalmology 1988;95:86–89.

57. Johnson TE, Hidayat A: Clinicopathological Correlation. Saudi Bulletin Ophthalmol 1988;3:29–30.

58. Johnson TE, Nasr AM, Nalbandian RM, Cappelen-Smith J: Enchondromatosis and hemangioma (Maffucci's syndrome) with orbital involvement. Am J Ophthalmol 1990;110:153–159.

59. Johnson TE, Senft SH, Nasr AM, Bergqvist G, Cavender JC: Pediatric orbital tumors in Saudi Arabia. Orbit 1990;9:205–215.

60. Johnson TE, Weatherhead RG, Nasr AM, Siqueira EB: Ectopic (Extradural) meningioma of the orbit. A report of two cases in children. J Pediatr Ophthalmol Strabismus 1993;30:43–47.

61. Jones DB, Steinkuller PG: Microbial preseptal and orbital cellulitis. In: Duane TD (ed). Clinical Ophthalmology. Philadelphia, Harper & Row Publishers, Inc., 1990, Vol 4, Chapter 25.

62. Jordan DR, Tse DT: Herniated orbital fat. Can J Ophthalmol 1987;22:173–177.

63. Kapoor S, Kapoor MS, Aurora AL, et al.: Orbital hemangiopericytoma: A report of a three year old child. J Pediatr Ophthalmol Strabismus 1978;15:40–42.

64. Kelly WM, Paglen PG, Pearson JA, San Diego AG, Soloman MA: Ferromagnetism of intraocular foreign body causes unilateral blindness after MR study. AJNR 1986;7:243–245.

65. Keltner JL, Satterfield D, Dublin AB, Lee BCP: Dural and carotid cavernous sinus fistulas. Diagnosis, management, and complications. Ophthalmology 1987;94:1585–1600.

66. Kennerdell JS, Dresner SC: The non-specific orbital inflammatory syndromes. Surv Ophthalmol 1984;29: 93–103.

67. Kennerdell JS, Maroon JC: Use of the carbon dioxide laser in the management of plexiform neurofibromas. Ophthalmic Surg 1990;21:138–140.

68. Kennerdell JS, Maroon JC, Malton M, Warren FA: The management of optic nerve sheath meningiomas. Am J Ophthalmol 1988;106:450–457.

69. Kersten RC, Kulwin DR, Levartovsky S, Tiradellis H, Tse DT: Management of lower-lid retraction with hard palate mucosa grafting. Arch Ophthalmol 1990;108: 1339–1343.

70. Kersten RC, Tse DT, Anderson RL, et al.: The role of orbital exenteration in choroidal melanoma with extrascleral extension. Ophthalmology 1985;92:436–442.

71. Kohn R, Hepler R: Management of limited rhino-orbital mucormycosis without exenteration. Ophthalmology 1985;92:1440–1444.

72. Krohel GB: Orbital cellulitis and abscess. In: Fraunfelder FT, Hampton Roy F (eds). Current Ocular Therapy 2. Philadelphia, WB Saunders, 1985.

73. Kushner BJ: Intralesional corticosteroid injection for infantile adnexal hemangioma. Am J Ophthalmol 1982;93; 496–506.

74. Kushner BJ: The treatment of periorbital infantile hemangioma with intralesional corticosteroid. Plast Reconstr Surg 1985;76:517–524.

75. Kushner BJ, Lemke BN: Bilateral retinal embolization associated with intralesional corticosteroid injection for capillary hemangioma of infancy. Letter to the editor. J Pediatr Ophthalmol Strabismus 1993;30:397–398.

76. Lee DA, Campbell RJ, Waller RR, et al.: A clinicopathologic study of primary adenoid cystic carcinoma of the lacrimal gland. Ophthalmology 1985;92:128–134.

77. Leone CR, Lloyd WC: Treatment protocol for orbital inflammatory disease. Ophthalmology 1985;92:1325–1331.

78. Moore AT, Buncic JR, Munro JR: Fibrous dysplasia of the orbit in childhood. Ophthalmology 1985;92:12–20.

79. Mottow LS, Jakobiec FA: Idiopathic inflammatory orbital pseudotumor in childhood. I. Clinical Characteristics. Arch Ophthalmol 1978;96:1410–1417.

80. Mottow-Lippa, Jakobiec FA, Smith M: Idiopathic inflammatory orbital pseudotumor in childhood. II. Results of diagnostic tests and biopsies. Ophthalmology 1981;88: 565–574.

81. Munirulhaq M: Orbital tumors in children. Orbit 1989;8:215–222.

82. Musarella M, Chan HSL, DeBoer G, et al.: Ocular involvement in neuroblastoma: prognostic implications. Ophthalmology 1984;91:936–940.

83. Ossoinig KC: Echographic differentiaion of vascular tumors of the orbit. Doc Ophthalmol 1981;29:283.

84. Panzo GJ, Tomsak RL: A retrospective review of 26 cases of dysthyroid optic neuropathy. Am J Ophthalmol 1983;96:190–194.

85. Parke DW, Font RL, Boniuk M, McCrary JA: 'Cholesteatoma' of the orbit. Arch Ophthalmol 1982; 100:612–616.

86. Parks SL, Glover TA: Benign mixed tumors arising in the palpebral lobe of the lacrimal gland. Ophthalmology 1990;97:526–530.

87. Price JC, Stevens DL: Hyperbaric oxygen in the treatment of rhino-cerebral mucormycosis. Laryngoscope 1980;90:737–747.

88. Rao NA, Font RL: Mucoepidermoid carcinoma of the conjunctiva. Cancer 1976;38:1699–1709.

89. Rakes SM, Yeatts RP, Campbell RJ: Ophthalmic manifestations of esthesio-neuroblastoma. Ophthalmology 1985; 92:1749–1753.

90. Robb RM: Refractive errors associated with hemangiomas of the eyelids and orbit in infancy. Am J Ophthalmol 1977;83:52–58.

91. Rootman J, Graeb DA: Vascular lesions. In: Rootman J

(ed). Diseases of the Orbit. A Multidisciplinary Approach. Philadelphia, JB Lippincott, 1988; 525–68.

92. Rootman J, Hay E, Graeb D, Miller R: Orbital-adnexal lymphangiomas. A spectrum of hemodynamically isolated vascular hamartomas. Ophthalmology 1986;93: 1558–1570.

93. Rootman J, McCarthy M, White V, Harris G, Kennerdell J: Idiopathic sclerosing inflammation of the orbit. A distinct clinicopathologic entity. Ophthalmology 1994; 101:570–584.

94. Rootman J, Nugent R: The classification and management of acute orbital pseudotumors. Ophthalmology 1982;89:1040–1048.

95. Rootman J, Robertson WD: Tumors. In: Rootman J (ed). Diseases of the Orbit, Philadelphia, JB Lippincott, 1988, pp. 281–480.

96. Rootman J, Robertson W, LaPointe JS: Inflammatory diseases. In: Rootman J (ed). Diseases of the Orbit. A Multidiscipinary Approach. Philadelphia, JB Lippincott, 1988, 143–204.

97. Rootman J, Robertson W, LaPointe JS, White V: Lymphoproliferative and leukemic lesions. In: Rootman J (ed). Diseases of the Orbit. A Multidisciplinary Approach. Philadelphia, JB Lippincott, 1988; 205–240.

98. Ruttum MS, Abrams GW, Harris GJ, Ellis MK. Bilateral retinal embolization associated with intralesional corticosteroid injection for capillary hemangioma of infancy. J Pediatr Ophthalmol Strabismus 1993;30:4–7.

99. Senft SH, Johnson TE, Nasr AM: Extraocular retinoblastoma in Saudi Arabia. Orbit 1993;12:19–26.

100. Sergott RC, Glaser JS: Graves' ophthalmology. A clinical and immunologic review. Surv Ophthalmol 1981;26: 1–21.

101. Sergott RC, Glaser JS, Charyulu K: Radiotherapy for idiopathic inflammatory orbital pseudotumor. Indications and results. Arch Ophthalmol 1981;99:853–856.

102. Shatz H: Benign orbital neurilemoma: Sarcomatous transformation in von Recklinhausen's disease. Arch Ophthalmol 1971;86:268–273.

103. Shields JA: Epithelial tumors of the lacrimal gland. In: Shields JA. Diagnosis and Management of Orbital Tumors. Philadelphia, WB Saunders, 1989; 259–274.

104. Shields JA: Fibrous connective tissue tumors. In: Shields JA. Diagnosis and Management of Orbital Tumors. Philadelphia, WB Saunders, 1989; 192–204.

105. Shields J: Histiocytic tumors and pseudotumors. In Shields J: Diagnosis and Management of Orbital Tumors. Philadelphia, WB Saunders, 1989; 378–388.

106. Shields JA: Optic nerve and meningeal tumors. In: Shields JA. Diagnosis and Management of Orbital Tumors. Philadelphia, WB Saunders, 1989; 170–191.

107. Shields JA: Peripheral nerve tumors of the orbit. In: Shields JA. Diagnosis and Management of Orbital Tumors. Philadelphia, WB Saunders, 1989; 152–157.

108. Shields JA: Vasculogenic tumors and malformations. In: Shields JA. Diagnosis and Management of Orbital Tumors. Philadelphia, WB Saunders, 1989; 132–134.

109. Shields JA: Secondary orbital tumors. In: Shields JA. Diagnosis and Management of Orbital Tumors. Philadelphia, WB Saunders, 1989; 341–377.

110. Shields JA, Bakewell B, Augsburger JJ, et al.: Classifica-

tion and incidence of space-occupying lesions of the orbit. A survey of 645 biopsies. Arch Ophthalmol 1984;120: 1606–1611.

111. Shields JA, Bakewell B, Augsburger JJ, Donoso LA, Bernadino V: Space-occupying orbital masses in children. A review of 250 consecutive biopsies. Ophthalmology 1986;93:379–384.

112. Shields CL, Shields JA, Peggs M: Tumors metastatic to the orbit. Ophthalmic Plast Reconstr Surg 1988;4:73–80.

113. Shorr N, Seiff SR: Central retinal artery occlusion associated with periocular corticosteroid injection of juvenile hemangioma. Ophthalmic Surg 1986;17:229–231.

114. Sibony PA, Krauss HR, Kennerdell JS, Maroon JC, Slamovits TL: Optic nerve sheath meningiomas. Clinical manifestations. Ophthalmology 1984;91:1313–1324.

115. Stewart WB, Krohel GB, Wright JE: Lacrimal gland and fossa lessions: An approach to diagnosis and management. Ophthalmology 1979;86:886–895.

116. Tabbara KF, Kersten R, Daouk N, Blodi FC: Metastatic squamous cell carcinoma of the conjunctiva. Ophthalmology 1988;95:318–321.

117. Thawley SE: Wegener's granulomatosis: unusual indication for orbital decompression. Laryngoscope 1979;89: 145–154.

118. Trokel SL, Hilal SK: Recognition and differential diagnosis of enlarged extraocular muscles in computed tomography. Am J Ophthalmol 1979;87:503–512.

119. Tychsen L, Tse DT, Ossoinig K, Anderson R: Trochleitis with superior oblique myositis. Ophthalmology 1984;91: 1075–1079.

120. Tse DT: Management of thyroid-related eyelid retraction. In: Wright KW, Tse DT (eds). Oculoplastic Surgery. Philadelphia, JB Lippincott, 1992.

121. von Noorden GK: Orbital cellulitis following extraocular muscle surgery. Am J Ophthalmol 1972;74:627–629.

122. Watters EC, Wallar PH, Hiles DA, Michaels RH: Acute orbital cellulitis. Arch Ophthalmol 1976;94:785–788.

123. Weatherhead RG: Pseudo-proptosis. A clinical classification of causes. Orbit 1989;8:113–115.

124. Weatherhead RG: Wolfring dacyops. Ophthalmology 1992;99:1575–1581.

125. Weisman JS, Hepler RS, Vinters HV: Reversible visual loss caused by fibrous dysplasia. Am J Ophthalmol 1990;110:244–249.

126. Wharam M, Beltangady M, Hays D, Heyn R, et al.: Localized orbital rhabdomyosarcoma. An interim report of the Intergroup Rhabdomyosarcoma Study Committee. Ophthalmology 1987;94:251–254.

127. William S, Char DH, Dillon WP, Lincoff N, Moseley M: Ferrous intraocular foreign bodies and magnetic resonance imaging. Am J Ophthalmol 1988;105:398–401.

128. Wilson WB: Meningiomas of the anterior visual system. Surv Ophthalmol 1981;26:109–127.

129. Wilson ME, Parker PL, Chavis RM: Conservative management of childhood orbital lymphangioma. Ophthalmology 1989;96:484–490.

130. Wright JE: Factors affecting the survival of patients with lacrimal gland tumours. Can J Ophthalmol 1982;17:3–9.

131. Wright JE, McNab AA, McDonald WI: Optic nerve glioma and the management of optic nerve tumours in the young. Br J Ophthalmol 1989;73:967–974.

132. Wright JE, Stewart WB, Krohel GB: Clinical presentation and management of lacrimal gland tumours. Br J Ophthalmol 1979;63:600.

133. Youssefi B: Orbital tumors in children. J Pediatr Ophthalmol Strabismus 1969;6:177–181.

134. Zimmerman LE: Squamous cell carcinoma and related lesions of the bulbar conjunctiva. In: Boniuk M (ed). Ocular and Adnexal Tumors: New and Controversial Aspects. St. Louis, CV Mosby, 1964; 49–74.

135. Zimmerman LE, Font RL: Ophthalmologic manifestations of granulocytic sarcoma (myeloid sarcoma or choroma). Am J Ophthalmol 1975;80:975–990.

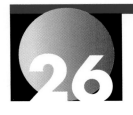

26 Periorbital and Orbital Injuries

Delyse R. Buus, David T. Tse

■ EYELID LACERATIONS

Eyelid lacerations are a common manifestation of periorbital trauma. Significant morbidity due to epiphora, ptosis, lagophthalmos, and lid malposition may result if not properly repaired. Motor vehicle accidents, altercations, and dog bites account for a large percentage of these eyelid injuries. An avulsing force on the eyelid is more likely to create a tear through the medial canthal tendon than through the stronger fibrous tarsal plate. The canalicular system lies superficially in the medial aspect of the eyelid and can easily be traumatized. Transection of the canaliculus should be suspected in any eyelid laceration occurring medial to the punctum.

The levator aponeurosis extends vertically from Whitnall's ligament to the anterior surface of the tarsal plate and lies deep to the orbital septum and the preaponeurotic fat pad. Injury to this important structure should always be suspected in any transverse upper lid laceration, especially if orbital fat is visible in the wound. Exploration of the levator aponeurosis through the wound should be undertaken in anyone with upper lid laceration and ptosis. Ptosis will result if a levator defect is not recognized or repaired. In amblyogenic age children with trauma to the upper eyelid, every effort should be made to assure the integrity of the levator aponeurosis, so as to avoid the development of ptosis.

Assessment

The assessment of a lid laceration must first include evaluation and treatment of systemic, neurologic, orbital, and ocular injuries. Associated systemic injuries may require consultation and treatment. If necessary, eyelid repair may be delayed for 24 to 48 hours until other more urgent nonocular injuries are treated.

Before applying eye drops or rendering any form of treatment, an accurate visual acuity must be recorded. Without a pretreatment documentation of acuity, an unrelated vision problem such as amblyopia may later be attributed to the treatment. In an unconscious patient, pupillary reaction must be carefully assessed. Pupillary response may be the only objective clue to the integrity of the visual pathway in this situation. This should be followed by a thorough eye examination to exclude any occult intraocular injuries. Intraocular injuries must take priority over lid lacerations. The fornices also should be inspected for retained foreign bodies and dislodged contact lenses. In massively swollen lids or severe lacerations, concomitant bony fractures may be present and appropriate radiographic studies should be considered. Before one attempts to repair eyelid and periocular lacerations, the patient's tetanus status must be inquired, and tetanus prophylaxis should be administered if appropriate. Finally, document all facial injuries with photographs whenever possible.

When lacerations involve the medial third of the lid, the integrity of the canalicular system must be established. If transected, an attempt at primary anastomosis should be made. Cut ends of the canaliculus can often be visualized by gently separating the wound edges. If this is not confirmatory, a Bowman probe should be passed to assess the integrity of the canaliculus. Another method of finding the proximal cut end of the involved canaliculus is to pass a pigtail probe through the other intact canaliculus.

Repair of Lid and Canalicular Laceration

The primary repair of eyelid and *canalicular lacerations* offers the best opportunity for restoring function and appearance. Late reconstructions are more difficult and rarely as satisfactory as a meticulous initial closure.

Repair of lid lacerations may be performed under local or general anesthesia, depending on the age of the patient, the extent of the lacerations, and associated injuries. Copious irrigation and removal of foreign particles reduces the risk of infection and traumatic tattooing. Debridement should be minimized, as the vascularity of the eyelid will often allow healing of ischemic or crushed tissues. Wound edges may retract creating the appearance of substantial tissue loss, but this is rare. Avulsed tissues should be replaced whenever possible and may remain viable as late as 24 hours after injury.

The first step in eyelid repair is reapproximation of anatomic landmarks such as the canaliculi, lid margins, medial and lateral canthal tendons, and brows. The remaining skin edges will then be more easily realigned.

An attempt at repairing the transected canaliculus should always be made, as it cannot be predetermined which individual will remain asymptomatic with a single functioning canaliculus. The first step in canalicular repair is identification of the proximal (medial) cut end of the canaliculus by direct visualization with loupes or a microscope. A Crawford silicone stent is passed through the punctum and then through the transected end of the canaliculus to bridge the lacerated area. The probe is advanced into the sac, then turned and aimed toward the nasolacrimal duct. The probe is retrieved under the inferior turbinate (see Lacrimal Section on the technique of silicone intubation, Chapter 24). The opposite canaliculus is intubated, and the ends of the stent are retrieved and tied in the nasal cavity.

If the medial end of the canaliculus cannot be identified visually, a *pigtail probe* passed through the opposite intact canaliculus will emerge from the transected end (Fig. 26–1) (1). The pigtail probe also may be used to place a silicone stent within the canalicular system (also see Chap. 24). The stent placed with a pigtail probe does not involve intubation into the nose and thus avoids potential injury to this uninvolved portion of the lacrimal system. The pigtail probe is advanced from the intact system until it emerges from the cut end of the canaliculus (Fig. 26–1). A 5-0 Prolene suture is passed through the eye of the probe and pulled back through the system (Fig. 26–2). In the same manner, the Prolene suture is passed through the remaining portion of the canaliculus distal (lateral) to the laceration. A piece of 0.6-mm diameter silicone tubing is then threaded over the suture and advanced into the canalicular system (Fig. 26–3). The transected edges of the canaliculus are reapproximated with several interrupted 7-0 nylon su-

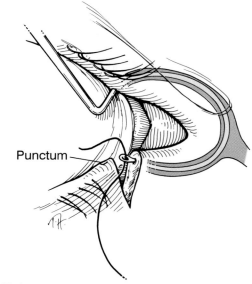

Figure 26–1.
The proximal cut end of the transected canaliculus is identified by passing a pigtail probe through the intact canaliculus. A Prolene suture is passed through the eye of the probe.

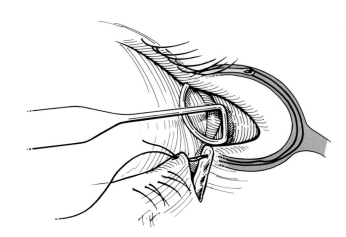

Figure 26–2.
The probe is rotated in a retrograde fashion, pulling the Prolene suture through the canalicular system.

tures. The medial canthal tendon is realigned with interrupted 5-0 Vicryl sutures (Fig. 26–4). The stent is trimmed and the suture ends tied together. Tying the Prolene suture within the lumen of the silicone stent unites the ends of the tubing (Fig. 26–5). The ends of the tubing and the suture knot are then rotated into the intact canaliculus. The orbicularis layer is closed with several interrupted 5-0 Vicryl sutures, followed by skin closure with 6-0 nylon (Fig. 26–6). Silicone stents placed through the system are essential to prevent stenosis and closure at the repair site.

Lid margin lacerations require precise reapproxima-

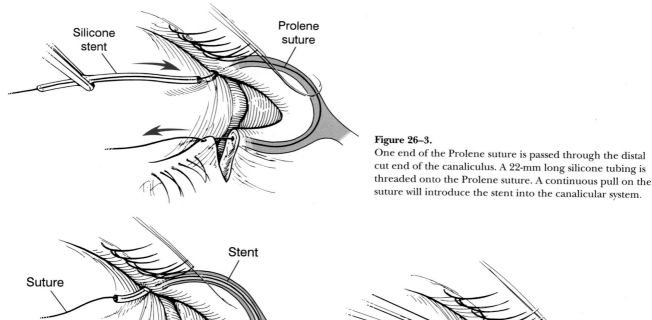

Figure 26–3.
One end of the Prolene suture is passed through the distal cut end of the canaliculus. A 22-mm long silicone tubing is threaded onto the Prolene suture. A continuous pull on the suture will introduce the stent into the canalicular system.

Figure 26–4.
A silicone stent bridging the wound.

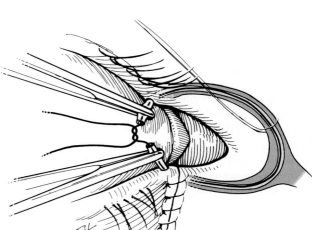

Figure 26–5.
The ends of the Prolene sutures are tied to unite the ends of the silicone stent.

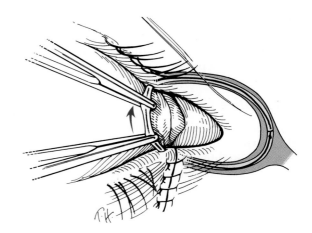

Figure 26–6.
The doughnut stent is rotated 180° to position the anastomosis within the common canaliculus.

tion of the tarsal plate to avoid notching (8). If the tarsal laceration is irregular, the edges may be trimmed so that the tarsal borders are sharp and perpendicular to the lid margin. Up to one third of the posterior lamella may be lost without compromising a primary closure. However, if the edges cannot be brought together easily, a lateral cantholysis becomes necessary. The edges of the tarsal plate are realigned with 3 to 4 interrupted 5-0 Vicryl sutures on a spatula needle (5). The sutures are passed in a lamellar fashion to avoid full-thickness passage, which could lead to corneal abrasion (Fig. 26–7). Closure of the lid margin is accomplished by a vertical mattress suture. A 5-0 silk suture is passed into a meibomian gland opening perpendicular to the lid margin about 3 mm from the cut edge; it exits through the tarsal plate 3 mm from the lid margin. The needle then enters the opposite tarsus 3 mm from the lid margin and exits from a meibomian gland opening 3 mm from the wound edge. The suture is passed back through the lid margin in a near-to-near fashion, entering and exiting through a meibomian gland orifice 1 mm from the cut edge (Fig. 26–8). Tying of the vertical mattress suture everts the lid margin. Puckering of the wound edges is a desirable ef-

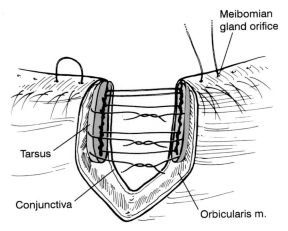

Figure 26–7.
5-0 Vicryl sutures uniting the tarsal plate.

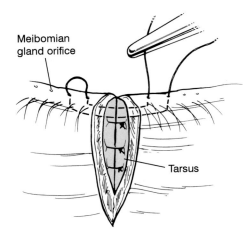

Figure 26–8.
Vertical mattress suture to align the lid margin.

fect that minimizes postoperative lid margin notching. The lash margin is realigned with a 7-0 nylon suture (Fig. 26–9). The ends of these sutures are left long and tied away from the wound with a suture to avoid contact with the cornea. The edges of the orbicularis muscle layer are closed with 6-0 Vicryl sutures. The skin is reapproximated with 7-0 nylon sutures (Fig. 26–10).

Exploration of *upper eyelid lacerations* is best performed under local anesthesia to assist in identification of the levator aponeurosis. The wound edges are gently retracted and the orbital septum identified. The orbital septum may be opened fully to expose the underlying orbital fat if necessary. The preaponeurotic fat pad is a key landmark to look for in any eyelid repair, since the levator aponeurosis is situated beneath this structure. The identity of the levator aponeurosis can be verified by asking the patient to look up while grasping the edge of the aponeurosis with a forceps. One should feel a tug on the forceps if the aponeurosis is engaged. The aponeurosis is repaired or reattached onto the tarsal plate with 6-0 Vicryl or silk sutures. It is not necessary to close the orbital septum.

Postoperative Care

Postoperatively, antibiotic ointment is applied for 1 week, at which time nonmarginal skin sutures are removed. Lid margin sutures are removed 2 weeks following the repair. The silicone stent remains in place for 4 to 6 months. Systemic antibiotics should be considered if the wound is contaminated or caused by dog bites, if closure is delayed, or if the patient is diabetic or immunocompromised. Amoxicillin with clavulanic acid (Augmentin) covers penicillinase resistant gram-positive cocci, anaerobes, and gram-negative organisms.

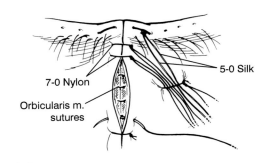

Figure 26–9.
Eyelash margin is aligned with a 7-0 nylon suture.

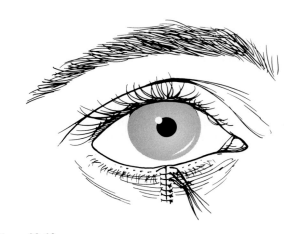

Figure 26–10.
Skin closure is achieved with 7-0 nylon sutures. The lid margin sutures can be secured away from the corneal surface.

■ ORBITAL BLOWOUT FRACTURE

Orbital fractures are a relatively common form of periorbital injury. Although any bone surrounding the orbit may be fractured, the thin bones of the orbital floor and medial orbital wall are most vulnerable. The most common site for a blowout fracture is the thin part of the maxillary bone (0.5-mm thick) in the posterior medial aspect of the floor. In addition, the very thin ethmoid bone (0.25-mm thick) along the medial wall of the orbit may be involved (9). Due to the relative thickness of the orbital rim, it is often spared in orbital fractures. The term "blowout fracture" refers specifically to a fracture of an orbital wall in the presence of an intact orbital rim.

It is believed that the mechanism of blowout fracture is a sudden increase in intraorbital pressure applied in an anterior-posterior direction toward the apex. The pressure is dissipated 90° to the line of force by the "blowout" of the thin orbital bones. Recent evidence suggested that an orbital floor blowout fracture can also occur from a blow directed to the orbital rim, causing buckling of the thin bones within the orbit. Incarceration of any portion of the fine connective tissue system of the orbit will produce tethering of the extraocular muscles through the mechanism of fat and fascial entrapment.

Orbital fractures may also occur as extensions of more complex midfacial fractures such as LeFort II and III fractures, zygomatic fractures, and orbital roof fractures. Less commonly, orbital fractures may result from penetrating injury to the orbit. Ocular injuries occur in up to 32% of individuals with orbital blowout fractures. Associated ocular injuries include: corneal abrasion, hyphema, iritis, lens dislocation, secondary glaucoma, cataract, vitreous hemorrhage, commotio retinae, retinal detachment, and ruptured globe.

Assessment

Diplopia, numbness of the cheek and teeth, and pain within the orbit are common symptoms suggestive of an orbital blowout fracture in patients who have sustained blunt periorbital trauma. Corroborative clinical findings associated with orbital fractures are eyelid ecchymosis and edema, restricted ocular motility, enophthalmos, hypo-ophthalmos, and subcutaneous or orbital emphysema (Figs. 26–11 and 26–12). Injury to the maxillary division of the trigeminal nerve may result in hypesthesia of the ipsilateral cheek, upper incisors, and the tip of the nose. Anisocoria is another subtle finding associated with blowout fracture. This is due to injury to the parasympathetic fibers coursing along the inferior division of third nerve to the inferior oblique muscle, interrupting the path to the ciliary ganglion. This sign is more indicative of a posterior floor fracture.

Plain radiographs will identify 70% to 80% of orbital fractures and are helpful in the initial evaluation of the patient with periorbital injuries. The information provided is often presumptive rather than definite. However, CT with direct or reconstructed coronal views will permit the most accurate assessment of fracture configuration, orbital volume increase, and relation of the inferior extraocular muscles to the fracture. Information regarding abnormalities of the orbital soft tissues also will be provided.

Not all orbital fractures will require repair. The indications for surgical intervention are: (1) persistent diplopia on primary gaze in the presence of a positive forced duction test and after resolution of orbital edema; (2) persistent diplopia on downgaze in the presence of a positive forced duction test and after resolution of orbital edema; (3) enophthalmos of more than 2 to 3 mm in the absence of residual orbital edema; and (4) significantly displaced fracture in which eventual enophthalmos will likely occur. Occasionally, diplopia in upgaze may constitute an indication for surgical repair because of occupational demand, such as a pilot, professional athlete, or a car mechanic who needs to look up while working under the car. Indications for conservative observation may include: (1) minimal diplopia with good motility; (2) no CT evidence of tissue incarceration; (3) absence of significant enophthalmos and hypo-ophthalmos; and (4) small bony defect.

The optimal time for surgery is within 2 to 3 weeks of the injury when the incarcerated tissues are most easily released (6). Initially, the need for surgery may be difficult to assess due to orbital edema and hemorrhage, which may restrict motility and conceal enophthalmos. The decision regarding surgery is therefore usually delayed 7 to 10 days until edema has subsided. Further delay is appropriate if there are ocular or systemic injuries, or if there is continuing improvement in motility.

Orbital floor fractures may cause disturbances in vertical gaze if the inferior rectus muscle or adjacent fat is entrapped in the defect. Medial wall fractures are more commonly associated with enophthalmos, but abduction deficits may be seen if entrapment of the medial rectus has occurred (10). Patients with diplopia should be followed closely until there is no further improvement in motility. In some cases, CT will demonstrate entrapment of a muscle within the bony defect. However, entrapment may not always be apparent radiographically. The muscle may be tethered indirectly by incarcerated orbital septae and fat without appearing distorted or displaced (Fig. 26–13). A forced duction test should help to differentiate a paretic from a restrictive motility disturbance when the CT findings are equivocal.

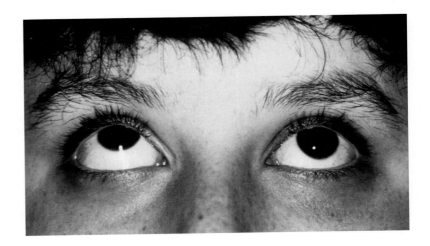

Figure 26–11.
Limitation of left eye in upgaze due to entrapment of orbital tissue within the floor defect.

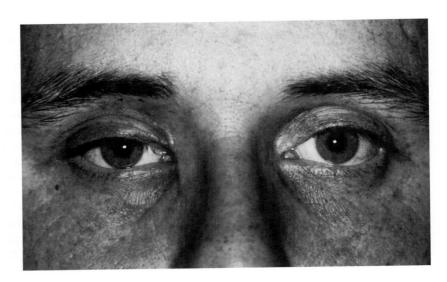

Figure 26–12.
Right sided enophthalmos with superior sulcus deformity and pseudoptosis due to a large medial wall fracture.

Prolapse of orbital fat through a fracture into an adjacent sinus causes a shift in orbital volume, which may lead to enophthalmos. The risk is greatest in individuals with fractures involving more than 50% of an orbital wall. Enophthalmos may not become fully apparent for weeks or months after the injury, at which time surgery is more difficult and the outcome less satisfactory. Early repair is recommended in patients with radiographic evidence of large fractures even though enophthalmos may not yet be apparent. If the fracture appears less extensive, the patient should be followed closely and the fracture repaired if 2 mm or more of enophthalmos develops.

Treatment

Initially, the patient with an orbital fracture should be instructed to avoid nose blowing, which could result in orbital cellulitis or emphysema. Oral antibiotics are recommended for patients with medial wall fractures, as cellulitis is more likely to occur in this group. In selected cases, a short course of oral prednisone for 1 week will facilitate resolution of orbital edema and permit earlier assessment of motility and enophthalmos.

Surgical repair is performed under general anesthesia. The orbital rim is most often approached through a transcutaneous infralash incision or a transconjunctival incision (7, 10). An orbital floor blowout fracture with concomitant low medial wall involvement can be approached through the lower eyelid, but more extensive medial wall fractures require a frontoethmoidal incision for adequate exposure. When the infralash approach is chosen, a surgical plane is developed between the orbicularis and the orbital septum and followed to the inferior orbital rim. The transconjunctival approach requires a lateral canthotomy and inferior cantholysis for adequate exposure. The lower lid retractors and conjunctiva are disinserted from the inferior border of the tarsal plate to provide access to the preseptal plane. Sharp dissection within this plane is carried inferiorly until the orbital rim is identified. The periosteum is incised at the orbital rim and elevated off of the orbital

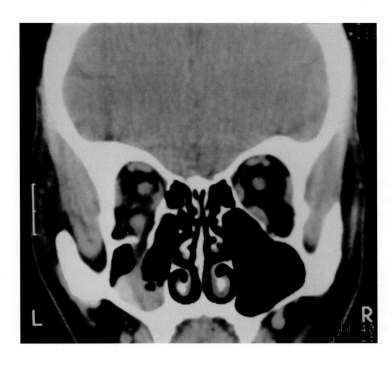

Figure 26–13.
Coronal CT scan of the orbits demonstrating disruption of the left orbital floor. There is distortion of the inferior rectus muscle and incarceration orbital tissue within the bony defect.

floor until the fracture site is identified. The subperiosteal elevation is extended backward until the area of the blowout fracture is identified. Prolapsed soft tissues are carefully elevated from the defect by using a Freer elevator and orbital retractors. It is essential to identify all the edges of the fracture, particularly the posterior rim, before covering the defect with an implant. The continuity of the orbital floor is restored by placing a 0.5- to 0.6-mm thick Supramid implant. The Supramid implant should be fashioned in a triangular shape with rounded corners. Furthermore, it should be large enough not only to cover the defect but also the entire orbital floor. The implant should bridge over the bony defect and rest on the stable adjacent portions of the floor. The base of the triangular shaped implant should rest tightly behind the inferior orbital rim. Besides using alloplastic teflon or Supramid sheet, autogenous cranial bone can also be used. For large floor fractures, titanium and vitallium micromesh plating systems can be utilized to provide a rigid scaffolding across the defects. These plates can be fixed to the orbital rim and autogenous or alloplastic materials placed over them. They are well tolerated and not associated with an increased risk of infection. Verification that the incarcerated tissue is released from the fracture site may be obtained by pulling on a preplaced traction suture passed under the insertion of inferior rectus muscle. There should be no movement of the implant during this traction test. The periosteum is then closed with several interrupted 5-0 Vicryl sutures. The infraciliary skin incision is reapproximated with a 7-0 nylon running suture. If the floor was approached through the lateral canthus, the lateral canthal tendon is reapproximated with 5-0 Vicryl suture.

The conjunctiva is closed with a running 6-0 fast absorbing plain suture.

Intraoperative complications of orbital floor exploration include hemorrhage, optic nerve ischemia from implant impingement, extraocular muscle or nerve injury and failure to free the entire entrapped muscle or connective tissue.

Postoperative Complications

Postoperative complications include residual diplopia, residual enophthalmos, ectropion, lid retraction, infection, hemorrhage, implant migration or extrusion, lymphedema, infraorbital nerve hypesthesia, and lacrimal duct obstruction. Infraorbital nerve hypesthesia due to the initial injury or secondary to intraoperative manipulation will usually resolve with time. Diplopia may persist or increase after surgery due to cicatricial changes in the muscle and orbital tissues, or due to release of a paretic muscle. Postoperative diplopia should be followed for at least 6 months before considering any strabismus surgery. Blindness was noted at an incidence of 1 in 1500.

The ophthalmologist may be involved in the assessment and repair of the orbital component of more extensive facial fractures. Zygomatic fractures involve the lateral orbital rim, the zygomatic arch, and inferior orbital rim, and are frequently referred to as tripod fractures. If a tripod fracture is displaced, it may result in trismus, displacement of the lateral canthal angle, and flattening of the cheek. Entrapment of orbital tissues may also occur. Open reduction and internal fixation are required to reduce the displaced zygomatic fracture.

Fractures of the orbital roof require prompt attention by a neurosurgeon due to the risk of associated intracranial injury, cerebrospinal fluid leak, and meningitis. LeFort II and III fractures are complex fractures of the maxillary, nasal, and orbital bones, which are best treated in conjunction with an otolaryngologist or facial plastic surgeon.

Postoperative Care

Following surgery, patients are hospitalized overnight, and the vision is checked frequently to allow early detection of optic nerve compromise due to hemorrhage or migration of the orbital implant. It is unnecessary to place a patch over the operated eye, so that the physician and nursing staff can watch for signs of progressive proptosis in the event of postoperative retrobulbar hemorrhage. Additionally, this will enable the patient to help monitor the vision and to alert the physician to any sudden change in acuity. Ice packs are applied for several days, and broad spectrum oral antibiotics are continued for 5 to 7 days. Nose blowing is discouraged.

■ ORBITAL FOREIGN BODIES

Orbital foreign bodies are infrequently encountered in periorbital trauma. They may produce a variety of signs and symptoms depending on the size, location, and composition of the retained material (4).

An orbital foreign body may result from any penetrating injury to the orbit. Projectiles are the most common cause, but penetrating injuries by substances that fragment or splinter during removal may also result in deposition of foreign matter within the orbit. In many cases, foreign bodies may be safely retained within the orbital fat. However, if the foreign body is large and abuts the optic nerve or extraocular muscles, visual dysfunction, diplopia, or pain may result.

The soft tissue response to a foreign body will vary depending on its composition. Stone, glass, and most metals are inert and, in the absence of infection, are well tolerated within the orbital fat. In contrast, pure copper is often poorly tolerated due to its tendency to incite an acute inflammatory response. Copper alloys such as brass and bronze are usually less reactive and in some cases may be well tolerated for an extended period of time. Vegetable matter is often associated with a chronic inflammatory response that may result in late abscess and fistula formation.

Assessment

Penetration of the orbit may be accompanied by injury to the globe or adjacent intracranial structures. A complete ocular and neurologic examination is the first priority in evaluating the patient with an orbital foreign body. Eye injuries should be treated promptly, and neurosurgical consultation should be arranged if intracranial involvement is suspected. Initial findings associated with an intraorbital foreign body may include edema, hemorrhage, proptosis, and pain. A mass may be palpable if the foreign body is large or located in the anterior orbit. Diplopia or decreased vision may be present if injury to the extraocular muscles or optic nerve has occurred. Delayed findings include orbital abscesses, fistulas, migration, and extrusion of the foreign material.

Identification and localization of a foreign body is best accomplished by CT scanning (Fig. 26–14). An MRI may provide further information regarding low density foreign bodies once it has been established that no magnetic material is present. The composition of the foreign body should be determined by history and by inspection of samples, whenever possible.

Treatment

In the acute setting, broad spectrum systemic antibiotics and tetanus prophylaxis should be administered. Cultures of the entrance wound or of the foreign body, if removed, will help guide antibiotic therapy. In the case of a long-standing foreign body with a fistulous tract, cultures of the exudate should be taken.

Orbital foreign bodies need not be removed if they are small, inert, smoothly contoured, and not causing compressive injury to the globe, optic nerve, or extraocular muscles. Foreign bodies in the posterior aspect of the orbit are particularly difficult to locate, and removal may be more hazardous than leaving the object in place. Removal should be considered if the object is large and irregular, is a nidus for infection, or is causing pain or compressive injury to the orbital contents. Copper and organic material should be removed due to their tendencies to incite acute and chronic inflammations, respectively.

Foreign bodies may be approached through an entrance wound, a fistulous tract, or via a standard approach to the appropriate orbital compartment. Localization may be facilitated by fluoroscopy, endoscopy, ultrasonography, or foreign body magnet.

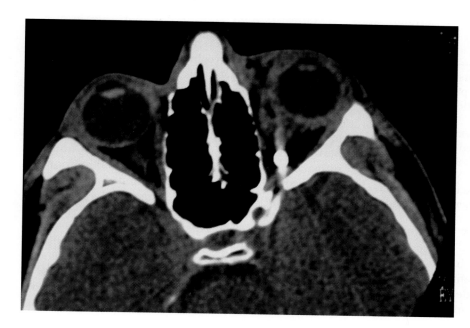

Figure 26–14.
Axial CT scan of an orbital BB. Pellet remained in orbit without causing any symptoms or functional impairment.

■ ORBITAL HEMORRHAGE

An orbital hemorrhage is a space-occupying lesion occurring within a cavity with limited potential for volume expansion. An expanding volume of blood within a confined orbit will lead to an increase in intraorbital and intraocular pressure. Increased intraocular pressure results from direct compression of the eye by the expanding hematoma and an elevated venous outflow pressure within the orbit. Visual loss results from compression of the optic nerve and central retinal artery.

The most common cause of an orbital hemorrhage is blunt trauma or a penetrating injury to the orbit. Intraorbital hemorrhage from retrobulbar injection following blepharoplasty or orbital surgery is a well-recognized complication encountered in ophthalmology (3, 11). Inadvertent entry into the orbit during sinus surgery can lead to the development of an expanding hematoma (2). Spontaneous bleeding from an orbital lymphangioma is a biological feature of the lesion. Aspirin use, hypertension, and unrecognized clotting abnormalities are common contributing factors to postoperative orbital hemorrhages.

Assessment

The most important step in the initial evaluation of a patient with an orbital hemorrhage is the accurate assessment of visual function. In a cooperative patient, visual acuity, color vision, and peripheral visual fields should be checked when possible. Pupillary reaction, intraocular pressure, and the status of the central retinal artery should be appraised promptly. Dilation of the pupil permits better evaluation of retinal perfusion, but impairs continued checks for the development of an afferent pupillary defect. However, if only the involved pupil is pharmacologically dilated, then assessment of an afferent pupillary defect can still be made by observing the direct and consensual pupillary responses of the uninvolved eye (reverse testing mechanism).

A hemorrhage may occur within the orbit or in the extraperiorbital (subperiosteal) space. An expanding hemorrhage developing within the orbit tends to spread diffusely within the orbital fat, causing intense pain, proptosis, decreased vision, motility disturbance, and subconjunctival hemorrhage. Funduscopic examination may show central retinal artery pulsation or occlusion, optic disc edema, and chorioretinal folds.

Treatment

Most orbital hemorrhages will not require treatment and will resolve within several weeks. However, if any compromise in visual function is detected, measures to relieve optic nerve compression, reduce intraocular pressure, and to promote retinal perfusion should be initiated without delay (Table 26–1). Recovery of vision is unlikely if retinal ischemia persists for more than 2 hours. Computed axial tomography or MRI should be performed to identify underlying pathology and to distinguish an extraperiosteal hemorrhage from a diffuse intraorbital hemorrhage. A localized extraperiosteal hemorrhage may be surgically drained or aspirated. Treatment should not be delayed by orbital imaging if vision is compromised.

TABLE 26–1
Treatment of Orbital Hemorrhage

1. Monitor intraocular pressure and retinal perfusion
2. Open traumatic or surgical wounds if present
3. Identify and cauterize any visible bleeders
4. Normalize blood pressure
5. Initiate medical treatment (timolol, acetazolamide, mannitol) if retinal perfusion is compromised
6. Lateral canthotomy and inferior cantholysis for persistent retinal ischemia
7. Orbital decompression if unresponsive to prior measures
8. Systemic steroids if evidence of optic nerve compromise is present

Visual acuity, pupillary reaction, intraocular pressure, and posterior pole perfusion status will guide the urgency and extent of treatment needed. First, surgical or traumatic wounds should be opened to allow drainage of blood. The systemic blood pressure should be normalized as hypertension will promote continued bleeding. However, precipitous lowering of blood pressure may have a deleterious effect on optic nerve perfusion. If the intraocular pressure is elevated, topical timolol 0.5%, intravenous acetazolamide (500 mg) and mannitol (1 to 2 g/kg over 20 minutes) should be given to decrease intraocular pressure and enhance retinal perfusion. If there is continued evidence of impaired retinal perfusion, a lateral canthotomy and inferior cantholysis should be performed without delay. This maneuver will provide a partial decompression of the orbit. In the rare event that these measures fail to restore perfusion to the posterior pole, an orbital decompression is required. High-dose systemic steroids (methylprednisolone 30 mg/kg intravenous loading dose, followed by a maintenance dose of 15 mg/kg every 6 hours for 48 to 72 hours) may be given to promote optic nerve recovery.

■ TRAUMATIC OPTIC NEUROPATHY

Traumatic optic neuropathy is an uncommon form of orbital injury. It is diagnosed when a direct or indirect injury to the optic nerve results in partial or complete loss of optic nerve function. Traumatic optic neuropathy occurs in approximately 3% of patients sustaining maxillofacial trauma. Up to 50% of these individuals will have a permanent reduction in visual acuity. Motor vehicle accidents, bicycle injuries, and falls are the most common causes of traumatic optic neuropathy.

Traumatic optic neuropathy may result from direct or indirect injury to the optic nerve. Direct injury refers to optic nerve damage resulting from a penetrating orbital wound. Indirect injury results when the force of a distant blow is transmitted to the optic nerve through bone compression or sudden soft tissue movement. Any section of the nerve may be involved, but the intracanalicular portion is most commonly affected by indirect injury. During blunt forehead trauma, deformation of the orbital bone is concentrated in the area of the optic canal. Because the optic nerve is relatively fixed within the optic canal, it is particularly susceptible to shearing and compression with bone deformation. Fractures of the optic canal may occur, but compression of the optic nerve by displaced bone fragments is probably uncommon.

Visual loss may be instantaneous or delayed. Primary injury occurs at the moment of impact and results in irreversible optic nerve injury due to disruption of axons and supportive vasculature. Secondary injury occurs subsequent to the moment of impact. Vasospasm and swelling of the optic nerve may lead to increased ischemia and further axonal loss, particularly within the confines of the optic canal. The goal of treatment in traumatic optic neuropathy is to minimize the delayed component of optic nerve injury.

The physical findings will vary depending on the location of the optic nerve injury. Anterior injuries are those that occur distal to the entry of the central retinal artery into the nerve. This type of injury results in vascular changes on funduscopic examination. An anterior transection of the optic nerve results in the findings of a central retinal artery occlusion with retinal edema and a cherry red spot. A contusion injury may lead to retinal hemorrhages due to venous obstruction. An avulsion of the optic nerve from the globe causes hemorrhage within the retina and vitreous, often in a ring-like configuration. Posterior injuries occur proximal to the entrance of the central retinal artery into the nerve. Injuries in this location are often without funduscopic abnormalities, although disc edema has been reported due to hemorrhage within the optic nerve sheath.

Assessment

Evaluation of the patient with traumatic optic neuropathy is often difficult due to the presence of concurrent injuries. Loss of consciousness is common, and many individuals will have associated systemic and neurologic injuries. Collaboration with neurology and the appropriate surgical specialties is required to assess all injuries and to prioritize treatment.

The diagnosis of traumatic optic neuropathy requires the findings of decreased vision and the presence of an afferent pupillary defect following a direct or indirect orbital trauma. The visual acuity is often less than 20/400, but milder degrees of visual loss may be seen. The absence of significant intraocular pathology supports the diagnosis of traumatic optic neuropathy. A complete assessment of acuity, visual field and pupillary response should be performed if possible. When it is considered safe to dilate the pupils, a funduscopic examination is important to rule out intraocular causes of visual loss. The periorbital area should be evaluated for fractures, hemorrhages, and foreign bodies, which may compromise optic nerve function.

Neuroimaging is recommended whenever traumatic optic neuropathy is suspected. Fractures of the sphenoid sinus, superior orbital rim, and optic canal are often seen in association with traumatic optic neuropathy and are best demonstrated by computed axial tomography. Identification of orbital hemorrhages, optic nerve sheath hemorrhages, and subperiosteal hematomas is also important, as these may require appropriate surgical intervention. In some cases, MRI may be helpful in providing additional soft tissue detail.

Treatment

Treatment of traumatic optic neuropathy is controversial (12). In the past, intervention was believed to be most appropriate for those individuals with delayed visual loss. More recently, reports of recovered vision in patients with no light perception immediately following trauma have prompted a more aggressive approach to treatment. Therapeutic modalities available are high-dose corticosteroids, optic canal decompression, and optic nerve sheath fenestration.

The use of high-dose corticosteroid therapy has been widely accepted due to the benefits demonstrated in the treatment of spinal cord injuries. At very high doses, corticosteroids limit vasospasm and edema, which may result in delayed ischemic injury.

Surgical decompression of the optic nerve may be performed transphenoidally or transcranially. The optic canal shares its medial wall with the ethmoid and sphenoid sinuses, and removal of this bone may reduce compression of the intracanalicular optic nerve by edema, hemorrhage, and bone fragments. Optic nerve sheath fenestration creates an opening in the dura and arachnoid of the intraorbital portion of the optic nerve,

TABLE 26–2
Treatment of Traumatic Optic Neuropathy

1. Initiate intravenous solumedrol 30 mg/kg followed by 5.4 mg/kg/hr for 48 hours.
2. Consider optic nerve decompression if no response after 48 hours IV steroid therapy.
3. If vision improves on methylprednisolone, switch to oral prednisone after 48 hours and taper rapidly.
4. If vision deteriorates with prednisone taper, reinstitute intravenous methylprednisolone and consider optic nerve decompression.
5. If disc edema and an enlarged optic nerve are suggestive of optic nerve sheath hematoma, consider optic nerve sheath fenestration.

releasing subarachnoid fluid collection. Improvement in vision has been reported using this technique to drain optic nerve sheath hematomas.

The standard of care in the treatment of traumatic optic neuropathy has not yet been established. The protocol presented here (Table 26–2) is adapted from a large prospective clinical trial, which provides one rational stepwise approach to therapy (12).

In the absence of medical contraindications, most patients with traumatic optic neuropathy should be treated initially with high-dose corticosteroids, including those with immediate visual loss. Exceptions are patients with avulsion or transaction of the optic nerve, which will not respond to treatment. Methylprednisolone (Solumedrol) is administered intravenously with an initial dose of 30 mg/kg followed by a continuous infusion of 5.4 mg/kg per hour. Treatment should begin as promptly as possible and is continued for 48 hours. If there is no response to methylprednisolone, optic nerve decompression is discussed with the patient. If there is improvement with steroid therapy, the patient is switched to oral prednisone, which is rapidly tapered while closely monitoring visual function. If recovered vision worsens during attempted steroid taper, intravenous solumedrol is reinstituted, and optic nerve decompression is offered. Patients with optic nerve sheath hematomas as evidenced by visual dysfunction, disc edema, and a radiographically enlarged intraorbital optic nerve may benefit from optic nerve sheath fenestration. Treatment of traumatic optic neuropathy is unlikely to be effective if initiated more than 1 week after injury.

■ REFERENCES

1. Busse H, Steinkoogler FJ, Fries J: Ring intubation of lacerated canaliculi lacrimales. Orbit 1985;4:73–75.
2. Buus DR, Tse DT, Farris, BK: Ophthalmic complications of sinus surgery. Ophthalmology 1990;97:612–619.
3. Castronuevo S, Krohel GB: Orbital Hemorrhage. In: Linberg JV (ed). Oculoplastic and Orbital Emergencies. Connecticut, Appleton and Lange. 1990; 145–154.
4. Cooper WC, Haik BG: Management of orbital foreign

bodies. In: Della Rocca RC, Nesi FA, Lisman RD (eds). Ophthalmic Plastic and Reconstructive Surgery. St. Louis, CV Mosby, 1987; 523–531.

5. Divine RD, Anderson RL: Techniques in eyelid wound closure. Ophthalmic Surg 1982;13:283.

6. Hawes MJ, Dortzbach RK: Surgery on orbital floor fractures: Influence of time of repair and fracture size. Ophthalmology 1983;90:1066–1070.

7. Kersten RC, Kulwin DR: Orbital Blowout Fractures. In: Tse DT (ed). Color Atlas of Ophthalmic Surgery, Oculoplastic Surgery. Philadelphia, JB Lippincott, 1992; 35–48.

8. Kulwin DR, Kersten RC: Eyelid laceration repair. In: Tse DT (ed). Color Atlas of Ophthalmic Surgery, Oculoplastic Surgery. Philadelphia, JB Lippincott, 1992; 27–34.

9. Lemke BN, Della Rocca RC: Osteology. In: Surgery of the Eyelids and Orbit: An Anatomical Approach. Norwalk, Connecticut: Appleton and Lange, 1990; 9–39.

10. Leone CR, Lloyd WC, Rylander G: Surgical repair of medial wall fractures. Am J Ophth 1987;97:349–356.

11. Spoor TC: Orbital Hemorrhages. In: Spoor TC, Nesi FA (eds). Management of Ocular, Orbital and Adnexal Trauma. New York, Raven Press, 1988; 351–562.

12. Steinsaper KD, Goldberg RA: Traumatic optic neuropathy. Surv Ophthalmol 1994;38:487–518.

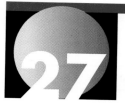

27 Congenital Eyelid Anomalies, Eyelid Malposition, and Blepharoptosis

Melissa Lynn Meldrum, David T. Tse

■ CONGENITAL ANOMALIES

Ankyloblepharon

Ankyloblepharon is a congenital adherence of the palpebral margins that may vary from a single filamentous band to an extensive adhesion of the entire lid margins. This condition represents an alteration in the orderly sequence of growth in which there was an incomplete separation of the fused lids. The usual site of fusion is the lateral canthus, but the inner canthus also may be involved. Medial ankyloblepharon may cause punctal occlusion and alter tear outflow, resulting in epiphora. This condition is frequently associated with a mild degree of symblepharon and often gives an appearance of pseudostrabismus. Treatment consists of simple separation of the lids with scissors. If the adhesion is extensive, marginal graft or suturing the conjunctival edge with the skin may be necessary to prevent readhesion.

Epicanthus

This is a congenital fold of skin over the medial canthus, which covers the caruncle. It may produce a pseudostrabismus appearance. Four separate types have been described: epicanthus superciliaris; epicanthus palpebralis; epicanthus tarsalis; and epicanthus inversus. In epicanthus superciliaris, the skinfold originates superiorly from the skin just below the brow and terminating

over the lacrimal sac. Epicanthus palpebralis is formed by the skinfold arising in the upper eyelid and extending to the lower lid. Epicanthus tarsalis, the typical Mongolian fold, arises from the superior tarsal fold and continues to the inner canthus. *Epicanthus inversus* is similar to epicanthus tarsalis, but arises from the lower lid and extends upward to partially camouflage the medial canthus. This form is a component of the blepharophimosis syndrome (Fig. 27–1). In Caucasians, epicanthus commonly disappears in early childhood as the bridge of the nose widens. When treatment is required, it is best delayed until 4 to 5 years of age. The basic defect consists of a vertical shortening of skin at the medial canthus. A realignment of skin can be achieved by any number of vertical skin lengthening methods, such as the double Z-plasty, Y to V-plasty, Mustarde's technique (14), and the five-flap procedure (3).

Coloboma

A lid coloboma is a full-thickness developmental defect that may involve the upper eyelid, the lower eyelid, or both. The edges of the defect may be adherent to the bulbar conjunctiva and cornea. A dermolipoma may be present adjacent to the defect. The cornea usually tolerates the exposure well, if the Bell's reflex is present and lubricant is applied diligently. If exposure ker-

TABLE 27–1
Clinical Characteristics of Ptosis

	Involutional Ptosis	Congenital Ptosis
Lid crease	Higher than normal	absent or indistinct
Lid position on downgaze	Lower than normal lid	Higher than normal lid
Levator Function	normal	generally decreased
Extraocular muscle function	normal	superior rectus function may be abnormal
Synkinetic movement	absent	may be present in Marcus-Gunn jaw winking
Other eyelid abnormalities	absent	may be present in blepharophimosis syndrome

atopathy becomes problematic, surgical closure of the defect will be necessary. The edges of the colobomatous defect are freshened and an end-to-end anastomosis is accomplished in the same manner as for repair of a full-thickness vertical lid laceration. The tarsal plate substance is usually present, permitting an anatomic closure. For a large defect, a lateral canthotomy and cantholysis may be necessary to achieve closure. Any reconstructive technique requiring a prolonged period of lid fusion, such as a tarsoconjunctival flap, will predispose to the development of amblyopia and is thus discouraged.

Epiblepharon, blepharophimosis, congenital entropion, congenital distichiasis, and congenital ptosis will be discussed in more detail in the following eyelid malposition section.

Cryptophthalmos

Failure of the eye lid to differentiate, with fusion of the upper and lower lids. Eye lid skin fuses with the cornea, which is usually abnormal. Cryptophthalmos can be unilateral, bilateral, complete, or partial, and may be inherited usually autosomal dominant. Surgical separation of the lids almost always fails because the lid and cornea fuse as one.

Euryblepharon

Sagging or drooping of the lower eye lid inferiorly away from the globe, especially involving the lateral half of the lid. There is inferior displacement of the lateral canthus and shortening of the lower eye lid skin. Euryblepharon is often mistaken for congenital ectropion which is very rare. Surgical repair of euryblepharon includes relaxing the lower lid skin with a skin graft, and tightening the lower lid and lateral canthus.

■ EYELID MALPOSITION

Blepharoptosis

Blepharoptosis, defined as drooping of the upper eyelid, is a common ophthalmologic condition. The normal upper lid margin rests between 1 to 3 mm below the superior limbus on primary gaze. An eyelid margin falling below this level, especially if it is asymmetrical when compared with the fellow lid, is described as ptotic. Although the diagnosis is easily made, determination of the underlying cause can sometimes be difficult. Therefore, a stepwise approach in the evaluation of a patient with ptosis is essential.

Patient Evaluation

The approach to a patient with a ptotic eyelid begins with a good history. An important categorical distinction in the evaluation is whether the problem is congenital or acquired. When the history is not reliable, old photographs are invaluable in making this distinction. Congenital ptosis is a developmental abnormality of the levator muscle with or without superior rectus involvement. The parents will relate a constant, nonprogressive drooping of the eyelid since birth. A history of birth trauma to the lid may suggest a cause different than the typical developmental dystrophy of the levator muscle. In this situation, levator aponeurosis disinsertion accounts for eyelid malposition. One also must keep in mind that aponeurogenic ptosis on a congenital basis may be present in a child. Neurogenic ptosis from a third nerve palsy or a Horner's syndrome, mechanical ptosis induced by a lid hematoma, chronic progressive external ophthalmoplegia (CPEO), or myogenic ptosis may be considered in the pediatric population. Acquired ptosis has many causes, including trauma, cataract surgery, and neurologic or systemic diseases. Clinical history will help differentiate between these types. For example, a history of general body fatigue associated with double vision and levator muscle weakness would suggest a neuromuscular disorder such as myasthenia gravis, myotonic dystrophy, or more rarely multiple sclerosis; whereas a history of progressive ptosis in a healthy elderly individual may indicate simple involutional ptosis. Family history is important in cases of myotonic dystrophy or blepharophimosis (a form of congenital ptosis), which are dominantly inherited. The history also will help guide the physical examination.

Examination

A complete eye examination, including dilation, should be performed on all patients. Visual acuity assessment is especially important in children, as ptosis-induced occlusion amblyopia may be present. Amblyopia should be corrected with patching of the sound eye before any surgical consideration. If the pupil is covered by the ptotic lid, more prompt surgical intervention may be necessary. A pupil examination and motility evaluation are important when ruling out a third nerve palsy as the potential cause of ptosis. In addition, during motility evaluation, superior rectus function should always be assessed in cases of congenital ptosis, as 5% to 10% of patients may have ipsilateral weakness of this muscle. In these cases, the superior rectus weakness like that of the levator muscle results from developmental dystrophy of the muscle. It is explained by the close embryologic association between the levator and the superior rectus muscle. The other extraocular muscles are not affected. During slit-lamp examination, the presence of iris heterochromia may be suggestive of congenital Horner's syndrome.

Lid measurements commonly used are measurements of the palpebral fissure, marginal light reflex distance, and levator function. Palpebral fissure is a measure of the distance between the upper and lower lid margins on primary gaze. In ptosis evaluation, palpebral fissure is a less reliable factor, as lower eyelid malposition will affect fissure aperture. Marginal light reflex is the distance between the upper lid margin and the corneal light reflex in primary gaze. This measurement is clinically more relevant as it is reflective of the amount of visual obstruction affected by the abnormal upper lid position. Levator function is the quantitative measurement of the amount of upper eyelid excursion from downgaze to upgaze. Care should be taken to eliminate any brow contribution in augmenting the lift of the ptotic lid. The brow elevation action should be blocked manually by the examiner's thumb while the levator function is quantitated. In congenital ptosis, levator function is typically poor, while in involutional ptosis, it is frequently normal. Accurate assessment of levator function is important in determining etiology and in the planning of surgical correction.

Position of the eyelid crease and fold should be noted, as patients with levator aponeurosis disinsertion typically present with a higher crease. Dynamic movement of the eyelids, the absence or presence of lid lag, lagophthalmos, or Bell's reflex also should be appraised. Jaw-winking ptosis can be elicited by having the infant suck on a bottle or the patient chew or move the jaw from side to side. Finally, the eyelid and the anterior orbit should be palpated to exclude the presence of any space-occupying lesion imparting a mechanical effect on the eyelid. Based on a good history and a thorough examination, an accurate etiologic diagnosis of ptosis can be derived.

A cover-uncover test should be performed to unveil any pseudoptosis associated with a vertical strabismus. Typically, a patient with pseudoptosis will demonstrate varying degrees of ptosis in the presence of a vertical strabismus. When the fixating hypertropic eye is occluded, the "ptosis" disappears as the hypotropic eye elevates to assume fixation. In this situation, muscle alignment is needed first before reevaluating the position of the eyelid.

Congenital Ptosis

Congenital ptosis comprises a group of cases in which the ptosis is due to a developmental dystrophy of the levator muscle, characterized by fibrosis and deficiency in striated muscle fibers (5). The condition may be associated with anisometropia, strabismus, and amblyopia. This group also will include those cases in which ptosis is a feature of blepharophimosis syndrome, double elevator palsy, and synkinetic jaw wink. In rare instances, an aponeurotic defect is affiliated with congenital ptosis.

The clinical hallmarks of congenital ptosis are mild to moderate ptosis, poor levator function, and a higher position of the ptotic eyelid on downgaze. This "tethering" of the upper eyelid on downgaze is related to fibrosis and dystrophic changes of the levator muscle and aponeurosis. These changes produce shortening of the levator muscle, hence a higher eyelid position on downgaze and reduced function of the levator. Generally, the upper eyelid crease is not well defined. The condition is usually unilateral but may be asymmetrically bilateral in an otherwise healthy child. A type of bilateral, autosomal-dominant ptosis is seen in *blepharophimosis*. There is horizontal shortening of the palpebral fissures in the presence of normal eyelid structures. The clinical features of blepharophimosis syndrome are telecanthus, epicanthus inversus, ptosis, and ectropion of the lateral portion of the lower lids (Fig. 27–1). In female patients with this syndrome, primary amenorrhea has been reported (18).

Initial evaluation of a child with congenital ptosis should include a complete eye examination with particular attention to visual acuity and ocular motility. In a

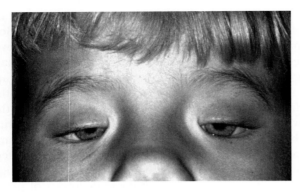

Figure 27–1.
A young child with blepharophimosis syndrome. Notice telecanthus, epicanthus inversus, and ptosis.

series of congenital ptosis cases, Anderson and Baumgartner (1) found a 20% incidence of amblyopia, of which 3% was directly attributable to the droopy eyelid. In the past, chin elevation posturing was considered a sign of fusion in a child with ptosis, thus indicating a low risk for amblyopia. However, MuCulloch and Wright (13) showed that chin elevation to maintain binocular vision does not rule out the presence of significant amblyopia. Once amblyopia is detected, the condition should be treated aggressively by patching of the sound eye.

A thorough motility examination also is essential. In a series of 113 cases, Anderson and Baumgartner (1) found 36 cases (31%) to have strabismus; of these 36 cases, 3% of cases were believed to be caused by ptosis that disrupted binocular function.

Treatment of congenital ptosis in most cases is surgical. Its timing depends on visual function. In general, if the visual axes are not obscured by the ptotic lids, it is best to defer repair until the child is 3 to 4 years old. Earlier intervention becomes necessary when occlusion amblyopia threatens visual acuity. At an older age, a more definitive procedure based on reliable and reproducible measurements of the levator function can be planned. The surgical procedure is determined by the amount of levator function present and the severity of the ptosis. Function is typically categorized as poor (less than 4 mm), fair (5 to 7 mm), and good (more than 8 mm). In cases of severe ptosis and less than 2 mm of levator function, suspension of the lid to the frontalis muscle is the procedure of choice. In mild cases with good function, advancement of the levator aponeurosis usually will yield good results. When ptosis is more severe and levator function is between 2 and 4 mm, suspension of the tarsal plate to the Whitnall's ligament will provide adequate elevation.

The concept of the *frontalis sling* procedure is to transfer the elevating function of the ptotic eyelid to the frontalis muscle. To achieve this, the lid is directly suspended to the brow using various materials. In older

children with sufficient limb length, the sling material of choice is autogenous fascia lata, as it is permanent and well tolerated. In very young children in whom the fascia lata is not well developed, synthetic materials such as Supramid suture, Goretex, silicone, or Mersilene mesh have been used. Because the sling material has little elasticity, a tethering effect on downgaze, lagophthalmos, and adynamic movement of the lid are expected postoperatively.

Concurrent anatomic abnormalities such as in blepharophimosis may require medial canthal tendon plication and canthoplasties. Occasionally, a transnasal wire may be needed to shorten the intercanthal distance if significant telecanthus is present. Physiologic defects, such as jaw-winking ptosis, will require transection of the levator muscle as well as frontalis suspension. In this syndrome, misdirected nerve fibers from the trigeminal nerve elevate the ptotic lid above its normal position when the muscles of mastication are activated.

Indications for frontalis suspension include: (1) congenital ptosis with poor to absent levator function; (2) jaw-winking synkinetic ptosis; (3) blepharophimosis syndrome; (4) failed levator resection; (5) congenital or acquired third nerve palsy; (6) myopathy; (7) trauma; and (8) congenital fibrosis syndrome. Ptosis with good to excellent levator function constitutes a contraindication for this procedure. Following frontalis suspension, some degree of lagophthalmos is expected. In children, this can be managed with simple lubrication. However, in patients with limited upgaze or poor Bell's reflex (patients with superior rectus weakness, third nerve palsies, or chronic external ophthalmoplegia), the surgeon must avoid overcorrection to minimize exposure keratopathy.

Fair or good levator function will allow the use of a levator aponeurosis resection alone or a procedure that attaches the levator directly to the Whitnall's ligament. Because levator aponeurosis resection in children needs to be performed under general anesthesia, a formula is used to determine the amount of levator aponeurosis resection. For patients with at least 8 mm of levator function, a rule of thumb is 3 to 4 mm of aponeurosis resection per millimeter of ptosis. An alternative formula employed by the authors to determine the amount of aponeurosis advancement in unilateral congenital ptosis with good function is the following: Amount of aponeurosis advancement (mm) = [Difference in levator function (mm) + Difference in eyelid fissure (mm)] + 3 (mm).

In children with poor function ptosis in which maximum aponeurosis advancement cannot effect sufficient lid elevation, a frontalis sling or Whitnall's sling will be required. Whitnall's sling is a good surgical alternative if parents wish to avoid bilateral eyelid surgery.

A major disadvantage of the Whitnall's sling procedure is the tendency for the lid to sag with time. If the

Whitnall's sling procedure fails to achieve permanent or satisfactory lid elevation, a frontalis suspension will be required.

Acquired Ptosis

The causes of acquired ptosis are diverse, but the vast majority of cases are aponeurogenic. Acquired ptosis can be classified into four categories: aponeurogenic, neurogenic, myogenic, and mechanical. Traumatic ptosis may be viewed as a separate category but in fact is a subcategory of each of the four categories. The distinction between each category is made based on history and physical examination. The list of specific diagnoses is broad, and only those most commonly encountered will be reviewed here.

Aponeurogenic Ptosis

Aponeurogenic ptosis is caused by involutional or disinsertional changes of the levator aponeurosis. This is often seen in elderly patients in whom ptosis developed after cataract surgery. The clinical triad of levator *aponeurosis disinsertion* consists of good levator function, a high lid crease, and the ptotic lid assuming a lower position on downgaze. The eyelid crease is formed by the fenestrating fibers from the levator aponeurosis inserting under the skin. When the levator aponeurosis is disinserted, the fenestrating fibers are pulled superiorly, creating a crease at a higher level. The levator function is normal because there is no intrinsic flaw in the levator muscle itself. Because the aponeurosis is disinserted from the tarsal plate, the ptotic lid is lower on downgaze. In contrast, the ptotic eyelid in congenital ptosis assumes a higher position on downgaze because of fibrosis of the levator muscle and aponeurosis. Another clinical clue of levator disinsertion is a bluish discoloration on the central portion of the ptotic lid. This is the cornea showing through the area of dehiscence above the superior tarsal margin.

The remainder of the eye examination, including pupillary examination and motility, should be normal. If a patient gives a history of fluctuation in ptosis throughout the day or diplopia, tests for *fatigability* and an edrophonium (Tensilon) test should be administered to rule out myasthenia gravis.

The aponeurotic surgery is the most direct approach in correcting the most common defect in involutional ptosis, aponeurosis rarefaction or disinsertion. This external approach also is the preferred method for myogenic or neurogenic ptosis with adequate levator function. The procedure is often performed under local anesthesia so that lid height and contour can be adjusted intraoperatively.

Neurogenic

Third Nerve Palsy. The oculomotor nerve innervates the levator of the upper lid, superior, inferior, medial rectus muscles, and the inferior oblique. A third nerve palsy, therefore, will result in complete ptosis and a "down and out" eye position. Parasympathetic innervation to the pupil accompanies the third nerve for much of its course. Depending on the cause of the injury, a fixed and dilated pupil also may be seen.

In evaluating ptosis resulting from presumed oculomotor palsy, the history and examination should be approached carefully and systematically. Time course of presentation, history of pain around the eye, or a history of severe headaches are important. Inquiry should be made into possible associated systemic conditions, including diabetes and hypertension. A careful cranial nerve examination should be performed to aid in localization of the pathology. Pupillary response should be assessed by the physician personally since this information is critically important in deciding the urgency of the condition.

Damage of the third nerve may occur anywhere on its course from the brain to the orbit. The oculomotor nerve nucleus, actually a complex with many subnuclei, is located in the rostral mesencephalon. The levator portion lies centrally and is a single subnucleus that supplies the levator of both sides. The superior rectus subnuclei have crossed projections, while the other subnuclei innervate the ipsilateral side. A lesion of the levator portion of the third nerve nucleus alone will therefore result in bilateral ptosis. If the entire nucleus is involved, one would see contralateral superior rectus palsy, bilateral ptosis, and ipsilateral medial rectus, inferior rectus and inferior oblique palsies. Third nerve palsies at this level are very rare.

From the nucleus, the third nerve travels through the subarachanoid space, lying parallel to the posterior communicating artery. Aneurysms of this artery are the most common cause (95% of patients) of third nerve palsies with pupillary involvement. Onset of the palsy occurs abruptly secondary to rapid aneurysm distention and bleeding. Pain always accompanies the event. Diabetic third nerve palsies present in a similar fashion. However, pupillary involvement occurs in fewer than 10% of patients. Diabetic palsies result from microinfarcts of the nerve with demyelination. In a diabetic palsy, recovery of function with remyelination should occur within 3 months. If the examination is unchanged in 3 months, an imaging study should be performed to rule out other causes, such as an aneurysm or tumor.

The nerve also can be injured by tumors or meningitis as it passes through the subarachanoid space. A tumor-induced palsy would have a more gradual presentation and would not be associated with significant pain. Meningitis-induced palsies would be accompanied by involvement of other cranial nerves.

On the course to the orbit, the oculomotor nerve passes through the cavernous sinus, which is a common area of damage. Pituitary tumors, inflammatory diseases (Tolosa-Hunt), or carotid-cavernous sinus fistulas may result in a third nerve palsy at this level. Clinically, damage can be localized to the cavernous sinus by careful evaluation of the other cranial nerves. Since the oculomotor nerve is in close proximity to nerves IV, V, and VI in the cavernous sinus, damage at this level will involve these nerves in varying degrees.

After the third nerve passes through the cavernous sinus, it enters the orbit through the superior orbital fissure and divides into superior and inferior divisions. The superior division contains the superior rectus and levator innervation while the inferior division carries innervation to the inferior oblique, inferior rectus, and medial rectus muscles. Blunt trauma to the lateral orbital wall may lead to posterior bony displacement and compression of cranial nerves traversing through the superior orbital fissure. Ptosis and ophthalmoplegia are common presentations.

Treatment of ptosis resulting from a third nerve palsy is difficult. Typically, levator function is minimal to absent and the eye is virtually immobilized in a combined hypotropic and exotropic position. Strabismus surgery should be performed first to correct diplopia. Following ocular alignment, the lid can then be elevated with a conservative frontalis sling procedure. Because upgaze is limited in these patients, lagophthalmos and exposure may be problematic.

Horner's Syndrome. The classic Horner's syndrome, or oculosympathetic paresis, consists of the triad of mild ptosis, miosis, and anhidrosis. Horner's syndrome results from damage of the sympathetic innervation to the eye and face. Ptosis is the result of paresis of the Muller's muscle, a sympathetically innervated smooth muscle situated beneath the levator aponeurosis. In the upper lid, this muscle accounts for 2 to 3 mm of lid elevation. The Muller's muscle in the lower lid conjoins with the capsulopalpebral fascia to become the retractors. Loss of sympathetic tone to the Muller's muscle results in the lower lid assuming a higher position relative to the inferior limbus. The slightly elevated lower lid margin has been referred to as "upside-down ptosis." The miotic pupil, due to paresis of the iris dilator muscle, is quite variable, depending on the location, completeness, and chronicity of the defect along the sympathetic pathway. Due to denervation of sweat and vasoconstrictor fibers distributed to the face, the ipsilateral face becomes warm, hyperemic, and unable to perspire (anhidrosis). Another clinical feature is the apparent, rather than real enophthalmos. The patient frequently describes the involved eye as looking "smaller." The narrowed interpalpebral fissure is attributable to the upper lid ptosis and elevation of the lower lid.

Damage to the sympathetic innervation may occur anywhere along the chain of three neurons that connect the brain to the Muller's muscle (see Chapter 11, for Horner's syndrome).

Myogenic

Myasthenia Gravis. Myasthenia gravis is characterized by fluctuating weakness of muscle function, with extraocular and oropharyngeal involvement seen most commonly. Myasthenia is an autoimmune disease in which antibodies are produced to the motor endplates with concomitant loss in the number of acetylcholine receptors at the neuromuscular junctions of skeletal muscle. The result is muscular weakness and fatigue.

Ocular findings including ptosis and diplopia are the presenting symptoms in up to 75% of patients with myasthenia gravis (17). The disease may progress to involve other muscle groups and may even be life-threatening. The majority of patients with ocular myasthenia evolve into a generalized state, most within the first 12 months (6). Thymic enlargement is seen in the majority of these patients, and a thymoma is present in 10% to 15% of patients (6). Thymectomy will often result in improvement of symptoms.

Treatment of ptosis associated with myasthenia gravis is primarily medical. The definitive diagnosis is first made with the Tensilon (edrophonium) test. A small test dose of 0.1 to 0.2 mg is given intravenously, and the patient is observed for the characteristic side effects of tearing, flushing, abdominal cramping, and arrhythmias. If the patient tolerates the test dose, the full remaining dose of 0.8 to 0.9 mg may be given slowly. However, some investigators believe continuing in 0.2-mg increments is preferable to the bolus approach to avoid paradoxical responses to the medicine. Atropine should always be available to reverse any side effects. A positive Tensilon test will result in improvement in strabismus or resolution of the ptosis. If the test is negative and the suspicion for myasthenia gravis remains high, a blood assay for antiacetylcholine receptor antibodies may be obtained. This assay is positive in the majority of patients with generalized symptoms and in half of those with ocular myasthenia (8). If a diagnosis of myasthenia gravis is made, the patient can be treated with a longer-acting anticholinesterase (Mestinon). The dose is titrated to alleviate the patient's symptoms while producing the fewest side effects. Steroids are used alone or in conjunction with Mestinon by some clinicians.

Surgery for the ptosis caused by myasthenia may be necessary if medication is ineffective and conservative treatment such as lid crutches are not acceptable. The surgery of choice is a limited levator resection, taking care to avoid lagophthalmos as these patients may have poor orbicularis tone.

Chronic Progressive External Ophthalmoplegia.
Chronic progressive external ophthalmoplegia (CPEO) is an ocular disorder characterized by slowly progressive ptosis and ophthalmoplegia without complaints of double vision. The condition begins in adolescence and progresses slowly over many years to severe ptosis. Muscle biopsy reveals the ragged red fibers. Systemic abnormalities may be associated with CPEO, as in the retinal pigmentary changes and cardiac conduction abnormalities of Kearns-Sayre. A related but pathologically dissimilar condition is oculopharyngeal dystrophy. This disease also is characterized by slowly progressive ophthalmoplegia, but the disease begins later in life (fifth to sixth decade) and is accompanied by weakness of the pharyngeal musculature.

Treatment of ptosis associated with CPEO is difficult, as these patients often have poor orbicularis tone and Bell's phenomenon. Nonsurgical treatment, such as lid crutches, is advocated by many. If surgery is undertaken, a very conservative approach must be planned and the lid raised only to clear the pupil. The patient must understand that if severe exposure develops, the lid may need to be lowered. The surgical procedure of choice depends on the amount of levator function present. Moderate to good function may allow for a levator resection whereas poor function necessitates a frontalis sling.

Mechanical Ptosis

Mechanical ptosis may develop secondary to scarring from burn injuries or diseases that can cause severe conjunctival cicatricial changes in the lids such as Stevens-Johnson syndrome or ocular pemphigoid. Large orbital tumors and lid lesions may induce mechanical ptosis. Classic examples include neurofibromas, lymphomas, or hemangiomas of the upper lid, but a large basal cell carcinoma on the lid also may produce mechanical ptosis. Treatment of the underlying pathology is the first step in reversing mechanical ptosis.

Ectropion

Ectropion is a condition commonly encountered in clinical practice. The pathogenesis of ectropion varies. Frueh and Schoengarth (9) succinctly summarized the evaluation and treatment of the six elements of pathology that may be present in an ectropic eyelid. These factors include: (1) horizontal lid laxity; (2) medial canthal tendon laxity; (3) punctal malposition; (4) vertical tightness of the skin; (5) orbicularis paresis secondary to seventh nerve palsy; and (6) lower eyelid retractor disinsertion.

The presence of each factor is determined by clinical examination. One or more of these components may be present in an ectropic eyelid. Proper recogni-

tion of the underlying anatomic defect will enable the surgeon to select the appropriate surgical procedure for correction. There are many procedures described for the treatment of each of these eyelid malpositions. In this section, only one technique will be recommended for each of the conditions.

Horizontal Lid Laxity. Horizontal lid laxity (Fig. 27–2) is most likely a result of stretching of the lateral and medial canthal tendons rather than actual elongation of the tarsal plate. This produces a redundancy in the lid tissues, causing the lid margin to fall away from the globe. Horizontal lid laxity can be corrected surgically by a number of procedures. One popular method is full-thickness excision of a wedge of eyelid tissue and closing the defect primarily. One disadvantage of this method of horizontal lid shortening is that it often leads to lateral canthal deformities such as blunting of the lateral canthal angle. Additionally, a block resection technique often exaggerates the laxity of the medial and lateral canthal tendon and may produce a horizontally narrowed palpebral fissure. More importantly, surgical correction is not aimed at the underlying pathology, namely, stretching of the lateral canthal tendon.

In correcting this element of lid malposition, the *"lateral tarsal strip"* procedure advocated by Anderson and Gordy (2) is preferred. In this technique, the eyelid is shortened at the lateral canthal end of the lid. The advantages of this technique are: (1) surgery is directed at correcting the anatomical defect; (2) there are no marginal lid sutures; (3) the danger of lid notching or misdirected lashes irritating the cornea is avoided; (4) canthal malposition and lid shortening may be corrected simultaneously; (5) the procedure can be performed quickly; and (6) the almond-shaped canthal angle is preserved.

The procedure also is useful in correcting eyelid laxity and canthal malposition in an anophthalmic socket. This technique provides immediate lid strength, allow-

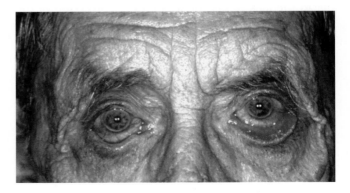

Figure 27–2.
Severe ectropion due to combined medial canthal tendon and lateral canthal tendon laxity.

ing it to support weight, as is needed when there is an ocular prosthesis.

Medial Canthal Tendon Laxity. Medial canthal tendon laxity is detected by observing the lateral displacement of the lower punctum with lateral traction on the nasal eyelid. When the lower punctum is no longer aligned vertically with the upper punctum and can be displaced to the nasal limbus when the eye is in primary position, the medial canthal tendon should be repaired. It is unusual to find medial canthal tendon laxity alone without concomitant lateral canthal laxity. If both elements of lid pathology are present, the medial canthal laxity should be corrected first before proceeding with the horizontal shortening procedure. The aim of medial canthal tendon plication is to restore the anatomic position of the inferior punctum, so that it is in apposition with the globe and tear lake. The technique of medial canthal tendon plication involves the exposure of the tendon, anchoring the lid nasally and posteriorly, and protecting the inferior canaliculus.

Punctal Malposition. The inferior punctum is normally in apposition with the globe and in vertical alignment with the superior punctum. Occasionally, punctal eversion without horizontal eyelid laxity or anterior lamellae cicatrix can be seen. The exact cause of this condition is unclear, but dehiscence or disinsertion of the lower eyelid retractors along the medial lid may be contributory. If punctal eversion is severe and the patient is symptomatic, surgical correction will be necessary to return the punctum to its normal anatomic position. A common approach is excision of tarsus, conjunctiva, and eyelid retractors as a horizontal, fusiform wedge at the lower margin of the tarsal plate. The conjunctiva is closed with three or four 7-0 absorbable sutures. However, inadequate punctal inversion and recurrent punctal ectropion are frequent drawbacks of a simple ellipse closure. Failure to unite the lower eyelid retractors to the tarsal plate and lack of a cicatrix to maintain the punctum in an inverted position are factors contributing to the lack of precise and lasting correction of the condition. A modification of the simple closure technique is preferred (19), which emphasizes the union of the lower eyelid retractors, not just to the conjunctiva but to the tarsal plate, and the formation of a cicatrix to help keep the punctum in its normal anatomical alignment. This technique can be combined with a horizontal shortening procedure of the eyelid, if laxity of the lower lid accompanies the punctal eversion; if not, it can be performed alone.

Vertical Tightness of the Skin. Cicatricial ectropion is caused by abnormal vertical shortening of the anterior lamella, which pulls the lid away from the globe. Conditions that cause excessive scarring or shrinkage in the skin or subcutaneous tissue (e.g., trauma, skin disease, burns) can cause ectropion. If lid retraction is due to one vertical line of scar tissue, a Z-plasty can be performed. However, if vertical tightness of the skin is diffuse, a full-thickness skin graft is indicated.

Orbicularis Paresis Secondary to Seventh Nerve Palsy. Ectropion is common in seventh cranial nerve palsies due to lack of orbicularis tone. To correct the lower lid position, the lateral tarsal strip procedure is recommended since it provides an immediate support to the paretic lower eyelid. In some cases, palpebral spring or lid-loading with a gold weight in the upper lid helps to augment lid closure and minimizes exposure.

Lower Eyelid Retractors Disinsertion. The lower eyelid retractors refer to both the capsulopalpebral fascia and the Muller's muscle. The capsulopalpebral fascia originates as the capsulopalpebral head with delicate attachments to the inferior rectus muscle and tendon. The capsulopalpebral head divides into two portions as it extends around and fuses with the sheath of the inferior oblique muscle. Anterior to the inferior oblique muscle, the two portions of the capsulopalpebral head rejoin to form the Lockwood's ligament. The fascial tissue anterior to the Lockwood's ligament is termed the capsulopalpebral fascia. A large portion of the capsulopalpebral fascia proceeds anteriorly to insert on the inferior fornix and to form the Tenon's capsule on the globe. The rest of the capsulopalpebral fascia then proceeds upward to insert onto the inferior margin and anterior and posterior surface of the tarsal plate (11).

Disinsertion of the retractors of the lower eyelid may manifest either as ectropion or entropion. Differential vector forces between the anterior and posterior lamella often determines whether ectropion or entropion will result (Fig. 27–3). Lower eyelid retractors disinsertion in the absence of horizontal laxity or anterior lamella shortage is the most difficult element of an ectropic eyelid to recognize clinically. In patients with lower eyelid retractors disinsertion or dehiscence, there are four clinical clues one should seek. These clinical clues are similar to those found in an entropic eyelid: (1) Deeper inferior fornix (the capsulopalpebral fascia sends attachments to the inferior fornix. When the retractors are disinserted, it pulls the inferior fornix inward, thereby deepening the inferior fornix). (2) Higher resting lower lid position (because the retractors are no longer attached to the inferior margin of the tarsal plate, when the involved eyelid is pulled out of its ectropic position, it often has a higher resting position of the lid margin). (3) Diminished lower eyelid excursion on downgaze (due to absence of attachment of the retractors to the tarsal plate). (4) A horizontal infratarsal red band at the edge of the disinserted retractors (This red band is thought to be the orbicularis muscle fibers

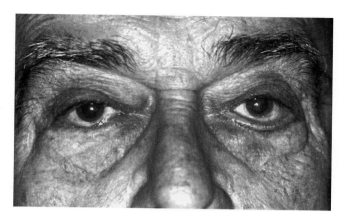

Figure 27–3.
Retractors disinsertion manifesting as entropion in one lid and ectropion in another.

showing through the area of retractors disinsertion. However, this sign is often not useful as the inferior fornix is commonly injected as the result of chronic lid eversion).

Occasionally, tarsal ectropion, a striking and unusual form of ectropion may be seen. In these patients, the lid is completely everted, with the tarsal plate turned essentially upside down. The palpebral conjunctiva is turned outward, and the lower border of the tarsus is flipped upward to the level of the inferior limbal margin. Putterman (15) corrected this condition by reattaching the disinserted Muller's muscle and capsulopalpebral fascia to the inferior tarsus via an anterior approach. Wesley (21) described an internal approach in which a wedge of redundant conjunctiva was excised and the retractors reattached to the inferior tarsal edge. An alternative treatment method, analogous to the medial spindle technique in correcting punctal ectropion may be used. For this procedure, a transconjunctival approach is used, but without excision of any forniceal conjunctiva. The looping passage of the fornix sutures through full-thickness eyelid and the formation of an in-

flammatory cicatrix, produce a vector force that helps to effect and maintain an inward rotation of the lid margin. The key to success in this method is to unite the lower eyelid retractors, not just the conjunctiva, to the tarsal plate, as the retractors are responsible for the inversion effect. Horizontal shortening is commonly required as well.

Entropion

Entropion is the inturning of the lid margin toward the globe, resulting in corneal irritation from the skin and lashes. Entropion can be classified into three basic groups: congenital, involutional, and cicatricial. Primary congenital entropion is an exceedingly rare developmental anomaly, while the involutional variety remains one of the most common eyelid conditions encountered in practice. The cicatricial variety, although uncommon, is by far the most challenging to treat.

Congenital Entropion and Epiblepharon. Congenital entropion is characterized by inversion of the eyelid margin, causing corneal irritation. This should not be confused with epiblepharon (Fig. 27–4), which is characterized by a redundant horizontal pretarsal skinfold pressing the lashes against the globe. Clinically, true congenital entropion is identified by an absence of lower eyelid crease and limited retraction on downgaze. The popular belief is that pretarsal orbicularis muscle hypertrophy is the etiology of lid margin rotation. However, more recently, the lower eyelid retractors disinsertion has been implicated (20). Therefore, once congenital entropion is recognized, surgical exploration of the retractors is indicated and the disinserted retractors should be reattached onto the tarsal plate.

In contrast, exploration of the retractors is not indicated in a patient with epiblepharon. Epiblepharon is the inturning of normal eyelashes in the nasal one-third of the eyelid, induced mechanically by an abnormal

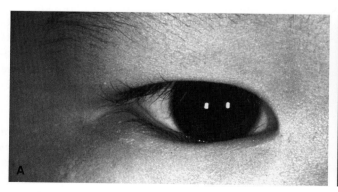

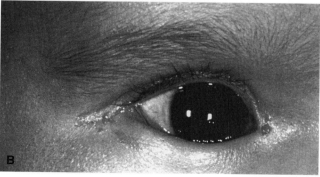

Figure 27–4.
A, Epiblepharon characterized by redundant pretarsal skin pressing the lashes against the cornea. The tarsal plate is in an upright position. **B,** Congenital entropion demonstrating inturning of the lower lid margin. The tarsal plate is not in an upright position.

skinfold. The lid margin itself is in the normal upright position. Epiblepharon may be caused by a lack of fenestrating fibers from the retractor aponeurosis inserting under the skin. This lack of subcutaneous adhesion accounts for the absent lower lid crease, permitting the lid fold to roll superiorly toward the lid margin. Epiblepharon generally causes conjunctival irritation and reflexive tearing. Corneal damage is uncommon since the misdirected lashes in infants are fine and soft. This condition is usually bilateral and more commonly seen in Asians. Most children with epiblepharon tend to outgrow the condition as their facial structures change. However, in symptomatic individuals, surgical correction may be indicated. Surgical management consists of excising a strip of pretarsal skin and orbicularis muscle below the lash line. An absorbable suture is used to close the skin edges. The absorbable suture provokes the formation of an inflammatory cicatrix under the eyelash line, preventing superior migration of the preseptal skin. It also eliminates the necessity to remove the suture in an infant.

Involutional Entropion. In involutional entropion, similar to involutional ectropion, several elements of pathology may be present. These factors include: (1) horizontal laxity of the eyelid tissues (medial and lateral canthal tendons); (2) overriding of the preseptal orbicularis; (3) dehiscence/disinsertion of the lower eyelid retractors; and (4) relative enophthalmos related to some atrophy of orbital fat.

The presence of each factor is determined by clinical examination. One or more of these components may be present in an entropic eyelid. Proper recognition of the underlying anatomic defect will enable the surgeon to select the appropriate surgical procedure for correction. Indications for surgical correction are based on symptoms and physical findings. The constant mechanical rubbing of the eyelashes against the ocular surface results in symptoms of persistent foreign body sensation, conjunctival injection, tearing, and discharge. This can often lead to secondary stromal scarring, corneal thinning, and vascularization. There are many procedures developed for the treatment of each of these eyelid malpositions. In this section, one technique will be recommended for each of the elements.

Horizontal Lid Laxity. A common element of pathology encountered in an entropic eyelid is horizontal lid laxity. Horizontal laxity may manifest either as entropion or ectropion of the lower eyelid. Differential vector forces between the anterior lamella and the posterior lamella often determine whether entropion or ectropion will result. A generalized horizontal laxity of the lower eyelid is present if there is sagging of the margin below the inferior limbus, when the lid is pulled out of its entropic position. This also can be demonstrated

when the eyelid margin can be pulled more than a centimeter away from the globe, and it fails to snap back against the globe. After the examiner has determined that horizontal laxity is present, it must be determined whether it is due to laxity of the medial canthal tendon or to stretching of the lateral canthal tendon. Normally, the inferior punctum is in vertical alignment with the upper punctum. If the inferior punctum can be displaced to the nasal limbus when the eye is in primary position, medial canthal tendon laxity is present and should be repaired. The aim of medial canthal tendon plication is to restore the anatomic position of the inferior punctum, so that it is in apposition with the globe and tear lake. If lateral canthal tendon laxity coexists, then a horizontal lid tightening procedure is needed (i.e., the lateral tarsal strip procedure).

Overriding of the Preseptal Orbicularis. This condition has been commonly referred to as acute *spastic entropion* (16). It is most frequently seen after intraocular surgery, chronic ocular irritation or inflammation, and often occurs in patients who have unrecognized involutional lid changes preoperatively. This condition is most likely due to the preseptal orbicularis muscle moving upward to a position overriding the pretarsal orbicularis, inducing inward rotation of the eyelid margin. The acute entropion usually resolves when the irritation/entropion cycle is broken by treating both the underlying cause and the entropion. Clinically, forceful squeezing of the eyelids will reproduce an immediate inversion of the lid margin. If the clinician is unable to reproduce it while the patient is in an upright position, placing the patient in a supine position by putting the examination chair in a flat position will bring out the spastic entropion. Taping the inturned eyelid to evert the margin will afford temporary relief for some patients. A quick and useful surgical technique for this condition is the fornix sutures technique (16). This procedure is particularly useful for debilitated or nursing home patients who are unable to undergo a more prolonged surgical procedure. One should aim for a slight overeversion of the lid margin when tying the sutures. The use of full-thickness sutures is quick, easily performed, and gives immediate relief, but its relatively high recurrence rates limits its usefulness for a permanent correction. A more permanent correction may be achieved by combining the fornix suture technique with a lid-tightening procedure.

Retractors Disinsertion Entropion. Another element of pathology present in an entropic eyelid is retractors disinsertion. Disinsertion of the lower eyelid retractors from the inferior tarsal border renders the eyelid unstable, thus predisposing it to the development of either ectropion or entropion. Again, the differential vector forces between the anterior and posterior lamella often determine whether ectropion or entropion will result. The readers should review the lower eyelid anatomy and the clinical clues for detection of retractors disinsertion in the ectropion section.

Direct repair of the disinserted retractors is analogous to the aponeurotic repair of ptosis of the upper eyelid (7). Intraoperative adjustment of lid contour and function ensures a more predictable result. Overzealous shortening or advancement of the retractors will exaggerate the eversion effect, leading to eyelid retraction and scleral show. If this occurs, the wound is opened and the retractor aponeurosis is resutured to a lower level on the tarsal plate.

In patients with involutional entropion and concomitant horizontal laxity, a horizontal eyelid tightening procedure such as the lateral tarsal strip procedure can be performed.

Orbital Enophthalmos. A decrease in orbital volume due to trauma, a phthisical globe, enucleation, or relative enophthalmos secondary to aging changes can lead to suboptimal support for the eyelid. This eyelid malposition problem can best be corrected by addressing the underlying pathology. If the lack of volume is secondary to anophthalmos, a secondary orbital implant, orbital floor implant or augmented prosthesis may be used. In the case of a phthisical globe, enucleation with implant and prosthesis may be indicated.

Cicatricial Entropion. Cicatricial entropion is caused by shrinkage of the tarsal conjunctival surface or shortening of the posterior lamella of the eyelids. This occurs as the result of pemphigoid, trauma, chemical burns, infection, and Stevens-Johnson syndrome, or following enucleation.

A cicatricial etiology for entropion should be suspected if resistance to downward traction on the lid is encountered and if horizontal traction on the lid does not temporarily improve the entropion. Difficulty of lid eversion may be present. Inspection of the conjunctival fornices invariably will reveal symblepharon, lid margin keratinization, and metaplasia of the meibomian gland openings.

The procedure of choice for correction of cicatricial entropion is the marginal rotational procedure (22). The surgical aim is to sever the vertical cicatricial scar band in the posterior lamella and mechanically evert the lid margin along the longitudinal axis. This eversion technique also can be used for upper eyelid cicatricial entropion (4).

■ TRICHIASIS AND DISTICHIASIS

Trichiasis is defined as normal lashes that have a normal location in the anterior lamella but are misdirected and rub against the cornea and conjunctiva. Although trichiasis may be present at birth, it is much more commonly acquired. Trichiasis is often the result of chronic blepharitis, trachoma, cicatricial pemphigoid, and Stevens-Johnson syndrome. Trauma with vertical eyelid lacerations or alkaline burns also can induce misdirected lashes.

Trichiasis should be distinguished from distichiasis, which implies an accessory row of abnormal lashes emanating from the meibomian gland orifices. Distichiasis is commonly a congenital disorder, with autosomal dominant inheritance and variable expressivity. This is a developmental anomaly in which a complete pilosebaceous unit is located within the posterior lamella. This anomaly represents a failure of primary epithelial differentiation into a sebaceous gland rather than metaplasia of the meibomian gland itself. The condition may involve only a few lashes or the entire lid margin.

Distichiasis also can be an acquired condition, occurring in cases of Stevens-Johnson syndrome, toxic epidermal necrolysis, cicatricial pemphigoid, and chemical and physical injuries of the eyelids. Distichiasis is associated with congenital lymphedema, chemosis and elephantiasis (23). It has been postulated that immunologic, chemical, and physical stimuli provoke metaplastic changes within the meibomian glands, resulting in aberrant formation of hair follicles.

Patients with distichiasis and trichiasis present with similar symptoms of a watery, red, and irritated eye. The discomfort is caused by the offending lashes rubbing on the cornea and conjunctiva, resulting in corneal irritation and abrasion. In more severe cases, corneal damage may progress to ulceration and perforation.

The treatment of distichiasis and trichiasis are similar and based on the extent of lid involvement. If the affected area is limited to a few lashes, simple periodic epilation or electrolysis may suffice. More extensive involvement limited to a localized area of the lid may be treated by focal cryotherapy application. Care must be taken in darkly pigmented patients due to the risk of skin depigmentation following cryotherapy. Diffuse lid involvement may require more extensive cryotherapy treatment. For distichiasis, If the aberrant lashes are too numerous and diffuse, the eyelid is split into anterior and posterior lamellae and the offending lash follicles within the tarsal plate are treated with cryotherapy. This treatment method spares cryodestruction to the anterior lamella lash follicles and skin melanocytes. Diffuse trichiasis associated with posterior cicatrix can be effectively treated with a tarsal fracture/marginal rotation procedure (4, 22).

■ EYELID RETRACTION

Thyroid eye disease is the most frequent cause of eyelid retraction. Other less common causes are trauma, surgery, seventh cranial nerve palsy, congenital lid retraction, Parinaud's dorsal midbrain syndrome, Parkinson's disease, cirrhosis, and myasthenia gravis.

Retraction of the eyelids is one of the most common ophthalmic manifestations of Graves' disease. This malposition may occur with or without exophthalmos and is responsible for functional and cosmetic problems in many patients with thyroid-related eye disease. The etiology of eyelid retraction in Graves' disease is not clearly understood, but several factors seem to be contributory. In the upper lid, these factors include: (1) Müller's muscle overreaction due to sympathetic stimulation; (2) levator contraction due to degeneration and thickening of the levator muscle and/or the aponeurosis; (3) levator adhesions to the orbicularis muscle and orbital septum; and (4) overreaction of the levator-superior rectus complex in response to a hypophoria produced by fibrosis and retraction of the inferior rectus.

In the lower eyelid, fibrosis of the inferior rectus exerting a retraction action on the lower eyelid via its capsulopalpebral head appears to be more influential than adrenergic stimulation of the Müller's muscle.

Surgical treatment of eyelid retraction is usually reserved for patients whose endocrine status and eyelid height have been stable for at least 6 months to 1 year, and in whom retraction causes significant exposure keratopathy, lagophthalmos, chronic conjunctival injection, and cosmetic imperfection.

A number of surgical procedures have been described to bring the retracted upper eyelid downward. These included: levator tenotomy or recession, Müller's muscle resection or myectomy, and combined levator tenotomy and müllerectomy. The aponeurotic approach for eyelid recession described by Harvey and Anderson (10) is anatomically, surgically, and physiologically sound. In this technique, the Müller's muscle is completely extirpated, the lateral horn of the levator severed, and the aponeurosis recessed. Additionally, this anatomic approach is similar to that used in aponeurotic ptosis surgery.

Repair of the retraction of the lower lid requires disinsertion of the lower lid retractors from tarsus via a conjunctival approach. An interpositional graft must then be placed in the space between the retractors and tarsus. Ideally, the graft material should be stiff enough to support the lower lid, essentially propping it into a better position next to the globe. Hard palate (12) is ideally suited as a graft material because it is stiff, autologous, and lined by mucous membrane, which can be used as a conjunctival substitute. The graft must be sutured into position, carefully burying all suture material so it does not abrade the cornea.

■ REFERENCES

1. Anderson RL, Baumgartner A: Amblyopia and ptosis. Arch Ophthalmol 1980; 98: 1068–1069.
2. Anderson RL, Gordy DD: The tarsal strip procedure. Arch Ophthalmol 1979; 97: 2192–2196.
3. Anderson RL, Nowinski TS: The five-flap technique for blepharophimosis. Arch Ophthalmol 1989; 107: 448–452.
4. Ballen PH: A simple procedure for the relief of trichiasis and entropion of the upper lid. Arch Ophthalmol 1964; 72: 239–240.
5. Berke RN, Wadsworth JAC: Histology of the levator muscle in congenital and acquired ptosis. Arch Ophthalmol 1955; 53: 413–428.
6. Wyngaarden J, Smith L, Bennett C (eds). Cecil Textbook of Medicine. WB Saunders, 1988; 2285–2287.
7. Dryden RM, Leibsohn J, Wobig J: Senile entropion: pathogenesis and treatment. Arch Ophthalmol 1978; 96: 1883–1885.
8. Evoli A, Tonali P, Bartoccioni E, Lo Monaco M: Ocular myasthenia: diagnostic and therapeutic problems. Acta Neurol Scand 1988; 77: 31–35.
9. Frueh BR, Schoengarth LD: Evaluation and treatment of the patient with ectropion. Ophthalmology 1982; 89: 1049–1054.
10. Harvey JT, Anderson RL: The aponeurotic approach to eyelid retraction. Ophthalmology 1981; 88: 513–524.
11. Hawes MJ, Dortzbach RK: The microscopic anatomy of the lower eyelid retractors. Arch Ophthalmol 1982; 100: 1313–1318.
12. Kersten RC, Kulwin DR, Levartovsky S, Tiradellis H, Tse DT: Management of lower lid retraction with hard palate mucosa grafting. Arch Ophthalmol 1990; 108: 1339–1343.
13. McCulloch DL, Wright KW: Unilateral congenital ptosis: compensatory head posturing and amblyopia. Ophthalmic Plast Reconstr Surg 1993; 9: 196–200.
14. Mustarde JC: Epicanthal folds and problems of telecanthus. Trans Ophthal Soc UK 1963; 83: 397–411.
15. Putterman AM: Ectropion of the lower eyelid secondary to Muller's muscle-capsulopalpebral fascia detachment. Am J Ophthalmol 1978; 85: 814–817.
16. Quickert MH, Rathbun E: Suture repair of entropion. Arch Ophthalmol 1971; 85: 304–305.
17. Seybold ME: Myasthenia gravis: a clinical and basic science review. JAMA 1983; 250: 2516–2521.
18. Townes PL, Muechler EK: Blepharophimosis, ptosis, epicanthus inversus and primary amenorrhea: a dominant trait. Arch Ophthalmol 1979; 97: 1664–1666.

19. Tse DT: Surgical correction of punctal malposition. Am J Ophthalmol 1985; 100: 339–341.

20. Tse DT, Anderson RL: Aponeurosis disinsertion in congenital entropion. Arch Ophthalmol 1983; 101: 436–440.

21. Wesley RE: Tarsal ectropion from detachment of the lower eyelid retractors. Am J Ophthalmol 1982; 93: 491–495.

22. Wies FA: Spastic entropion. Trans Am Acad Ophthalmol-Otolaryngol 1955; 59: 503–506.

23. Kolin T, Johns KJ, Wadlington WB, Butler MG, Sunalp MA, Wright KW: Hereditary lymphedema and distichiasis. Arch Ophthalmol 1991; 109(7): 980–981.

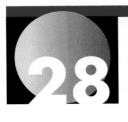

28 Eyelid Tumors

Steve Gilberg, David T. Tse

Proper recognition of the clinical characteristics and knowledge of the biologic behavior of eyelid lesions are important in their management. The eyelids provide essential protective mechanisms against glare, infection, foreign particles, and trauma, and are crucial in the distribution of precorneal tear film. When this unique anatomic structure is altered, the result can be ocular discomfort, decreased vision, and even loss of the eye. A permanent alteration in the delicate lid–globe relationship can result from the destructive growth of a malignant lesion or the improper management of a benign lesion. Surgical excision of periocular tumors requires attention to several principles: (1) an understanding of the biologic behavior of the lesion; (2) complete eradication of the tumor followed by lid reconstruction; (3) render protection to the globe; (4) maintain a functional lacrimal drainage system; and (5) cosmesis.

■ DISTINGUISHING FEATURES OF MALIGNANT AND BENIGN EYELID LESIONS

In assessing an eyelid lesion, attempts should be made to determine the lesion's malignant potential. A prolonged history of sun exposure should arouse suspicion of actinically induced lesions such as melanoma, squamous, or basal cell carcinoma. Patients of light complexion are more likely to develop malignant skin lesions, whereas it is uncommon to find basal, squamous cell carcinoma, or melanoma in darkly pigmented individuals. A history of basal or squamous cell carcinoma on the face, neck, or forearm suggests a threshold level of exposure in the past and a greater predisposition toward additional lesions.

The presence of a lesion that has remained unchanged for many years suggests a benign process, whereas one that is of recent onset and demonstrates new changes may indicate either an inflammatory process or a malignant lesion. If the patient is uncertain as to the duration or previous size of a lesion, review of old photographs may be helpful. A lesion that bleeds spontaneously or frequently also may provoke suspicion of a malignant process.

Ophthalmologists are afforded an excellent method of detailed observation of lesions of the eyelid with the slit-lamp biomicroscope. This illuminated, highly magnified image enables the observer to assess the numerous fine details of a lesion. The lesion should first be examined undisturbed and then with surface crusting or discharge removed. A central ulcer, rolled edges, and telangiectatic vessels traversing a lesion are more characteristic of a basal cell carcinoma. By transillumination, one can determine whether a lesion is cystic or solid, with most cystic tumors being of benign origin. Examination of structures adjacent to or incorporated within the lesion also can provide clues to the biologic activity of the lesion. Malignant processes through their destructive growth disturb the normal anatomic relationship of the meibomian orifices to the eyelid margin and can cause loss or misdirection of lashes.

After examination of the lesion, assessment of the lymphatic drainage system of the eyelid is essential. Tumor spread follows the normal anatomic lymphatic channels with the outer two thirds of the upper and outer one third of the lower lid draining into the ipsilateral preauricular nodes. The medial one third of the upper lid and the medial two thirds of the lower lid drain into the ipsilateral submandibular nodes. The cervical lymphatic chain and supraclavicular nodes also should be assessed for possible involvement. In patients with known lid tumors exhibiting metastatic potential, such as melanoma, sebaceous cell carcinoma, squamous cell carcinoma, or Merkle cell tumor, the ipsilateral lymph nodes should always be palpated during each follow-up examination.

■ INDICATIONS FOR BIOPSY

Any suspicious lesion on the eyelid possessing characteristics suggestive of a malignant process should be considered for biopsy. The changes clinicians should look for in an eyelid lesion include: (1) a skin growth that increases in size and appears pearly, translucent, tan, brown, black, or multicolored; (2) a mole, birthmark, or any brown spot that changes in size, thickness, texture, and is irregular in outline; (3) a pigmented lesion that appears after age 21 and is larger than 6 mm; (4) a spot or sore that continues to itch, hurt, crust, scab, erode, or bleed; and (5) an open sore that does not heal within 3 weeks. Some cutaneous malignancies may mimic benign lesions in appearance, and the only method of accurate diagnosis is biopsy.

■ METHODS OF BIOPSY

Excisional

A biopsy is a necessary component of the management plan of all patients with lesions suspicious for malignancy. If there is clinical certainty of the benign nature of a lesion, an excisional biopsy, removing the lesion in its entirety, can be undertaken. Pathologic examination of the specimen will either confirm its benign nature or, if it is found to be malignant, assess the completeness of excision.

Incisional

If malignancy cannot be excluded clinically, an incisional biopsy is usually performed. An incisional biopsy obtains a portion of the lesion to confirm histologically its malignant nature before more definitive treatment. When obtaining an incisional biopsy, be sure that the surgical sample includes not only pathology, but also a rim of adjacent normal tissue. Many diseases produce nonspecific "endstage" changes centrally but diagnostic features may be present only at the leading edge of the lesion. The surgeon should have some idea about the suspected pathologic diagnosis of a lesion and biopsy accordingly. For example, the base of a keratoacanthoma may be indistinguishable from a squamous cell carcinoma; submit the entire lesion so that the pathologist can section through the cup-shaped crater, a clue that may aid the pathologist in the correct interpretation. After confirmation of a malignant tumor, definitive excision and reconstruction can then be planned.

Eyelid tumors may present a challenge in obtaining adequate biopsy material without disturbing the normal anatomic relationship of the eyelid and globe. Excessive tissue removal can lead to ectropion, punctal malposition, and cosmetic deformity. In the majority of small biopsies (3 to 4 mm), the excision bed will heal well by secondary intention. Lesions involving the lid margin, peripunctal region, or those exceeding 1 cm in size may require more careful closure.

For lesions posterior to the lash line, a shave biopsy with a microsurgical blade or sharp Westcott scissors following the contours of the lid margin is useful. Gentle cautery should be applied sparingly to avoid damage to the lash follicles lying more anteriorly.

■ BENIGN EYELID LESIONS

It is not uncommon to refer to most benign-appearing eyelid tumors under the global catch phrase "papilloma." Frequently, clinicians apply this term to numerous lesions, including skin tags, warts, seborrheic and actinic keratoses. The term papilloma should be reserved for pathologic description of lesions with microscopic papillomatous changes. By applying more precise terms to many of the benign eyelid lesions encountered, clinicians will become more proficient at recognition.

■ EPITHELIAL ORIGIN

Squamous Cell Papilloma

Squamous papilloma is a broad term applied to several lesions that display a variable clinical appearance but share a common histologic characteristic of benign hyperplasia of the squamous epithelium of the epidermis. This lesion is the most common benign eyelid tumor and has frequently been referred to as a skin tag. Clinically, squamous papilloma may present in various forms: mushroom shape, flat or sessile, polypoid, or with a corrugated surface. Some may show extreme hyperkeratosis (clinical leukoplakia), forming a cutaneous horn. The most common ones appear as flesh-colored, pedunculated or sessile (broad base) in appearance (Fig. 28–1). Occasionally, clinicians have used the term verruca vulgaris to describe squamous papillomas with a corrugated surface. A true verruca vulgaris typically appears as a filiform wart and must have identifiable viral inclusions. Histologically, a squamous papilloma has finger-like projections covered by acanthotic epithelium and hyperkeratosis. They usually overlie a fibrovascular core derived from the dermis. Simple surgical excision with histopathologic examination is the treatment of choice.

Pseudoepitheliomatous Hyperplasia

Pseudoepitheliomatous hyperplasia tends to occur in areas of chronic inflammation such as in granulomas and ulcers, in stasis dermatitis, lupus vulgaris, and in basal cell carcinomas. This benign cutaneous lesion usually displays a rapid growth phase and presents as an elevated, ulcerative lesion, similar in appearance to a basal or squamous cell carcinoma. In fact, this lesion is often misdiagnosed as a malignancy because of its resemblance to carcinoma. Other causes include burns, radiation, and insect bites (37). Histologically, the thickened epidermis protrudes downward into the dermis. This microscopic feature should be distinguished from a squamous cell carcinoma, in which the lobules of downward protruding epidermis have invasive, infiltrating edges. In pseudoepitheliomatous hyperplasia, the edges of the lesion appear to push down into the dermis, rather than invade into it. Frequently, pseudoepitheliomatous hyperplasia is a finding secondary to other cutaneous pathology, such as overlying a malignant lymphoma or granular cell tumor. It also is seen with cutaneous blastomycosis. The degree of pseudoepitheliomatous hyperplasia seen with cutaneous blastomycosis may mimic squamous cell carcinoma both clinically and histologically. Treatment involves excision including, when possible, the inciting lesion. Therapy should be directed toward the predisposing disorder.

Keratoacanthoma

Keratoacanthoma is a solitary benign epidermal tumor that occurs predominately on sun-exposed white skin of middle-aged and elderly patients. This lesion typically starts as an erythematous maculopapular mass. Within a few weeks it grows into a firm, dome-shaped, violaceous, indurated nodule with a central keratin-filled crater (Fig. 28–2). It tends to grow rapidly over 6 to 8 weeks, attaining a maximum size of 2 cm in diameter and 1 cm in height. A lesion may persist for several years but characteristically undergoes spontaneous regression within weeks to several months. It often involutes with minimal

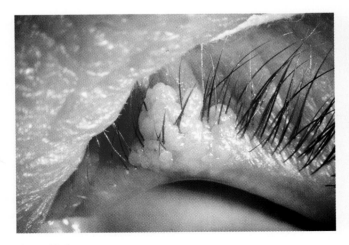

Figure 28–1.
Squamous papilloma.

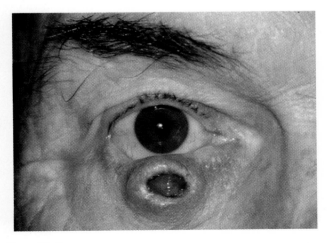

Figure 28–2.
Keratoacanthoma.

residual scarring. Recurrences are rare. The clinical features of abrupt onset and rapid growth followed by spontaneous involution are so distinctive for this lesion that the diagnosis is virtually assured when both of these characteristics are present. Squamous cell carcinoma may have a similar clinical appearance but generally lacks the distinctive history of a rapid growth pattern. Keratoacanthomas may occur in patients with xeroderma pigmentosum, in immunosuppressed individuals, organ transplant recipients, and as a component of the Muir-Torre syndrome.

The nature of treatment must be made only after careful evaluation and biopsy examination to rule out a true squamous cell carcinoma. An excisional biopsy is recommended, but if not feasible, a generous elliptical incisional biopsy from normal skin to normal skin through the center of the lesion should be obtained. A simple punch biopsy is insufficient. Without the overall architectural pattern of the lesion, pathologists may have difficulty distinguishing between this lesion and squamous cell carcinoma. The pathology involves thickening of the epidermis with downward protrusion into the dermis; the deep edge lacks the infiltrative advancing zone characteristic of squamous cell carcinoma. Intraepithelial microabscesses and inflammation at the base are frequently present.

Surgical excision is the treatment of choice for keratoacanthomas situated in the periocular region. It is simultaneously diagnostic and curative. Other treatment measures include cryosurgery, electrodesiccation and curettage, radiation, intralesional steroids, and topical or intralesional 5-fluorouracil.

Seborrheic Keratosis

A seborrheic keratosis is generally a verrucous, round or ovoid, variably raised, light brown to black, sharply demarcated papule or plaque. This benign epidermal lesion usually ranges in dimension from a few millimeters to several centimeters and appear to be "stuck on" to the surface of the skin (Fig. 28–3). The surface of the lesion typically displays a greasy or waxy appearance. Close inspection of the surface may show numerous grooves, often referred to as "cerebriform" in character. Seborrheic keratoses are most commonly situated on the face, neck, and trunk. They usually occur in elderly and middle-aged individuals. A common analogue of seborrheic keratosis in black adults and many Asians is called dermatosis papulosa nigra. A rare association has been noted in which sudden appearance of multiple, large seborrheic keratoses over a short period of time may be considered a marker of internal malignancy.

Microscopically, the lesion is composed of small, benign, epithelioid cells with a tendency to form pseudocysts within the mass of the lesion. Hyperkeratosis, acanthosis, and papillomatosis are observed, but each of these elements may predominate in specific lesions. Sharply demarcated keratin plugs are characteristic, and pigmentation is variable. The management of this lesion is mainly for cosmesis and diagnosis and is easily achieved by surgical excision. Since the epidermal proliferation occurs predominately outward rather than into the dermis, the base of the lesion is sharply demarcated. This feature permits its removal with a shave excision. Cryoablation, curettage, and electrodessication also are effective treatment methods.

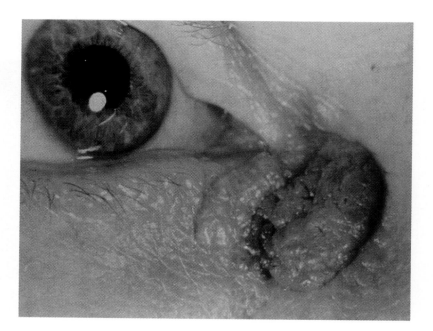

Figure 28–3.
Seborrheic keratosis over the medial canthus displaying a rough, cerebriform surface architecture and a stuck-on appearance.

Inverted Follicular Keratosis

Inverted follicular keratosis is a variant of pseudoepitheliomatous hyperplasia and presents as a wart-like keratotic nodule or cutaneous horn. Originally it was believed to arise from hair follicles—hence the term. Histologic examination reveals suprabasilar acantholysis with swirls of benign squamous cells (squamous eddy) just above this zone. It is associated with exuberant hyperkeratosis and may be considered a cause of "cutaneous horn." Most dermatopathologists now believe that inverted follicular keratosis is a form of irritated seborrheic keratosis. Surgical excision must be complete; otherwise recurrence is likely.

Actinic (Senile) Keratosis is a precursor to squamous cell carcinoma. (See squamous cell carcinoma.)

Dermoid Cyst

Dermoid cysts are congenital sequestrations of surface ectoderm comprising elements of both the epidermis and skin appendage structures such as hair, sweat gland, or sebaceous glands. A dermoid cyst is a choristomatous malformation—a growth that originates during embryogenesis from tissue elements that normally are not present in the location of the lesion. It has been postulated that surface ectoderm is trapped along lines of embryonic closure, such as in a bony suture. Dermoid cyst is the most common benign orbital tumor encountered in the pediatric population, typically discovered shortly after birth. The superficial subcutaneous dermoid, usually appears as a smooth, freely movable, painless nodule situated beneath the lateral brow. The lesion is not attached to the skin, but a pedicle is affixed to the bone at the frontozygomatic suture line. They also may present along the medial periocular region. Deep orbital dermoids typically present in adolescence or adult life, when slow cystic expansion leads to globe displacement and proptosis. Sharply marginated orbital wall defect adjacent to the lesion is a characteristic finding on computed tomography (CT). Some deep dermoids may erode through orbital bones and extend into temporalis fossa, sinus, or even the intracranial cavity. Microscopically, dermoid cysts are lined by stratified squamous epithelium with adnexal elements in the wall. The lumen is filled with keratinous debris and sebaceous material. Complete surgical excision with preservation of the lining is recommended, as spillage of the cystic contents can incite a foreign body granulomatous inflammation reaction in the surrounding tissues.

Epidermoid Cyst

An epidermoid cyst is characterized clinically by its cheesy content, which is keratin derived from the hyperkeratotic squamous epithelial lining of the cyst. Most of these cysts are derived from plugged hair follicles or inclusions of squamous epithelial cells that have been displaced into a subcutaneous location. They are slow-growing, elevated, round benign tumors of varying size. A key clinical feature is the movable skin overlying the lesion. With rupture of the cyst, a considerable foreign-body reaction results. Malignant degeneration is rare, but squamous cell and basal cell carcinomas arising from epidermoid cysts have been reported. Histologically, an epidermoid cyst is distinguished from a dermoid cyst by the absence of adnexal structures in the enclosing wall.

Epidermal Inclusion Cysts

Epidermal inclusion cysts appear as yellow, solitary, nontender intracutaneous or subcutaneous nodules measuring 2 to 5 mm in diameter (Fig. 28–4). They may result from aberrant invagination of surface epidermis after trauma in which nests of epithelium are deposited

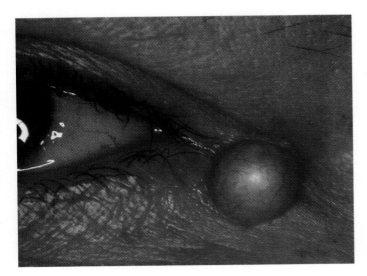

Figure 28–4.
An intracutaneous epidermal inclusion cyst.

within the dermis. Histologically, the cyst wall is lined by keratinized stratified squamous epithelium with a keratin-filled lumen. Adnexal structures are absent. The keratin is somewhat greasy (and malodorous), and the greasy contents of these cysts has led to the misnomer of "sebaceous cyst." There is nothing related to the sebaceous apparatus with these cysts. A cyst may rupture spontaneously, eliciting a granulomatous response and sometimes secondary infection. One should wait for the inflammation to subside before attempting to remove the cyst. Complete removal of the entire cyst wall is required for permanent cure.

Cutaneous melanocytic lesions arise from three cell sources: nevus cells, deep dermal melanocytes, and epidermal melanocytes. All are derived from neural crest cells. The morphologic characteristics of melanocytes and nevus cells are similar; however, nevus cells show a characteristic focal collection of nests and lack dendritic processes. Lesions composed of nevus cells are the pigmented nevi and may occur in the epidermis or within the dermis. Those formed from epidermal melanocytes give rise to the acquired melanoses. Lesions originating from dermal melanocytes develop into blue nevi and oculodermal melanocytosis. Both nevus cells and melanocytic lesions may undergo malignant transformation.

■ MELANOCYTIC ORIGIN

Nevus Cell Nevi

Characteristic topographic features generally will permit an accurate clinical prediction to coincide with the three histologic subtypes. Histologically, nevi are classified as junctional, compound, or intradermal depending on the location of the nevus cells in the skin.

Junctional Nevi

Junctional nevus cells are found in nests at the junction of the basal epidermis layer and the dermis and represent the earliest stage in the evolution of the nevus. The dermis is not involved. Clinically, junctional nevi are flat, oval or round, well-demarcated, light to dark brown, hairless macules that can gradually enlarge to 2 to 6 mm in size (Fig. 28–5). Because of their junctional activity, there is a low potential for malignant conversion to cutaneous melanoma.

Compound Nevus

The nevus cells are found at the dermal–epidermal junction and also in the dermis, creating subepithelial nests. The compound nevus shows features of both junctional and intradermal nevi. These lesions are more common than the junctional nevi and appear as a slightly raised, smooth-surfaced, and well-defined

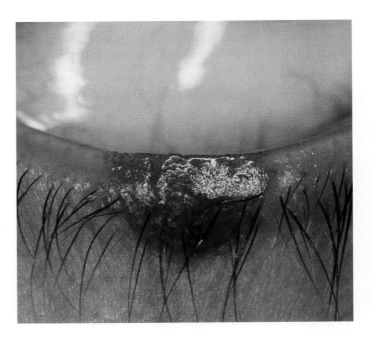

Figure 28–5.
A flat, well-circumscribed, brownish junctional nevus.

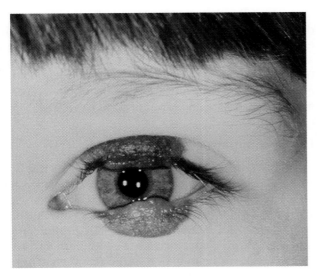

Figure 28–6.
A kissing compound nevus.

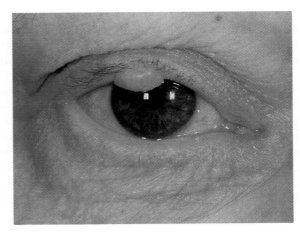

Figure 28–7.
A flesh-colored, raised intradermal nevus with hairs on surface.

round papule or nodule. It has a soft or velvety feel to palpation, and dark brown-black pigmentation is visible on the surface. Coarse hair may project from the surface of the compound nevi. As with a purely junctional nevus, the compound nevus has a low malignant potential; the melanoma arises from the junctional component.

Most congenital nevi are of compound variety. The "kissing" nevus with mirror-image configuration involving apposed portions of the upper and lower lids is a compound nevus (Fig. 28–6). During embryogenesis, excessive numbers of precursor melanocytes merge in the fused lid skin, creating the appearance of kissing congenital nevi upon separation of the lids.

Intradermal Nevus

Intradermal nevi show little or no junctional activity, with discrete nests of nevus cells lying exclusively within the upper dermis. They are commonly found on the eyelid margin and are more prevalent in adults. The posterior aspect of marginal eyelid nevus characteristically molds to the conjunctival surface of the globe. The lesion is commonly dome-shaped, sessile, pedunculated, or even polypoid. The skin markings become indistinct and pigmentation is decreased to a light brown or flesh tone color (Fig. 28–7). Intradermal nevus frequently exhibit a surface vascular pattern due to the surrounding of the intradermal nevus cells by fibrovascular septa. Fine vellus hairs may be present on the surface. These lesions do not undergo malignant transformation.

Nevus lesions of the eyelid away from the lid margin can be excised. Those of the eyelid margin may be

shaved off. Deep excisions into the eyelid margin are generally unnecessary as malignant changes usually commence at the junctional zone of the epithelium and not in the deeper dermis layer.

Dermal Melanocytes

The blue nevus and the nevus of Ota comprise this group of melanocytic lesions. These lesions have a characteristic bluish color, owing to light scattering by dermal melanin particles (Tyndall effect).

Blue Nevi

These lesions are generally present at birth and arise from localized proliferation of dermal melanocytes that have been arrested during embryogenesis in the dermis before reaching the epidermis. The blue nevus is a dome-shaped, round, well-circumscribed, 3 to 8 mm, dark bluish nodules. It rarely exceeds 1 cm in diameter, and malignant transformation does not occur. Histologically, the nevus cells are haphazardly arranged deep in the dermis and are typically spindle-shaped. Treatment is usually surgical excision.

Nevus of Ota (Congenital Oculodermal Melanocytosis)

This is a specific form of congenital melanosis characterized by periocular skin melanocytosis in conjunction with ipsilateral ocular melanocytosis (melanosis oculi). Hyperpigmentation of the affected tissue is produced by increased population of heavily pigmented melanocytes within the tissue. Not only are the conjunctiva, sclera, and episclera involved, but the uveal tract is diffusely thickened by the uveal melanocytes.

There is similar bluish hyperpigmentation of the eyelid and facial skin, in areas supplied by the ophthalmic and maxillary divisions of the trigeminal nerve. The mandible, oral and nasal mucosa, tympanic membrane, and dura may be affected.

This lesion is commonly seen in Asians and African-Americans. Eighty-five percent of reported cases are among Japanese. This condition predominantly affects females, and unilateral involvement is the rule. Bilateral cases have been reported. In the majority of cases, pigmentation becomes visible during the first few months of life, while in others, it is not evident until puberty or during pregnancy. The skin lesion is typically flat, blotchy blue or blue-gray in color, with irregular and indistinct borders. The lesion typically enlarges and darkens in response to hormonal stimulation. The eye is involved in 60% of cases. Slate-gray or bluish pigmentation of the episclera is commonly observed. In patients with this condition, malignant transformation to melanoma has been reported in 4.5% of cases, with the uveal tract being the most common site of malignancy (19). Because of the depth and diffuse distribution of the dermal melanocytes, surgical excision is difficult. Most patients use cover-up cosmetics. Occasionally, these congenital melanocytic lesions can be extremely large requiring complicated excision and reconstruction (11).

Epidermal Melanocytes

Epidermal melanocytes produce three common benign lesions; all are flat and nonpalpable.

Freckles (Ephelides)

An ephelis is a small (1 to 3 mm), well-circumscribed, red-brown or tan macule that appears in childhood and darkens with sun exposure. Histologically, the color is due to increased pigmentation in the basal layer of the epidermis. This layer contains large melanocytes but without increased numbers. The melanin is derived from abnormal, genetically determined, hyperactive melanocytes that release the pigment upon ultraviolet light stimulation. Ephelis requires no treatment.

Lentigo Simplex

Lentigo simplex can be found anywhere on the body and are not affected by sun exposure. They are flat, brown to black, and measure 1 to 2 mm in diameter. They are larger than freckles and clinically indistinguishable from junctional nevi. Histologically, lentigo simplex shows an increased number of basal melanocytes, with elongation of the rete pegs. There is no potential for neoplastic transformation and these lesions do not require treatment. Multiple facial lentigines may suggest Peutz-Jeghers syndrome, which is characterized by intestinal polyps and occult visceral tumors.

Lentigo Senilis

Lentigo senilis is observed in more than 90% of elderly whites and appears as a dark-brown macule with an irregular border. They resemble flat seborrheic keratoses and occur largely on sun-exposed areas such as the forehead and the dorsum of the hands. Histologically, there is hyperpigmentation and an increased number of basal epithelial melanocytes, which are amorphous and without atypia. Cryotherapy is effective; however, treatment of these lesions is usually unnecessary.

■ TUMORS OF ADNEXAL ORGIN

The eyelids contain numerous adnexal structures, including sebaceous glands, sweat glands, and hair follicles. Benign tumors arising from these structures may occur in the eyelid.

Sebaceous Glands

Sebaceous Hyperplasia/Sebaceous Adenoma

The group of benign sebaceous gland tumors includes senile sebaceous hyperplasia and true sebaceous adenoma. The former occurs on the face of older patients in which dermal sebaceous glands may undergo hypertrophy and hyperplasia. This entity affects mainly the scalp, forehead, cheek, temple, and sebaceous glands of the eyelid. The lesion is a small yellow papule with a central depression and may be solitary or multiple. Sebaceous hyperplasia also may occur in the meibomian glands, presenting as a single or multilobulated, slightly umbilicated yellow nodule arising from the meibomian glands. If the area of involvement is diffuse, the eyelid may become thickened, inducing mild lid margin ectropion. Sebaceous hyperplasia may be seen as an isolated entity or in association with tuberous sclerosis where they present chiefly over the malar eminence. Histologically, one or several hyperplastic mature sebaceous glands with normal architecture oriented around a central dilated duct is seen. These lesions may be excised or removed by electrodesiccation.

Sebaceous adenoma is exceedingly rare on the eyelid. When present, it is usually solitary and appears as a smooth, firm, waxy yellow, superficial epidermal nodule in older patients. The primary significance of this lesion is that it may be a cutaneous marker for internal malignancy. The association of cutaneous keratoacanthomas or sebaceous tumors with visceral malignancy, particularly colonic adenocarcinoma, is known as the Muir-Torre syndrome. There is a reported 40% incidence of internal malignancy in patients with one or more benign cutaneous sebaceous tumors. It appears that a patient with even one benign sebaceous tumor anywhere on the body may presage the possibility of future internal malignancy.

Milia

Milia are intracutaneous retention cysts originating from occlusion of pilosebaceous structures. They usually spontaneously occur as multiple, firm, white, globoid lesions under the thin epidermis. The umbilicated center seen clinically corresponds to the occluded orifice. The superficial keratin cysts are typically small, measuring 1 to 3 mm in diameter. They are commonly found on the eyelids, cheeks, and nose. Although milia do not cause symptoms, patients frequently request removal for cosmetic reasons. Histologically, the lesions display a dilated hair follicle filled with keratin. Treatment includes excision, cauterization, or topically applied trichloroacetic acid.

Sebaceous Cysts

Sebaceous cysts are similar to milia but are larger and result from occlusion of the pilosebaceous unit or Zeis glands. Sebaceous cysts are clinically indistinguishable from epidermal inclusion cysts. They are less common than epidermal inclusion cysts and tend to occur in areas containing numerous hair follicles such as the brow. These cysts may remain quiescent or grow to considerable size. Meibomian gland cysts are customarily observed in the eyelids. These retention cysts usually develop secondary to an inflammatory or neoplastic process involving the lid margin. The growth of a meibomian cyst is limited by the fibrous tarsal substance and may undergo degenerative changes. The treatment of choice is surgical excision of the cyst with its enclosing walls.

Sweat Gland Lesions

Syringoma

This common skin lesion is a benign tumor of eccrine origin and occurs predominantly on and just beneath the lower lids in adolescent and middle-aged females. The lid margins are usually spared. Syringomas also may occur on the cheeks, chest, neck, and axilla. They generally present as multiple, small (1 to 3 mm), flesh-colored, smooth surfaced papules (Fig. 28–8). They are often bilateral, have a waxy appearance, and may be suggestive of xanthelasma. They can be distinguished from xanthelasma by virtue of the younger age of onset and their lack of confluence to produce a plaque. The tumors are of cosmetic importance only. In addition to syringoma, the differential diagnosis of multiple, bilateral, small nodular lesions in the periocular region include trichoepithelioma, basal cell nevus syndrome, milia, and dermatosis papulosa nigra. Histologically, syringomas are composed of compressed ducts within the

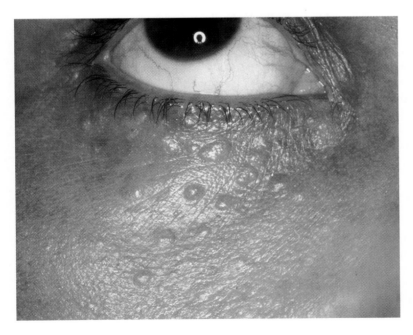

Figure 28–8.
Multiple, small, skin-colored syringomas on lower lid and cheek.

dermis, which have the characteristic "tadpole-like" configuration due to squeezing by the dense hyalinized fibrous stroma. Occasionally, it may be mistaken for a breast duct carcinoma. The lesions may be surgically excised or treated by a carbon dioxide laser for cosmetic reasons (57).

Pleomorphic Adenoma (Mixed Tumor of the Sweat Glands, Chondroid Syringoma)

These lesions are believed to arise from the sweat glands of the skin and are rarely seen in the eyelids. Clinically, they appear as an intradermal, multilobulated mass. Histopathologically, they are identical to the pleomorphic adenomas of the lacrimal gland. They are composed of tubular structures lined by a double layer of epithelial cells embedded in a mucoid stroma. Chondroid metaplasia often exists.

Eccrine Acrospiroma (Clear Cell Hidradenoma)

Histochemical and electron microscopic studies have established the eccrine origin of this unusual benign tumor of the eyelid. It appears as a solitary, nodular or cystic deep dermal mass. The overlying skin is flesh-colored, reddish-blue (secondary to hemorrhage), thickened or verrucous. The surface may ulcerate and discharge a serous material. Few lesions are painful. Histopathologically, the tumor is composed of one or more lobules of glycogen-rich cells with characteristic small ductal lumina as seen in eccrine sweat glands. The glycogen-rich clear cells also gave rise to the term of clear cell hidradenoma. Excision is recommended because malignant variants have been reported.

Adenoma of the Glands of Moll (Apocrine Adenoma)

These are extremely rare tumors of the apocrine glands of Moll. They occur more commonly on the scalp. When present on the eyelid, they appear as solitary, raised nodules. Histopathologically, cystic invaginations (villus-like projections) extend into the dermis. They are lined by a double layer of cells composed of luminal high columnar cells and outer myoepithelial cells and exhibit decapitation secretion.

Hidrocystoma (Sudoriferous Cyst, Ductal Cyst of Sweat Gland Origin)

Sudoriferous cysts are divided into two types: apocrine hidrocystoma or eccrine hidrocystoma. The apocrine hidrocystoma develops from a blocked excretory duct of a gland of Moll. These lesions are filled with clear or milky fluid and typically appear as 1- to 3-mm solitary, translucent, cystic nodules situated along the lid mar-

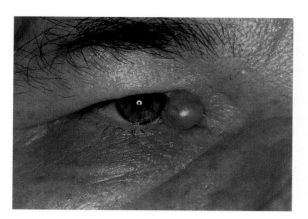

Figure 28–9.
An apocrine hidrocystoma on medial upper lid.

gins (Fig. 28–9). Most of the cysts are clear and transmit light well, compared with epidermal inclusion cysts and cystic basal cell carcinomas. Microscopically, the dermis displays several large cystic spaces lined by double rows of secretory cells. The papillary projection of the inner layer demonstrates characteristic decapitation secretion of the apical portion of the cells. The fluid within the cyst may appear more turbid than in eccrine hidrocystomas because the contents of the cyst contains cytoplasmic debris. Local excision is the treatment of choice.

Eccrine hidrocystomas commonly occur in the eyelids and are regarded as ductal retention cysts. The cyst contains watery fluid within the lumen and has a similar clinical appearance as an apocrine hidrocystoma. Histopathologically, the dermis has only one cyst cavity and is lined by a single or double layer of cuboidal epithelium.

Hair Follicle Lesions

Trichoepithelioma (Brooke's Tumor)

Trichoepithelioma is a rare benign epidermal tumor that represents a hamartoma of immature hair matrix cells. This tumor may occur as a solitary lesion or as multiple nodules in a dominantly inherited variety. They are usually multiple, rounded, slightly elevated, firm, skin-colored nodules ranging from 2 to 8 mm in diameter (Fig. 28–10). These lesions usually affect the face, neck, trunk, and may be found on the eyelids. Trichoepitheliomas tend to appear after puberty and gradually increase in size and number. Because there may be telangiectasia on the surface of the lesions, they may be mistaken for basal cell carcinoma. Microscopically, the lesion has a typical histologic appearance of numerous horn cysts composed of a fully keratinized center surrounded by basal cell epithelioma-like cells. These horn cysts represent abortive attempts at hair shaft formation. Occasionally, there may be rupture of a cyst with for-

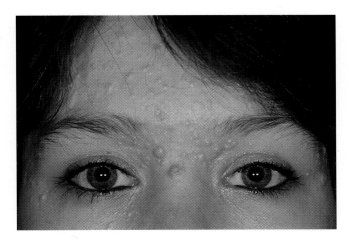

Figure 28–10.
Trichoepithelioma.

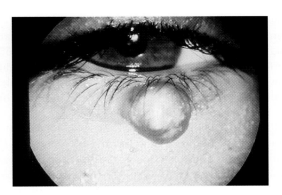

Figure 28–11.
Pilomatrixoma.

eign-body giant cell reaction and calcium deposition. Trichoepithelioma can be distinguished from basal cell carcinoma because of the presence of primitive hair structures, absence of mitosis, horn cysts, and a minimal inflammatory infiltrate. Malignant transformation of trichoepithelioma into basal cell carcinoma occurs rarely (82). Treatment involves complete excision.

Trichofolliculoma

This hamartoma is an uncommon but distinctively characteristic benign tumor that appears on the face or neck. It typically occurs as a small, dome-shaped, flesh-colored nodule with a diagnostic tuft of white hair protruding from the central pore. Histologically, the cystic cavity is lined by keratinized stratified squamous epithelium from which numerous primordial hair follicles arise. Many of these are well-developed and contain a central hair shaft, which can be well visualized when the section is viewed with polarized light. The follicles are surrounded by concentric lamellae of fibrous tissue.

Trichilemmoma

This is a benign tumor stemmed from the outer root sheath of the hair follicle. It usually appears in adults as a small flesh-colored nodule resembling a verrucous papule. Multiple trichilemmomas are seen in patients

with Cowden's disease (multiple hamartoma syndrome). The significance of Cowden's disease lies in its value as a marker for the eventual development of thyroid or breast disease. Treatment is simple surgical excision.

Pilomatrixoma (Calcifying Epithelioma of Malherbe)

Malherbe's calcifying epithelioma is a benign skin tumor originating from hair matrix cells. Forty percent of the lesions are first noted in patients 10 years of age or younger, and an additional 20% of the lesions occur in young adults. The tumor usually occurs on the face, arms, neck, eyelid, brow, or the zygomatic region. They commonly present as a nontender, solitary subcutaneous nodule with a reddish-purple hue and subepithelial patches of yellow discoloration (Fig. 28–11). The average size of lesion is 10 mm or less, and the consistency ranges from firm to cystic. Characteristically, the lesion is not adherent to the underlying deep structures, but it is adherent to an intact overlying skin containing multiple telangiectatic vessels. Microscopic examination shows a layer of intact keratinized stratified squamous epithelium overlying a well-circumscribed subepithelial tumor. Centrally, islands of epithelial cells surrounded by aggregates of basophilic shadow cells can be seen. Most lesions contain calcium granules that may occasionally induce a foreign body granulomatous inflammatory reaction. Surgical excision is the procedure of choice.

■ VASCULAR BENIGN TUMORS

Capillary Hemangioma

Capillary hemangiomas generally appear during the first few weeks of life and frequently involve the eyelid. They are estimated to occur in 1 of every 200 live births.

Typically, the lesion exhibits a reddish-purple color, is elevated, and has a soft consistency with small surface invaginations. Most of these lesions are superficial with a predilection for the head and neck region. More deeply located lesions may have only a slight violaceous color or impart no color change to the overlying skin at all, making diagnosis more difficult. Approximately 75% of the lesions involve the orbit. Histologic examination shows that these lesions consist of multiple lobules of capillaries separated by fibrous septa. The endothelial cells are surrounded by pericytes.

Rapid growth is common in the early stages but usually ceases by 1 year. These tumors may become large enough to obstruct the visual axis and cause deprivation amblyopia or astigmatic errors. Approximately 75% of the lesions resolve spontaneously by 7 years of age with excellent cosmetic results. Generally, involution is accompanied by fading of the color of the lesion from reddish to a dull grayish-red with wrinkling of the overlying skin (crepe paper). Regression of the capillary hemangioma is accompanied by thickening of the fibrous septa and replacement of the tumor lobules by adipose tissue.

Capillary hemangiomas of the eyelid should be treated when they lead to functional compromise of the visual system or are extremely disfiguring. The current treatment of choice is intralesional injection of a combination of triamcinolone (40 mg/ml) and betamethasone (6 mg/ml) (42). Steroids are mixed in a 50:50 combination and approximately 2 ml of mixture is injected with a 27-G needle throughout the lesion. Regression should begin within 2 weeks and continue for 4 months. If the lesion responds initially but is still unacceptable, a repeat treatment after 2 to 4 months may be beneficial. The exact mechanism of the therapeutic effect of intralesional steroids is unknown, but possible sensitization of the capillary bed to circulating catecholamines is postulated.

Complications of intralesional steroid injection include central retinal artery occlusion, orbital hemorrhage, visual loss, eyelid necrosis, linear subcutaneous atrophy, and adrenal suppression. Therefore, use of steroids solely for cosmetic reasons in children requires extensive discussion of all potential complications with the parents before treatment.

Cavernous Hemangioma

Cavernous hemangiomas usually arise within the orbit proper but occasionally may be found in the eyelid. This eyelid lesion is less commonly seen than capillary hemangioma of the lid. It is usually seen as an isolated lesion in adults but also may be seen as part of the meningocutaneous angiomatosis (Sturge-Weber) syndrome as the nevus flammeus or port wine stain skin lesion. The skin discoloration ranges from light pink to violet, and the skin texture is usually normal. Cavernous hemangiomas are composed of large vascular channels in a fibrous stroma. The superficial eyelid cavernous hemangiomas are usually well circumscribed but are not encapsulated. They are usually isolated from the systemic arterial circulation and may undergo secondary degenerations such as calcification and fibrosis. It is not unusual to see thrombosis and phlebolith formation secondary to blood stagnation.

A cavernous hemangioma of the eyelid may be surgically removed or it may respond to cryotherapy, radiation, or sclerosing agents. Recently, the port wine stain of Sturge-Weber has been effectively treated with a tunable dye laser (73). By selecting an appropriate wavelength that preferentially absorbs hemoglobin, the vascular component of the lesion is coagulated. Adjacent damage to normal tissues is reduced by spreading treatments over several sessions, and by "painting" the tissue with nonoverlapping applications. As laser energy penetrates only a few millimeters of the skin, thinner lesions tend to have a better response. A persistent postoperative pink appearance can be camouflaged by the applications of cosmetics.

Pyogenic Granuloma

Pyogenic granulomas of the eyelid may be seen after trauma or surgery or may be formed over inflammatory lesions. It is commonly seen after spontaneous drainage of a chalazion. They typically are seen as a rapidly growing, red pedunculated or sessile conjunctival mass. The term pyogenic granuloma is a misnomer because it is neither pyogenic nor a granuloma. Histologically, it consists of an exuberant proliferation of granulation tissue with proliferating capillaries and endothelial cells. An associated inflammatory cell infiltrate is usually seen at the base. Local excision is the treatment of choice.

Lymphangioma

These lesions are usually congenital and may involve the eyelid, conjunctiva, and orbit. They usually manifest later than capillary hemangiomas. The orbital component may lead to spontaneous bleeding that presents as a subconjunctival hemorrhage, a diffuse hematoma of the eyelid, or even as severe acute proptosis. Formation of blood cysts (chocolate cysts) may occur and tend to resorb spontaneously. They do not involute like capillary hemangiomas and may progressively enlarge. The tumor consists of dilated anastomosing lymphatic channels lined by endothelium. It contains well-developed lymphoid follicles with germinal centers. The tumor characteristically has infiltrating extensions and is without a capsule, making these lesions extremely difficult to excise. Conservative management is recommended unless vision is threatened directly by the tumor or orbital hemorrhage (81). The argon laser appears to be effective in debulking the lymphangioma with minimal blood loss (36).

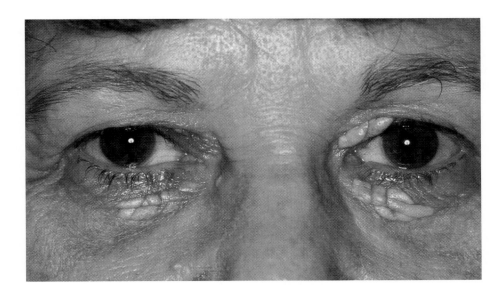

Figure 28–12.
Xanthelasmas. Bilateral flat yellow plaques with superonasal eyelid predilection.

■ XANTHOMATOUS LESIONS

Xanthelasma

Xanthelasma is a form of cutaneous xanthomatosis characterized by the deposition of lipid-laden histiocytes in the dermis of the eyelid skin. They result from hyperlipidemia, either due to a primary genetic defect or secondary to defective metabolism of lipids. The vast majority of patients with this cutaneous disorder show no evidence of metabolic abnormality. However, in 30% to 40% of patients with xanthelasma, a lipid abnormality can be demonstrated, particularly hyperlipidemia types II and III in which serum cholesterol is elevated. Type II hypercholesterolemia is an autosomal-dominant condition in which there is a defect in the receptor mechanism for low density lipoproteins. Low density lipoproteins accumulate so that the cholesterol level is high. Type III hyperlipidemia is associated with accumulation of chylomicrons, pre-beta lipoproteins, and intermediate lipoproteins. The cholesterol and triglyceride levels are elevated. Xanthelasma is also associated with secondary hyperlipidemias. Disorders contributing to secondary hyperlipidemia include primary biliary cirrhosis, nephrotic syndrome, chronic pancreatitis, diabetes mellitus, and myxedema.

Xanthelasmas usually occur in middle-aged and elderly patients, often females. The lesions typically commence near the inner canthi of upper eyelids. The lipids are deposited as slightly elevated, yellowish, confluent, and sharply demarcated plaques that are usually bilateral (Fig. 28–12). The extent of the disease varies from a few lesions of pinhead size to extensive involvement of both upper and lower lids. They are asymptomatic but can cause a significant cosmetic blemish.

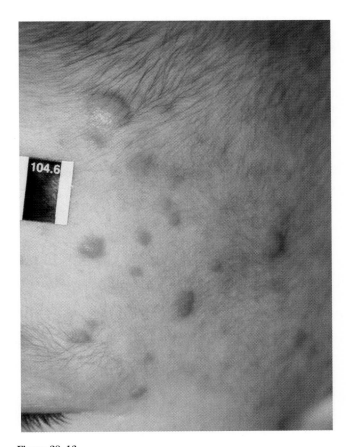

Figure 28–13.
Juvenile xanthogranuloma: multiple raised, orange nodules that later regressed.

Histologically, the superficial dermis is packed with diffuse deposits of foamy, lipid-laden histiocytes. There is an absence of inflammation or fibrosis. Treatment consists of full-thickness skin excision to include the orbicularis muscle layer or surface tissue vaporization with the carbon dioxide laser (26). Large xanthelasmas may require skin grafting to avoid lid retraction. An alternative treatment method is the topical application of 75% trichloroacetic acid. Recurrence can occur with any of the treatment modalities.

Juvenile Xanthogranuloma (Nevoxanthoendothelioma)

Juvenile xanthogranuloma (JXG) is a benign histiocytic proliferation of unknown etiology, occurring predominantly in infants and young children. They are usually limited to the eyes and skin. Juvenile xanthogranuloma may present as an isolated lesion or in groups and have a predilection for the skin of the head, neck, and extremities. The skin lesions typically present as dome-shaped, elevated, sharply demarcated nodules of yellow or orange color, varying from 5 to 10 mm in diameter (Fig. 28–13). Spontaneous regression takes place over several years and is generally completed by adolescence.

Ocular and adnexal juvenile xanthogranulomas may occur without generalized cutaneous involvement. These lesions can affect the conjunctiva, iris, or ciliary body, and there have been rare instances of orbital involvement reported. The iris lesion normally appears as a salmon or darkly pigmented nodule in which the fragile vessels can rupture, causing a spontaneous hyphema with secondary glaucoma and uveitis.

Histopathologically, a histiocytic infiltration intermixed with lymphocytes, eosinophils, and multinucleated Touton giant cells is observed.

■ INFLAMMATORY EYELID LESIONS

Herpes Zoster

Herpes zoster is caused by a DNA-virus and most frequently involves skin supplied by the ophthalmic division of the trigeminal nerve. Clinically, the dermatitis usually begins as a vesicular eruption in the distribution of the frontal branch of the ophthalmic nerve, involving the forehead and eyelids, and typically respecting the midline. Marked pain is the main feature. Severe inflammatory reaction may be seen, and the base of these lesions may appear hemorrhagic. With involvement of the nasociliary branch, iritis and keratitis may occur. The eruptive vesicular stage is followed by spontaneous drying and crusting.

Treatment consists of symptomatic relief of pain. The administration of oral acyclovir has shown great promise in reducing the incidence of postherpetic neuralgia. It is most effective when given within 72 hours of the onset of disease. In immunocompetent individuals, 800 mg five times daily for 10 days is recommended. Warm compresses are applied to keep the skin clean. Evaluation of the eye is essential in herpes zoster to detect anterior uveitis, corneal involvement, secondary glaucoma and reduced corneal sensation. Long-term control of chronic pain from postherpetic neuralgia may include tricyclic antidepressants, capsaicin cream or carpamazepine. Skin grafting to the lids may be required to reduce cicatricial ectropion as a result of anterior lamella shortage.

Molluscum Contagiosum

Molluscum contagiosum is a self-limited, mildly contagious dermatologic disease caused by a large filterable DNA virus of the poxvirus group. Humans are the only known host, and the contagion is presumed to be transmitted directly. The lesions occur more commonly in children, appearing particularly on the face and trunk. Patients with eczema are prone to this infection. The lesions are shiny flesh-colored, discrete dome-shaped papules that may vary in size from 1 to 5 mm in diameter. The individual molluscum has a diagnostic central umbilication, from which cheesy debris can be expressed (Fig. 28–14). They also tend to occur on the eyelid or along the lid margins. They are usually not inflamed and often remain asymptomatic. Occasionally, they may produce a toxic follicular conjunctivitis sec-

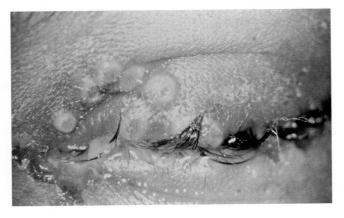

Figure 28–14.
Multiple lid nodules of molluscum contagiosum with typical umbilicated center. A follicular conjunctivitis may accompany this viral infection.

ondary to shedding of viral particles into the conjunctival fornix. Lesions on the lid margin can be inconspicuously hidden by eyelashes and only to be discovered while searching for the cause of an unexplained chronic follicular conjunctivitis. The recalcitrant follicular conjunctivitis and keratitis cannot be effectively treated until the molluscum is eradicated.

Lesions of the lid margin can be treated by shave excision followed by curettage to remove residual virus infected cells and cauterization of the base. The lesion may be excised or treated with cryotherapy. The application of chemical caustics, such as trichloroacetic acid or aqueous phenol also can be effective. Once eliminated, they rarely recur.

Histologically, the lesion consists of hyperplastic epithelial cells that grow downward into the underlying dermis as multiple lobules. The nuclei are compressed and displaced to the periphery of the cell by the homogeneous eosinophilic intracytoplasmic inclusion bodies (molluscum bodies) above the level of the basal cells. As the inclusion matures and contains increasing numbers of virus, the staining characteristic of the inclusion bodies changes to basophilic at the level of the granular cell layer. The increased basophilia is due to a greater uptake of hematoxylin stain by the nucleic acid.

Chalazion

A chalazion is a chronic inflammatory granuloma of a meibomian gland. It appears to be caused by alterations in secretions with retention of secretory material due to obstruction of the ducts. The condition is associated with seborrhea, chronic blepharitis, and acne rosacea. Chalazia originating in the Zeis sebaceous glands are termed "external chalazia"; those in the meibomian glands of the tarsus are termed "internal chalazia."

Clinically, the lesion presents with soft tissue swelling, erythema, and a firm nodule. As the gland fills with oily secretions, it increases in size over weeks. The lesion most commonly is seen to bulge externally through the skin and less commonly through the conjunctiva. It may remain contained within the tarsus or break through anteriorly beneath the skin or on the conjunctival side, inducing pyogenic granuloma formation. The chalazion also may present as an acutely inflamed, tender nodule causing significant adjacent tissue reaction. This results from bacterial infection, usually Staphylococcus, and may be associated with a tender preauricular lymph node. Such lesions frequently rupture spontaneously through the conjunctival surface. Rarely they may extend anteriorly through the tarsus and perforate the cutaneous surface of the eyelid. During the acutely inflamed stage, medical treatment consists of warm compresses and topical antibiotic ointment. Systemic antibiotic is indicated when adenopathy is present or when infection may evolve into cellulitis.

When the chalazion does not respond to more conservative medical management after 2 weeks, or when the lesion is large and symptomatic, surgical excision is indicated. Local anesthesia is injected subcutaneously around the lesion and into the conjunctival fornix. A chalazion clamp is applied and the eyelid everted. A vertical tarsal incision 2 to 3 mm from the lid margin is made. The secretions and granulomatous tissue are curetted and the lining removed by sharp dissection. Electrocautery may be applied judiciously to prevent bleeding. A steroid-antibiotic ointment is instilled and a mild pressure bandage applied for 2 to 3 hours. The antibiotic ointment is continued 3 to 4 times a day for 1 week.

Local injection of corticosteroids has been shown to be effective in treating chalazion. It is particularly suitable for lesions located near the lacrimal drainage system. A volume of 0.5 ml of 5 mg/ml triamcinolone acetonide may be injected directly into the core of the chalazion. Steroid injections should be avoided in pigmented individuals as they may cause skin depigmentation or persistent subcutaneous deposits, particularly with the depot form of medication.

Marginal chalazia are more difficult to excise because of the possibility of postoperative lid notching and should be treated conservatively for a longer period of time. Refractory marginal chalazia may respond to steroid injection, and this treatment may be considered before surgical drainage to avoid possible surgically induced lid notching.

It should be emphasized that any atypical or recurrent chalazion must be regarded as a possible neoplastic lesion and should be biopsied. Basal cell carcinoma, squamous cell carcinoma, and adenocarcinoma of the meibomian glands all have been mistaken for chalazia. Histologically, the essential reaction is that of an epithelioid and giant cell response to liberated fat from the meibomian glands.

■ MALIGNANT EYELID LESIONS

Cutaneous carcinoma is the most common malignancy in the United States. About 500,000 people in this country are treated annually for basal or squamous cell carcinoma of the skin (4, 70). Approximately 5% to 9% of all skin cancers arise in the eyelids. The most common malignancies of the periocular region are basal, squamous, and sebaceous cell carcinoma and malignant melanoma. Among immunosuppressed patients, Kaposi's sarcoma is being recognized with increasing frequency. Management of any malignant eyelid lesion requires an early and accurate diagnosis followed by total eradication of the tumor and reconstruction of the eyelid for restoration of both function and cosmesis.

Basal Cell Carcinoma

Basal cell carcinoma is by far the most common malignant tumor involving the ocular adnexa, accounting for 90% of all eyelid malignancies and 20% of all lid tumors. In the United States, basal cell carcinoma develops in approximately 400,000 people annually (70). The tumor primarily involves the lower lid (50% to 66%) and medial canthus (25% to 30%). The upper eyelid (15%) and lateral canthus (5%) are less commonly involved.

Actinic damage is an important factor in the genesis of basal cell carcinoma as it is in most other epithelial tumors of the skin. Unlike squamous cell carcinoma, there is no precursor lesion for basal cell carcinoma. Individuals of fair complexion are particularly susceptible to the effects of ultraviolet radiation. Basal cell carcinoma is rare among black individuals. Most patients with basal cell carcinoma are between 50 and 80 years of age, with 5% to 15% between the ages of 20 and 40 years. The appearance of a single isolated basal cell carcinoma in an adolescent should suggest a forme fruste of the basal cell nevus syndrome.

Approximately 10% of patients with a history of radiation treatment to the head for management of acne, hirsutism, eczema, and psoriasis subsequently develop cutaneous neoplasms within the treatment field. The median interval between radiation exposure and development of carcinoma is approximately 21 years. Two-thirds of radiation-induced skin cancers are basal cell carcinoma and one-third squamous cell carcinoma (13).

Patients with immune dysfunction have an increased risk of developing malignant skin tumors. Individuals with lymphoma, leukemia, or those having undergone renal transplantation have an elevated risk of developing squamous cell carcinoma of the skin (8, 60, 78, 79). In contrast, patients with acquired immunodeficiency syndrome experience a greater risk of basal cell carcinoma (48).

Clinical Appearance

Basal cell carcinoma is a tumor with varied clinical and histologic manifestations. The most common clinical presentations include the nodular, noduloulcerative, pigmented, cystic, morpheaform or sclerosing, and superficial varieties.

The typical nodular basal cell carcinoma appears as a firm, pearly, dome-shaped nodule, displaying multiple

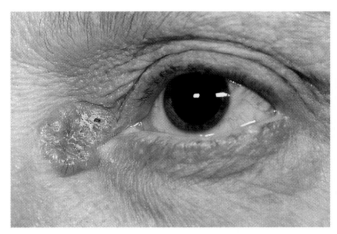

Figure 28–15.
Basal cell carcinoma: A nodular lesion with central ulceration, rolled, "pearly" margin, and telangiectatic vessels.

telangiectatic vessels coursing over its borders (Fig. 28–15). The overlying epithelial surface that has not ulcerated is usually smooth in appearance. A hyperkeratotic or surface crust, typical of benign and malignant squamous lesions, is generally not seen with basal cell carcinomas. Some lesions may bleed spontaneously and without pain after minimal trauma. With increasing radial growth, the interior of the tumor may outgrow its blood supply, leading to central ulceration. Eventually, this may appear as a slowly enlarging ulcer, leading to the common noduloulcerative variant with characteristic rolled and indurated borders.

Histologically, basal cell carcinoma is composed of solid lobules of small, regularly shaped cells with basophilic and scanty cytoplasm. The most distinctive histopathologic feature of this tumor is peripheral palisading or "picket fence" formation of peripheral nuclei at the edge of the mass.

Pigmented basal cell carcinomas are rare and account for less than 10% of basal cell cancers removed. They are similar to the nodular type basal cell carcinomas with respect to age, sex, location, duration, and rate of recurrence. Melanin pigmentation may occur in all types of basal cell carcinomas with the possible exception of the morpheaform type. These lesions are sometimes misdiagnosed as pigmented nevi or malignant melanomas.

Cystic basal cell carcinoma may develop with mucin accumulation or degenerative necrosis within solid lobules of proliferating basaloid cells. There is no particular biologic import associated with the cystic variety, except that they may be difficult to differentiate from an innocuous, benign epithelial inclusion cyst or apocrine hidrocystoma. Morpheaform or sclerosing basal cell carcinoma appear as a flat, waxy, poorly demarcated pale colored, indurated plaque. Ulceration, rolled edges, and crusting are conspicuously absent, whereas telangiectasia is prominent. If situated along the lid margin, the tumor can masquerade as a localized, chronic blepharitis. Histologically, the morpheaform type basal cell carcinoma is characterized by discrete, elongated islands of basaloid cells encased in a dense fibrous stroma beneath an intact epidermis. These finger-like cords of tumor may project deep into the dermis and connective tissue, beyond the area of suspected clinical involvement. This variety of basal cell carcinoma is especially invasive and is more likely to infiltrate the orbit.

Incompletely excised morpheaform tumors are ten times more likely to recur than the nodular type (17). This type of tumor is best managed by the Mohs micrographic technique, with its exacting histologic tissue margin control and tissue sparing properties.

Superficial basal cell carcinoma is a less common variety that is found on the trunk, but also may arise on the eyelids. These flat superficial lesions appear as erythematous, scaly patches with well-defined pearly borders. They enlarge very slowly, with little tendency to invade or ulcerate. These lesions often are mistaken for psoriatic plaques or Bowen's disease.

Biologic Behavior

Regardless of histologic type, basal cell carcinoma is usually only locally invasive. If neglected, uncontrolled tumor growth can infiltrate nearby structures including the orbit, paranasal sinuses, and cranial cavity. Tumor deaths due to direct intracranial extension of basal cell carcinoma may occur.

Basal cell carcinomas rarely metastasize, with an incidence estimated to be less than 0.1% (77). The common sites of metastasis are the regional lymph nodes, followed by lung, bone, skin, liver, spleen, and adrenal gland. Mean survival after appearance of metastasis is 1.6 years.

Treatment

An incisional biopsy of any suspicious eyelid lesion is required to establish a definitive histologic diagnosis before complete excision and repair. It is not uncommon for the tumor, particularly if it is of the morpheaform variety to have subclinical extensions that prohibit planned excisional biopsy without monitoring of margins. If it is anticipated that a graft or flap will be required to repair the defect, microscopically controlled examination of the surgical margins must be used to avoid delay in clinical detection of potential recurrent tumor beneath the flap.

In simple surgical excisions, Doxanas and Green reported a 27% incomplete excision rate of basal cell carcinomas. Of these incompletely excised tumors, only 25% recurred (17). This low rate of recurrence is believed to be secondary to the surgical trauma inducing local stimulation of the immune system (2).

A variety of treatment modalities have been used in the management of periocular basal cell carcinomas. Treatment success is dependent on several variables, including location, size, growth pattern of the tumor, and immune status of the patient (14, 32). Surgical excision, cryosurgery, radiotherapy, and Mohs micrographic surgery have been reported to achieve 5-year cure rates of 90% or greater. Currently, the best available treatment options are surgical excision with standard frozen section control or Mohs micrographic surgery. Reports suggest 5-year cure rates using these two forms of treatment in excess of 95%.

Mohs' Micrographic Surgery. The fresh frozen tissue technique of micrographic surgery, an adaptation of Mohs' original fixed tissue technique, was developed to maximize both examination of tumor margins and conservation of tissue in the periocular region. This painstakingly detailed resection is best accomplished by dermatologists trained in Mohs' micrographic technique. The Mohs' fresh tissue technique involves first the removal of the gross mass of the tumor plus a small peripheral margin of normal tissue. A thin layer of tissue, approximately 2 mm thick, is further excised from the entire base and edges of the wound. The specimen is divided into portions that fit on a glass slide, and the edges are carefully marked with different colored dyes to maintain orientation. Frozen sections in the horizontal plane are obtained from the under surface of each of these specimens. Locations of residual tumor are marked on a map and only those areas are subsequently re-excised. Using this system of mapping, the exact location of residual tumor is known. Surgical resection is continued until there is a microscopically proved tumor-free plane. Once this plane has been achieved, the eyelid defect is then reconstructed by the surgeon on the same or following day.

Mohs' micrographic technique is considered by many to be the standard against which other forms of excisional surgery are compared. Mohs' surgery is firstly limited in its availability because of the special training required by dermatologists to acquire the skills necessary. In addition, Mohs' surgery conceptually cannot adequately manage noncontiguous tumors that are sometimes seen with infiltrative morpheaform basal cell carcinoma or multicentric sebaceous cell carcinoma. Finally, there is debate whether Mohs' surgery can adequately assess margins of lentigo maligna with frozen sections due to the difficulty of interpretation and that a modification of the technique requiring delayed examination of permanent sections may be necessary.

Frozen Section Control. Excision of basal cell carcinoma using frozen section control also can yield excellent results. Cure rates of 99% to 100% have been reported (58, 61). Frozen section control of tumor margins is performed by noting the clinical boundaries of the tumor edges and excising an additional 3-mm cuff of normal appearing tissue. Each of the margins is then examined by a pathologist, and if no tumor cells are noted, immediate repair is undertaken.

Cryosurgery. For tumors with well-defined borders, cryosurgery can be an alternative to excisional surgery. Cryotherapy is useful for small lesions but is less effective for larger and deeply invasive tumors. Lesions greater than 10 mm in diameter treated by cryotherapy have a reported cure rate of only 85% for the nodular variety and 82% for the infiltrative type. Complications of cryotherapy include depigmentation, hyperpigmentation, lid notching, hypertrophic scar, pseudoepithelial hyperplasia, ectropion, punctal and canalicular stenosis, and lash loss (22).

Ionizing Radiation Therapy. A basic tenant of cancer surgery is to obtain tumor-free margins. As techniques insuring the adequacy of tumor-free margins have become more popular and available, radiation therapy is less frequently used today to treat primary basal cell carcinomas. With the use of Mohs micrographic technique and its low 2% or less risk of recurrence, surgeons have been able to use more complicated reconstructive techniques using skin flaps that previously were considered too thick and might prevent early discovery of recurrence of tumor. However, for individuals with multiple medical problems, elderly patients unable to tolerate surgical resection, or for patients in whom surgery would result in extensive disfigurement with potential loss of useful ocular function, radiation therapy can serve as an acceptable alternative.

Radiotherapy applications for treatment of basal cell carcinoma use dosing regimens varying from 3400 to 6500 cGy with fractions of 250 to 650 cGy (20, 25, 44). Protection of the globe during treatment is achieved by customized lead shields. The 5-year tumor control rate of 92% to 95% for periocular basal cell carcinomas treated by radiation therapy is slightly less than those associated with histologically monitored surgical excisions (20, 44).

Side effects and complications of radiotherapy include skin atrophy, ectropion, entropion, nasolacrimal duct stenosis, keratitis, conjunctival keratinization, cataract formation, loss of eyelashes, and globe perforation. Radiation-induced atrophy and vascular damage to skin may compromise potential use as flaps for future reconstruction. Ocular protection and administration by a well-trained radiation therapist can reduce many of these complications.

Chemotherapy. In patients with extensive, widespread skin cancer that cannot be managed by standard meth-

ods of treatment, chemotherapy can be considered an alternative. Chemotherapy can lead to remission of the tumor or induce shrinkage of the lesion such that other forms of treatment or less radical surgery can be used. Successful use of systemic cisplatin and doxorubicin in the treatment of selected cases of large and deeply invasive basal cell and squamous cell carcinomas of the periorbital region have been reported (49, 50).

Recurrence

Tumor recurrence may be related to histologic characteristics of the basal cell carcinoma, anatomic site, and failure of cure by the type of previous primary treatment, specifically nonsurgical modalities. With regard to tumor type, incompletely excised nodular basal cell carcinoma have been found to recur in only 8% of cases, whereas ulcerative and morpheaform basal cell carcinomas have recurrence rates of 60% and 75%, respectively (17).

Anatomically, basal cell carcinomas situated in the medial canthal region are more likely to be deeply infiltrative than those arising from the central lid margin (55, 56). This propensity for deep penetration of a medial canthal tumor has been believed to be related to the proximity to the embryologic fusion planes. Tumors located in this high-risk zone can invade deeply and gain access to the orbit. Recently, however, the concept of embryologic fusion planes of the midface has been challenged by Wentzell and Robinson when they were unable to demonstrate distinct anatomical planes in cadaver dissections (80).

The type of previous treatment of basal cell carcinomas can adversely affect therapeutic success of recurrent lesions. Recurrent lesions tend to be more aggressive and have a higher rate of recurrence than primary tumors, and previously irradiated tumors recur at a higher rate than lesions treated by other means (66).

The majority of recurrent basal cell carcinomas occur within 5 years of primary excision, and patients should be followed routinely within this period. Additional, the development of a basal cell carcinoma of the skin indicates a threshold level of actinic exposure has been surpassed and the patient is at risk for further lesions of the eyelid and other areas exposed to the sun. A new basal cell carcinoma will develop in 20% to 30% of patients within 1 year of having been treated for the initial lesion; by the fifth year, an additional basal cell carcinoma will develop in 36% (67).

Basal Cell Nevus Syndrome (Gorlin's Syndrome)

The basal cell nevus syndrome is an uncommon, autosomal-dominant, multisystem disorder with high penetrance and variable expressivity. In its fullest expression, the disease complex is characterized by the following features: multiple nevoid basal cell carcinomas, odontogenic keratocysts of the jaw, congenital skeletal anomalies, ectopic calcification of the falx cerebri, and pitting of the hands and feet. A diagnosis may be established by the presence of any two of these characteristics and is supported by a positive family history. Males and females are affected with equal frequency, and the condition is most commonly found in whites. Genetic counseling is an important aspect of patient management, as are frequent examinations to avoid potentially disfiguring and lethal complications.

Systemic Manifestations

Multiple basal cell carcinomas that appear early in life are one of the hallmarks of basal cell nevus syndrome. These cutaneous tumors usually present as pigmented or flesh-color smooth, round papules between the second and third decades of life, although they may develop in the first few years of life. During childhood, such lesions remain quiescent until puberty, when they increase in number and demonstrate more rapid and invasive growth behavior. Their distribution is widespread, unlike the more common acquired basal cell carcinomas that typically develop in the sun-exposed areas. The central facial region and trunk are most often affected; the scalp, neck, and extremities also may be involved. Approximately 50% of the affected patients exhibit basal cell carcinomas, which may number from a few to several hundred.

Jaw cysts are found in about 70% of patients and often appear in the first decade of life. Symptoms of pain, swelling, drainage, and displacement of teeth provide the basis of the presenting complaint in half of the cases. The cysts arise in the mandible twice as frequently as the maxilla. Surgical removal of the cysts is the treatment of choice.

Various developmental skeletal anomalies are common but nonspecific manifestations of the basal cell nevus syndrome. Skeletal abnormalities include bifurcating ribs, partial agenesis of ribs, and synostosis. Spine deformities such as kyphoscoliosis, spina bifida, and hemivertebrae also can be found.

Ectopic calcification is present in 80% of patients, especially of the falx cerebri, sacrotuberous tissues, subcutaneous tissues, and even the basal cell carcinomas themselves. Pitting of the palms and soles, a unique feature of basal cell nevus syndrome, appears as an erythematous cutaneous depressions measuring 2 to 3 mm in diameter and consist of focal areas of defective keratinization.

Ophthalmic Manifestations

The most common and serious ophthalmic manifestation in basal cell nevus syndrome is basal cell carcinomas of the eyelids and periocular structures. The cutaneous tumors are multiple and are microscopically indistinguishable from the actinically induced basal cell carcinomas. Orbital hypertelorism and an associated lateral displacement of the medial canthi are found in a majority of patients. These features, coupled with prominent supraorbital ridges, frontoparietal bossing, a broad nasal root, and mild mandibular prognathism, produce a characteristic facies.

Treatment

The potentially invasive and destructive nature of large numbers of basal cell carcinomas may lead to disfigurement and considerable ocular morbidity. Ionizing radiation therapy is contraindicated because of its increased mutagenic potential in these patients. Curettage and electrocoagulation treatment and cryosurgery can be useful in small lesions. For large, invasive, or recurrent lesions, the Mohs micrographic excision technique is recommended. An experimental method of chemoprevention of basal cell carcinoma and multiple keratoacanthomas with long-term administration of systemic isotretinoin has been reported. For patients in whom conventional modes of therapy had either failed or cannot be applied, photodynamic therapy may be considered. Photodynamic therapy is a new treatment technique in which hematoporphyrin derivative (HpD), a photosensitizer, is administered intravenously. This drug is preferentially retained by malignant tissues and initiates a cytotoxic reaction when exposed to red light (630 nm) generated by a dye laser. Normal tissues adjacent to a tumor retain HpD to a much lesser degree and are thus spared damage from the light-induced reaction.

Squamous Cell Carcinoma

Squamous cell carcinoma is a malignant neoplasm of keratinizing cells of the epidermis. It constitutes approximately 9% of all periocular cutaneous tumors and is considered the second most common eyelid malignancy. Squamous cell carcinoma of the eyelids is a potentially lethal tumor that can invade the orbit by direct or perineural extension, spread to regional lymph nodes, as well as metastasize to distal sites. Actinic keratoses and Bowen's disease are considered premalignant lesions. In addition, cutaneous squamous cell carcinoma also may arise from radiation dermatoses, burn scars, and inflammatory lesions (13).

Premalignant Lesions: Actinic Keratosis

Actinic keratosis is the most common precancerous skin lesion. Affected individuals are usually elderly with a fair complexion and a history of chronic sun exposure. Actinic keratoses tend to increase in number with age, and often develop on the face, forearm, scalp, and dorsum of the hands. They are typically round, flat, scaly, keratotic plaques with an erythematous base, measuring only few millimeters in diameter. Occasionally, these lesions have a nodular, horny, or even wart-like appearance. On palpation, these lesions have the texture of fine sandpaper.

Risk of malignant transformation from a single actinic keratosis lesion has been estimated to be less than 0.24% per year (38). Although the risk per lesion per year may be low, a patient with several actinic keratoses followed over a 10-year period may have an expected risk of malignant transformation of 16.9% (39). Squamous cell carcinomas arising from actinic keratoses are believed to be less aggressive and possess lower metastatic potential than squamous cell carcinoma arising de novo. Treatment of periocular actinic keratoses is dependent on size and location of the lesions. Small lesions not involving the eyelid may be observed. An incisional or excisional biopsy may be performed to establish a definitive diagnosis. With histologic confirmation of actinic keratosis, the remainder of the lesion may be treated with excision or cryotherapy.

Bowen's Disease

Bowen's disease is synonymous with carcinoma in situ of the skin. In contrast to most squamous epithelial proliferative lesions occurring predominantly on sun-exposed areas, these lesions may appear in nonexposed regions of the body with relatively high frequency. Bowen's disease also may involve the oral mucosa, nail beds, conjunctiva, and the urogenital area.

Bowen's disease produces a wide variety of clinical appearances. Typically, a patient presents with an isolated, slightly elevated, erythematous lesion with well-demarcated borders that fails to heal. The lesion has the appearance of a second degree burn, does not bleed or itch, and is devoid of hairs. The average diameter is about 1.3 cm, a size much larger than a typical actinic keratoses. In Bowen's disease, full-thickness epidermal cellular atypia and loss of polarity of the immature, neoplastic epithelial cell are the constant cytologic findings. The histopathologic hallmark of this condition is the lack of penetration of cancerous cells into the dermis. The basement membrane remains intact with 5% of Bowen's disease lesions progressing to invasive squamous cell carcinoma. Complete surgical excision is usually curative.

Squamous Cell Carcinoma

Like basal cell carcinomas, the majority of squamous cell carcinomas develop in fair complexioned, elderly individuals with a history of chronic sun exposure. The average age of presentation is 70 years of age. However, primary squamous cell carcinoma may be seen in young patients who are immunosuppressed (31). Individuals with lymphoma, leukemia, or those who have undergone renal transplantation also have an elevated risk of developing squamous cell carcinoma of the skin (8, 60, 78, 79). In young patients, the presence of cutaneous squamous cell carcinomas also should suggest the possibility of an underlying genetic predisposition such as XP or albinism.

The most frequent conditions mistaken for squamous cell carcinoma are inverted follicular keratosis, benign keratosis, keratoacanthoma, pseudoepitheliomatous hyperplasia, and basal cell carcinoma.

Clinical Presentation

Squamous cell carcinoma affects the lower eyelid more commonly than the upper eyelid, with a propensity for lid margin involvement. These tumors vary in presentation and there are no distinctive clinical features that can reliably establish the diagnosis of squamous cell carcinoma. They often present as painless plaques or nodules with variable degree of scale, crust, and ulceration (Fig. 28–16). Surface crusting is characteristic because of a tendency for these malignant cells to form keratin. They also may appear as papillomatous growths, cutaneous horns, or cysts along the lid margin. The pearly translucent border and superficial network of telangiec-

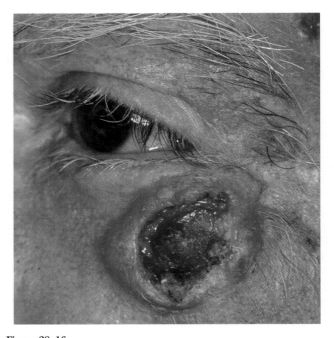

Figure 28–16.
Squamous cell carcinoma: a large noduloulcerative tumor with an indurated border and a granular ulcer bed covered with a thick crust. Note the actinic changes in the adjacent area.

tasia, features frequently associated with basal cell carcinomas, are lacking in squamous cell carcinomas.

Biologic Behavior

Squamous cell carcinomas proliferate more rapidly than basal cell carcinomas, with a mean duration from onset to time of diagnosis of nine to 12 months. Unlike basal cell, squamous cell carcinoma has greater potential for regional lymph node and distant metastases. The more anaplastic the tumor is, the greater the likelihood of metastases or local recurrence after treatment. Regional lymph node involvement varies from a low of 1.3% to as high as 21.4%. An increased risk of tumor spread is associated with larger lesions and those with greater depth of invasion (23). Finally, tumors arising in areas of previous radiation therapy or osteomyelitic cutaneous fistulas have higher rates of metastases, 20% and 44%, respectively, than actinically induced squamous cell carcinomas of the skin (18).

Squamous cell carcinoma of the eyelid can gain entrance into the orbit by direct contiguous extension. Alternatively, tumor cells can spread locally along fascial planes, perichondrium, lymphatics, blood vessels, or nerve sheaths. Perineural spread of squamous cell carcinoma via branches of the trigeminal or supraorbital nerves can lead to invasion of the orbit or intracranial cavity. Infiltration of the trigeminal nerve can mimic the clinical appearance of tic douloureux (75). Tumor invasion of motor nerves of the orbit can cause ophthalmoplegia (68). Direct or perineural extension of squamous cell carcinoma is best treated by orbital exenteration and resection of involved lymph nodes combined with palliative radiation and chemotherapy. Overall, prognosis is generally poor (71).

Treatment

The preferred method of management of primary periocular squamous cell carcinoma is surgical excision with microscopic monitoring of tissue margins. The ensuing defect is then immediately reconstructed.

Similar to the treatment of basal cell carcinoma, radiation therapy may be considered an alternative primary treatment in patients with contraindications to surgery or refusing surgical excision. Most protocols for radiation therapy use doses greater than that for treatment of basal cell carcinomas (65). Radiotherapy also can provide palliation for patients with orbital tumor extension and known metastatic disease. Cryotherapy also can be offered to individuals who refuse surgery or are poor surgical candidates. This form of treatment may be considered for well demarcated tumors less than 10 mm in diameter, that do not involve the conjunctival fornix, medial canthus, or bone.

Topical or systemic chemotherapy has limited application and is best reserved as adjuvant therapy in advanced disease or in individuals with multiple recurrent carcinomas related to XP (46). The use of cisplatin alone or in combination with doxorubicin have provided encouraging results for advanced disease (50). Curettage and electrodessication should not be used in the treatment of squamous cell carcinoma in the periocular region.

Xeroderma Pigmentosum

Xeroderma pigmentosum (XP) is a rare, autosomal-recessive disorder with an estimated incidence of approximately 1 per 1,000,000 persons. This condition is characterized by sun sensitivity and a defective repair mechanism for ultraviolet-induced DNA damage in skin cells. Radiation in the ultraviolet spectrum of sunlight induces damage to nuclear DNA by creating dimers between two adjacent pyrimidine molecules. In normal individuals, this defect is repaired by a series of enzymatic steps. However, in patients with XP, the initial step in this reparative process is flawed.

Patients with XP experience cutaneous and ocular abnormalities, including the development of neoplasia at an early age. The skin cancers develop at a frequency more than 1000 times that in the general population. In addition, some patients with XP may have progressive neurologic degeneration.

Cutaneous Abnormalities

Patients afflicted with this condition demonstrate an acute sun sensitivity in early childhood. The initial sign is often an abnormal skin reaction, resembling sunburn, in infants with only minimal sun exposure. Freckles, dry and scaly skin, hypopigmentation, cutaneous atrophy, and telangiectasia may develop in the first several years of life. Eventually, premalignant actinic keratoses form in sun-damaged areas. It has been reported that basal cell or squamous cell carcinomas develop in 45% of patients by age 8 years, with 97% of the lesions occurring on the face, head, or neck (Fig. 28–17). This young age of onset for first skin neoplasm is nearly 50 years younger than that of the United States general population. Malignant melanoma was encountered in 5% of patients. Other types of cutaneous neoplasms were reported, including keratoacanthoma, fibrosarcoma, and angiosarcoma. Two thirds of patients die of either metastatic disease or infection before the age of 20.

Ocular Abnormalities

Ophthalmic manifestations of XP are confined to the ocular and periocular tissues frequently exposed to the insult of ultraviolet radiation. These include the skin of

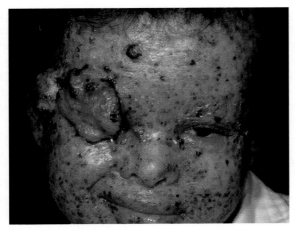

Figure 28–17.
A large squamous cell carcinoma involving the right upper eyelid, brow, and the zygomatic arch region in a young child with xeroderma pigmentosum. Cicatricial ectropion with secondary conjunctival keratinization and exposure keratopathy affecting the left eye.

the eyelids, interpalpebral zone of the bulbar conjunctiva, cornea, and iris. Common ocular symptoms are photophobia, lacrimation, serous or mucopurulent discharge, and reflexive blepharospasm.

Like skin elsewhere, the eyelids demonstrate similar characteristic dermal changes in xeroderma pigmentosum. In addition to cutaneous neoplasms, madarosis and eyelid malpositions are frequently encountered. The most common eyelid manifestation of the disease is progressive atrophy of the lower lid. The process begins at the lid margin with progressive shrinkage of the anterior lamella, evolving to a total loss of the eyelid. This can lead to exposure, conjunctival inflammation, symblepharon formation, and corneal ulceration.

The conjunctiva, especially in the interpalpebral fissure, is dry and hyperemic with areas of pigment deposition and keratin formation. Pingueculae, pseudopterygia, phylctenules, and epithelial hyperplasia are benign lesions that also may be encountered. Squamous cell carcinoma of the conjunctiva is seen in approximately 13% of patients.

Neurologic Abnormalities

Abnormal neurologic findings can consist of progressive mental deterioration, hearing loss, hyporeflexia, ataxia, and quadriparesis. Microcephaly and delayed secondary sexual development also have been described.

Treatment

Treatment of XP lies in avoidance of sun exposure and protection from ultraviolet light with liberal use of sunscreen lotion. Frequent examinations and early detection of cutaneous and ocular malignancies are essential. Isolated basal cell carcinomas may be managed by conventional excisional methods. Dermabrasion, dermatome shaving, and excision followed by skin grafting of affected facial areas (excluding the periocular region) are surgical options for those with multiple basal cell carcinomas. Recently, high-dose oral isotretinoin was found to be effective in the chemoprophylaxis of skin cancers in patients with XP. However, the withdrawal of therapy resulted in a rapid reversal of the chemoprophylactic effect.

Sebaceous Cell Carcinoma

Sebaceous cell carcinoma is considered the third most common eyelid malignancy, after basal and squamous cell carcinomas. This neoplasm accounts for approximately 1% of all eyelid tumors and 4.7% of all malignant epithelial eyelid lesions (1, 16, 28). It is a potentially lethal tumor that must be recognized early as morbidity and mortality associated with this malignancy approaches that of malignant melanoma. The incidence of regional metastases is 17% to 28% (51) with a 10-year actuarial tumor death rate of 28% (64). A key factor for this high mortality is delay in establishing a correct diagnosis, as this malignancy is notorious for masquerading as other benign lid conditions such as blepharoconjunctivitis, blepharitis, and chalazion.

Sebaceous cell carcinoma tends to affect persons between the fifth and ninth decades of life, with most diagnoses made in the seventh decade. Women are affected 1.5 to 2 times more often than men. Most sebaceous carcinomas arise from the meibomian glands of the eyelid, but they also may arise from other sebaceous glands of the ocular adnexa including the glands of Zeis at the lid margin, sebaceous glands embedded in the caruncle and brow, and those associated with fine hair follicles throughout the skin surface of the lids.

The upper eyelid is more frequently involved than the lower lid contrary to what is seen with basal cell carcinoma. Separate upper and lower eyelid primaries occur in 6% to 8% of cases, and likely represent multicentric origin rather than contiguous spread from one lid to the other (16, 54).

Etiology

The etiology of most cases of sebaceous carcinoma of the eyelid is unknown, but rarely it may be seen in children who have received prior radiation treatment for tumors such as retinoblastoma or cavernous hemangioma of the face (45, 69).

Clinical Presentation

Sebaceous cell carcinoma of the eyelid frequently exhibits variable and deceptive clinical presentations that

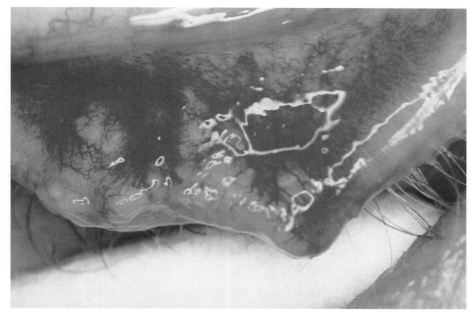

Figure 28–18.
Sebaceous carcinoma of the meibomian glands of the lower lid. Note the multiple subconjunctival yellow nodules, destruction of the lid margin, and loss of lashes. The sebaceous secretions of the tumor cells bring about an intense tarsoconjunctival inflammation.

results from its multiple anatomic sites of origin and different patterns of growth. The most common presentation is a slowly enlarging, firm, and painless mass affecting the tarsal plate or the lid margin. These lesions exhibit varying degrees of yellow coloration due to the presence of lipid within the mass (Fig. 28–18). The presence of yellow color excludes other malignant tumors, such as squamous cell or basal cell carcinoma in which lipid is characteristically absent. Lesions originating from the glands of Zeis appear as small, yellowish nodules located at the lid margin anterior to the gray line. Tumors arising from sebaceous glands of the caruncle usually appear as a subconjunctival, multilobulated yellow mass.

The sebaceous carcinoma nodule can be mistaken clinically for a chalazion because of its location in the tarsus, yellow color, and nodular appearance. It is generally rock hard and nonmobile, while a chalazion has a rubbery consistency and is not adherent to the overlying skin. As the neoplastic nodule within the tarsal plate enlarges, it may erupt toward the eyelid skin to initiate the intraepidermal growth phase, wherein the sebaceous cells spread diffusely throughout the epidermis. This "pagetoid" epidermal invasion, mimicking Paget's disease of the breast, is a distinctive feature of sebaceous carcinomas. Clinically, the lid is diffusely thickened and the skin appears indurated. With further tumor spread through the lid, loss of lashes can occur. These surface skin changes have frequently been misdiagnosed as blepharitis or dermatitis. Similarly, the tumor may erupt onto the conjunctiva and propagate within the conjunctival epithelium. These malignant cells migrate along the conjunctival epithelium, extend onto the epibulbar surface and corneal epithelium, resulting in intense conjunctival inflammation and superficial keratitis. This severe conjunctival inflammation is believed

to be induced by sebaceous secretions from the intraepithelial tumor cells (33). Hence, the unique characteristic of pagetoid skin or conjunctival involvement by this tumor can cause an irritated red eye, commonly masquerading as conjunctivitis or blepharoconjunctivitis. Sebaceous cell carcinoma also can mimic leukoplakia, ocular pemphigoid, squamous cell carcinoma of the conjunctiva, and carcinoma in situ.

A unique characteristic of sebaceous cell carcinoma is the multicentric development of lesions within the same or opposing eyelid. The simultaneous development of noncontiguous tumors within the same eyelid makes the application of standard tissue margin control techniques less reliable than with other tumors such as basal or squamous cell carcinoma.

Treatment

Any cases of unilateral external ocular inflammation that are long-standing and refractory to medical therapy should be viewed with a high index of suspicion for occult sebaceous carcinoma. A full-thickness eyelid biopsy of the most involved area followed by direct closure is recommended. The pathologist should be alerted in advance of the clinician's suspicion so as to optimize handling and examination of the specimen. If the initial biopsy is negative and the external inflammatory condition persists or worsens, a repeat biopsy is indicated.

After histologic confirmation of sebaceous carcinoma, the surgeon must evaluate the extent of possible pagetoid involvement on the bulbar conjunctiva. Nondirected or map conjunctival biopsies (63) are taken in all four quadrants and examined by permanent sections to avoid misinterpretation of subtle intraepithelial spread as can occur with frozen sections. If the bulbar conjunctiva is extensively involved and reconstruction is not possible, exenteration is recommended. It is important to examine the opposing eyelid for suspicious areas which also should be subjected to full-thickness biopsy. If both upper and lower eyelids are involved by tumor without involvement of the conjunctiva, it is possible, although technically difficult, to remove both eyelids and reconstruct the defect. Concomitant involvement of both eyelids as well as the conjunctiva requires exenteration.

In cases of nodular sebaceous carcinoma, Folberg and co-workers recommend visible tumor be excised with a 5-mm margin of clinically normal tissue. The margins are assessed by frozen section, and additional tissue is taken until the margins are free of tumor. The eyelid defect is repaired the following day after permanent sections have been evaluated to confirm the absence of tumor cells at the margins.

If the tumor is confined to one eyelid but there is evidence of pagetoid spread, removal of the entire eyelid and resection of involved conjunctiva is recommended. Lisman and colleagues have used cryotherapy rather than surgical excision in the management of diffuse intraepithelial pagetoid spread involving the bulbar conjunctiva in patients refusing exenteration (47). It also has been suggested that wide excision of the primary lid tumor under frozen section control, with or without cryotherapy, might be an alternative to exenteration in one eyed patients or those refusing disfiguring surgery (35). The role of radiation in treating sebaceous carcinoma appears to be adjunctive rather than primary.

Prognosis

Factors that worsen prognosis include (1) duration of symptoms greater than 6 months before diagnosis, (2) vascular and lymphatic infiltration, (3) orbital extension, (4) poor tumor differentiation, (5) multicentric origin, (6) intraepithelial carcinomatous changes of the conjunctiva, cornea or skin, and (7) location of the tumor in the upper eyelid. Factors leading to an improved prognosis are (1) early diagnosis (before 6 months) and (2) wide and complete excision (28).

Approximately 9% to 36% of treated sebaceous carcinomas recur with orbital invasion occurring in 6% to 17% of all cases. Regional lymph nodes are the most common site of metastases, found in 17% to 28% of patients. It is important to note that cervical and supraclavicular nodes may be involved without evidence of intervening preauricular or submandibular enlargement. Remote metastatic sites include the lungs, liver, skull, and brain.

Merkel Cell Carcinoma (Trabecular Carcinoma)

Merkel cells are believed to be of neural crest origin and are found in the basal layer of the epidermis adjacent to hair shafts and axon terminals. These specialized epidermal cells may function as slowly adapting mechanoreceptors mediating the sense of touch and direction of hair movement (39).

Merkel Cell Carcinomas

Merkel cell carcinoma is a rare but particularly aggressive primary malignant neoplasm of the skin. Most tumors occur in elderly patients, with a mean age of 66 to 73 years (30). The tumor is found almost exclusively in whites. The majority of these tumors arise in the head and neck region. The periocular region is rarely affected, with the first cases involving the eyelid reported only recently in the early 1980s (3, 38, 43).

Clinical Presentation

Merkel cell carcinoma usually presents as a rapidly growing, firm, nontender, dome-shaped solitary dermal skin nodule. The tumor is typically red in color, with hues ranging from pink to violaceous and purple. The surface of the tumor is smooth, shiny, and may contain multiple telangiectatic vessels (Fig. 28–19). It may clinically resemble an amelanotic melanoma, a primary cutaneous lymphoma, or an angiomatous lesion. The overlying epidermis is usually intact, but ulceration and involvement of the hair follicles may be observed.

Histopathology

Merkel cell carcinoma originates from the papillary dermis and often extends into the subcutaneous tissue. The neoplasm has no capsule and the cells are tightly arranged in interconnecting trabecular cords separated from each other by connective tissue strands. Included

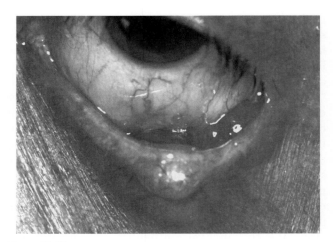

Figure 28–19.
Merkel cell carcinoma: a violaceous, telangiectatic nodular lesion on the lower lid margin with some loss of lashes. A similar nodular mass extended to the fornix.

in the histologic differential diagnosis of these poorly differentiated round cell tumors are lymphoma, metastatic small cell carcinomas, and carcinoid tumors. Special stains to further characterize the lesion may be helpful, but electron microscopy and immunohisto-chemical studies are needed to conclusively establish the diagnosis. Meticulous systemic workup to exclude other primary tumors is mandatory when confronted with a possible diagnosis of Merkel cell carcinoma.

Treatment

Localized Disease. Localized disease requires prompt and aggressive initial treatment for favorable outcome. Wide surgical excision of the primary Merkel cell tumor is recommended, however complete removal is difficult due to frequent extensions through lymphatic channels. Local recurrence develops in 30% to 40% of patients within 1 year of initial diagnosis despite apparent complete excision of the primary tumor (5, 74). Radiation may be used as primary treatment in patients unable to tolerate surgery or in tumors encroaching on vital structures (40, 62). Surgical excision with adjunctive local radiotherapy may be superior to either treatment alone, even when a wide excision has been performed (10). Early metastasis is almost always to the regional lymph nodes with initial hematogenous spread occurring in less than 2% of patients. If resected lymph nodes contain metastatic tumor, radiotherapy should be administered in a wide field to include the primary site, the soft tissue surrounding the lymphadenectomy, and the intervening regional lymphatic drainage areas.

Extraregional Disease. Chemotherapy using a combination of drugs active against small cell carcinoma of the lung is recommended in the treatment of unresectable disease in patients with Merkel cell carcinoma (5, 21). Tumor regression as a result of chemotherapy is often dramatic. However, once the disease progresses, the clinical course often deteriorates rapidly (21).

Malignant Melanoma

Malignant melanoma represents approximately 5% of all cutaneous cancers. It has been estimated that an American's current lifetime risk for developing cutaneous melanoma is 1 in 128 (27). Despite its relatively low incidence, almost two thirds of all deaths from cutaneous cancer are due to malignant melanomas (41). The majority of cutaneous melanomas appear to develop de novo without antecedent melanocytic nevi.

Primary cutaneous malignant melanomas of the eyelid skin are extremely rare, comprising 1% of all eyelid malignancies. There are four commonly accepted clinicopathologic forms of cutaneous melanoma: lentigo maligna melanoma, superficial spreading melanoma, nodular melanoma, and acral lentiginous melanoma.

As the latter type has never been reported to involve the eyelids, it will not be discussed further.

Lentigo Maligna Melanoma

Lentigo maligna (Hutchinson's melanotic freckle) is considered the premalignant lesion of lentigo maligna melanoma. Lentigo maligna melanoma represents 10% of all cutaneous melanomas but accounts for 91% of head and neck melanomas (7).

Lentigo maligna usually presents as a flat, nonpalpable, tan to brown macule with irregular borders. Within the lentigo maligna lesion, areas of gray and white discoloration may be seen. It occurs predominantly on sun-exposed facial skin of elderly individuals. The lesion slowly increases in size by centrifugal spread or (radial) growth for many years. Histologically, the atypical melanocytes remain intraepithelial and do not involve the dermis. After a period of radial spread, invasion (vertical growth) into the dermis occurs, leading to the development of lentigo maligna melanoma.

Clinically, invasive areas are marked by nodule formation and flecks of dark brown or black pigmentation (Fig. 28–20). It is estimated that the incidence of malignant transformation of lentigo maligna is between 25% and 30% (12). Once malignant transformation occurs, local and distant metastasis, although rare, can occur. For lentigo maligna and lentigo maligna melanoma, surgical excision with careful histologic examination of the margins is the treatment of choice and the only method confirming that the lesion has been removed completely.

Superficial Spreading Melanoma

Superficial spreading melanoma is considered the most common variant of melanoma, accounting for 70% of cutaneous melanomas. Unlike lentigo maligna and lentigo maligna melanoma, superficial spreading melanoma primarily involves nonexposed skin surfaces. Clinically, its location on the nonexposed skin surfaces and a more rapid rate of growth are the distinguishing features of this tumor. The hallmark of this lesion is a round macular lesion with haphazard shades of tan, black, or red. The border is often notched by focal regression or asymmetric tumor growth. As the vertical growth phase continues, focal nodules can be palpated and skin markings disappear. They may be amelanotic and are extremely rare on the eyelids.

Nodular Melanoma

Nodular melanoma constitutes 15% of all cutaneous melanomas. These pigmented papules or nodules with discrete edges typically appear over the course of a few

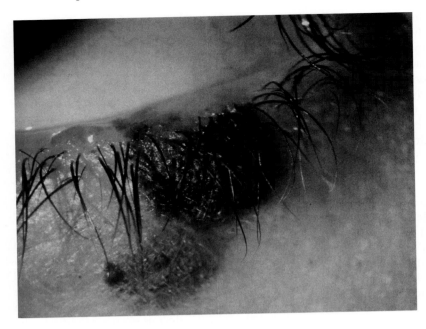

Figure 28–20.
Malignant melanoma of the lower eyelid. Note irregular borders, nodularity, and various shades of pigmentation within the lesion.

months and occur primarily on sun-exposed areas of the head, neck, and trunk. Nodular melanomas also may be amelanotic and are extremely rare on the eyelids. They arise without a clinically apparent radial growth phase; the vertical growth phase is often the initial and only growth phase of this variant of melanoma (34).

Treatment

A patient with a suspected eyelid melanoma should have a careful slit-lamp examination to exclude con-junctival involvement. As eyelid malignant mela-nomas have a propensity for regional lymph node metastasis, careful palpation of the preauricular and submandibular lymph nodes is essential. An incisional biopsy should be performed on all pigmented eyelid lesions suspected of being a melanoma. With histo-logic confirmation, Mohs micrographic excision is recommended to assure total resection (9, 83) fol-lowed by immediate reconstruction of the defect. Fol-low-up by an oncologist is necessary for monitoring of potential metastatic disease.

◼ KAPOSI SARCOMA

Kaposi sarcoma is a malignant vascular tumor that de-velops on skin, mucous membranes, lymph nodes, and visceral organs. The incidence of Kaposi sarcoma has in-creased with the advent of the acquired immune defi-ciency syndrome (AIDS). Kaposi occurs in approxi-mately 24% to 35% of AIDS patients (6, 29).

Clinical

The prevalence of ophthalmic Kaposi sarcoma in AIDS patients has been estimated at 10% to 24% (59, 72). Ophthalmic Kaposi sarcoma is usually localized to the eyelids, conjunctiva, caruncle, and lacrimal sac. The eyelid lesion presents either as a flat or raised, non-tender, purple-red nodule. It may be mistaken for a pyogenic granuloma, hemangioma, lymphoma, or ma-lignant melanoma. The eyelid tumor mass is capable of causing ocular irritation, recurrent hemorrhage, trichiasis, and visual obstruction. Conjunctival Kaposi sarcoma typically presents as a discrete, dark reddish mass on the bulbar or palpebral conjunctiva, with the inferior fornix more frequently involved (72). The le-sion often resembles a subconjunctival hemorrhage. All spontaneous subconjunctival hemorrhages in pop-ulations at risk for AIDS should be regarded with sus-picion.

Histopathology

The tumor is characterized by atypical spindle-shaped cells with prominent ovoid nuclei, interspersed with multiple slit-like vascular channels. The stroma contains dense collagenous connective tissue, extravasated ery-throcytes, and hemosiderin pigment.

Treatment

AIDS-related Kaposi sarcoma is a multifocal disease in which one cannot expect cure with excision of isolated lesions. As Kaposi sarcoma of the conjunctiva and eyelid are slow-growing and rarely invasive, their treatment may be unnecessary and observation more appropriate for lesions not causing functional or cosmetic problems (72). Indications for treatment include cosmetically disturbing lesions, ocular discomfort, or visual obstruction by the lesion (72). For patients with localized, well-delineated conjunctival or eyelid lesions, surgical excision is the best treatment option. Patients with large lesions that would require extensive reconstruction are best treated with radiation therapy. Cryotherapy also has been reported to be effective in treating lid or epibulbar lesions not easily excised (82). In cases of advanced disease, the use of chemotherapeutic agents has also been advocated (24). Subconjunctival injection of alpha-interferon has been reported to be efficacious in treating localized conjunctival Kaposi sarcoma.

■ SUMMARY

Skin cancers of the periocular region present challenges in diagnosis and management to both ophthalmologists and dermatologists. The protective function of the eyelids can be endangered by the potential destructive effects of malignant tumors of the skin. Proper recognition and understanding of the biologic behavior of each tumor discussed in this chapter are essential in the prevention of potential devastating ocular complications. The goals in the management of any malignant eyelid lesion are to establish an early diagnosis, to effect a permanent cure by total eradication of the tumor, and preserve or restore both eyelid function and cosmesis.

■ REFERENCES

1. Aurora A, Blodi F: Lesions of the eyelids: a clinicopathological study. Surv Ophthalmol 1970; 15: 94–104.
2. Beard C: Management of malignancy of the eyelids. Am J Ophthalmol 1981; 92: 1–6.
3. Beyer C, Goodman M, Dickersin R, Dougherty M: Merkel cell tumor of the eyelid. Arch Ophthalmol 1983; 101: 1098–1101.
4. Boring C, Squires T, Tong T: Cancer statistics. Cancer 1991; 41: 5–19.
5. Bourne R, O'Rourke M: Management of Merkel cell tumor. Austral New Zeal J Surg 1988; 58: 971–974.
6. Centers for Disease Control: Update: Acquired Immunodeficiency Syndrome. In: United States: MMWR, 1986; 35: 17–21.
7. Clark WJ, Elder D, Guerry D, Epstein M, Greene M, Van Horn M: The development and subsequent cellular evolution of the primary human cutaneous melanomas. Hum Pathol 1984; 15: 1147–1165.
8. Cohen C: Multiple cutaneous carcinomas and lymphomas of the skin. Arch Dermatol 1980; 116: 687–689.
9. Coleman W, Davis R, Reed R, Kremetz E: Treatment of lentigo maligna and lentigo maligna melanoma. J Dermatol Surg Oncol 1980; 6: 476–479.
10. Cotlar A, Gates J, Gibbs F: Merkel cell carcinoma: Combined surgery and radiation therapy. Am Surg 1986; 52: 159–164.
11. Cruz O, Patrinely J, Stal S, Font R: Periorbital giant congenital melanocytic nevus. Arch Ophthalmol 1992; 110: 562–563.
12. Davis J, Pack G, Higgins G: Melanotic freckles of Hutchinson. Am J Surg 1967; 113: 457–463.
13. Dix C: Occupational trauma and skin cancer. Plast Reconstruct Surg 1960; 26: 546.
14. Dixon A, Lee S, McGregor D: Factors predictive of recurrence of basal cell carcinoma. Am J Dermatopathol 1989; 11: 222–232.
15. Dodson J, DeSpain J, Hewett J, Clark D: Malignant potential of actinic keratoses and the controversy over treatment. Arch Dermatol 1991; 127: 1029–1031.
16. Doxanas M, Green W: Sebaceous gland carcinoma: review of 40 cases. Arch Ophthalmol 1984; 102: 245–249.
17. Doxanas M, Green W, Iliff C: Factors in the successful surgical management of basal cell carcinoma of the eyelids. Am J Ophthalmol 1981; 91: 726–736.
18. Doxanas M, Illif W, Illif N, Green W: Squamous cell carcinoma of the eyelids. Ophthalmology 1987; 94: 538–541.
19. Dutton J, Anderson R, Schelper R, et al.: Orbital malignant melanoma and oculodermal melanocytosis. Ophthalmology 1984; 91: 497.
20. Fitzpatrick P, Thompson G, Easterbrook W: Basal and squamous cell carcinoma of the eyelids and their treatment by radiotherapy. J Radiat Oncol Biol Physiol 1984; 10: 449–454.
21. Feun L, Savaraj N, Legha S: Chemotherapy for metastatic Merkel cell carcinoma. Review of the M.D. Anderson Hospital's experience. Cancer 1988; 62: 683–685.
22. Fraunfelder F, Zacarian S, Limmer B: Cryosurgery for malignancies of the eyelid. Ophthalmology 1980; 87: 461–465.
23. Friedman H, Cooper P, Wanebo H: Prognostic and therapeutic use of microstaging of cutaneous squamous cell carcinoma of the trunk and extremities. Cancer 1985; 56: 1099–1105.
24. Gelmann E, Longo D, Lane H: Combination chemotherapy of disseminated Kaposi's sarcoma in patients with the

acquired immune deficiency syndrome. Am J Med 1987; 82: 456.

25. Gladstein A: Efficacy, simplicity and safety of X-ray therapy of basal cell carcinoma of the periocular skin. J Dermatol Surg Oncol 1978; 4: 586–593.

26. Gladstone G, Beckman H, Elson L: CO2 laser excision of xanthelasma lesions. Arch Ophthalmol 1985; 103: 440.

27. Harris M, Roses D: Malignant melanoma: Treatment. In: Friedman R, ed. Cancer of the Skin. Philadelphia: Saunders, 1991: 177–197.

28. Harvey J, Anderson R: Management of meibomian gland carcinoma. Ophthal Surg 1982; 13: 53–61.

29. Herman D, Palestine A: Ocular manifestations of Kaposi's sarcoma. Ophthal Clin North Am 1988; 1: 73–80.

30. Hitchcock C, Bland K, Laney R: Neuroendocrine (Merkel cell) carcinoma of the skin. Its natural history, diagnosis, and treatment. Ann Surg 1988; 207: 201–207.

31. Hoxtell E, Mandel J, Murray S: Incidence of skin carcinoma after renal transplantation. Arch Dermatol 1977; 113: 436–438.

32. Jacobs G, Rippey J, Altini M, Dent M: Prediction of aggressive behavior in basal cell carcinoma. Cancer 1982; 49: 533–537.

33. Jakobiec F: Tumors of the lids. In: Symposium on diseases and Surgery of the Lids, Lacrimal Apparatus and Orbit. St. Louis: CV Mosby, 1982: 288–292.

34. Jakobiec F: Tumors of the eyelids. In: Transactions of the New Orleans Academy of Ophthalmology: Symposium on Diseases of the Lids, Lacrimal apparatus and Orbit. St. Louis: Mosby, 1982.

35. Kass L, Hornblass A: Sebaceous carcinoma of the ocular adnexa. Surv Ophthalmol 1989; 33: 477–490.

36. Kennerdell J, Maroon J, Garrity J, Abla A: Surgical management of orbital lymphangioma with carbon dioxide laser. Am J Ophthalmol 1986; 102: 308–314.

37. Kincaid M, Green W, Hoover R: Iododerma of the conjunctiva and skin. Ophthalmology 1981; 88: 1216.

38. Kirkham N, Cole M: Merkel cell carcinoma: a malignant neuroendocrine tumor of the eyelid. Br J Ophthalmol 1983; 67: 600–603.

39. Kivela, AT, Tarkkanen A: The Merkel cell and associated neoplasms in the eyelids and periocular region. Surv Ophthalmol 1990; 35: 171–187.

40. Knox S, Kapp D: Hyperthermia and radiation therapy in the treatment of recurrent Merkel cell tumors. Cancer 1982; 62: 1479–1486.

41. Kopf A, Bart R, Rodriquez-Sains R, Ackerman A: Malignant Melanoma. New York: Masson, 1979.

42. Kushner B: Intralesional corticosteroid injection for infantile adnexal hemangioma. Am J Ophthalmol 1982; 93: 496–506.

43. Lamping K, Fischer M, Vareska G: A Merkel cell tumor of the eyelid. Ophthalmology 1983; 90: 1399–1402.

44. Lederman M: Radiation treatment of cancer of the eyelids. Br J Ophthalmol 1976; 60: 794–805.

45. Lemos L, Santa Cruz D, Baba N: Sebaceous carcinoma of the eyelid following radiation therapy. Am J Pathol 1978; 2: 305–311.

46. Lippman S, Shimm D, Meyskens FJ: Nonsurgical treatments for skin cancer: Retinoids and alpha-interferon. J Dermatol Surg Oncol 1988; 14: 862–869.

47. Lisman R, Jakobiec F, Small P: Sebaceous carcinoma of the eyelids. Ophthalmology 1989; 96: 1021–1026.

48. Lobo D, Chu P, Grekin R, Berger T: Nonmelanoma skin cancers and infection with the human immunodeficiency virus. Arch Dermatol 1992; 128: 623–627.

49. Luxenberg M, Guthrie TJ: Chemotherapy of eyelid and periorbital tumors. Trans Am Ophthalmol Soc 1985; 83: 162–180.

50. Luxenberg M, Guthrie TJ: Chemotherapy of basal cell and squamous cell carcinoma of the eyelids and periorbital tissues. Ophthalmology 1986; 93: 504–510.

51. Maniglia A: Meibomian gland adenocarcinoma of the eyelid with neck metastasis. Laryngoscopy 1978; 88: 1421–1426.

52. Marks P, Foley P, Goodman G: Spontaneous remission of solar keratoses: the case for conservative management. Br J Dermatol 1986; 115: 649–655.

53. Martin H, Strong E, Spiro R: Radiation induced skin cancer of the head and neck. Cancer 1970; 25: 61–70.

54. McCord C, Cavanagh H: Microscopic features and biologic behavior of eyelid tumors. Ophthal Surg 1980; 11: 671–681.

55. Mohs F, Lathrop T: Modes of spread of cancer of skin. Arch Dermatol 1952; 66: 427–439.

56. Mora R, Robins P: Basal-cell carcinomas in the center of the face: Special diagnostic, prognostic and therapeutic considerations. J Dermatol Surg Oncol 1978; 4: 315–321.

57. Nerad J, Anderson R: Carbon dioxide laser treatment of eyelid syringomas. Ophthal Plast Reconstruct Surg 1988; 2: 91–94.

58. Older J, Quickert M, Beard C: Surgical removal of basal cell carcinoma of the eyelids utilizing frozen section control. Trans Am Acad Ophthalmol Otolaryngol 1975; 79: 658–663.

59. Palestine A, Rodrigues M, Macher A, Chan C: Ophthalmic involvement in acquired immunodeficiency syndrome. Ophthalmology 1984; 91: 1092–1099.

60. Penn I, Halgrimson C, Starzl T: De novo malignant tumors in organ transplant recipients. Transplant Proceedings 1971; 3: 773–778.

61. Perlman G: Basal cell carcinoma of the eyelids. Surg Forum 1975; 26: 540–542.

62. Pople I: Merkel cell tumor of the face successfully treated with radical radiotherapy. Eur J Surg Oncol 1988;14: 79–81.

63. Putterman A: Conjunctival map biopsy to determine pagetoid spread. Am J Ophthalmol 1986; 102: 87–90.

64. Rao N, McLean J, Zimmerman L: Sebaceous carcinoma of the eyelid and caruncle: correlation of clinicopathologic features with prognosis. In: Jakobiec F, ed. Ocular and Adnexal Tumors. Birmingham: Aesculapius, 1978: 461–476.

65. Reifler D, Hornblass A: Squamous cell carcinoma of the eyelid. Surv Ophthalmol 1986; 30: 349–365.

66. Robbins P, Rodriguez-Sains R, Rabinovitz H, Rigel D: Mohs surgery for periocular basal cell carcinomas. J Dermatol Surg Oncol 1985; 11: 1203–1207.

67. Robinson J: Risk of developing another basal cell carcinoma. A 5-year prospective study. Cancer 1987; 60: 118.

68. Rootman J, Robertson W: Tumors. In: Rootman J, ed. Diseases of the Orbit. Philadelphia: Lippincott, 1988: 281–480.

69. Schlernitzauer D, Font R: Sebaceous cell carcinoma of the eyelid following radiation therapy for cavernous hemangioma of the face. Arch Ophthalmol 1977; 95: 2203–2204.

70. Scotto J, Fears T, Fraumeni JJ: The incidence of non-melanoma skin cancer in the United States. In: National Institute of Health, 1983.

71. Shields J: Secondary orbital tumors. In: Diagnosis and Management of Orbital Tumors. Philadelphia: Saunders, 1989: 347–348.

72. Shuler J, Holland G, Miles S, Miller B, Grossman I: Kaposi sarcoma of the conjunctiva and eyelids associated with the acquired immunodeficiency syndrome. Arch Ophthalmol 1989; 107: 858–862.

73. Tan O, Carney J, Margolis R, et al.: Histologic responses of port-wine stains treated by argon, carbon dioxide and tunable dye lasers. A preliminary report. Arch Dermatol 1986; 122: 1016–1022.

74. Tennvall J, Bjáarkland A, Johansson L, Ákerman M: Merkel cell carcinoma: management of primary, recurrent and metastatic disease. A clinicopathological study of 17 patients. Eur J Surg Oncol 1989; 15: 1–9.

75. Trobe J, Hood I, Parsons J: Intracranial spread of squamous carcinoma along the trigeminal nerve. Arch Ophthal 1982; 100: 608–611.

76. Visser O, Bos P: Kaposi's sarcoma of the conjunctiva and CMV retinitis in AIDS. 1986; 64: 77.

77. Von Domarus H, Van Scott E, Johnson W: Metastatic basal cell carcinoma, Report of 5 cases and review of 170 cases in the literature. J Am Acad Dermatol 1984; 10: 1043.

78. Walder B, Robertson M, Jeremy D: Skin cancer and immunosuppression. Lancet 1971; 2: 1282–1283.

79. Weimar V, Ceilley R, Gocken J: Aggressive biologic behavior of basal and squamous cell cancers in patients with chronic lymphocytic leukemia or chronic lymphocytic lymphoma. J Dermatol Surg Oncol 1979; 5: 609–614.

80. Wentzell J, Robinson J: Embryologic fusion planes and the spread of cutaneous carcinoma: A review and reassessment. J Dermatol Surg Oncol 1990; 16: 1000–1006.

81. Wilson M, Parker P, Chavis R: Conservative management of childhood orbital lymphangioma. Ophthalmology 1989; 96: 484–489.

82. Wolken S, Spivey B, Blodi F: Hereditary adenoidcystic epithelioma (Brooke's tumor). Am J Ophthalmol 1968; 68: 26–34.

83. Zitelli J, Mohs F, Larson P, Snow S: Mohs micrographic surgery for melanoma. Dermatol Clin 1989; 7: 833–843.

VII Ocular Inflammation

Section Editor: Narsing A. Rao

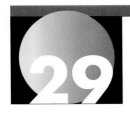

29 Uveitis: Introduction and Classification

Ramana S. Moorthy, Narsing A. Rao

The uveal tract consists of the iris anteriorly, ciliary body in the middle, and choroid posteriorly (see anatomy section). Inflammation of any of these structures is known generally as uveitis; the anatomic division of the uveal tract serves as the basis for classifying uveitis entities, namely *anterior, intermediate, posterior,* and *panuveitis* (Table 29–1).

Patients with acute anterior uveitis present with photophobia, pain, redness, tearing, and decreased vision in the affected eye. There is rapid onset of symptoms. When examined, patients often have reduced visual acuity, depending on the intensity of intraocular inflammation and secondary corneal, lenticular, and retinal changes. There is perilimbal flush caused by dilation of circumcorneal conjunctival vessels, and there may be collections of inflammatory cells on the posterior cornea, called keratic precipitates. The sine qua non of anterior uveitis is the presence of inflammatory cells and protein in the aqueous humor. The intensity of both *cell and flare* (from presence of protein) is graded from 1+ to 4+ and is discussed in the next chapter (Table 30–1). Chronic anterior uveitis often develops in a more insidious manner, and patients may experience decreased vision or may see the physician for a routine evaluation, with minimal or no complaints. On examination, the eye may appear quiet but show evidence of past episodes of uveitis. This evidence may include pigmented keratic precipitates, moderate to dense aqueous flare with variable amounts of cells, posterior synechiae (areas where the iris has become adherent to the anterior lens capsule), and posterior subcapsular cataract. When large keratic precipitates ("mutton fat") are present with nodules on the iris, the inflammation is

said to be granulomatous; if these iris nodules or mutton fat keratic precipitates are absent, the uveitis is called nongranulomatous. Thus, anterior uveitis may be subdivided into acute or chronic and granulomatous or nongranulomatous.

Inflammation of the midsegment, the ciliary body, and pars plana presents in an insidious manner. The patient will experience floaters and/or reduced vision of gradual onset, but the eye will typically appear quiet. The anterior chamber may have a few cells that have spilled over from the vitreous. Inflammatory cells will be present in the vitreous and may be graded from 1+ to 4+ depending on the clarity of fundus view with indirect ophthalmoscopy (see next chapter). Macular edema may be present on examination of the fundus, especially if vision is reduced. This can be confirmed by fluorescein angiography. In addition, peripheral retinal venules may exude inflammatory cells around their walls, making them appear sheathed on fundus examination. Exudation also occurs from the vessels of the ciliary body and produces mounds of inflammatory exudate on the pars plana, which with time becomes white, fibrotic, and gliotic, thus earning the name "snow banks." These are typical findings in patients with intermediate uveitis.

In this discussion, the posterior segment refers to the retina and choroid. Patients with posterior segment inflammation (posterior uveitis) present with reduced vision and floaters of rapid or insidious onset. Pain, photophobia, redness, and tearing are characteristically absent. On examination, vision may be profoundly reduced if the macula, papillomacular bundle, or optic nerve are involved by inflammation. When the retina or

TABLE 29–1
CLASSIFICATION OF UVEITIS ENTITIES

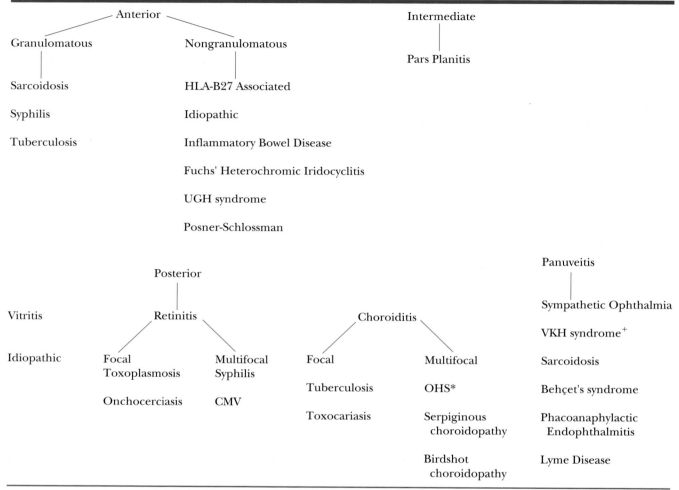

*OHS = Ocular histoplasmosis syndrome
+Vogt-Koyanagi-Harada syndrome

choroid are inflamed, inflammatory cells spill into the vitreous. Metamorphopsia, micropsia, or macropsia are hallmarks of macular changes due to cystoid macular edema, exudative retinal detachment, or subretinal neovascularzation. Inflammation of the retinal vessels is marked by sheathing, irregularity, and focal narrowing of venules and arterioles. In addition, there may be vitreous cells and reduced vision from macular edema or ischemia. Exudation of inflammatory cells along the vessel walls may take the form of small white fluffy balls or an appearance similar to that of candle wax drippings. Diffuse ischemia may result in retinal neovascularization in the posterior pole including the optic disc or in the periphery. These features may be confirmed by fluorescein angiography.

Retinitis is characterized by whitening of the retina, retinal thickening, irregular feathery borders that make

the transition between normal and inflamed retina difficult to distinguish, and sheathing of overlying and adjacent retinal vessels. Vitreous inflammation may be severe. As the inflammation resolves, the margins of the diseased retina become well-defined and discrete, and the retina becomes less thick. The underlying retinal pigment epithelium may proliferate or become atrophic. Finally, the vitreous cells gradually disappear.

Choroidal inflammation is marked by pale yellow to creamy white lesions beneath the retina and pigment epithelium, and the overlying retinal vessels may be unafffected. The choroidal lesion may be small (e.g., only one quarter disc diameter) to several disc diameters. Inflammation may extend from the choroid to involve the overlying retina and vitreous. The choroidal inflammatory foci also may disrupt the pigment epithelium and allow exudation of fluid from the choroid, which results in exudative retinal detachment. As the choroidal inflammation resolves, the overlying retina, pigment epithelium, and choroid degenerate, leaving an atrophic scar with variable amounts of pigmentation.

The etiology of the uveitis is often important in its management, in assessing prognosis, and in ruling out or identifing potentially curable infectious entities. In some patients, the uveitis may be induced by trauma or by infectious agents such as *Toxoplasma gondii,* while in others it is believed to represent an autoimmune process. The latter in many instances is classified as idiopathic uveitis.

The role of autoimmunity in the pathogenesis of uveitis was first explored by Hess and Römer (4), who demonstrated an antibody response to retinal photoreceptors, and by Elschnig (2), who proposed an autoimmune etiology for sympathetic ophthalmia. Since that time, several retinal and choroidal proteins have been identified that can induce uveitis or uveoretinitis in laboratory animals (1, 3, 5, 6–8). These antigens, which include retinal soluble (S-antigen) protein, interphotoreceptor retinoid binding protein (IRBP), and rhodopsin, induce intraocular inflammations that are known as experimental autoimmune uveitis (EAU); in these conditions, the inflammation is primarily a cell-mediated (T-cell) immune response directed against the tissue that contains the antigens. T-helper cells (CD4-positive) are primarily responsible and predominate histopathologically in the choroidal infitrates early in the course of the disease (3). Humoral immunity also may play a role in the development of uveitis, particularly in the breakdown of the blood–ocular barrier (5). The EAU model and other experimental models induced by retinal pigment epithelial, uveal, and skin melanins (8) have been helpful in elucidating the pathogenesis of uveitis and in developing newer therapies. However, the role of retinal proteins in the induction of uveitis in humans is not yet clear, but these antigens may play a role in perpetuation of uveal and retinal inflammation.

■ REFERENCES

1. Hess C, Römer P: Experimentelle Untersuchungen über Antikörper gegen Netzhautelemente. Arch f Augenheilkd 1906: 54: 13–52.
2. Elschnig A: Studien zur sympathischen Ophthalmie. 2. Die antigene Wirkung des Augenpigmentes. Albrecht von Graefes Arch Ophthalmol 1910: 76: 509–546.
3. Wacker WB, Donoso LA, Kalsow CM, Yankeelov JA Jr, Organisciak DT: Experimental allergic uveitis. Isolation, characterization, and localization of a soluble uveitopathogenic antigen from bovine retina. J Immunol 1977: 119: 1949–1958.
4. Rao NA, Wacker WB, Marak GE Jr: Experimental allergic uveitis: Clinicopathologic features associated with varying doses of S antigen. Arch Ophthalmol 1979: 97: 1954–1958.
5. Nussenblatt RB, Kuwabara T, de Monasterio FM, Wacker WB: S-antigen uveitis in primates: A new model for human disease. Arch Ophthalmol 1981: 99: 1090–1092.
6. Gery I, Mochizuki M, Nussenblatt RB: Retinal specific antigens and immunopathogenic processes they provoke. Prog Retinal Res 1986: 5: 75–109.
7. Marak GE Jr, Shichi H, Rao NA, Wacker WB: Patterns of experimental allergic uveitis induced by rhodopsin and retinal rod outer segments. Ophthalmic Res 1980: 12: 165–176.
8. Broekhuyse RM, Kuhlmann ED, Winkens HJ: Experimental autoimmune anterior uveitis (EAAU). III. Induction by immunization with purified uveal and skin melanins. Exp Eye Res 1993: 56: 575–583.

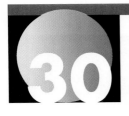

Approach to the Uveitis Patient

Ramana S. Moorthy, Narsing A. Rao

As with the clinical evaluation of all ophthalmic patients, a thorough ocular and systemic history is of utmost importance. In addition, in the evaluation of patients with uveitis, the following questions should be asked (5, 7):

Symptoms: Has there been pain, redness, and photophobia (characteristic of acute anterior uveitis), or has there been only loss of vision associated with floaters, as in pars planitis or posterior uveitis? More chronic uveitis syndromes are generally not associated with redness or pain.

Duration: Did symptoms begin suddenly or have a gradual onset? Have there been previous similar episodes in one or both eyes?

Treatment: What medications are currently being used or have been used in the past to treat the uveitis? How effective were they?

Ocular History: Has there been trauma or surgery in either eye? This may be particularly important in cases of sympathetic ophthalmia.

Systemic Disorders: Is there any history of collagen vascular diseases, inflammatory bowel disease, immunodeficiency syndromes (AIDS, etc.), sarcoidosis, tuberculosis, or syphilis?

Medications: Is the patient taking any medication that may suppress the immune system?

Personal/Social History: Are there any domestic or exotic pets at home? Has the patient ingested any raw or undercooked meat? This is important in cases of toxoplasmosis. Has there been any history of intravenous drug abuse, sexual promiscuity, homosexuality, sexually transmitted disease, or blood transfusion? These questions may help rule in AIDS or syphilis.

Geographic/Travel: Does the patient live in an area where certain diseases are endemic, such as Lyme disease, coccidioidomycosis, histoplasmosis, or tuberculosis? What is the patient's ethnic origin? This information is helpful when Vogt-Koyanagi-Harada or Behçet's syndrome are suspected.

Family History: A family history of collagen vascular disease or contagious disease, such as tuberculosis, may help in establishing the cause of uveitis.

Review of Systems: Dermatologic symptoms such as rashes, sores, nodules, alopecia, vitiligo, or poliosis often are associated with various uveitic syndromes. Complaints of arthralgias, back pain, joint stiffness, or swelling may help establish a diagnosis of collagen vascular disease. Respiratory symptoms such as cough, shortness of breath, or sputum production could be compatible with tuberculosis or sarcoidosis. Gastrointestinal symptoms such as diarrhea, recurrent abdominal pain, or melena may suggest inflammatory bowel disease. Oral aphthous ulcers suggest Behçet's syndrome, as do genitourinary symptoms such as genital ulceration. Dysuria and balanitis suggest Reiter's syndrome. Neurologic symptoms of headache, meningismus, tinnitus, or hearing loss often can be seen in Vogt-Koyanagi-Harada syndrome.

■ PHYSICAL EXAMINATION

The physical examination should be used to determine the degree, nature, and location of the inflammation. If visual loss or other symptoms are present, the physical examination should be directed toward determining the causes.

Visual Acuity

The best-corrected Snellen acuity should be determined. Knowledge of the cause of reduced vision may influence the choice of treatment. For instance, a patient with pars planitis with decreased visual acuity from cystoid macular edema may require periocular steroids; however, the same is not true if the visual loss were due to posterior subcapsular cataract.

External Examination

Acute anterior uveitis may be associated with diffuse conjunctival or episcleral injection. Deep limbal vessels may be injected, thereby producing "ciliary flush." The lacrimal gland may be enlarged in sarcoidosis. Poliosis (whitening) of eyelashes or vitiligo (loss of normal skin pigmentation) of skin around eyelids may be present in patients with Vogt-Koyanagi-Harada syndrome.

Slit-Lamp Biomicroscopy

A systematic approach to the slit-lamp examination is essential. The conjunctiva may reveal tiny translucent nodules in sarcoidosis. The cornea may show epithelial dendrites, stromal scars, or edema in herpetic eye disease. Keratic precipitates (KPs) may be present on the endothelium. Small- to medium-sized KPs suggest nongranulomatous inflammation (Fig. 30–1), whereas larger, greasy "mutton fat" KPs suggest granulomatous inflammation (Fig. 30–2). As KPs become more chronic, they shrink, flatten, and become pigmented (Fig. 30–3). The distribution of KPs is usually in a base down (Arlt's) triangle involving the inferior half of the cornea. Exceptions to this include herpetic keratouveitis and Fuchs' heterochromic iridocyclitis (FHI), both of which have diffuse distribution of KPs. In addition, FHI is associated with characteristic stellate KPs.

The hallmark of anterior uveitis is the presence of flare (increased aqueous protein concentration, Tyndall effect) and inflammatory cells in the anterior cham-

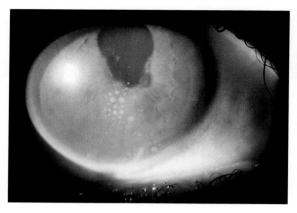

Figure 30–2.
Large and small keratic precipitates (A) are observed in granulomatous uveitis. Slit-lamp photograph shows location of these precipitates (B).

ber. The grading system for both flare and cells is shown in Table 30–1. Increased vascular permeability and breakdown of the blood–aqueous barrier results in leakage of protein and cells into the anterior chamber. If protein leakage is severe, a plasmoid aqueous results. Similarly, large numbers of inflammatory cells may settle into the bottom of the anterior chamber and form a hypopyon.

Sectoral atrophy of the iris often is seen in herpetic keratouvetis. Iris nodules may be seen in granulomatous inflammatory diseases. When they occur on the pupillary margin, they are called Koeppe nodules; Busacca nodules are situated away from the pupillary margin. Histopathologically, these represent focal collections of lymphocytes and epithelioid cells within the iris stroma. The pupillary margin can become stuck to the anterior lens capsule and form posterior synechiae, which may result in iris bombe and pupillary block. Fine pupillary

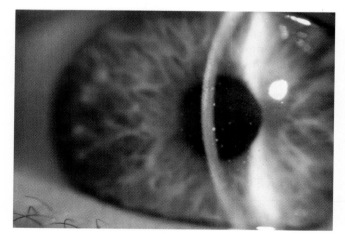

Figure 30–1.
Small keratic precipitates (A) are noted in nongranulomatous anterior uveitis. Note the location of keratic precipitates with slit lamp photography (B).

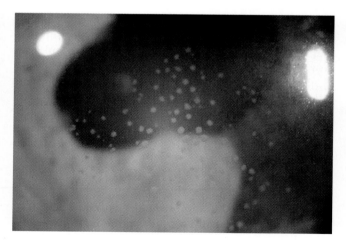

Figure 30–3.
Pigmented keratic precipitates in a patient with chronic anterior uveitis.

TABLE 30–1
Grading of Anterior Chamber Cell and Flare
and Vitreous Activity

	Grade	Definition (Wide Beam, Narrow Slit)
Anterior Chamber[1]		
Cells	0	No cells/field
	trace	0–5 cells/field
	1+	5–10 cells/field
	2+	10–20 cells/field
	3+	20–50 cells/field
	4+	>50 cells/field
Flare	0	Complete absence
	1+	Faint/Barely Detectable
	2+	Moderate—Iris Details Visible
	3+	Marked—Iris Details Hazy
	4+	Intense—Coagulated Aqueous and Fibrin
Vitreous[2]		
Cells/Opacities	0	No Opacities
	1+	Few fine and coarse opacities
		Fundus details clear
	2+	Scattered opacities
		Fundus details slightly obscured
	3+	Many opacities
		Fundus details markedly obscured
	4+	Dense opacities
		Fundus—No view

[1] Kimura, S.J., Thygeson, P., Hogan, M.J.: Signs and symptoms of uveitis. I. Anterior Uveitis. Am. J. Ophthalmol., 47:155–170, 1959.
[2] Kimura, S.J., Thygeson, P., Hogan, M.J.: Signs and symptoms of uveitis. II. Classification of the posterior manifestations of uveitis. Am. J. Ophthalmol., 47:171–176, 1959.

membranes may result in pupillary occlusion and may prevent the pupil from moving (pupillary seclusion). Peripheral anterior synechiae between the iris and cornea also may form, resulting in angle closure. Severe inflammation may cause dilation of normal iris stromal vessels, which should not be mistaken for rubeosis iridis, an uncommon complication of uveitis.

■ DIFFERENTIAL DIAGNOSIS

After a careful history and physical examination, the physician should attempt to generate a list of entities for a differential diagnosis. This may be done using the "naming-meshing" system of Smith and Nozik (18). A complete categorization and description of the uveitis entity

Pigment on the anterior lens capsule suggests previous inflammatory episodes. Patients with long-standing inflammation or those receiving long-term corticosteroid therapy may have posterior subcapsular cataracts. Pseudophakic patients with lens-related uveitis should be examined for retained lens fragments or the haptics of a lens implant chafing the peripheral iris. Pockets of posterior capsular opacification may suggest sequestered *Proprionobacterium acnes*.

The vitreous cavity should be assessed after adequate dilation of the pupil. "Snowball" opacities are seen in pars planitis and in sarcoidosis. Spillover of cells from the anterior chamber into the anterior vitreous is quite common in severe anterior uveitis. The grading of posterior vitreous cells can be done with a Hruby lens or Goldmann contact lens. Grading of vitreous cells is shown in Table 30–1. Severe intraocular inflammation can result in retinal edema, cyclitic membranes, traction bands, vitreous strands, and retinal detachment.

Gonioscopy and Intraocular Pressure

Inflammation can cause either an increase or a decrease in intraocular pressure. The pressure may be low from shutdown of aqueous humor production if the ciliary body is inflamed. Intraocular pressure may be elevated if inflammatory cells and debris clog the trabecular meshwork or if peripheral anterior synechiae are present; other mechanisms that can cause an increase in pressure include swollen trabecular meshwork ("trabeculitis"), corticosteroid-induced glycosaminoglycan deposition in the trabecular meshwork, and angle closure from pupillary block or from ciliary body swelling that blocks the aqueous outflow. Gonioscopy should be performed in cases of elevated intraocular pressure to determine if peripheral anterior synechiae or angle closure are present. Fine iris vessels that cross the angle in FHI may be seen with gonioscopy.

Fundus examination by indirect ophthalmoscopy and contact lens is essential in the uveitis patient. The retina should be examined for the presence of disc edema or hypermia, vascular sheathing, perivascular exudates, cystoid macular edema, foci of retinitis or choroiditis, serous, tractional, or rhegmatogenous retinal detachment, pigmented or atrophic scars, or pars plana exudates ("snowbanks").

for the patient should be organized into one statement. Categorization is based on age, race, and sex of patient followed by anatomic, which part of the uveal tract is involved, and clinical description of uveitis, namely granulomatous or nongranulomatous, unilateral or bilateral, and acute, chronic, or recurrent. Historical and nonophthalmic clinical data also may be integrated into the description. Once the entity is named, the pattern of uveitis exhibited is matched with a list of potential entities that share similar characteristics. Those entities that closely match are ranked high; those that do not match are ranked low. This approach may be integrated with a "tailored" laboratory investigation.

■ LABORATORY INVESTIGATIONS

The importance of excluding infectious and potentially curable causes served as the impetus for the laboratory evaluation of uveitis patients. Establishing the cause of uveitis in a given patient is important, but the search often can be unrewarding. A "shotgun" approach is expensive and unfruitful. Based on the clinical picture, however, many entities may be ruled out, and the laboratory investigations may be "tailored" (19). Laboratory evaluation may be classified into noninvasive and invasive techniques. Noninvasive techniques include serologic evaluation, skin tests, and radiography, such as chest, computerized tomography, magnetic resonance imaging, or gallium radionuclide scanning. Invasive testing includes conjunctival biopsy, anterior chamber paracentesis, vitreous biopsy, and choroidal and chorioretinal biopsy.

The first episode of mild, unilateral, nongranulomatous uveitis may not require work-up; however, recurrent episodes of anterior uveitis, initial episodes of bilateral anterior uveitis, any intermediate uveitis, posterior uveitis, panuveitis, or chronic anterior uveitis of more than 6 weeks' duration should be evaluated using the tailored approach.

Serologic markers that are commonly obtained during the evaluation of a uveitis patient include antinuclear antibody (ANA) titer; angiotensin converting enzyme (ACE) level; Venereal Disease Research Laboratory (VDRL) or rapid plasma reagin (RPR) test; fluorescent treponemal antigen antibody (FTA-ABS) titer or microhemagglutinin assay—*Treponema pallidum* (MHA-TP); Lyme antibody (IgM and IgG) titers; human leukocyte antigens (HLA) A29, B5, and B27 and others; enzyme-linked immunosorbent (ELISA) tests for toxoplasma or toxocara titers; and complete blood count.

Antinuclear antibody results are helpful in cases of anterior uveitis and sclerouveitis. In particular, up to 90% of patients with pauciarticular juvenile rheumatoid arthritis (JRA) with associated uveitis will have an elevated ANA level (6). Patients with collagen vascular diseases, such as systemic lupus erythematosus (SLE), also may have an elevated ANA level. ANA also should be considered in the work-up of patients with scleritis. The a*ngiotensin-converting enzyme* level may be elevated in 60% to 90% of patients with sarcoidosis, especially those with pulmonary involvement (16, 22), but other pulmonary or liver diseases also may cause falsely elevated ACE lev-

els. This test should be considered in any patient with granulomatous uveitis. Any patient with anterior, posterior, or panuveitis who is unresponsive to corticosteroid therapy should have testing to rule out syphilis and Lyme disease. *VDRL and RPR* are screening tests for syphilis that may become negative after adequate treatment. False-positive results occur in SLE, rheumatoid arthritis, hepatitis, pregnancy, leprosy, and malaria (3). *FTA-ABS or MHA-TP* are confirmatory tests for past or present syphilis that may remain positive for life. However, Lyme disease, SLE, and pregnancy may give false-positive results (3). *Lyme IgG and IgM* antibodies should be considered in patients with panuveitis who are not responsive to corticosteroid therapy and in whom the disease is associated with history of exposure to tick bites in endemic areas (21).

Specific *HLA antigens* may be tested to confirm or exclude suspected diagnoses. HLA-A29 is positive in 80% to 90% of cases of birdshot choroidopathy (8, 11). Patients of Asian or Mediterranean descent with retinal vasculitis associated with hypopyon iritis should have HLA-B5 testing to substantiate the diagnosis of Behçet's disease (19). Patients with HLA-B27–associated diseases such as ankylosing spondylitis, Reiter's syndrome, inflammatory bowel disease, or psoriatic arthritis often develop acute, fibrinous or hypopyon iritis; this is especially true for young men with these conditions (19). Antitoxoplasma antibody titers are elevated in patients with toxoplasma retinochoroiditis. Antitoxocara antibody titers using the ELISA method should be obtained in children with posterior pole or peripheral granuloma or diffuse endophthalmitis (4, 13); titer level of greater than or equal to 1 to 8 is very sensitive and specific. A complete blood count is useful for detecting leukemia or lymphoma that may masquerade as a uveitis and for monitoring uveitis patients who are receiving systemic immunosuppressive therapy.

Radiographic studies that may prove helpful include chest x-ray, gallium scan, sacroiliac joint films, computed tomography scans, and magnetic resonance imaging. Chest radiography should be considered in patients with granulomatous uveitis, as the presence of hilar adenopathy or calcified granulomas suggests sarcoidosis or tuberculosis, respectively. When chest radiography is normal in suspected cases of sarcoidosis, a gallium scan may show evidence of uptake in the repiratory tract or parotid and lacrimal glands (12, 14).

Young males who have acute anterior uveitis and who test positive for HLA-B27 should have sacroiliac joint radiography, which may show evidence of ankylosing spondylitis (15). Computed tomography or magnetic resonance imaging should be performed on patients older than 55 years who have apparent idiopathic vitritis. This is recommended to exclude primary intraocular and central nervous system lymphoma.

Fluorescein angiography is valuable in many cases for evaluating the nature of retinal inflammation and visual loss. Staining of retinal and choroidal lesions, the optic disc, vessels, and subretinal fluid associated with serous retinal detachments is useful in differentiating various uveitis entities. Assessment of cystoid macular edema in pars planitis and birdshot retinochoroidopathy is essential for the management of patients with these diseases. Ultrasonography is invaluable when media opacities such as corneal edema, cataract, posterior synechiae, and vitreous opacities obscure visualization of the posterior segment. Vitreous opacities, retinal detachment, choroidal thickening, and intraocular masses may readily be detected by b- and a-mode ultrasonography, which also may help in the diagnostic evaluation of the uveitis patient.

Skin testing to exclude the possibility of tuberculosis is particularly important in patients with uveitis that is unresponsive to corticosteroid therapy. If greater than 10 mm of induration is present after intradermal injection of 0.1 ml of single-strength purified protein derivative (PPD), prior exposure to tuberculosis is likely. This should lead to further evaluation and a possible trial of antituberculous therapy. Controls for skin tests with ubiquitous environmental antigens, such as candida or trichophyton, should be used to assess anergy. Patients with human immunodeficiency virus infection/AIDS or sarcoidosis may be anergic.

Invasive testing includes primarily diagnostic biopsy of various intraocular tissues. Biopsy of suspicious conjunctival nodules may be very helpful in establishing the diagnosis of sarcoidosis but does not correlate with the presence of anterior uveitis (10). "Blind" conjunctival biopsies are not recommended because of their low yield; anterior chamber paracentesis is not routinely performed and is of limited clinical value, but it may be used to correlate systemic and aqueous antibody titers in cases of toxoplasmosis (2) and other infectious uveitis entities. Recently, Aouizerate and collegues (1) detected DNA sequence specific for *Toxoplasma gondii* in aqueous humor using the polymerase chain reaction technique. Vitreous biopsy via pars plana vitrectomy with accurate cytopathologic evaluation is crucial in establishing the diagnosis of intraocular lymphoma (20). Chorioretinal biopsy is reserved for cases in which the cause of progressive retinitis or choroiditis cannot be determined by clinical examination, serologic evaluation, or by vitreous biopsy. Martin et al. (9) suggest three indications for chorioretinal biopsy: (1) macular-threatening lesions unresponsive to therapy, (2) suspicion of malignancy, or (3) suspicion of an infectious etiology. This procedure is performed usually in the eye that is more severely affected, often one with very poor vision and visual prognosis, and requires pars plana vitrectomy followed by lamellar scleral dissection, diathermy, and excision of the retinochoroid layer (9). In addition to advanced vitreoretinal techniques, this specialized technique requires careful pathologic evaluation of the excised specimen with light and electron microscopy, immunohistochemistry, in situ molecular or polymerase chain reaction (PCR), and tissue culture to determine the cause of posterior uveitis (17). With this array of invasive and noninvasive laboratory testing, the cause of uveitis may be determined in up to 60% of cases. The caveat to remember in the work-up of any patient with uveitis is that the knowledge of the cause of the intraocular inflammation should influence the treatment of the patient and/or allow the physician to communicate to the patient about long-term prognosis or systemic implications.

■ REFERENCES

1. Aouizerate F, Cazenave J, Poirier L, et al.: Detection of Toxoplasma gondii in aqueous humour by the polymerase chain reaction. Br J Ophthalmol 1993; 77: 107–109.
2. Desmonts G: Definitive serological diagnosis of ocular toxoplasmosis. Arch Ophthalmol 1966; 76: 839–853.
3. Felman YM, Nikitas JA: Syphilis serology today. Arch Dermatol 1980; 116: 84–89.
4. Hagler WS, Pollard ZF, Jarrett WH, Donnelly EH, et al.: Results of surgery for ocular *Toxocara canis*. Ophthalmology 1981; 88: 1081–1086.
5. Hogan MJ, Kimura SJ, Thygeson P: Signs and symptoms of uveitis. I. Anterior uveitis. Am J Ophthalmol 1959; 47: 155–170.
6. Kanski JJ: Juvenile arthritis and uveitis. Surv Ophthalmol 1990; 34 : 253–267.
7. Kimura SJ, Thygeson P, Hogan MJ: Signs and symptoms of uveitis. II. Classification of the posterior manifestations of uveitis. Am J Ophthalmol 1959; 47: 171–176.
8. Le Hoang P, Donnefort N, Foucault C, et al.: Association between HLA-A29 antigen and birdshot retinochoroidopathy. Acta XXV Concilium Ophthalmologicum. Proceedings of the XXVth International Congress of Ophthalmology, Rome, May 1986.
9. Martin DF, Chan CC, de Smet MD, et al.: The role of chorioretinal biopsy in the management of posterior uveitis. Ophthalmology 1993; 100: 705–714.

10. Nichols CW, Eagle RC Jr, Yanoff M, Menocal NG, et al.: Conjunctival biopsy as an aid in the evaluation of the patient with suspected sarcoidosis. Ophthalmology 1980;87: 287–291.

11. Nussenblatt RB, Mittal KK, Ryan SJ, Green WR, Maumenee AE, et al.: Birdshot retinochoroidopathy associated with HLA-A29 antigen and immune responsiveness to retinal S-antigen. Am J Ophthalmol 1982; 94: 147–158.

12. Nussenblatt RB, Palestine AG: Uveitis: Fundamentals and clinical practice. Chicago: Year Book Medical Publishers, 1989a: 206–207.

13. Nussenblatt RB, Palestine AG, Blodi F, Brancato R, Cristini G, et al., eds: Uveitis: Fundamentals and Clinical Practice. Chicago: Year Book Medical Publishers, 1989b: 347.

14. Palestine AG, Nussenblatt RB, Chan CC: Treatment of intraocular complications of sarcoidosis. Ann NY Acad Sci 1986; 465: 564–574.

15. Rao NA, Forster DJ, Augsburger JJ: The Uvea: Uveitis and Intraocular Neoplasms. Textbook of Ophthalmology, In: Vol 2. Podos SM, Yanoff M, eds. New York: Gower Medical Publishing, 1992: 2.16–2.18.

16. Rømer FK, Schmidt P, Geday H: Angiotensin-converting enzyme in uveitis and sarcoidosis. Acta Ophthalmol 1980; 58: 243–249.

17. Rutzen AR, Ortega-Larrocea G, Dugel PU, Chong LP, Lopez PF, Rao NA: Retinal and choroidal biopsy in intraocular inflammation: A clinicopathologic study. Tr Am Ophthalm Soc 1994; XCII: 431–458.

18. Smith RE, Nozik RA: Uveitis: A Clinical Approach to Diagnosis And Management. 2nd ed. Baltimore: Williams and Wilkins, 1989a: 23–26.

19. Smith RE, Nozik RA: Uveitis: A Clinical Approach to Diagnosis and Management. 2nd ed. Baltimore: Williams and Wilkins, 1989b: 34–41.

20. Whitcup SM, de Smet MD, Rubin BI, et al.: Intraocular lymphoma: clinical and histopathologic diagnosis. Ophthalmology 1993; 100: 1399–1406.

21. Winward KE, Smith JL, Culbertson WW, Paris-Hamelin A: Ocular Lyme borreliosis. Am J Ophthalmol 1989; 108: 651–657.

22. Weinreb RN, Kimura SJ: Uveitis associated with sarcoidosis and angiotensin converting enzyme. Trans Am Ophthalmol Soc 1979; 77: 280–293.

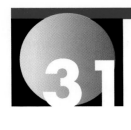

31 Therapy and Complications of Uveitis

Ramana S. Moorthy, Narsing A. Rao

Many factors play a role in determining whether a patient with uveitis should be treated and when and how the treatment should be delivered. The mere presence of inflammation in the eye is not, in itself, an indication for treatment. For example, a patient with Fuchs' heterochromic iridocyclitis does not require corticosteroid therapy despite anterior chamber cells, as this entity does not respond to such therapy. Similarly, treatment should not be given to a patient with pars planitis, visual acuity of 20/25, and a normal macula. A patient with juvenile rheumatoid arthritis with chronic flare and no cells may require treatment only with mydriatic agents. Thus, knowledge of the natural history and type of uveitis entity is essential in determining when and how to treat. The treatment can be divided into two types: nonspecific treatment, which includes cycloplegic agents, corticosteroids, and other anti-inflammatory or immunosuppressive agents; and specific treatment, which includes antimicrobial agents for the management of toxoplasmic retinochoroiditis.

■ NONSPECIFIC TREATMENT

Cycloplegic Agents

These medications are used to reduce ciliary spasm and pain in acute uveitic entities and to prevent development of posterior synechiae. Stronger mydriatic agents with a longer duration of action, such as homatropine, scopolamine, or atropine, are required to break synechiae if these have recently formed. Shorter-acting agents, such as tropicamide and phenylephrine, may be used to keep the pupil mobile and to prevent synechiae formation, especially in cases of severe anterior segment inflammation.

■ CORTICOSTEROIDS

Corticosteroids nonspecifically suppress the immune response. They inhibit the cyclo-oxygenase and lipoxygenase pathways, decrease complement levels, inhibit release of vasoactive peptides, decrease histamine content, inhibit neutrophil chemotaxis, decrease numbers of local and circulating monocytes, decrease interleukin production, and decrease macrophage activity (1).

Corticosteroids may be given by topical, periocular, and systemic routes. Although several different preparations for each type of delivery are available, physicians should become familiar with two or three preparations and use these more frequently. Topical steroids are used in anterior uveitis. Treatment usually consists of prednisolone 1% every 1 to 2 hours, with administration slowly tapered according to response. Complications of use include intraocular pressure elevation, cataract formation, potentiation of existing infection, and perforation if corneal or scleral thinning is present.

Periocular corticosteroids may be delivered in the posterior sub-Tenon's space or in the retroseptal space (1). This route is used in cases of severe anterior uveitis, intermediate uveitis, posterior uveitis (noninfectious), and cystoid macular edema (CME). Corticosteroids also may be delivered into the subconjunctival space, but this route is avoided when repeat injections are planned because white, chalky vehicle depositions are unsightly; moreover, the subconjunctival route may be more apt to produce intraocular pressure elevations and jeopardize the tissue if future intraocular surgery (especially glaucoma surgery) is planned. A depot of approximately 40 mg of triamcinolone is given to adults, and 20 mg is given to children. Complications include those described for topical steroids and ptosis, scarring of the conjunctiva, worsening of infectious uveitis, accidental ocular perforation and intracular injection, subconjunctival or retrobulbar hemorrhage, and systemic absorption.

Systemic corticosteroids are given for cases of severe anterior uveitis, especially bilateral intermediate uveitis, noninfectious posterior uveitis, panuveitis, and CME. Prednisone is the preferred agent. Recommended dosage is 1 to 1.5 mg/kg/day; this is tapered slowly and generally maintained at low doses for several weeks. An example of a slow taper would be 80 mg of predniosone daily for 1 week or until response, 60 mg daily for 1 week, 50 mg daily for 1 week, 40 mg daily for 1 to 2 weeks, and if the inflammation continues to respond or has become quiet, begin reducing the dose by 5 mg each week until 10 mg/day is reached. At this point, if the inflammation is still controlled, every other day dosing with taper at 2-week intervals is prescribed, and the prednisone may be stopped when a dose of less than 5 mg every other day is reached. A slow taper in severe cases is essential to prevent recurrences. Complications, however, in addition to those of topical agents, include increased appetite, weight gain, peptic ulcers, sodium and fluid retention, osteoporosis, aseptic necrosis of the hip, hypertension, diabetes mellitus, menstrual irregularities, mental status changes including psychosis, exacerbation of infections, impaired wound healing, and acne (1). Intravenous high-dose corticosteroids (i.e., 1 gm/day of Solu-Medrol) may be given for 3 to 4 days in cases of severe, sight-threatening noninfectious panuveitides, such as Behçet's syndrome, when acute inflammatory suppression may be essential to preserve eyesight (13). In general, corticosteroids should be used judiciously to reduce autoimmune-induced tissue damage only after infectious etiologies for uveitis have been ruled out or after infections have been adequately covered with appropriate antibiotics.

Cytotoxic and Cytostatic Immunosuppressive Agents

Cases of uveitis that are unresponsive to corticosteroids and that are severe and sight-threatening or associated with intolerable corticosteroid side effects warrant the use of cytotoxic or cytostatic agents (7). The absolute indications for these agents include Behçet's syndrome, Vogt-Koyanagi-Harada syndrome, sympathetic ophthalmia, and rheumatoid sclerouveitis. Relative indications include pars planitis, retinal vasculitis with central vascular leakage, severe chronic iridocyclitis and panuveitis, and juvenile rheumatoid arthritis-related iridocyclitis, although the latter is controversial because of the young age of these patients. Cytotoxic agents exert their influence on lymphocytes by inhibiting the proliferation of clones via interruption of DNA synthesis at various stages. Available agents include azathioprine and methotrexate, which inhibit purine ring biosynthesis, and alkylating agents such as cyclophosphamide and chlorambucil, which cross-link DNA. There are myriad side effects and complications associated with the use of these agents (Table 31–1). A rheumatologist, oncologist, or internist is an essential member of the team in the management of these complex cases.

Cytostatic agents include cyclosporin A and FK506. Cyclosporine is a naturally occurring product of the fungus *Tolypocladium inflatum*. This agent has a more specific role in inhibiting inflammation than do corticosteroids or cytotoxic agents. It prevents T-cell activation by inhibiting expression of receptors on T-lymphocytes that recognize the DR antigen found on antigen presenting cells. This leads to inhibition of interleukin (IL)-2 production as well as inhibition of IL-2 receptor expression. This agent has been shown to be effective in the treatment of specific uveitis entities such as Behçet's and VKH syndrome. Cyclosporine is usually begun at a dosage of 5 mg/kg/day orally. Titration to higher doses must be done with close monitoring of renal function. The risk of nephrotoxicity increases with doses greater than 5 mg/kg/day (2). The main side effects of cyclosporine are dose-dependent nephrotoxicity in up to 75% of patients and hypertension in 25% (7). Dosage must be reduced if serum creatinine levels increase by more than 20% to 30%, or the renal tubular damage may become irreversible. Other common side effects are paresthesias, hypertrichosis, gastrointestinal upset, gingival hyperplasia, anemia, and elevated sedimentation rate (7). Trough levels of the drug should be maintained between 100 and 400 ng/ml. Patients receiving this medication should be followed closely by an internist, oncologist, or rheumatologist.

FK506, a new cellular immunosuppressant, is isolated from the broth of *Streptomyces tsukubaensis*. This agent has been found to be efficacious in treatment of transplant rejection, and, because of its close relation-

TABLE 31–1
Immunosuppressive Medications in Uveitis

Drug	Mechanism of Action	Indications	Side Effects
Azathioprine	Purine synthesis inhibitor	VKH, SO, Behçet's, Scleritis	Myelosuppression Secondary infections and neoplasias
Chlorambucil	Slowest Alkylating Agent	VKH, SO, Behçet's, Vasculitis	Myelosuppression Secondary infections and neoplasias
Cyclophosphamide	Alkylating Agent cross links DNA	Behçet's, VKH, SO, Scleritis, Vasculitis	Hemorrhagic Cystitis Myelosuppression Secondary infections and neoplasias
Methotrexate	Purine analog	Scleritis, JRA, Refractory Uveitis, SO	Stomatitis/Gastritis Myelosuppression Secondary infections and neoplasias
Colchicine	Microtubule Inhibitor	Behçet's—Reduces recurrences	GI irritation and bleeding
Cyclosporine	T-Cell Inhibitor	Behçet's, VKH, SO, Vasculitis, Scleritis	Nephrotoxicity Hypertrichosis Gingival Hyperplasia Tremor/Myopathy Neuropathy Myelosuppression Secondary infections and neoplasias
FK506	T-cell Inhibitor like CyA	Same as CyA	Same as CyA

ship to cyclosporin A, has been effective in the treatment of experimental autoimmune uveitis. Like cyclosporine, FK506 has been shown to operate as a prodrug that binds endogenous intracellular receptors, the immunophilins, and the target protein complexes, protein phosphatase and calcineurin (18). FK506 was used in the treatment of S-antigen induced uveitis (EAU) in primates (6). It prevented the development of uveitis even 3 weeks after immunization with S-antigen when immunopathogenic mechanisms of uveitis had fully developed. Furthermore, the inflammation in primates was inhibited at doses less than 0.125 mg/kg/day (6). FK506 was shown to be more potent than cyclosporin A since it suppressed EAU in rats at much lower doses (14). An initial multicenter clinical trial of FK506 indicated promising results (15). An initial dose of FK506 0.05 mg/kg/day reduced inflammation in 22% of cases, 0.1 mg/kg/day reduced inflammation in 50% of cases, and 0.2 mg/kg/day reduced inflammation in all cases receiving this dose, but was associated with nephrotoxicity. Renal impairment was seen in 30% of patients,

mostly in those patients receiving 0.2 mg/kg/day of FK506. In nearly half of these cases of nephrotoxicity, the increase in serum creatinine was dose-dependent and was reversible. Other side effects included tremor, nausea, hyperglycemia, and chest discomfort. Nearly 70% of patients receiving FK506 had no side effects. Currently, a daily dose of 0.1 to 0.15 mg/kg is deemed appropriate for the treatment of intraocular inflammation, and trough levels of the drug in whole blood should be less than 20 ng/ml (15). Further clinical studies are needed to determine the role of FK506 in the treatment of various uveitis entities.

Nonsteroidal Anti-inflammatory Drugs

Most presently available nonsteroidal anti-inflammatory drugs exert their effects by inhibition of the cyclooxygenase pathway of arachidonic acid. Although such topical and oral agents may have some role in the treatment of aphakic CME and scleritis, respectively, their role in the mangement of uveitis is unclear.

■ COMPLICATIONS

The major sight-threatening complications of uveitis are cataracts, glaucoma, CME, retinal detachment, subretinal neovascularization, and band keratopathy. If untreated or inappropriately treated, eyes with uveitis may become phthisical.

Cataract

Cataracts occur in patients with uveitis as a direct result of the inflammation, as well as secondary to treatment for the inflammation (corticosteroid treatment). Anterior subcapsular cataracts occur when extensive posterior synechiae form and result in necrosis of the underlying lens epithelium and opacification. Inflammation in the posterior chamber may result in posterior migration of equatorial lens epithelial cells and their subsequent proliferation and degeneration. This, in turn, results in posterior subcapsular cataracts, the most common type of cataract seen in uveitis. Cataracts are especially common in uveitis associated with juvenile rheumatoid arthritis (9, 10, 20), Fuchs heterochromic iridocyclitis (5, 11, 12), pars planitis (19), and VKH syndrome (16).

Patients with uveitis and cataracts should have minimal or no inflammation before removal of the cataract. Some investigators recommend that the minimal inflammatory state should be controlled for 3 months without flareups; after 3 months, cataract surgery may be safely planned. Oral steroid pulse of 40 to 60 mg of prednisone given daily for 5 to 7 days preoperatively and topical steroid drops administered every 1 or 2 hours may stabilize inflammation in the immediate postoperative period and are recommended. The cataract may be removed by extracapsular cataract extraction or phacoemulsification. If extensive vitritis or vitreous debris is present, a simultanous pars plana vitrectomy should be performed. If extensive posterior synechiae are not present, a posterior chamber intraocular lens may be placed in the bag. In the presence of extensive posterior synechiae, an intraocular lens probably should not be placed, especially if there is chronic persistent inflammation. Postoperatively, steroids may be rapidly tapered according to inflammatory response (4, 8).

Glaucoma

Intraocular pressure elevation may occur in uveitic eyes from inflammatory cells and debris that clog the trabecular meshwork, peripheral anterior synechiae, forward rotation of the lens–iris diaphragm, or posterior synechiae with iris bombé that results in angle closure, inflammation of the trabecular beams ("trabeculitis"), or rubeosis. In addition, corticosteroids, oral and topical, may cause elevation of intraocular pressure, probably by inducing the deposition of glycosaminoglycans (GAGs) in the trabecular meshwork. Topical steroids use may result in intraocular pressure elevation in susceptible individuals as early as 2 weeks after initiation of therapy. However, elevation usually occurs 4 to 6 weeks after therapy is started. Glaucoma is commonly seen in Fuchs' Heterochromic Iridocyclitis (FHI) (12), VKH syndrome (3), uveitis associated with juvenile rheumatoid arthritis (20), and Pössner-Schlossman syndrome.

Therapy should be directed toward control of intraocular inflammation with simultaneous use of aqueous suppressants, beta-blockers, and carbonic anhydrase inhibitors, if necessary. Of course, if the intraocular pressure elevation is steroid-induced, corticosteroids should be tapered. Miotic agents are contraindicated in inflamed eyes, as they may exacerbate inflammation and synechia formation. Surgical peripheral iridectomy should be performed in cases of pupillary block. Iris specimens from surgical iridectomies also may be used for histopathologic confirmation of the cause and diagnosis of the uveitis entity. Laser iridotomies often close off in eyes with uveitis; however, large laser iridotomies may be attempted when systemic problems preclude formal intraocular surgery. If glaucoma cannot be controlled medically, trabeculectomy with 5-fluorouracil or mitomycin should be performed. If this fails, a Molteno or similar seton should be used. Cyclocryotherapy or cyclophotocoagulation is reserved for the most severe cases, as these procedures increase the risk of eventual hypotony and phthisis bulbi.

Cystoid Macular Edema

Cystoid macular edema is a major cause of limited visual acuity in patients with uveitis and should be suspected in patients with uveitis and decreased vision, metamorphopsia, or both. Examination with biomicroscopy using a 90- or 60-diopter (D) lens or fundus contact lens is important. Fluorescein angiography also is essential, especially in cases where CME is not clinically apparent. Although it may occur with any severe anterior or posterior uveitis, it is seen most commonly in patients with intermediate uveitis (pars planitis), birdshot chorioretinopathy, and retinal vasculitis. CME should be treated early, and low-dose acetazolamide may be helpful in some patients. However, because intraocular inflammation needs to be controlled, corticosteroids are the first line of therapy. Typically, 40 mg of triamcinolone acetate may be given in the posterior sub-Tenon's space; this injection is repeated every 2 weeks. Failure of vision to improve or CME to resolve after 4 injections is usually an indication for systemic corticosteroid therapy. If this is unsuccessful, pars plana vitrectomy or systemic immunosuppressive therapy may be considered.

Retinal Detachment

Serous retinal detachments are seen in posterior scleritis, sympathetic ophthalmia, and VKH syndrome. Intense choroidal inflammation results in exudation of fluid from the choroid into the subretinal space, but this usually responds well to systemic or periocular corticosteroids. Tractional retinal detachments may be seen in toxocariasis, pars planitis, or toxoplasma retinochoroiditis. Intense vitreous inflammation can lead to organization of the vitreous and formation of traction bands. These are usually treated surgically if the macula becomes detached. Rhegmatogenous retinal detachments occur if severe retinitis results in retinal necrosis and subsequent hole or tear formation. These are classically seen in cytomegalovirus retinitis and acute retinal necrosis syndrome. Treatment of tractional retinal detachments that involve the macula and rhegmatogenous retinal detachments requires scleral buckling, often in addition to complex vitreoretinal surgery with intraocular gas or silicone oil retinal tamponade.

Subretinal Neovascularization

Chronic choroidal inflammation results often in destruction of the overlying retinal pigment epithelium and Bruch's membrane. This structural change, along with various angiogenic factors liberated by the inflammation, may result in growth of neovascular membranes from the choroid. This complication is seen in presumed ocular histoplasmosis syndrome and in chronic recurrent VKH syndrome (17). If sight is threatened, angiographic identification and photocoagulation should be performed.

Band Keratopathy

Band keratopathy (9, 10, 20) is commonly caused by chronic uveitis entities, especially iridocyclitis associated with juvenile rheumatoid arthritis (Fig. 31–1). Pathologically, calcium is deposited in Bowman's membrane in the interpalpebral zone (possibly due to differences in pH). If this is visually significant, calcium may be removed by epithelial debridement and application of topical 1% to 2% EDTA.

Hypotony and Phthisis Bulbi

Chronic inflammation of the ciliary body, which leads to atrophy of the ciliary epithelium, increased uveoscleral

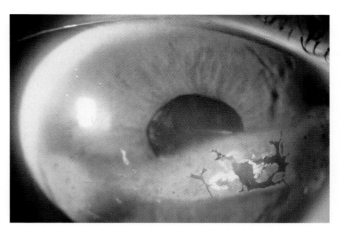

Figure 31–1.
Band keratopathy in a patient with juvenile rheumatoid arthritis with chronic anterior uveitis.

outflow, and cyclitic membrane formation with ciliary body and retinal detachments, results in hypotony. In chronically inflamed eyes, other changes include breakdown of the blood–aqueous barrier and altered aqueous composition, which result in reduced nutritional supply to anterior segment structures. Corneal endothelial decompensation with edema and vascularization result. Chronic angle closure from peripheral anterior synechiae, rubeosis, and cataract formation often follow. The ciliary body and choroid become chronically edematous. The retina also becomes edematous, may detach, and may be thrown into folds. Cyclitic membranes and epiretinal membranes may form. Disc edema and eventual optic atrophy occur. When structural disorganization occurs with metaplastic changes of the retinal pigment epithelium and other tissues, along with scleral thickening, the eye becomes "square" shaped. This change is called *phthisis bulbi*. Pars plana vitrectomy with removal of cyclitic membranes in chronically hypotonous eyes may prevent the gradual downhill course to phthisis.

■ REFERENCES

1. Biswas J, Rao NA: Management of intraocular inflammation. In: Ryan SJ, ed. Retina, Vol 2. St Louis: CV Mosby 1989: 139–146.
2. Feutren G, Mihatsch MJ: For the Int. Kidney Biopsy Registry of Cyclosporine in Autoimmune Diseases. Risk factors for cyclosporine-induced nephropathy in patients with autoimmune diseases. N Engl J Med 1992; 326: 1654–1660.
3. Forster DJ, Rao NA, Hill RA, Nguyen QH, Baerveldt G: Incidence and management of glaucoma in Vogt-Koyanagi-Harada syndrome. Ophthalmology 1990; 97(Suppl): 143.
4. Foster CS, Fong LP, Singh G: Cataract surgery and in-
traocular lens implantation in patients with uveitis. Ophthalmology 1989; 96: 281–288.
5. Franceschetti A: Heterochromic cyclitis (Fuchs' syndrome). Am J Ophthalmol 1955; 39: 50–58.
6. Fujino Y, Mochizuki M, Chan CC, et al.: FK506 treatment of S-antigen induced uveitis in primates. Curr Eye Res 1991; 10: 679–690.
7. Hemady R, Tauber J, Foster CS: Immunosuppressive drugs in immune and inflammatory ocular disease. Surv Ophthalmol 1991; 35: 369–385.
8. Hooper PL, Rao NA, Smith RE: Cataract extraction in uveitis patients. Surv Ophthalmol 1990;35:120–144.

9. Kanski JJ, Shun-Shin GA: Systemic uveitis syndromes in childhood: An analysis of 340 cases. Ophthalmology 1984; 91: 1247–1252.

10. Key SN III, Kimura SJ: Iridocyclitis associated with juvenile rheumatoid arthritis. Am J Ophthalmol 1975; 80: 425–429.

11. Kimura SJ, Hogan MJ, Thygeson P: Fuchs' syndrome of heterochromic cyclitis. Arch Ophthalmol 1955; 54: 179–186.

12. Liesegang TJ: Clinical features and prognosis in Fuchs' uveitis syndrome. Arch Ophthalmol 1982; 100: 1622–1626.

13. Minakawa R, Ohno S, Hirose S, et al.: Clinical manifestation of Vogt-Koyanagi-Harada's disease. Jpn J Clin Ophthalmol 1985; 39: 1249–1253.

14. Mochizuki M, Kawashima H: Effects of FK506, 15-deoxyspergualin, and cyclosporine on experimental autoimmune uveoretinitis in the rat. Autoimmunity 1990; 8: 37–41.

15. Mochizuki M, Masuda K, Sakane T, et al.: A multicenter clinical open trial of FK 506 in refractory uveitis, including Behçet's disease. Japanese FK 506 Study Group on Refractory Uveitis. Tranplant Proc 1991; 23: 3343–3346.

16. Moorthy RS, Buddi R, Smith RE, Rao NA: Incidence and management of cataracts in Vogt-Koyanagi-Harada syndrome. Am J Ophthalmol 1994; 118: 197–204.

17. Moorthy RS, Chong LP, Smith RE, Rao NA: Subretinal neovascular membranes in Vogt-Koyanagi-Harada syndrome. Am J Ophthalmol 1993a; 116: 164–170.

18. Schreiber SL, Crabtree GR: The mechanism of action of cyclosporin A and FK506. Immunol Today 1992; 13: 136–142.

19. Smith RE: Pars planitis. In: Ryan Sl, ed. Retina, Vol 2. St. Louis: CV Mosby 1989: 637–645.

20. Wolf MD, Lichter PR, Ragsdale CG: Prognostic factors in the uveitis of juvenile rheumatoid arthritis. Ophthalmology 1987; 94: 1242–1248.

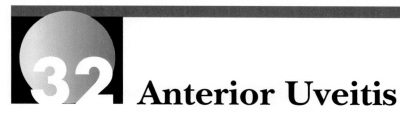

32 Anterior Uveitis

Ramana S. Moorthy, Narsing A. Rao

Entities associated with inflammation that involves primarily the anterior uvea may be termed anterior uveitis, iritis, or iridocyclitis. Specific anterior uveitis entities include HLA-B27 related iridocyclitis, juvenile rheumatoid arthritis (JRA), herpetic kerato-uveitis, Fuchs' heterochromic iridocyclitis, syphilis, tuberculosis, intraocular lens associated uveitis, Posner-Schlossman syndrome, traumatic iridocyclitis, and idiopathic anterior uveitis.

◼ HLA-B27 RELATED UVEITIS

HLA-B27 haplotype-related iridocyclitis is a common type of anterior uveitis. Approximately 50% of patients who present with an acute anterior uveitis, if tested, are found to be HLA-B27 positive (1–3). Of this group, more than half will have some type of spondyloarthropathy that is otherwise seronegative (3), such as ankylosing spondylitis (AS), Reiter's syndrome, and psoriatic arthropathy. Other systemic associations with HLA-B27 include Crohn's disease, Whipple's disease, and ulcerative colitis, which are together called inflammatory bowel diseases (IBD). IBD may have connective tissue, joint, and intraocular manifestations. Hence, it is apparent that the HLA-B27 haplotype may predispose individuals to systemic, as well as intraocular inflammations, although the way in which the haplotype functions in this capacity is still unclear.

Up to 90% of patients who have AS are described as HLA-B27 positive (4, 5). AS tends to affect men in the third to fourth decades of life, but it also occurs in women and children. There is a strong familial predisposition to AS since the HLA-B27 haplotype is inherited. The sacroiliac joints are primarily involved but peripheral joints may also become arthritic. Symptoms of sacroiliac joint involvement may be gradual in onset, and may affect the lower, as well as the upper back. Pain, stiffness, localized tenderness, muscle spasms, and sciatica are common complaints. Up to 25% of AS patients develop iridocyclitis (4).

Reiter's syndrome also tends to affect young men, usually between the ages of 15 and 35. The characteristic triad of Reiter's syndrome consists of arthritis, urethritis, and conjunctivitis. In one large study, 98% of patients developed arthritis, 74% developed urethritis, and 58% developed conjunctivitis. (6) Other oral and genital lesions include keratoderma blennorrhagicum or balanitis circinata, respectively. The arthritis will affect the upper and lower extremities, as well as the sacroiliac joints, in up to 20% of patients (6). Urethritis is usually nonspecific and not associated with bacterial infection, but may be accompanied by cystitis or prostatitis. The ocular involvement is usually in the form of conjunctivitis, often with a follicular reaction, mucopurulent discharge, and occasionally with preauricular adenopathy. Some patients develop a nongranulomatous iritis. Other ocular manifestations include keratitis and episcleritis. The etiology of Reiter's syndrome is unknown, but there is some association with bacillary dysentery. Organisms such as Shigella, Yersinia, Chlamydia, Mycoplasma, Ureaplasma ureolyticum, and Salmonella have all been implicated as possible causes of Reiter's syndrome. More than two-thirds (67 to 90%) of patients with Reiter's syndrome are HLA-B27 positive (6–7).

Psoriatic arthritis tends to affect individuals in their third to fourth decades, unlike the other HLA-B27-associated disorders. A history of psoriatic skin changes associated with destructive arthropathy of the small joints of the hands and feet, sacroiliitis, and spondylitis are common in this disorder. HLA-B27 is expressed in up to 60% of these patients (5). A small number of these patients develop an anterior uveitis that is similar in nature to HLA-B27-associated iridocyclitis.

Inflammatory bowel diseases are enthropathic arthropathies that have rheumatologic manifestations, and include ulcerative colitis, Crohn's disease, and Whipple's disease. Patients with IBD who express the HLA-B27 haplotype have a higher incidence of sacroiliac joint involvement and iridocyclitis, further implicating a genetic link to these disorders (5). The ocular manifestations of IBD are varied. Any of the ocular tissues can become inflamed, resulting in conjunctivitis, corneal infiltrates, episcleritis, scleritis, vitritis, or optic neuritis. The most common of these changes is nongranulomatous iridocyclitis, which occurs in up to 11% of patients (8–9). Ocular inflammation may parallel intestinal or articular disease. It has been reported that in some patients with ulcerative colitis, colectomy results in resolution of the ocular disease; however, this may not prevent recurrences of ocular inflammation (10). Patients with Whipple's disease may respond to treatment with systemic tetracycline.

Clinical Features

The iridocyclitis seen with HLA-B27 disease is usually of acute onset and characterized by a red, "hot" eye. Usually only one eye is involved, but over many years, the other eye may also become involved. Males in their second to third decades are more commonly affected. Patients with acute anterior uveitis who express HLA-B27 tend to be much younger than those who do not. Symptoms include severe pain, redness, tearing, photophobia, and decreased vision. The inflammation is characteristically severe and nongranulomatous, often with a fibrinous exudate, formation of a hypopyon (Figure 32–1) and posterior synechiae. Multiple small keratic precipitates may be seen. Vitritis is variable and limited to the anterior vitreous, and represents "spill over" inflammation from the anterior segment. Cystoid macular edema may be present. Recurrences are common in this disorder, but the initial episode is the most severe. Recurrences may occur as often as once every 3 to 6 months or as infrequently as every 3 years. Despite the eventual bilateral involvement, usually only one eye is involved at a time, and in those cases with simultaneous

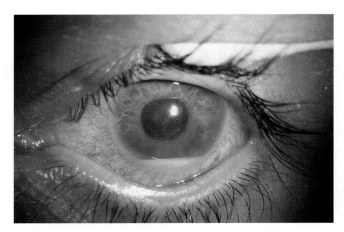

Figure 32–1.
Acute anterior uveitis with hypopyon in a HLA-B27 positive patient.

bilateral involvement, one eye is predominantly involved.

Patients who present with typical, recurrent, acute and severe anterior uveitis, particularly young males with a history of back pain, arthralgias, or gastrointestinal symptoms, should be tested for the presence of HLA-B27 haplotype. Although it does not change the approach to the management, a positive test does allow counseling of the patient regarding the prognosis as well as the nature of the course of this disease. Associated systemic symptoms must be appropriately investigated by an internist or rheumatologist.

The differential diagnosis of acute recurrent anterior uveitis includes infectious, as well as noninfectious disorders. However, with the appropriate history and clinical presentation, the differential diagnosis can be narrowed.

The prognosis of HLA-B27-associated iridocyclitis is good when acute episodes are treated early. However, in one large retrospective study of a series of uveitis patients, those who were HLA-B27 positive tended to have more complications than those who were HLA-B27 negative, including cataracts, glaucoma, posterior synechiae, and cystoid macular edema. But final visual acuity did not differ between the two groups (3).

Patients with acute HLA B27-related iridocyclitis should be treated with frequent topical corticosteroid drops, often every hour or every half hour, with intense cycloplegia initially to break posterior synechiae. In particularly severe cases of anterior segment inflammation, especially in the presence of a hypopyon or cystoid macular edema, periocular steroids or a short course of high dose oral prednisone with a rapid taper may be effective in reducing the inflammation and augmenting topical therapy. Most patients with Whipple's disease can be treated with systemic tetracycline, which may improve the ocular disease.

Juvenile Rheumatoid Arthritis (JRA)

Juvenile chronic arthritis includes many different spondyloarthropathies of unknown etiology. A subset of diseases called JRA is of special interest to the ophthalmologist. JRA accounts for 70% of all cases of juvenile chronic arthritis (11), and is the most common disorder associated with iridocyclitis in the pediatric age group. JRA may be subdivided into four groups of diseases; Still's disease, polyarticular JRA, pauciarticular early onset JRA, and late onset JRA.

Systemic onset JRA or Still's disease accounts for 20% of all cases of JRA. Patients who present with Still's disease are often less than 5 years of age, with systemic manifestations such as fever, rash, lymphadenopathy, and hepatosplenomegaly. These patients tend not to develop iridocyclitis; they account for a little less than 6% of all JRA patients who have uveitis (12, 13, 14, 15).

Polyarticular JRA, in which five or more joints are involved, accounts for forty percent of all JRA cases. Thirty percent of these patients are negative for rheumatoid factor. A preponderance of females are affected by this disease, and the arthritis occurs more commonly in the rheumatoid factor positive group. Approximately seven to fourteen percent of JRA patients with uveitis fall into this group (12, 13, 14, 15).

The pauciarticular group may be subdivided into early-onset and late-onset forms, and comprises approximately 40% of all patients with JRA: 25% with early onset and 15% with later onset (7,16). Up to 80% of patients with early-onset disease are females, while the later-onset disease is more common in males. Typically, fewer than 5 joints are involved, and in the early-onset form the knee, ankle, or elbow are usually involved. In the late-onset form, the sacroiliac joints are involved. Iridocyclitis is more common in the early-onset variety, with 20 to 40% of these patients developing chronic iridocyclitis, compared with 10 to 20% of the later onset group. Rheumatoid factor is negative in both groups. However, up to 60% of patients with the early-onset disease are positive for antinuclear antibody (ANA). Patients with late-onset disease are not typically ANA positive. Additionally, the late-onset variety does have a 75% incidence of HLA-B27 positivity (17). These 2 forms of JRA are associated with iridocyclitis comprising between 78 and 91% of JRA patients with uveitis (12, 13, 14, 15).

The clinical features typically include bilateral nongranulomatous chronic anterior segment inflammation associated with white, quiet eyes. The only exception to this are those patients who have late-onset pauciarticular disease and who express the HLA-B27 antigen. Typically, patients with JRA-associated uveitis are asymptomatic, and are discovered to have inflammation only on routine slit lamp examination (11). The anterior chamber reaction is variable, associated with small keratic precipitates, posterior synechia, and anterior vitreous cells. Often, chronicity of the inflammation is marked by the presence of cells in the anterior chamber and in the anterior part of the vitreous, calcific band keratopathy, and the development of a cataract (Figure 32–2). Patients with active or inactive inflammation may show flare in the anterior chamber. However, only the presence of cells suggests active inflammation. Patients with JRA tend to develop uveitis within the first 7 years after the diagnosis, although some patients with JRA have developed uveitis as much as 20 years after the diagnosis of JRA. Little correlation is thought to exist between the severity and activity of the joint disease and the eye disease. Risk factors for development of uveitis in JRA patients include being female, pauciarticular onset, and the presence of antinuclear antibodies (11, 14).

Patients who present with anterior uveitis during childhood should have laboratory evaluation for presence of serum antinuclear antibodies and HLA-B27, as well as an erythrocyte sedimentation rate. A complete evaluation by a pediatrician is essential. Appropriate radiographic studies to assess joint involvement is also important.

The differential diagnosis of JRA should include sarcoidosis, which can present in a similar fashion. The value of serum angiotensin converting enzyme in the pediatric age group is less clearcut than in adults (18). A chest radiograph may be useful in showing hilar lymphadenopathy in sarcoidosis.

Course and Prognosis

Owing to the insidious nature of the intraocular inflammation associated with JRA, patients are often seen late in the course of the disease, when complications such as

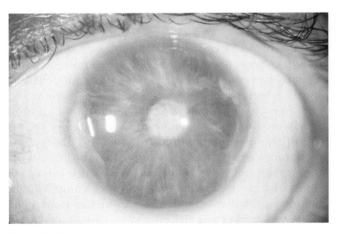

Figure 32–2.
Peripheral band keratopathy and cataract in a patient with JRA-associated chronic uveitis.

cataract, glaucoma, or band keratopathy have already developed. Early detection and management with topical corticosteroid drops and mydriatics are useful and essential in reducing the long-term complications of JRA. Over 50% of patients with JRA-related uveitis develop band keratopathy (19), 30% can develop cataracts (14), and up to 22% develop glaucoma (11, 12, 14, 15). Hypotony and phthisis bulbi may occur if the uveitis is not managed properly (11).

The treatment of JRA-associated uveitis is directed towards control of intraocular inflammation by means of topical corticosteroids and mydriatics. Short-acting mydriatics are preferred to long-acting agents to keep the pupil mobile and avoid development of posterior synechiae. Topical corticosteroids may be used frequently, up to 1 drop every hour or every 2 hours during acute exacerbations, and tapered according to response of inflammation. The presence of continuous flare alone does not require treatment with topical steroids. Flare suggests long-term breakdown of the blood-aqueous barrier, which allows proteins to leak into the anterior chamber; this is not uncommon in longstanding cases of inactive uveitis. Using corticosteroids in situations in which there are no cells in the anterior chamber, may enhance the development of glaucoma and cataracts. When topical corticosteroids are ineffective in controlling a patient's intraocular inflammation, posterior sub-Tenon's injections of depo-corticosteroid may be useful. Systemic corticosteroids are of limited utility because of the associated stunting of growth and development that may occur with the use of these agents (11); so the risks may outweigh the benefits. This is also true for cytotoxic agents. Glaucoma may be controlled medically with topical beta blockers and systemic carbonic anhydrase inhibitors, but it must be kept in mind that patients taking salicylates for their arthritis can develop severe metabolic acidosis if given carbonic anhydrase inhibitors (11). In addition, miotics should not be used in eyes with intraocular inflammation, since these agents may worsen the inflammation.

The surgical treatment of JRA-associated complications has been problematic. It is recommended that cataracts be removed by the extracapsular phascoemulsification technique combined with a pars plana vitrectomy (11, 20). This approach has shown to be of most benefit in visual rehabilitation of these patients. Dissection of the peripheral vitreous base, as well as cyclitic membranes when possible, is important in the intraoperative management of these patients, since it reduces the risk of phthisis bulbi. Postoperative complications include pupillary membrane formation, hypotony, glaucoma, and cystoid macular edema (11, 20). Aphakic patients with JRA who have undergone lensectomy and pars plana vitrectomy should be left aphakic. However, the management of unilateral aphakia in children is difficult and challenging. Contact lens correction of aphakia and aggressive treatment of amblyopia is essential.

Glaucoma has a poor prognosis in patients with JRA-associated uveitis. Up to one-third of these cases may progress to no light perception (13). Standard filtering surgery is of little benefit in these cases (21). Trabeculodialysis offers a better chance of success, with adequate control of pressure achieved in up to 60% of cases in one study (11). Tube shunts or drainage devices, however, may offer even better success rates in the management of glaucoma.

Band keratopathy can be managed by scraping of the corneal epithelium and the use of a topical calcium chelator, such as EDTA, to remove calcium from Bowman's membrane.

Fuchs' Heterochromic Iridocyclitis (FHI)

FHI is an important, and often overlooked cause of anterior uveitis in middle-aged adults. It accounts for approximately 2 to 5% of all cases of anterior uveitis in this age group (22). The etiology and pathogenesis of FHI remain unclear, but it may represent an autoimmune reaction against pigment present within the iris.

Typically, FHI is characterized by heterochromia of the iris (Figure 32–3), diffuse atrophy of the iris stroma, stellate fine keratic precipitates scattered throughout the endothelial surface of the cornea, and mild anterior segment inflammation with moderate numbers of cells that may spill over into the anterior vitreous (23, 24, 25, 26). In the majority of patients, it is a unilateral condition. The eye with the lighter colored iris is usually the involved eye. However, 7 to 15% of patients have bilateral involvement without heterochromia. Other variations include unilateral involvement with no heterochromia and "paradoxical" inflammation in the darker colored eye (27, 28). Involvement of the darker colored eye is particularly common in blue-eyed patients, in whom loss of the anterior iris stroma exposes underlying pigment epithelium and results in a darker

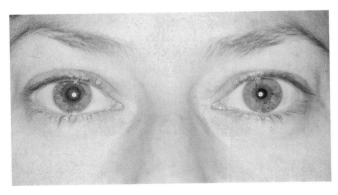

Figure 32–3.
A 32-year-old female with Fuchs' heterochromic iridocyelitis. Note light-colored right iris.

appearance to the iris, the so called paradoxical heterochromia. It is best to show heterochromia in bright sunlight. Despite the variability of heterochromia, iris atrophy is a characteristic feature (27). Stellate keratic precipitates, which are scattered throughout the surface of the corneal endothelium instead of simply in Arlt's triangle, are also characteristic of FHI (24, 26, 27). Because there is atrophy of the iris stroma, the iris vessels are prominent. Gonioscopy reveals abnormal appearing iris vessels crossing the angle, vessels that may lead to rare, spontaneous hyphema (27). In addition, it was found that patients with FHI who undergo ocular surgery may develop a hyphema postoperatively. There are no typical symptoms of anterior uveitis such as redness, pain, or photophobia in these patients. Most patients present with reduced vision secondary to cataract (27), which develop in approximately 50% of patients with FHI. Between 16 and 59% of patients develop glaucoma of the open-angle type (23, 24, 27).

No laboratory tests are indicated in typical cases of FHI. In atypical cases, however, evaluation for other causes of anterior uveitis is important.

The differential diagnosis of FHI includes herpetic keratouveitis, which may be associated with diffuse keratic precipitates and iris stromal atrophy. Other causes of heterochromia, such as iris melanoma and congenital Horner's syndrome, should also be ruled out (28). Intermediate uveitis, when the cells spill over into the anterior chamber, can mimic FHI since these patients may not have any symptoms of acute anterior uveitis.

The cellular reaction in the anterior segment is often unresponsive to corticosteroids. Corticosteroid therapy is, therefore, not warranted, and may in fact exacerbate the complications associated with FHI, including cataracts and glaucoma. After a week of intensive topical therapy, if the anterior segment inflammation does not respond to treatment, it is essential to taper the topical medications quickly. Treatment of complications of FHI are intriguing. Cataract surgery typically is not associated with any greater risk than in patients without FHI (29). Patients tend to tolerate intraocular lens implantation well. Postoperative complications include hyphema, vitreous hemorrhage, glaucoma, and progressive vitreous opacification. Patients with glaucoma associated with FHI may have serious problems with intraocular pressure control. In one study, medical therapy adequately controlled intraocular pressure in only thirty percent of the patients (27). Those remaining required surgical treatment and less than sixty percent of them had adequate control of intraocular pressure after surgery, with or without medications (27).

Herpetic Iridocyclitis. Herpes simplex (HSV) and herpes zoster (HZV) viruses can each produce an anterior uveitis. Typically, the uveitis is secondary to keratitis. However, the uveitis may be present without any evidence of corneal involvement. Uveitis can also occur with herpes zoster ophthalmicus (HZO). Herpetic iridocyclitis can be acute, recurrent, or chronic.

HSV iridocyclitis is usually seen in association with stromal or disciform keratitis, but may be occasionally seen with only dendritic epithelial keratitis or with no active corneal disease (30, 31). Examination of the cornea reveals fine diffuse keratic precipitates. Anterior segment reaction is variable but may be intense enough to produce a hypopyon. Posterior synechiae and sectoral iris atrophy with transillumination defects may also be present in prolonged or recurrent cases. Patients who present with disciform stromal scars of the cornea and anterior segment inflammation should be suspected of having HSV uveitis. It is thought that the anterior segment inflammation may represent either virus replication within the iris or immune reaction to viral antigen (30,32).

Herpes zoster anterior uveitis is usually seen in conjunction with HZO (33–34). Anterior segment inflammation can occur at any time during the course of the disease. The uveitis results from vascular occlusion, and the subsequent ischemia from a vasculitis mediated by the HZV. Ischemia of the iris vessels and sectoral iris stromal atrophy (Figure 32–4) may also occur. Stromal atrophy is much more common in HZV than in HSV. Clinical findings include the presence of fine keratic precipitates which may or may not be associated with a (micro-)dendritic or stromal keratitis, a variable amount of anterior segment cells that may be numerous enough to produce a hypopyon, and occasionally a combination of hypopyon and hyphema (34). In addition, posterior synechiae may also be found. Cultures of the aqueous humor rarely reveal virus. Pathologically, the inflammation is nongranulomatous initially, but may become granulomatous with chronicity (35).

Complications of uveitis and keratouveitis include the development of stromal scarring, which often limits

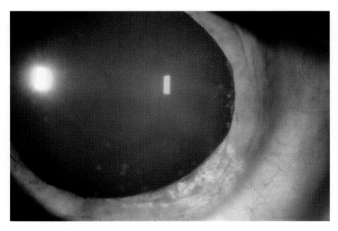

Figure 32–4.
Chronic herpes zoster anterior uveitis. Pigmented keratic precipitates and segmental iris atrophy is present.

visual acuity significantly, and glaucoma, typically from trabeculitis caused by either HSV or HZV. Trabeculitis results in a reduction in aqueous outflow facility and causes intraocular pressure elevation (32). The glaucoma associated with herpetic iridocyclitis is often difficult to control.

Laboratory investigations in herpetic iridocyclitis are of little value. Antibody levels to HSV and HZV are not useful since an increased rate of positivity exists in the majority of the general adult population. The presence of corneal epithelial disease is helpful in making the diagnosis, but if the epithelial disease is not characteristic of herpes, cultures and scrapings of the epithelium may be helpful. Electron microscopy of the epithelial scraping is useful in identifying virus particles.

Because of the exquisite sensitivity of HSV to topical antivirals such as trifluorothymidine, these medications are indicated in the treatment of HSV keratouveitis. If epithelial involvement is present, steroids should not be used alone, since they may enhance virus replication in the cornea and worsen the epithelial disease. HZO should be treated acutely with oral acyclovir, 600 to 800 mg 5 times daily for 10 days, to reduce the long-term complications. Recurrent epithelial disease, stromal keratitis, or even recurrent iridocyclitis in patients with HSV keratouveitis may be an indication for the use of systemic acyclovir (36). Currently, the effectiveness of oral acyclovir in preventing recurrences in patients with keratouveitis is under study. Corticosteroids in HZO are used mainly to reduce postherpetic neuralgia, but these should definitely be avoided in immunocompromised individuals.

■ SYPHILIS

Syphilitic uveitis accounts for less than 1% of all cases of uveitis (37). In acquired syphilitic infection, iridocyclitis is a common ocular manifestation (38) that occurs in the secondary stages of the illness. Iridocyclitis can be granulomatous or nongranulomatous. Dilated capillary loops within the iris, called roseata, appear as red nodular lesions within the iris stroma. Posterior segment involvement can include vitritis, chorioretinitis, vasculitis, optic papillitis, or neuroretinitis. An acute posterior placoid form of chorioretinitis has also been reported (39). Involvement of the optic nerve results eventually in optic atrophy. Most of the damage is probably a result of direct infection of the tissues by treponemal organisms, which may be shown by darkfield examination (38,40). Immune reaction to treponemal antigens may also be responsible for intraocular inflammation.

Laboratory testing is essential in patients with this infectious and potentially treatable cause of anterior uveitis. Serologic tests may be divided into two types: namely, those tests for recent, active infection, such as venereal disease research laboratory (VDRL) and rapid plasma reagin (RPR) tests, and tests of past infections (antibodies to treponemal organisms) such as fluorescent treponemal antibody (FTA-ABS) and microhemagglutination assay for Treponema pallidum (MHA-TP). Interpretation of serologic tests for syphilis is often confusing. A negative VDRL and FTA indicate no evidence of syphilis or early primary syphilis. A positive VDRL and a negative FTA-ABS suggest early primary syphilis, in which case the test needs to be repeated to rule out a false-positive VDRL. A false-positive VDRL test can be the result of various other conditions, including systemic lupus erythematosus (SLE), rheumatoid arthritis, hepatitis, pregnancy, leprosy, and malaria. Following the levels of VDRL titers in the serum may be

useful if early primary syphilis is suspected. A negative VDRL and a positive FTA suggests adequately treated syphilis or tertiary syphilis. If neurosyphilis is suspected, evaluation of VDRL titers in spinal fluid is indicated. A positive VDRL and a positive FTA suggests recently treated, untreated, or inadequately treated syphilis, and it is recommended that the tests be repeated. Decreased titers of VDRL on the repeat test suggests adequate treatment; increasing VDRL titers suggest possible reinfection. In a large series of patients with ocular syphilis, the VDRL was positive in only 68% of patients, whereas all were FTA-ABS positive (41).

Differential diagnosis of syphilitic uveitis includes other causes of both granulomatous and nongranulomatous anterior uveitis. Purified protein derivative (PPD) skin test, chest radiograph, and serum angiotensin converting enzyme levels should be obtained to rule out tuberculosis and sarcoidosis. ANA, HLA-B27, and rheumatoid factor should be obtained to rule out rheumatologic disease, which may give false–positive VDRL test results. In addition, if syphilis is truly suspected, because of the AIDS epidemic, tests for HIV infection should also be done on these patients (41).

The treatment of syphilis depends on the stage of the disease. Primary, secondary, or latent stages of less than 1 year duration should be treated with benzathine penicillin, 2.4 million units, given once intramuscularly (42). An alternative treatment at this point is doxycycline, 100 mg by mouth twice daily for 2 weeks. Late stages of syphilis present for more than 1 year, with or without associated cardiovascular gumma, and late latent lesions should be treated with intramuscular benzathine penicillin, 2.4 million units weekly for 3 weeks. Another option is doxycycline, 100 mg orally twice daily for 4 weeks. Treatment for neurosyphilis and congenital

TABLE 32–1
Treatment of Syphilis[1]

Type of Syphilis	Drug of Choice and Dosage
Congenital	1. Penicillin G 50,000 U/kg IM or IV QD 8–12 h × 10–14 days
	2. Procaine penicillin G 50,000 U/kg IM QD × 10–14 days
Early—<1 yr Duration	1. Penicillin G 2.4 million units IM × 1
Primary, Secondary, or	2. or erythromycin 500 mg po QID × 2 weeks
Latent	3. or doxycycline 100 mg po bid × 2 weeks
Late—>1 yr Duration	1. Penicillin G 2.4 million units IM QD week × 3
Cardivascular/gummatous	2. Doxycycline 100 mg po bid × 4 weeks
No Neurosyphilis	
Neurosyphilis	1. Penicillin G 2 to 4 million units IV QD 4 hr × 10–14 days
	2. or procaine penicillin G 2.4 million units IM QD day + probenecid 500 mg po QID × 10–14 days

[1] Medical Letter on Drugs and Therapeutics. 36:1–6, 1994.

syphilis is outlined in Table 32–1. Patients who are allergic to penicillin may be treated with doxycycline. Erythromycin may also be used. In addition, early primary and secondary cases may be treated with 250 mg of ceftriaxone by intramuscular injection given daily for 10 days.

Patients who present with anterior uveitis that is unresponsive to corticosteroids should be worked up for syphilis. Prognosis for vision is good since uveitis is typically treatable and curable with adequate antibiotics. Prolonged inflammation that is untreated or inadequately treated may result in glaucoma or irreversible optic atrophy. Syphilitic infections can be much more aggressive in immunocompromised patients who are HIV positive, and should be treated aggressively.

■ TUBERCULOSIS

Tuberculosis (TB) was a major cause of uveitis in the past, but today it accounts for less than 1% of all cases of uveitis (37). However, the AIDS epidemic has again brought TB into the limelight as an important cause of uveitis. TB affects nearly all ocular tissues with a granulomatous inflammatory process. Corneal infections may manifest as phlyctenulosis or interstitial keratitis (40). Granulomatous iridocyclitis, usually chronic, may be present. Vitritis, retinal periphlebitis, solitary or multiple choroidal tubercles, and panuveitis are also manifestations of posterior segment tuberculous infection. Involvement may also be seen in miliary TB, in which multiple choroidal infiltrates are present. Patients without pulmonary disease may have evidence of tuberculous ocular inflammation. Like syphilis, TB uveitis is caused by the organism directly or from hypersensitivity reactions to mycobacterial antigens.

Patients suspected of having TB uveitis should have a purified protein derivative (PPD) skin test and chest radiograph. The interpretation of a positive PPD test is controversial. However, it is clear that patients who have not had a previous BCG vaccination, and who have a positive PPD, should be assumed to be recent converters. Patients who have had previous BCG (Bacille Cal-mette-Guerin) vaccinations or who live in areas where TB may be endemic should have cautious interpretations of positive PPD tests. Typically, patients who have had distant past BCG vaccinations will not mount a positive PPD skin test years after the vaccination. Thus, a positive PPD skin test should indicate again either recent exposure to the bacillus, or to antigens of the bacillus. In endemic areas, the degree of positivity (greater than the standard 10 mm induration for single strength PPD) of the skin reaction should be used to determine if treatment is warranted. In addition, further confusion results in skin test interpretation in immunocompromised patients in whom the cell-mediated immune response may be dampened. As a result, patients who are immunocompromised, or perhaps some patients with sarcoidosis, may have a negative PPD despite active infection. This condition is also seen in patients on systemic corticosteroids or in patients who have severe miliary TB, a situation in which the organisms have overwhelmed the immune response of the host.

Syphilis and sarcoidosis should be ruled out when TB is suspected. The treatment of TB uveitis should be managed by an internist in conjunction with an ophthalmologist. Typically, isoniazid is used in combination

TABLE 32–2
Treatment of Tuberculosis and Confirmed Tuberculous Uveitis

Drug	Usual Adult Dosage	Duration	Side Effects
Isoniazid	300 mg QD	6 months	Hepatotoxicity (esp. >40 yo)
Rifampin	600 mg QD	6 months	Hepatotoxicity, GI, thrombocytopenic purpura Orange color to body fluids
Ethambutol	15 mg/kg/day	6 months	Optic neuritis
Pyrazinamide	500 mg tid	6 months	Hepatitis, hyperuricemia, GI, arthralgias
Streptomycin	15 mg/kg/d IM (max 1 gm)	6 months	Ototoxicity, vestibular damage Reduce dosage if >40 yo or reduced renal function

In endemic areas use three or four drug combinations especially if drug-resistant strains are present.

with rifampin for 6 months, in addition to pyrazinamide, which is given for the first 2 months. If pyrazinamide is not used, isoniazid and rifampin should be given for 9 months (see Table 32–2). If TB is endemic to the patient's area of residence, if the patient is immunocompromised, or if the TB is drug resistant, 3 or perhaps 4 agents may be needed concomitantly for 6 to 9 months for adequate treatment. For patients in nonendemic areas who have a positive PPD and a negative chest radiograph, it is suggested that a trial of isoniazid alone for 2 to 3 weeks be given to see if any intraocular inflammation improves (43). Improvement would suggest TB as the causative agent. Similar to other anterior uveitis entities, topical corticosteroids and mydriatic agents may be needed to control severe anterior segment inflammation.

The course and prognosis of TB uveitis is similar to syphilitic uveitis. Once the cause has been established, the use of anti-TB medications usually controls the intraocular inflammation and may result in a cure.

■ INTRAOCULAR LENS INDUCED UVEITIS (UVEITIS-GLAUCOMA-HYPHEMA [UGH] SYNDROME)

In the past, the use of intraocular lens implants in the anterior chamber often resulted in intraocular inflammation. Additionally, intraocular inflammation was often worsened by the use of certain materials in the manufacture of these lenses, and by surface contaminants on these lenses introduced during surgery or during manufacturing (44). It is assumed the lens materials and contaminants initiate the complement cascade, with subsequent release of chemotactic factors, oxygen free radicals, and inflammatory mediators into the anterior chamber, resulting in anterior segment inflammation (45). Polymethylmethacrylate (PMMA) has been shown to activate complement in vitro (45), and it appears that both nylon and polypropylene are potent activators of complement, as well (46). PMMA seems a weaker complement activator than polypropylene (20). The stimulation of inflammatory cascades is, of course, less important when the intraocular lens is implanted in the capsular bag; however, in vitro studies have shown sulcus fixation of either PMMA lenses or polypropylene lenses can cause the optics to chafe the iris and ciliary body, resulting in breakdown of the blood-aqueous barrier and subsequent inflammation (44). One special variant of intraocular lens-related uveitis is the uveitis-glaucoma-hyphema *(UGH) syndrome.* This was commonly seen with anterior segment intraocular lenses that were rigid and whose haptics eroded into the iris root (44). UGH syndrome is uncommon today, but can occur after posterior chamber intraocular lens implantation. It is characterized by recurrent bouts of inflammation that may be severe enough to produce a hypopyon, chafing of the iris and ciliary body that produces hyphema, and intraocular pressure elevation during exacerbation of inflammation; all of which necessitates removal of the intraocular lens.

Intraocular lens associated uveitis typically presents as persistent postoperative inflammation in the anterior segment. Keratic precipitates, corneal edema, hypopyon, anterior vitreous cells, and cystoid macular edema are often present. In these forms of uveitis, it is important to rule out indolent infectious causes of postoperative inflammation, including Propionibacterium acnes, Staphylococcus epidermidis, or other low-grade pathogens. Additionally, examination of the anterior chamber may reveal remnants of cortical lens material, which can also induce postoperative inflammation. If Propionibacterium acnes endophthalmitis is suspected, vitrectomy, cultures of vitreous specimen and posterior capsule, and injection of intraocular vancomycin and amikacin should be performed. The treatment consists of the judicious use of topical and periocular steroids, as well as mydriatic agents. The presence of uveitis, glaucoma, and hyphema often neccessitate removal of the intraocular lens. If excessive cortical material remains and incites inflammation, it should be removed. If low-grade endophthalmitis is suspected, especially if inflammation is waxing and waning, or is unresponsive to corticosteroids, a pars plana vitrectomy with or without capsulectomy, aerobic and anaerobic cultures of vitreous and capsule, and injection of intravitreal antibiotics is recommended.

POSNER-SCHLOSSMAN SYNDROME

Glaucomatocyclitic crisis, also known as Posner-Schlossman syndrome (47), is an entity that occurs in young to middle-aged adults and is characterized by unilateral attacks of elevated intraocular pressure associated with signs of anterior uveitis. Intraocular pressure may acutely reach levels of 40 to 60 mm Hg, resulting in blurring of vision, halos, and mild to moderate discomfort. The cornea may show mild epithelial edema. The pupil is mildly dilated in the affected eye. Fine keratic precipitates and a mild cellular reaction in the anterior chamber and anterior vitreous may also occur. Gonioscopy reveals an open angle between attacks (48). Attacks may last anywhere from several hours to several weeks. This disease has a benign and self-limiting course and does not result in visual field changes after the attacks (48), making surgical intervention unnecessary. Some of these eyes, however, do develop chronic open-angle glaucoma.

Treatment is necessary only during attacks. Topical β-blockers or mild miotics (such as 0.5% to 2% pilocarpine) are used to control intraocular pressure. Topical corticosteroids can control inflammation if given 2 to 4 times daily. Strong miotics or mydriatic agents aggravate symptoms and should be avoided (48).

TRAUMATIC IRIDOCYCLITIS

Blunt trauma to the eye can disrupt the blood-aqueous barrier and disperse pigment into the anterior chamber. An anterior chamber inflammatory reaction results, often preceeded by symptoms of photophobia and mild pain. Inflammation is self-limited and may be treated with cycloplegics alone if the inflammation is mild. In severe cases, topical corticosteroids are often helpful in reducing uveitis and the associated symptoms. In any case of blunt eye trauma, the globe should be examined for traumatic dislocation of the lens, angle recession, cyclodialysis, choroidal rupture, and rupture of the globe.

KAWASAKI'S DISEASE

Kawasaki's disease (49) is an acute exanthematous disease of children who are typically less than 5 years of age. The etiology is unknown. Anterior uveitis may occur in this systemic illness along with conjunctival injection, acute nonsuppurative cervical lymphadenopathy, macular rash, myocarditis, pericarditis, and coronary artery aneurysms. The uveitis is nongranulomatous and bilateral. Presence of uveitis may aid in diagnosis since it occurs in most patients with the disease. The uveitis occurs during the first week of the illness, is self-limited, and only occasionally calls for treatment with topical corticosteroids and cycloplegics. Other syndromes such as streptococcal and staphylococcal toxin-mediated diseases may also cause uveitis and must be ruled out.

IDIOPATHIC ANTERIOR UVEITIS

Approximately 40% of patients that present to a uveitis clinic with iridocyclitis have no associated systemic condition (50). Without an apparent etiologic basis for the uveitis, these cases are labeled idiopathic. Some authorities include in this group those patients who are HLA-B27 positive but who have no other evidence of HLA-B27-related disease (e.g., ankylosing spondylitis, Reiter's syndrome, or inflammatory bowel disease). These patients present with acute, extensive, or recurrent inflammation, keratic precipitates, posterior synechiae, and secondary cystoid macular edema. Patients respond well to topical corticosteroids and have a reasonably good visual prognosis. Severe cases may need periocular or short-term systemic corticosteroids. Repeat laboratory investigations may be done periodically in an attempt to detect an associated systemic condition.

■ REFERENCES

1. Smith RE, Nozik RA. Uveitis: a clinical approach to diagnosis and management. 2nd ed. Baltimore: Williams & Wilkins, 1989a: (34–41).

2. Rothova A, Kijlstra A, Buitenhuis HJ, van der Gaag R, Feltkamp TEW. HLA-B27 associated uveitisùa distinct clinical entity? In: Saari KM, ed. Uveitis update. Amsterdam: Excerpta Medica, 1984: (91–95).

3. Rothova A, Van Veenendall WG, Linssen A, Glasius E, Kijlstra A, De Jong PTVM. Clinical features of acute anterior uveitis. Am J Ophthalmol 1987; 103: 1(37–14)5.

4. Brewerton DA, Caffrey M, Nicholls A, Walters D, James DCO. Acute anterior uveitis and HL-A 27. Lancet 1973; 2: 9(94–99)6.

5. Resnick D, Niwayama G. Diagnosis of bone and joint disorders. 2nd ed. Philadelphia: WB Saunders, 1988; 2: 11(03–12)51.

6. Lee DA, Barker SM, Su WPD, Allen GL, Liesegang TJ, Ilstrup DM. The clinical diagnosis of Reiter's syndrome: ophthalmic and nonophthalmic aspects. Ophthalmology 1986; 93: 3(50–35)6.

7. Smith RE, Nozik RA. Uveitis: a clinical approach to diagnosis and management. 2nd ed. Baltimore: Williams & Wilkins, 1989b: 1(71–17)9.

8. Hopkins DJ, Horan E, Burton IL, Clamp SE, de Dombal FT, Goligher JC. Ocular disorders in a series of 332 patients with Crohn's disease. Br J Ophthalmol 1974; 58: 7(32–73)7.

9. Wright R, Lumsden K, Luntz MH, Sevel D, Tauelove SC. Abnormalities of the sacro-iliac joints and uveitis in ulcerative colitis. Q J Med 1965; 34: 2(29–23)6.

10. Baiocco PJ, Gorman BD, Korelitz BI. Uveitis occurring after colectomy and ileal-rectal sleeve anastomosis for ulcerative colitis. Dig Dis Sci 1984; 29: 5(70–57)2.

11. Kanski JJ. Juvenile arthritis and uveitis. Surv Ophthalmol 1990; 34: 2(53–26)7.

12. Key SN III, Kimura SJ. Iridocyclitis associated with juvenile rheumatoid arthritis. Am J Ophthalmol 1975; 80: 4(25–42)9.

13. Kanski JJ, Shun-Shin GA. Systemic uveitis syndromes in childhood: an analysis of 340 cases. Ophthalmology 1984; 91: 12(47–12)52.

14. Wolf MD, Lichter PR, Ragsdale CG. Prognostic factors in the uveitis of juvenile rheumatoid arthritis. Ophthalmology 1987; 94: 12(42–12)48.

15. Chylack LT Jr, Bienfang DC, Bellows AR, Stillman JS. Ocular manifestations of juvenile rheumatoid arthritis. Am J Ophthalmol 1975; 79: 10(26–10)33.

16. Cassidy JT, Levinson JE, Bass JC, et al. A study of classification criteria for a diagnosis of juvenile rheumatoid arthritis. Arthritis Rheum 1986; 29: 2(74–28)1.

17. Nussenblatt RB, Palestine AG. Uveitis: fundamentals and clinical practice. Chicago: Year Book, 1989a: 1-52.

18. Weinreb RN, Tessler H. Laboratory diagnosis of ophthalmic sarcoidosis. Surv Ophthalmol 1984; 28: 6(53–66)4.

19. Smiley WK. The eye in juvenile rheumatoid arthritis. Trans Ophthalmol Soc UK, 1974; 94: 8(17–82)9.

20. Hooper PL, Rao NA, Smith RE. Cataract extraction in uveitis patients. Surv Ophthalmol 1990; 35: 1(20–14)4.

21. Beauchamp GR, Parks MM. Filtering surgery in children: barriers to success. Ophthalmology 1979; 86: 1(70–18)0.

22. Smith RE, Nozik RA. Uveitis: A clinical approach to diagnosis and management, 2nd ed. Baltimore: Williams & Wilkins, 1989d: 2(09–21)2.

23. Franceschetti A. Heterochromic cyclitis (Fuchs' syndrome). Am J Ophthalmol 1977; 39: (50–58).

24. Kimura SJ, Hogan MJ, Thygeson P. Fuchs' syndrome of heterochromic cyclitis. Arch Ophthalmol 1955; 54: 1(79–18)6.

25. Fuchs E. Über Komplikationen der Heterochromie. Z Augenheilkd 1906; 15: 1(91–21)2.

26. Kimura SJ. Fuchs' syndrome of heterochromic cyclitis in brown-eyed patients. Trans Am Ophthalmol Soc 1978; 76: (76–89).

27. Liesegang TJ. Clinical features and prognosis in Fuchs' uveitis syndrome. Arch Ophthalmol 1982;100: 16(22–16)26.

28. Nussenblatt RB, Palestine AG. Uveitis: fundamentals and clinical practice. Chicago: Year Book, 1989b: 1(76–17)9.

29. Gee SS, Tabbara KF. Extracapsular cataract extraction in Fuchs' heterochromic iridocyclitis. Am J Ophthalmol 1989; 108: 3(10–31)4.

30. O'Connor GR. Recurrent herpes simplex uveitis in humans. Surv Ophthalmol 1976; 21: 1(65–17)0.

31. Nussenblatt RB, Palestine AG. Uveitis: Fundamentals and clinical practice. Chicago: Year Book, 1989d: 4(16–42)9.

32. Smith RE, Nozik RA. Uveitis: A clinical approach to diagnosis and management, 2nd ed. Baltimore: Williams & Wilkins, 1989c: 2(04–20)8.

33. Womack LW, Liesegang TJ. Complications of herpes zoster ophthalmicus. Arch Ophthalmol 1983; 101: (42–45).

34. Cobo M, Foulks GN, Liesegang T, et al. Observations on the natural history of herpes zoster ophthalmicus. Curr Eye Res 1987; 6: 1(95–19)9.

35. Hedges TR III, Albert DM. The progression of the ocular abnormalities of herpes zoster: histopathologic observations of nine cases. Ophthalmology 1982; 89: 1(65–17)7.

36. Cobo LM, Foulks GN, Liesegang T, et al. Oral acyclovir in the therapy of acute herpes zoster ophthalmicus: an interim report. Ophthalmology 1985; 92: 15(74–15)83.

37. Henderly DE, Genstler AJ, Smith RE, Rao NA. Changing patterns of uveitis. Am J Ophthalmol 1987; 103: 1(31–13)6.

38. Nussenblatt RB, Palestine AG. Uveitis: fundamentals and clinical practice. Chicago: Year Book, 1989c: 3(27–33)5.

39. Gass JDM, Braunstein RA, Chenoweth RG. Acute syphilitic posterior placoid chorioretinitis. Ophthalmology 1990; 97: 12(88–12)97.

40. Smith RE, Nozik RA. Uveitis: a clinical approach to diagnosis and management, 2nd ed. Baltimore: Williams & Wilkins, 1989e: 2(13–22)1.

41. Tamesis RR, Foster CS. Ocular syphilis. Ophthalmology 1990; 97: 12(81–12)87.

42. _____: Treatment of sexually transmitted diseases. Med Lett Drugs Ther. 1990; 32:(5–1)0.

43. Schlaegel TF Jr, Weber JC. Double-blind therapeutic trial of isoniazid in 344 patients with uveitis. Br J Ophthalmol 1969; 53:4(25–42)7.

44. Apple DJ, Mamalis N, Loftfield K. Complications of intraocular lenses. A historical and histopathological review. Surv Ophthalmol 1984; 29:(1–5)4.

45. Mondino BJ, Nagata S, Glovsky MM. Activation of the alternative complement pathway by intraocular lenses. Invest Ophthalmol Vis Sci 1985; 26:9(05–90)8.

46. Tuberville AW, Galin MA, Perez HD, Banda D, Ong R, Goldstein IM. Complement activation by nylon- and polypropylene-looped prosthetic intraocular lenses. Invest Ophthalmol Vis Sci 1982; 22:7(27–73)3.

47. Posner A, Schlossman A. Syndrome of unilateral recurrent attacks of glaucoma with cyclitic symptoms. Arch Ophthalmol 1948; 39: 5(17–53)5.

48. Schlossman A. Glaucomatocyclitic crisis (Posner-Schlossman syndrome). In: Fraunfelder FT, Roy FH, eds. Current ocular therapy. 3rd ed. Philadelphia: WB Saunders, 1990: 558.

49. Puglise JV, Rao NA, Weiss RA, et al. Ocular features of Kawasaki's disease. Arch Ophthalmol 1982; 100: 11 (01–11)03.

50. Rao NA, Forster DJ, Augsburger JJ. The uvea: uveitis and intrauveal neoplasms. Textbook of Ophthalmology, New York: Gower Medical Publishing, 1992; 2: 5.1(8–5).19.

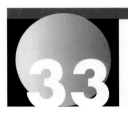

33 Intermediate Uveitis

Ramana S. Moorthy, Narsing A. Rao

Intermediate uveitis includes various entities that are characterized by cells in the anterior vitreous but without iridolenticular adhesions or external signs of uveitis. Pars planitis, multiple sclerosis, sarcoidosis, and Lyme disease are important entities that present with the clinical features of intermediate uveitis. Among these, pars planitis, also known as cyclitis, peripheral uveitis, peripheral cyclitis, chronic cyclitis and vitritis, is a relatively common entity in young adults and children of either sex (1, 2, 3). It accounts for up to 15% of all uveitis cases (1).

■ PARS PLANITIS

In pars planitis, symptoms usually consist of floaters or decreased vision if cystoid macular edema is present. There is usually no pain or photophobia. In 80% of the cases the inflammation is bilateral, but often asymmetric or unilateral in the early stages. Clinical findings include inflammatory cells and snowball opacities in the vitreous (Figure 33–1), especially inferiorly, and whitish-appearing inflammatory exudates along the pars plana, inferiorly (Figure 33–2), which may be visible on scleral depression. Associated with these pars plana exudates are areas of local retinal periphlebitis. Cystoid macular edema (Figure 33–3) is often present (4).

The disease may be benign and self-limited with only rare recurrences, become chronic and indolent, or it may follow a course with numerous associated complications (2, 5) the most common of which are cataracts and cystoid macular edema (6). Visual acuity of less than 20/40 is caused by cystoid macular edema (CME) in up to 76% of eyes. Pars planitis may also result in band keratopathy, glaucoma, vitreous organization and tractional retinal detachment, vitreous hemorrhage, and macular dragging from peripheral vitreous organization (2,6–7). The presence of vitreous opacities in chronic cases may also result in decreased vision.

Laboratory testing is often not useful in these cases. Little is known about the pathogenesis of intermediate uveitis, although various infectious agents, as well as immune deviations, have been implicated in the development of pars planitis. Most recently a novel protein, P 36, a 36 kD protein, has been isolated by Western blot technique in the sera of patients who have intermediate uveitis (8). However, it is unclear whether this protein plays a role in the pathogenesis of this uveitis.

The differential diagnosis includes multiple sclerosis, Lyme disease and sarcoidosis, all of which may present with signs of intermediate uveitis. Syphilis should also be ruled out in cases of pars planitis.

Because of the chronic, indolent nature of the disease, treatment of pars planitis should generally not be undertaken unless vision drops below 20/40, cystoid macular edema is present, or severe vitreous inflammation develops. Treatment can be divided into four steps (1,9):

1. Use of periocular corticosteroids in the form of posterior sub-Tenon's injections of 40 mg of triamcinolone given every 2 weeks. Patients who are intolerant of periocular injections can be treated with oral

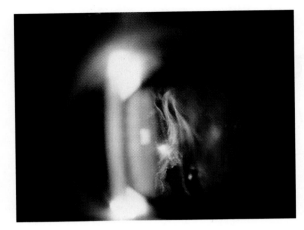

Figure 33–1.
Vitreous opacities in a patient with pars planitis.

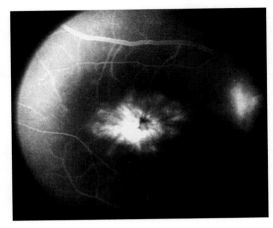

Figure 33–3.
Typical fluorescein angiographic features of cystoid macular edema in a patient with pars planitis.

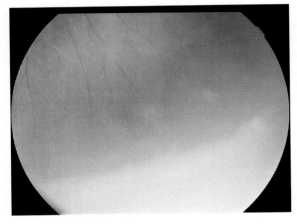

Figure 33–2.
Organizing vitreous exudate at pars plana inferiorly.

corticosteroids, with the initial dose in the range of 20 to 60 mg a day.

2. If the disease process cannot be controlled by sub-Tenon's deposteroids or with oral corticosteroids, or if the patient is intolerant of corticosteroids, cryotherapy of the vitreous base may be considered.

Cryotherapy of the vitreous base is usually recommended when there is neovascularization of the pars plana exudate or peripheral retina and no evidence of tractional retinal detachments. It has been shown recently, however, that the presence of peripheral neovascularization may predispose to the development of tractional and rhegmatogenous retinal detachments after cryotherapy. Laser photocoagulation for peripheral neovascularization may be useful if there is evidence of neovascularization in association with the pars plana exudate.

3. If cryotherapy fails to prevent progression of the inflammation, therapeutic pars plana vitrectomy, to remove vitreous debris, may reduce the macular edema.

4. If the previous measures fail, immunosuppressive agents such as cyclosporine, azathioprim, or cyclophosphamide may be used to reduce the inflammation and the cystoid macular edema. Controlled treatment trials and studies of these various agents are needed to further define which is the best method of treatment of pars planitis.

■ INTERMEDIATE UVEITIS IN ASSOCIATION WITH MULTIPLE SCLEROSIS

Patients with multiple sclerosis may develop signs and symptoms of intermediate uveitis. It has been reported that 5 to 10% of patients with multiple sclerosis have evidence of intermediate uveitis, retinal periphlebitis, or some form of intraocular inflammation (10). But the presence of intermediate uveitis alone does not imply that the diagnosis of multiple sclerosis should be sought.

■ REFERENCES

1. Smith RE. Pars planitis. In: Ryan SJ, ed. Retina. St. Louis: CV Mosby, 1989; 2: 637–45.

2. Brockhurst RJ, Schepens CL, Okamura ID. Uveitis II. Peripheral uveitis: clinical description, complications and differential diagnosis. Am J Ophthalmol 1960; 49: 1257–1266.

3. Welch RB, Maumenee AE, Wahlen HE. Peripheral posterior segment inflammation, vitreous opacities, and edema of the posterior pole: pars planitis. Arch Ophthalmol 1960; 64: 540–549.

4. Henderly DE, Haymond RS, Rao NA, Smith RE. The significance of the pars plana exudate in pars planitis. Am J Ophthalmol 1987; 103: 669–671.

5. Smith RE, Godfrey WA, Kimura SJ. Chronic cyclitis I: course and visual prognosis. Trans Am Acad Ophthalmol Otolaryngol, 1973: 77: OP760-OP768.

6. Smith RE, Godfrey WA, Kimura SJ. Complications of chronic cyclitis. Am J Ophthalmol 1976;82:277–282.

7. Aaberg TM. The enigma of pars planitis [Editorial]. Am J Ophthalmol 1987; 103: 828–830.

8. Bora N, Gobleman CL, Cirrito TP, et al. Correlation of serum and plasma P-36 with active pars planitis. ARVO abstract. Invest Ophthalmol Vis Sci 1993; 34: 973.

9. Kaplan HJ. Intermediate uveitis pars planitis, chronic cyclitis: a four-step approach to treatment. In: Saari KM, ed. Uveitis update. Amsterdam: Excerpta Medica, 1984; 169–172.

10. Giles CL. Peripheral uveitis in patients with multiple sclerosis. Am J Ophthalmol 1970; 70: 17–19.

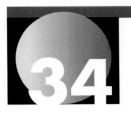

Posterior Uveitis

Ramana S. Moorthy, Narsing A. Rao

■ OCULAR TOXOPLASMOSIS

Ocular toxoplasmosis is the most common cause of posterior uveitis, accounting for up to 50% of cases (1). It is caused by the intracellular protozoan, Toxoplasma gondii, for which the definitive host is the cat; humans are intermediate hosts.

Toxoplasma infections in humans occur either after ingestion of sporozoites that are shed in cat feces and remain viable in the soil for many years, or by ingestion of encysted forms of the organism, the so-called bradyzoite, in undercooked meat. The latter is the most common source of infection in humans, and has a propensity to infect the cardiac muscle and neural tissues, including the retina. The encysted form can remain dormant in these particular tissues for years, and then reactivate because of changes in host factors. Changes in immunity of the host can result in rupture of the encysted forms; this releases the sporozoites, which transform into actively proliferating tachyzoites that may then cause reactivation of the infection.

Ocular toxoplasmosis can be the result of congenital infection or acquired infection, although the majority of toxoplasma infections of the eye are congenital. In 40% of the cases, congenital infection is passed on by a previously asymptomatic female who becomes infected and subsequently infects the fetus via placental transmission (2). In most cases, infants born with toxoplasmosis are asymptomatic, however, congenital systemic disease (encephalomyelitis, hepatosplenomegaly, and retinochoroiditis), or isolated congenital ocular disease (retinochoroiditis) can occur rarely (2A). The neural tissues are particularly susceptible to infection in the first trimester. Toxoplasmosis retinochoroiditis usually

presents in older children or adults caused by a reactivation of congenital retinal lesions.

Newly acquired toxoplasma infections in humans occur in six forms: the exanthematous, the influenzal, meningoencephalitic, ocular, visceral, and lymphadenopathic varieties. Typically, most immunocompetent patients who acquire the disease present with a mononucleosis-like illness accompanied by fever, lymphadenopathy, and malaise. The eyes are not commonly affected in this instance. In patients with AIDS, however, toxoplasma retinochoroiditis can be the presenting form of a newly acquired infection, and can have a devastating course that occasionally progresses to orbital cellulitis, despite treatment (3). This will be discussed in a later section (see Chapter 38).

Clinical Features

Patients with toxoplasma infections caused by reactivation of congenital retinal lesions have symptoms of floaters or reduced vision, either from direct involvement of the optic disc or macula, or from dense vitritis. There is usually no pain or redness in the eye. In severe cases, there may be inflammation of the anterior segment, resulting in keratic precipitates, flare and cells in the anterior chamber, and formation of posterior synechiae. Characteristically, fundus examination reveals focal retinochoroiditis (whitening of the retina and choroid) with overlying inflammation in the vitreous. In most cases, only one eye is involved. There is usually evidence of old congenital toxoplasma scars (densely pigmented chorioretinal scars) in the same eye

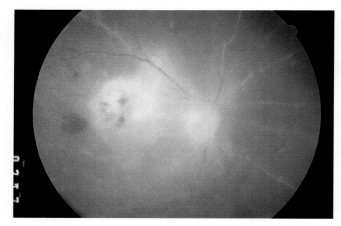

Figure 34–1.
Retinal vascular sheathing and retinochoroiditis from Toxoplasma gondii infection.

or in the fellow eye. The appearance of the white retinal lesions with overlying marked vitritis has been termed the "headlight in a fog" appearance when viewed by indirect ophthalmoscopy. An active retinochoroiditis is often seen as a whitish lesion at the edge of an old pigmented toxoplasmosis scar (i.e., satellite lesion). If there is no evidence of adjacent pigmented chorioretinal scar, the focus of retinochoroiditis in some patients may suggest a newly acquired infection. Adjacent retinal vessels, particularly the veins, may be sheathed (Figure 34–1). Typically, lesions of toxoplasma retinochoroiditis involve the inner retinal layers, although the outer retinal layers may be involved exclusively (4). For cases in which the outer retinal layers are involved, the overlying vitreous inflammation may be absent or minimal initially, but will increase as the infection progresses.

Patients with AIDS often have devastating infections from toxoplasma, with a larger area of necrotizing retinochoriditis than in immunocompetent individuals. Intraocular inflammation is variable and correlates to the CD4 (T-helper lymphocyte) count. Patients with AIDS and ocular toxoplasmosis often have concurrent CNS involvement. Most patients have reactivation of past infections, but up to 25% of cases of toxoplasma retinochoriditis in AIDS patients are acquired (3).

Laboratory Investigation

In the majority of patients the diagnosis of toxoplasma retinochoriditis is a clinical one. In uncertain cases, however, serologic testing is useful, including enzyme-linked immunosorbent assay (ELISA) of antibodies against toxoplasma. A positive IgM titer suggests recently acquired infection, while a positive IgG titer alone indicates reactivation of old infection. It is important to realize that many individuals who have no evidence of ocular toxoplasmosis may have positive IgG titers. Thus, a positive IgG titer does not necessarily confirm the diagnosis. However, in a patient with clinical features suggestive of toxoplasma retinochoroiditis, any positive titer may be significant. These tests must be done on undiluted serum, since many laboratories report titers of less than 1:16 or 1:32 as negative. The Sabin-Feldman dye test used in the past is not used today, since it needs live toxoplasma organisms. Patients with congenital toxoplasmosis may show intracranial calcification on CT scans.

Pathologic Assessment

Toxoplasma infection of the eye primarily involves the retina, usually with secondary choroiditis. Tachyzoites and bradyzoites within cysts may be found within the retina (Figure 34–2), which often undergoes necrotic change. In the chronic stage, RPE hyperplasia is noted at the margin of the necrotic retina.

Differential Diagnosis

The differential diagnosis of toxoplasma retinochoroiditis is limited in most instances, and in immunocompetent individuals the appearance is characteristic. In immunocompromised individuals, differential diagnosis should include other forms of necrotizing retinitis, including CMV retinitis, progressive outer retinal necrosis, and syphilis.

Treatment

Toxoplasma retinochoroiditis is a self-limiting intraocular inflammation in most immunocompetent individuals. Peripheral lesions of the retina are usually not sight threatening, and because of the self-limited course, do not need to be treated. However, when lesions occur within the temporal arcades, or are close to the disc or macula, treatment is indicated. The following table (Table 34–1) lists the guidelines for treatment of ocular toxoplasmosis. A combination of sulfadiazine and

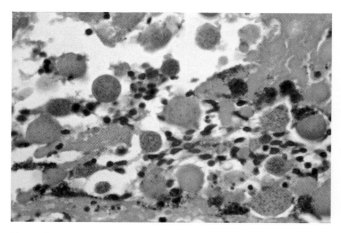

Figure 34–2.
Multiple cysts of Toxoplasma gondii in the necrotic retina.

TABLE 34–1
Treatment for Ocular Toxoplasmosis

Drug	Mechanism of Action	Dosage	Side Effects
Pyrimethamine	Inhibits DHF Reductase (DHF = dihydrofolate)	25 mg po BID	Myelosuppression—Base line CBC and QD wk
Sulfadiazine	Inhibits folate metabolism	2 g loading dose 1 g po QID	Rash, Stevens-Johnsons syndrome
Clindamycin	Kills toxoplasma organisms	300 mg po QID	Pseudomembranous colitis/GI distress
Prednisone	Decreases inflammation Lesions threatening macula or optic nerve	1–1.5 mg/kg/d	See side effects of corticosteroids

Note: 1. Folinic acid—5 mg po QD to BID should be given with pyrimethamine as citrovorum rescue
    2. Patients with AIDS—Avoid corticosteroids, may need three antibiotics, indefinite maintenance on two or three drugs at one-half of usual doses.
    3. Congenital toxoplasmosis—pyrimethamine 1 mg/kg/QD 3 days and sulfadiazine 50–100 mg/kg/d po × 3 weeks
        —use corticosteroids if sight-threatening lesions
    4. Begin antibiotics and steroids together and taper steroids before antibiotics. Continue antibiotics for 2 weeks longer. Thus, total course of treatment lasts 4–6 weeks.

pyrimethamine is the treatment of choice; folinic acid is given concurrently to counteract the myelosuppressive effects of pyrimethamine. Clindamycin may be used in place of pyrimethamine in patients who are allergic to sulfa medications (5). This regimen also avoids the bone marrow toxicosis of pyrimethamine. Since clindamycin can cause pseudomembranous colitis, the drug should be discontinued in patients who develop diarrhea. Prednisone (1 to 1.5 mg/kg/day) can also be given to patients who have lesions that threaten the optic nerve or the macula. Generally, antitoxoplasma medication should be continued for 4 to 6 weeks. Steroids should be tapered quickly after the first 2 weeks, and depo-steroids injections into the sub-Tenon's space should be avoided. Systemic corticosteroids are not indicated in patients who are immunocompromised.

Course and Prognosis

Most cases of toxoplasma retinochoroiditis in immunocompetent individuals resolve spontaneously once the host immune system controls the infection. Macular lesions or optic nerve lesions, however, may result in irreversible visual loss. When posterior segment inflammation spills into the anterior segment, complications of anterior uveitis, glaucoma, and cataract may develop. Exudative, tractional, and rhegmatogenous retinal detachments can occur when the inflammation of the posterior segment is severe. In addition, subretinal neovascularization may also occur since Bruch's membrane and the RPE are often disrupted adjacent to the toxoplasma chorioretinal scar. These retinal complications are rare, however.

■ TOXOCARIASIS

Toxocara canis, the dog round worm, is the most common nematode ocular infection in the United States. It is present in up to 80% of puppies 2 to 6 months of age, and may be found in public parks and playgrounds (6). The dog is the definitive host for this nematode, which has a complete life cycle within the dog; in the human, however, it has an incomplete life cycle. Typically, the child ingests soil that contains ova of toxocara. The ova then hatch in the small intestine and pass through the intestinal wall into various tissues, causing a syndrome of visceral larva migrans (VLM). These larvae may settle in the liver, lung, brain and eye, resulting in various clinical manifestations. In the dog, the worms make their way through the trachea or are swallowed and pass into the intestine; the ova of these nematode are then excreted into the soil (6). This does not occur in humans.

Clinical Features

Once patients have developed VLM, characterized by fever, cough, malaise, anorexia, and seizures, a generalized leukocytosis and eosinophilia develops. Patients are most commonly boys between 6 months and 3 years of age (6). Often a history of pica can be elicited. Ocular manifestations develop simultaneously or even several years after the episode of VLM. Patients with ocular toxocara are usually asymptomatic, and often, no history of VLM is elicited. Ocular manifestations take 3 forms: posterior pole granuloma (7), peripheral granuloma, and diffuse endophthalmitis. The death of the worm may result in severe intraocular inflammation; thus, antihelminthics should be avoided once the worm has entered the eye.

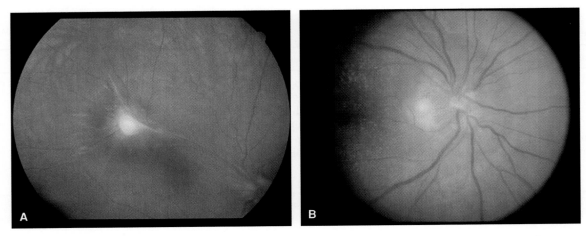

Figure 34–3.
A, Toxocara granuloma with traction on the optic disc. **B,** Juxtapapillary nematode granuloma.

The posterior pole granuloma is seen in patients 6 to 14 years of age (8), and takes the form of an elevated white mass in the posterior pole with associated vitritis. Some dragging of the temporal arcade vessels may occur (Figure 34–3). In addition, tractional bands within the vitreous may extend to the optic nerve or macula, in which case the patient may have leukocoria or decreased vision.

The peripheral granuloma form tends to present at a later age, sometimes when the patient is as old as 40 (8). In these cases the eye is quiet, but the patient often complains of mildly reduced vision, and in some cases floaters. On examination, there may be a peripheral traction band connected to the disc and arising from a peripheral granuloma, often located inferiorly. These granulomas can be extensive. Retinal pigment epithelial clumping and migration take place alongside the tractional band. Macular heterotopia may result from these tractional bands. In some patients the peripheral granuloma may appear similar to the snowbanks seen in pars planitis. However, snowbanks and pars planitis are bilateral, whereas toxocara granulomas are typically unilateral.

The diffuse endophthalmitis form is usually seen in younger patients, between 2 and 9 years of age (8). The eye is quiet externally, but there may be spillover anterior segment inflammation from the vitreous with keratic precipitates, posterior synechiae, or hypopyon. The vitreous is hazy and cyclitic membranes may be present. Retinal detachment and a yellow-white mass in the retina are seen on ophthalmoscopy. Vision is severely affected in these individuals and leukocoria is the presenting sign. Other manifestations unusual for toxocariasis include diffuse unilateral subacute neuroretinitis (DUSN), described by Gass and colleagues (9). Optic nerve papillitis, retinal detachment, peripheral keratitis, and conjunctivitis have also been reported (6).

Pathologic Assessment

The characteristic lesion of ocular toxocariasis is a localized granulomatous inflammation that surrounds the dead larvae consisting of eosinophils, epithelioid cells, lymphocytes, and plasma cells. The area of inflammatory response is often much larger than the larva. In some enucleated globes it is difficult to show the larval remnants, and multiple sections of the lesion may be needed to detect the necrotic larva.

Laboratory Tests

The most reliable test for this infection is the detection of antibodies to toxocara organisms using the ELISA technique. Any titer greater than 1:8 is considered diagnostic of toxocariasis (6). If serum is negative, some ophthalmologists advocate the use of aqueous or vitreous taps for antibody testing, which may be positive, even if the serum is negative (10). Paracentesis of intraocular fluid may show eosinophils. Echography may be useful in showing peripheral granulomas and in differentiating them from retinoblastoma or persistent hyperplasia of primary vitreous (PHPV) and other causes of leukocoria (11, 12). There is no need to examine the stool specimen for ova and parasites because these are not found in human feces.

Differential diagnosis for any patient with ocular toxocariasis should include the various causes of leukocoria: retinoblastoma, PHPV, Coat's disease, retinopathy of prematurity, toxoplasmosis, and intermediate uveitis. Toxocara endophthalmitis is commonly misdiagnosed as retinoblastoma (6).

Treatment

Peripheral lesions are usually associated with minimal intraocular inflammation and do not require treatment.

Posterior pole lesions and cases with endophthalmitis should be treated with systemic or periocular steroids (6). The role of antihelminthics, such as thiabendazole and diethylcarbazine, is not clear, but if used, they should be given with corticosteroids, since death of the organism causes severe inflammation.

Laser photocoagulation of larva that are near the fovea or disc has been advocated to kill the organism (13, 14). However, this may again incite severe intraocular inflammation. Surgical intervention is indicated for complications associated with inflammation including cataract, glaucoma, cyclitic membranes, retinal detachment, or traction on the macula (6,15). Lesions involving the macula or optic disc have a poor prognosis; peripheral granulomas have a better prognosis if the macula is uninvolved.

■ OCULAR HISTOPLASMOSIS SYNDROME (OHS)
(see Retina, Chapter 59)

Histoplasma capsulatum is found in temperate climates throughout the world. It is endemic in the Ohio and Mississippi river valleys and some parts of the Mid-Atlantic states. Humans become infected by inhaling spores of the histoplasma organisms in windblown soils and aerosolized pigeon droppings. A mild influenza-like illness develops but is usually self-limited and resolves. Occasionally the organisms may disseminate into various organs during the initial illness, including the liver, spleen, and eyes, particularly the choroid.

Clinical Features

Signs of ocular histoplasmosis have been found in up to 13% of individuals in endemic areas (16). Approximately 1 in 1000 patients in such areas develop macular disease (17). Patients are usually between 20 and 50 years of age. OHS is uncommon in blacks. There appears to be an association of HLA-B7 in patients with disciform scarring and histo spots (18,19). Patients usually have no symptoms such as photophobia, redness, or pain, and there is an absence of anterior chamber or vitreous cellular reaction (20). The characteristic triad of findings of OHS consist of multiple punched-out atrophic choroidal scars, peripapillary atrophy and pigmentation, and macular scars with associated maculopathy (Figure 34–4). The maculopathy may consist of an active choroidal neovascular membrane (CNVM), atrophic scar, or disciform scar.

Macular atrophic scars predispose to the development of subretinal neovascular membrane, which is the common cause of the visual loss (21). Patients usually complain of sudden decrease in central vision, metamorphopsia, or a central scotoma. There is often a serous and hemorrhagic retinal detachment, retinal pigment epithelial detachment, and an underlying CNVM. A disciform scar may eventually develop, and central vision can be permanently lost if the CNVM is untreated. Rarely has spontaneous improvement in visual acuity been reported (22). In a few patients, visual loss may be the result of reactivation of choroiditis near the macula (21), but this is rare, as well.

Laboratory Tests

Laboratory testing has little use in OHS because of the characteristic appearance of this syndrome. The incidence of histoplasma exposure in areas where this dis-

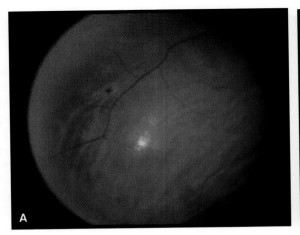
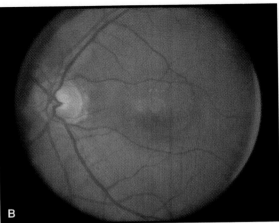

Figure 34–4.
A, Peripheral punched-out choroidal lesion in a case of presumed ocular histoplasmosis. **B,** Fundus changes in presumed ocular histoplasmosis. Note macular scar with focal retinal hemorrhage.

ease is endemic makes the skin test nondiagnostic; up to 90% of patients in these areas may be skin test positive. Furthermore, a skin test can reactivate macular lesions (20). Fluorescein angiography may be useful in detecting subretinal neovascular membranes so that laser photocoagulation can be done.

Pathologic Assessment

Histoplasma capsulatum, although detected in histopathologic sections, has not been cultured from eyes with OHS. Histopathologically, choroidal lesions exhibit scarring, lymphocytic infiltration, and chorioretinal adhesions. In a few cases, necrotizing granulomas have been noted. It is in these necrotic areas that Histoplasma capsulatum has been found.

Differential Diagnosis

Entities that look like presumed ocular histoplasmosis include scleral crescent associated with myopic chorioretinal atrophy in myopic degeneration. Multifocal choroiditis, punctuate inner choroidopathy, and subretinal fibrosis associated with multifocal choroiditis, may appear similar to OHS, but all these entities have cells in the vitreous. Birdshot chorioretinopathy has less propensity for the development of choroidal neovascular membranes; the lesions are usually deeper, and they occur in older patients.

Treatment

Patients who have macular atrophic form of presumed ocular histoplasmosis should be monitored with an Amsler grid. Any new metamorphopsia or decreased visual acuity or scotomas should be followed up with examination and fluorescein angiography to determine if a CNVM exists. The Macular Photocoagulation Study (MPS) has clearly shown benefit in the treatment of ex-

trafoveal subretinal neovascular membranes greater than 200 microns from the center of the foveal avascular zone with argon green laser, and juxtafoveal membranes between 1 and 199 microns from the center of the foveal avascular zone using krypton red (23–24). Using this approach, and with a 3-year follow-up, the MPS showed that only 7% of treated patients with extrafoveal CNVMs had greater than 6 lines of visual loss, compared with 19% of control subjects without treatment (23). Similarly, for juxtafoveal subretinal neovascularization treated with krypton laser photocoagulation, at 1 year 25% of control subjects, versus 7% of treated patients, had lost 6 lines of vision (24). The recurrence of subretinal membranes within 5 years after laser has been shown by the MPS study to be approximately 26% (25). In cases of subfoveal subretinal neovascular membranes, there is no clear-cut evidence to support any single approach. It is thought that because reactivation of CNVMs may represent an immune response, subfoveal membranes can be treated with corticosteroids. But periocular and systemic corticosteroids have resulted in limited success. Recently, submacular surgery to remove CNVMs has been beneficial in several patients.

Course and Prognosis

In the absence of macular involvement, OHS is benign and self-limited. The main determinant of final visual acuity is the presence of macular subretinal neovascular membranes, particularly subfoveal neovascular membranes. Recurrence of subretinal membrane may be increased as much as 26% within 5 years of laser photocoagulation (25). Patients with a disciform scar in one eye have a 25% chance of developing subretinal neovascular membrane in the fellow eye over a 3-year period if the fellow eye shows macular changes (26). Occasionally, subretinal neovascular membranes may develop de novo, without preexisting macular scars (27).

■ ACUTE RETINAL NECROSIS SYNDROME

The acute retinal necrosis (ARN) syndrome is a viral retinitis that usually presents clinically with signs of posterior uveitis. This entity was first described by Urayama in 1971 (28). It was not until 1982, however, that Culbertson and coworkers (29) showed herpes virus particles in the retina of a patient with ARN. Since that time, herpes zoster virus, herpes simplex virus, and cytomegalovirus have all been implicated in its pathogenesis (30, 31, 32).

Clinical Features

ARN by definition occurs in immunocompetent individuals of either sex and of any age, although most pa-

tients are in the 3rd to 5th decade of life. Symptoms include photophobia, pain, and blurring of vision, although the onset is typically insidious. Signs of anterior and posterior uveitis develop, and keratic precipitates, anterior segment flare and cell, and varying degrees of vitritis can be seen. The hallmark of this disease, however, is the peripheral retinal necrosis. An occlusive retinal vasculitis that involves both arteries and veins is associated with the peripheral lesions. Typically, the peripheral lesions begin in one quadrant (Figure 34–5A), but eventually become circumferential. As the disease progresses, these peripheral lesions extend more posteriorly. An intense vitritis is often present, as

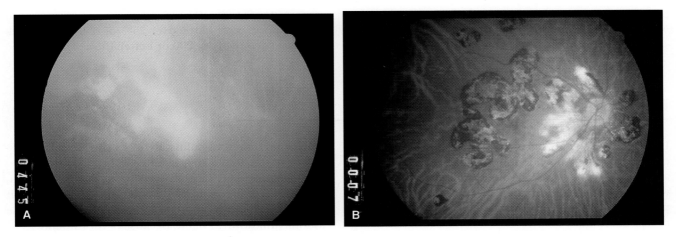

Figure 34–5.
A, Peripheral retinal necrosis in a patient with ARN. **B,** Chorioretinal scars around the disc and in the posterior pole characteristic of serpiginous choroidopathy.

are optic disc edema and macular edema. The combination of vitritis, macular edema, and disc edema results in a profound reduction in visual acuity.

Laboratory Investigations

The diagnosis of ARN is made on clinical appearance. Serum antibody titers to HSV or HZV virus may be supportive of the diagnosis. However, these antibody titers may not be elevated with isolated ocular involvement, or may be falsely elevated in patients who have previously been exposed to these relatively common viruses. If diagnosis is in doubt, a diagnostic vitrectomy and retinal biopsy are often helpful in demonstrating viral inclusions by electron microscopy within retinal tissue (33) and elevated intraocular antibody titers (34). Cultures from vitreous specimens are often negative, and should not be interpreted as evidence against acute retinal necrosis (30).

Differential Diagnosis

In the immunocompetent individual, there are few diseases that appear similar to acute retinal necrosis, although retinal vasculitis and Behçet's disease can mimic ARN. In the immunocompromised patient, progressive outer retinal necrosis, syphilitic retinitis, and CMV retinitis, as well as toxoplasma retinochoroiditis, can appear similar to ARN. The diagnosis of ARN, however, by definition, should be restricted to immunocompetent individuals.

Pathologic Assessment

Histopathologically, acute retinal necrosis is characterized by full thickness retinal necrosis, choroiditis, and vitritis. Eosinophilic intranuclear inclusions are present

in various cells and 80 to 100 nm size particles may be shown on electron microscopy. Both of these findings are characteristic of the herpes viruses. Virus particles are typically found in the inner retina in transition zones between areas of necrosis and uninvolved retina (33).

Treatment

It is recommended that approximately 1.5 grams per square meter per day of acyclovir be given intravenously for 7 to 21 days, after which oral acyclovir, 400-600 mg 5 times a day may be given for 4 to 6 weeks more (35). Although this regimen significantly reduces the retinitis, it does not affect the vitritis, development of retinal detachment, or subsequent involvement of the contralateral eye. Corticosteroids may be used also, beginning 48 hours after the initiation of intravenous acyclovir. Oral corticosteroids, prednisone 1 mg/kg/day, help to reduce intraocular inflammation. Scatter photocoagulation to create a new ora may be helpful in preventing retinal detachment that involves the posterior pole (36).

Course and Prognosis

The active retinitis usually lasts 4 to 6 weeks, and typically leaves significant retinal destruction with retinal atrophy, retinal pigment epithelial changes, and vitreous organization. It is this vitreous organization that results in tractional and rhegmatogenous retinal detachments late in the course of the disease. Rhegmatogenous detachments occur in up to 75% of patients, as early as 2 months after the onset of the disease (37–38). Contralateral eye involvement has been reported in up to

36% of cases of ARN within the first 6 weeks after involvement of the first eye (38). The involvement of the second eye, however, may be delayed by many years in some instances (39). The visual prognosis of untreated cases is poor, with a little over 25% of such eyes retaining visual acuity of 20/200 or better (33).

■ RETINAL VASCULITIS

Inflammation involving retinal blood vessels, arteries, or veins can be subdivided into retinal vasculitis associated with Behçet's disease, with rheumatologic diseases, with systemic vasculitides and Eales' disease, or as idiopathic retinal vasculitis. All of the diseases with which retinal vasculitis is associated are listed in the following table (Table 34–2).

Clinical Findings

Patients who have retinal vasculitis present with reduced vision, floaters, scotoma, and some loss of visual field. They typically do not have much pain unless there is accompanying anterior segment inflammation. The eye is quiet. Fundus examination reveals involvement of the arteries, veins, or both. There is segmental or diffuse sheathing and luminal narrowing of the inflamed vessels. There may be exudation around these paravascular areas of sheathing, with associated vitreous inflammation. When occlusion of the vasculature occurs, such as in hyperviscosity syndromes and hemoglobinopathies, areas of retinal ischemia, infarction, hemorrhage, or neovascularization develop. These characteristics are particularly true for autoimmune vascular diseases and idiopathic retinal vasculitis. Behçet's disease will be discussed in detail in a later chapter.

Eales' disease is rare in the United States. In India, however, it is a common disorder among young adult males (40). It is thought to be a hypersenstivity response to some unknown antigen. Because of the endemicity of tuberculosis in India and the increased rate of PPD positivity in patients with Eales' disease, tuberculosis has been implicated as a causative factor; however, this has not been proven (41). Most patients present with reduced vision and vitreous hemorrhage; in most cases it is bilateral. The disease produces an obliterative perivasculitis that involves the venules, and usually starts in multiple quadrants in the periphery. Arteriolar involvement is unusual. The occlusive venulitis results in peripheral retinal ischemia and retinal neovascularization. Intraretinal hemorrhages are not common. Neovascularization can occur rapidly from the ischemic retina.

Laboratory Investigations

Laboratory investigations need to be particularly extensive in patients with retinal vasculitis. In general, these should include workup for rheumatologic collagen vascular diseases, as well as infectious etiologies. However, many instances require a thorough history and physical examination with review of systems to tailor the approach of the workup. For example, patients who have oral aphthous ulcerations should be evaluated for Behçet's disease. Additionally, patients who present with evidence of discoid lupus rashes on the face or glomerulonephritis should be evaluated for SLE. Patients who have obliterative peripheral retinal periphlebitis and who come from areas where tuberculosis is endemic should be evaluated for tuberculosis, as well as for Eales' disease. Fluorescein angiography is helpful in documenting the extent of vascular involvement, degree of capillary nonperfusion, and presence of neovascularization. Staining of vessel walls or leakage from vessels may indicate active vasculitis.

Differential Diagnosis

Retinal vasculitis includes a vast array of disorders that can produce similar pictures. These are presented in Table 34–2.

TABLE 34–2
Conditions Associated with Retinal Vasculitis

Behçet's syndrome
Collagen vascular diseases
Wegener's granulomatosis
Systemic lupus erythematosis
Polyarteritis nodosa
Polymyositis/Dermatomyositis
Sarcoidosis
Multiple Sclerosis
Inflammatory Bowel Disease
Syphilis
Tuberculosis
Intermediate Uveitis
Toxoplasmosis
Acute Retinal Necrosis
Cytomegalovirus retinitis
Birdshot Retinochoroidopathy
Eales' disease
Idiopathic

Treatment

The treatment of retinal vasculitis depends on the cause. In cases of infectious processes, such as syphilis and tuberculosis, antimicrobials are useful. However, when immune mechanisms are implicated in the vasculitis, it is necessary to use corticosteroid therapy, often systemically. In addition, certain entities, such as Behçet's disease or idiopathic retinal vasculitis, often demand the use of cytotoxic agents or cytostatic agent, such as cyclosporine. In addition, E*ales' disease,* in particular, is an entity where the peripheral nonperfusion can be treated with scattered photocoagulation guided by fluorescein angiography. This will result in regression of neovascularization and will reduce the complications of Eales' disease, namely vitreous hemorrhage and tractional and rhegmatogenous retinal detachments.

■ GEOGRAPHIC (SERPIGINOUS) CHOROIDOPATHY (see Retina, Chapter 59)

This entity is also called geographic *helicoid peripapillary choroiditis.* The etiology is unknown; some ophthalmologists believe it is inflammatory, and others believe that it is a degenerative disease (42, 43). It affects males and females equally, most of whom are approximately 47 years of age. The condition is often bilateral, but asymmetric. Patients present with progressive, dense, paracentral and central scotomas. Typically, the lesions start at the disc and spread in a serpiginous fashion with centripetal extensions (Figure 34–5B). Lesions are usually in the superficial choroid and can involve the retinal pigment epithelium. They can also become multifocal and noncontiguous when recurrent. The active areas are characterized by grey-white changes in the retinal pigment epithelium with overlying retinal edema. These usually occur at the edge of previous atrophic lesions. Progression of retinal damage can be asymptomatic unless the macula is involved (43, 45). Recurrences can occur from weeks to years after onset, and some patients have an associated vitritis or anterior uveitis.

In most instances the diagnosis is based on clinical appearance. Fluorescein angiography is helpful in revealing areas of active geographic choroiditis, since the active edges often show early blockage and late staining in a "brush fire" type of pattern. Atrophic lesions are hyperfluorescent from diffuse staining of underlying sclera. Serial fundus photography is essential in documenting progression of the disease (44). Pathologically, aggregates of lymphyocytes are seen in the choroid, with focal damage to the choriocapillaris and RPE atrophy.

Treatment

Corticosteroid therapy to reduce inflammatory activity is indicated in patients with progressive lesions that threaten the macula. Periocular steroids are often useful because of the asymmetric involvement of one eye. Immunosuppressive agents such as cyclosporine may be used.

Course and Prognosis

Serpiginous choroidopathy is usually progressive. Macular involvement occurs in up to 88% of patients and results in poor vision (43,45). In 1 study, over 50% of patients had reactivation over a 5-year period. Additionally, up to 25% of patients develop subretinal neovascular membranes (42,44) that need to be treated with laser photocoagulation when they are sight threatening.

■ RUBELLA RETINOPATHY (See Chapter 21)

Rubella can cause chorioretinitis. Patients present during childhood with congenital rubella syndrome manifest by mental retardation, microcephaly, deafness, cataracts, and "salt and pepper" pigmentary retinopathy. Histopathologically, there is no evidence of inflammation or vasculopathy in the choroid or retina (46). Choroidal neovascularization may complicate the late clinical course of rubella retinopathy.

■ BRUCELLA UVEITIS

Brucella, a gram negative rod, is transmitted to humans in infected tissues and milk from cattle, pigs, and dogs. This bacteria may cause acute or chronic, granulomatous or nongranulomatous anterior uveitis, intermediate uveitis, and vitritis (47). Diagnosis is made on the basis of clinical suspicion, serology, and confirmed, if possible, by culture. Treatment is with oral tetracycline.

■ OPHTHALMOMYIASIS INTERNA

Larvae of animal bot flies can enter the eye directly and enter the subretinal space creating "railroad track"-type changes in the retina (48). Late optic atrophy may occur. If the larva dies in the subretinal space, inflammatory scarring may occur. If the organism enters the vit-reous, variable, at times intense, inflammation results as the organism dies. Control of the inflammation with corticosteroids and eventual surgical removal of the larva by vitrectomy if the inflammation cannot be controlled, is the treatment of choice.

■ ONCHOCERCIASIS

Onchocerciasis (49) is an infection caused by the nematode, Onchocerca volvulus, that is transmitted to humans in equatorial Africa and Central and South America by the bite of the Simulium or blackfly. These flies breed in marshland adjacent to the large riverbeds common in these areas. Blindness is the major source of morbidity from this infection and is one of the leading causes of blindness in the world. Microfilariae gain access to the systemic circulation and travel to the eye. They may lodge in the cornea and result is a severe, sclerosing, interstitial keratitis. Anterior segment inflammation occurs. The microfilarae may be visualized in the anterior chamber by slit lamp examination. As the microfilariae die, inflammation increases. With anti-helminthic treatment, intraocular and systemic inflammation can become severe. In some cases, treatment itself may cause death, severe, acute systemic inflammation called Mazzottti's reaction. Posterior segment manifestations include variable amounts of chorioretinal scarring, pigment alteration and atrophy, choroidal neovascular membranes, and optic atrophy. Diagnosis is made by skin biopsy of subcutaneous nodules or by visualizing microfilariae in the eye. Treatment is with suramin or diethylcarbamazine; however, the newer antihelminthic ivermectin only needs to be administered once yearly, and has been successful in eradicating the nematode from infected humans without inducing severe host inflammatory response.

■ CYSTICERCOSIS

Cysticercus cellulosae (50), a larva of the pork tapeworm, Taenia solium, invades the eye through the systemic circulation after humans ingest undercooked pork. It is the most common larval tapeworm to invade the eye. It is endemic in Africa, Southeast Asia, and Central and South America. The most common clinical ocular sign is a white, subretinal mass after the parasite has lodged in the subretinal space. Subretinal fibrous proliferation and vitritis may result as the larva grows and moves. The larva may enter the vitreous through a rent in the retina. Death of the intraocular parasite results in severe panuveitis from release of parasitic toxins which may cause phthisis bulbi. Diagnosis is made by direct visualization of the larva in the eye. Indirect hemagglutinin titers against C. cellulosae in serum may be diagnostic if more than 1:64. Since death of the worm can induce severe panuveitis, medical therapy is not useful in the treatment of the intraocular larva. Pars plana vitrectomy with early and complete removal of the larva is the treatment of choice.

■ DIFFUSE UNILATERAL SUBACUTE NEURORETINITIS (DUSN) (see Retina, Chapter 59)

DUSN (51) should be considered in any case of unilateral "wipeout" syndrome involving the fundus. DUSN is caused by a round worm, possibly Baylisascaris or Ancylostoma species. Patients may present with floaters and decreased vision in one eye. There is often mild vitritis with patchy retinal pigment epithelial and chorioretinal atrophy which becomes diffuse and eventually results in optic atrophy with attenuated retinal arterioles. Diagnosis is made by meticulous search for the elusive subretinal roundworm. Treatment using laser photocoagulation of the worm before foveal involvement has been successful.

■ CATERPILLAR HAIRS

Airborne caterpillar hairs may land on the eye and by rubbing and blinking can make their way into the anterior chamber and subretinal space (52). In the anterior chamber they can induce an intense anterior uveitis. They can migrate in the subretinal space leaving tracks of retinal pigment epithelial atrophy and subretinal scars. The caterpillar hairs in the anterior chamber or vitreous should be surgically removed. Laser barrier treatment may be useful in preventing migration of the subretinal hair into the macula. Topical and periocular corticosteroids and cycloplegics may be used to reduce intraocular inflammation.

■ REFERENCES

1. Smith RE, Nozik RA. Uveitis: a clinical approach to diagnosis and management. 2nd ed. Baltimore: Williams & Wilkins, 1989a: 128–134.
2. Nussenblatt RB, Palestine AG. Uveitis: fundamentals and clinical practice. Chicago: Year Book, 1989b: 336–354.
2A. Dunn SA, Schwartz D, Brinkley J, Wright KW. Congenital toxoplasmosis presenting as an isolated chorioretinitis in the neonate. J Ped Ophthal Strab, 1988, Vol. 25 No. 1, P30–32.
3. Moorthy RS, Smith RE, Rao NA. Progressive ocular toxoplasmosis in patients with acquired immunodeficency syndrome. Am J Ophthalmol 1993; 115: 742–747.
4. Doft BH, Gass JDM. Outer retinal layer toxoplasmosis. Graefes Arch Clin Exp Ophthalmol 1986; 224: 78–82.
5. Lakhanpal V, Schocket SS, Nirankari VS. Clindamycin in the treatment of toxoplasmic retinochoroiditis. Am J Ophthalmol 1983; 95: 605–613.
6. Shields JA. Ocular toxocariasis: a review. Surv Ophthalmol 1984; 28: 361.
7. Wilder HC. Nematode endophthalmitis. Trans Am Acad Ophthalmol Otolaryngol 1950; 55: 99–109.
8. Smith RE, Nozik RA. Uveitis: a clinical approach to diagnosis and management. 2nd ed. Baltimore: Williams & Wilkins, 1989b:135–140.
9. Gass JDM, Gilbert WR Jr, Guerry RK, Scelfo R. Diffuse unilateral subacute neuroretinitis. Ophthalmology 1978; 85: 521–545.
10. Felberg NT, Shields JA, Federman JL. Antibody to Toxocara canis in the aqueous humor. Arch Ophthalmol 1981; 99: 1563–1564.
11. Shields JA, Stephens RF. Ultrasonography in pediatric ophthalmology. In: Harley RD, ed. Pediatric ophthalmology. 2nd ed. Philadelphia: WB Saunders, 1983; 1: 145–154.
12. Wan WL, Cano MR, Pince KJ, Green RL. Echographic characteristics of ocular toxocariasis. Ophthalmology 1991; 98: 28–32.
13. Fitzgerald CR, Rubin ML. Intraocular parasite destroyed by photocoagulation. Arch Ophthalmol 1974; 91: 162–164.
14. Raymond LA, Gutierrez Y, Strong LE, Wander AH, Buten R, Cordan D. Living retinal nematode filarial-like destroyed with photocoagulation. Ophthalmology 1978; 85: 944–949.
15. Hagler WS, Pollard ZF, Jarrett WH, Donnelly EH. Results of surgery for ocular Toxocara canis. Ophthalmology 1981; 88: 1081–1086.
16. Davidorf FH, Anderson JD. Ocular lesions in the earth day, 1970, histoplasmosis epidemic. Int Ophthalmol Clin 1975; 153: 51–60.
17. Smith RE, Ganley JP. An epidemiologic study of presumed ocular histoplasmosis. Trans Am Acad Ophthalmol Otolaryngol 1971; 75: 994–1005.
18. Godfrey WA, Sabates R, Cross DE. Association of presumed ocular histoplasmosis with HLA-B7. Am J Ophthalmol 1978; 85: 854–858.
19. Braley RE, Meredith TA, Aaberg TM, Koethe SM, Witkowski JA. The prevalence of HLA-B7 in presumed ocular histoplasmosis. Am J Ophthalmol 1978; 85: 859–861.
20. Smith RE, Nozik RA. Uveitis: a clinical approach to diagnosis and management. 2nd ed. Baltimore: Williams & Wilkins, 1989c: 141–145.
21. Gass JDM, Wilkinson CP. Follow-up study of presumed ocular histoplasmosis. Trans Am Acad Ophthalmol Otolaryngol 1972; 76: 672–694.
22. Jost BF, Olk RJ, Burgess DB. Factors related to spontaneous visual recovery in the ocular histoplasmosis syndrome. Retina 1987; 7: 1–8.
23. Macular Photocoagulation Study Group. Argon laser photocoagulation for ocular histoplasmosis: results of a randomized clinical trial. Arch Ophthalmol 1983; 101: 1347–1357.
24. Macular Photocoagulation Study Group. Krypton laser photocoagulation for neovascular lesions of ocular histoplasmosis: results of a randomized clinical trial. Arch Ophthalmol 1987; 105: 1499–1507.
25. Macular Photocoagulation Study Group. Persistent and recurrent neovascularization after krypton laser photocoagulation for neovascular lesions of ocular histoplasmosis. Arch Ophthalmol 1989; 107: 344–352.
26. Nussenblatt RB, Palestine AG. Uveitis: fundamentals and clinical practice. Chicago: Year Book, 1989c: 379–387.
27. Ryan SJ Jr. De novo subretinal neovascularization in the histoplasmosis syndrome. Arch Ophthalmol 1976; 94: 321–327.
28. Urayama A, Yamada N, Sasaki Y, et al. Unilateral acute uveitis with retinal periarteritis and detachment. Jpn J Clin Ophthalmol 1971; 25: 607–619.
29. Culbertson WW, Blumenkranz MS, Haines H, Gass JDM, Mitchell KB, Norton, EWD. The acute retinal necrosis syndrome: part 2: histopathology and etiology. Ophthalmology 1982; 89: 1317–1325.
30. Freeman WR, Thomas EL, Rao NA, et al. Demonstration of herpes group virus in acute retinal necrosis syndrome. Am J Ophthalmol 1986; 102: 701–709.

31. Jabs DA, Schachat AP, Liss R, Knox DL, Michels, RG. Presumed varicella zoster retinitis in immunocompromised patients. Retina 1987; 7: 9–13.

32. Chess J, Marcus DM. Zoster-related bilateral acute retinal necrosis syndrome as presenting sign in AIDS. Ann Ophthalmol 1988; 20: 431–435.

33. Culbertson WW, Blumenkranz MS, Pepose JS, Stewart JA, Curtin VT. Varicella zoster virus is a cause of the acute retinal necrosis syndrome. Ophthalmology 1986; 93: 559–569.

34. Sarkies N, Gregor Z, Forsey T, Darougar S. Antibodies to herpes simplex virus type I in intraocular fluids of patients with acute retinal necrosis. Br J Ophthalmol 1986; 70: 81–84.

35. Blumenkranz MS, Culbertson WW, Clarkson JG, Dix R. Treatment of the acute retinal necrosis syndrome with intravenous acyclovir. Ophthalmology 1986; 93: 296–300.

36. Han DP, Lewis H, Williams GA, Mieler WF, Abrams GW, Aaberg TM. Laser photocoagulation in the acute retinal necrosis syndrome. Arch Ophthalmol 1987; 105: 1051–1054.

37. Fisher JP, Lewis ML, Blumenkranz M, et al. The acute retinal necrosis syndrome: part 1: clinical manifestations. Ophthalmology 1982; 89: 1309–1316.

38. Clarkson JG, Blumenkranz MS, Culbertson WW, Flynn HW Jr, Lewis ML. Retinal detachment following the acute retinal necrosis syndrome. Ophthalmology 1984; 91: 1665–1668.

39. Pepose JS. Acute retinal necrosis syndrome. In: Ryan SJ, ed. Retina. St Louis: CV Mosby, 1989; 2: 617–623.

40. Das T, Biswas J, Kumar A, et al. Eales' disease. Ind J Ophthalmol 1994; 42: 3–18.

41. Ashton, N. Pathogenesis and aetiology of Eales's disease. In: Pandit YK ed: XIX International Congress of Ophthalmology. Bombay: The Times of India Press, 1962: 828.

42. Laatikainen, L, Erkkilä, H: A follow-up study on serpiginous choroiditis. Acta Ophthalmol, 1981: 59: 707-718.

43. Maumenee, AE: Clinical entities in "uveitis": An approach to the study of intraocular inflammation. XXVI Edward Jackson Memorial Lecture. Am J Ophthalmol, 1970: 69: 1-27.

44. Nussenblatt, RB, Palestine, AG: Uveitis: Fundamentals and clinical practice. Chicago: Year Book, 1989a, 309-314.

45. Weiss, H, Annesley, WH, Jr, Shields, JA, Tomer, T, Christopherson, K: The clinical course of serpiginous choroidopathy. Am J Ophthalmol, 1979: 87:133-142.

46. Krill, AE. Retinal diseases of rubella. Arch Ophthalmol.,1967: 77: 445.

47. Tabbara, KF: Brucellosis and nonsyphilitic treponemal uveitis. Int Ophthalmol Clin, 1990: 30: 294.

48. Gass, JDM: Stereoscopic Atlas of Macular Diseases, 3rd ed. St. Louis: CV Mosby, 1987, 480-483.

49. Taylor, HR, Dax, EM: Ocular Onchocerciasis. In Tabbara KF, Hyndiuk RA eds: Infections of the eye. Boston, Little Brown, 1986.

50. Cano, MR: Ocular Cysticercus. In Schachat AP, Murphy RP, Patz A eds: Retina. Vol. 2. St. Louis , CV Mosby, 1989, 583-587.

51. Gass, JDM: Stereoscopic Atlas of Macular Diseases, 3rd ed. St. Louis: CV Mosby, 1987, 470-475.

52. Raspiller, A, Lepori, JC, George, JL: Choriorétinopathie par migration de poils de chenilles. Bull Mém Soc Fr Ophtalmol, 1984: 95: 153-156.

35 White Dot Syndromes

Ramana S. Moorthy, Narsing A. Rao

White dot syndromes are a group of entities that must be considered in patients who have multifocal choroiditis or who have deep retinal, retinal pigment epithelial, or superficial choroidal lesions. The lesions are typically white to yellowish, not elevated, and may not be associated with significant vitreous inflammation. The five main white dot syndromes to be discussed are recurrent multifocal choroiditis and panuveitis (MFC), multiple evanescent white dot syndrome (MEWDS), acute retinal pigment epitheliitis, acute posterior multifocal placoid pigment epitheliopathy (APMPPE), and birdshot retinochoroidopathy.

Multifocal choroiditis and panuveitis, which is on a continuum with punctate inner choroidopathy and subretinal fibrosis/uveitis syndrome, occurs in females more commonly than in males (3:1) (1, 2, 3, 4, 5, 6, 7); average age of onset is between 20 and 40. Epstein-Barr virus was implicated in early reports, since these patients had elevated anti-Epstein-Barr viral antibody titers (8, 9). The results could not be reproduced by other investigators. Thus, the etiology of MFC remains unclear. Clinically, patients present with mild to severe reduction in vision, with the more severe reduction secondary to cystoid macular edema or subretinal neovascularization. Up to two-thirds of patients may have anterior chamber inflammation, which is usually mild (4). Synechiae may occur, but are rare. Almost all patients have vitritis, and peripapillary pigment atrophy occurs in up to a third of them (1, 2, 3, 4, 5, 6, 7). Typically, there are several punched-out lesions in the periphery

that may become equatorial and appear in circumferential lines. They are usually 50–350 microns in diameter, yellow to gray, and are at the level of the retinal pigment epithelium. These lesions may be confused with POHS, although vitritis is absent in POHS. In up to 80% of these patients the lesions are bilateral (1, 2, 3, 4, 5, 6, 7). One-third of the patients will develop subretinal neovascular membranes, which may involve the fovea and cause significant reduction in the vision, resulting in macular disciform scars (5). Cystoid macular edema develops in some patients, especially when the vitritis is chronic. Some patients develop progressive subretinal fibrosis. Fluorescein angiograms reveal acute lesions to be hypofluorescent early and hyperfluorescent late. Punched-out lesions often appear as window defects that reveal underlying choroidal and perhaps late scleral staining. Epstein-Barr virus titers may be checked, particularly in patients with active disease; but these may be unreliable because of the ubiquitous nature of unrelated EBV exposure and past infections. These tests include antiviral capsid antigen antibody (VCA IgM and IgG), early antibody (EA), and anti-Epstein-Barr nuclear antigen antibody (EBNA). Positive VCA IgG and EA suggest past infection, and stay positive for life. Positive VCA IgM and EBNA imply active or chronic infection (10). The visual prognosis is good unless subretinal neovascular membranes or fibrosis develop. Also see Retina section in Chapter 59 and **Table 59-3** for list of White Dot syndromes.

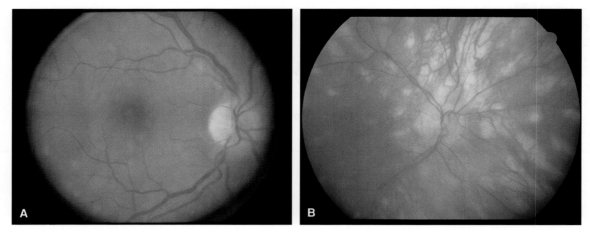

Figure 35–1.
A, Note multiple tiny lesions in the posterior pole of a patient with multiple evanescent white dot syndrome. **B,** Multiple radiating choroidal lesions in birdshot choroidopathy.

■ MULTIPLE EVANESCENT WHITE DOT SYNDROME (See Chapter 59)

Multiple evanescent white dot syndrome was reported first by Jampol and Sieving in 1984 (11, 12). The overwhelming majority of patients are female; the average age is approximately 25, with a range of 17 to 38 years (11, 12). The pathogenesis is unclear, but it is considered postviral retinal pigment epithelial inflammation with secondary retinal and photoreceptor damage. Clinically, 40-50% of patients will have a viral prodrome (11, 12). Visual acuity can range from 20/40 to 20/200, and patients often complain of photopsias. Up to 80% of patients have some vitreous cells, usually rare to 1-11, 12; there is usually no anterior chamber reaction. In 90% of cases the condition is unilateral (11, 12). On fundus examination, multiple 100 to 200 micron-sized white dots are seen at the level of the retinal pigment epithelium or deep retina, often in the posterior pole (Figure 35–1a). These changes are seen as the course of MEWDS progresses (11). Fluorescein angiography reveals early hyperfluorescence of the lesions with late staining. Disc edema may be present and disc leakage is often present (11). Characteristically, the electroretinogram (ERG) shows a reduced a-wave and reduced early receptor potentials, implying photoreceptor dysfunction. This returns to normal upon resolution. The prognosis is excellent: up to 80% of patients have 20/20 or better vision within 10 weeks of the onset of symptoms. Photopsias and large blind spots may last for many months, even in the absence of fundus changes. It is felt that the idiopathic blind spot enlargement syndrome or

big blind spot syndrome and MEWDS represent two different ends of the spectrum of the same disease. Up to 10% of patients have recurrences in the same eye, or develop MEWDS in the other eye (11, 12). As the disease is usually self-limiting, no therapy is required.

Retinal Pigment Epitheliitis

Retinal pigment epitheliitis affects males and females equally, usually in their 20s (13–14). The etiology is unknown but is suspected to be viral (14). Clinically, these patients present with sudden mildly decreased vision, 20/20 to 20/70, typically unilateral (13–14). On examination there are usually 2 to 4 clusters of dark grey spots, sometimes in a honeycomb pattern; surrounding the spots is a hyperpigmented halo. These spots are typically at the level of the retinal pigment epithelium. The halo decreases with time and the lesions are easily missed. The spots usually surround the macula. On fluorescein angiography the dots are hypofluorescent with a hyperfluorescent halo, which may become even more hyperfluorescent with time (14). Electrooculogram abnormalities may be found in the acute stage of the disease, but normalize when the disease is inactive; the ERG is normal (14). Prognosis is good, with resolution of symptoms in 6 to 12 weeks. Cystoid macular edema and subretinal neovascular membrane do not usually complicate this disease and vision returns to normal within 1 to 3 months.

■ ACUTE POSTERIOR MULTIFOCAL PLACOID PIGMENT EPITHELIOPATHY (APMPPE) (see Retina, Chapter 59)

APMPPE occurs in young individuals, usually under the age of 30; males and females are affected equally. There is a viral prodrome in up to one-third of patients (15–17). Patients present with rapid, bilateral decrease in vision, in one-third of the cases to worse than 20/100. A decrease in color vision also occurs. On clinical examination, classic yellow-white, creamy infiltrates at the level of the retinal pigment epithelium and inner choroid are noted. Patients usually begin to develop retinal pigmentary changes within 1 to 2 weeks after the onset of symptoms. Lesions may be approximately the size of the optic disc, and can become confluent. New lesions continue to appear in the first 3 weeks after the onset of symptoms, suggesting some evolution of this disease. Papillitis, retinal vasculitis, macular edema, and superficial hemorrhages may be present in rare instances (15, 16, 17). There is seldom anterior segment cells or vitreous cells. Once the lesions begin to resolve, significant RPE mottling and depigmentation is seen. Fluorescein angiography reveals active lesions that block early and then stain late. The EOG may be diminished in the acute stage of the disease, reflecting the involvement of the retinal pigment epithelium (15). No treatment exists for this condition and it is self-limited. Prognosis is good, with up to 90% of patients regaining 20/30 or better vision. Residual symptoms have been described in up to three-quarters of patients (16). Only rarely do subretinal neovascular membranes complicate the continuous pigment epithelial changes that occur in this disease.

■ BIRDSHOT CHORIORETINOPATHY

This syndrome was first reported by Ryan and Maumenee in 1980 (18). It has also been called vitiliginous choroiditis and salmon-patch chorioretinopathy. Typically, patients are older at onset than for the other white dot syndromes, with an average age of 52 years; females are more commonly affected than males. It is rare in nonwhites (8). Up to 90% of patients are HLA-A29 positive (8). The pathogenesis of this syndrome is unknown, but hypersensitivity reactions to certain retinal antigens and the association of HLA-A29 antigen expression imply a defect in immunoregulation that may be genetically modulated. Clinically, patients present with symptoms of floaters and blurred vision. Most patients have bilateral disease. On external examination the eye is quiet. A few patients have anterior segment inflammation, and up to 80% have some vitreous cells and opacities (8, 18, 19). On fundus examination, the lesions are creamy white to yellow, 1/4 to 1 disc diameter in size, and found in the midperiphery. Usually flat, they appear to be located deep in the retina and involve adjacent superficial choroid. The spots tend to radiate from the disc (Figure 1B). Cystoid macular edema is a common sequelae (8,18). Fluorescein angiography show the cystoid macular edema and often retinal vascular staining. The lesions themselves, however, do not show any altered fluorescence. The ERG shows a diminished B-wave amplitude and prolonged implicit time (8).

Laboratory Evaluation

Fluorescein angiography is useful in confirming cystoid macular edema. In addition, HLA-A29 positivity is increased in this disease and the presence of this antigen should be sought with HLA typing (8).

The prognosis is variable. Some patients maintain reasonably good visual acuity, while others experience progressive visual loss associated with optic atrophy and severe degeneration of the outer retina and inner choroid.

Treatment

Treatment of this entity is usually with systemic and periocular steroids, but is reserved for patients who have cystoid macular edema with reduction in visual acuity to less than 20/40. Immunosuppressives may be used in steroid-resistant cases. Cyclosporine may be helpful (8). Some patients develop choroidal neovascular membranes that may require laser photocoagulation.

■ REFERENCES

1. Morgan, CM, Schatz, H: Recurrent multifocal choroiditis. Ophthalmology, 1986: 93: 1138-1147.
2. Dreyer, RF, Gass, JDM: Multifocal choroiditis and panuveitis. A syndrome that mimics ocular histoplasmosis. Arch Ophthalmol, 1984: 102: 1776-1784.
3. Watzke, RC, Packer, AJ, Folk, JC, Benson, WE, Burgess, D,

Ober, RR: Punctate inner choroidopathy. Am J Ophthalmol, 1984: 98: 572-584.

4. Nozik, RA, Dorsch, W: A new chorioretinopathy associated with anterior uveitis. Am J Ophthalmol, 1973: 76: 758-762.

5. Doran, RML, Hamilton, AM: Disciform macular degeneration in young adults. Trans Ophthalmol Soc UK, 1982: 102: 471-480.

6. Palestine, AG, Nussenblatt, RB, Parver, LM, Knox, DL: Progressive subretinal fibrosis and uveitis. Br J Ophthalmol, 1984: 68: 667-673.

7. Cantrill, HL, Folk, JC: Multifocal choroiditis associated with progressive subretinal fibrosis. Am J Ophthalmol, 1986: 101: 170-180.

8. Nussenblatt, RB, Palestine, AG: Uveitis: Fundamentals and clinical practice. Chicago: Year Book, 1989: 291-308.

9. Tiedeman, JS: Epstein-Barr viral antibodies in multifocal choroiditis and panuveitis. Am J Ophthalmol, 1987: 103: 659-663.

10. Spaide, RF, Sugin, S, Yannuzzi, LA, De Rosa, JT: Epstein-Barr virus antibodies in multifocal choroiditis and panuveitis. Am J Ophthalmol, 1991: 112: 410-413.

11. Jampol, LM, Sieving, PA, Pugh, D, Fishman, GA, Gilbert, H: Multiple evanescent white dot syndrome. I. Clinical findings. Arch Ophthalmol, 1984: 102: 671-674.

12. Sieving, PA, Fishman, GA, Jampol, LM, Pugh, D: Multiple evanescent white dot syndrome. II. Electrophysiology of the photoreceptors during retinal pigment epithelial disease. Arch Ophthalmol, 1984: 102: 675-679.

13. Krill, AE, Deutman, AF: Acute retinal pigment epitheliitus [sic]. Am J Ophthalmol, 1972: 74: 193-205.

14. Deutman, AF: Acute retinal pigment epitheliitis. Am J Ophthalmol, 1974: 78: 571-578.

15. Gass, JDM: Acute posterior multifocal placoid pigment epitheliopathy. Arch Ophthalmol, 1968: 80: 177-185.

16. Smith, VC, Pokorny, J, Ernest, JT, Starr, SJ: Visual function in acute posterior multifocal placoid pigment epitheliopathy. Am J Ophthalmol, 1978: 85: 192-199.

17. Ryan, SJ, Maumenee, AE: Acute posterior multifocal placoid pigment epitheliopathy. Am J Ophthalmol, 1972: 74: 1066-1074.

18. Ryan, SJ, Maumenee, AE: Birdshot retinochoroidopathy. Am J Ophthalmol, 1980: 89: 31-45.

19. Gass, JDM: Vitiliginous chorioretinitis. Arch Ophthalmol, 1981: 99: 1778-1787.

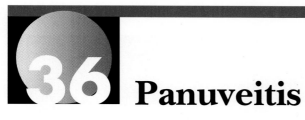

36 Panuveitis

Ramana S. Moorthy, Narsing A. Rao

■ SARCOIDOSIS

Sarcoidosis is a granulomatous, systemic disease of unknown etiology. It affects blacks 10 times more commonly than whites and is more common in females (1). It can, however, affect all races. Seen primarily in adults between the ages of 20 and 50, sarcoidosis can also be seen in children and the elderly.

Clinical Features

Systemic manifestations of sarcoidosis include interstitial lung disease, lymphadenopathy, skin lesions, especially erythema nodosum, and arthritis. In children with sarcoidosis, erythema nodosum and arthritis are often the presenting symptoms (2).

Ocular involvement occurs in up to 38% of patients with sarcoidosis, and is more common in blacks than whites (1, 3, 4). Ocular manifestations include dry eye or enlarged lacrimal gland; conjunctival nodules; anterior, posterior, and panuveitis; retinal vasculitis; papillitis and optic neuritis. Up to two-thirds of patients with ocular involvement have anterior segment inflammation (3, 5) characterized by mutton fat keratic precipitates with variable amounts of anterior segment flare and cells. The iris may exhibit granulomas (Figure 36–1) which results in a chronic iridocyclitis. Acute exacerbations may also occur. Conjunctival granulomas are present concurrently in up to 17% of patients, and lacrimal gland involvement occurs in up to 26% of cases (3–5).

Posterior uveitis or panuveitis is seen in up to 25% of patients with sarcoidosis (3, 4, 5). Findings include retinal vasculitis (Figure 36–2) and periphlebitis with exudation, which results in the so-called candle wax dripping ("taches de bougie"). Snowball opacities and

vitreous cells that arise from the candle wax drippings may accumulate in the inferior vitreous cavity. Chorioretinitis, choroidal nodules, and retinal pigment epithelial changes can occur secondary to granulomatous inflammation of the choroid (Figure 36–3). Optic disc neovascularization and retinal neovascularization occur if occlusive periphlebitis has caused peripheral retinal ischemia. Subretinal neovascularization is uncommon. Peripheral granulomas of the choroid appear in a circumferential pattern in the midperiphery. These nodules vary in size from approximately one-quarter disc diameter to one disc diameter. As the acute phase of choroiditis resolves, these granulomas leave in their wake an area of retinal pigment epithelial and choroidal atrophy. Papillitis (Figure 36–4), retrobulbar neuritis, optic atrophy, and disc edema can also occur in sarcoidosis. Approximately 33% of patients who have posterior segment disease have central nervous system involvement as well (6).

Laboratory Evaluation

Investigations to confirm or exclude the diagnosis of sarcoidosis should include serum angiotensin converting enzyme (ACE) level and a chest radiograph. The ACE level is a mark of total body granuloma load, and is elevated in up to 90% of patients with sarcoidosis (7). ACE is, however, not specific for sarcoidosis; it can be elevated in patients with other granulomatous inflammations and in patients who have pulmonary and liver disease. In addition, the ACE level may be reduced by corticosteroid treatment (7, 8). Lysozyme level in the serum may also be elevated in sarcoidosis, and tends to

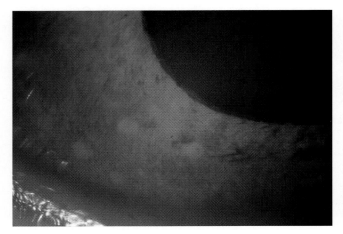

Figure 36–1.
A patient with sarcoidosis showing granulomas in the iris stroma.

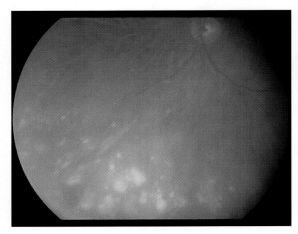

Figure 36–3.
Retinal pigment epithelial changes in sarcoidosis.

parallel the ACE level. Chest radiographs disclose hilar adenopathy, parenchymal involvement, or interstitial fibrosis in up to 80% of patients with sarcoidosis (9). If the ACE level is elevated and the chest radiograph is normal, a gallium scan of the head, neck, and chest region may be of value in determining if there is involvement by sarcoidosis in these regions. Gallium uptake occurs in areas where granulomatous inflammation is present, and this tends to be a more sensitive measure of inflammatory activity in sarcoidosis than chest radiography (10). Skin testing may reveal anergy, which is common in these patients. Anergy suggests some defect in cell-mediated immunity. Reduced numbers of T-helper cells in the circulation, and accumulations of these cells in areas of inflammation suggest that cellular immune mechanisms play a key role in the pathogenesis of sarcoidosis (11). Additional laboratory evaluation should include biopsy of suspicious nodules of the skin, conjunctiva, and lacrimal glands, which may show non-

caseating granulomas characteristic of sarcoidosis (7,12).

Differential Diagnosis

It is important to rule out other causes of granulomatous inflammation, particularly tuberculosis and syphilis. In cases of acute iridocyclitis, HLA B27-associated disease should also be ruled out. In children, juvenile rheumatoid arthritis-associated iridocyclitis may appear similar to sarcoidosis, and in these cases, serum ANA titers should be obtained (2).

Treatment

Corticosteroids are the mainstay of treatment of ocular sarcoidosis. Topical corticosteroids are often effective and in many cases are all that is necessary for control of anterior segment inflammation. Panuveitis or posterior uveitis, however, calls for the use of periocular or sys-

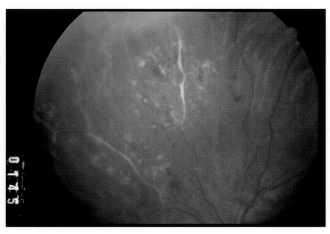

Figure 36–2.
Retinal vasculitis and hemorrhages in sarcoidosis.

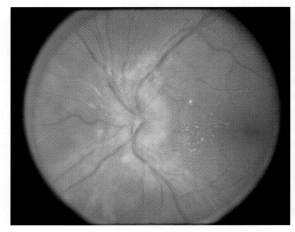

Figure 36–4.
Papillitis in a patient with sarcoidosis.

temic corticosteroids. The management of associated systemic sarcoidosis is the realm of a qualified internist.

Prognosis

Ocular sarcoidosis usually follows a chronic course, although younger patients often develop acute inflamma-tion. This responds well to topical corticosteroids, however, and these patients actually have a better visual prognosis. Patients with chronic iridocyclitis and panuveitis have a relatively poorer prognosis, (5) and many develop complications such as cataracts, glaucoma, and cystoid macular edema and optic atrophy (4).

■ BEHÇET'S SYNDROME

Behçet's syndrome is an occlusive vasculitis of unknown etiology. It is a systemic disorder that is rare in the United States, and much more common in the countries along the old silk route traveled by Marco Polo. These regions include the Mediterranean, the Middle East, and the Far East, especially Japan. In some of these countries, Behçet's syndrome accounts for up to 20% of all cases of uveitis (13).

Clinical Features

Behçet's syndrome affects primarily young adults between the ages of 20 and 40. The classic triad of this syndrome consists of recurrent aphthous ulceration of the mouth, ocular lesions including hypopyon iritis and retinal vasculitis, and genital ulcerations. In additon, a fourth "major" criterion for the diagnosis of Behçet's is skin lesions, including erythema nodosum, cutaneous thrombophlebitis, and hyperirritability of skin (14). In the complete form of Behçet's, all four of the above major criteria are present at some time during the course of the disease. The incomplete form is said to exist if only 3 of the major criteria are present, or if ocular lesions are present in addition to 1 other major criterion. Aphthous ulcers are the most common presenting major criterion, and were seen in 98% of cases in 1 large study (13). These usually heal within a week, but are recurrent. Skin lesions may be seen in up to 90% of patients, and genital lesions in up to 80% of patients. Important minor criteria include arthritis in up to 50% of cases and central nervous system involvement, including brainstem, meningoencephalitic, and confusional syndromes in 42% (15). It is interesting that most patients who have neuro-Behçet's do not have ocular involvement (16).

Ocular manifestations occur in up to 70% of patients, but are the presenting complaint in less than a quarter of patients with Behçet's (13, 14). Anterior uveitis is seen more often in women than in men, and can present with signs of hypopyon iritis. The hypopyon is usually transient and is seen in only a third of the cases of iridocyclitis (13). The episodes of iridocyclitis last for several weeks. Posterior segment involvement is more common in men (17). Typically, retinal involvement is in the form of an occlusive vasculitis that may affect the arteries, the veins, or both (Figure 36–5). White infiltrates may be present in the inner retina, associated with intraretinal hemorrhages. In addition, perivascular sheathing may be intense. A mild to moderate degree of vitritis may also be seen. Recurrent attacks are associated with large areas of capillary nonperfusion and subsequent development of retinal neovascularization (17).

Laboratory Investigations

Over half of Behçet's patients of Japanese and Mediterranean origin are HLA B5 (subset HLA-BW 51) positive (18), so this test is often useful in the diagnosis of Behçet's syndrome. Skin abrasion tests may be done to show dermatographia. A skin puncture can result in pustule formation, the so-called Behçet skin test.

Differential Diagnosis

The retinitis and the retinal necrosis seen in Behçet's can mimic viral retinitis. Other causes of retinal vasculitis, including rheumatologic disorders, sarcoidosis, and

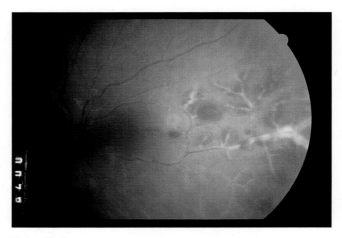

Figure 36–5.
Retinal vasculitis and hemorrhages in a patient with Behçet syndrome.

idiopathic retinal vasculitis, should also be included in the differential diagnosis.

Treatment

Treatment of Behçet's syndrome in the acute phase consists of topical corticosteroids and mydriatic agents for the anterior uveitis, and periocular and systemic corticosteroids for severe posterior segment manifestations. Unfortunately these medications tend to lose their effectiveness with time. Colchicine, 0.6 mg administered orally twice daily, may also be useful in limiting the acute flare-ups of the disease. This medication inhibits leukocyte migration and chemotaxis. The majority of patients with Behçet's however, will require immunosuppressive therapy (19, 20). Recently, cyclosporine has been shown to be effective in combination with decreased dose systemic corticosteroids in controlling inflammation in steroid-resistant cases (21). Cyclosporine may be begun at 5 mg/kg/day orally, and continued for 4 to 6 weeks, along with initally higher doses of systemic corticosteroids, with a gradual taper of the steroids. This dosage of cyclosporine reduces the potential nephrotoxic effects of the medicine. Medications such as chlorambucil, 6-12 mg/day, and azathioprine, between 1 and 2.5 mg/day, in combination with decreased dose systemic corticosteroids, are also effective in controlling Behçet's disease (19, 20). It is essential with all immunosuppressive medications to closely monitor the systemic status of the patient with the assistance of an internist.

Prognosis

Untreated Behçet's syndrome has a poor prognosis and is a blinding condition. Recurrent anterior uveitis can result in cataract and glaucoma, while posterior segment inflammation associated with obliterative vasculitis can result in destruction of the retina, macular ischemia, and eventual optic atrophy. Secondary neovascularization of the retina and iris with neovascular glaucoma is also seen. The retinal neovascularization can bleed and produce vitreous hemorrhage, vitreous traction, and retinal detachments (18). Despite new immunosuppressive treatments, severe complications still occur.

■ SYMPATHETIC OPHTHALMIA

Sympathetic ophthalmia (SO) is a bilateral, granulomatous panuveitis that is seen after penetrating ocular injury or intraocular surgery. It is an uncommon condition that affects less than 1% of patients with penetrating ocular injuries and 0.01% who have undergone intraocular surgery (22–24), but it is a potentially blinding condition.

The etiology of sympathetic ophthalmia is unknown; however, it is thought that a genetically predisposed host incites a cell-mediated immune response against an intraocular antigen, possibly retinal proteins, uveal tissue, or melanin (25, 26). This immune response then results in prolonged granulomatous inflammation in both eyes.

Clinical Features

Sympathethic ophthalmia affects individuals of all ages. There is no sex predilection, but because ocular trauma is much more common in males, fewer females are affected (27). Most cases (60%) occur after penetrating ocular injuries; the remainder are seen after surgical procedures (30%), and subsequent to perforated corneal ulcers (10%) (27, 28). Typically, inflammation develops as early as 4 to 8 weeks after the insult, although the interval from trauma to onset of inflammation can be as short as 5 days or as long as 42 years (28). Most cases occur less than 1 year after the inciting injury (27). Inflammation is often present in the injured eye (exiting eye) at the time of the insult, but it is the uninjured eye that develops the sympathizing inflammation at a later date. Patients present with pain, photophobia, and decreased vision or loss of accommodation in the sympathizing eye. The inflammation is granulomatous in nature, with mutton fat keratic precipitates, iris nodules, cell and flare in the anterior chamber, and Dalen-Fuchs' nodules that represent aggregates of epithelioid cells at the level of Bruch's membrane. These Dalen-Fuchs' nodules can be scattered diffusely throughout the fundus. Retinal detachment, optic atrophy or optic disc edema are present in many cases (27). Occasionally, sympathetic ophthalmia may have systemic manifestations similar to Vogt-Koyanagi-Harada (VKH) syndrome. These include cerebrospinal fluid pleocytosis, meningismus, skin manifestations such as alopecia and vitiligo, poliosis, and dysacusis.

The diagnosis of sympathethic ophthalmia is a clinical one, although fluorescein angiography may aid in the diagnosis. This typically shows changes similar to VKH syndrome, with multiple areas of pinpoint fluorescein leakage at the level of retinal pigment epithelium, with pooling of dye in the subretinal fluid in cases in which serous retinal detachments are present.

Pathologic Assessment

Histologic changes of sympathetic ophthalmia are identical in both the exciting and the sympathizing eyes

(29). A diffuse granulomatous inflammation is seen in the uveal tract, with sparing of the choriocapillaris. Dalen-Fuchs' nodules are present in approximately one-third of the eyes (27). These represent collections of lymphocytes, histiocytes, and altered pigment epithelial cells just internal to Bruch's membrane, and are seen also in VKH syndrome and sarcoidosis. Patients with sympathethic ophthalmia may also develop phacoana-phylactic endophthalmitis in the exciting eye (25).

Treatment

Early enucleation of an injured eye that has no salvage-able vision is the best way to prevent sympathetic oph-thalmia. The decision to enucleate an eye that has been severely injured and that has irreversible visual loss is an easy one. However, in cases in which the eye has useful vision and can be salvaged, most ophthalmologists ad-vocate not enucleating because of the low incidence of sympathetic ophthalmia. It has been suggested by many that enucleation, if it is to be done, should be com-pleted within 2 weeks of the injury. Once inflammation develops in the fellow eye, however, the early use of top-ical, as well as systemic and periocular corticosteroids, is recommended. Although these medications can be ta-pered after several weeks, inflammation may persist and become prolonged. Corticosteroid therapy has been shown to improve visual outcome in up to 75% of cases, with final visual acuities of 20/50 or better (27, 30, 31). In patients intolerant of long-term corticosteroid ther-apy or with inflammation resistant to corticosteroid therapy, the use of cytotoxic agents or cyclosporine is recommended. There is controversy as to whether or not it is advisable to enucleate the exciting eye once sympathethic ophthalmia has begun. Some studies have shown that enucleation of the exciting eye (e.g., the eye that sustained trauma) within 2 weeks after the appear-ance of inflammation may improve the prognosis of the sympathizing eye (27,31). Other reports, however, have shown that there is no benefit in removing the exciting eye before, during, or after the development of sympa-thethic ophthalmia (32).

Course and Prognosis

Sympathetic ophthalmia has a devastating outcome if not aggressively treated. Complications are common: cataracts develop in 47% of cases, glaucoma in 43%, ex-udative retinal detachments in 25%, and severe chori-oretinal scarring in 25%; recurrent inflammation oc-curs in up to 60% of patients (30).

■ VOGT-KOYANAGI-HARADA SYNDROME (VKH)
(see Retina, Chapter 59)

The VKH syndrome is a bilateral, granulomatous panu-veitis associated usually with dermatologic and neuro-logic manifestations. Vogt in 1906, and Koyanagi, in 1929, reported an iridocyclitis associated with poliosis, vitiligo, and dysacusis. In 1926, Harada described a syn-drome of serous retinal detachments and cerebrospinal fluid (CSF) pleocytosis associated with a posterior uveitis. Bruno and and McPherson, in 1949, consoli-dated the findings of Vogt, Koyanagi, and Harada into a spectrum of disease known as Vogt-Koyanagi-Harada syndrome.

Clinical Features

VKH syndrome is seen typically in darkly pigmented races, including Orientals, Hispanics, American Indi-ans, Asian Indians, and Blacks (33–39). It affects both sexes, but is seen more commonly in females (38–40). This is particularly true in the Hispanic population, in which there is nearly a 3 to 1 ratio of females to males that are affected (38). Most patients are between the ages of 20 and 50. (38) However, a child of 7 years of age has been described with the disease (42). Although oc-ular manifestations are fairly consistent from one racial group to another, extraocular manifestations appear to vary widely between Japanese and Hispanics: Hispanics usually do not develop the extraocular manifestations of vitiligo, alopecia, and poliosis (39, 41, 43, 44), but do de-velop meningismus and CSF pleocytosis (41).

Clinically, the syndrome can be divided into four dis-tinct phases (38). The first phase or the prodromal phase, is characterized by a flulike illness associated with meningismus and headache, as well as tinnitus and dysacusis. The second, or uveitic phase is associated with acute onset of iridocyclitis, vitritis, optic disc edema, and multiple serous retinal detachments (Figure 36–6). The inflammation is typically granulomatous. This is the point in time at which most patients present to the oph-thalmologist, because of a sudden loss of vision, pain, and photophobia. The third, or convalescent phase is associated with subsidence of the uveitis, but with a de-pigmentation of the skin (vitiligo), which may be peri-ocular, a whitening of the eyelashes (poliosis), as well as a diffuse depigmentation of the choroid. Alopecia is also common at this point. Perilimbal vitiligo, referred to as Sugiura's sign, is seen often along with fundus pig-mentary changes (39). The depigmentation of choroid results in the so-called "sunset glow" appearance of the fundus (Figure 36–7). Typically in the inferior periph-ery of the retina, well circumscribed yellow-white

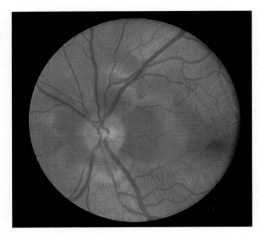

Figure 36–6.
Multiple serous detachment of the retina in VKH syndrome.

punched-out chorioretinal scars, probably representing resolved Dalen-Fuchs'nodules, are found. These can be similar to those seen in sympathetic ophthalmia. Finally, the fourth phase has been reported recently as a continuous recurrent inflammatory phase characterized by primarily anterior segment inflammation. The major ophthalmic complications of VKH syndrome occur most often in this phase of the illness.

Laboratory Investigations

There is an increased incidence of HLA DR4 antigen in Japanese patients (45), and recent studies have shown that the DR4 *0401 gene is particularly highly associated with VKH syndrome in Japanese patients (46). However, no specific serologic tests are available to help make the diagnosis of VKH syndrome. The diagnosis is usually a clinical one, but is aided by two ancillary stud-

ies: fluorescein angiography and ultrasonography. Fluorescein angiography typically reveals multiple pinpoint areas of hypofluorescence at the level of the RPE that tend to leak fluorescein into the subretinal space (47). In addition, late disc staining and pinpoint areas of hyperfluorescence that do not increase in size have also been reported (48).

Standardized echography can be beneficial in making the diagnosis (49). Echographic findings include low-to-medium reflective choroidal thickening, most marked in the posterior pole and peripapillary area and tapering to the periphery, serous retinal detachments, scleral and episcleral thickening, and mild to moderate vitreous opacities. The presence of meningismus and headache suggest neurologic involvement. MRI may show areas of unidentified bright objects within the white matter, suggestive of inflammatory lesions (38), and CSP pleocytosis with more than 3 mononuclear cells/mm (3) may also be present. These latter tests are merely supportive of the diagnosis.

Pathologic Assessment

Histopathologically, the VKH syndrome is characterized by a diffuse, granulomatous inflammation of the entire uveal tract. It is similar to sympathethic ophthalmia. In cases of chronic VKH syndrome the inflammation involves the choriocapillaris and there are chorioretinal scars.

Etiology

The etiology of VKH syndrome is unknown. However, several theories have been proposed. These include a possible role of uveal melanin as an inciting agent resulting in autoimmunity to uveal melanocytes, genetic predisposition in an individual with the HLA DR4 antigen, and abnormalities in immune regulation (39). Since inflammation tends to be more intense in the peripapillary choroid, where choroidal melanocytes predominate, this theory of autoimmunity to uveal melanocytes may explain the pathogenesis of the VKH syndrome (50).

Treatment

Systemic corticosteroids are the mainstay of treatment for VKH syndrome. Prednisone, given orally at a dosage of 60-200 mg/day depending on the severity of the inflammation, results in a rapid resolution of serous retinal detachments and disc edema within 1 to 2 weeks. Frequent topical application of corticosteroids and topical mydriatic agents is also useful for associated anterior segment inflammation. The key in the management of this illness is to continue high dose corticosteroids for approximately 2 weeks, with a grad-

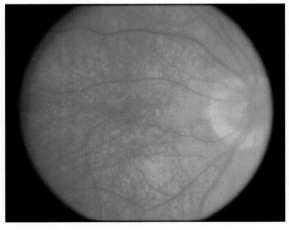

Figure 36–7.
A patient with chronic VKH syndrome showing features of "sunset glow" fundus.

ual taper over a period of 4 to 6 months. It is important not to wean the patient off steroids less than 3 months after the onset of symptoms (38,51), since this may increase the incidence of recurrent anterior segment inflammation and its associated complications (38,51). However, if there is recurrent anterior segment inflammation, cytotoxic or cytostatic agents may be necessary, in addition to corticosteroids, to control inflammation; in these cases, agents such as azathioprine, cyclophosphamide, and cyclosporin are appropriate (52). Because of the associated systemic complications of these medications, patients must be monitored closely by an internist while on such immunosuppressive therapy. An increase in cells in the aqueous humor or vitreous cavity, decline in vision, or recurrence of neurologic symptoms usually heralds an increase in disease activity, which necessitates more aggressive therapy.

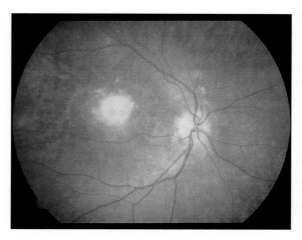

Figure 36–8.
Macular scar from subretinal neovascularization in chronic VKH syndrome.

Course and Prognosis

Most patients who are treated appropriately with corticosteroid therapy have a relatively benign course after the disease begins to respond. A slow and gradual taper of corticosteroids is essential since a rapid taper may predispose the patient to recurrent anterior segment inflammation (38). If this occurs, the complications of

VKH syndrome can be devastating; cataracts develop in approximately 38% of patients (53), glaucoma in up to 30% of patients (54), and subretinal neovascularization (Figure 36–8), a major cause of severe visual loss, in up to 10% of patients (55). Other causes of visual loss include optic atrophy and severe RPE alterations.

■ LENS-INDUCED UVEITIS

Lens-induced intraocular inflammation can be characterized into three different disorders, namely phacoanaphylactic endophthalmitis, phacotoxic uveitis, and phacolytic glaucoma.

Phacoanaphylactic endophthalmitis is a severe granulomatous intraocular inflammation that develops after traumatic or spontaneous disruption of the lens. The lens protein acts as an antigen and the inflammation is thought to be a localized arthus reaction to the exposed lens material. This inflammation is seen occasionally after extracapsular catract surgery, and is an immune-mediated reaction to retained lens material. It can also occur after traumatic rupture of the lens capsule. Patients present with severe pain, redness, and photophobia. Mutton fat keratic precipitates, severe anterior segment reaction, possibly with hypopyon, and posterior synechiae are often seen (56). It is usually unilateral and the diagnosis is based on history and clinical examination.

Phacotoxic uveitis occurs after surgery or trauma in which lens protein has been exposed in the eye. The inflammation may be of sudden or delayed onset. There is anterior segment flare and cells, small keratic precipitates, and occasionally synechiae formation. This inflammation, however, is nongranulomatous (56).

Phacolytic glaucoma occurs in situations where there is a hypermature, Morgagnian cataract. There is liquefaction of the cortex and a settling of the brunescent dense nucleus in the capsular bag. The liquified protein subsequently leaks through the capsular bag into the anterior segment. Macrophages then migrate into the anterior segment, phagocytose the lens protein, and obstruct the trabecular meshwork, which results in glaucoma (56). Histopathologically, these macrophages are seen to be laden with eosinophilic lens protein.

Pathologic Assessment

Phacoanaphylactic endophthalmitis is a zonal granulomatous inflammatory reaction that surrounds the exposed lens material. This inflammation consists of polymorphonuclear leukocytes, around which is a zone of macrophages, epithelioid cells, and giant cells. An outermost layer of lymphocytes, plasma cells and macrophages is also present. The iris and ciliary body are infiltrated by the mononuclear cells. Phacotoxic uveitis histopathologically is a nonspecific inflammatory reaction with lymphocytes, neutrophils, and occasional giant cells (56). In phacolytic glaucoma, macrophages laden with the eosinophilic lens protein are seen within the anterior chamber and in the trabecular meshwork.

Treatment

Topical and systemic corticosteroids suppress inflammation in each of these entities. However, the definitive treatment in phacoanaphylactic endophthalmitis and phacotoxic uveitis involves removal of all remaining native lens material. This should be done after the inflammatory reaction has subsided. Corticosteroids should be continued for several days after surgery and then tapered slowly. If the inflammation is controlled early and the lens material removed, the prognosis is generally good. Phacolytic glaucoma demands prompt extraction of the cataract, which usually results in rapid normalization of intraocular pressure.

■ LYME DISEASE

Lyme disease is a tick-borne spirochetal illness that is caused by Borrellia burgdorferi (57). It is transmitted to humans by the bite of a deer tick, Ixodes dammini. This particular deer tick is common in the eastern United States. In the western United States, Ixodes pacificus has been implicated in the pathogenesis of this disease. Clinical manifestations of Lyme disease can be characterized into three stages:

1. Stage I occurs a month after the initial tick bite and is manifested by erythema chronicum migrans, constitutional symptoms, and ocular findings (58), usually conjunctivitis (58, 59). The patient may also have headaches, stiff neck, malaise, fever, and lymphadenopathy. Occasionally a fever may occur.

2. Stage II follows 1 to 4 months after infection, and is manifest by neurologic, musculoskeletal, cardiac, and ocular abnormalities. Up to 30 to 40% of patients develop neurologic disease, taking the form of encephalitis, meningitis, and Bell's palsy; 8% of patients develop myocarditis and heart block (60, 61). Stage II ocular manifestations of Lyme disease include keratitis, iritis, pars planitis, vitritis, panophthalmitis, and optic neuritis (60, 61).

3. Stage III usually has its onset more than 5 months after the initial infection and is characterized by interstitial keratitis, chronic meningitis, chronic arthritis, adult respiratory distress syndrome, and chronic atrophic skin changes (60, 61). In one series, the most common uveitic finding was inflammation resembling pars planitis (62). However, unlike cases of true pars planitis, patients with Lyme uveitis have granulomatous keratic precipitates with posterior synechiae formation.

Laboratory Evaluation

Antibody titers to Borellia burgdorferi should be obtained using indirect immunofluorescent assay or ELISA. Only 40 to 60% of patients with Lyme disease have elevated antibody titers (63, 64). Both IgG and IgM titers should be obtained. However, the Lyme IgM is negative in early stage I. It should be noted that patients with Lyme disease may have false–positive syphilis serology, with RPR or VDRL being positive. Syphilis serology should, however, be obtained, because of the similarity of syphilitic ocular disease to Lyme disease. It is important to correlate the laboratory findings with the clinical picture before deciding on the mode of treatment.

Treatment

Recommended treatment for Lyme disease consists of tetracycline, the drug of choice, followed by erythromycin or penicillin. Patients who do not respond to the initial treatment may require alternative or combination therapy. Doxycycline is also used in the treatment of this condition. In addition, efforts to reduce the incidence of disease with pesticide spraying have met with some limited success. Neurologic complications of Lyme disease should be treated with intravenous ceftriaxone and/or penicillin G (65, 66).

■ REFERENCES

1. Siltzbach, LE, James, DG, Neville, E, et al.: Course and prognosis of sarcoidosis around the world. Am J Med, 1974: 57:847-852.
2. Lindsley, CB, Godfrey, WA: Childhood sarcoidosis manifesting as juvenile rheumatoid arthritis. Pediatrics, 1985: 76:765-768.
3. Obenauf, CD, Shaw, HE, Sydnor, CF, Klintworth, GK: Sarcoidosis and its ophthalmic manifestations. Am J Ophthalmol, 1978: 86:648-655.
4. Jabs, DA, Johns, CJ: Ocular involvement in chronic sarcoidosis. Am J Ophthalmol, 1986: 102:297-301.
5. James, DG, Neville, E, Langley, DA: Ocular sarcoidosis. Trans Ophthalmol Soc UK, 1976: 96:133-139.
6. Gould, H, Kaufman, HE: Sarcoid of the fundus. Arch Ophthalmol, 1961: 65:453-456.
7. Weinreb, RN, Tessler, H: Laboratory diagnosis of ophthalmic sarcoidosis. Surv Ophthalmol, 1984: 28:653-664.
8. Weinreb, RN, Kimura, SJ: Uveitis associated with sar-

coidosis and angiotensin converting enzyme. Am J Ophthalmol, 1980: 89:180-185.

9. Smith, RE, Nozik, RA: Uveitis: A Clinical approach to diagnosis and management, 2nd ed. Baltimore: Williams & Wilkins, 1989b: 184-188.

10. Nosal, A, Schleissner, LA, Mishkin, FS, Lieberman, J: Angiotensin-I-converting enzyme and gallium scan in noninvasive evaluation of sarcoidosis. Ann Intern Med, 1979: 90:328-331.

11. Hunninghake, GW, Crystal, RG: Pulmonary sarcoidosis: A disorder mediated by excess helper T-lymphocyte activity at sites of disease activity. N Eng J Med, 1981: 305:429-434.

12. Nichols, CW, Eagle, RC, Jr, Yanoff, M, Menocal, NG: Conjunctival biopsy as an aid in the evaluation of the patient with suspected sarcoidosis. Ophthalmology, 1980: 87:287-291.

13. Mishima, S, Masuda, K, Izawa, Y, Mochizuki, M, Namba, K: The eighth Frederick H. Verhoeff Lecture. Behçet's disease in Japan: Ophthalmologic aspects. Trans Am Ophthalmol Soc, 1979: 77:225-279.

14. Shimizu, T, Ehrlich, GE, Inaba, G, Hayashi, K: Behçet disease (Behçet syndrome). Semin Arthritis Rheum, 1979: 8:223-260.

15. Lesser, RS, DeHoratius, RJ: Miscellaneous clinical manifestations, part III: Neuro-Behçet, systemic amyloidosis, lymphoreticular system. In: Plotkin, GR, Calabro, JJ, O"Duffy, JD (eds):Behçet's disease: A contemporary synopsis. Mount Kisco NY: Futura, 1988: 281-293.

16. Inaba, G: Clinical features of neuro-Behçet's syndrome. In Recent Advances in Behçet's Disease. Edited by T. Lehner, C.G. Barnes. London, Royal Society of Medicine Services, 1986, 235-246.

17. Imai, Y: Studies on prognosis and symptoms of Behçet's disease in long-term observation. Jpn J Clin Ophthalmol, 1971: 25:661-695.

18. Nussenblatt, RB, Palestine, AG: Uveitis: Fundamentals and clinical practice. Chicago: Year Book, 1989a: 212-247.

19. Yazici, H, Pazarli, H, Barnes, CG, et al: A controlled trial of azathioprine in Behçet's syndrome. N Engl J Med, 1990: 322:281-285.

20. Smith, RE, Nozik, RA: Uveitis: A clinical approach to diagnosis and management, 2nd ed. Baltimore: Williams & Wilkins, 1989c: 189-193.

21. Nussenblatt, RB, Palestine, AG, Chan, CC, Mochizuki, M, Yancey, K: Effectiveness of cyclosporin therapy for Behçet's disease. Arthritis Rheum, 1985: 28: 671-679.

22. Liddy, BSL, Stuart, J: Sympathetic ophthalmia in Canada. Can J Ophthalmol, 1972: 7:157-159.

23. Holland, G: Über Indikation und Zeitpunkt der Entfernung eines verletzten Auges. Klin Monatsbl Augenheilkd, 1964: 145:732-740.

24. Allen, JC: Sympathetic ophthalmia: a disappearing disease. JAMA, 1969: 209:1090.

25. Chan, CC: Relationship between sympathetic ophthalmia, phacoanaphylactic endophthalmitis, and Vogt-Koyanagi-Harada disease. Ophthalmology, 1988: 95:619-624.

26. Rao, NA, Robin, J, Hartmann, D, Sweeney, JA, Marak, GE, Jr: The role of the penetrating wound in the development of sympathetic ophthalmia: Experimental observations. Arch Ophthalmol, 1983: 101:102-104.

27. Lubin, JR, Albert, DM, Weinstein, M: Sixty-five years of sympathetic ophthalmia: A clinicopathologic review of 105 cases (1913-1978). Ophthalmology, 1980: 87:109-121.

28. Green, WR: Inflammatory diseases and conditions of the eye. In Ophthalmic Pathology: An Atlas and Textbook. Vol. 3, 3rd ed. Edited by W.H. Spencer. Philadelphia, WB Saunders, 1986, 1792-2013.

29. Easom, HA, Zimmerman, LE: Sympathetic ophthalmia and bilateral phacoanaphylaxis: A clinicopathologic correlation of the sympathogenic and sympathizing eyes. Arch Ophthalmol, 1964: 72:9-l5.

30. Makley, TA, Jr, Azar, A: Sympathetic ophthalmia: A long-term follow-up. Arch Ophthalmol, 1978: 96:257-262.

31. Reynard, M, Riffenburgh, RS, Maes EF: Effect of corticosteroid treatment and enucleation on the visual prognosis of sympathetic ophthalmia. Am J Ophthalmol, 1983: 96:290-294.

32. Winter, FC: Sympathetic uveitis: A clinical and pathologic study of the visual result. Am J Ophthalmol, 1955: 39:340-347.

33. Vogt, A: Frühzeitiges Ergrauen der Zilien und Bemerkungen über den sogenannten plötzlichen Eintritt dieser Veränderung. Klin Monatsbl Augenheilkd, 1906: 45:228-242.

34. Koyanagi, Y: Dysakusis, Alopecia und Poliosis bei schwerer Uveitis nicht traumatischen Ursprungs. Klin Monatsbl Augenheilkd, 1929: 82:194-211.

35. Harada, E: Clinical observations of nonsuppurative choroiditis. Acta Soc Ophthalmol Jpn, 1926: 30:356.

36. Bruno, MG, McPherson SD Jr: Harada's disease. Am J Ophthalmol, 1949: 32:513-522.

37. Smith, RE, Nozik RA: Uveitis: A clinical approach to diagnosis and management, 2nd ed. Baltimore: Williams & Wilkins, 1989a: 162-165.

38. Moorthy, RS, Inomata H, Rao NA: The Vogt-Koyanagi-Harada syndrome. Surv Ophthalmol, (in press), 1994b.

39. Sugiura, S: Vogt-Koyanagi-Harada disease. Jpn J Ophthalmol, 1978: 22:9-35.

40. Nussenblatt, RB, Palestine, AG: Uveitis: Fundamentals and clinical practice. Chicago: Year Book, 1989b: 274-290.

41. Beniz, J, Forster, DJ, Lean, JS, Smith, RE, Rao, NA: Variations in clinical features of the Vogt-Koyanagi-Harada syndrome. Retina, 1991: 11: 275-280.

42. Forster, DJ, Green, RL, Rao, NA: Unilateral manifestation of the Vogt-Koyanagi-Harada syndrome in a 7-year-old child. Am J Ophthalmol, 1991: 111:380-382.

43. Ohno, S, Char, DH, Kimura, SJ, O'Connor, GR: Vogt-Koyanagi-Harada syndrome. Am J Ophthalmol, 1977: 83:735-740.

44. Snyder, DA, Tessler, HH: Vogt-Koyanagi-Harada syndrome. Am J Ophthalmol, 1980: 90:69-75.

45. Ohno, S: Immunological aspects of Behçet's and Vogt-Koyanagi-Harada's diseases. Trans Ophthalmol Soc UK, 1981: 101:335-34l.

46. Islam, SMM, Numaga, J, Fujino, Y, et al: Role of HLA DRB1 genotypes in Vogt-Koyanagi-Harada disease. ARVO abstract. Invest Ophthalmol Vis Sci, 1993: 34:1103.

47. Kanter, PJ, Goldberg, MF: Bilateral uveitis with exudative retinal detachment: Angiographic appearance. Arch Ophthalmol, 1974: 91:13-19.

48. Brinkley, JR, Dugel, PU, Rao, NA: Fluorescein angiographic findings in the Vogt-Koyanagi-Harada syndrome.

49. Forster, DJ, Cano, MR, Green, RL, Rao, NA: Echographic features of the Vogt-Koyanagi-Harada syndrome. Arch Ophthalmol, 1990: 108:1421-1426.

50. Inomata, H, Kato, M: Vogt-Koyanagi-Harada disease. In Handbook of Clinical Neurology. Vol 56. Edited by Vinken, PJ, Bruyn, GW, Klawans, HL, McKendall, RR, Amsterdam, Elsevier, 1989, 611-626.

51. Rubsamen, PE, Gass, JDM: Vogt-Koyanagi-Harada syndrome: Clinical course, therapy, and long-term visual outcome. Arch Ophthalmol, 1991: 109:682-687.

52. Nussenblatt, RB, Palestine, AG, Chan, CC: Cyclosporin A therapy in the treatment of intraocular inflammatory disease resistant to systemic corticosteroids and cytotoxic agents. Am J Ophthalmol, 1983: 96:275-282.

53. Moorthy, RS, Buddi, R, Smith, RE, Rao, NA: Prevalence and management of cataracts in Vogt-Koyanagi-Harada syndrome. Am J Ophthalmol (in press), 1994a.

54. Forster, DJ, Rao, NA, Hill, RA, Nguyen, QH, Baerveldt, G: Incidence and management of glaucoma in Vogt-Koyanagi-Harada syndrome. Ophthalmology, 1993: 100:613-618.

55. Moorthy, RS, Chong, LP, Smith, RE, Rao, NA: Subretinal neovascular membranes in Vogt-Koyanagi-Harada syndrome. Am J Ophthalmol, 1993: 116:164-170.

56. Smith, RE, Nozik, RA: Uveitis: A clinical approach to diagnosis and management, 2nd ed. Baltimore: Williams & Wilkins, 1989d: 198-203.

57. Centers for Disease Control and Prevention: Lyme disease–Connecticut. M.M.W.R., 37:1-3, 1988.

58. Steere, AC, Bartenhagen, NH, Craft, JE, et al: The early clinical manifestations of Lyme disease. Ann Intern Med, 1983: 99:76-82.

59. Bruhn, FW: Lyme disease. Am J Dis Child, 1984: 138:467-470.

60. Aaberg, TM: The expanding ophthalmologic spectrum of Lyme disease. Am J Ophthalmol, 1989: 107:77-80.

61. Winterkorn, JMS: Lyme disease: Neurologic and ophthalmic manifestations. Surv Ophthalmol, 1990: 35:191-204.

62. Winward, KE, Smith, JL, Culbertson, WW, Paris-Hamelin, A: Ocular Lyme borreliosis. Am J Ophthalmol, 1989: 108:651-657.

63. Schwartz, BS, Goldstein, MD, Ribeiro, JM, Schulze, TL, Shahied, SI: Antibody testing in Lyme disease: A comparison of results in four laboratories. JAMA, 1989: 262:3431-3434.

64. Duffy, J, Mertz, LE, Wobig, GH, Katzmann, JA: Diagnosing Lyme disease: The contribution of serologic testing. Mayo wClin Proc, 1988: 63:1116-1121.

65. Steere, AC: Lyme disease. N Engl J Med, 1989: 321:586-596.

66. Dattwyler, RJ, Halperin, JJ, Volkman, DJ, Luft, BJ: Treatment of Lyme borreliosis–randomised comparison of ceftriaxone and penicillin. Lancet, 1988: 1:1191-1194.

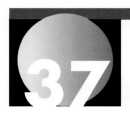

37 Masquerade Syndromes

Ramana S. Moorthy, Narsing A. Rao

Many noninflammatory entities can mimic either anterior or posterior uveitis. Many of these noninflammatory entities are neoplastic, although some are not (Table 37–1). It is important that a patient with uveitis be examined for the possibility of a masquerade syndrome that may be confounding the diagnosis.

■ INTRAOCULAR LYMPHOMA

Primary intraocular lymphoma, previously called reticulum cell sarcoma (1, 2), should be considered in any patient over the age of 50 with a vitritis of unexplained etiology, particularly if this vitritis is unresponsive to corticosteroids. Clinically, patients present with bilateral and often asymmetric vitritis (3). They may have some blurring of vision and complain of floaters. There is usually no pain or redness in the eyes. Up to 80% of patients with intraocular lymphoma have involvement of the central nervous system (4, 5), but the eye may be the only organ that is involved. Ocular presentation is typically that of a vitritis (6); the pathognomonic presentation is that of multiple, discrete, yellow-white subretinal and subpigment epithelial masses (Figure 37–1), although this presentation may not be that common.

Pathologic Assessment

Vitreous aspirates often reveal poorly differentiated large mononuclear cells with hyperchromatic nuclei (Figure 37–2) mixed with necrotic cells. In enucleated globes or in chorioretinal biopsy specimens, the poorly differentiated neoplastic cells are found in the subretinal and subpigment epithelial space; the choroid usually contains infiltrates of inflammatory cells.

Diagnosis

A diagnosis can be made in 95% of the cases, by showing malignant cells in vitreous aspirates (3). Computer-ized tomography (CT) or magnetic resonance imaging scans are particularly important to rule out CNS involvement. Cerebrospinal fluid cytology may be helpful in cases with associated CNS lymphoma. The differential diagnosis should include other causes of posterior uveitis; typically, intraocular lymphoma is a diagnosis of exclusion, but must always be considered in patients over the age of 50 with a vitritis.

Treatment

Lymphomas involving the eye and brain should be referred to a tertiary cancer center for appropriate management. The recommended treatment, the Sloan-Kettering protocol, utilizes external beam radiation to the eyes and CNS, with high dose intravenous, and intrathecal methotrexate via the Ommaya reservoir and high dose systemic Ara C. This particular Sloan-Kettering protocol has resulted in the highest rate of disease remission and prolonged survival (3,7).

Prognosis

The prognosis of intraocular lymphoma has changed drastically because of the new modalities of treatment. Average survival has increased from 26 months after diagnosis to as much as 10 years. The worst prognosis is in patients who have symptomatic CNS disease in association with intraocular lymphoma.

TABLE 37–1
Masquerade Syndromes–Clinical Findings and Diagnosis[1]

Anterior Segment	Age	Signs of Inflammation	Diagnostic Tests and Examinations
Retinoblastoma	<15	Flare, cells, pseudohypopyon	Aqueous tap, ultrasound, fundus exam
Leukemia	<15	Flare, cells, iris mass	Peripheral blood smear, bone marrow biopsy
Intraocular foreign body	Any	Flare, cells	Radiography, ultrasonography
Malignant Melanoma	Any	Flare, cells	Ultrasonography, fluorescein angiography
Juvenile xanthogranuloma	<15	Hyphema, flare, cells	Skin exam, iris biopsy
Rhegmatogenous retinal detachment	Any	Flare, cells, pigment in vitreous	Indirect ophthalmoscopy w/scleral depression
Posterior Segment			
Retinitis pigmentosa	Any	Vitreous cells	ERG, EOG, family history, visual fields
Primary B-cell intraocular Lymphoma	>60	Vitreous cells, RPE infiltrates Retinal hemorrhages and exudates	Vitreous biopsy
Malignant melanoma	>20	Vitreous cells and hemorrhage Exudative retinal detachment	Ultrasound, fluorescein angiography
Multiple sclerosis	>20	Periphlebitis and vitritis	Neurologic examination

[1] From Section 3, Ophthalmology Basic and Clinical Science Course, American Academy of Ophthalmology.

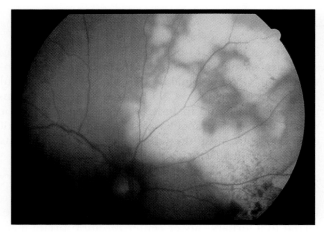

Figure 37–1.
Subretinal and subretinal pigment epithelial infiltrates of lymphoma cells.

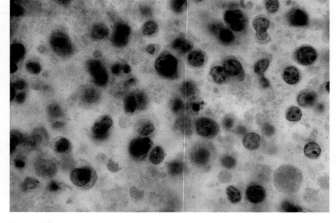

Figure 37–2.
Vitrectomy specimen showing lymphoma cells with hyperchromatic large nuclei and prominent nucleoli.

■ UVEAL MELANOMA

Malignant melanoma can cause signs of intraocular inflammation. Iris heterochromia, anterior segment flare and cell, and elevated intraocular pressure can result if there is invasion of the trabecular meshwork by the tumor. Vitreous cells and exudative retinal detachment and shifting retinal fluid may also be seen (8). Sponta- neous necrosis of the tumor may result in vitreous hemorrhage and intense inflammatory reaction with elevated intraocular pressure (melanomalytic glaucoma) (9). In these instances, ultrasonography is useful in making the diagnosis of uveal melanoma.

■ RETINOBLASTOMA

Retinoblastoma should be ruled out in any case of intraocular inflammation in a child under the age of 5. Occasionally, the retinoblastoma may present with neoplastic cells in the anterior chamber, which simulate hypopyon (pseudohypopyon) (10). An endophthalmitic or panophthalmitic picture may be seen with endophytic tumors. When tumors spread subretinally, they are called exophytic, and may be associated with serous retinal detachments. Ultrasound and CT scanning may show calcification within the eye, a sign suggestive of retinoblastoma. In children with retinoblastoma, levels of lactate dehydrogenase are often greater in aqueous than in serum. Although useful in the diagnosis of retinoblastoma, anterior chamber paracentesis carries the risk of spreading tumor cells outside the eye. The treatment of retinoblastoma is discussed elsewhere in the text.

■ LEUKEMIA

Acute and chronic leukemia can involve any structures in the eye. Conjunctival masses, heterochromia and thickening of the iris, and anterior segment inflammation, with collections of cells in the anterior chamber, occasionally combined with a hyphema, and elevated intraocular pressure may all be signs of leukemic infiltration (11, 12). Retinal involvement can include infiltration of the retina by leukemia cells, vascular tortuosity and dilation, retinal hemorrhages associated with vascular obstruction, and occasionally peripheral retinal neovascularization from ischemia (11). Even though leukemic infiltration in the choroid is common, rarely are these infiltrates detected on clinical examination. However, these infiltrates are known to cause serous retinal detachments. Fluorescein angiography may reveal a picture similar to VKH syndrome (11). Leukemia should be suspected in any person under the age of 15 with intraocular inflammation, and appropriate hematologic investigations should be carried out.

■ MISCELLANEOUS ENTITIES

Chronic peripheral retinal detachments can produce intraocular inflammation, in which case the vitreous cells are usually pigmented. Retained intraocular foreign bodies can also produce anterior and posterior segment inflammation; iron and copper produce particularly devastating inflammation. Juvenile xanthogranuloma, which occurs in children under the age of 1 year, can present with anterior segment cell and flare; however, those patients often present with spontaneous hyphemas. Biopsy of the skin lesions or iris may be needed to confirm the diagnosis. These lesions have characteristic Touton-type giant cells admixed with histiocytes and other inflammatory cells.

Retinitis pigmentosa (Figure 37–3) can be associated with vitreous cellular reaction. This diagnosis is made by history, clinical examination, and electrophysiologic testing.

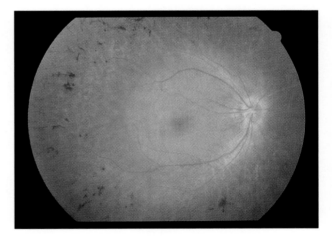

Figure 37–3.
A patient with retinitis pigmentosa who presented initially with cells in the vitreous cavity.

■ REFERENCES

1. Taylor, CR, Russell, R, Lukes, RJ, Davis, RL: An immunohistological study of immunoglobulin content of primary central nervous system lymphomas. Cancer, 1978: 41: 2197-2205.

2. Warnke, R, Miller, R, Grogan, T, et al: Immunologic phenotype in 30 patients with diffuse large-cell lymphoma. N Engl J Med, 1980: 303: 293-300.

3. Char, DH, Ljung, BM, Miller, T, Phillips, T: Primary in-

traocular lymphoma (ocular reticulum cell sarcoma) diagnosis and management. Ophthalmology, 1988: 95:625-630.

4. Minckler, DS, Font, RL, Zimmerman, LE: Uveitis and reticulum cell sarcoma of brain with bilateral neoplastic seeding of vitreous without retinal or uveal involvement. Am J Ophthalmol, 1975: 80: 433-439.

5. Barr, CC, Green, WR, Payne, JW, Knox, DL, Jensen, AD, Thompson, RL: Intraocular reticulum-cell sarcoma: Clinicopathologic study of four cases and review of the literature. Surv Ophthalmol, 1975: 19: 224-239.

6. Lang, GK, Surer, JL, Green, WR, Finkelstein, D, Michaels, RG, Maumenee, AE: Ocular reticulum cell sarcoma. Clinicopathologic correlation of a case with multifocal lesions. Retina, 1985: 5: 79-86.

7. Valluri, S, Moorthy, RS, Khan, A, Rao, NA: Combination treatment of intraocular lymphoma. Retina (in press).

8. Char, DH: Diagnosis of choroidal melanoma. In Retina. Vol. 1. Edited by S.J. Ryan. St. Louis, CV Mosby, 1989, 647-662.

9. Fraser, DJ Jr, Font, RL: Ocular inflammation and hemorrhage as initial manifestations of uveal malignant melanoma: Incidence and prognosis. Arch Ophthalmol, 1979: 97: 1311-1314.

10. Shields, JA, Augsburger, JJ: Current approaches to the diagnosis and management of retinoblastoma. Surv Ophthalmol 1981: 25: 347-372.

11. Kincaid, MC, Green, WR: Ocular and orbital involvement in leukemia. Surv Ophthalmol, 1983: 27: 211-232.

12. Ridgway, EW, Jaffe, N, Walton, DS: Leukemic ophthalmopathy in children. Cancer, 1976: 38: 1744-1749.

38 Ophthalmic Manifestations of AIDS

Ramana S. Moorthy, Narsing A. Rao

Acquired immune deficiency syndrome (AIDS) is a retroviral induced programmed cell death of the cell-mediated arm of the immune system that results in multiple opportunistic infections and neoplastic diseases, and that eventually leads to death. This syndrome has caused enormous human suffering in the last decade and has steadily increased in incidence (1). Ophthalmic manifestations of AIDS have been described in up to 70% of patients (2), and include external manifestations involving the cornea, conjunctiva, and eye lids, as well as infectious uveitic entities. Several of these entities are described below.

■ KAPOSI'S SARCOMA

Kaposi's sarcoma is the most common anterior segment lesion seen in AIDS; it occurs in 30% of all patients with AIDS (6). Involvement of the eyelids, conjunctiva, and, more rarely, the orbit occurs in 20% of patients with AIDS associated systemic Kaposi's sarcoma (7). Three stages of ocular adnexal Kaposi's sarcoma have been described (8). Stage I and Stage II tumors are patchy and flat, with less than 3 mm of elevation; these have been present for less than 4 months. Stage III tumors are nodular, elevated, greater than 3 mm in height, and have been present for greater than 4 months. The etiology of these tumors is thought to be an infectious process related to HIV (9).

Histopathologically, Stage I tumors consist of thin, dilated vascular channels, often filled with erythrocytes. There are usually no mitotic figures and no spindle cells or slit spaces are seen. A moderate mononuclear cell infiltrate may be present. Stage II lesions have plump fusiform cells lining thin, dilated empty vascular channels. No mitotic cells are seen. A sparse inflammatory infiltrate consisting of macrophages and lymphocytes may be present and there may be foci of immature spindle cells and early slit vessels. Stage III lesions are characterized by large, dense aggregates of spindle cells with hyperchromatic nuclei and variable number of mitotic figures. Between the spindle cells are slit spaces, which may contain erythrocytes, but few inflammatory cells (8).

Treatment

Treatment of ocular adnexal Kaposi's sarcoma may be necessary for cosmesis and to relieve functional difficulties, including foreign body sensation, recurrent erosions, tear film abnormalities, and obstruction of the visual axis (Fig. 38–1). Tumors confined to the bulbar conjunctiva that are Stage I or II can be excised surgically, leaving 1 to 2 mm tumor-free margins (10). Stage III lesions of the bulbar conjunctiva should be surgically excised after the delineation of feeder vessels by fluorescein angiography (10). Stage I and II Kaposi's sarcoma of the eyelid can be treated with cryotherapy (10). Stage III Kaposi's sarcomas call for external beam radiation therapy; however, when merely palliation is desired in cases of Stage III lesions involving the lid, cryotherapy can be employed to avoid radiation-related complications (10).

■ MICROSPORIDIAL KERATOCONJUNCTIVITIS

Microsporidia are obligate intracellular protozoan parasites that infect numerous hosts. Microsporidia have been implicated in human diarrhea, cholangitis, sinusitis, urinary tract infections, and respiratory tract infections in patients with AIDS (3). Recently, these organisms have been implicated also in keraconjunctivitis in these patients (3, 4). The causative agent is Encephalitozoon hellem.

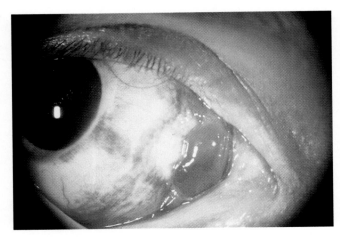

Figure 38–1.
Kaposi's sarcoma arising in the conjunctiva.

Clinical Features

Typically, patients present with intermittent redness of the eye associated with photophobia, foreign body sensation, decreased vision, and dryness. Clinical examination reveals punctate epithelial keratopathy (3, 4). The process is frequently bilateral. The microsporidia may be identified in conjunctival or corneal scrapings, swabs, or biopsies (3, 4).

Pathologic Assessment

Histopathologically, the microsporidia appear as gram positive spores in the superficial conjunctiva. There is associated acute inflammation consisting predominantly of polymorphonuclear leukocytes. Intraepithelial spores are often found. In addition, immunofluorescent staining of corneal and conjunctival biopsies for E. hellem is also useful for identification of these organisms (3, 4).

Treatment

The treatment of choice for microsporidial keratoconjunctivitis is topical fumagillin (5). This is obtained in a dry powder form with 23 mg of fumagillin per gm of dry powder. A suspension of the powder, 3 mg per cc in sterile saline, is usually made. This is filtered through 0.22 um cellulose acetate filter paper and transferred to sterile dropper bottles. The treatment should be given frequently, every hour initially for the first week (5). This usually results in a cure. The frequency of the administration may be reduced to every 2 hours after the first week, and then slowly tapered. Patients may need indefinite maintenance doses of topical fumagillin twice daily (5).

■ MOLLUSCUM CONTAGIOSUM

Molluscum contagiosum lesions are caused by the molluscum virus, which is a DNA virus of the pox virus family. Virus particles are often shed into the conjunctival cul de sac, which produces a follicular conjunctivitis that can persist until the lid margin lesion heals and no more particles are shed. These are umbilicated lesions of the skin are 2 to 3 mm in diameter (11). In healthy individuals, they are typically unilateral lesions; in patients with AIDS, however, they are usually multiple, bilateral, and recurrent (11). If symptoms of follicular conjunctivitis or other functional difficulties exist, surgical excision with cryotherapy at the base is useful.

■ HERPES ZOSTER OPHTHALMICUS

Any patient under the age of 45 who presents with herpes zoster ophthalmicus (Figure 38–2) should be investigated for possible HIV infection. Typically, a vesicular rash develops over the distribution of the ophthalmic division of the trigeminal nerve, in a dermatomal distribution. An associated conjunctivitis, keratitis (characterized by multiple dendrites), and anterior uveitis are common findings (2, 12). Sector iris atrophy often oc-

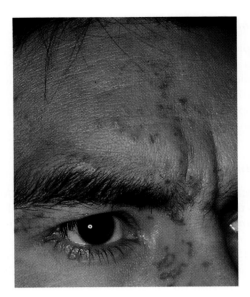

Figure 38–2.
Ophthalmic zoster in an HIV infected individual.

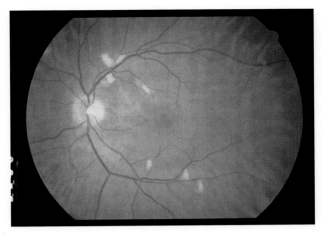

Figure 38–3.
HIV retinopathy is characterized by the presence of multiple cotton-wool spots.

curs. These patients should receive intravenous acyclovir to prevent dissemination of the zoster infection (2). Dissemination of zoster virus may result in progressive outer retinal necrosis. Systemic corticosteroids should be avoided. Topical acyclovir ointment (5%) can be used for the skin lesions, and topical trifluorothymidine for corneal lesions.

■ HIV RETINOPATHY

HIV retinopathy is the most common ocular complication of AIDS, and is found in up to 70% of such patients (13, 14). This retinopathy includes cotton wool spots (Figure 38–3), superficial and deep retinal hemorrhages, and microaneurysms (15). It is thought that virus-related vascular alterations occur in one or both of two ways: (1) immune complex-mediated occlusive vasculopathy; (2) endothelial cell abnormalities that result from HIV infection of these cells leading to irregularity and obstruction of the capillary lumen (16). The retinopathy is not sight threatening, and its prognostic significance is unclear. These microvascular changes may be evanescent and recur in other areas of the retina.

■ CYTOMEGALOVIRUS RETINITIS (CMV)

Retinitis caused by CMV is the most common ocular opportunistic infection in patients with AIDS; it occurs in up to 40% of patients with AIDS (13, 14, 17). In a recent retrospective study of 100 patients with AIDS, the median time between the diagnosis of AIDS and the development of CMV retinitis was 9 months (18). A CD4 lymphocyte count of less than 50 cells per mm (3) has been associated with an increased risk of development of CMV retinitis (19). Nearly all patients will have CD4 counts of less than 50, and often less than 20 cells per mm (3, 19). CMV is transmitted venereally, typically in patients who are homosexual or bisexual. Infected individuals may shed the virus chronically in urine or oral secretions. Unlike immunocompetent individuals, immunocompromised patients have severe morbidity and mortality associated with CMV infection.

Clinical Features

Well-established CMV retinitis is easy to recognize as a typical "pizza pie" appearance of retinal necrosis with intraretinal hemorrhages, typically along the temporal arcade vessels (Figure 38–4). There is usually an abrupt transition from normal to necrotic retina. Vitreous inflammation is minimal. Retinitis that occurs in the periphery may not have retinal hemorrhages, but may show marked granularity with necrosis of the retina. As the retinitis progresses, more retinal hemorrhages de-

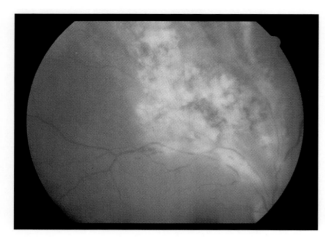

Figure 38–4.
Typical features of CMV retinitis.

velop, more retinal necrosis occurs, and the typical clinical picture then unfolds. After treatment, lesions usually become flatter, more granular, and often appear greyish. The preretinal and intraretinal hemorrhages disappear. Healing occurs from the center of the lesion outward, so the atrophic granular appearance spreads from the central areas of necrosis towards the periphery of the lesion. It is important to realize that reactivation of the retinitis (Figure 38–5) occurs at the borders of the lesions, and not in the central areas. Assessment of activity at the borders of existing lesions is thus most important for tracking progression of disease (11). Perivascular sheathing may often be seen adjacent to areas of active retinitis. Occasionally, multifocal retinitis is seen initially, with multiple patches of retinitis in the mid-periphery of one eye. In addition, patients may present with a picture of acute, frosted retinal periphlebitis in the midperiphery, which may then progress to classic retinal necrosis with intraretinal hemorrhages (20).

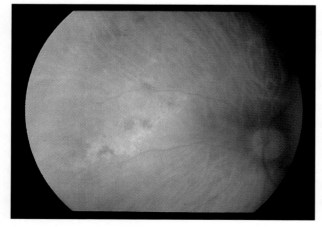

Figure 38–5.
Reactivated CMV infection in the retina.

Pathologic Assessment

Histopathologically, there is full-thickness retinal necrosis. Cytomegalic cells containing eosinophilic intranuclear and basophilic cytoplasmic inclusions are seen (6). Virus particles may be seen by electron microscopy. Localization of viral DNA may be carried out by in situ molecular hybridization.

Treatment

The treatment of CMV retinitis in patients with AIDS requires the use of specific antiviral agents, namely ganciclovir or foscarnet. Both are effective in the treatment of CMV retinitis, with response rates increased as much as 100% (21, 22, 23, 24). It has been shown by the Studies of the Ophthalmic Complications of AIDS (SOCA) treatment trials that the use of foscarnet, along with other retroviral agents, may be more beneficial to AIDS patients in prolonging survival than is ganciclovir (25). However, it was found that both are effective agents in treating CMV retinitis. The median survival time is variable, but has increased significantly over the past 5 years. It has been stated that patients who do not receive treatment die within 6 weeks. Those who are unresponsive to ganciclovir usually succumb in 1 month, compared with 3.1 months for those who respond partially, and 10 months in patients who respond completely to ganciclovir treatment (17). Furthermore, there are now anecdotal descriptions of patients who, having been treated for CMV retinitis for 2 to 3 years, are still alive (26).

Ganciclovir is given intravenously beginning at an induction dose of 5 mg/kg/dose, twice daily for 2 weeks, followed by a maintenance dose of 5 mg/kg/day. This can be given daily or switched to weekdays only at 6 mg/kg/day. A continuous indwelling central venous catheter is necessary for administration of ganciclovir. The use of colony stimulating factors, such as granulocyte colony stimulating factor (GCSF) or granulocyte-monocyte colony stimulating factors (GMCSF), has allowed the infectious disease specialist to increase dosages of ganciclovir and to avoid the associated myelosuppression, which is the main side effect of ganciclovir, thus providing more aggressive treatment of CMV in patients with AIDS. Myelosuppression may take the form of neutropenia or thrombocytopenia (17). This can be exacerbated by zidovudine (AZT), an antiretroviral used to treat HIV infection. Foscarnet calls for intravenous induction therapy, usually at 60 mg/kg/dose given 3 times daily. This induction dose is given for 2 weeks and then maintenance may be kept at between 90 and 120 mg/kg/day. Toxic side effects of foscarnet include nephrotoxicity and abnormalities in calcium, magnesium, and potassium metabolism, which occur in up to 30% of patients (27, 28, 29, 30). Seizures also occur in up to 10% of patients receiving foscarnet (31).

Despite a remarkable initial response to treatment, relapses occur in up to 50% of patients, typically 6 to 8 weeks after beginning induction therapy (17). Virtually all patients will have a relapse if there is no maintenance therapy after induction therapy. Many investigators have shown that, given a long enough period of time, all patients will relapse, despite maintenance therapy (11). If relapse occurs on maintenance therapy, reinduction of the same medication should be tried again for 2 weeks, followed by higher maintenance doses. The concomitant use of GCSF and GMCSF may be necessary. In addition, if relapse occurs a second time on maintenance therapy, the alternate medication should be used. Finally, if relapse occurs a third or fourth time on a single agent regimen, both agents should be used together. Induction can be with either ganciclovir or foscarnet, while maintenance doses of the other medication are continued. Subsequently, after induction, maintenance doses of both ganciclovir and foscarnet should be continued indefinitely.

Recent evidence suggests that CMV retinitis can be treated also with an intravitreal ganciclovir implant. This polymer device contains a reservoir of ganciclovir that slowly releases the drug into the vitreous cavity. This has been effective in the treatment of new, untreated CMV retinitis in controlled studies (32). However, it is unclear whether intravitreal ganciclovir therapy will be as effective as intravenous therapy in reducing mortality associated with CMV infection in AIDS (32). In a recent randomized, controlled clinical trial evaluating the safety and efficacy of a ganciclovir implant, Martin and colleagues (33) randomized 26 patients (30 eyes) with previously untreated peripheral CMV retinitis to immediate treatment with ganciclovir implant or deferred treatment. The median time to progression of retinitis was 15 days in the deferred treatment group compared with 226 days in the immediate treatment group (p < 0.00001) (33). They described postoperative complications of late retinal detachments or tears in 8 patients. Visceral CMV disease developed in 31% of patients. The estimated risk of development of CMV retinitis in the fellow eye was 50% at 6 months. In addition, the median survival time for these patients was 295 days (33). The authors concluded that the ganciclovir implant is effective in the treatment of CMV retinitis but that fellow eyes are likely to develop CMV retinitis and visceral CMV infections may develop in some patients (33). This clinical trial was the first to clearly establish the safety and efficacy of the ganciclovir implant in the treatment of CMV retinitis. This device provides another alternative route by which ganciclovir may be delivered. It may be particularly useful for patients who cannot tolerate systemic antiviral therapy, or those patients receiving concomitant zidovudine, which may increase myelosuppression.

Prognosis and Complications

A recent study of 22 patients with CMV retinitis revealed a mean survival of 16.7 months (26). Visual acuity was no light perception (NLP) in 49% of treated eyes after a mean of 15 months of patient survival. Retinal detachments, which occur in 29 to 33% of patients with CMV retinitis (26, 34), are managed with pars plana vitrectomy and long-term silicone oil tamponade.

■ PROGRESSIVE OUTER RETINAL NECROSIS (PORN)

PORN is a syndrome found in patients with AIDS that is somewhat similar to the acute retinal necrosis syndrome observed in immunocompetent patients (35, 36, 37, 38). It is characterized by acute necrotizing retinitis with variable vitreous and anterior segment inflammation. This syndrome is thought to be caused by a member of the herpes virus family; varicella zoster virus and herpes simplex virus type I have been identified in retinal biopsies using the polymerase chain reaction technique (35–38). Patients typically present with mutiple punctate areas of outer retinal necrosis that are scattered throughout the midperiphery. These areas of necrosis become confluent and involve mainly the outer retina, and spare the retinal blood vessels (Figure 38–6). However, unlike acute retinal necrosis, early in the course of the disease, clinically it appears that only the outer retina is involved. The disease is unilateral at onset, but can become bilateral over time. Another form of this ill-

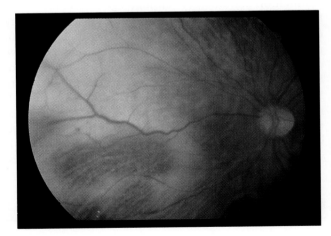

Figure 38–6.
Progressive outer retinal necrosis (PORN) in an HIV infected individual.

ness, involving primarily the macula with a central perifoveal lesion, has also been described (39). Its course is similar to the classic variety of progressive outer retinal necrosis. Retinal hemorrhages are uncommon and the retinal vasculature is characteristically spared. Virtually all patients develop retinal detachments (39), and severe optic atrophy may also ensue. Patients, as a rule, have poor final visual acuity; in a recent series of cases, despite aggressive antiviral therapy, many patients lost vision completely in one or both eyes (39).

Treatment of progressive outer retinal necrosis is often unsuccessful; it is often resistant to all available antivirals and is relentlessly progressive. PORN is usually unresponsive to acyclovir, minimally responsive to ganciclovir or foscarnet alone, and moderately responsive initially to a combination of ganciclovir and foscarnet (35, 36, 37, 38, 39). The combination of systemic ganciclovir and foscarnet, along with intravitreal ganciclovir supplementation, has been somewhat successful in slowing the progression of PORN. Retinal detachments are treated as in CMV retinitis, with pars plana vitrectomy and long-term silicone oil tamponade.

■ TOXOPLASMA RETINOCHOROIDITIS

Toxoplasmosis is the most common nonviral intracranial infection seen in AIDS. Ocular toxoplasmosis, however, is relatively uncommon. Like toxoplamosis in immunocompetent patients, the majority of ocular toxoplasma infections in AIDS appear to be reactivation of preexisting scars; however, a much greater percentage of patients with AIDS develop primary ocular toxoplasma infections. Some reports suggest that up to 25% of toxoplasma retinochoridifis is a primary acquired infection in patients with AIDS (40). At autopsy, approximately 40% of patients with AIDS have been found to have intracranial toxoplasma abcesses (41), so it is important to do a complete neurologic evaluation, including magnetic resonance imaging scanning and lumbar puncture to evaluate patients who present with ocular toxoplasmosis. Unlike immunocompetent individuals who have ocular toxoplasma retinochoroiditis, patients with AIDS tend to have larger areas of retinochoroiditis with a greater degree of retinal necrosis which may or may not be adjacent to an old toxoplasma chorioretinal scar. Ocular inflammation is variable and depends on the patient's total lymphocyte count. In addition, the inflammation may be severe enough to extend into the orbit, and thereby produce a panophthalmitis (42). Clinically, toxplasma retinochoroiditis (Figure 38–7) can mimic CMV retinitis, syphilitic retinitis, or progressive outer retinal necrosis. Laboratory evaluations may not be helpful since serum titers of antitoxoplasma antibodies, including IgG and IgM, may not be elevated. It is important to use undiluted serum in the determination of these titers. The presence of any titer in a patient with AIDS is suggestive of toxoplasma retinochoroiditis when the diagnosis is in question. In some instances,

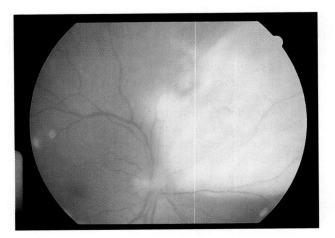

Figure 38–7.
Reactivated toxoplasma retinochoroiditis.

chorioretinal biopsy may be essential in making the diagnosis.

Treatment

Unlike patients who are immunocompetent, patients with AIDS and toxoplasma retinochoroiditis should be treated with a combination of pyrimethamine, sulfadiazine, and, if necessary, clindamycin in doses that are similar to those used in immunocompetent individuals. However, patients with AIDS will require long-term maintenance therapy to prevent reactivation of disease. In addition, steroids should be avoided in the treatment of patients with AIDS and toxoplasma infections (42).

■ SYPHILITIC CHORIORETINITIS

Ocular syphilis has become more prevalent with the increased prevalence of AIDS. Clinical presentations of ocular syphilis include uveitis, optic neuritis, and retinitis (43, 44, 45). Associated dermatologic and central nervous system manifestations are uncommon. In addition, an acute syphilitic, posterior placoid chorioretinitis has also been described in patients with AIDS (45). These patients usually present with vitritis and bilateral large, solitary placoid, pale yellow, subretinal lesions with evidence of central fading and a pattern of RPE mottling. Fluorescein angiography shows early hypofluorescence followed by late hyperfluorescence of the yellow lesions. Associated shallow exudative retinal detachments may also be seen. Like toxoplasma retinochoroiditis, syphilitic chorioretinitis in patients with AIDS tends to follow a more aggressive course than in patients who are immunocompetent (43), and a more severe retinal necrosis may occur. Because of this, treatment of these patients should be more aggressive. The treatment regimen recommended for primary and secondary syphilis in immunocompetent individuals is thought to be inadequate in patients with AIDS. Thus, all patients with AIDS and ocular syphilis should be treated with the neurosyphilis protocol, which consists of 12 to 24 million units of aqueous crystalline penicillin G intravenously for 10 days. This should be followed by 2.4 million units a week of intramuscular benzathine penicillin G for 3 weeks (11).

■ HISTOPLASMOSIS

Disseminated histoplasmosis is a life-threatening infection in patients with AIDS, and ocular lesions can accompany disseminated disease (46, 47). These lesions typically are creamy white intraretinal and subretinal infiltrates that vary between one sixth to one quarter disc diameter in size. There may be scattered intraretinal hemorrhages. The retinal infiltrates typically have distinct borders, and histopathologically are located superficially and deep in the retina. The infiltrates contain histoplasma organisms in all layers including choriocapillaris and inner choroid; the retinal lesions may be perivascular. Ocular histoplasmosis should be considered in the differential diagnosis of any retinochoroiditis in patients with AIDS. This is particularly important in regions in which histoplasmosis is endemic.

■ INFECTIOUS MULTIFOCAL CHOROIDITIS

Infectious multifocal choroiditis can be caused by Pneumocystis carinii, Cryptococcus neoformans, and Mycobacterium avium-intracellulare. P. carinii choroiditis is seen most often in patients who are receiving aerosolized pentamidine treatments. Aerosolized pentamidine is helpful in preventing a recurrence of P. carinii pneumonia, but the drug, deposited mainly in the lungs, does not reach therapeutic concentrations systemically, and thus does not prevent disseminated infection (48). Accordingly, patients being treated with this medication may have a higher incidence of choroiditis and disseminated pneumocystis infection. Fundus changes characteristic of Pneumocystis carinii include elevated plaque-like, yellow-white lesions in the choroid (Figure 38–8) without any vitritis or anterior segment inflammation (48, 49). These lesions typically are hyperfluorescent late in fluorescein angiography. Patients may be only minimally symptomatic. In patients with disseminated lesions of P. carinii, chest radiography, arterial blood gas, liver function tests, and CT scanning of the abdomen must be done in consultation with an infectious disease specialist. The patient must receive a 3-week course of intravenous trimethoprim and sulfamethoxazole. Systemic administration of pentamidine may be substituted in patients who are allergic to sulfa medications. Most lesions disappear by 12 weeks, leaving only mild retinal pigment epithelial granularity.

C. neoformans choroiditis may be seen before the development of meningoencephalitic and systemic symptoms in patients with AIDS. The clinical pattern of choroiditis is similar to that of pneumocystis infections (50). Patients who have C. neoformans meningitis de-

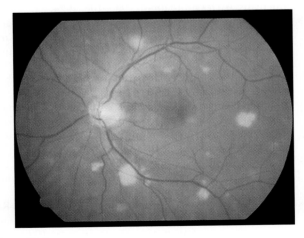

Figure 38–8.
Multiple choroidal lesions of disseminated Pneumocystis carinii infection.

velop obstructive hydrocephalus and can develop papilledema. This may eventually subside with treatment of the intracranial infection and the hydrocephalus, but will leave significant optic atrophy and visual loss. Optic nerve sheath decompression has been used for cryptococcal papilledema associated with progressive visual loss, but has met with limited success (51).

Mycobacterium-avium intracellulare and other atypical microbacteria can also produce a multifocal choroiditis similar to that of Pneumocystis carinii. Again, however, there is evidence of disseminated systemic infection and pulmonary infection that may predispose these patients to the development of infectious multifocal choroiditis (52). Patients should be treated with appropriate systemic antimycobacterial agents by an infectious disease specialist.

As noted previously, multifocal choroiditis in patients with AIDS has several etiologies, so it is important that the ophthalmologist obtain an exhaustive workup for disseminated infections in such patients. In these instances, ophthalmologists, working closely with infectious disease specialists, may play a life-saving role by early diagnosis and appropriate treatment of these infectious entities.

■ RIFABUTIN-INDUCED UVEITIS

Rifabutin has been associated with a hypopyon uveitis, iritis, and anterior vitritis in patients taking the drug for Mycobacterium Avium complex prophylaxis (53). The response appears not to be dose-dependent and has been described in patients taking less than 600 mg/day, although dose escalation trials have shown predictable increase in intensity of intraocular inflammation with doses greater than 1200 mg/day. Treatment consists of discontinuation of the drug and hourly topical steroids and mydriatics with gradual taper based on response to treatment over several weeks.

■ REFERENCES

1. Centers for Disease Control and Prevention.: HIV/AIDS surveillance report. Atlanta, CDCP, 1: December 1990.
2. Frangieh, GT, Dugel, PU, Rao, NA: Ocular manifestations of acquired immunodeficiency syndrome. Curr Opin Ophthalmol, 1992: 3:228-235.
3. Schwartz, DA Visvesvara, GS, Diesenhouse, MC, et al: Pathologic features and immunofluorescent antibody demonstration of ocular microsporidiosis (Encephalitozoon hellem) in seven patients with acquired immunodeficiency syndrome. Am J Ophthalmol, 1993: 115: 285-292.
4. Pepose, JS: Patient with AIDS presents with keratoconjunctivitis. Arch Ophthalmol, 1990: 108: 1224.
5. Diesenhouse, MC, Wilson, LA, Corrent, GF, Visvesvara, GS, Grossniklaus, HE, Bryan, RT: Treatment of microsporidial keratoconjunctivitis with topical fumagillin. Am J Ophthalmol, 1993: 115: 293-298.
6. Rao, NA, Biswas, J: Ocular pathology in AIDS. Ophthalmol Clin North Am, 1988: 1: 63-72.
7. Shuler, JD, Holland, GN, Miles, SA, Miller, BJ, Grossman, I: Kaposi sarcoma of the conjunctiva and eyelids associated with the acquired immunodeficiency syndrome. Arch Ophthalmol, 1989: 107: 858-862.
8. Dugel, PU, Gill, PS, Frangieh, GT, Rao, NA: Ocular adnexal Kaposi's sarcoma in acquired immunodeficiency syndrome. Am J Ophthalmol, 1990a: 110: 500-503.
9. Ensoli, B, Nakamura, S, Salahuddin, SZ, et al: AIDS-Kaposi's sarcoma-derived cells express cytokines with autocrine and paracrine growth effects. Science, 1989: 243: 223-226.
10. Dugel, PU, Gill, PS, Frangieh, GT, Rao, NA: Treatment of ocular adnexal Kaposi's sarcoma in the acquired immune deficiency syndrome. Ophthalmology, 1992: 99: 1127-1132.
11. Dugel, PU, Rao, NA: Ocular infections in the acquired immunodeficiency syndrome. Int Ophthalmol Clin, 1993: 33(1): 103-127.
12. Cobo, M, Foulks, GN, Liesegang, T, et al: Observations on the natural history of herpes zoster ophthalmicus. Curr Eye Res, 1987: 6: 195-199.
13. Holland, GN, Pepose, JS, Pettit, TH, Gottlieb, MS, Yee, RD, Foos, RY: Acquired immune deficiency syndrome: ocular manifestations. Ophthalmology, 1983: 90: 859-873.
14. Pepose, JS, Holland, GN, Nestor, MS, Cochran, AJ, Foos, RY: Acquired immune deficiency syndrome: Pathogenic mechanisms of ocular disease. Ophthalmology, 1985: 92: 472 484.
15. Friedman, AH: The retinal lesions of the acquired immune deficiency syndrome. Trans Am Ophthalmol Soc, 1984: 82: 447-491.
16. Pomerantz, RJ, Kuritzkes, DR, De La Monte, SM,: Infection of the retina by human immunodeficiency virus type I. N Engl J Med, 1987: 317: 1643-1647.
17. Jabs, DA, Enger, C, Bartlett, JG: Cytomegalovirus retinitis and acquired immunodeficiency syndrome. Arch Ophthalmol, 1989: 107: 75-80.
18. Holland, GN, Sison, RF, Jatulis, DE, et al: Survival of patients with the acquired immune deficiency syndrome after development of cytomegalovirus retinapathy. Ophthalmology, 1990: 97: 204-211.
19. Kupperman, BD, Petty, JG, Richman, DD, Mathews, WC, Fullerton, SC, Freeman, WR: Cross-sectional prevalence of CMV retinitis in AIDS patients: correlation with CD4

counts. ARVO abstract. Invest Ophthalmol Vis Sci, 1992: 33: 750.

20. Rabb, MF, Jampol, LM, Fish, RH, Campo, RV, Sobol, WM, Becker, NM: Retinal periphlebitis in patients with acquired immunodeficiency syndrome with cytomegalovirus retinitis mimics acute frosted retinal periphlebitis. Arch Ophthalmol, 1992: 110: 1257-1260.

21. Collaborative DHPG Treatment Study Group: Treatment of serious cytomegalovirus infections with 9-(1,3-dihydroxy-2-propoxymethyl)guanine in patients with AIDS and other immunodeficiencies. N Engl J Med, 1986: 314: 801-805.

22. Henderly, DE, Freeman, WR, Causey, DM, Rao, NA: Cytomegalovirus retinitis and response to therapy with ganciclovir. Ophthalmology, 1987: 94: 425-434.

23. Holland, GN, Sidikaro, Y, Kreiger, AE, et al: Treatment of cytomegalovirus retinopathy with ganciclovir. Ophthalmology, 1987: 94: 815-823.

24. Jabs, DA, Newman, C, De Bustros, S, Polk, BF: Treatment of cytomegalovirus retinitis with ganciclovir. Ophthalmology, 1987a: 94: 824-830.

25. Studies of Ocular Complications of AIDS Research Group in Collaboration with the AIDS Clinical Trials Group. Mortality in patients with the acquired immunodeficiency syndrome treated with either foscarnet or ganciclovir for cytomegalovirus retinitis. N Engl J Med, 1992: 326: 213-220.

26. Roarty, JD, Fisher, EJ, Nussbaum, JJ: Long-term visual morbidity of cytomegalovirus retinitis in patients with acquired immune deficiency syndrome. Ophthalmology, 1993: 100: 1685-1688.

27. Walmsley, SL, Chew, E, Read, SE, et al: Treatment of cytomegalovirus retinitis with trisodium phosphonoformate hexahydrate (foscarnet). J Infect Dis, 1988: 157: 569-572.

28. Lehoang, P, Girard, B, Robinet, M, et al: Foscarnet in the treatment of cytomegalovirus retinitis in acquired immune deficiency syndrome. Ophthalmology, 1989: 96: 865-874.

29. Jacobson, MA, O'Donnell, JJ, Mills, J: Foscarnet treatment of cytomegalovirus retinitis in patients with the acquired immunodeficiency syndrome. Antimicrob Agents Chemother, 1989: 33: 736-741.

30. Palestine, AG, Polis, MA, De Smet, MD, et al: A randomized, controlled trial of foscarnet in the treatment of cytomegalovirus retinitis in patients with AIDS. Ann Intern Med, 1991: 115:665-673.

31. Jabs, DA: Treatment of cytomegalovirus retinitis—1992. Arch Ophthalmol, 1992: 110:185-187.

32. Anand, R, Font, RL, Fish, RH, Nightingale, SD: Pathology of cytomegalovirus retinitis treated with sustained release intravitreal ganciclovir. Ophthalmology, 1993: 100:1032-1039.

33. Martin, DF, Parks, DJ, Mellow, SD, et al. Treatment of cytomegalovirus retinitis with an intraocular sustained-release ganciclovir implant. A randomized controlled clinical trial. Arch Ophthalmol, 1994: 112:1531-1539.

34. Freeman, WR, Henderly, DE, Wan, WL, et al: Prevalence, pathophysiology, and treatment of rhegmatogenous retinal detachment in treated cytomegalovirus retinitis. Am J Ophthalmol, 1987: 103:527-536.

35. Freeman, WR, Thomas, EL, Rao, NA, et al: Demonstration of herpes group virus in acute retinal necrosis syndrome. Am J Ophthalmol, 1986: 102:701-709.

36. Jabs, DA, Schachat, AP, Liss, R, Knox, DL, Michels, RG: Presumed varicella zoster retinitis in immunocompromised patients. Retina, 1987b 7:9-13.

37. Chess, J, Marcus, DM: Zoster-related bilateral acute retinal necrosis syndrome as presenting sign in AIDS. Ann Ophthalmol, 1988: 20:431-435.

38. Forster, DJ, Dugel, PU, Frangieh, GT, Liggett, PE, Rao, NA: Rapidly progressive outer retinal necrosis in the acquired immunodeficiency syndrome. Am J Ophthalmol, 1990: 110:341-348.

39. Margolis, TP, Lowder, CY, Holland, GN, et al: Varicella-zoster virus retinitis in patients with the acquired immunodeficiency syndrome. Am J Ophthalmol, 1991: 112:119-131.

40. Holland, GN, Engstrom, RE, Jr, Glasgow, BJ, et al: Ocular toxoplasmosis in patients with the acquired immunodeficiency syndrome. Am J Ophthalmol, 1988: 106:653-667.

41. Hénin, D, Duyckaerts, C, Chaunu, MP, et al: Étude neuropathologique de 31 cas de syndrome d'immuno-dépression acquise. Rev Neurol (Paris), 1987: 143:631-642.

42. Moorthy, RS, Smith, RE, Rao, NA: Progressive ocular toxoplasmosis in patients with acquired immunodeficiency syndrome. Am J Ophthalmol, 1993: 115:742-747.

43. Tamesis, RR, Foster, CS: Ocular syphilis. Ophthalmology, 1990: 97:1281-1287.

44. Passo, MS, Rosenbaum, JT: Ocular syphilis in patients with human immunodeficiency virus infection. Am J Ophthalmol, 1988: 106:1-6.

45. Gass, JDM, Braunstein, RA, Chenoweth, RG: Acute syphilitic posterior placoid chorioretinitis. Ophthalmology, 1990: 97:1288-1297.

46. Specht, SC, Mitchell, KT, Bauman, AE, Gupta, M: Ocular histoplasmosis with reitinitis in a patient with acquired immune deficiency syndrome. Ophthalmology, 1991: 98:1356-1359.

47. Macher, A, Rodrigues, MM, Kaplan, W, et al: Disseminated bilateral chorioretinitis due to Histoplasma capsulatum in a patient with the acquired immunodeficiency syndrome. Ophthalmology 1985: 92:1159-1164.

48. Dugel, PU, RAO, NA, Forster, DJ, Chong, LP, Frangieh, GT, Sattler, F: Pneumocystis carinii choroiditis after long-term aerosolized pentamidine therapy. Am J Ophthalmol, 1990b: 110:113-117.

49. Rao, NA, Zimmerman, PL, Boyer, D, et al: A clinical, histopathologic, and electron microscopic study of Pneumocystis carinii choroiditis. Am J Ophthalmol, 1989: 107:218-228.

50. Carney, MD, Combs, JL, Waschler, W: Cryptococcal choroiditis. Retina, 1990: 10:27-32.

51. Cohen, DB, Glasgow, BJ: Bilateral optic nerve cryptococcosis in sudden blindness in patients with acquired immune deficiency syndrome. Ophthalmology, 1993: 100:1689-1694.

52. Morinelli, EN, Dugel, PU, Riffenburgh, R, Rao, NA: Infectious multifocal choroiditis in patients with acquired immune deficiency syndrome. Ophthalmology, 1993: 100:1014-1021.

53. Jacobs, DS, Piliero, PJ, Kuperwaser, MG, et al: Acute uveitis associated with rifabutin use in patients with human immunodeficiency virus infection. Am J Ophthalmol, 1994:118:716-722.

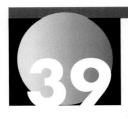

39 Episcleritis and Scleritis

Ramana S. Moorthy, Narsing A. Rao

The sclera is composed of collagen bundles of various sizes and shapes that are not uniformly oriented, unlike the cornea (1). The inner layer of the sclera becomes confluent with the suprachoroidal and the supraciliary lamellae of the uveal tract. Peripheral to the scleral stroma, the episclera, which consists of dense vascular connective tissue, merges with the scleral stroma; anteriorly, it blends with Tenon's capsule. The surface of Tenon's capsule is covered by conjunctiva. The vascular structures overlying the sclera include conjunctival vessels, the most superficial, and the deeper superficial episcleral vessels that are within Tenon's capsule. It is this superficial episcleral plexus that becomes maximally dilated in cases of episcleritis. The deepest vascular plexus lies directly on top of the sclera, and becomes maximally congested in eyes with scleritis. Topical phenylephrine drops may reduce injection of conjunctival and superficial episcleral vessels, but not of the deep scleral vessels.

■ EPISCLERITIS

Episcleritis is a benign, self-limited but often recurrent disorder that affects young adults. It is not usually associated with a systemic disorder (2), although it can occasionally occur in association with gout or after herpes zoster infection. Episcleritis never evolves into a true scleritis.

Clinical Features

There are two types of episcleritis, nodular episcleritis and simple episcleritis (1). Both are associated with symptoms of mild discomfort and redness, extreme tenderness to the touch, and some tearing. In simple episcleritis, the redness is usually sectoral or diffuse (Figure 39–1); in the nodular variety it is localized to the area that surrounds the nodular thickening of the episclera. After recurrent episodes of episcleral inflammation, the superficial lamellae of the sclera may rearrange themselves and become more translucent as the collagen fibers become more organized and more parallel, but this should not be mistaken for thinning of the sclera. Treatment of episcleritis is usually with topical nonsteroidal antiinflammatory agents and topical corticosteroids. The episcleritis usually responds over the course of several days to 2 weeks. Unresponsive cases should be treated with systemic indomethacin, 50 mg twice daily.

The differential diagnosis of episcleritis includes other entities that may be associated with episcleral and conjunctival vascular injection, namely keratoconjunctivitis sicca, mild rosacea related keratoconjunctivitis, inflamed pinguecula, and bulbar conjunctival abrasion. These entities may be differentiated by ophthalmic examination and ancillary testing.

■ SCLERITIS (see Retina, Chapter 59)

Scleritis can be classified into anterior and posterior varieties. Anterior scleritis can be further subclassified into nonnecrotizing, nodular, diffuse, and necrotizing varieties, with and without clinically apparent inflam-

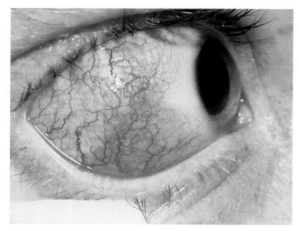

Figure 39–1
Marked injection of episcleral tissue in episcleritis.

mation (1, 3). It tends to affect patients between 20 and 60 years of age and predominantly affects females. Systemic associations are more common in cases of scleritis than in episcleritis. In a large series of over 800 patients with scleritis, an associated systemic disorder was found in all patients with necrotizing scleritis without clinically apparent inflammation (scleromalacia perforans), in 50% with nodular and necrotizing disease, in 33% with diffuse anterior disease, and in only 10% with posterior scleritis. (1) Severe polyarticular rheumatoid arthritis is the most common cause of scleromalacia perforans (1, 3, 4). Up to 40% of patients with necrotizing scleritis have other connective tissue disorders; at least 20% of patients with diffuse anterior nodular scleritis have rheumatoid arthritis or some other connective tissue disorder. Approximately 12% of patients with diffuse anterior and nodular scleritis have ankylosing spondylitis, although all of these percentages are variable, depending on the series (3, 4, 5, 6). Nearly 15% of patients with scleritis have a previous history of herpes zoster ophthalmicus. Other conditions that have been implicated in scleritis include syphilis, tuberculosis, gout, and Reiter's disease.

Clinical Manifestations

Patients present with an intensely painful eye with photophobia and tearing. There is often violaceous injection of the scleral vessels, but pain is the dominant feature (1), and is the reason why most patients seek the advice of an ophthalmologist. The only exception to this is necrotizing scleritis without clinically apparent inflammation, which may not cause pain. The pain in scleritis is often localized, but may bore into the jaw, sinuses, and temple, and may be severe enough to prevent sleep. The violaceous injection of the eye on clinical examination may have a bluish-red hue, in contrast to the more fire red appearance of episcleritis.

Initially, the nodular form of scleritis may resemble

nodular episcleritis, but scleral edema is often present and helps to distinguish these two entities. In the diffuse form of scleritis, there is more significant involvement of the entire sclera anteriorly. There is loss of the normal radial pattern of blood vessels in the conjunctiva and episclera as the entire episcleral and deep scleral tissues become inflamed.

Anterior necrotizing scleritis with inflammation is the most severe form, and presents with pain and redness (Figure 39–2). There may be a marked bluish-red hue to the injection. In addition, there may be significant thinning of the sclera and associated anterior uveitis is often present. Vision-threatening complications are particularly common in this entity, and include cataract, keratitis, keratolysis, and secondary glaucoma.

Scleromalacia perforans usually occurs in females with sero-positive polyarticular rheumatoid arthritis of a long-standing and severely debilitating nature. This ocular condition starts with a yellowish-white necrotic scleral patch (Figure 39–3) that eventually enlarges, allowing the underlying uvea to prolapse through the thin and atrophic sclera. Spontaneous perforation is rare, unless the intraocular presssure is increased.

Posterior scleritis represents 20% of all cases of scleritis (7), but is often misdiagnosed. It is associated with systemic disorders in less than 10% of cases. Clinically, these patients present choroidal effusions, serous retinal detachments, and choroidal detachments (7). Occasionally, there may be chorioretinal folds associated with the posterior scleritis and which may be mistakenly diagnosed as choroidal tumors. Macular edema and optic disc edema are also common findings. Proptosis and motility disturbances can occur with posterior extension of the inflammation.

Laboratory Evaluation

Laboratory evaluation of patients with scleritis should include a complete blood count with differential, ery-

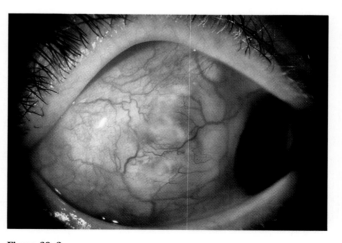

Figure 39–2.
Diffuse necrotizing anterior scleritis with marked inflammation.

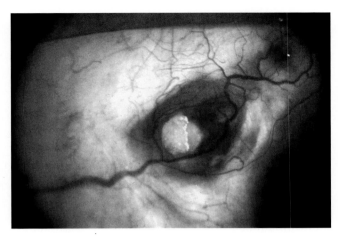

Figure 39–3.
Necrotizing scleritis with minimal inflammation that developed after cataract surgery in a patient with rheumatoid arthritis.

throcyte sedimentation rate, antinuclear antibody, rheumatoid factor, circulating immune complexes and LE cell preparation; serum uric acid levels may also be useful. Serologic test for syphilis should also be done. Extensive workup of patients with episcleritis is generally not necessary unless the inflammation is recurrent or bilateral.

Radiologic evaluation should include chest radiograph and sacroiliac joint films. Other joints can also be evaluated, especially if symptomatic, to rule out processes such as gout, rheumatoid arthritis, and sarcoidosis. B-scan ultrasonography is invaluable in the diagnosis of posterior scleritis since it shows a thickened sclero-choroid layer with a large gap between the scleral and the episcleral tissue, particularly at the junction of the optic nerve and globe where it is called the "T" sign. Associated choroidal and serous retinal detachments may also be noted (7).

Anterior segment fluorescein angiography may be useful in showing areas of scleral nonperfusion in necrotizing scleritis, but is not routinely used or needed to make the diagnosis of scleritis (1, 2, 3, 4, 5, 6, 7, 8). In posterior scleritis, however, fluorescein angiography may reveal multiple pinpoint areas of leakage that eventually expand and stain fluid in the subretinal space (7). Late disc staining is often seen. This picture is similar to that seen in Vogt-Koyanagi-Harada syndrome, sympathetic ophthalmia, and lupus choroidopathy (9).

Treatment

Scleritis is often accompanied by severe pain that may prevent sleep. Topical corticosteroids may provide some relief, but are not potent enough to reduce the scleral inflammation in most instances. Occasionally, they are useful as an adjunct to systemic therapy, when attacks are mild, or in-between attacks. Periocular injection of corticosteroids are contraindicated since these

can result in thinning of the sclera. Because of the relatively increased incidence of cataract and glaucoma, topical corticosteroids should be used sparingly.

Oral nonsteroidal antiinflammatory agents are useful in suppressing inflammation in most varieties of nodular or diffuse scleritis and posterior scleritis (1, 2, 3, 4, 5, 6, 7). Initially increased dosages are called for. The medication should be continued until the inflammation decreases and then stopped abruptly once the inflammation is gone. Pain, tenderness, episcleral and scleral injection, and intraocular involvement are excellent parameters for monitoring disease activity. There are several choices in nonsteroidal antiinflammatory agents, although some appear to work more effectively than others. The most commonly used agent is ibuprofen, which is given in doses of 400 to 800 mg 3 times daily. Oral diclofenac can also be used in 75 mg doses 2 or 3 times daily. Perhaps the most effective nonsteroidal antiinflammatory agent is indomethacin, 25 to 75 mg 2 or 3 times daily, depending upon the severity of inflammation. If response is to occur, it will be within 2 or 3 days after the initiation of treatment. The side effects of nonsteroidal antiinflammatory agents, particulary indomethacin, include irritation of the gastrointestinal tract, which can lead to gastric and duodenal ulcers, renal papillary tip necrosis with long-term use ultimately resulting in renal insufficiency, and defective platelet aggregation resulting in prolonged bleeding time. With the awareness of these complications, oral nonsteroidal medications can be safely used in the management of these patients.

Systemic corticosteroid therapy is useful in severe scleritis (anterior and posterior) or necrotizing scleritis. When there are areas of vascular closure in the scleral circulation that are detected on slit lamp examination or fluorescein angiography, systemic steroids are mandatory (8). Prednisone, 60 to 80 mg, is administered daily for the first several days. Response is often dramatic, occurring within 2 days of initiating treatment. Tapering of the corticosteroids should be slow and gradual after the first week. Prednisone may be decreased from the initial dose of 60 to 80 mg to approximately 40 mg daily. This dose should be maintained for 1 or 2 weeks, followed by a slow taper, approximately 2.5 to 5 mg per week, until a maintenance dose of 10 to 20 mg is attained. If treatment is not effective in controlling inflammation or if breakthrough inflammation occurs during a taper, it may be necessary to administer intravenous methylprednisolone, 100 to 250 mg every 6 hours. Again, tapering should be slow. If the scleritis is unresponsive to steroid therapy, immunosuppressive therapy should be considered.

Immunosuppresive therapy is considered essential in the control of inflammation associated with necrotizing scleritis. Systemic disorders associated with necrotizing scleritis are shown in Table 39–1. Because of the associated inflammatory changes in other parts of the

TABLE 39–1
Systemic Disorders Associated With Necrotizing Scleritis

1. Rheumatoid arthritis–especially scleromalacia perforans
2. Relapsing polychondritis
3. Wegener's granulomatosis
4. Polyarteritis nodosa
5. Systemic lupus erythematosus

body, it may be necessary to place these patients on a combination of corticosteroids and immunosuppressive agents. In most instances, we have opted to treat these patients with a combination of corticosteroids and cyclosporine. Cyclosporine has relatively fewer systemic side effects than do other immunosuppressive agents, and it is tolerated well by younger patients.

Cyclosporine is typically administered at a dosage of 5 mg/kg/day, along with prednisone in the dose range of 20 to 40 mg a day. As detailed previously, cyclosporine levels should be obtained every 2 weeks, along with systemic evaluation by an internist. Other agents that have been found useful in the treatment of necrotizing scleritis are oral azathioprine and cyclophosphamide. In our experience, cyclophosphamide is perhaps the immunosuppressive agent that is best suited for management of necrotizing scleritis, but it does, however, have major systemic side effects, the most important of which are bone marrow toxicosis, secondary neoplasias, and hemorrhagic cystitis. Cyclophosphamide is typically begun at 1 to 2 mg/kg/day and gradually increased until the scleral inflammation is controlled. Most immunosuppressives take 2 to 4 weeks to have an effect in the periocular area. Accordingly, it is necessary to maintain adequate levels of corticosteroids to suppress inflammation, while the immunosuppressive levels are increased. Because of the serious systemic side effects associated with all immunosuppressive medications, it is essential that an internist who is familiar with their use be involved in the care of these challenging patients.

Surgical therapy typically has no role in cases of scleritis. If there is active inflammation, medical therapy is the mainstay of treatment. Once the inflammation has resolved, scleral necrosis and thinning may be apparent with uveal prolapse. Particularly in cases of scleromalacia perforans or when necrotizing scleritis has quieted, it may be necessary to place scleral allografts over the areas of the scleral thinning to prevent perforation. Peripheral keratolysis or progressive corneal thinning may also need to be treated with lamellar keratoplasty (1).

Complications and Prognosis

Glaucoma occurs in up to 5% of patients with scleritis (1) and can be related to the use of corticosteroids. Occasionally, however, episcleral venous pressure will be increased, and will cause an elevation in the intraocular pressure (10). In addition, angle closure can also occur in these patients. Treatment of glaucoma secondary to scleritis is often complicated, and calls for the use of topical beta blockers, along with oral acetazolamide. If medical therapy fails to control intraocular pressure, trabeculectomy or tube shunt implant may be necessary (11).

Cataracts can develop secondary to the anterior segment inflammation or to corticosteroid use. Cataract extraction should be undertaken with great caution; only when the scleritis has been quiet for more than 3 months under adequate immunosuppressive and steroid therapy, without recurrences, should surgery be attempted. There is danger of cataract surgery reactivating the scleritis and causing necrosis at the wound (Figure 39), which can result in complications such as wound leak and endophthalmitis (12, 13). Preoperative systemic corticosteroid therapy with continuation of immunosuppressive therapy is necessary before cataract extraction. We also recommend that prednisone be given 40 to 60 mg daily, for 1 week before cataract surgery. Steroids may be gradually tapered once the surgery has been completed successfully. Retinal detachment can occur in patients with scleritis; exudative retinal detachments are especially common in patients with posterior scleritis.

The prognosis of scleritis is variable. Most patients who have nonnecrotizing scleritis that is nodular or diffuse retain reasonably good visual acuity. Necrotizing scleritis with inflammation, however, can be difficult to control, even with a combination of steroids and immunosuppressives. Up to 25% of such patients will have a decrease in visual acuity of two or more Snellen lines over a 3-year period (1). There is an increased mortality rate associated with necrotizing anterior scleritis and scleromalacia perforans. If untreated, nearly all cases of scleritis will progress to at least some scleral thinning and scleral defect. In necrotizing scleritis, the condition may be progressive and particularly painful. It can lead to destruction of the entire eye because of associated complications. Patients with posterior scleritis have reasonably good visual outcome since systemic nonsteroidal antiinflammatory agents and corticosteroids often quell the inflammation and associated exudative retinal detachments (7).

■ REFERENCES

1. Watson P: Diseases of the sclera and episclera. In Duane's Clinical Ophthalmology, Vol. 4, Chapter 23. Edited by Tasman W, Naeger EA. Lippincott-Raven: Philadelphia, 1992, 1–43.

2. Watson PG, Bovey E: Anterior segment fluorescein angiography in the diagnosis of scleral inflammation. Ophthalmology, 1985: 92:1–11.

3. Watson PG, Hayreh SS: Scleritis and episcleritis. Br J Ophthalmol, 1976: 60:163–191.

4. McGavin DDM, Williamson J, Forrester JV, et al: Episcleritis and scleritis. A study of their clinical manifestations and association with rheumatoid arthritis. Br J Ophthalmol, 1976: 60:192–226.

5. Lyne AJ, Pitkeathley DA: Episcleritis and scleritis: Association with connective tissue disease. Arch Ophthalmol, 1968: 80:171–176.

6. Sevel D: Necrogranulomatous scleritis: Clinical and histologic features. Am J Ophthalmol, 1967: 64:1125–1134.

7. Benson WE: Posterior scleritis. Surv Ophthalmol, 1988: 32:297–316.

8. Meyer PAR, Watson PG: Low dose fluorescein angiography of the conjunctiva and episclera. Br J Ophthalmol, 1987: 71:2–10.

9. Moorthy RS, Inomata H, Rao NA: The Vogt-Koyanagi-Harada syndrome. Surv Ophthalmol, 1994 (in press).

10. Wilhelmus KR, Grierson I, Watson PG: Histopathologic and clinical associations of scleritis and glaucoma. Am J Ophthalmol, 1981: 91:697–705.

11. Watson PG, Grierson I: The place of trabeculectomy in the treatment of glaucoma. Ophthalmology, 1981: 88:175–196.

12. Bloomfield SE, Becker CG, Christian CL, Nauheim JS: Bilateral necrotising scleritis with marginal corneal ulceration after cataract surgery in a patient with vasculitis. Br J Ophthalmol, 1980: 64:170–174.

13. Salamon SM, Mondino BJ, Zaidman GW: Peripheral corneal ulcers, conjunctival ulcers, and scleritis after cataract surgery. Am J Ophthalmol, 1982: 93:334–337.

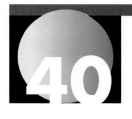

40 Endophthalmitis

Ramana S. Moorthy, Narsing A. Rao

Endophthalmitis refers to intraocular inflammation that involves the intraocular cavities. It is usually caused by an infectious agent. Less often, noninfectious stimuli such as retained lens material and, in some instances, toxic substances introduced into the eye during cataract surgery, may produce endophthalmitis; such intraocular inflammations are known as sterile endophthalmitis.

Infectious agents can gain access into the eye directly from periocular tissues and skin, or hematogenously from other infected tissues. Endophthalmitis can be divided into three varieties: postoperative, traumatic, and endogenous. Hematogenous spread of an infectious agent into the eye, termed endogenous endophthalmitis, is much less common than traumatic endophthalmitis or postoperative endopthalmitis. Bleb-associated endophthalmitis after filtering surgery is included under the category of postoperative endophthalmitis. Extension of infections from microbial keratitis, wound leaks, wound infections, and suture removal fit into a miscellaneous category, but most of these are considered to be postoperative. Damage to the ocular structures occurs not only from the toxins released by the microorganisms, but also from the inflammatory response produced by the host. Retina and anterior segment structures may be directly injured, or vitreous organizations can lead to retinal detachment. Organisms that produce exotoxins and endotoxins, and organisms that are virulent, have the worst prognosis. These include coagulase-positive *Staphylococcus aureus*, *Streptococcus species*, *Bacillus species* and various gram-negative organisms, including *Pseudomonas species*, *Serratia marcesens*, and *Proteus species*. The more indolent infections are typically the result of *Staphyloocccus epidermis* and *Propionibacterium acnes*.

The sources of bacteria in postoperative infections are the lids and conjunctiva, because many of these bacteria are commensals of these tissues. Lacrimal outflow system infections, especially those as a result of *Streptococcus pneumoniae* or contaminated glaucoma medications, can also contribute to postoperative endophthalmitis. Introduction of the etiologic agent occurs during surgery; however, manifestations may be delayed from 24 hours up to 2 years after surgery. Preoperative evaluation of the lacrimal system for silent dacrocystitis and of the lids for blepharitis, proper sterile technique, and sterilization of the conjunctival sac before surgery, are important in preventing endophthalmitis. In addition, prophylactic topical antibiotics may be given preoperatively to reduce bacterial colony counts. Using povidone solution, 5 to 10% for 5 to 10 minutes just before surgery, reduces bacterial colony counts on the lid margins and conjunctiva. Careful draping and isolation of the lids and lashes from the surgical field is essential. Traditional postoperative antibiotics given prophylactically in the subconjunctival space (e.g., gentamicin 20 mg) have no proven efficacy in preventing endophthalmitis. In addition, the use of intravenous antibiotics that have been advocated for penetrating ocular injuries, and topical antibiotics used in patients with filtering blebs, is controversial.

The overall incidence of postoperative endophthalmitis is 1 in 1000 (1). Bleb-associated endophthalmitis occurs in 1% of patients. Posttraumatic endophthalmitis occurs in 3 to 8% of patients (1). Endogenous endophthalmitis is much less common (2). Pain and decreased vision are the most important symptoms of endophthalmitis. On examination, decreased vision, hypopyon (Figure 40–1), and vitritis are the classic triad of findings. Diffuse conjunctival injec-

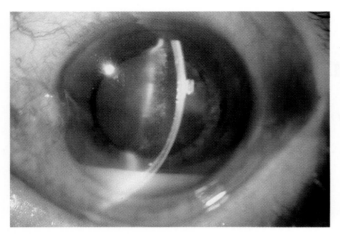

Figure 40–1.
Hypopyon in endogenous endophthalmitis.

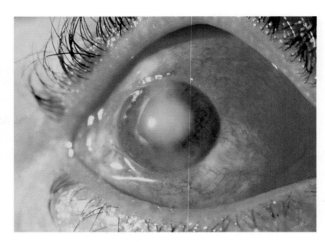

Figure 40–2.
Bleb-associated endophthalmitis.

TABLE 40–1
Exogenous Endophthalmitis—Etiology

Type	Causative Organism	Time of Onset After Surgery	Surgery (Intravitreal)	Antibiotics
Acute Postoperative				
Mild	S. epidermidis	1–14 days	AC/Vit tap No PPV	Amikacin Vancomycin
Severe	S. aureus, Streptococcus sp. Gram negatives	1–4 days	AC/Vit tap PPV	Amikacin Vancomycin
Chronic postoperative	P. acnes S. epidermidis Fungus	2 weeks–2 years	AC/Vit tap PPV(esp. fungus)	Vancomycin Amphotericin
Posttraumatic	S. epidermidis B. cereus and sp.	1–5 days (fungi–longer)	AC/Vit tap PPV	Amikacin Vancomycin
Associated Filtering bleb	S. pneumoniae H. influenzae	Anytime	AC/Vit tap PPV	Amikacin Vancomycin

From: Section 9. Basic and Clinical Science Course. American Academy of Ophthalmology. AC = anterior chamber; Vit = vitreous; PPV = pars plana vitrectomy.

tion, lid edema, corneal edema, and retinal vascular sheathing are often present. When a hypopyon develops without vitritis during the early postoperative period (1 to 4 days), the inflammation may be sterile and the patient may be closely observed without surgical intervention. However, suspicion of an infectious etiology must be increased when such a hypopyon develops.

TABLE 40–2
Dosage of Intravitreal Antibiotics

Antibiotic	Concentration	Dose (cc)
Vancomycin	1 mg/0.1 cc	0.1
Amikacin	400 mcg/0.1 cc	0.1
Gentamicin	100 mcg/0.1 cc	0.1
Ceftazidime	2.2 mg/0.1 cc	0.1
Amphotericin	5 mcg/0.1 cc	0.1

■ POSTOPERATIVE ENDOPHTHALMITIS

Acute postoperative endophthalmitis occurs 1 day to 2 weeks after intraocular surgery. The longer the dura-tion of surgery or the more complicated the surgery, the more likely endophthalmitis will occur. Clinically, delineation of those endophthalmitides that develop gradually, from those that develop acutely and have a fulminant course, is vital. Mild cases are less painful than severe cases, and these patients often have vision of 20/400 or better. The etiologies of postoperative endophthalmitis are shown in Table 40–1. *S. epidermidis* is the most common cause of endophthalmitis in this group (1). Patients with mild cases can be treated with anterior segment and vitreous paracentesis and cultures, and with intravitreal injection of antibiotics. Typically, vancomycin combined with amikacin, gentamicin, or ceftazidime are the preferred intravitreal antibiotics. The dosages for intravitreal antibiotics are given in Table 40–2.

Patients with mild cases of endophthalmitis have a good prognosis, with 80% of eyes attaining final visual acuity of 20/40 or better. Severe postoperative endophthalmitis that occurs 1 to 4 days after surgery, and with loss of vision to approximately 20/400, is typically the result of *S. aureus, S. species,* or gram-negative organisms (1, 3). These patients have a much poorer prognosis (1, 3). They require anterior segment paracentesis, a complete vitrectomy, and administration of intravitreal antibiotics. In addition, topical antibiotics and intravenous antibiotics should be given. Topical, periocular, and intraocular corticosteroids can also be used to curb the inflammatory host-mediated damage to ocular tissues. If an intraocular lens is present, it need not be removed unless visualization is hampered during vitrectomy. Only 20% of patients in this group attain vision of 20/40 or better (1,3).

Chronic postoperative endophthalmitis typically develops from 2 weeks to 2 years after surgery. Signs and symptoms are mild-to-minimal and of gradual onset. Patients may have minimal inflammation of the conjunctiva, vision may be only mildly affected, and pain may be minimal; they may complain of floaters. On examination, a small hypopyon and mild vitritis may be present, and keratic precipitates may be present on the cornea. *S. epidermidis* can present within 6 weeks of surgery with nongranulomatous inflammation. Fungal endophthalmitis typically begins 1 to 3 months after surgery and

is usually caused by Candida (1, 3). *P. acnes* usually develops 3 months or more after extracapsular cataract extraction surgery (4). This infection characteristically results in mutton fat keratic precipitates which imply granulomatous inflammation. Small hypopyon, mild vitritis, and plaques on the posterior capsule are also characteristic (4), and there may be residual lens material in the capsular bag. For chronic postoperative endophthalmitis with mild anterior segment inflammation, and unclear etiology, treatment initially is with frequent topical corticosteroids. If this does not improve the inflammation or results in waxing and waning of inflammation, diagnostic anterior chamber and, possibly, vitreous paracentesis should be done, and Gram and Giemsa stains, fungal, aerobic, and anaerobic cultures of aspirates should be obtained. *P. acnes* often requires up to 2 weeks of incubation for growth to take place (4). Identification of this organism needs adequate samples, necessitating a vitrectomy with biopsies of the posterior capsule(4). Fungal endophthalmitis calls for a pars plana vitrectomy, intravitreal amphotericin B, 5 $\mu\mu$g / 0.1cc, and topical and systemic antifungal medications.

Endophthalmitis associated with filtering blebs (Figure 40–2) usually occurs when organisms gain access to the eye through a leaking bleb; however, intact blebs that are thin can also predispose to these infections. The most common causes of these infections are *S. pneumoniae* and *Hemophilus influenzae.* The rate of infection developing after glaucoma surgery and filtering blebs is approximately 1%(1, 3). There may be a prodrome of bacterial conjunctivitis-like symptoms with conjunctival discharge before the onset of endophthalmitis, after which there is rapid progression of infection with pain and severe loss of vision. A pars plana vitrectomy and anterior chamber paracentesis with cultures of fluids, followed by intravitreal, subconjunctival, and intravenous antibiotics are essential to control the infection. Prognosis for visual acuity is poor because of the virulent organisms responsible for the endophthalmitis in these situations; only 25% of patients will achieve vision of better than 20/400 (1, 3).

■ TRAUMATIC ENDOPHTHALMITIS

Endophthalmitis occurs in 3 to 8% of patients with penetrating ocular injuries(1, 3). If an intraocular foreign body is present, the incidence is even higher. *Bacillus cereus* accounts for almost 25% of the cases of traumatic endophthalmitis (1, 3). This has a rapid and severe course once it takes hold in the eye, and visual loss often leads to blindness or enucleation. This infectious agent is most commonly found in soil, and thus, soil-contaminated penetrating ocular injuries, especially if associated with foreign bodies, are common causes of *Bacillus*

endophthalmitis. B. cereus is sensitive to both clindamycin and vancomycin. The appropriate management is anterior chamber paracentesis and vitrectomy with cultures. Intravitreal vancomycin 1 mg, clindamycin 200 $\mu\mu$g, and amikacin 400 $\mu\mu$g is suggested. Broad spectrum coverage can be obtained with vancomycin and amikacin, and clindamycin can be added or substituted for amikacin if Bacillus is suspected. Intravenous, topical, and subconjunctival antibiotics can also be given concurrently. In addition, prompt removal of the intraocular foreign body is vital. Fungal endophthalmitis should be suspected and treated if plant or organic intraocular or periocular debris is present. Intraocular foreign bodies not associated with infection do not require intravitreal administration of prophylactic antibiotics. But if infection is suspected, injection of intravitreal antibiotics can be essential in preserving vision.

■ ENDOGENOUS ENDOPHTHALMITIS

Endogenous endophthalmitis occurs from blood transmission of infections arising at sites far removed from the eye, such as infected intravenous lines, heart valves, kidney, and bone. Patients who are immunosuppressed, chronically ill, immediately postoperative, or postpartum are most predisposed to these infections (2). Occasionally, both eyes may simultaneously be affected (2). Patients present with pain and decreased vision; there is often a hypopyon and vitritis. The most common organisms are *S. species*, associated with endocarditis; *S. aureus*, associated with cutaneous infections; and *B. cereus*, associated with intravenous drug abuse (2). The most common gram-negative organisms are *Nisseria meningitidis* and *Hemophilus influenzae* (2). Enteric organisms, such as *E. coli* and *Klebsiella species*, can also cause endogenous endophthalmitis.

Fungal endogenous endophthalmitis is typically caused by Candida, followed by Aspergillus (2). Candida infections are usually seen in patients who are immunosuppressed and on continuous hyperalimentation with intravenous lines. Apergillus infections are seen in patients with a history of intravenous drug abuse. Up to 12% of patients with candidemia eventually develop endophthalmitis (2). Patients with fungal endogenous endophthalmitis typically present with focal and multifocal chorioretinitis, granulomatous, or nongranulomatous inflammation with keratic precipitates, hypopyon, and vitritis. Vitritis consists of cellular aggregates and large chunks of floating debris. In these patients, the etiology of the endophthalmitis is known because of a characteristic history of sepsis and positive bacterial or fungal blood cultures. If the agent is unknown, blood cultures for bacteria and fungus should be obtained. In addition, diagnostic anterior chamber paracentesis and vitreous paracentesis should be done if necessary.

Treatment of endogenous endophthalmitis requires intraocular, as well as systemic antibiotics. Gram-positive bacteria can be treated with intraocular vancomycin and intravenous nafcillin. Gram-negative infections can be treated with intraocular amikacin and intravenous gentamicin or ceftriaxone. Endogenous *Candida endophthalmitis*, without disseminated fungemia, can be treated with pars plana vitrectomy and intraocular amphotericin and oral ketoconazole. If disseminated fungal infection is present, intravenous amphotericin or oral fluconazole may be needed. Intravenous amphotericin therapy should be administered with the guidance of an internist since this agent is nephrotoxic, and the close monitoring of serum creatinine is important.

Treatment

A vitrectomy should be done in most cases of endophthalmitis, especially if severe inflammation is present. Intravitreal antibiotics, along with topical, subconjunctival, and intravenous antibiotics, are the cornerstones of therapy. In the presence of severe intraocular inflammation, intraocular, periocular, and topical corticosteroids are also useful in limiting host-mediated damage to ocular tissue.

Differential Diagnosis

The differential diagnosis of endophthalmitis includes other causes of severe anterior segment and posterior segment inflammation. Severe anterior uveitis may present with hypopyon, particularly in patients with positive HLA-B27. Retained lens material can cause sterile intraocular inflammation. Microbial keratitis can present with hypopyon without intraocular infection. Occasionally, intraocular tumors, especially retinoblastoma, may be associated with a pseudohypopyon and vitreous cells. The most important feature distinguishing infectious endophthalmitis from other causes of intraocular inflammation, is that the vitritis seen in endophthalmitis is progressive and out of proportion to the anterior segment findings of inflammation. When the diagnosis is in doubt, anterior chamber paracentesis and vitreous aspiration should be done and intraocular antibiotics should be given.

Prognosis

The prognosis of patients with endophthalmitis depends on the causative organisms. Typically, patients who have postoperative endophthalmitis have a good final visual acuity if inflammation is mild and caught early. If the preoperative visual acuity is only mildly reduced, final visual acuity may be good. Patients who have bleb-associated endophthalmitis have a poorer prognosis, since most of these infections are the result of *S. species* (1, 3). Traumatic endophthalmitis has a poor prognosis since the majority of the infections are because of *B. cereus* (1, 3). Endogeneous endophthalmitis has a variable prognosis because of the wide variety of causative organisms (2), but early diagnosis and appropriate treatment may be sightsaving as well as lifesaving.

■ REFERENCES

1. Flynn, HW, Jr, Pflugfelder, SC, Culbertson, WW, Davis, JL: Recognition, treatment, and prevention of endophthalmitis. Semin Ophthalmol, 1989: 4:69–83.
2. Greenwald, MJ, Wohl, LG, Sell, CH: Metastatic bacterial endophthalmitis: A contemporary reappraisal. Surv Ophthalmol, 1986: 31:81–101.
3. Mandelbaum, S, Forster, RK: Infectious endophthalmitis. In Focal Points: Clinical Modules for Ophthalmologists, Module 9 San Francisco, American Academy of Ophthalmology, 1983.
4. Zambrano, W. Flynn, HW, Jr, Pflugfelder, SC, et al: Management options for Propionibacterium acnes endophthalmitis. Ophthalmology, 1989: 96:1100–1105.

VIII Glaucoma

Section Editors: **G. A. Cioffi**
E. M. Van Buskirk

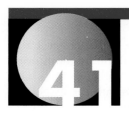

41 Introduction: What Is Glaucoma?

G. A. Cioffi, E. M. Van Buskirk

■ DEFINITION OF GLAUCOMA

In the United States between 1.5 and 2 million people have been diagnosed with glaucoma, and an estimated 1 million additional individuals have the disease but have not been diagnosed (20,29). The prevalence of glaucoma increases with age, and 0.5 to 2% of the population, over the age of 40 years, has glaucoma. Glaucoma accounts for approximately 10% of the blindness in this country. Between 5000 and 6000 people become legally blind from the disease each year (21). In 1977, almost 500 million dollars was spent on direct health care costs for glaucoma, with the loss in productivity in the work place being almost fourfold that amount (35).

In antiquity, "glaucoma" referred to the watery, green appearance of the blind glaucomatous eye. This description likely referred to the cloudy edematous cornea or the cataractous, crystalline lens associated with acute angle-closure glaucoma. In the years since the original description of glaucoma, many redefinitions and subclassifications have emerged. Most definitions of glaucoma have included elevated intraocular pressure as a fundamental component, and most classifications have primarily focused on the intraocular pressure, aqueous humor dynamics, and anomalies of each (1,11,31). However, elevation of intraocular pressure is not found in all forms of glaucoma. In fact, only one characteristic finding is common to all the classifications and definitions of glaucoma. The single common denominator unifying all the definitions and classifications of the entity known as glaucoma, is a characteristic optic neuropathy resulting in a specific pattern of visual field loss. All definitions share this abnormality of the optic nerve as the essential component to make the diagnosis. Therefore, the term glaucoma has actually come to refer to a group of diseases which are unified by this common denominator: glaucomatous optic neuropathy. A historical perspective helps to elucidate the development of our present day conceptions of the disease and our knowledge of its etiology.

■ HISTORY OF GLAUCOMA

In 1818, Demours, and subsequently McKenzie, associated increased intraocular pressure and the disease known as glaucoma (6,17). Von Graefe described the optic neuropathy associated with glaucoma in 1857, with further descriptions within the same year by Jaeger and Schnabel (34). Recognition of the optic neuropathy had to await the development of the ophthalmoscope by von Helmholtz in the 1850s (36). Jaeger defined glaucoma as an intrinsic optic neuropathy, while Von Graefe principally believed that glaucoma was a neuropathy induced by increased intraocular pressure. However, even Von Graefe's original description of glaucoma included three forms: acute inflammatory glaucoma, chronic glaucoma associated with increased intraocular pressure, and amaurosis with excavation of the optic nerve head, associated with normal intraocular pressure. Acute inflammatory glaucoma likely referred to acute angle-closure glaucoma with elevated intraocular pressure. Chronic glaucoma associated with increased intraocular pressure, most likely incorporated the various forms of chronic glaucoma in which intraocular pressure remains elevated. However, the category of amaurosis with excavation, as originally described by Von Graefe, was glaucoma without elevated intraocular pressure. Von Graefe later recanted this assertion, claiming that all forms of glaucoma are associated with elevated intraocular pressure.

With the development of accurate tonometry, between the 1880s and the early 1900s, more exact measurements of intraocular pressure could be obtained (18,30). Before the twentieth century, physicians primarily relied on digital palpation to determine the ocular tension. As better methods for the assessment of the aqueous humor dynamics and intraocular pressure became available, the association between intraocular pressure and glaucoma received increasing emphasis. The measurement of intraocular pressure became the most easily obtainable clinical sign of glaucoma. Large epidemiologic studies were easily done by monitoring this accurately measured variable. With repeated measurements, the majority of patients with the associated optic neuropathy were found to have increased intraocular pressure (2,22). Because of this, most classifications of glaucoma became focused primarily on the etiology of the increased intraocular pressure and various aspects of the aqueous humor dynamics.

However, recent studies have reexamined this concept of glaucoma as a disorder of aqueous humor dynamics and increased intraocular pressure. Many patients, afflicted with glaucomatous optic nerve damage and vision loss, never exhibit increased intraocular pressures above the statistically normal range (8). With the further understanding that intraocular pressure is but one, albeit important, risk factor for the development of glaucomatous optic neuropathy, new definitions and classifications have begun to emerge. These classifications focus not only on intraocular pressure but also on specific etiologic mechanisms of glaucomatous optic nerve damage.

■ GLAUCOMATOUS OPTIC NEUROPATHY

Characteristic ophthalmoscopic findings of the optic nerve in glaucoma include focal atrophy of the neuroretinal rim, especially in the inferior and superior temporal regions (see Clinical Testing: Optic Nerve Head Evaluation). Concurrent deepening of the physiologic cup occurs with progression of glaucomatous optic neuropathy. Loss of the peripapillary nerve fiber bundles, as well as peripapillary atrophy, are also typical findings of glaucomatous optic neuropathy. Associated defects in visual function occur with the progression of glaucomatous optic neuropathy. Early visual field loss is characterized by increased variability and a generalized reduction in sensitivity of the visual field. Focal deficits, resulting from the loss of nerve fiber bundles, result in the most typical glaucoma visual field defects. (See Clinical Testing: Perimetry) These include arcuate scotomas, peripheral nasal defects, and paracentral scotomata.

■ INTRAOCULAR PRESSURE AND GLAUCOMA

Intraocular pressure can be accurately measured in most individuals. Epidemiologic studies have shown that the mean intraocular pressure level of normal adults is between 15mm Hg and 18mm Hg (15,16). Approximately 95% of normal individuals will have intraocular pressures between 10 and 22mm Hg. The ease of intraocular pressure monitoring has made it a convenient clinical tool to screen for glaucoma.

Of all the clinical risk factors assessed in a person suspected of having glaucoma, increased intraocular pressure is the most likely to predict the eventual development of glaucomatous optic neuropathy. Nearly all individuals will develop glaucomatous optic neuropathy if the intraocular pressure remains sufficiently elevated for an extended period of time. Studies have shown asymmetric, and more extensive visual field loss and glaucomatous optic nerve damage in eyes with the higher intraocular pressures, when compared with the contralateral eyes of individuals (5). Laboratory animal studies have also shown that increased intraocular pressure causes glaucomalike optic neuropathy. Increased intraocular pressure in nonhuman primates creates an optic neuropathy which is both clinically and histopathologically similar to the glaucomatous optic nerve damage seen in humans (26). Increased intraocular pressure also impairs axoplasmic flow of the optic nerve in primate and nonprimate models (27). This may contribute to neuronal death. Finally, the extracellular matrix of the optic nerve, both in cell culture and in vivo in laboratory animal models, has been altered by changes in the tissue pressure, which may underlie the structural changes seen in glaucomatous optic neuropathy (19, 28). The view that glaucomatous optic neuropathy is a pressure-induced neuropathy is supported by these clinical and laboratory findings.

■ OCULAR HYPERTENSION AND "LOW TENSION" GLAUCOMA

As outlined previously, elevated intraocular pressure, or ocular hypertension, is a risk factor for the development of glaucoma. Yet many individuals manifest this risk factor and never develop glaucoma. The prevalence of ocular hypertension (intraocular pressure above the statistical norms) in the general population varies greatly in different geographic locations, but approximately 3 to 8% of the United States population exhibits intraocular pressures consistently above 22mm Hg, without concurrent optic nerve damage (13, 24). Studies have shown that each year, between 0.5 and 1% of individuals with ocular hypertension will develop glaucomatous optic nerve damage and visual function deficits (10, 37). Other studies have examined the possible benefits of prophylactic lowering of the intraocular pressure in ocular hypertensives to prevent or delay the development of glaucoma. These studies remain almost evenly divided on the benefit or lack of benefit of prophylactic therapy. A national, multi-center, collaborative study is presently underway to examine the efficacy of such therapy (25). This study will enhance our understanding of the relationship between intraocular pressure and glaucoma.

As already described, increased intraocular pressure is a major risk factor for the development of glaucomatous optic nerve damage. However, many patients never exhibit statistically elevated intraocular pressure but develop progressive glaucomatous optic nerve damage. Approximately one-sixth of patients with glaucoma consistently have intraocular pressures below 22mm Hg (1,12). In addition, many patients with a history of increased intraocular pressure continue to progress despite maximal reduction of the intraocular pressure, even after filtration operations. Even in patients with diagnosed glaucoma, studies have shown that at least 50% have normal intraocular pressures on a single screening measurement (33). Therefore, intraocular pressure alone is a poor indicator of the presence of disease.

The development of glaucomatous optic neuropathy in patients with statistically normal intraocular pressure results in a paradox if glaucoma is defined by elevation of intraocular pressure. Glaucomatous optic neuropathy occurring in an eye without intraocular pressure elevations is referred to as "low tension glaucoma." Many believe that the optic nerves of such individuals are more susceptible to pressure damage, even within the normal range. Therefore, the original definition of glaucoma is modified to accommodate the disease low tension glaucoma.

This simplistic revision of the definition of glaucoma is faulty for two reasons. First, the artificial dichotomy between low or normal intraocular pressure and elevated intraocular pressure is based on incorrect statistical assumptions. Intraocular pressures between 21 and 24mm Hg are commonly used as an upper limit of normal. This is based on the assumption that intraocular pressures are distributed in a Gaussian distribution, with a mean of approximately 16mm Hg (15,16). Two standard deviations above the mean is approximately 22mm Hg and, therefore, considered to be the upper limit of "normal." However, intraocular pressures are not distributed in a Gaussian fashion. Instead, they are skewed to the right (4). Therefore, defining a particular pressure level as normal or abnormal cannot be based on these statistical assumptions. Second, basing the definition of a disease on a single risk factor will always result in a flawed or inappropriate definition. As described in the next section, there are a variety of risk factors for the development of glaucoma of which intraocular pressure is only one. If instead, the definition of glaucoma is based on characteristic optic nerve changes with concomitant visual field loss (removing intraocular pressure from the definition), low tension glaucoma becomes part of the overall spectrum of glaucoma, in which intraocular pressure likely plays a smaller role and other risk factors are more important. This new definition has the added benefit of encouraging investigation into other risk factors and establishment of new therapies to prevent vision loss in patients with glaucoma but low intraocular pressures.

■ RISK FACTORS IN THE DEVELOPMENT OF GLAUCOMA

Many risk factors are associated with the development of glaucomatous optic neuropathy, including some common systemic disorders (Table 41–1). These include diabetes mellitus, systemic hypertension, peripheral vascular disease and migrainous syndromes (3, 9, 14). Studies examining familial patterns in the development of glaucoma, as well as the association of many congenital disorders with glaucoma, indicate hereditary factors are involved in some glaucoma patients (32). Others have reported vasospastic disorders, such as Raynaud's-like phenomenon and migraine headaches, to be more frequent in individuals with glaucoma, especially in the subset with low intraocular pressures (7, 23). Factors other than intraocular pressure are believed to be involved in the development of glaucoma, especially in patients who never exhibit pressure elevations, and likely, to varying degrees, in all glaucoma patients.

TABLE 41–1

Risk Factors for the Development of Glaucomatous Optic Neuropathy

Elevated Intraocular Pressure
Cup-to-Disc Ratio Assymetry
Myopia
African Ancestry
Positive Family History of Glaucoma
Increased Age
History of Migraine Headaches
Contralateral Retinal Vein Occlusion
Systemic Hypertension
Diabetes Mellitus
Peripheral Vascular Disease

■ REFERENCES

1. American Academy of Ophthalmology. Preferred Practice Patterns. Primary open-angle glaucoma. San Francisco, American Academy of Ophthalmology, 1989: 1–27.

2. Armaly, MF: On the distribution of applanation pressure. I. Statistical features and the effect of age, sex, and family history of glaucoma. Arch Ophthal 1965, 73:11.

3. Becker, B: Diabetes mellitus and primary open-angle glaucoma. Am J Ophthal 1971, 71:1.

4. Colton, T, Ederer, F: The distribution of intraocular pressures in the general population. Surv Ophthal 1980, 25:123.

5. Crichton, A., Drance, SM, Douglas, GR and Schulzer, M: Unequal intraocular pressure and its relation to asymmetric visual field defects in low-tension glaucoma. Ophthalmology 1989, 96:1312.

6. Demours. Traite des maladies des yeux, Paris, 1818, 1:470.

7. Drance, SM, Douglas GR, Wijsman, K, et al: Response of blood flow to warm and cold in normal and low-tension glaucoma patients. Am J Ophthal 1988, 105:35.

8. Flammer, J, Gasser, P, Prunte, C, and Yao, K: The probable involvement of factors other than intraocular pressure in the pathogenesis of glaucoma. In Drance, SM (ed.): Applied Pharmacology of the Glaucomas, Baltimore, Williams & Wilkins, 1993.

9. Goldberg, I, Hollows, FC, Kass, MA, Becker, B: Systemic factors in patients with low-tension glaucoma. Br J Ophthal 1981, 65:56.

10. Hart, WM Jr, Yablonski, M, Kass, MA, Becker, B: Multivariate analysis of the risk of glaucomatous visual field loss. Arc Ophthal 1979, 97:1455.

11. Hoskins, HD, Jr., Kass, M: Becker-Shaffer's Diagnosis and Therapy of the Glaucomas, ed. 6, St. Louis, CV Mosby, 1989: 2.

12. Kahn, HA, and Milton, RC: Alternative definitions of open-angle glaucoma. Effect on prevalence and associations in the Framingham Eye Study. Arch Ophthalmol 1980, 98:2172.

13. Kolker, AE, Becker, B: Ocular hypertension vs. open-angle glaucoma: a different view. Arch Ophthal 1977, 95:586.

14. Leighton, DA, Phillips, CI: Systemic blood pressure in open-angle glaucoma. low tension glaucoma, and the normal eye. Br J Ophthal 1972, 56:447.

15. Leydhecker, W, Akiyama, K, Neumann, HG: Der intraokulare Druck gesunder menschlicher Augen. Klin Monatsbl Augenheilkd 1958, 133:662.

16. Loewen, U, Handrup, B, Redeker, A: Results of a glaucoma mass screening program. Klin Monatsbl Augenheilkd 1976, 169:754.

17. Mackenzie, W: Glaucoma. A Practical Treatise of the Disease of the Eye. London, Longman, Rees, Orme, Brown & Green, 1830: 580.

18. Maklakoff, A: L'ophtalmotonometrie. Arch Ophthalmol. Paris 1885, 5:159.

19. Morrison, JC, Cork, LC, Dunkelberger, GR, Brown, A, and Quigley, HA: Aging changes of the rhesus monkey optic nerve. Invest Ophthalmol Vis Sci 1990, 31:1623.

20. National Center for Health Statistics: Prevalence of selected impairments, United States, July 1963-June 1965, Rockville, MD., 1968. Vital and health statistics, Series 10: data from National Health Survey No. 48 (DHEW Pub. No PHS 1000)

21. National Center for Health Statistics: Office visits to ophthalmologists: national ambulatory medical survey, DHEW Pub No. PHS 79–1250, Rockville, MD, 1976.

22. Perkins, ES: Glaucoma screening from a public health clinic. Br J Ophthal 1965, 1:417.

23. Phelps, CD, Corbett, JJ: Migraine and low-tension glaucoma: a case-control study. Invest Ophthal Vis Sci 1985, 26:1105.

24. Phelps, CD: Ocular hypertension: to treat or not to treat? Arch Ophthal 1977, 95:588.

25. Ocular Hypertension Treatment Study (EY-93–01), National Institutes of Health, Bethesda MD.

26. Quigley, HA, Addicks, EM: Chronic experimental glaucoma in primates. II. Effect of extended intraocular pressure elevation on optic nerve head and axonal transport. Invest Ophthal Vis Sci 1980, 19:137.

27. Quigley, HA, Anderson, DR: The dynamics and location of axonal transport blockade by acute intraocular pressure elevation in primate optic nerve. Invest Ophthalmol 1976, 15:606.

28. Quigley, HA, Dorman-Pease, ME, Dunkelberger, GR, and Brown, A: Changes in collagen and elastin in the optic nerve head in chronic human and experimental monkey glaucoma. ARVO abstracts. Supplement to Invest Ophth Vis Sci, Philadelphia, Lippincott-Raven 1990, 554.

29. Roden, DR: The prevalence and cost of glaucoma detection and treatment. Proceedings of the first national glaucoma conference, National Society to Prevent Blindness, Tarpon Springs, FL, 1980.

30. Schiotz, HJ: Ein neues tonometer. Arch Augenheilkd 1905, 52:401.

31. Shields, MB(ed.): Textbook of Glaucoma, ed. 2, Baltimore, Williams & Wilkins, 1987:1.

32. Shin, DH, Becker, B, Kolker, AE: Family history in primary open-angle glaucoma. Arch Ophthal 1977, 95:598.

33. Sommer, A., Tielsch JM, Katz, J, Quigley, HA, Gottsch, JD, Favitt, J, Singh, K and Baltimore Eye Survey Research Group: Relationship between intraocular pressure and primary open angle glaucoma among white and black Americans. Arch Ophthalmol 1991, 109:1090.

34. Van Buskirk, EM, Cioffi, GA: Glaucomatous optic neuropathy. Am J Ophthalmol 113:4, 447–452.

35. Vision Research, A national plan, Report of the advising eye council, 1:12–13.

36. Von Helmholz, H: Beschreibung eines Augen-Spiegels zur Untersuchung der Netzhaut im lebenden Auge. Berlin, A. Forstner, 1851 (description of an ophthalmoscope for examining the retina of the living eye. Hollenhorst, RW, trans) Arch Ophthalmol 1951, 46:565.

37. Wilensky, JT, Podos, SM, Becker, B: Prognostic indicators in ocular hypertension. Arch Ophthal 1974, 91:200.

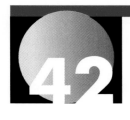

Pathogenesis of Glaucoma

G. A. Cioffi, E. M. Van Buskirk

◼ GLAUCOMATOUS OPTIC NEUROPATHY

This section summarizes the major ideas concerning the development of glaucomatous optic neuropathy. Complete descriptions of the clinical findings associated with glaucomatous optic neuropathy and the general anatomy of the optic nerve are found later in the text (see Clinical Testing: Optic Nerve Head Evaluation and Anatomy: Optic Nerve).

Factors intrinsic or extrinsic to the optic nerve, alone or in combination, may affect the health of the optic nerve. Extrinsic factors that may contribute to the development of glaucomatous optic neuropathy include the intraocular pressure and the systemic cardiovascular status. Intrinsic factors would include the composition of the support tissues of the optic nerve and the vascular anatomy and physiology within the nerve. Individual optic nerves may possess anomalies of these intrinsic characteristics which result in or heighten the susceptibility to glaucomatous optic neuropathy. Other individuals may possess optic nerves that develop glaucomatous damage primarily from extrinsic insult. Thus, a spectrum of factors should be considered in each individual case of glaucoma.

Intraocular pressure plays a major role in the development of glaucomatous optic neuropathy for most subjects. One hypothesis of the etiology of glaucoma proposes that neuronal damage results from mechanical pressure on the optic nerve. This idea focuses primarily on increased intraocular pressure and its deleterious effects on the extracellular matrix and glial support tissues of the optic nerve. The hypothesis suggests there is direct, mechanical insult which results from intraocular pressure increased above a tolerable threshold. The intraocular pressure causes backward

bowing, stretching, and compression of the support tissues within the optic nerve (19). The primary site of this mechanical distortion and secondary neural damage is the lamina cribrosa (Figure 42–1). Misalignment of the laminar cribrosa's fenestrae and compression of the laminar connective tissue plates results in the inhibition of axoplasmic flow within the axons of the ganglion cells. Interruption of axoplasmic flow or direct mechanical compression causes death of the nerve cells resulting in glaucomatous optic neuropathy.

This extrinsic, pressure-induced hypothesis of glaucomatous optic neuropathy is supported by laboratory models of glaucoma and by clinical and histologic examinations of human glaucomatous eyes. Increased intraocular pressure in nonhuman primate models causes obstruction of axoplasmic flow in the laminar region (20). Histology in primate eyes shows posterior bowing of the lamina with compression of the connective tissue plates and distortion of the laminar fenestrae, resulting from increased intraocular pressure. Transverse sections through the lamina cribrosa have documented increased size of the laminar fenestrae in the superior and inferior poles of the optic nerve. These regional differences of the lamina cribrosa may account for asymmetric mechanical damage of the axons within the various regions (21). In early glaucomatous optic neuropathy, damage of the ganglion cell axons occurs primarily in the superior and inferior regions of the optic nerve. Histology shows nonuniform distribution with increased numbers of large ganglion cell axons in the inferior and superior poles of the optic nerve. Large ganglion cell axons appear to be preferentially damaged early in glaucomatous optic neuropathy (22). This apparent in-

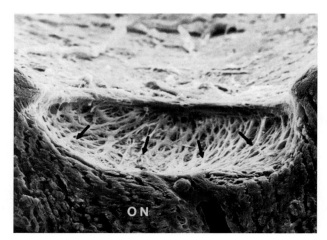

Figure 42–1.
Bowing of Lamina Cribrosa of a Glaucomatous Optic Nerve (trypsin digest): Note the posterior bowing of the lamina cribrosa, with compression of the laminar connective tissue plates. (Courtesy of John Morrison, MD) ON: Optic Nerve (ON), Arrows: Lamina Cribrosa)

creased susceptibility of the large cell axons may be the result of the relative distribution of these axons within the regions of the optic nerve, which are primarily distorted by mechanical forces. Other glial support tissues within the optic nerve also show changes in glaucomatous optic neuropathy. Extracellular matrix components, including elastin fibers of the lamina cribrosa, are altered in glaucomatous eyes and in experimental models of glaucoma (14). These changes may be the result of, or response to, increased intraocular pressure and mechanical stress, and may be associated with axonal death in glaucoma.

A second hypothesis proposes that, primarily, the development of intraneural ischemia and its consequences lead to the development of glaucomatous optic neuropathy. This idea proposes that vascular perfusion of the neural tissue within the optic nerve is deficient in glaucoma. Vascular perfusion is dependent on arterial blood pressure, venous outflow, tissue pressure surrounding the vasculature, autoregulation, and local and regional vasomodulators. An insufficiency or abnormality of any or all of these components may result in regional ischemia (9). This vascular hypothesis suggests that elevated intraocular pressure results in increased tissue pressure within the optic nerve tissue surrounding the vasculature (12). This causes vascular collapse and decreased neural perfusion, resulting in glaucomatous optic neuropathy.

However, increased tissue pressure is only one possible cause of decreased vascular perfusion. Glaucoma patients are more likely to have systemic vascular disorders including diabetes mellitus, systemic hypertension, peripheral vascular disease, and vasospastic syndromes (see Introduction: Risk Factors in Glaucoma). These as-

sociations between extrinsic vascular factors and glaucoma support a vascular etiology in the development of glaucomatous optic neuropathy. Studies have also shown that individuals with glaucoma and low blood pressure more commonly develop visual field defects (9). Also, patients with glaucoma, but with normal intraocular pressures, are more likely to have systemic vascular disorders than the general population. Neural damage in both these instances may be the result of decreased arterial blood flow.

In laboratory studies, axoplasmic flow of the ganglion cell axons is obstructed by interrupting the short posterior ciliary artery circulation to the optic nerve (16). This may lead to ganglion cell death similar to that found in mechanical compression. In addition, clinical findings in anterior ischemic optic neuropathy, especially when associated with temporal arteritis, may be similar to those found in glaucoma. Optic nerve cupping and pallor are found in both diseases.

Autoregulatory mechanisms within regional vascular beds are thought to accommodate changes in arterial blood pressure in normal individuals. Deficient autoregulation of the optic nerve vasculature may result in decreased optic nerve perfusion in glaucoma patients (2). Changes in fluorescein angiography have also supported a vascular component in the development of glaucomatous optic neuropathy. Hypoperfusion and fluorescein filling defects in the optic nerve, especially in the superior and inferior poles, occur in glaucomatous eyes (13). Vascular watershed zones may exist within the optic nerve, and these zones may increase the optic nerve's susceptibility to ischemic insult (11). These intrinsic vacular factors (anomalies of autoregulation and vacular anatomy) may contribute to glaucomatous optic neuropathy.

Glaucomatous optic neuropathy seems to derive from many potential sources working independently or in concert. A combination of the various intrinsic and extrinsic factors may contribute to varying degrees in each individual. Any examples of how these factors interact could be hypothesized. Increases in intraocular pressure with mechanical distortion of the optic nerve results in increased tissue pressure on the microvasculature of the optic nerve and decreased perfusion of the neuronal tissue may result. Also, mechanical distortion of the laminar cribrosa fenestrae could directly compromise ganglion cell axons, rendering them more susceptible to damage from an insufficient vascular supply. Further studies examining changes in the compliance and structure of the optic nerve, resulting from increased intraocular pressure, should increase our understanding of the mechanical component of the development of glaucomatous optic neuropathy. Greater understanding of autoregulatory mechanisms and regional and systemic vasomodulation may also shed light on the possible contribution of the vascular system in glaucomatous optic neuropathy. Finally, immunologic studies examining the relationship between immunologic disorders and glaucomatous optic neuropathy may add another dimension and increase our understanding of the etiology of glaucomatous optic nerve damage (8).

■ AQUEOUS HUMOR DYNAMICS AND INTRAOCULAR PRESSURE ELEVATION

The level of intraocular pressure is dependent upon the rate of production of aqueous humor, the resistance of aqueous humor outflow, and the absorption by the episcleral venous system. Aqueous humor is produced in the ciliary processes of the ciliary body. The aqueous humor derives from the plasma within the capillary network of the ciliary processes. The production of aqueous humor appears to be the result of diffusion, ultrafiltration, and active transport (23). Active transport or secretion involves the transport of water-soluble substances across the cell membranes and is not dependent on the hydrostatic pressure within the capillary network. Ultrafiltration, however, is pressure-dependent and results in water and water-soluble substances flowing from the plasma component of the blood into the posterior chamber. Passive diffusion results in lipid soluble substances, passing through the lipid portions of the cell membranes along a concentration gradient. Debate persists over the exact mechanism of aqueous humor formation and how each of these three mechanisms contribute.

For aqueous humor to be formed, fluid derived from the ciliary processes capillaries must cross both the pigmented and nonpigmented layers of epithelium (7, 15, 18, 25). The capillaries of the ciliary processes are fenestrated, allowing access of the plasma to the ciliary processes' stroma. The tight junctions of the nonpigmented epithelial cells act as the blood-aqueous barrier. It seems that these metabolically active, nonpigmented epithelial cells are primarily responsible for the active transport and formation of aqueous humor (18). The nonpigmented epithelial cells have many mitochondria and pinocytotic vesicles, indicating increased metabolic activity and fluid transport. The high surface area of the ciliary processes provides ample area for aqueous humor production and release into the posterior chamber. Normal aqueous humor flow rates, as measured by fluorophotometry or tonography, are approximately 1.8 to 3.0 microliters per minute (18). The entire volume of the anterior chamber is replaced approximately every 2 hours. The aqueous humor is derived from the plasma, but it has two important compositional differences; the normal aqueous humor is almost devoid of protein and has a marked excess of ascorbate (5). Ascorbic acid is found in concentrations 10 to 15 times higher in the aqueous than in the plasma. Increased amounts of protein may be seen in the aqueous humor as a response to trauma or disease. This may result from breakdown of the blood aqueous barrier or from abnormal production of protein in the anterior segment of the eye.

In the normal eye, aqueous humor produced by the ciliary body is released into the posterior chamber, flows between the anterior surface of the lens and posterior surface of the iris through the pupil and into the anterior chamber (Figure 42–2). Aqueous humor outflow from the anterior chamber is principally through the trabecular meshwork and into Schlemm's canal. Schlemm's canal empties into intrascleral collection channels, and eventually into intrascleral, episcleral, and conjunctival aqueous veins. This pathway is known as "conventional" outflow and is responsible for at least 90% of the aqueous humor outflow (4, 7). The remaining aqueous humor exits the eye by the "unconventional," or uveoscleral, outflow system. Unconventional outflow of aqueous humor from the anterior chamber is through the ciliary muscle into the suprachoroidal space (6). This fluid exits the eye either through the sclera or is absorbed by adjacent vasculature of the choroid. The unconventional outflow system is not well

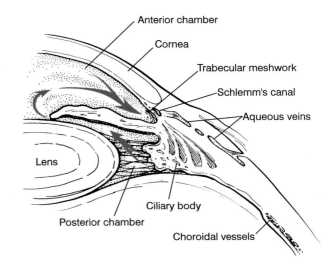

Figure 42–2.

Aqueous humor production and flow: Aqueous humor is produced by the ciliary body and released into the posterior chamber. In the normal eye, aqueous humor flows from the posterior chamber, between the lens and the iris, through the pupil and into the anterior chamber. Most of the aqueous humor outflow is through the trabecular meshwork (conventional outflow pathway).

understood in humans. Uveoscleral outflow is thought to be intraocular pressure-independent.

The trabecular meshwork lies within the anterior chamber angle between the scleral spur and Schwalbe's line (see Gonioscopy: Normal Anterior Chamber Angle). The scleral spur is an infolding of the sclera, into which the anterior longitudinal fibers of the ciliary muscle insert. Schwalbe's line is the junction between the trabecular meshwork and the posterior extent of Descemet's membrane and the corneal endothelial layer. The trabecular meshwork may be divided into three sec-

tions: the uveal meshwork, the corneoscleral meshwork, and the juxtacanalicular meshwork (10) (Figure 42–3a and 42–3b). The trabecular meshwork acts as a porous sieve between the anterior chamber and Schlemm's canal. The uveal meshwork is adjacent to the aqueous humor of the anterior chamber and is composed of branching, uveal trabeculae which span from the peripheral iris root to Schwalbe's line. The corneoscleral meshwork consists of sheetlike trabeculae with small perforations. The openings within the uveal meshwork are considerably larger than the openings within the

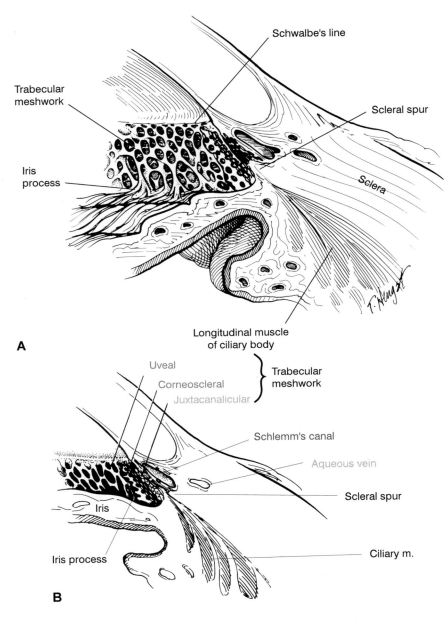

Figures 42–3a and 3b.
Anterior Chamber Angle and Trabecular Meshwork: The trabecular meshwork lies in the anterior chamber angle and extends from the base of the iris to the peripheral cornea. (Figure 42–3a) Aqueous humor flows through the trabecular meshwork into Schlemm's canal. The trabecular meshwork is composed of three layers: the uveal meshwork, the corneoscleral meshwork, and the juxtacanalicular meshwork (Figure 42–3b).

sheets of the corneoscleral meshwork. Between the corneoscleral meshwork and Schlemm's canal, lies loosely organized, connective tissue: the juxtacanalicular meshwork. This is composed of multiple layers of connective tissue with the last layer constituting the inner wall of Schlemm's canal. Schlemm's canal is an endothelial-lined channel, much like the venous system. The trabecular meshwork and Schlemm's canal are present for the 360° of the anterior chamber angle. However, Schlemm's canal is often a discontinuous canal. Intrascleral aqueous veins were originally described by Ascher (3) and connect Schlemm's canal to the episcleral and conjunctival venous system. Most of these episcleral and conjunctival veins drain posteriorly via orbital veins into the cavernous sinus.

The exact mechanism by which aqueous transits from the anterior chamber into Schlemm's canal is not known. The uveal and corneoscleral meshwork behave as a metabolically active, porous filter to the aqueous, and provide a network which may become enmeshed with particulate debris or cells, resulting in outflow obstruction and elevated intraocular pressure. Fluid enters Schlemm's canal by passing through the porous outer layers of the juxtacanalicular tissue, and then passing through the wall of Schlemm's canal and the endothelial layer. Some propose that transcellular transport of aqueous through the wall of Schlemm's canal is via giant vacuoles (26). Micropores have also been shown within the inner wall of Schlemm's canal, through which aqueous may pass (24). The juxtacanalicular meshwork and inner wall of Schlemm's canal is likely the principal site of aqueous outflow resistance. Extracellular matrix components, such as locally synthesized and regulated proteoglycans, glycoproteins and hyaluronic acid, appear to constitute a major source of outflow resistance before Schlemm's canal (1). Abnormalities in the turnover of these extracellular components may increase the aqueous humor outflow resistance, resulting in some forms of glaucoma. Changes in the structure of the trabecular meshwork itself also may contribute to increased outflow resistance. Mechanical change of the meshwork from trauma, intratrabecular debris, or collagenous scar tissue, all may decrease outflow of aqueous humor. The *Goldmann*

equation is used to quantify the intraocular pressure and its relationship to the production and outflow of aqueous humor:

$$P_o = (F/C) - P_v$$

where P_o is the pressure of the undisturbed eye (mm Hg), F is the rate of aqueous humor formation (μl/min), C is the facility of outflow (μl/min/mm Hg), and P_v is the episcleral venous pressure (mm Hg). Therefore, the intraocular pressure depends on rate of aqueous humor formation, absorption through the episcleral venous system, and outflow resistance through the trabecular meshwork (7, 15, 18). The rate of aqueous formation depends on the integrity of the blood-aqueous barrier, the circulation and blood pressure within the ciliary body, and diurnal, possibly hormonal, controls. The rate of aqueous humor formation is typically less during sleep. Aqueous formation also decreases with age, with anterior segment inflammation, and with some forms of surgery. A variety of drugs have also been developed to decrease aqueous humor formation and lower the intraocular pressure. Episcleral venous pressure is relatively constant in most eyes and ranges between 8 to 12mm Hg. In some disease entities, episcleral venous pressure (P_v) may be elevated, resulting in an elevation of intraocular pressure (Po). Reflux of blood into Schlemm's canal in these disorders may also increase intraocular pressure by reducing facility of outflow of aqueous humor.

Intraocular pressure is maintained within the range of 10 to 21mm Hg in most normal eyes (17). Intraocular pressure and aqueous humor formation vary throughout the day in all eyes. Seasonal variations of aqueous humor production have also been shown to result in changes of the intraocular pressure. Most individuals have their highest daily intraocular pressure shortly after awakening in the morning. In normal individuals, intraocular pressure may vary as much as 4 to 6mm Hg throughout the day. Individuals with glaucoma often exhibit larger fluctuations in intraocular pressure, because their decreased outflow reserve results in an inability to handle variations in the rate of aqueous production.

■ REFERENCES

1. Acott TS, Westcott M, Passo MS, Van Buskirk EM: Trabecular meshwork glycosaminoglycans in human and cynomolgus monkey eyes. Invest Ophthal Vis Sci 1985, 26:320.

2. Anderson, DR: The mechanisms of damage of the optic nerve. Paper presented at the meeting of the Glaucoma Committee of the International Ophthalmology Congress, Quail Lodge, CA, Oct 28–29, 1982.

3. Ascher, KW: The Aqueous Veins, Biomicrosopic Study of the Aqueous Humor Elimination, Charles C Thomas, Springfield, IL, 1961.

4. Ashton, N: The exit pathway of the aqueous. Trans Ophthal Soc UK 1960, 80:397.

5. Becker, B: Chemical composition of human aqueous humor. Effects of acetazolamide. Arch Ophthal 1957, 57:793.

6. Bill, A, Phillips, CI: Uveoscleral drainage of aqueous humor in human eyes. Exp Eye Res 1971, 12:275.

7. Brubaker, RF: The flow of aqueous humor in the human eye. Trans Am Ophthal Soc 1982, 80:391.

8. Cartwright MJ, Crajewski AL, Friedberg ML, Anderson DR, Richards DW: Immune-related disease and normal tension glaucoma: a case control study. Arch Ophthalmol 1992; 110;500.

9. Drance, SM: Some factors in the production of low tension glaucoma. Br J Ophthalmol 1972, 56:229.

10. Fine, BS: Structure of the trabecular meshwork and the canal of Schlemm. Trans Am Acad Ophthal Otol 1966, 70:777.

11. Hayreh, SS: Blood supply of the optic nerve head and its role in optic atrophy, glaucoma, and oedema of the optic disc. Br J Ophthalmol 1969, 53:721.

12. Hayreh, SS: Pathogenesis of optic nerve damage and visual field defects in glaucoma. Doc Ophthalmol Proc Series 1980, 22:89.

13. Hayreh, SS: Pathogenesis of optic nerve damage and visual field defects in glaucoma. Doc Ophthalmol Proc Series 1980, 22:89.

14. Hernandez, MR, Luo, XX, Igoe, F, and Neufeld, AH: Extracellular matrix of the human lamina cribrosa. Am J Ophthalmol 1987, 104:567.

15. Krupin, T, Wax, M, Moolchandani, J: Aqueous production. Trans Ophthal Soc UK 1986, 105:156.

16. Levy, NS: The effect of interruption of the short posterior ciliary arteries on slow axoplasmic transport and histology within the optic nerve of the rhesus monkey. Invest Ophthal 1976, 15:495.

17. Leydhecker W, Akigama K, Neuman HG: Der intraoculare druckgesunder menschlicher augen. Klin Monatsbl Augenheilkd 1958, 133:662

18. Macri, JF, Cevario, SJ: The formation and inhibition of aqueous humor production. Arch Ophthal 1978, 96:1664.

19. Quigley, HA, Hohman, RM, Addicks, EM, Massof, RW, and Green, WR: Morphologic changes in the lamina cribrosa correlated with neural loss in open-angle glaucoma. Am J Ophthalmol 1983, 95:673.

20. Quigley, HA, and Addicks, EM: Chronic experimental glaucoma in primates. II. Effect of extended intraocular pressure elevation on optic nerve head and axonal transport. Invest Ophthalmol Vis Sci 1980, 19:137.

21. Quigley, HA, and Addicks, EM: Regional differences in the structure of the lamina cribrosa and their relation to glaucomatous optic nerve damage. Arch Ophthalmol 1981, 99:137.

22. Quigley, HA, Sanchez, RM, Dunkelberger, GR, et al: Chronic glaucoma selectively damages large optic nerve fibers. Invest Ophthalmol Vis Sci 1987, 23:913.

23. Richardson, KT: Cellular response to drugs affecting aqueous dynamics. Arch Ophthal 1973, 89:65.

24. Segawa, K: Pores of the trabecular wall of Schlemm's canal. Ferritin perfusion in enucleated human eyes. Acta Soc Ophthal Jap 1970, 74:1240.

25. Smith, RS, Rudt, LA: Ultrastructural studies of the blood-aqueous barrier, 2. The barrier to horseradish peroxidase in primates, Am J Ophthal 1973, 76:937.

26. Tripathi, RC: Ultrastructure of the trabecular wall of Schlemm's canal in relation to aqueous outflow. Exp Eye Res, 1968, 7:335.

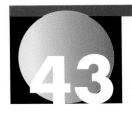

43 Clinical Testing and Examination Techniques in Glaucoma

G. A. Cioffi, E. M. Van Buskirk

■ TONOMETRY

Introduction

Until the introduction of the Maklakov tonometer in the late nineteenth century, intraocular pressure was estimated by digital palpation of the globe (41). Over the past century, many additional tonometers have been developed. With the development of the Schiotz tonometer in 1905, tonometry became relatively accurate and widely available (54). Today, a variety of mechanical and electronic tonometric devices are available, but all exploit one of two principles to measure the intraocular pressure, indentation, or applanation. Indentation tonometry measures the amount of deformation or indentation of the front surface of the globe produced by a fixed amount of force. Applanation tonometers apply a variable amount of force to the corneal surface, to produce a fixed amount of deformation or flattening. The Goldmann-type applanation tonometers are the current standard for tonometry throughout the world.

Indentation Tonometry

The Schiotz tonometer is the primary indentation tonometer used to measure intraocular pressure (54). The principles of indentation tonometry are elucidated by a description of the Schiotz tonometer. The *Schiotz tonometer* uses a series of weights, varying from 5.5 to 15 gm, which are attached to a plunger. The plunger rests on the corneal surface and the Schiotz tonometer mea-

sures the amount of indentation produced by the attached weight. The amount of indentation depends on the weight attached to the plunger, the ocular rigidity and intraocular pressure. Increasing the plunger weight, decreasing the ocular rigidity or decreasing the intraocular pressure, results in a higher reading on the Schiotz scale. The scale readings are inversely related to the intraocular pressure, and a conversion table is provided with the instrument. The conversion tables convert the reading to an intraocular pressure value (millimeters of mercury). In the late 1940s and the early 1950s, Friedenwald calculated several sets of conversion tables. These tables have become the standard for Schiotz tonometry (22, 23).

The accuracy of the Schiotz tonometer depends on several factors (3). The most accurate conversion is the table developed by Friedenwald in 1948, which uses an average value for the ocular rigidity. However, the variability in ocular rigidity of different individuals is a significant source of error for indentation tonometry. Hyperopic eyes typically have higher than average ocular rigidity and therefore, give a falsely high intraocular pressure measurement. Conversely, highly myopic eyes have lower than average ocular rigidity; hence, the Schiotz tonometer underestimates the intraocular pressure in these eyes. Alterations in intraocular blood volume, corneal topography abnormalities, and the changes of aqueous humor dynamics created by the indentation tonometer, also contribute to inaccuracies in measuring the intraocular pressure with this technique.

Applanation Tonometry

As previously mentioned, applanation tonometry uses a variable amount of force to produce a fixed amount of flattening of the corneal surface. Applanation tonometry is based on the Imbert-Fick principle, which states that the external force (F) exerted to a sphere, equals the pressure inside this sphere (P) times the area (A) which is flattened or "applanated" by the external force ($F = P \times A$) (25, 44). This principle is valid only for an ideal, dry, thin-walled sphere. The *Imbert-Fick* principle has been modified for use in applanation tonometry to account for the corneal thickness and the moisture on the surface of the cornea. The tips on all Goldmann-type tonometers are standardized to applanate a 3.06 mm diameter of the cornea, which standardizes the area of applanation. This standardized area of applanation has been calculated so that resistance of flattening of the cornea created by the thickness of the cornea is essentially negated by the capillary attraction of the tear film between the tonometer tip and the cornea.

To measure the intraocular pressure with a Goldmann tonometer, a topical anesthetic and fluorescein are instilled in the tear film to enhance visualization of contact between the tonometer and the corneal surface. A cobalt blue light on the slit lamp is used to illuminate the fluorescein and the biprism of the applanator. The applanation tip is brought into gentle contact with the front surface of the cornea. The tear meniscus at the margin between the applanation tip and the cornea is visualized through the slit lamp. The tip of the applanation device contains two beam-splitting prisms which optically convert the circular point of contact between the tonometer and the cornea into two semicircles. A variable amount of force can be applied to the tonometer tip to create the desired amount of flattening of the

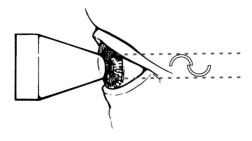

Figure 43–1.
Applanation Tonometry: The tip of an applanation tonometer flattens the cornea and the observer's view through the biprism. The meniscus between the tonometer tip and cornea is converted into two semicircles by the biprism. The applanation force is adjusted to align the inner edges of the semicircles as shown.

corneal surface. The force of applanation is adjusted so that the inner edge of the semicircles meet and the intraocular pressure is read from a scale on the applanation instrument. By adjusting the overlap of the semicircles, the desired area of applanated cornea is achieved (Figure 43–1). The scale on the tonometer is in grams of force and must be multiplied by 10 to convert to millimeters of mercury.

Applanation tonometry displaces much less aqueous humor from the anterior chamber than indentation tonometry and is largely unaffected by variations of scleral rigidity. However, like indentation tonometry, applanation tonometry also has sources of potential error. Excessive or inadequate amounts of sodium fluorescein in the tear film cause inaccurate tonometric measurements. Incorrect alignment of the semicircles and corneal scarring or edema may result in inaccurate measurements. Regular (especially greater than four diopters) or irregular corneal astigmatism may lead to inaccurate readings with applanation tonometry. With regular astigmatism, errors can be minimized by rotating the dividing line of the biprisms to 45° from the major axis of the astigmatism.

■ OTHER TYPES OF TONOMETRY

Other types of applanation tonometers include the *Perkins* and Draeger tonometers (15, 45). These are handheld instruments which use the same principles and techniques as conventional Goldmann tonometry and are often useful for examinations in the operative suite or for individuals who cannot sit at a slit lamp. Another applanation tonometer, the *MacKay-Marg*, applanates a smaller area of the cornea and may be useful in eyes with extensive corneal scarring (40). A recently developed tonometer, the Tonopen, incorporates a

small, strain gauge in the tip which touches the cornea and calculates the intraocular pressure electronically (36). This computer-based, pen-shaped tonometer collects and averages multiple readings which are presented on a digital display. Another tomometer, the pneumotonometer uses an air pressurized tip to sense the force required to distort the surface of the cornea (19). Because of the small size of the pneumotonometer tip, it is also useful in eyes with corneal scarring. The pneumotonometer, MacKay-Marg, and Tonopen accurately measure the intraocular pressure in patients wearing soft contact lenses. Goldmann applanation tonometry is not useful in this setting because contact between the applanation device and the contact lens distorts the readings.

■ GONIOSCOPY

Introduction

Gonioscopy is an examination technique used to visualize the structures of the anterior chamber angle. Mastering the various techniques of gonioscopy is crucial in the evaluation of the pathophysiology of aqueous humor outflow obstruction and the diagnosis of the various glaucomas. Gonioscopic lenses are required to visualize the chamber angle because, under normal conditions, light reflected from the angle structures undergoes total internal reflection at the tear-air interface. At this interface, the refractive index difference is increased and the critical angle (approximately 46°) is reached. Thus, light is totally reflected back into the corneal stroma. This prevents direct visualization of the angle structures. All gonioscopy lenses eliminate the tear-air interface by placing a plastic or glass surface adjacent to the front surface of the eye. The small space between the lens and cornea is filled by the tears, saline solution, or a clear viscous substance.

Direct and Indirect Gonioscopy

There are two broad categories which describe all the various gonioscopy techniques: indirect gonioscopy and direct gonioscopy (7) (Table 43–1). Mastering several gonioscopic techniques assists in the diagnosis of the various types of outflow obstruction. All direct gonioscopy lenses provide direct visualization of the chamber angle (e.g., light reflected directly from the chamber angle is visualized). Therefore, with direct gonioscopy lenses, the observer has an erect view of the angle structures (Figure 43–2). The most commonly used direct gonioscopy lens is the Koeppe lens (32). This lens

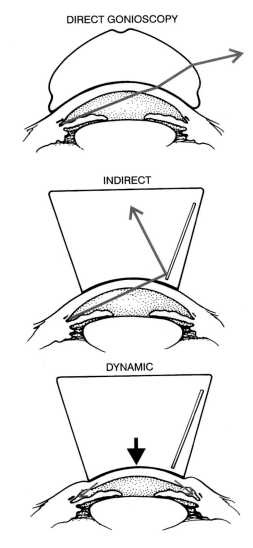

Figure 43–2.
Direct and Indirect Gonioscopy: Gonioscopic lenses eliminate the tear-air interface and total internal reflection. With direct lenses, the light ray reflected from the anterior chamber angle is observed directly, whereas with indirect lenses the light ray is reflected by a mirror within the lens. Posterior pressure with an indirect lens forces open an appositionally closed or narrow anterior chamber angle (dynamic gonioscopy).

TABLE 43–1
Most Common Gonioscopy Lenses

> **Direct Lenses**
> Koeppe
> Barkan
> Swan–Jacob
> Thorpe
> Layden
>
> **Indirect Lenses**
> Goldmann one- or three-mirror
> Zeiss four-mirror
> Sussman four-mirror
> Posner four-mirror
> Ritch four-mirror (trabeculoplasty)

is placed on the cornea and saline solution is used to fill the space between the cornea and the lens. The saline acts as an optical coupler between the two surfaces. Direct gonioscopy is most easily done with the subject in a supine position. A handheld binocular microscope or an operating microscope is typically used to illuminate and visualize the chamber angle through the direct gonioscopic lenses. Direct gonioscopy with a Koeppe lens is useful in the operating room for examinations under anesthesia of the infant eye, because it provides a panoramic view of the chamber angle. Other direct gonioscopy lenses include the Swan-Jacob and the Barkan lenses, which are frequently used for goniotomy surgery. Modifications incorporated in these lenses allow easy access of the goniotomy knife at the time of surgery. Direct gonioscopy is essential when completing goniotomies, because it provides an erect orientation of the chamber angle.

Indirect gonioscopy is more frequently used in the clinician's office. With indirect gonioscopy, a contact lens with an internal mirrored surface is used (7, 21, 56). Light reflected from the chamber angle passes into the lens and is reflected by the mirrored-surface within the lens to the observer (Figure 43–2). Because an internal mirror is present in all indirect gonioscopy lenses, the image seen by the observer is both inverted and shifted from right to left. These lenses are commonly referred to as "gonioprisms" and may have between one and four internal mirrors. Many gonioprisms, such as the Goldmann lens, require a viscous optical coupler between the lens and the cornea to fill the domed space over the cornea. Indirect gonioscopy is used with the subject in an upright position, with illumination and magnification provided by a slit lamp. These lenses provide clear visualization of the anterior chamber angle structures and may be modified with antireflective coatings for use during laser procedures.

The Sussman, Posner, and Zeiss four-mirror gonioprisms allow all four quadrants of the chamber angle to be visualized without manipulation of the lens. These lenses also allow the examiner to use the subject's tear film as the optical coupler between the cornea and the lens. The lenses are easy to use and provide the ability to do dynamic gonioscopy. With dynamic gonioscopy, gentle pressure is placed on the cornea and aqueous humor is forced into the chamber angle (Figure 43–2). The posterior diameter of most gonioprisms is smaller than the corneal diameter, and posterior pressure can be used to force open a narrowed chamber angle. Dynamic gonioscopy may be misleading in the inexperienced hand, because undue pressure on the cornea may distort the chamber angle or may give the observer the false impression of an open angle in an eye with appositional closure. With all indirect gonioscopy techniques, the observer may enhance visualization of the chamber angle by positioning the subject's eye (having the subject look towards the mirror) or by applying pressure with the posterior surface of the lens to provide more complete evaluation of the chamber angle. However, caution must be used not to induce artificial opening or closing of the anterior chamber angle with these techniques.

■ CLINICAL APPEARANCE OF THE NORMAL ANTERIOR CHAMBER ANGLE

Gonioscopy allows visualization of the anterior chamber angle structures, the principal site of aqueous humor outflow from the eye. Beginning with the iris root and preceding anteriorly towards the peripheral cornea, the following structures may be observed when the chamber angle is completely open: iris root, ciliary body band, scleral spur, posterior trabecular meshwork, anterior trabecular meshwork, Schwalbe's line, and peripheral cornea (Figure 43–3). A variety of grading systems have been described for evaluation of the anterior chamber angle structures. These grading systems have strived to standardize the gonioscopic description from one observer to another and for serial examinations by a single observer. However, a quadrant-by-quadrant, narrative description of the chamber angle is usually easier, more descriptive, and may also be used to document serial gonioscopic findings.

The ciliary body band is the most anterior portion of the ciliary body and is visible at the insertion of the iris root into the ciliary body. The ciliary body band is often difficult to see in the hyperopic eye but is wide and easily seen in the myopic eye. It typically is grayish-white in color. Just anterior to the ciliary body band is the scleral spur. This is the point of attachment of the longitudinal, anterior ciliary muscle fibers to the sclera. It typically is whitish unless covered with pigment granules, as in pigment dispersion syndrome, or after traumatic pigment dispersion. Often, small iris processes, originating at the base of the iris, will connect to the scleral spur.

The trabecular meshwork is just anterior to the scleral spur. The meshwork is usually lightly pigmented, but may be almost free of pigmentation in young patients or in patients with little ocular pigmentation. The posterior portion of the trabecular meshwork becomes darker with age. This portion of the trabecular meshwork is the principal functional portion of the trabecular meshwork (primary site of aqueous humor outflow). Iris processes, fine iris fibers extending from the pe-

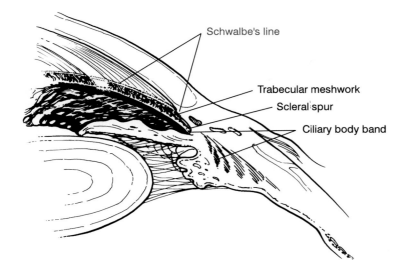

Figure 43–3.
Gonioscopic View of a Normal Anterior Chamber Angle: The structures of the anterior chamber angle include the iris root, the ciliary body band, the scleral spur, the trabecular meshwork, Schwalbe's line, and the peripheral cornea. Iris processes may extend from the peripheral iris to the trabecular meshwork and Schwalbe's line.

ripheral iris, may also insert into the trabecular meshwork or even anterior to the trabecular meshwork to Schwalbe's line (Figure 43–3).

Schwalbe's line represents the junction between the anterior trabecular meshwork and the peripheral cornea. It is a slightly elevated ridge and may be white or pigment covered.

A convenient gonioscopic technique to determine the position of Schwalbe's line is the parallelopiped or corneal light wedge technique. The parallelopiped technique allows the observer to determine the exact junction of the cornea and the trabecular meshwork. The observer uses a narrow slit beam of light and oblique illumination. On the peripheral cornea, light reflecting from both the anterior and posterior surfaces of the cornea is seen. The posterior point at which these slits of light converge is Schwalbe's line. Posterior to Schwalbe's line, only one slit beam of light is seen. This technique is helpful to establish landmarks, especially in lightly pigmented eyes, in which pigment deposition does not detail the various angle structures.

Frequently, blood vessels are seen in the anterior chamber angle and concern arises of the possibility of angle neovascularization (59). Several types of blood vessels in the anterior chamber angle may be normal. Large loops from the peripheral arterial circle of the iris may emerge from the iris in front of the ciliary body band. These vessels are described as "serpentine" and typically course circumferentially within the iris. Small, radial vessels may also be seen, especially in eyes with lightly pigmented irides. These vessels, because of their small size, more closely resemble anterior segment neovascularization. They are differentiated from neovascularization because they do not progress, hemorrhage, or extend further anterior than the scleral spur.

■ OPTIC NERVE HEAD EVALUATION

Direct examination of the optic nerve provides concrete anatomic confirmation of its integrity and a basis for therapeutic and diagnostic decisions. A variety of techniques are available to view the optic nerve head appearance. These techniques, alone or in concert, allow the clinician to evaluate the optic nerve and monitor its status.

Ophthalmoscopy (Direct and Indirect)

Clinical evaluation of the optic nerve may be done by direct or indirect ophthalmoscopy. Direct ophthalmoscopy provides a highly magnified erect view through an undilated pupil. The red-free filter within most indirect ophthalmoscopes provides better illumination of the peripapillary nerve fiber layer and aids in its evaluation. However, the direct ophthalmoscopic view may be limited by miosis, or even small media opacities. Direct ophthalmoscopy is also limited because it is monocular and cannot provide stereopsis and three-dimensional evaluation of the nerve. Binocular indirect ophthalmoscopy is useful in eyes with dilated pupils and offers a stereoscopic, three-dimensional view. However, the lack of magnification with indirect ophthalmoscopy often makes it impossible to document subtle changes of the optic nerve. A useful instrument for examining the optic nerve is the monocular indirect ophthalmoscope. This instrument provides less magnification than the direct ophthalmoscope yet has sufficient clarity and magnification to observe subtle changes of the optic nerve. The monocular indirect ophthalmoscope provides excellent visualization through miotic pupils and is less affected by media opacities than direct ophthalmoscopy.

Slit Lamp Examination and Fundoscopic Lenses (Binocular Biomicroscopy)

The most definitive method of clinical optic nerve head evaluation is binocular biomicroscopy. This technique provides a highly magnified stereoscopic view of the optic nerve and retina. In binocular biomicroscopy, the slit lamp is used with an auxiliary fundus lens to examine the optic nerve. Handheld, noncontact lenses include the 78 diopter and 90 diopter lenses (52). The Hruby lens (-55 diopters) is also a noncontact lens which is mounted to the slit lamp. These lenses provide excellent magnification and stereopsis, and many slit lamps contain red-free filters for better illumination and detection of the peripapillary nerve fiber layer.

Fundus contact lenses may also be placed on the corneal surface, and the slit lamp is used to visualize the optic nerve through these lenses. Fundus contact lenses often provide the best view of the optic nerve and may aid in stabilization of the patient's eye during the evaluation. Clear visualization of the optic nerve head with these lenses generally requires a pupillary diameter of at least 3 mm (50). With binocular biomicroscopy, the apparent cup size appears larger than with monocular examination techniques. Detailed drawings of the optic nerve head and peripapillary area should be made using these lenses. These drawings can be used to document and follow glaucomatous optic neuropathy.

Photography

Two-dimensional fundus photography is often used to document the optic nerves and for serial comparison over time in individuals with glaucoma (27, 57). Color photography typically offers better evaluation of the optic nerve, but a variety of black and white photographic techniques are also used. Special techniques have been developed to provide high resolution photographic images of the peripapillary nerve fiber layer, allowing identification of the nerve fiber layer atrophy, or "drop out," associated with glaucoma (2, 24). Red-free illumination of the fundus enhances contrast and resolution of striations within the nerve fiber layer. Photography with high-resolution film, a narrow band interference filter, and a wide-angle camera affords the best visualization of the nerve fiber layer.

Color stereoscopic photography is the most frequently used method to document and follow glaucomatous optic neuropathy (14, 57). Stereoscopic photography provides three-dimensional imaging of the optic nerve and allows evaluation of the depth of the cup and height of the surrounding nerve fiber layer. In stereophotography, two photographs of the optic nerve head are taken and the stereoscopic effect is obtained by shifting the camera position between the two photographs. Pairs of stereophotographs may be taken simultaneously with two separate cameras, or independently with a single camera in sequence, using a prefixed angulation. Special viewers allow stereo pairs to be observed simultaneously. Stereophotographs should be obtained in all individuals with glaucoma and in individuals suspected of having glaucoma. These photographs should be taken at the initial examination to act as a baseline documentation and as a source for future comparison of the status of the optic nerve. Serial stereophotographs may be taken intermittently to provide documentation of progression or allow extended visual comparisons with previously acquired images.

Computerized Optic Nerve Head Analysis

Stereoscopic photography was used in the development of the early optic nerve head analysis systems, in which computerized analysis of the disk contour and cup pallor were established (55). These techniques have largely been abandoned because of the development of confocal scanning laser ophthalmoscopy, with its ability to image the optic nerve and peripapillary retina, in three dimensions (12, 58). Scanning confocal laser ophthalmoscopy remains in its developmental stages but holds promise for future analysis of the changes in three-dimensional morphology of the optic nerve associated with glaucomatous optic neuropathy. Other technologies have been developed to measure the peripapillary nerve fiber layer thickness, but these techniques remain investigational.

The Clinical Appearance of the Normal Optic Nerve Head

The morphologic appearance of the optic nerve head allows the clinician to detect and monitor the glaucomatous optic neuropathy. A knowledge of the normal optic nerve head appearance must underlie recognition of glaucomatous optic neuropathy (48). The insertion of the optic nerve into the globe is nasal to the posterior pole of the eye. The optic nerve is primarily composed of the axons of the retinal ganglion cell, glial tissue, and vascular elements (see Anatomy: The Optic Nerve Head). The optic nerve "head" or "disk" refers to the anterior surface of the optic nerve, vertically oval in shape, seen on funduscopic examination (Figure 43–4). The neural retinal tissue of the optic nerve has a pinkish-orange appearance, is slightly convex toward the observer, and is composed primarily of the ganglion cell axons (nerve fibers). The abrupt angulation of the nerve fibers as they exit the eye results in a central de-

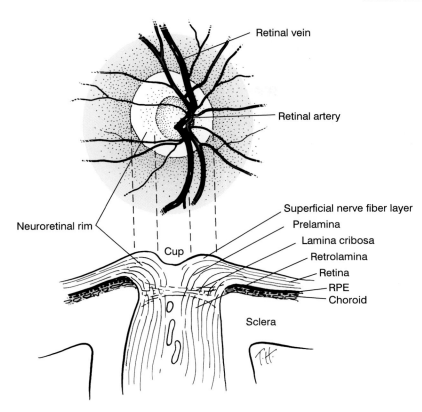

Retinal vein

Retinal artery

Superficial nerve fiber layer
Prelamina
Lamina cribosa
Retrolamina
Retina
RPE
Choroid

Neuroretinal rim

Cup

Sclera

Figure 43–4.
Normal optic nerve (anterior optic nerve head and transverse view, right eye): note the central cup, neuroretinal rim, retinal vessels, four divisions of anterior optic nerve (superficial nerve fiber layer, prelaminar region, lamina cribrosa, retrolaminar region).

pression devoid of nerve fibers, known as the "cup." The cup is more pale than the surrounding neural tissue. In eyes with larger cups, often the fenestrations of the lamina cribrosa may be seen as grayish spots in the base of the depression. The central retinal artery and the central retinal vein emerge from the optic nerve cup, usually from the nasal side. The central cup is vertically oval in shape, similar to, but smaller in size than the overall optic nerve.

Frequently, clinicians describe the cup-to-disk ratio, which is a comparison of the horizontal or vertical cup diameter with the horizontal or vertical disk diameter, respectively. The normal vertical cup-to-disk ratio is often greater than the horizontal cup-to-disk ratio. The vertical cup-to-disk ratio is typically between 0.1 and 0.4, although as many as 5% of normal individuals will have cup-to-disk ratios larger than 0.6 (10, 20, 48). There is a wide range of normal for both the size of the cup-to-disk ratio and the shape of the optic nerve and physiologic central cup. The cup-to-disk ratio and size of the optic nerve head is normally symmetric between the two eyes. Asymmetry of the cup-to-disk ratio of more than 0.2 occurs in less than 1% of normal individuals (20). Increased size of the physiologic cup may be a familial trait, and it is also seen with high myopia. Individuals with high myopia often have an oblique insertion of the optic nerve into the globe, which results in a tilted appearance to the optic nerve head. In general, blacks

have larger cup-to-disk ratios and optic nerve head size, compared with whites. (11)

The Clinical Appearance of Glaucomatous Optic Neuropathy

Glaucomatous optic neuropathy is the final common denominator of all forms of glaucoma. Characteristic changes in the clinical appearance of the optic nerve head are associated with glaucomatous optic neuropathy and correlate with the anatomic findings seen by histology in eyes with glaucomatous damage (37,49,33) (see Anatomy: The Optic Nerve and Pathogenesis: Glaucomatous Optic Neuropathy). Initial changes of the glaucomatous optic nerve head may include focal erosion of the neural retinal rim, secondary to localized atrophy of nerve fibers, or overall enlargement of the cup-to-disk ratio, secondary to diffuse thinning of the neural retinal rim (Figures 43–5, 43–6, and 43–7). Focal erosions most typically occur at the superior and inferior temporal poles of the optic nerve in early glaucomatous optic neuropathy. Thinning of the neural retinal rim with development of a focal "notch" extension of the cup into the neural retinal rim may be seen. With diffuse atrophy, the overall cup enlarges, and the depth of the central cup increases (Figures 43–6 and 43–7). As previously mentioned, significant asymmetry of the cup-to-disk ratio between the two eyes is infrequent in

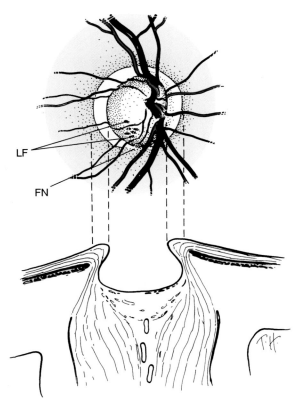

Figure 43–5.
Glaucomatous optic nerve: (anterior optic nerve head and transverse view, right eye). Note the thinning and undermining of inferior neuroretinal rim and focal notching (FN) of inferior neuroretinal rim, enlarged central cup with visible laminar fenestrae (LF), nasal shift of retinal vessels and peripapillary atrophy.

healthy subjects and may represent early asymmetric atrophy of the optic nerves.

Laminar trabeculations or pores are seen as grayish dots in the base of the physiologic cup, even in the nor-

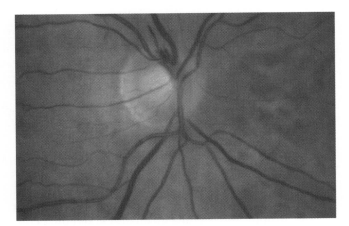

Figure 43–6.
Glaucomatous Optic Nerve: Moderately enlarged cup with peripapillary atrophy. Note the nerve fiber layer hemorrhage at the superior margin of the optic nerve. (Right Eye)

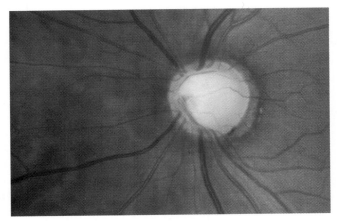

Figure 43–7.
Glaucomatous Optic Nerve: Advanced cupping with diffuse thinning and undermining of the neuroretinal rim, nasalization of the retinal vessels and loss of the normal nerve fiber layer striations (left eye).

mal eye (43). With glaucomatous optic neuropathy, neural atrophy results in more extensive exposure of the underlying lamina and may reveal more laminar pores. As the neural rim atrophies, the central cup enlarges and appears more pale. However, pallor is typically a late sign of an increase in the cup size. Estimation of cup-to-disk ratios, focal erosions, or diffuse neural retinal atrophy based only on pallor, are usually erroneous and greatly underestimate the extent of the glaucomatous optic neuropathy.

The *nerve fiber layer* radiating from the neural retinal rim to the surrounding peripapillary retina has a fine, striated appearance, created by the bundles of axons. In the healthy eye, the nerve fiber layer bundles have a plush, refractile appearance. Red-free examination provides the best visualization of the striations within the nerve fiber layer (1,60). Since the nerve fiber layer undergoes some natural depopulation and loss of turgor with aging, its clinical examination may become less reliable after the age of 60. With glaucomatous optic neuropathy, both diffuse and localized defects may be seen in the peripapillary nerve fiber layer. With diffuse loss of the nerve fiber layer, the normal luster is lost and the striations disappear. Localized loss of nerve fibers may occur early in glaucoma, especially at the superior and inferior poles of the optic nerve. Localized or slit-like defects appear as darkened areas with lack of the normal striations and have a dull reflection compared with the surrounding nerve fiber layer. Peripapillary nerve fiber layer defects are often associated with focal notching of the neural retinal rim.

Small hemorrhages may occur at the neural retinal rim or in the peripapillary nerve fiber layer in as many as one-third of glaucoma patients at some time during the course of their disease (18, 26) (Figure 43–6). The appearance of these hemorrhages is a valuable and ominous clinical sign of progression. With nerve fiber layer atrophy, "baring" of the peripapillary blood vessels also occurs (61). These vessels appear more prominent as they are less obscured by the surrounding nerve fiber layer. The vessels may have a sheathed appearance, resulting from the nerve fiber layer death and draping of the internal limiting membrane over the bared vessels.

In advanced glaucomatous optic neuropathy, extensive atrophy of the neural retinal rim, with a cup-to-disk ratio nearing 1.0, may occur. The optic nerve develops a chalk-white appearance with baring of the lamina. Posterior bowing of the lamina cribrosa produces a deep appearing cup and circumferential expansion of the cup behind the plane of the retina, leading to undermining of the optic nerve edge. The undermining of the neural retinal rim results in the classic "bean pot" configuration seen in late glaucomatous optic neuropathy. Nasalization of the central retinal artery and central retinal vein occurs, since these vessels lose their tissue support and lie adjacent to the nasal neural retinal rim. The nasal neural retinal rim is most often preserved until late in the disease. The temporal branches of the central retinal vessels typically course along the eroded superior and inferior neural retinal rim of the enlarged cup and may disappear beneath the undermined rim.

■ PERIMETRY

Introduction

Assessment and monitoring of the visual function in glaucoma currently relies heavily on evaluation of the visual field. The visual field is the portion of space visible to the fixating eye at a given time. Descriptions of visual field abnormalities in disease date back as far as the time of Hippocrates. In the early 1800s, techniques for accurate assessment of the visual field were described by Young and Purkinje (46, 63). During the mid-to-late 1800s, Von Graefe and Bjerrum developed techniques to measure and document both the normal and glaucomatous visual fields (8, 29). Bjerrum is largely credited with the development of the tangent screen and multiple isopter: kinetic perimetry. Later, a variety of techniques to access the visual field were developed which could concentrate on small portions of the central field or evaluate the full extent of the normal visual field. During the early twentieth century, work by Ronne, Traquair and Goldmann, as well as others, led to the development of standardized hemispheric projection perimetry (28, 51, 62). In this technique, a large perimetric bowl is used to project different light stimuli onto various areas of the subject's visual field. Contributions by Armaly, Drance, and others led to better definitions of the normal visual field and visual field changes to be expected in glaucoma (4, 5, 6, 16, 39).

Static and Kinetic Perimetry

By the mid-1900s, two types of bowl perimetric techniques had been popularized: static and kinetic presentations of the test target. Adaptations of these techniques are still used today. Static perimetry uses a stationary light stimulus of variable intensity which may be increased until the subject recognizes the stimulus. The stimulus may be presented at various points in the visual field. Kinetic perimetry uses a moving stimulus of fixed intensity, moved at a steady rate from outside the visual field into the seeing area, at which point it is perceived by the subject. The subject is asked to indicate the point at which the test stimulus is first seen. When the kinetic visual field is plotted, a line connecting the locations at which a particular stimulus is seen, is known as an isopter. Delayed reaction time on the part of the subject may falsely constrict the kinetic isopters of the visual field. The person administering the test must be cognizant of the subject's ability to react and modify the technique accordingly. Manual kinetic perimetry provides valuable information in multiple clinical settings.

Aulhorn and Harms provided eloquent descriptions of the differences and similarities between static and kinetic testing (5,6) (Figure 43–8). In the late 1960s and early 1970s, many investigators began to further standardize visual field assessment. This led to the development of automated, static perimetry which currently dominates visual field testing in glaucoma.

Automated, static perimetry allows the assessment of specific points within the visual field using static stimulus presentation controlled by computer. Developments of the past decades have sought to maximize the information provided by static perimetry while minimizing testing time. Static perimetry is less dependent upon reaction time of the subject than kinetic perimetry is, because adjustments in the time between presentations are made, depending upon the previous reaction times of each individual subject. However, static perimetry may be time-consuming, as well as exhausting, for the subject. Kinetic perimetry is usually more rapid, but it is often less reproducible and accurate.

Subjects with poor fixation, decreased visual acuity, and limited attentiveness often do better with manual kinetic perimetry than with automated static perimetry. Automation by computer has allowed static threshold perimetry to become practical in the clinical setting. Computerized stimulus presentation allows bracketing above and below the threshold of detection for each point in the visual field. Currently, stimuli can be pre-

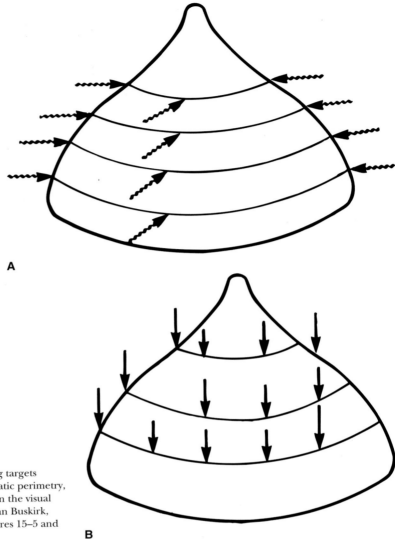

Figure 43–8.
Kinetic and Static Perimetry: In kinetic perimetry, moving targets define the isopters of the visual field (Figure 43–8a). In static perimetry, sensitivity of retina is determined at multiple points within the visual field (Figure 43–8b). (Reprinted by permission of E.M Van Buskirk, Clinical Atlas of Glaucoma, WB Saunders, 1986, p37, figures 15–5 and 15–6)

sented, and the subject's responses recorded while the perimeter monitors fixation. Computerization also has allowed better data storage and analysis for comparison with age-matched, normal populations. Although automated kinetic perimetry has been developed, it has not gained broad clinical acceptance.

■ THE VISUAL FIELD – NORMAL AND GLAUCOMATOUS

If perimetric testing is to be useful in the management and diagnoses of glaucoma, it must detect glaucomatous visual field defects, quantify the size and depth of defects within a visual field, and allow sequential comparison. To obtain these objectives, perimetric testing relies heavily on an understanding of the normal visual field for comparison.

The normal visual field extends approximately 100° temporally, 60° nasally and superiorly, and 70° inferiorly (31). The eloquent description of the visual field by *Traquair* as "an island of vision surrounded by a sea of blindness" provides a unique three-dimensional mental image of the visual field (62) (Figure 43–9). Light sensitivity is greatest at the fovea and decreases with greater degrees of eccentricity from fixation. This peripheral decrease of sensitivity is what led to Traquair's classic analogy of the visual field to an island of vision. The sloping contour of the hill or island of vision results from this variable sensitivity. The blind spot is a "bottomless" scotoma, reflecting the complete lack of light

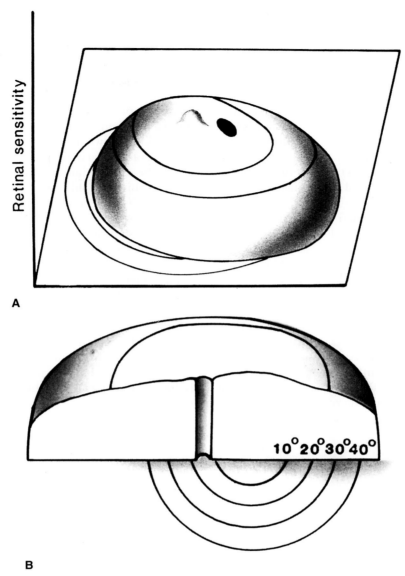

A

B

Figure 43–9.
Traquair's Island of Vision: Three-dimensional island of vision (Figure 43–9a) and a transected view to illustrate the blind spot (Figure 43–9b)
The peak of the island of vision represents the highest point of retinal sensitivity: the fovea. (Reprinted by permission of E.M. Van Buskirk,
Clinical Atlas of Glaucoma, WB Saunders, 1986, p.37, Figures 15–1 and 15–2)

sensitivity at the optic nerve. Beyond the limits of the peripheral visual field, the light sensitivity decreases to zero. The peak of the contour represents the fovea, the point of highest sensitivity.

With increased age, the normal overall sensitivity of visual field decreases. Currently, automated perimeters use large sets of age-matched, normative data for comparison of the visual field in individuals with glaucoma. These normal population data sets provide a baseline for comparison of the visual field. The data sets are used to appropriately remodel the shape of normal "hill of vision" for populations of differing ages. Many factors, other than age, influence the shape of the hill of vision as tested by perimetry: patient attentiveness, fixation,

cooperation, and visual acuity. All may alter the visual field assessment.

Generalized decrease in sensitivity and increase in variability are the hallmarks of early glaucomatous visual field loss (16,38). However, generalized reduction of sensitivity of the visual field and increased variability of the visual field are difficult to quantify. The visual field changes may result from a variety of other etiologies, including aging and media opacities. Individuals suspected of having glaucoma are often elderly, and cataractous change of the crystalline lens is common. These factors contribute to the difficulty in assessing early visual field loss in glaucoma and illustrate the lack of specificity of these early visual field changes.

The onset of clinically detectable visual field loss varies for individual optic nerves. Studies which examined the number of optic nerve fibers lost before the occurrence of reproducible visual field defects (as measured with manual kinetic testing) have shown as much as 40% loss of the nerve fibers before defects were observed (47). Redundancy in the visual system may protect against clinically detectable visual function loss until later in the disease. With progression of the glaucomatous optic nerve damage, profound generalized loss or discrete localized loss of the neural function results in more reproducible and distinguishable visual field defects.

The most characteristic visual field defects associated with glaucoma are related to localized loss or impairment of the retinal nerve fiber bundles (9, 13, 17, 30, 42). The anatomy of the retinal nerve fiber layer as it enters the optic nerve accounts for the patterns of the visual field defects seen in glaucoma (see Anatomy: The Optic Nerve). Nerve fiber bundle loss results in the most definitive and reproducible visual field defects seen in early glaucoma. Nerve fiber bundle defects include arcuate or Bjerrum defects, nasal step defects, temporal wedge defects, and paracentral scotomas. (Figures 43–10, 43–11, and 43–12). An arcuate scotoma extends from the blind spot and arches above or below fixation. These defects occur within an area 10° to 20°

from fixation and may become larger and more dense over time. A full, arcuate scotoma arches completely from the blind spot, around fixation, ending at the nasal raphe. These scotomas typically "fan out" as they extend nasally. This corresponds to the anatomy of the nerve fiber layer fanning out from the superior and inferior temporal optic nerve. Arcuate scotomas may begin as, or extend to, small localized defects within 10° of fixation, known as paracentral scotomas.

Loss of the nerve fiber layer is often asymmetric between the superior and inferior retinal nerve fibers. Because of this, a steplike defect may occur in the nasal visual field where the nerve fibers meet along the nasal raphe. Superior visual field loss more typically precedes inferior visual field loss and may result in a superior nasal step scotoma. Nasal steps may occur outside the central 30° of the visual field in as many as 10% of glaucoma patients. Because of this, central visual field testing may result in a delay in diagnosis. Another potential visual field scotoma associated with loss of nerve fiber bundles, is the temporal sector defect. In approximately 2 to 3% of individuals with glaucoma, nerve fibers extending nasally from the disk are damaged early in the disease. This results in a temporal visual field loss, which is difficult to detect if only the central 24° or 30° of visual field is monitored.

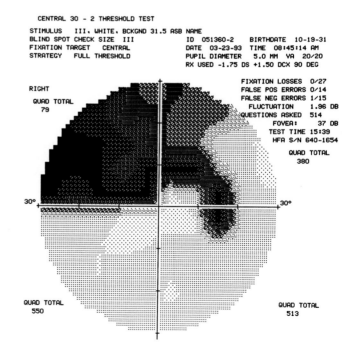

Figure 43–10.
Glaucomatous Visual Field, Arcuate Scotoma: Superior scotoma extending from the physiologic blind spot, arching above central fixation and ending at the nasal horizontal meridian (right eye visual field).

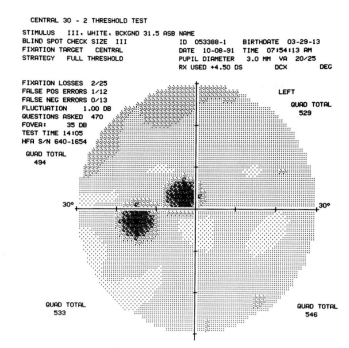

```
CENTRAL 30 - 2 THRESHOLD TEST
STIMULUS   III, WHITE, BCKGND 31.5 ASB NAME
BLIND SPOT CHECK SIZE III            ID  053388-1  BIRTHDATE  03-29-13
FIXATION TARGET   CENTRAL            DATE  10-08-91  TIME  07:54:13 AM
STRATEGY   FULL THRESHOLD            PUPIL DIAMETER   3.0 MM  VA  20/25
                                     RX USED +4.50 DS     DCX        DEG

FIXATION LOSSES  2/25
FALSE POS ERRORS 1/12                                 LEFT
FALSE NEG ERRORS 0/13                                QUAD TOTAL
FLUCTUATION   1.00 DB                                    529
QUESTIONS ASKED  470
FOVEA:    35 DB
TEST TIME 14:05
HFA S/N 640-1654

QUAD TOTAL
   494

30°                                                      30°

QUAD TOTAL                                         QUAD TOTAL
   533                                                546
```

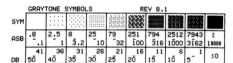

```
GRAYTONE SYMBOLS              REV 8.1
SYM     │ ::: │ :::: │     │     │     │▨▨▨│███│███│███│███│
ASB  .8 │2.5 │8    │25  │79  │251 │794│2512│7943│ ≥ │
     .1 │  1 │3.2  │10  │32  │100 │316│1000│3162│10000│
     41 │ 36 │ 31  │ 26 │ 21 │ 16 │11 │ 6 │ 1 │   │
DB   50 │40  │35   │30  │25  │20  │15 │10 │5  │ ≤0 │
```

DEVERS EYE INSTITUTE
GLAUCOMA SERVICE
1040 NW 22ND AVE.
SUITE 320
PORTLAND, OR. 97210
HUMPHREY INSTRUMENTS
A CARL ZEISS COMPANY

Figure 43–11.
Glaucomatous Visual Field, Paracentral Scotoma: Dense superior scotoma adjacent to central fixation (left eye visual field).

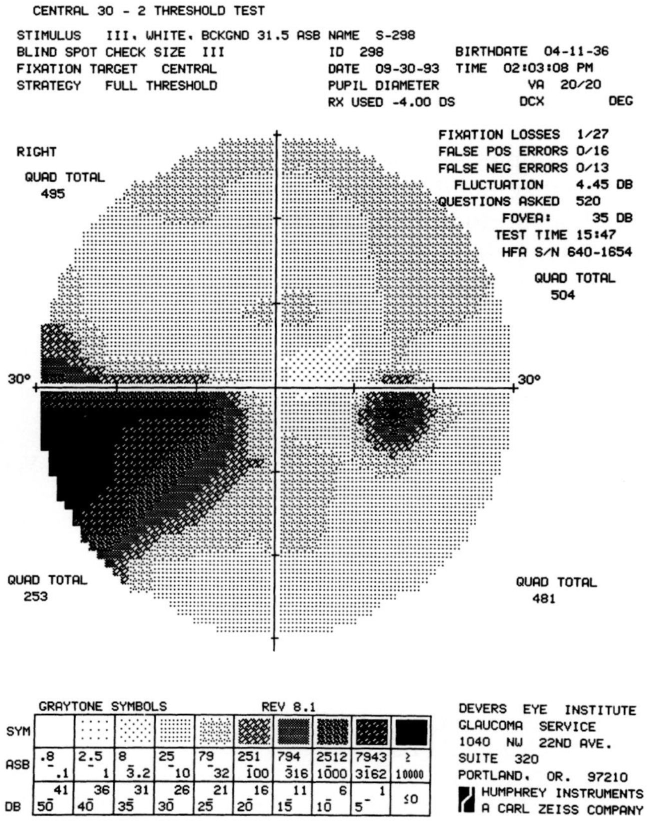

```
CENTRAL 30 - 2 THRESHOLD TEST
STIMULUS   III, WHITE, BCKGND 31.5 ASB NAME  S-298
BLIND SPOT CHECK SIZE III            ID  298       BIRTHDATE  04-11-36
FIXATION TARGET   CENTRAL            DATE  09-30-93  TIME  02:03:08 PM
STRATEGY   FULL THRESHOLD            PUPIL DIAMETER          VA  20/20
                                     RX USED -4.00 DS     DCX        DEG

                                     FIXATION LOSSES  1/27
RIGHT                                FALSE POS ERRORS 0/16
QUAD TOTAL                           FALSE NEG ERRORS 0/13
   495                               FLUCTUATION   4.45 DB
                                     QUESTIONS ASKED  520
                                     FOVEA:    35 DB
                                     TEST TIME 15:47
                                     HFA S/N 640-1654

                                                  QUAD TOTAL
                                                     504

30°                                                      30°

QUAD TOTAL                                         QUAD TOTAL
   253                                                481
```

```
GRAYTONE SYMBOLS              REV 8.1
SYM     │ ::: │ :::: │     │     │     │▨▨▨│███│███│███│███│
ASB  .8 │2.5 │8    │25  │79  │251 │794│2512│7943│ ≥ │
     .1 │  1 │3.2  │10  │32  │100 │316│1000│3162│10000│
     41 │ 36 │ 31  │ 26 │ 21 │ 16 │11 │ 6 │ 1 │   │
DB   50 │40  │35   │30  │25  │20  │15 │10 │5  │ ≤0 │
```

DEVERS EYE INSTITUTE
GLAUCOMA SERVICE
1040 NW 22ND AVE.
SUITE 320
PORTLAND, OR. 97210
HUMPHREY INSTRUMENTS
A CARL ZEISS COMPANY

Figure 43–12.
Glaucomatous Visual Field, Nasal Step: Inferior scotoma extending to the nasal horizontal meridian. Asymmetric loss of superior and inferior visual field results in a nasal step (right eye visual field).

■ SHORT WAVE LENGTH AUTOMATED PERIMETRY

Short wave length automated perimetry (or blue-on-yellow perimetry), is a promising technology that may diagnose glaucomatous visual field loss earlier than traditional white-on-white perimetry (34,53). Short wave length automated perimetry utilizes a yellow background with a blue test stimulus. Short wave length automated perimetry uses the same test strategies and presentation patterns as standard automated perimetry. Recently, investigators have noted that short wave length automated perimetry identifies initial visual field defects in ocular hypertensives 3 to 5 years before standard automated perimetry. Defects localized with short wave length automated perimetry correspond to nerve fiber bundle defects similar to those seen later in the disease with standard automated perimetry. Longitudinal studies of ocular hypertensives have documented that more than 50% of individuals with short wave length automated perimetry deficits go on to develop typical glaucomatous visual field deficits on the standard perimetry within 5 years (35). One of the concerns with short wave length automated perimetry is that ocular media transmission losses produced by yellowing of the crystalline lens may decrease the test's reliability. The validity and long-term importance of short wave length automated perimetry is currently being investigated.

■ OTHER PERIMETRIC TESTS

Many new perimetric tests have been developed in recent years. These include high pass resolution perimetry, scotopic perimetry, motion threshold perimetry, pattern discrimination perimetry, and temporal modulation perimetry. These forms of perimetry are still being investigated for their usefulness in the diagnosis of glaucoma. Because of the specialized instrumentation needed for these techniques, most are not commercially available or commonly used at this time.

■ OTHER PSYCHOPHYSICAL TESTS

Other psychophysical tests are also being investigated in the management and diagnosis of glaucoma. Patterned electroretinography (PERG) is one such test that has shown some promise in the early diagnosis of glaucoma (35, 53). However, because of the expensive instrumentation, the long test times, and the need for skilled testing personnel, the use of PERG is limited at this time. This test is sensitive to ganglion cell and optic nerve dysfunction but is nonspecific for glaucoma. Animal models of glaucoma have shown PERG deficits in nonhuman primates with elevated intraocular pressure, optic nerve cupping, and subsequent histologic changes similar to that found in human glaucoma (35). Longitudinal human studies with PERG have also shown abnormalities 1 to 4 years before abnormalities seen on standard perimetry.

■ REFERENCES

1. Airaksinen PJ, France SM, Douglas GR, et al: Diffuse and localized nerve fiber loss in glaucoma. Am J Ophthal 1984, 98:566.
2. Airaksinen PJ, Nieminen H: Retinal nerve fiber layer photography in glaucoma. Ophthalmology 1985, 92:877.
3. Anderson DR, Grant WM: Re-evaluation of the Schiotz tonometer calibration. Invest Ophthal 1970, 9:430.
4. Armaly MF: Ocular pressure and visual fields, Arch Ophthalmol 1969, 81:25.
5. Aulhorn E and Harms H: Early visual field defects in glaucoma, Glaucoma symposium, Tutzing Castle 1966, Basel, 1967, Karger
6. Aulhorn E and Harms H; Visual perimetry. In: Handbook of sensory physiology vol 7, New York 1972, Springer Verlag.
7. Becker S: Clinical Gonioscopy—A Text and Stereoscopic Atlas. CV Mosby, St. Louis, 1992.
8. Bjerrum JP: Om en tilfojelse til saedvanlige synsfeltundersogelse samt om synfeltet ved glaucokom, Nord Ophthal Tidsskr, Kjobenh 1889, 2:144.
9. Brais P, Drance SM: The temporal field in chronic simple glaucoma. Arch Ophthal 1976, 88:518.
10. Carpel EF, Engstrom PF: The normal cup-disk ratio. Am J Ophthal 1981, 91:588.
11. Chi T, Ritch R, Stickler D, et al: Racial differences in optic nerve head parameters. Arch Ophthal 1989, 107:836.

12. Cioffi GA: Optic nerve head analysis in the 1990's. J Glauc 1993, 2(2)77.

13. Damgaard-Jensen L: Vertical steps in isopters at the hemiopic border—in normal and glaucomatous eyes. Acta Ophthal 1977, 55:111.

14. Donaldson DD: A new camera for stereoscopic fundus photography. Arch Ophthal 1965, 73:253.

15. Draeger J: Simple hand applanation tonometer for use on the seated as well as on the supine patient. Am J Ophthal 1966, 62:1208.

16. Drance SM: The early field defects in glaucoma. Invest Ophthal 1969, 8:84.

17. Drance SM: The glaucomatous visual field. Invest Ophthal 1972, 11:85.

18. Drance SM, Fairclough M, Butler DM, Kottler MS: The importance of disc hemorrhage in the prognosis of chronic open angle glaucoma. Arch Ophthal 1977, 95:226.

19. Durham DG, Bigliano RP, Masino JA: Pneumatic applanation tonometer. Trans Am Acad Ophth Otol 1965, 69:1029.

20. Fishman RS: Optic disc asymmetry. A sign of ocular hypertension. Arch Ophthal 1970, 84:590.

21. Forbes M: Gonioscopy with corneal indentation. Arch Ophthal 1966, 76:488.

22. Friedenwald JS: Some problems in the calibration of tonometers. Am J Ophthal 1948, 31:935.

23. Friedenwald JS: Tonometer calibration: an attempt to remove discrepancies found in the 1954 calibration scale for Schiotz tonometers. Trans Am Acad Ophthal Otol 1957, 61:108.

24. Frisen L: Photography of the retinal nerve fibre layer: an optimized procedure. Br J Ophthal 1980, 64:641.

25. Goldmann H, Schmidt TH: Uber applanationstonometrie. Ophthalmologica 1957, 134:221.

26. Gloster J: Incidence of optic disc hemorrhages in chronic simple glaucoma and ocular hypertension. Br J Ophthal 1981, 65:452.

27. Gloster J, Parry DG: Use of photographs for measuring cupping in the optic disc. Br J Ophthal 1974, 58:850.

28. Goldmann H: Grundlagen exakter Perimetrie, Ophthalmologica 1945, 109:57.

29. Graefe, A von: Uber die Untersuchung des gestichtsfeldes bei amblyopischen Affectionen, Graefes Arch Klin Exp Ophthalmol 1856, 2:258.

30. Harrington DO: The Bjerrum scotoma. Trans Am Ophthal Soc 1964, 62:324.

31. Harrington DO: The Visual Fields. A Textbook and Atlas of Clinical Perimetry, 5th ed. CV Mosby, St. Louis, 1981.

32. Hetherington J Jr: Koeppe lens gonioscopy. In: Controversy in Ophthalmology, Brockhurst FJ, Boruchoff SA, Hutchinson BT, Lessel S, Eds. WB Saunders. Philadelphia 1977, p. 142.

33. Hitchings RA, Spaeth GL: The optic disc in glaucoma. I. Classification. Br J Ophthal 1976, 60:778.

34. Johnson CA, Adams AJ and Lewis RA: Automated perimetry of short-wavelength sensitive mechanisms in glaucoma and ocular hypertension. Preliminary findings. Perimetry Update 1988/89, Kugler and Ghedini, New York, 1989, 31.

35. Johnson CA, Adams AJ and Casson EJ: Short-wavelength-sensitive perimetry (SWSP) can predict which glaucoma suspects will develop visual field loss. Progress in biomedical Optics: Proceedings of Ophthalmic Technologies II, SPIE Publications, 1992, vol 1644:230.

36. Kao SF, Lichter PR, Bergstrom TJ, et al: Clinical comparison of the Oculab Tono-Pen to the Goldmann applanation tonometer. Ophthalmology 1987, 94:1541.

37. Kirsch RE, Anderson DR: Clinical recognition of glaucomatous cupping. Am J Ophthal 1973, 75:442.

38. Langerhorst CT, Van den Berg TJ, Greve EL: Is there general reduction of sensitivity in glaucoma? Internat Ophthal 1989, 13:31.

39. Lynn JR, and Tate GW: Computer controlled apparatus for automatic visual field examination, US patent 3,883,234, issued May 1975.

40. Mackay RS, Marg E: Fast, automatic, electronic tonometers based on an exact theory. Acta Ophthal 1959, 37:495.

41. Maklakoff A: L'ophthalmotonometrie. Arch Ophthmol. Paris 1885, 5:159.

42. Mikelberg FS, Drance SM: The mode of progression of visual field defects in glaucoma. Am J Ophthal 1984, 98:443.

43. Miller KM, Quigley HA: The clinical appearance of the lamina cribrosa as a function of the extent of glaucomatous optic nerve damage. Ophthalmology 1988, 95:135.

44. Moses RA: The Goldmann applanation tonometer. Am J Ophthal 1958, 46:865.

45. Perkins ES: Hand-held applanation tonometer. Br J Ophthal 1965, 49:591.

46. Purkinje JE: Beobachtungen und Versuche zur physiologie der sinne, Berlin, G Reimer 1825, 2:6.

47. Quigley HA, Addicks EM, Green WR: Optic nerve damage in human glaucoma. III. Quantitative correlation of nerve fiber loss and visual field defect in glaucoma, ischemic neuropathy, papilledema, and toxic neuropathy. Arch Ophthal 1982, 100:135.

48. Quigley HA, Brown AE, Morrison JC, Drance SM: The size and shape of the optic disc in normal human eyes. Arch Ophthal 1990, 108:51.

49. Read RM, Spaeth GL: The practical clinical appraisal of the optic disc in glaucoma: the natural history of cup progression and some specific disc-field correlations. Trans Am Acad Ophthal Otol 1974, 78:255.

50. Repka MX, Uozato H, Guyton DL: Depth distortion during slitlamp biomicroscopy of the fundus. Ophthalmology 1986, 93(S):47.

51. Ronne H: Ueber des Geischtfeld beim Glaukom, Klin Monatsbl Augenheilk 1909, 47:12.

52. Rosenwasser, GOD, Tiedeman JS: A stable slit lamp mounting device for 90 D lens use in non-contact ophthalmoscopy. Ophthalmic Surg 1986, 17:525.

53. Sample PA and Weinreb RN: Color perimetry for assessment of primary open angle glaucoma. Investigative Ophthal and Vis Sci, 1990, 31:1869.

54. Schiotz HJ: Ein neues tonometer. ARch Augenheilkd 1905, 52:401.

55. Schwartz B: New techniques for the examination of the optic disc and their clinical application. Trans Am Acad Ophthal Otol 1976, 81:227.

56. Schwartz B: Slit lamp gonioscopy. In: Controversy in Ophthalmology, Brockhust, RJ, Boruschoff SA, Hutchinson BT, Lessell S, eds. WB Saunders, Philadelphia, 1977, p. 146.

57. Sharma NK, Hitchings RA: A comparison of monocular and stereoscopic photographs of the optic disc in the identification of glaucomatous visual field defects. Br Ophthal 1983, 67:677.

58. Shields MB: The future of computerized image analysis in the management of glaucoma. Am J Ophthal 1989, 108:315.

59. Shihab ZM, Lee P-F: The significance of normal angle vessels. Ophthal Surg 1985, 16:382.

60. Sommer A, Quigley HA, Robin AL, et al: Evaluation of nerve fiber layer assessment. Arch Ophthal 1984, 102:1776.

61. Sutton GE, Motolko MA, Phelps CD: Baring of a circulinear vessel in glaucoma. Arch Ophthal 1983, 101:739.

62. Traquair HM: Introduction to clinical perimetry, London, 1927, Kimpton.

63. Young T: The Baerian Lecture. On the mechanism of the eye. Philos Trans R Soc Long (Biol) 1801, 91:23.

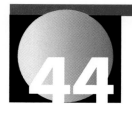

44 Anatomy of the Optic Nerve

G. A. Cioffi, E. M. Van Buskirk

■ THE OPTIC NERVE

The optic nerve is the connection between the neurosensory retina and the lateral geniculate body. The nerve is primarily composed of neural fibers (the retinal ganglion cell axons), glial cells and extracellular matrix supportive tissue, and vascular elements (1, 6, 9, 11, 13). The optic nerve "head" refers to the anterior surface of the optic nerve seen during funduscopic examination (see Clinical Testing, Figures 43–6 and 43–7). The neural component of the optic nerve is composed of approximately 1.2 to 1.5 million axons. The intraorbital optic nerve is divided into two components: the anterior optic nerve and the posterior optic nerve. The anterior optic nerve extends from the retinal surface to the posterior aspect of the globe. The posterior optic nerve transits the orbit from the globe to the optic canal. The diameter of the optic nerve head and anterior portion of the optic nerve is approximately 1.5 mm (10). The optic nerve expands to approximately 3 to 4 mm in diameter upon exiting the globe. This increase in diameter is accounted for by glial tissue, the leptomeninges (optic nerve sheath), and the beginning of the axonal myelination.

Retinal ganglion cell axons, or *"nerve fibers,"* converge radially to form the optic nerve as they abruptly turn posteriorly to exit the eye through the lamina cribrosa. The nerve fibers enter the optic nerve from the retina in a characteristic pattern (Figure 44–1). Fibers entering the superior and inferior temporal aspects of the optic nerve are termed "arcuate" nerve fibers and originate from the peripheral retina, taking an arcuate course around the macula to enter the nerve (18, 19). These are the fibers most susceptible to damage in early glaucomatous optic neuropathy. Fibers originating from the macular region, or the "papillomacular fibers," occupy approximately one-third of the temporal optic nerve. Arcuate nerve fibers originate either superior to or inferior to the median raphe and arch above or below the fovea. Papillomacular fibers take a more direct course from the macular and perimacular region to the optic nerve. Other nerve fibers from the superior, inferior, and nasal retina radially converge at the nerve as shown in Figure 44–1.

The anterior optic nerve may be divided conveniently into four anatomic regions (1, 16, 17) (Figures 44–2 and 44–3). The most anterior zone is the superficial nerve fiber layer region which is continuous with the nerve fiber layer of the retina. This region is primarily composed of the axons of the retinal ganglion cells in transition from the superficial retina to the neuronal component of the optic nerve. Immediately posterior to the nerve fiber layer is the prelaminar region, which lies adjacent to the peripapillary choroid. More posteriorly, the laminar region is continuous with the sclera and is composed of the lamina cribrosa, a structure consisting of fenestrated, connective tissue lamellae which allow the transit of neural fibers through the scleral coat (6, 16, 17). Finally, the retro-laminar region lies posterior to the lamina cribrosa, is marked by the beginning of axonal myelination, and is surrounded by the leptomeninges of the central nervous system.

The lamina cribrosa is composed of a series of fenestrated sheets of connective tissue and elastic fibers. This layer provides the main support for the optic nerve as it exits the eye and penetrates the scleral coat. The beams of connective tissue are composed primarily of collagen and other extracellular matrix components,

591

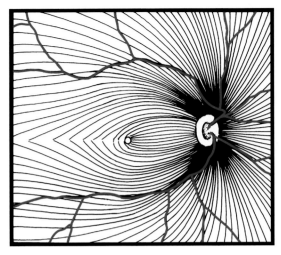

Figure 44–1.
Nerve Fiber Layer Organization: The retinal nerve fibers (ganglion cell axons) converged at the optic nerve. Arcuate fibers extend from the temporal retina above and below the fovea to the optic nerve. Papillomacular fibers take a more direct rout to the optic nerve.

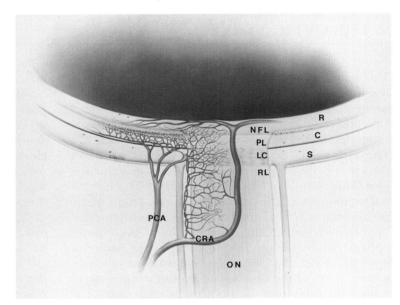

Figure 44–2.
Anterior Optic Nerve Vasculature: Arterial supply to the anterior optic nerve and peripapillary choroids. Lamina Cribrosa (LC), Superficial Nerve Fiber Layer (NFL), Prelamina (PL), Retrolamina (RL), Cranial Retinal Artery (CRA), Optic Nerve (ON), Choroid (C), Posterior Ciliary Artery (PCA), Retina (R), Sclera (S). (Reprinted by permission of G.A. Cioffi, The Glaucomas, eds. Ritch R, Shields MB, Krupin T, Mosby, 1996, p178, Figure 8–2).

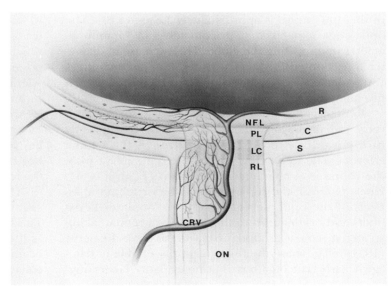

Figure 44–3.
Anterior Optic Nerve Vasculature: Venous drainage of the anterior optic nerve and peripapillary choroid. Lamina Cribrosa (LC), Nerve Fiber Layer (NFL), Prelamina (PL), Retrolamina (RL), Choroid (C), Optic Nerve (ON), Central Retinal Vein (CRV), Vortex Vein (VV). (Reprinted by permission of G.A. Cioffi, The Glaucomas, eds. Ritch R, Shields MB, Krupin T, Mosby, 1996, p 183, Figure 8–12).

such as elastin, laminin, and fibronectin. These connective tissue beams are perforated by various size fenestrations through which the neural component of the optic nerve passes. Central, larger fenestrae allow transit of the central retinal artery and central retinal vein. The fenestrations within the lamina are, histologically, larger superiorly and inferiorly as compared with the temporal and nasal aspects of the optic nerve. Supposedly, these regional differences in the fenestrae play a role in the development of glaucomatous optic neuropathy. The fenestrations of the laminar cribrosa are often seen at the base of the optic nerve head cup on ophthalmoscopic examination. Between the optic nerve and the adjacent peripapillary tissue lies a rim of connective tissue, the border tissue of Elschnig (3). The connective tissue beams of the laminar cribrosa extend from this surrounding connective tissue border and are arranged in a series of parallel stacked plates.

■ VASCULATURE OF THE ANTERIOR OPTIC NERVE AND PERIPAPILLARY REGION

The vascular anatomy of the anterior optic nerve and peripapillary region has been extensively studied. The precise microvascular anatomy of this region remains difficult to ascertain owing to the small vessel caliber, the complex three-dimensional angio-architecture, and the relative inaccessibility of the tissue. A detailed knowledge of the microvascular supply and drainage of the optic nerve and peripapillary region must underpin any understanding of the possible role of the vascular system in glaucoma.

■ GENERAL ANATOMY OF THE ARTERIAL SUPPLY

The arterial supply of the anterior optic nerve is derived entirely from branches of the ophthalmic artery. One to five posterior ciliary arteries divide from the ophthalmic artery, itself a branch of the internal carotid artery, in the posterior orbit (1, 4, 13). Typically, between two and four posterior ciliary arteries course anteriorly before dividing into approximately 10 to 20 short posterior ciliary arteries, just before entering the posterior globe. Often, the posterior ciliary arteries separate into a medial and a lateral group before branching into the short posterior ciliary arteries. In addition, the long posterior ciliary arteries, which are also branches of the posterior ciliary arteries, course anteriorly along the outside of the globe before penetrating the sclera to supply the iris, ciliary body, and the anterior region of the choroid.

The short posterior ciliary arteries penetrate the sclera surrounding the optic nerve to supply the peripapillary choroid and the majority of anterior optic nerve. Some short posterior ciliary arteries course, without branching, through the sclera directly into the choroid; others divide within the sclera to provide branches to both the choroid and the optic nerve. Often a noncontinuous, arterial circle exists within the perineural sclera, known as the circle of Zinn-Haller (Figures 44–2 and 44–4). This structure is formed by the confluence of branches of the short posterior ciliary arteries. This arterial circle may completely encircle the optic nerve or may be interrupted along its course. This arterial circle provides multiple perforating branches into the various regions of the anterior optic nerve, to the peripapillary choroid, and to the pial arterial sys-

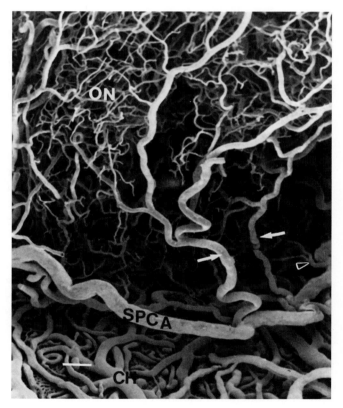

Figure 44–4.
Primate Optic Nerve Vascular Corrosion Casting: Posterior view of the optic nerve vasculature entering the glove. The short posterior ciliary artery (SPCA) gives brances to the laminar (arrowhead) and the retrolaminar (arrows) regions. Optic Nerve (ON); Choroid (CH). (Reprinted by permission of Cioffi GA, J. Glaucoma, 3(S1):S45–54, 1994, Figure 8).

tem. The central retinal artery, also a posterior orbital branch of the ophthalmic artery, penetrates the optic nerve approximately 10 to 15 mm behind the globe.

The central retinal artery has few if any intraneural branches; the exception being an occasional small branch within the retro-laminar region.

REGIONS OF THE ANTERIOR OPTIC NERVE: ARTERIAL SUPPLY

Superficial Nerve Fiber Layer

The superficial nerve fiber layer is supplied principally by recurrent retinal arterioles branching from the central retinal artery. As the central retinal artery emerges from within the optic nerve, it branches into a superior and an inferior trunk. From these major trunks, as well as from more distal branches, small arterioles emerge to supply the superficial nerve fiber layer of the optic nerve and peripapillary retina (Figure 44–5). The capillary branches from these vessels are continuous with the retinal capillaries at the disk margin, but they also have posterior anastomoses with the prelaminar capillaries of the optic nerve. No direct choroidal or choriocapillaris contribution is observed in this region.

Prelaminar Region

The prelaminar region is principally supplied by direct branches of the short posterior ciliary arteries and by branches of the circle of Zinn-Haller, when it is present (Figure 44–2)(Figure 44–4). In eyes with a well-developed circle of Zinn-Haller, arterial branches emerge to supply both the prelaminar and laminar regions. Some investigators have described large choroidal arteries from the peripapillary choroid or from the choriocapillaris to the prelaminar region. There are branches from the circle of Zinn-Haller and from the short posterior ciliary arteries which course through the choroid and ultimately supply the optic nerve in this region. These vessels do not arise from the choroid but merely pass through it. The direct arterial supply to the prelaminar region arising from the choroidal vasculature is minimal. Several, small centripetal arteries or arterioles branch from the larger vessels of the peripapillary choroid, but no direct connection between the peripapillary choriocapillaris and the prelaminar region exists.

Laminar Region

The lamina cribrosa region also receives its blood supply from branches of the short posterior ciliary arteries, or from branches of the circle of Zinn-Haller; this is similar to the prelaminar region (Figures 44–2 and 44–4). These precapillary branches perforate the outer aspects of the lamina cribrosa before branching into an intraseptal capillary network. As in the prelaminar region, the larger vessels of the peripapillary choroid may con-

tribute occasional small arterioles to this region, although there is no connection between the peripapillary choriocapillaris and the capillaries of the optic nerve.

Retro-laminar Region

The retro-laminar region is also supplied by branches from the short posterior ciliary arteries, as well as the pial arterial branches (Figures 44–2 and 44–4). The pial

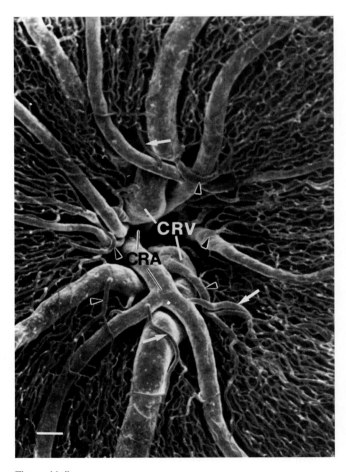

Figure 44–5.
Primate Optic Nerve Vascular Corrosion Casting: Anterior view of the optic nerve vasculature. The arterial supply (arrow) to the superficial nerve fiber layer derives from the central retinal artery (CRA) and the venous drainage (arrowhead) is via the central retinal vein (CRV). (Reprinted by permission of Cioffi GA, J Glaucoma, 3(S1):S45–54, 1994, Figure 3).

arteries originate from both the central retinal artery before it pierces the retrobulbar optic nerve and branches of the short posterior ciliary arteries more anteriorly. The central retinal artery may supply several small intraneural branches in the retro-laminar region. These small intraneural branches of the central retinal artery anastomose with the capillary network supplied by the pial and the short posterior ciliary arteries.

With the exceptions of the superficial nerve fiber layer branches of the central retinal artery, the occasional retro-laminar branches of the central retinal artery, and the small contribution of the choroidal vasculature to the prelaminar and laminar regions, the principal arterial supply to the anterior optic nerve is derived from the short posterior ciliary arteries.

Capillary Angio-architecture

The rich capillary beds of each of the four anatomic regions within the anterior optic nerve are anatomically confluent. These capillary interconnections unite the microvasculature along the length of the anterior optic nerve. Capillaries in the nerve fiber layer region are continuous with the retinal capillaries at the disk margin. More posteriorly, the capillaries of the nerve fiber layer region form a complicated plexus which interconnects with the capillaries of the prelaminar regions. The capillaries of the laminar region conform to the pattern of the connective tissue septae which compose the laminar supportive architecture. Capillaries in the laminar region are organized in the polygonal pattern of the laminar septae.

The arterioles along the periphery of the optic nerve have a limited smooth muscle layer surrounding the endothelial layer. The capillary network of the anterior optic nerve is composed of nonfenestrated vessels, similar to the capillaries of the retina. These capillaries are comprised of a single layer of tight-junctioned endothelial cells surrounded by supportive glial tissue and intermittent pericytes.

Venous Drainage

Remarkably, in view of the abundant arterial supply from many source vessels, the venous drainage of the anterior optic nerve is almost exclusively via a single vein, the central retinal vein. In the nerve fiber layer, blood is drained directly into the retinal veins which then join to form the central retinal vein (Figure 44–3). In the prelaminar, laminar, and retro-laminar regions, venous drainage also occurs via the central retinal vein or axial tributaries to the central retinal vein. Occasionally, small venules connecting the optic nerve and the peripapillary choroid can be identified, mainly within the prelaminar region.

Peripapillary Choroidal Microvasculature

The peripapillary choroid is primarily supplied by the short posterior ciliary arteries. The choroid is a rich vascular layer which nourishes the outer retina and retinal pigment endothelium. The outer choroid is composed of large nonfenestrated vessels, and the vessel caliber of the inner choroidal layers is smaller. The innermost layer of the choroid, the choriocapillaris, is composed of richly anastomotic, fenestrated capillaries beginning at the optic disk margin. The capillaries of the choriocapillaris are separate and distinct from the capillary beds of the anterior optic nerve. The arterial supply of the peripapillary choroid originates from branches of the short posterior ciliary arteries, either directly or via the arterial circle of Zinn-Haller. These branches supply the outer choroid and the choriocapillaris. Some branches from the circle of Zinn-Haller and short posterior ciliary arteries which ultimately supply the optic nerve, also course through the choroid. As previously mentioned, the peripapillary choroid may give off many small branches into the prelaminar and laminar region. Choroidal veins drain into the vortex venous system.

Variability of Vascular Patterns

There is marked inter-individual variation in the vascular patterns of the anterior optic nerve and peripapillary region. Among individuals, the predominant variability is observed in the arterial supply. The posterior ciliary arteries vary in number, distribution, and caliber. These arteries may be distributed only medially and laterally, or a third superior grouping may be present (5, 7, 8, 12, 15). The grouping of these vessels into lateral and medial groups could play a role in the clinical presentations subsequent to an ischemic insult. The distribution of the posterior ciliary arteries may explain the altitudinal visual field defects seen after anterior ischemic optic neuropathy, the nasal visual field loss seen in glaucoma, and the arcuate field loss seen in acute optic nerve infarction. These hypotheses rely heavily on physiologic inference from anatomic findings and thus, remain unproven.

■ REFERENCES

1. Anderson DR: Ultrastructure of human and monkey lamina cribrosa and optic nerve head. Arch Ophthal 1969, 82:800.

2. Anderson, DR. Vascular supply to the optic nerve of primates. Am J Ophthalmol 1970;70:341.

3. Anderson DR, Hoyt WF: Ultrastructure of intraorbital

portion of human and monkey optic nerve. Arch Ophthal 1969, 82:506.

4. Cioffi GA, Van Buskirk EM: Vasculature Anatomy of the Optic Nerve. In: The Glaucomas, Ritch R, Shields MR, Krupin T (ed) CV Mosby, St. Louis, Chapter 8, In Press.

5. Geijssen, HC. Studies on normal pressure glaucoma. New York: Kugler, 1991;pp 8–31.

6. Hayreh SS: Anatomy and physiology of the optic nerve head. Trans Am Acad Ophthal Otol 1974, 78:240.

7. Hayreh, SS. Anterior ischemic optic neuropathy. Arch Neurol 1981;38:675.

8. Hayreh, SS. Inter-individual variation in blood supply of the optic nerve head. Its importance in various ischemic disorders of the nerve head, and glaucoma, low-tension glaucoma and allied disorders. Doc Ophthalmol 1985;59:217.

9. Hernandez MR, Luo XX, Igoe F, Neufeld AH: Extracellu-arl matrix of the human lamina cribrosa. Am J Ophthal 1987, 104:567.

10. Jonas JB, Gusek GC, Guggenmoos-Holtzmann I, Naumann GOH: Size of the optic nerve scleral canal and comparison with intravital determination of optic disc dimensions. Graef's Arch Ophthal 1988, 226:213.

11. Kronfeld PC: Normal variations of the optic disc as observed by conventional ophthalmoscopy and their anatomic correlations. Trans Am Acad Ophthal Otol 1976, 81:214.

12. Lichter, PR, and Henderson, JW. Optic nerve infarction. Am J Ophthalmol 1978;85:302.

13. Liebermann MF, Maumenee AE, Green WR: Histologic studies of the vasculature of the anterior optic nerve. Am J Ophthal 1976, 82:405.

14. Minkler, DS. Histology of optic nerve damage in ocular hypertension and early glaucoma. Surv Ophthalmol 1989;33:401.

15. Olver, JM, Spalton, DJ, and McCartney, ACE. Microvascular study of the retrolaminar optic nerve in man: the possible significance in anterior ischaemic optic neuropathy. Eye 1990;4:7.

16. Quigley HA, Addicks EM: Regional differences in the structure,of the lamina cribroasa and their relationship to glaucomatous optic nerve damage. Arch Ophthalmol 1981, 99:137.

17. Radius, RL, and Gonzales, M. Anatomy at the lamina cribrosa in human eyes. Arch Ophthalmol 1981;99:2159.

18. Radius RL, Anderson DR: The course of axons through the retina and optic nerve head. Arch Ophthal 1979, 97:115.

19. Radius RL, Anderson DR: The histology of retinal nerve fiber layer bundles and bundle defects. Arch Ophthal 1979, 97:948.

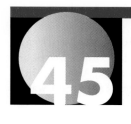

45 Clinical Manifestations of the Glaucomas

Open-Angle Glaucoma

G. A. Cioffi, E. M. Van Buskirk

■ PRIMARY OPEN-ANGLE GLAUCOMA

Primary open-angle glaucoma (POAG) is characterized by the development of glaucomatous optic neuropathy in an eye with a normal-appearing anterior chamber angle and absence of other ocular or systemic disorders which may account for the optic nerve damage. Most cases of primary open-angle glaucoma are associated with statistically elevated intraocular pressure. Primary open-angle glaucoma is also called chronic open-angle glaucoma or simple open-angle glaucoma. POAG is the most common form of glaucoma. It is typically a bilateral disease but may be asymmetric.

The prevalence of POAG is approximately 0.5 to 1% of the adult population in the United States (28). The prevalence of POAG increases sharply with increasing age. Individuals in the fifth decade of life have a prevalence of approximately 0.25%, while individuals in the ninth decade of life have a prevalence greater than 10%. Blacks have an increased risk of developing POAG as compared with whites (46). POAG in blacks is typically more severe and onset occurs at an earlier age.

Blacks have between a fourfold and sixfold increase in risk of developing POAG as compared with whites (76). There does not appear to be a sex predilection for POAG. The risk of developing POAG is greater in persons with a positive family history of glaucoma among close relatives. Diabetes mellitus and systemic hypertension have also been associated with an increased risk of developing POAG. Myopia is a risk factor for the development of POAG. As previously mentioned, elevation of intraocular pressure is one of the most significant risk factors for the development of POAG. The higher the intraocular pressure, the more likely that glaucomatous optic nerve damage will develop in POAG (56). Intraocular pressure fluctuations are greater in eyes with POAG than in normal eyes. The increase of intraocular pressure and the development of glaucomatous optic neuropathy typically progress slowly. Intraocular pressures in the range of 20 to 45mm Hg are most commonly found in POAG.

■ PATHOGENESIS OF POAG

A variety of theories have attempted to explain the elevation of intraocular pressure in POAG. The rate of aqueous humor production is normal in POAG, but aqueous humor outflow is decreased. However, the exact mechanism of outflow obstruction is not fully understood. Restriction of aqueous outflow within the trabecular meshwork or between the trabecular meshwork and Schlemm's canal are the most likely sites of obstruction. Although much of the resistance of normal outflow is created in the various layers of the trabecular meshwork, no consistent anatomic abnormalities have been identified in POAG eyes to explain the decrease in outflow facility. Narrowing of the intratrabecular spaces and occlusion of these spaces by abnormally produced substances may contribute to a decrease in outflow. Glycosaminoglycans have been reported to be more abundant in the trabecular meshwork in eyes with POAG and may mechanically block outflow at the level of the trabecular meshwork (3, 41). As previously noted, the transition area between the trabecular meshwork and Schlemm's canal, the juxtacanalicular connective tissue, is the point of highest outflow resistance. Abnormalities in the transit of aqueous humor across the inner wall of Schlemm's canal may contribute to intraocular pressure elevations in POAG. Physical alterations in Schlemm's canal itself, with possible collapse of the canal, also may contribute to outflow abnormalities. Immunologic abnormalities associated with increased gamma globulins and plasma cells in the trabecular meshwork of POAG patients have also been reported (9). These studies, among others, have raised the question of a possible immunologic or autoimmune mechanism in the development of POAG.

■ TREATMENT OF POAG

The medical and surgical options for the management of POAG are outlined in Glaucoma Therapy (Chapter 47). However, several important considerations should be noted when treating patients with POAG. In general, pressures in the high teens or low 20s are acceptable in patients with minimal optic nerve damage. In more advanced glaucomatous optic neuropathy cases, intraocular pressure levels should be reduced to lower levels to decrease the chance of glaucomatous optic nerve damage progression in these eyes with a minimum neural reserve.

When initiating medical therapy in POAG patients, a "one-eyed trial" is appropriate. Administering topical medications in one eye of a patient with bilaterally elevated intraocular pressure will allow the clinician to assess the efficacy of the therapy by comparing the intraocular pressures of the two eyes. This is done with the realization that some topical therapies have crossover effects (that these therapies will reduce intraocular pressure in the contralateral eye), but that intraocular pressure lowering is normally significantly greater in the treated eye, if the therapy is effective. Both aqueous humor suppressants and aqueous humor outflow enhancers may be used for this therapy. The one-eyed trial helps eliminate incorrect clinical assumptions of medical efficacy because of diurnal variations in the intraocular pressure. Laser trabeculoplasty is effective in patients with POAG and may be used in patients who poorly tolerate medical therapy or if medical therapy is insufficient. Surgical intervention is generally reserved for patients who fail medical and/or laser therapy. Surgical therapy should not be reserved as a last alternative in eyes with only severe glaucomatous optic neuropathy but should be instituted at any point in the therapeutic course in which other modalities have failed. Early or initial surgical intervention is recommended by some clinicians in lieu of medical or laser therapy.

The goal of intraocular pressure reduction is to slow or halt the progression of glaucomatous visual field loss and optic nerve damage. Intraocular pressure reduction alone may not stop progression, but it remains the mainstay of therapy and should be initiated in POAG. Some patients may have continued visual field loss despite maximal lowering of intraocular pressure. These patients obviate the need for new therapeutic modalities aimed at maintaining and protecting the optic nerve from progressive glaucomatous nerve damage. A pilot study of 25 glaucoma patients with normal intraocular pressures examined the use of calcium channel blockers to prevent visual field loss. Oral nifedipine showed some promise of protecting patients from loss of vision, and it was suggested that decreased vasospasm of the optic nerve vasculature may be responsible (1). More work in such therapeutic modalities is needed.

■ SECONDARY OPEN-ANGLE GLAUCOMA

Secondary open-angle glaucomas are characterized by glaucomatous optic neuropathy in eyes with elevated intraocular pressure, developmentally normal and open (not obstructed by the peripheral iris) anterior chamber angles, and the absence of systemic disorders which may account for the optic nerve damage. In secondary open-angle glaucoma, the aqueous outflow obstruction is the result of exogenous or intraocular factors, and not a primary abnormality of the trabecular meshwork, as is found in primary open-angle glaucoma.

Pigmentary Dispersion Syndrome and Pigmentary Glaucoma

Pigmentary dispersion syndrome was described approximately 50 years ago and is frequently associated with a secondary open-angle glaucoma (22). Pigmentary dispersion syndrome is classically seen in young, myopic males in the third and fourth decades of life. Melanin granules are dispersed throughout the aqueous humor. Acute dispersion may be exacerbated by pharmacologic pupillary dilation or physical activity. Melanin granules are also found adherent to the posterior surface of the cornea, oriented in a vertical pattern which is heavier centrally and inferiorly. The vertical arrangement of the adherence to the endothelial surface of the cornea is believed to be secondary to the aqueous humor convection currents in the anterior chamber. This posterior corneal pigmentation pattern is referred to as a *Krukenberg's spindle* (77). Pigment deposits also occur on the peripheral lens, the anterior iris surface, the lenticular zonules, and along the interface between the anterior vitreous and the posterior lens. Other clinical features of pigment dispersion syndrome include radial transillumination defects of the iris and abundant pigmentation in the anterior chamber angle. Pigmentary glaucoma is a form of secondary open-angle glaucoma, with elevated intraocular pressure resulting from the dispersion of pigment in the anterior segment of the eye. Although it was originally thought to be a rare form of secondary open-angle glaucoma, it is now recognized with increased frequency, especially in white males.

Melanin liberated from the pigmented epithelial layers of the posterior surface of the iris into the aqueous humor ultimately obstructs outflow through the trabecular meshwork. Several theories have been proposed concerning the cause of this pigment dispersion. Pigment dispersion is believed to occur because of mechanical rubbing between the peripheral iris and the packets of lenticular zonules. Some authors believe that there is an abnormality of the iris pigment epithelium resulting in inappropriate liberation of the pigment (65). Others have proposed that abnormalities of the anterior segment anatomy, with an abnormally deep anterior chamber and posterior bowing of the peripheral iris, account for the pigment dispersion (12). These anatomic anomalies result in the rubbing of the iris on the lens zonules. Supporters of this hypothesis point to gonioscopic findings of a posteriorly displaced peripheral iris in patients with pigmentary dispersion syndrome. Whatever the exact cause of the pigment dispersion, there is almost uniform agreement that increased intraocular pressure results from progressive outflow obstruction as pigment granules become enmeshed in the trabecular meshwork.

The differential diagnosis of pigmentary dispersion syndrome includes other secondary open-angle glaucomas and ocular disorders. Dispersion of pigment granules into the anterior chamber can result from ocular trauma, intraocular tumors, or after intraocular hemorrhage, during which breakdown products of blood may be confused with pigment granules. After blunt trauma, marked amounts of pigment may be seen floating in the anterior chamber. Intraocular tumors may also liberate pigment into the anterior chamber. Glaucomas associated with ocular trauma and intraocular tumors are discussed further in this text. Pseudoexfoliation glaucoma may appear clinically similar to pigmentary dispersion glaucoma, with pigment granules on the anterior surface of the iris, increased pigment in the anterior chamber angle, and a secondary open-angle glaucoma.

The management of pigmentary glaucoma includes standard antiglaucoma medications to suppress aqueous production or enhance aqueous outflow. In addition, Campbell suggested that miotics may mechanically reduce the contact between the peripheral iris and lens zonules, thereby eliminating progressive pigment dispersion (12). However, miotics should be used with caution because several authors have noted a higher-than-normal incidence of retinal detachments in patients with pigmentary dispersion syndrome. An association between lattice degeneration of the retina and pigment dispersion syndrome has been observed (94). Young myopic patients with pigmentary glaucoma tolerate miotic therapy poorly. Argon laser trabeculoplasty is effective in pigmentary dispersion glaucoma, especially in younger patients (22). When both medical and laser therapy fail, pigmentary dispersion glaucoma patients do well with filtration surgery. Antimetabolites as adjunctive therapy to the filtration surgery may improve success, because of the young age of this patient population.

■ PSEUDOEXFOLIATION SYNDROME AND GLAUCOMA

Pseudoexfoliation syndrome, characterized by deposits of white, fibrillar material on the anterior lens surface and throughout the anterior chamber, is associated with a secondary open-angle glaucoma. Vogt is credited, in the mid-1920s, with the original description of white flakes on the anterior surface of the lens being associated with glaucoma in some patients (83). He referred to this as "senile exfoliation" of the lens. Dvorak-Theobald recommended the term "pseudoexfoliation" of the lens capsule when referring to this syndrome to separate it from true exfoliation (20). The association of pseudoexfoliation syndrome and glaucoma varies throughout the world (66). In Sweden and Norway, over 60% of open-angle glaucoma patients have pseudoexfoliation syndrome. In the United States, this association falls well below 15%. The prevalence of pseudoexfoliation syndrome (without glaucoma) varies widely among reports and in various geographic regions. The prevalence of pseudoexfoliation syndrome in the United States is between 1 and 5% of the population and increases with age. In Scandinavian countries, however, pseudoexfoliation syndrome is found in over 50% of the population. No clear hereditary patterns have been identified in pseudoexfoliation syndrome. Throughout the world, women are found to have a slightly higher prevalence of the syndrome, but the incidence of glaucoma in the syndrome shows no sex predilection.

Most of the characteristic clinical findings associated with pseudoexfoliation syndrome are secondary to the deposit of a whitish, fibrillar material on the various structures of the anterior segment of the eye. Classically, the material is deposited on the central portion of the anterior lens capsule in a circular pattern with a surrounding clear zone (Figure 45–1). With pupillary dilation, this clear zone can be identified, and a second zone of deposition is seen on the peripheral lens surface and anterior surface of the zonules. The material deposited on the central surface of the lens may have scroll-like edges and appear much the same as true exfoliation of the lens. The more peripheral deposits on the anterior lens assume the radial orientation of the underlying zonular attachments to the lens. White flecks of the pseudoexfoliation material may also be seen on the pupillary margin of the iris, as well as on the anterior surface of the iris. Peripupillary iris atrophy is often present with loss of pigmentation and transillumination defects. Similar deposits may be found on the endothelial surface of the cornea and in the anterior chamber angle. Hypoperfusion and neovascularization of the iris have been reported in the late stages of pseudoexfoliation syndrome.

Iridodonesis and phacodonesis may also occur with this syndrome. Gonioscopic findings are noteworthy, not only for pseudoexfoliation deposits, but also for increased pigmentation of the angle structures. Pigmentation of the angle structures is usually patchy in pseudoexfoliation syndrome, as compared with the more uniform pigment distribution seen in pigmentary dis-

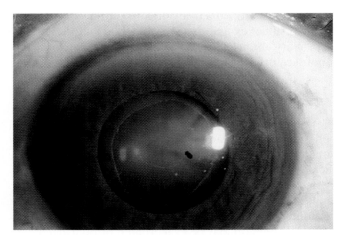

Figure 45–1.
Pseudoexfoliation Syndrome: Pseudoexfoliation material on the anterior surface of the lens. Note the fibrillar deposits centrally with a surrounding clear zone and the radial arrangement of the deposits on the peripheral lens.

persion syndrome. In addition, a line of pigment deposition anterior to Schwalbe's line is often present in pseudoexfoliation syndrome (Sampaolesis' line) (59, 66). Decreased density of corneal endothelial cells may be seen by specular microscopy in this syndrome. Intraocular pressure elevation may occur months to years after the discovery of pseudoexfoliation syndrome. Intraocular pressures tend to be greater in the eye with the more significant deposition of pseudoexfoliation material when the deposition is asymmetric. Clinical findings of pseudoexfoliation syndrome may be asymmetric between the two eyes, and although unilateral cases of pseudoexfoliation have been reported, most cases are bilateral.

The pseudoexfoliation material is a fibrillar protein with many characteristics of the connective and elastic tissues of basement membrane. Debate over the source of the pseudoexfoliation material continues. Some investigators think the material is derived from the lens epithelium, while others believe its source may be multifocal (59, 66). The material has been found in the basement membranes of the ciliary body, iris, trabecular meshwork, conjunctival vessels, and iris vessels, as well as on the lens surface. Although the actual source of the exfoliation material is not known, it is generally accepted that elevation of intraocular pressure results from obstruction of the trabecular meshwork by the fibrillar material. Some studies have suggested that there is also an underlying baseline deficiency of aqueous humor outflow in these eyes. Other investigators believe that pseudoexfoliative glaucoma is an ocular manifestation of a systemic disease.

The differential diagnosis of pseudoexfoliation syndrome includes true exfoliation of the lens and pigmentary glaucoma (see Pigmentary Dispersion Syndrome and Pigmentary Glaucoma). In 1917, Lindberg described a case of chronic glaucoma associated with exfoliative material on the anterior lens surface (43). It was later determined that the white flakes seen by Lindberg actually represented true exfoliation of the anterior lens capsule. True exfoliation of the anterior capsule of the crystalline lens appears as white, scroll-like projections, similar in appearance to pseudoexfoliation and capsular separation from the underlying lens. Also, it is typically secondary to infrared radiation exposure (glass blower's cataracts).

The management of glaucoma associated with pseudoexfoliation syndrome is generally the same as with any open-angle glaucoma. Some practitioners believe that medical therapy is more difficult in this syndrome. As with pigmentary dispersion syndrome, argon laser trabeculoplasty has been shown to be effective in these patients. Conventional filtration surgery also is effective. The long-term prognosis for control of the intraocular pressure is good in patients with pseudoexfoliation syndrome and glaucoma. Lens extraction is not necessary for the control of the glaucoma, as was once thought. Caution should be used when doing cataract extraction in patients with pseudoexfoliation syndrome. Up to a sevenfold increase in the incidence of vitreous loss has been noted during extracapsular cataract extraction in patients with pseudoexfoliation syndrome. Rupture of the posterior lens capsule also occurs more frequently in these patients. Zonular insufficiency and decreased capsular integrity are thought to contribute to these complications. Patients should be examined, preoperatively, for evidence of zonular dialysis and phacodonesis.

■ GLAUCOMA ASSOCIATED WITH INTRAOCULAR INFLAMMATION

Glaucoma associated with intraocular inflammation (inflammatory glaucoma) is a secondary open-angle glaucoma resulting from anterior segment inflammation and obstruction of aqueous humor outflow by inflammatory cells and debris (51,67). Although reduced intraocular pressure is commonly cited as a sign of acute anterior uveitis (iridocyclitis), intraocular inflammation often leads to severe elevation of the intraocular pressure and glaucoma. Iridocyclitis may reduce aqueous humor production and/or increase uveoscleral outflow, but it may also disrupt the blood-aqueous barrier of the ciliary processes. The latter leads to an outpouring of protein into the posterior chamber, with consequent increased aqueous humor viscosity and influx of associated plasma proteins and growth factors. Inflammatory cells activated by these factors may themselves obstruct the aqueous humor outflow pathways. Inflammatory debris, increased aqueous viscosity, and alterations with the extracellular matrix of the trabecular meshwork may also decrease aqueous humor outflow.

Many ocular inflammatory disorders result in a secondary inflammatory glaucoma with similar clinical characteristics. After bouts of anterior segment inflammation, pigment may be spattered on the inner surface of the meshwork, giving a dirty or muddy appearance. In other cases, the inflammatory precipitates that are commonly manifested on the cornea (keratic precipitates) may accumulate on the surface of the meshwork itself. These clumps of inflammatory cells may mechanically block the aqueous humor outflow. Inflammation of the trabecular meshwork (trabeculitis) may also occur without keratic precipitates and result in outflow obstruction. In more severe, particularly granulomatous, uveitides the trabecular meshwork may become occluded by peripheral anterior synechia, secondarily closing the chamber angle. In rare occurences, posterior synechiae (adhesions between the iris and lens), manifesting as an irregularly shaped pupil, may block aqueous flow into the anterior chamber, leading to iris "bombé" and secondary angle-closure glaucoma. Granulomatous uveitis, associated with sarcoidosis or tuberculosis, typically shows severe peripheral anterior synechiae and glaucoma. Other less severe uveitides may manifest with only a few cells in the anterior chamber, with a mild perilimbal erythematous flush, without synechiae or other gonioscopic abnormalities, and infrequently cause glaucoma. This is the more common appearance in nongranulomatous uveitis, particularly that associated with pars planitis in young adults.

Herpetic viruses (*Herpes simplex* and *Herpes zoster*) may result in anterior segment inflammation and secondary glaucoma (34, 51, 67). External signs (lid involvement, red eye, and skin lesions) may be minimal, even in cases of severe intraocular inflammation. Intraocular pressures should be monitored both initially and chronically, even when overt signs of the infection are missing. This is especially true for *Herpes zoster* ophthalmicus. The kerato-uveitis associated with both herpes viruses may be associated with hypopyon and severe acute intraocular pressure elevation, or chronic, low-grade inflammation and glaucoma. *Herpes zoster* kerato-uveitis usually manifests fewer peripheral anterior synechiae, but posterior synechiae and large geographic patches of stromal iris atrophy are typical with both *H. simplex* and *H. zoster*.

The therapy of glaucoma associated with inflammation should be directed primarily toward the uveitis itself. Corticosteroids or nonsteroidal antiinflammatory drugs form the mainstay of therapy. Ocular hypotensive agents may supplement antiinflammatory therapy. Aqueous humor secretory suppressants are usually most effective. Cholinergics typically exacerbate inflammation and should only be used as a last resort. Control of intraocular inflammation and resolution of secondary reduction of aqueous outflow may require several weeks of steroid therapy. The temptation to stop therapy prematurely, because of suspected pressure elevation from steroid response, should be avoided. Delayed intraocular pressure elevation is more likely the result of the amelioration of the inflammation, with subsequent increased aqueous production by the ciliary body and is not a true steroid response. Glaucoma associated with uveitis does not usually respond to argon laser trabeculoplasty. Filtration surgery may be used, but the intraocular inflammation should be minimized preoperatively, and the postoperative course should be supplemented with increased antiinflammatory drugs. Adjunctive antimetabolite therapy will greatly enhance filtration success.

Other Inflammatory Glaucomas

■ GLAUCOMATO-CYCLITIC CRISIS (POSNER-SCHLOSSMAN SYNDROME)

Glaucomato-cyclitic crisis *(Posner-Schlossman syndrome)* is an uncommon variety of uveitic glaucoma, manifesting in young or middle-aged adults with sudden attacks of acute intraocular pressure elevation, mild-to-moderate ocular pain, blurred vision, and corneal edema with rainbowlike halos around lights (58). Glaucoma in these patients may be confused with acute angle-closure glaucoma, but the differentiation is readily made based upon the absence of a closed-chamber angle on gonioscopic examination. Glaucomato-cyclitic crisis is typically unilateral, but subsequent attacks may occur in either eye. A mild anterior uveitis, with a few cells and flare, and occasional fine, keratic precipitates is common. The elevation of intraocular pressure is out of proportion to the severity of the intraocular inflammation. The chamber angle remains open despite a history of multiple attacks and typically remains free of peripheral anterior synechiae. These acute attacks are self-limited but may be reduced both in duration and severity, although not in frequency, with topical corticosteroids and aqueous secretory suppressants. Occasionally, a sustained intraocular pressure elevation develops between attacks, requiring filtration surgery.

■ FUCHS' HETEROCHROMATIC IRIDOCYCLITIS

An unusual and poorly understood variety of glaucoma is Fuchs' heterochromic iridocyclitis (42). It is usually unilateral, but may be bilateral, and is associated with inflammatory cells circulating in the anterior chamber. Affected eyes manifest signs of a mild anterior uveitis, with cells present in the aqueous humor and anterior vitreous humor. This inflammation is resistant to conventional antiinflammatory therapy with corticosteroids. The intraocular inflammation may intensify and resolve spontaneously. In unilateral cases, the affected eye is usually, but not always, hypochromic, relative to the fellow eye (see Figure 32–3). The iris depigmentation may be more evident in natural lighting. The iris manifests a thin, mottled, atrophic fibular appearance to the stroma, even in the absence of hypochromia. Fine, wispy blood vessels may extend from the iris into the trabecular meshwork but do not progress or lead to peripheral anterior synechiae. These vessels often bleed slightly into the chamber angle when the intraocular pressure is abruptly reduced during intraocular surgery. Perhaps the most characteristic feature of Fuch's heterochromic iridocyclitis is the extensive stellate-shaped keratic precipitates on the corneal endothelial surface that send long tendrils to contiguous deposits. Ipsilateral, visually significant cataracts commonly develop with or without corticosteroid therapy. Even after successful, uncomplicated cataract extraction, chronic glaucoma may compromise the ultimate visual result.

■ LUETIC INTERSTITIAL KERATITIS

Uveitis associated with luetic interstitial keratitis may also cause acute and chronic glaucoma. These may be related to exacerbation of the anterior uveitis associated with luetic keratouveitis. In congenital lues, the anterior segment is small, increasing the risk of angle-closure glaucoma. Luetic interstitial keratitis may also occur with a secondary open-angle glaucoma associated with irregular trabecular pigmentation and a glassy pretrabecular membrane, as sometimes occurs in other smoldering nongranulomatous uveitides.

■ EPISCLERITIS AND SCLERITIS

Episcleritis and scleritis are associated with an open-angle glaucoma in about 10% of cases, usually related to inflammation and edema in the trabecular meshwork and the intrascleral outflow pathways (91). Angle-closure glaucoma has been reported after pupillary dilation in predisposed eyes and from the edema of the ciliary body associated with posterior scleritis.

■ STEROID-INDUCED GLAUCOMA

Steroid-induced glaucoma is a secondary open-angle glaucoma in which transient or persistent elevations of intraocular pressure are noted after the administration of corticosteroids. In the 1950s and 1960s, there were several reports of increased intraocular pressure after corticosteroid administration. In 1950, McLean reported an increase in the intraocular pressure after the systemic administration of ACTH (47, 79). In subsequent years, other investigators showed increased intraocular pressure in both normal and glaucomatous eyes after administration of local corticosteroids (79). In 1963, Becker and Mills showed a rise in intraocular pressure in normal individuals after the topical administration of corticosteroids (79). In the same year, Armaly showed that aqueous humor outflow and formation were both decreased after long-term administration of topical dexamethasone (79). A rise in intraocular pressure occurred more frequently in elderly patients and was more pronounced in patients with a history of glaucoma or with a familial history of open-angle glaucoma. Subsequent studies described increases in intraocular pressure with systemically administered corticosteroids, topically applied dermalogic preparations of corticosteroids, sub-Tenon's injections of corticosteroids, and orally inhaled corticosteroids. Cantrill et al compared the intraocular pressure response of various topically applied corticosteroids. They found that dexamethasone 0.1% produced the greatest rise of intraocular pressure in their patients. Herschler found that the duration and severity of the pressure elevation was directly related to the decreasing solubility of the corticosteroid agent used.

The onset of glaucoma after corticosteroid administration typically occurs 3 to 4 weeks after initiation of the therapy but can occur within days. With the withdrawal of the steroid therapy, corticosteroid-induced intraocular pressure elevations typically resolve within days to weeks. However, protracted and persistent elevations of intraocular pressure after the withdrawal may occur.

The etiology of intraocular pressure elevation after corticosteroid administration is not fully understood. An impairment of the aqueous humor outflow facility is thought to play the major role in the pressure elevation. Investigators believe that an accumulation of glycosaminoglycans results in obstruction of the trabecular meshwork after corticosteroid administration.

The management of elevated intraocular pressure after corticosteroid administration is the same as that for primary open-angle glaucoma. Surgical intervention is rarely needed to control the intraocular pressure but may be used if maximally tolerated medications prove ineffective. Withdrawal of corticosteroid therapy is recommended, if possible, as the initial therapy.

■ INTRAOCULAR HEMORRHAGE: HYPHEMA-INDUCED, GHOST-CELL, AND SICKLE-CELL GLAUCOMAS

Intraocular hemorrhage may result in a secondary open-angle glaucoma. Intraocular bleeding usually occurs after injury or surgery but may occur spontaneously from neovascularization, tumors, or iris vascular tufts. Whatever the etiology, blood in the aqueous humor can obstruct the aqueous outflow pathways, leading to glaucoma. Hyphema from blunt injury or ocular contusion may manifest as a small layer of red blood cells in the inferior portion of the chamber angle, or may entirely replace the aqueous humor. Most intracameral hemorrhages clear spontaneously, but approximately 10 to 15% rebleed, usually within the first week. (23) Recurrent hemorrhage is more likely to completely fill the anterior chamber, leading to glaucoma and/or blood staining of the cornea.

Rebleeding most often occurs when blood in the anterior chamber clots or during clot retraction, 2 to 3 days after the initial hemorrhage. The blood may gradually be absorbed, or an intracameral clot associated with degenerative blood components may appear as a large, black mass, the so-called "eight-ball" hyphema. This is nearly always associated with severe elevation of the intraocular pressure (also see Chapter 64).

Small, fine vascular tufts may occur at the pupillary margin in an otherwise normal eye. These tufts may bleed spontaneously, leading to intermittent attacks of blurred vision and increased intraocular pressure. They can sometimes be obliterated with laser to prevent recurrent bleeding. Spontaneous hyphemas may also occur from iris neovascularization or from intraocular tumors, particularly with juvenile xanthogranuloma. In rare instances, they may also signal the presence of malignant melanoma.

The etiology of intraocular pressure elevation associated with hemorrhage is mechanical obstruction of the aqueous humor outflow pathways. Persistent intraocular hemorrhage gradually undergoes degeneration into a variety of breakdown products of the red blood cells. Red blood cell "ghosts" are khaki-colored, spherical, nonpliable degenerative red cell bodies that develop after long-standing vitreous hemorrhage (14). Degenerative erythrocytic forms, such as red blood cell ghosts or sickled red blood cells, are not as malleable as fresh erythrocytes and are more likely to obstruct aqueous humor outflow and cause glaucoma. The rigid red blood cell ghosts move into the anterior chamber but do not pass through the trabecular meshwork, leading to ghost cell glaucoma. They can be seen circulating in the anterior chamber as iridescent bodies or, when concentrated enough, present as a tan-colored pseudohypopyon in the inferior anterior chamber angle. Red blood cells with hemoglobin S tend to sickle in the relatively hypoxic environment of aqueous humor and become less pliable, leading to severe glaucoma, even with small hyphemas. Even a mild pressure rise to 25mm Hg for over 24 hours can result in optic nerve ischemia in patients with sickle cell trait (18). Other degenerative red blood cell fragments may be ingested by macrophages which themselves can obstruct the trabecular meshwork: a syndrome known as hemolytic glaucoma (13). Vitreous or aqueous aspirates usually show a variety of red cell products, macrophages, and red cell ghosts in such cases.

Management of patients with intraocular hemorrhage and secondary elevation of intraocular pressure should address both the etiology of the hemorrhage and reduction of the intraocular pressure. Anterior segment neovascularization may require retinal laser ablation (see Neovascular Glaucoma). Bed rest and systemic aminocaproic acid have been advocated to limit the possibility of rebleeding. Large, nonclearing anterior chamber hemorrhages associated with increased intraocular pressure may call for an anterior chamber washout to prevent corneal staining and control the intraocular pressure. Intraocular pressure elevations can usually be controlled with aqueous suppressant therapy, although filtration surgery may be needed (also see Ocular Trauma, Chapter 64).

■ ELEVATED EPISCLERAL VENOUS PRESSURE AND GLAUCOMA

Carotid-Cavernous Sinus Fistulas

Secondary open-angle glaucoma may result from an increase in the episcleral venous pressure (55, 60). Clinically, significantly dilated, tortuous and prominent episcleral veins characterize these eyes, and such findings may be mistaken for an infectious "red" eye. Proptosis and chemosis may also be present, especially with high flow carotid-cavernous sinus fistulas (see Figure 13–4) These patients often complain of hearing pulsations, and an ocular bruit may be heard by auscultation over the eye lid or temporal orbit. The chamber angle is usually open, often with blood reflux into Schlemm's canal. On rare occasions, neovascularization occurs, apparently on an ischemic basis resulting from arterial shunting. Trabecular outflow facility is normal unless blood reflux or other anomalies block the trabecular meshwork.

The aqueous humor exits the eye primarily by way of the trabecular meshwork, Schlemm's canal, and aqueous veins, which drain to the episcleral veins. Under most conditions, episcleral venous pressure is in the range of 8 to 12mm Hg, but may be increased under physiologic and pathologic conditions, leading to elevation of the intraocular pressure. Simple breath holding, Valsalva maneuvers, or compression of neck veins will transiently increase episcleral venous pressure. In-

creased episcleral venous pressure may occur pathologically from obstruction of orbital venous drainage, increased central venous pressure, arteriovenous fistulas or idiopathically. Idiopathic elevation of the episcleral venous pressure (see next section) may actually be secondary to low flow arteriovenous shunts in the posterior orbit or cavernous sinus, which cannot be seen by angiography. Although elevations of episcleral venous pressures typically range between 20 to 30mm Hg with these various pathologic conditions, the intraocular pressure frequently ranges between 40 to 60mm Hg. This suggests an additional outflow obstruction may be present.

■ OTHER CAUSES OF INCREASED EPISCLERAL VENOUS PRESSURE

Venous obstruction may occur with retrobulbar tumors, cavernous sinus thrombosis, or from distal obstruction associated with increased pressure in the superior vena cava. Most common is dysthyroid ophthalmopathy with orbital congestion, proptosis, lid retraction, and chemosis. Arteriovenous fistulas classically occur between the carotid artery and the cavernous sinus, especially after blunt or penetrating trauma. These typically are high flow shunts, usually of acute onset, and are associated with increased venous pressure, proptosis, chemosis, bruits over the orbit, and severe glaucoma. The majority of arteriovenous fistulas are traumatic in origin. However, those encountered in the ophthalmologist's office more typically are low-flow, low-volume shunts associated with other intracranial vessels and less prominent clinical findings. An idiopathic, sometimes familial, syndrome of prominent episcleral veins and glaucoma has

also been observed with no demonstrable arterialvenous shunt or other cause for the increased episcleral venous pressure (48). Sturge-Weber oculofacial hemangioma syndrome may also manifest increased episcleral venous pressure associated with episcleral hemangiomas and a secondary open-angle glaucoma (see Developmental Glaucomas: Phakomatoses).

Eyes with elevated intraocular pressure on the basis of increased episcleral venous pressure, are often resistant to conventional medical and laser glaucoma therapy, and often require trabeculectomy or other filtration surgery. Intraoperative or immediate postoperative uveal effusion and suprachoroidal hemorrhage are frequent because of the increased intraocular venous pressure. Prophylactic posterior sclerotomies, completed at the time of filtration surgery, may prevent the serious complication of suprachoroidal hemorrhage.

Angle-Closure Glaucoma

■ PRIMARY ANGLE-CLOSURE GLAUCOMA WITH PUPILLARY BLOCK

Primary angle-closure glaucoma refers to an increase in intraocular pressure secondary to iris apposition to the trabecular meshwork (16, 57). This apposition prevents aqueous humor outflow from the anterior chamber and may occur suddenly (acute angle-closure glaucoma), slowly over time (chronic angle-closure glaucoma), or intermittently (subacute angle-closure glaucoma). Pri-

mary angle-closure glaucoma derives from relative pupillary block. Relative pupillary block is an increased resistance to aqueous humor flow from the posterior chamber into the anterior chamber, through the pupil. Relative pupillary block is dependent on the contact between the lens and iris and is increased in eyes with narrow anterior segments, such as hyperopic eyes. The pressure in the posterior chamber is increased by pupillary block and pushes the peripheral iris forward (see Figure 32–3). The forward displacement or bowing of the peripheral iris leads to closure of the trabecular meshwork, and results in severe elevations in intraocular pressure, known as primary angle-closure glaucoma (Figure 32–4). Eyes with short axial lengths, small corneal diameters, and increased thickness of the crystalline lens are predisposed to increased pupillary block and angle-closure glaucoma. Relative pupillary block also increases with age as the lens thickens and the pupil becomes more miotic. Maximal pupillary block occurs in the middilated position; therefore, angle-closure may be exacerbated by pupillary dilation. In the middilated eye, the apposition between the lens and iris is substantial, and the peripheral iris is lax enough to be anteriorly displaced. Eyes in which the pupil has been pharmacologically dilated are most prone to increased pupillary block and acute angle-closure glaucoma as the medications begin to wear off and the pupil is in the middilated position. In the normal eye, there is apposition between the posterior surface of the iris and the anterior surface of the lens, but the resistance to aqueous humor flow into the anterior chamber is minimal.

Primary angle-closure glaucoma occurs much less frequently than primary open-angle glaucoma (approximate ratio 1:4–10). However, certain populations have a significantly increased risk of developing angle-closure glaucoma. Primary acute angle-closure is more common than open-angle glaucoma in the Eskimo population (19). As many as 2 to 3% of Eskimos over age 40 will have angle-closure glaucoma. Eskimo women have a twofold to threefold-increased risk of having the disease as compared with Eskimo men. Asians also have an increased risk for the development of angle-closure glaucoma. Conversely, certain populations rarely have angle-closure glaucoma, such as native Americans and Pacific Islanders (95). Subacute and chronic angle-closure glaucoma are more common than acute angle-closure glaucoma in blacks. Increased age, hyperopia, and a positive family history of angle-closure glaucoma all slightly increase the risk of angle-closure glaucoma.

Primary angle-closure glaucoma with relative pupillary block may occur acutely with a sudden attack of diminished vision, pain, nausea, emesis, and significantly elevated intraocular pressures. The cornea becomes edematous, and the anterior chamber shallows both peripherally and centrally. It is common to have intraocular pressures greater than 50mm Hg with this disorder. Typically, the eye becomes red with ciliary injection of the episcleral and conjunctival vessels, especially near the corneoscleral limbus. Subacute, primary angle-closure glaucoma with pupillary block refers to intermittent episodes of angle-closure glaucoma, typically less severe than acute angle-closure glaucoma. Patients may report episodes of blurred vision and halos around

lights, secondary to corneal edema. These attacks generally resolve within minutes to hours, and the eye may appear normal between attacks with the exception of a narrow or shallow anterior chamber angle. Chronic, primary angle-closure glaucoma with pupillary block is also known as "creeping angle-closure." Patients are usually asymptomatic with this disorder, although they may have other stigmata of glaucoma, including glaucomatous optic neuropathy and visual field loss. Intraocular pressures range from normal to highly elevated and are the result of prolonged narrowing of the anterior chamber angle with formation of peripheral anterior synechiae. This results from prolonged apposition of the iris to the trabecular meshwork, and the amount of pressure elevation depends on the extent of angle-closure.

The diagnosis of acute angle-closure glaucoma is often self-evident; increased elevations of intraocular pressure and a closed anterior chamber angle are present. When extensive corneal edema prohibits gonioscopic examination of the anterior chamber angle, acutely lowering the intraocular pressure often clears the corneal edema. Examination may also be enhanced by the application of glycerin to the anterior surface of the cornea after topical anesthesia. This will temporarily osmotically dehydrate and clear the cornea, enhancing the view of the anterior segment. Dynamic gonioscopy may be done to assess the extent of appositional versus synechial angle-closure (see Clincal Testing and Examination Techniques: Gonioscopy). Subsequent to acute angle-closure attacks, the iris may become significantly atrophic, pigment may be dispersed throughout the anterior segment, and glaukomflecken may be seen as white opacities on the anterior surface of the lens. Glaukomflecken represents necrotic

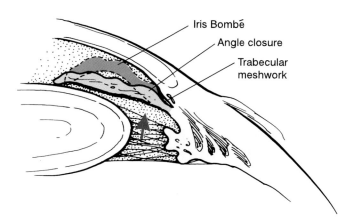

Figure 45–2.
Primary Angle-closure Glaucoma with Pupillary Block: Relative pupillary block causes increased pressure in the posterior chamber with a forward shift of the peripheral iris and closure of the anterior chamber angle. "Iris bombé" refers to an iris configuration with forward bowing of the peripheral iris.

damage of the anterior lens capsule. The severe pressure elevation seen with acute angle-closure attacks may cause optic nerve damage within hours to days. In chronic angle-closure glaucoma with pupillary block, gonioscopy reveals a narrowed inlet to the anterior chamber angle, with areas of peripheral anterior synechiae. Peripheral anterior synechiae are adhesions between the peripheral iris and trabecular meshwork or cornea. Portions of the anterior chamber angle may be appositionally closed, while other regions are narrow but open.

Angle-closure glaucoma may also occur secondary to posterior synechiae. Total synechiae formation between the iris and the anterior lens surface may create obstruction of aqueous flow into the anterior chamber resulting in an iris configuration, known as iris bombé (Figure 45–2). The peripheral iris appears to balloon into the anterior chamber causing angle-closure glaucoma. This typically follows chronic uveitis. Iris bombé configuration is also seen in primary angle-closure glaucoma if the relative pupillary block results in a large pressure differential between the anterior and posterior chambers. Secondary angle-closure glaucomas, such as angle-closure after a central retinal vein occlusion or angle-closure secondary to a posterior segment intraocular tumor, should be ruled out in all cases of angle-closure glaucoma. Examination of the fellow eye with gonioscopy should be done in all patients presenting with angle-closure glaucoma. Patients with a marked difference in the depth of the anterior chamber and the configuration of the anterior chamber angle between the two eyes should be suspected of having a secondary cause of angle-closure glaucoma.

■ TREATMENT

Therapy for angle-closure glaucoma was originally described by von Graefe in 1857 (85). He suggested the use of surgical iridectomy in patients with shallow anterior chambers and increased intraocular pressure. Iridectomy, either laser or incisional, remains the mainstay of therapy for angle-closure glaucoma (Figure 45–3). Medical therapy is used to lower the intraocular pressure and decrease the corneal edema before the iridectomy. Aqueous humor suppressants, such as topical beta-adrenergic blockers and carbonic anhydrase inhibitors, should be administered. Carbonic anhydrase inhibitors may be given orally or intravenously. Patients who are nauseated frequently will not tolerate oral medications and intravenous administration may be needed. Miotic therapy may be used in an attempt to break the relative pupillary block and pull the peripheral iris from the trabecular meshwork. However, miotics are often ineffective owing to total iris paralysis from pressure-induced ischemia. After reduction of the intraocular pressure, miotics may become more effective. Placement of an iridectomy is usually effective in alleviating pupillary block. The iridectomy allows an alternative flow pattern for the aqueous humor from the posterior chamber into the anterior chamber (Figure 45–3). It also allows equalization of pressure between the two chambers and promotes flattening of the peripheral iris away from the trabecular meshwork. Laser iridotomy has provided a safer alternative to the surgical iridectomy for this treatment.

Even after placement of an iridotomy, the intraocular pressure occasionally may not return to normal levels. This may be the result of prolonged appositional closure and trabecular meshwork damage or because of the formation of peripheral anterior synechiae. A persistent decrease in the outflow facility may necessitate continuous aqueous humor suppressant therapy. Prophylactic peripheral iridotomies are generally recommended in the contralateral eye of patients experiencing primary angle-closure glaucoma. Approximately 70% of these patients will experience angle-closure attacks in the fellow eye without this prophylaxis. Placement of iridotomies in patients with narrow anterior chamber angles, but no history of angle-closure glaucoma, is controversial. In general, in eyes with areas of appositional closure, prophylactic iridotomies are recommended to prevent acute angle-closure attacks. Therapy for subacute angle-closure glaucoma is similar to the therapy for acute angle-closure glaucoma. Chronic angle-closure glaucoma frequently requires

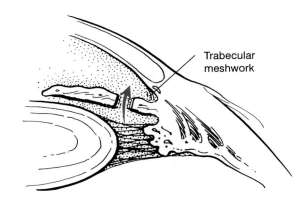

Figure 45–3.
Peripheral Iridotomy: The iridotomy allows equilibration of pressure between the anterior and posterior chambers, with flattening of the peripheral iris and opening of the anterior chamber angle.

subsequent medical therapy to control the intraocular pressure even after placement of an iridotomy. Typically, filtration procedures work well in individuals in whom the intraocular pressure is not controlled, despite maximally tolerated medical therapy. However, a higher incidence of postoperative flat anterior chambers and malignant glaucoma is seen in patients with chronic angle-closure glaucoma and extensive peripheral anterior synechiae. Angle-closure patients, in whom laser iridotomies are not effective in deepening the anterior chamber, are at a higher risk of postoperative aqueous humor misdirection and malignant glaucoma.

Many systemic medications carry warnings against their use in individuals with glaucoma. Angle-closure glaucoma is the concern of most of these warnings because of systemic anticholinergic or sympathomimetic activity which may cause pupillary dilation and exacerbate pupillary block. Individuals with narrow anterior chamber angles should be warned against the use of these medications because of this risk.

Other Varieties of Angle-Closure Glaucoma

■ PLATEAU IRIS CONFIGURATION AND SYNDROME

As many as 20% of individuals with angle-closure glaucoma never manifest classic pupillary block with peripheral displacement or bowing of the iris. Many of these individuals will have an abnormal, anatomic configuration of the anterior chamber: plateau iris configuration. Wand et al separated such individuals into two categories: plateau iris configuration and plateau iris syndrome (89). In plateau iris configuration, the central anterior chamber depth is normal and the iris plane is flat, but the peripheral iris is displaced posteriorly, creating a narrow inlet to the chamber angle. Prominent rolls of peripheral iris are present in these eyes and angle-closure with intraocular pressure elevation may occur. Relative pupillary block seems to play an important role in the pressure elevation associated with plateau iris configuration, because an iridotomy often results in chamber angle opening and pressure lowering. Plateau iris configuration is much more frequent than plateau iris syndrome.

In plateau iris syndrome, the iris plane is flat into the periphery, and there are multiple rolls of redundant peripheral iris which tend to occlude the chamber angle, especially with pupillary dilation. The diagnosis of plateau iris syndrome is made only when a subject has a patent iridotomy and acute angle-closure glaucoma continues to occur with pupillary dilation. Plateau iris syndrome is seen in individuals younger than the general population of primary angle-closure glaucoma and has no sex predilection. The primary therapy for plateau iris syndrome is prolonged miotic therapy and avoidance of pupillary dilation. Miotic therapy prevents the occlusion of the narrowed chamber angle by the peripheral rolls of iris. Argon laser iridoplasty (see Glaucoma Therapy: Laser) may be done in individuals in whom progressive angle-closure occurs, despite miotics and patent iridotomites. Surgical therapy is similar to that of primary angle-closure glaucoma.

■ MALIGNANT GLAUCOMA

Malignant glaucoma is another form of angle-closure glaucoma. Since its original description by von Graefe (84), malignant glaucoma has been known by many names (ciliary block glaucoma, direct lens block glaucoma, and aqueous misdirection syndrome). Malignant glaucoma almost always occurs after surgery, especially surgical procedures such as surgical iridectomy and trabeculectomy, for angle-closure glaucoma. It is estimated that approximately 1 to 4% of surgeries for angle-closure glaucoma will result in malignant glaucoma (17, 72, 73). In these eyes, the anterior chamber shallows or becomes flat with increased elevations of the intraocular pressure during the early postoperative period. This syndrome may be aggravated by miotics and is often relieved by cycloplegics (17). Frequently, malignant glaucoma will occur during the postoperative period upon the cessation of cycloplegic therapy. Malignant glaucoma has also been described in individuals without any previous history of surgery, in patients with retinopathy of prematurity, and after a central retinal vein occlusion (38, 44, 63).

Malignant glaucoma results when aqueous humor is misdirected into the posterior chamber of the eye causing hydration of the vitreous and pooling of aqueous humor within or posterior to the vitreous body. It is believed that the hyaloid face prevents the flow of aqueous humor into the anterior chamber. Anterior displacement of the lens-iris diaphragm or vitreous-iris diaphragm causes shallowing of the anterior chamber. Total closure of the anterior chamber angle may result, leading to increased elevations of intraocular pressure. B-scan ultrasonography is often helpful in the diagnosis of malignant glaucoma, since an echolucent pool of aqueous humor may be identified in the vitreous cavity. Compacted or compressed vitreous may also be imaged as an echogenic interface, just posterior to the lens. Anterior segment ultrasonography has shown anterior rotation of the ciliary body and forward movement of the lens-iris diaphragm. Laxity of the lens zonules may contribute to the anterior displacement of the lens.

The differential diagnosis for malignant glaucoma includes pupillary block glaucoma, choroidal detachments, suprachoroidal hemorrhage, and aqueous humor overfiltration syndrome after fistulizing procedures. These implications are discussed later in this section (see Complications Following Filtration Surgery). The therapy for malignant glaucoma includes aggressive cycloplegia and suppression of aqueous humor with carbonic anhydrase inhibitors and beta-adrenergic blockers. Hyperosmotic agents dehydrate the vitreous cavity, which allows deepening of the anterior chamber. Surgical disruption of the anterior hyaloid face, either with laser or incisional surgery, may be needed to prevent the vicious cycle of aqueous humor misdirection, vitreous hydration, anterior chamber shallowing, and subsequent obstruction of aqueous humor outflow.

■ NANOPHTHALMOS

Nanophthalmos is a rare disorder which is characterized by a small eye, with a shallow anterior chamber secondary to a relatively large crystalline lens (74). The lens is said to be of normal size, while the globe is too small. This anatomic configuration predisposes individuals to angle-closure glaucoma later in life. These eyes are typically highly hyperopic and have a small corneal diameter and shallow anterior chamber. Retinal pigmentary changes are common. An increased rate of uveal effusions with nonrhegmatogenous retinal detachments after any form of intraocular surgery, are seen. Angle-closure glaucoma in nanophthalmic eyes may initially be the result of a pupillary block mechanism, and a peripheral iridotomy may temporarily relieve the glaucoma. Later in life, secondary angle-closure glaucoma may occur because of enlargement of the crystalline lens and further narrowing of the anterior chamber, with closure of the chamber angle. In these cases, laser peripheral iridoplasty may open the anterior chamber angle and delay or prevent intraocular surgery. Conventional filtration surgery should be used only as a last resort in these eyes because of the increased incidence of serous uveal effusions and postoperative flat anterior chambers. Histologically, these eyes have thickened sclera. Scleral resections or vortex vein decompressions have been recommended to lessen postoperative complications.

■ RUBEOSIS IRIDES AND NEOVASCULAR GLAUCOMA

Neovascularization of the anterior segment of the eye may result in either open-angle glaucoma or angle-closure glaucoma. Glaucoma, associated with neovascularization of the anterior segment, most frequently occurs in individuals with diabetes mellitus or previous retinal vein occlusion (11, 29, 75). (Table 45–1). Rubeosis irides refers to the proliferation of new blood vessels within the anterior segment, usually at the pupillary margin or on the peripheral iris. These vessels are tufts of fibrovascular tissue which appear initially as a fine network, and may later progress into larger blood vessels which cover the entire surface of the iris and the entire anterior segment. Rubeosis irides may be distinguished from normal vessels by elevation above the iris, extensive proliferation, and propensity to hemorrhage (see Gonioscopy: The Normal Anterior Chamber Angle). Rubeosis irides is the sequelae of a variety of ocular and systemic disorders which may be categorized by their common features: intraocular/retinal ischemic disorders, extraocular ischemic disorders, continual inflammatory disorders, and other miscellaneous disorders (Table 45–1). Diabetic retinopathy is the most frequent cause of anterior segment neovascularization. Cases associated with this disorder comprise approxi-

TABLE 45-1
Most Common Etiologies of Anterior Segment
Neovascularization

Intraocular/Retinal Ischemic Disorders
Diabetic Retinopathy**
Retinal Vein Occlusion (Central or Branch)**
Retinal Artery Occlusion (Central or Branch)**
Chronic Retinal Detachment
Retinopathy of Prematurity
Sickle Cell Retinopathy
Radiation Retinopathy

Extraocular Ischemic Disorders (Ischemic Oculopathy)
Carotid Artery Occlusive Disease
Carotid Cavernous Fistula

Chronic Inflammatory Disorders
Coats's Exudative Retinopathy
Chronic Uveitis (Anterior or Posterior)
Retinal Vasculitis
Endophthalmitis
Lens-Induced Uveitis

Others
Intraocular Tumor (Melanoma, Retinoblastoma, Metastatic)
Trauma

** most common causes

mately one-third of all cases. Central retinal vein occlusions, especially the ischemic variety, account for approximately 25% of all cases of rubeosis irides (26). Other ischemic retinal diseases such as central retinal artery occlusion, branch retinal artery occlusion, and branch retinal vein occlusion are also frequent causes of rubeosis irides. Any form of continuous intraocular inflammation, such as endophthalmitis, trauma, lens-induced uveitis, or chronic retinal detachment, may also result in neovascularization of the anterior segment. Most researchers believe that angiogenic factors, produced by the ischemic retina or induced by chronic inflammation, result in neovascularization of the anterior segment. These factors are thought to diffuse from the posterior segment into the anterior segment, resulting in the new vessel growth. The diffusion of these factors may be enhanced by the removal of the crystalline lens, surgical disruption of the anterior segment, or removal of the vitreous.

Neovascular glaucoma is a potentially devastating consequence of rubeosis irides. Neovascular glaucoma may occur with either an open-anterior or closed-anterior chamber angle. In most cases, open-angle glaucoma occurs initially, with proliferation of fibrovascular

tissue in the anterior segment and possibly secondary hemorrhage, leading to a secondary open-angle glaucoma. Open-angle neovascular glaucoma may also occur without hemorrhage. With further proliferation of fibrovascular material in the anterior chamber angle, and contracture of myofibroblasts, the anterior chamber angle closes. Peripheral anterior synechiae form, and ectropion uveae may occur secondary to pulling of the anterior surface of the iris, by scarring and contracture in the chamber angle.

Individuals with neovascular glaucoma typically present with acute pain, decreased vision, a significantly red eye, and photophobia. There may be secondary corneal edema. Left untreated, these eyes frequently progress to blind, painful eyes with intractable glaucoma. After an ischemic event, such as a central retinal vein occlusion, eyes are most likely to develop neovascular glaucoma within 2 to 4 months, although the timing is variable. "Ninety day glaucoma" has been used to refer to eyes in which neovascular glaucoma develops approximately 3 months after a central retinal vein occlusion.

Therapy for neovascular glaucoma is principally aimed at eliminating the stimulus for anterior segment neovascularization. The overall visual prognosis for eyes with neovascular glaucoma is poor. However, it has greatly improved since the advent of panretinal photocoagulation for the treatment of diabetic and postvein occlusion ischemic retinopathy. Cyclocryotherapy of the retina may also be considered in eyes with media opacities. Medical antiglaucoma therapy may be considered in the open-angle variety of neovascular glaucoma, but its success is limited. If concomitant medical aqueous suppressants and panretinal photocoagulation can be instituted during the early rubeotic stage, progression to severe open-angle glaucoma or closed-angle glaucoma may be prevented. However, most cases of neovascular glaucoma necessitate surgical therapy. Trabeculectomy with adjunctive antimetabolite therapy may be considered in eyes in which an iridectomy may be done. If the rubeosis irides is too extensive to safely execute a surgical iridectomy at the time of trabeculectomy, a glaucoma seton tube implant or transscleral cyclodestructive procedure should be considered. Most filtration surgeries will fail if the stimulus of neovascularization is left unchecked. In rare instances, the neovascularization in the anterior segment may regress spontaneously after a filtration procedure. Some researchers have suggested that this results from filtration of the angiogenic factors out of the anterior segment. This hypothesis remains unproven. Direct goniophotocoagulation of rubeotic vessels within the chamber angle has also been promoted, but its success remains limited.

■ EPITHELIAL DOWNGROWTH AND FIBROUS INGROWTH

Epithelial downgrowth is an uncommon abnormality which may occur after any type of penetrating trauma, or as a complication of intraocular surgery, and may result in intractable angle-closure glaucoma (32,96). Epithelial downgrowth, most frequently seen after cataract surgery, occurs in approximately 0.01% of all cases (32). It has also been reported after penetrating keratoplasty and glaucoma filtration surgery. It is believed that epithelial cells from the conjunctiva invade the anterior segment of the eye through the wound site. Poor wound apposition or a postoperative wound leak increase the risk of epithelial invasion and downgrowth. These epithelial cells may cover the posterior surface of the cornea, the structures of the anterior chamber angle, and the anterior surface of the iris. Free floating epithelial cells are also seen circulating in the anterior chamber. This results in a secondary angle-closure glaucoma as the epithelial membrane contracts and closes the chamber angle.

Eyes with this complication typically have increased intraocular pressures, and a border of advancing epithelial cells is seen on the posterior surface of the cornea. This appears as a sharply demarcated, translucent membrane advancing across the posterior surface of the cornea, which occurs at a border between normal and edematous cornea. Epithelial growth on the anterior surface of the iris may also occur but is more difficult to visualize. Application of low energy, argon laser burns to the surface of the iris may help in the diagnosis. The laser burns result in a whitening of the epithelial cell layer, allowing its identification.

Fibrous ingrowth may also occur after penetrating trauma or with inadequate wound closure. Instead of epithelial cell invasion, fibroblastic scar and vascular tissue invade the anterior and posterior segments of the eye. Fibrous ingrowth may result in fibrovascular scar tissue proliferation throughout the entire globe, leading to phthisis bulbi.

Prognosis for visual rehabilitation in either epithelial downgrowth or fibrous ingrowth is poor. Many extensive surgical procedures, including penetrating keratoplasty with total iris resection and stripping of the epithelial cell layer from the anterior segment, have been reported. Continued problems with control of intraocular pressure are frequent, even after extensive removal of the epithelial or fibrous tissue. Conventional filtration surgery rarely works in this syndrome, since the epithelial cells which are circulating in the anterior chamber proliferate on the internal surface of the filtration bleb, resulting in bleb failure. Glaucoma seton implants are frequently used in addition to aqueous humor suppressants to control the intraocular pressure, with variable success. Any intraocular surgical procedure may stimulate more aggressive growth of the invading tissue and hasten the demise of the eye.

Other Syndromes and Ocular Abnormalities Associated with Glaucoma

■ IRIDO-CORNEAL ENDOTHELIAL SYNDROME

Clinical entities only recently ascribed to a single spectrum of disorders, the irido-corneal endothelial (ICE) syndrome, were described separately in the mid-twentieth century (99). These entities include Chandler's syndrome, essential iris atrophy, and the iris-nevus syndrome of Cogan-Reese. Although the individual clinical findings will vary slightly at first presentation, these disorders share an abnormality of the corneal endothelium, the anterior chamber angle, and the iris. Eventually, many of these eyes will develop glaucoma, with associated bullous keratopathy and corneal opacification. Initial presentation is most often in early-to-middle adulthood with corneal edema, ocular pain, varying degrees of corectopia, iris atrophy, and visual blurring (97, 99). These disorders are nearly always unilateral and are more common in women.

The underlying pathophysiologic anomaly with the ICE syndrome involves corneal endothelial degeneration with fine guttate-like changes resembling beaten silver, similar to, but finer than, the changes of Fuch's endothelial dystrophy. The corneal endothelium becomes more like an epithelial cell layer, with aggressive growth and multiple cell layer thickness. This anomalous endothelium migrates to the anterior chamber angle, over the trabecular meshwork, and onto the surface of the iris.

In Chandler's syndrome, the corneal changes predominate with only mild iris stromal atrophy and corectopia. Corneal edema tends to be severe, even at normal intraocular pressures, and often calls for corneal transplantation. In essential iris atrophy, the iris changes predominate with progressive stromal iris atrophy, which later develops through-and-through holes, marked corectopia, and polycoria. As the endothelial membrane contracts toward the chamber angle, it pulls the pupil with it, stretching the iris on the opposite side, leading to so-called "stretch holes." Eventually, little may be left of the iris except for a few stromal strands of the iris sphincter. Small round melt holes may also develop in unstretched areas of iris.

The Cogan-Reese iris-nevus syndrome manifests with corneal edema, iris atrophy, and angle changes similar to those typical of the other ICE disorders. In addition, these patients will develop multiple, discrete, pigmented nodules, or diffuse nevus-like areas on the iris surface. Histologically, these nodules are areas of iris stroma extruding through holes in the ectopic endothelial membrane, which covers the iris surface.

In actual clinical practice, the majority of ICE patients present somewhere between these classic extremes, with some findings of each entity (70, 97). With progressive peripheral synechiae, the intraocular pressure can be controlled initially with medical therapy, but filtration surgery often becomes necessary as aqueous humor outflow becomes further compromised. Postoperatively, endothelialization may also occur over a filtration fistula or within the bleb itself, resulting in compromise or filtration failure.

■ POSTERIOR POLYMORPHOUS DYSTROPHY

Posterior polymorphous dystrophy is a corneal dystrophy which may be associated with open-angle glaucoma (36). It manifests some of the signs of the iridocorneal endothelialization syndrome but also possesses distinctive features that distinguish it. It is nearly always bilateral and is often familial, being inherited in an autosomal-dominant fashion. Unlike the ICE syndrome, it is manifest from childhood but usually does not become clinically apparent until early adult life. It is primarily a disorder of the corneal endothelium, with craterlike defects visible with biomicroscopy. The lesions may become contiguous and appear as a tract across the endothelial surface of the cornea. Most patients have normal irides. Some may develop iridocorneal adhesions and about 15% develop elevated intraocular pressure, requiring glaucoma therapy.

■ IRIDOSCHISIS

Iridoschisis is an uncommon iris abnormality which is associated with glaucoma (64). Individuals normally present in the six or seventh decades of life, with bilateral defects of the inferior irides. The layers of the iris stroma actually separate, especially in the inferior quadrants. Glaucoma occurs in approximately 50% of individuals with iridoschisis. Glaucoma may be either open-angle or angle-closure glaucoma. Pigment dispersion into the anterior chamber angle is sometimes seen and may contribute to the decrease in outflow facility. Histopathologically, the iris stroma shows extensive atrophy. Corneal edema and abnormalities of the corneal endothelium are associated with this syndrome. Management of glaucoma associated with iridoschisis follows traditional guidelines for angle-closure or open-angle glaucoma.

■ GLAUCOMA ASSOCIATED WITH OCULAR TRAUMA AND ANGLE RECESSION

Any form of eye trauma may disrupt the aqueous humor outflow pathways and result in increased intraocular pressure. Blunt trauma distorts the spherical configuration of the multilaminate globe (15). Sudden shearing of one layer against another during a blunt injury may produce separation of the uveal tract at the chamber angle. In some cases, the disruption tears the root of the iris away from the ciliary body, manifesting as iridodialysis. In other cases, the ciliary body and iris together are separated from the sclera, leaving a gap or cyclodialysis cleft. In most cases, the attachments between the iridociliary body and the chamber angle are partially disrupted, leading to a configuration known as anterior chamber angle recession, or simply "angle recession." In angle recession, the ciliary body band appears many times wider than normal when viewed gonioscopically (Figure 45–4). The ciliary body band develops a slate-gray appearance, and in some cases, the bare white

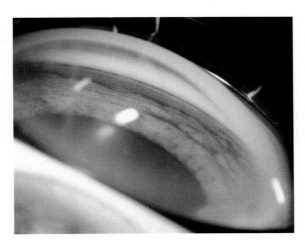

Figure 45–4.
Angle Recession: Note the widening of the ciliary body band.

the angle disruption is so extensive that it develops a cyclodialysis cleft, the traumatized eye may develop hypotony (see Ocular Hypotony). In either case, the eye may also exhibit disruption of the lenticular zonules with phakodonesis, lens subluxation, or dislocation. Long forgotten blunt trauma should be considered as a possible etiology in any unilateral glaucoma. The development of glaucoma after penetrating ocular trauma depends on the extent of injury, but is, in general, similar to that occurring with blunt trauma. Such injuries are often associated with severe inflammation, chronic peripheral anterior synechia from collapse of the anterior chamber, and lens disruption. Secondary angle-closure glaucoma may result.

Ocular contusion or angle-recession glaucoma should be managed as an open-angle glaucoma with conventional hypotensive medical agents. However, cholinergic agents are less likely to be effective in angle recession because of the disruption of the ciliary muscle. The success of argon laser trabeculoplasty is poor in angle recession glaucoma. If the conjunctiva is satisfactory, most cases respond well to conventional filtration surgery, although persistence of inflammation, lens injury, aphakia, and relative youth may indicate the need for adjunctive antimetabolite therapy or more extensive surgical procedures.

The aphakic eye in a young person with disruption of the anterior segment has a poor prognosis for filtration surgery. If no satisfactory site for conventional filtration surgery can be identified, a seton implant may be indicated. Eyes with poor visual potential are probably better managed with the less invasive cyclodestructive procedures.

sclera may be seen; but this is more typical of a traumatic cyclodialysis cleft. With traumatic disruption of the angle tissues, there is often a showering of pigment into the anterior chamber. This pigment tends to accumulate inferiorly in the angle, appearing spattered or as clumps over the surface of the trabecular meshwork. Associated inflammation may result in the development of peripheral anterior synechia within areas of recessed or nonrecessed angle. Depending on the extent of angle recession, damage to the trabecular meshwork may cause increased resistance to aqueous humor outflow, diminished outflow reserve, and intraocular pressure elevation. Although glaucoma commonly occurs early after injury, it may not become manifest for many years. If

■ CHEMICAL BURNS

Chemical burns to the eye may lead to extreme intraocular inflammation, collagenous contracture of the sclera, and disruption of the intrascleral aqueous outflow pathways. All are potential causes of acute or continual elevated intraocular pressures. With collagenous contracture, the scleral shrinkage may result in increased elevations of intraocular pressure. Such injuries, particularly alkali burns, can be profoundly destructive and cause vascular sclerosis leading to intractable glaucoma. These eyes respond poorly to medical and/or laser therapy, since the outflow obstruction is downstream from the trabecular meshwork.

In addition, severe conjunctival burns make conventional filtration surgery exceedingly difficult, necessitating filtration with antimetabolite therapy or a tube implant. Visual potential must be evaluated and cyclodestructive procedures considered. Caution should be used when considering ciliary destruction in eyes after severe chemical burns, because aqueous humor production may be decreased. This results from anterior segment ischemia and poor perfusion of the ciliary body. Overzealous cyclodestruction, in these cases, may result in total aqueous suppression and hypotony.

■ LENS-ASSOCIATED GLAUCOMA

Although cataractous changes of the crystalline lens commonly occur in elderly glaucoma patients, only under unusual circumstances do abnormalities of the lens directly lead to glaucoma (21). Some factors associated with angle-closure glaucomas can derive, in varying degrees, from the size or location of the crystalline lens. In classic angle-closure glaucoma, relative pupillary block occurs when the posterior chamber aqueous humor cannot escape between the lens and the pupillary margin to enter the anterior chamber. This process can become acutely exacerbated with sudden enlargement of the lens or if the lens-iris diaphragm has shifted forward, as sometimes occurs after occlusion of the central retinal vein. Even in the healthy eye, cataractous change and enlargement of the lens, with increase in iridolenticular touch and relative pupillary block, may result in angle-closure glaucoma. Dislocated or subluxed lenses also may migrate forward to become entrapped in the pupil, leading to angle-closure glaucoma. A lens may also dislocate entirely into the anterior chamber, causing inflammation and a reverse pupillary block, with the pupil compressed against the back surface of the lens. Spherophakia, as in Weill-Marchesani syndrome, may allow the small, spherical lens to become entrapped in the pupil, resulting in pupillary block and angle-closure glaucoma. Treatment for these problems is a peripheral iridectomy (laser or surgical) or lens extraction when indicated. Dislocated lenses may also become hypermature and develop a permeable capsule leading to phacolytic glaucoma.

A spectrum of glaucomas associated with a permeable or "leaky" lens capsule have been described (21, 49). These include phacolytic glaucoma, which is a lens-induced uveitis with secondary glaucoma, and obstruction of the trabecular meshwork by lens protein or particles of lens material. Phacolytic glaucoma classically presents in an eye with poor visual acuity and a long-standing mature or hypermature cataract (Figure 45–5) These eyes acutely develop increased intraocular pressures, pain, erythema, and corneal edema but have an open anterior chamber angle. The hypermature cataract, with its wrinkled leaky lens capsule, exudes

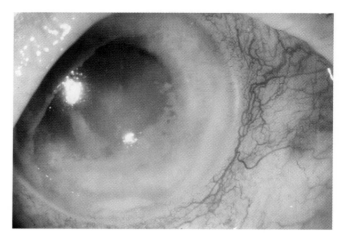

Figure 45–5.
Phacolytic Glaucoma: Significantly inflamed eye with layer of inflammatory cells in the inferior chamber angle and collections of macrophages on the anterior surface of the lens and iris.

proteinaceous material that circulates in the anterior chamber along with macrophages that have ingested lens material. A pseudo-hypopyon may be present, formed by the lens protein and macrophages. Conventional hypotensive and antiinflammatory therapy are almost always ineffective, but lens extraction usually relieves both the elevated intraocular pressure and the inflammation. Milder forms of inflammatory glaucoma associated with a permeable, but immature, lens may also occur. Phacoanaphylactic endophthalmitis is a largely histologic diagnosis describing an immune response to released lens protein via a lens capsular violation (21). Sensitization to lens proteins, which are normally immunologically sequestered in the lens capsule, is required. Polymorphonuclear leukocytes are liberated into the aqueous humor and anterior chamber. The resultant inflammation may cause an increased intraocular pressure.

■ GLAUCOMA AFTER CATARACT EXTRACTION

Virtually any of the varieties of glaucoma previously discussed may develop in an eye that has had cataract surgery, but some glaucomas are specifically associated with complications of cataract surgery (78). Retention of viscous aqueous substitutes, such as sodium hyaluronate, commonly used during cataract surgery, may temporarily obstruct the aqueous humor outflow pathways. In a similar fashion, retained lens material or red blood cells also may block aqueous humor outflow. These disorders are usually self-limited. Most chronic glaucomas after cataract surgery relate to prolonged inflammation (uveitis), wound abnormalities, postoperative flat anterior chambers, and peripheral anterior synechiae. Chronic uveitis may derive from retained lens material, prolonged intraocular surgery, uveal or vitreal incarceration within the wound, or loss of vitreous during surgery. Shallowing of the anterior chamber after cataract surgery may result from wound malposition and aqueous leak, choroidal detachment, pupillary block, aphakic malignant glaucoma, or suprachoroidal hemorrhage.

Excessive amounts of retained lens cortex after extracapsular cataract extraction may exacerbate postoperative glaucoma. This may lead to chronic postoperative uveitis, which by itself can result in glaucoma, or to direct outflow obstruction by the lens material. Although this material usually absorbs spontaneously, unacceptably increased intraocular pressures may call for evacuation of the retained material. With small amounts of retained lens cortical material, aqueous suppressants are usually sufficient to control the intraocular pressure, and corticosteroids may be added to lessen the inflammatory response. Long-standing uveitis associated with residual glaucoma may also respond to topical corticosteroids and hypotensive agents.

The uveitis-glaucoma-hyphema syndrome (UGH syndrome) has been reported with all varieties of intraocular lens implants after cataract extraction. It occurs most commonly with anterior chamber lenses but has also been associated with iris-supported and even posterior chamber intraocular lenses. The patient may have a history of uncomplicated cataract extraction but may later develop prolonged inflammation. Intraocular inflammation and intermittent hyphemas persist and recurrent episodes of elevated intraocular pressure and decreased vision occur. The UGH syndrome is secondary to mechanical rubbing of the intraocular lens on the iris, causing continuous pigment dispersion, producing a nidus for inflammation, and resulting in direct vascular trauma leading to intraocular bleeding. Elevated intraocular pressure is the result of outflow obstruction from prolonged inflammation, pigment dispersion, and anterior chamber hemorrhage. Most often, lens removal or repositioning is required, although corticosteroids and aqueous suppressants should be tried.

Intraocular lens placement, both in anterior and posterior chambers, may result in prolonged inflammation and progressive angle-closure without an accompanying UGH syndrome (35). Posterior chamber lenses may create progressive shallowing of the anterior chamber with closure of the chamber angle, especially anterior to the lens haptics. This is more commonly seen with sulcus-fixated posterior chamber intraocular lenses, as compared with lenses placed within the capsular bag. Anterior chamber lenses are much more likely to cause aqueous outflow insufficiency secondary to direct trabecular meshwork trauma and progressive angle-closure. Compromise of the anterior chamber angle and aqueous outflow occur not only at the site of the haptic placement into the chamber angle, but over months to years, may progress to close off distant sites of the anterior chamber angle. Especially with closed loop haptic anterior chamber lenses, progressive damage to the trabecular meshwork may occur. Placement of anterior chamber intraocular lenses is discouraged in patients with preexisting deficiency of aqueous outflow.

Wound leak and choroidal detachment are usually associated with an abnormally low or low-normal intraocular pressure. Pupillary block often has an elevated intraocular pressure, but in the presence of choroidal detachment or wound leak, the pressure may be normal or decreased. Malignant glaucoma or posterior entrapment of aqueous humor within or behind the vitreous body, and suprachoroidal hemorrhage are both associated with elevated intraocular pressure. The differential diagnosis is obvious with the large, dark choroidal detachments associated with suprachoroidal hemorrhage. When the posterior view is limited, secondary to corneal edema or other media opacities, ultrasonography may be useful in diagnosing a choroidal detachment and hemorrhage. With ultrasonography and malignant glaucoma, the vitreous humor may appear to be compacted against the posterior surface of an intraocular lens or the pupil, with relatively clear fluid behind the compacted vitreous (see Other Varieties of Angle-closure Glaucoma, Malignant Glaucoma). This condition may be correctable with anterior vitrotomy using the nd:YAG laser to provide an escape pathway, through the compacted vitreous, into the anterior chamber. A more complete discussion of the diagnosis and management of these disorders is found later in this section (see Complications of Filtration Surgery).

A shallow anterior chamber from any cause, if not corrected, may result in peripheral anterior synechiae and chronic glaucoma. Incarceration of iris or vitreous within the cataract wound may lead to continual inflammation or may serve as a route for ingrowing fibroblasts or epithelium, with resultant intractable glaucoma. Bleeding incisional vessels, fibrous ingrowth, or epithelial downgrowth all derive from wound malposition.

■ GLAUCOMA ASSOCIATED WITH INTRAOCULAR TUMORS

Intraocular tumors may cause either open-angle or closed-angle glaucoma. Metastatic tumors and malignant melanomas are the most frequent tumors associated with glaucoma, but hemangiomas, neurofibromas, and leukemia, among others, have been reported (71,98). Anterior segment tumors tend to invade the angle directly, while posterior segment masses more commonly lead to angle-closure glaucoma by anterior displacement of the lens-iris diaphragm. Neovascular glaucoma may also complicate intraocular tumors. Most iris nevi are benign, requiring only photographic documentation and careful follow-up for assessment of growth and possible chamber angle invasion.

The most common intraocular tumor in adults,

uveal melanoma, accounts for the majority of tumor-induced glaucomas (98). Expanding posterior segment melanomas can lead to angle-closure glaucoma by anteriorly displacing the vitreous, lens, ciliary body, and iris. Intraocular tumors should always be considered in any unilateral angle-closure glaucoma. Melanomas of the anterior segment, iris, or ciliary body are more likely to be associated with open-angle glaucoma. As mentioned, direct extension of tumors from the iris and ciliary body may infiltrate the anterior chamber angle. The trabecular meshwork may provide a template for rapid expansion of iris or ciliary body tumors, which can extend from a localized nidus to fill the entire trabecular meshwork, leading to a ring-shaped melanoma. Extension of an intraocular melanoma into the anterior chamber angle is a poor prognostic sign, often requiring enucleation.

Another rare melanoma-induced glaucoma is melanomalytic glaucoma (80, 98). This develops when necrotic tumors, usually of the ciliary body, release pigmented debris that is ingested by macrophages. Large, tumor-laden, densely pigmented macrophages are visi-ble circulating in the aqueous humor and become enmeshed in the interstices of the trabecular meshwork, leading to glaucoma. These behave similarly to other macrophage-induced glaucomas (e.g., phacolytic or hemolytic). The anterior chamber angle is open, but the trabecular meshwork is infiltrated with black pigmented material and pigment-laden macrophages, similar in appearance to pigmentary glaucoma. Melanomalytic glaucoma can be differentiated from pigmentary glaucoma by its unilaterality, lack of radially transillumination defects, and the large pigmented cells circulating in the anterior chamber. This is in contrast to the fine pigment granules of the pigment dispersion syndrome. Ocular tumors may be misdiagnosed as uveitis, rubeosis, or even primary angle-closure glaucoma. Long-standing visual loss, unilateral shallowing of the anterior chamber, unilateral irregular chamber angle pigmentation, or a poor view of the fundus all suggest the possibility of tumor. When media opacities obscure visualization of the fundus, transillumination and ultrasonography are diagnostically helpful.

Congenital, Infantile, Juvenile and Developmental Glaucoma

■ INTRODUCTION

Primary congenital or infantile glaucoma refers to glaucoma occurring at birth or shortly thereafter, in eyes with developmental abnormalities of the anterior chamber angle. These abnormalities result in decreased aqueous outflow and usually occur bilaterally. Primary juvenile glaucoma is similar to primary congenital glaucoma, except that it occurs later in childhood or even early adulthood. Other developmental glaucomas may also develop during early childhood. These are often associated with other ocular and systemic abnormalities. Childhood glaucomas may develop as the result of other ocular abnormalities, such as trauma, inflammation, or neoplasia. For a discussion of congenital cataracts with congenital glaucoma (see Chapter 21).

■ PRIMARY CONGENITAL-INFANTILE GLAUCOMA

Primary congenital glaucoma occurs at birth or within the first several months of life (88, 68). It is characterized by severe elevations of intraocular pressure, which when left untreated will cause stretching of the various support tissues of the eye and enlargement of the globe (buphthalmos). Primary infantile glaucoma occurs during childhood and may also result in buphthalmos, even with onset later in childhood, up to approximately 3 years of age. Some primary congenital glaucomas have a hereditary basis, most commonly an autosomal recessive pattern of inheritance with incomplete penetrance. At least 70% of congenital glaucoma cases are bilateral, and male children have a slightly higher prevalence.

The classic presentation of a child with primary congenital or infantile glaucoma is the triad of excessive epiphora, photophobia, and blepharospasm. The epiphora and photophobia are believed to be reactions to the corneal edema which results from the elevation of intraocular pressure. Blepharospasm is likely the result of photophobia. On clinical examination, these children may show marked corneal edema in one or both eyes and increased corneal diameter (Figure

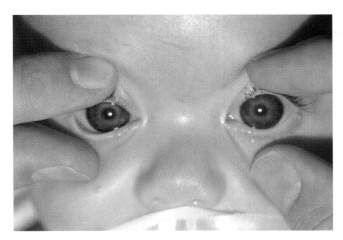

Figure 45–6.
Congenital Glaucoma: A 2-month-old child with bilateral corneal edema and enlarged corneas. The right corneal diameter is 12 mm and the left is 13 mm.

45–6). The normal, horizontal corneal diameter, at birth, is approximately 10.5 mm. Corneal diameters in excess of 12 mm are considered megalocorneas and a diagnostic evaluation for glaucoma should be done. Although corneal edema initially occurs secondary to increased intraocular pressure, with enlargement of the globe and stretching of the cornea, breaks in Descemet's membrane may occur, leading to central scarring of the cornea and persistent edema, despite lowering of intraocular pressure (88). These breaks in Descemet's membrane are usually oriented horizontally and are referred to as Haab's striae. Intraocular pressures greater than 20mm Hg, Haab's striae, and corneal diameters greater than 12 mm are diagnostic of congenital glaucoma. Optic nerve cupping and damage may not be evident on the initial examinations. With enlargement of the globe, patients show a large, myopic refractive error. Accurate gonioscopy and tonometry are critical for the diagnosis and ultimate management of congenital glaucoma. This may be accomplished in an office setting with some infants, especially those under the age of 3 to 4 months (81). However, examination under general anesthesia should not be postponed in infants when the office examination is insufficient.

At the time of an examination under anesthesia, several important measurements and evaluations should be done. Accurate corneal diameters should be obtained with a caliper. Tonometry is done at the earliest possible time after induction of general anesthesia, because all general anesthetics result in lowering of the intraocular pressure. Many clinicians prefer in-office examinations without sedation or under chloral hydrate sedation, which does not lower intraocular pressure to the same extent as inhaled general anesthetics. Direct gonioscopic lenses are preferred for examinations under anesthesia of the infant's eye. Koeppe, Barkan or

Swan-Jacob gonioscopy lenses allow excellent visualization of the anterior chamber angle. The anterior chamber angle in the normal child eye appears different from the adult eye. The trabecular meshwork typically has a nonpigmented homogenous appearance until late in childhood. The anterior chamber angle in a normal infant eye has a glassy appearance, and there may appear to be a membrane over the surface of the angle structures. In primary congenital-infantile glaucoma, the iris root shows a high insertion, but the chamber angle is open. Frequent iris processes and scalloping of the peripheral iris may also be seen. Lightly pigmented irides allow identification of many iris vessels, both centrally and peripherally. Dilated funduscopic examination in primary congenital-infantile glaucoma may reveal a variety of optic nerve findings. The optic nerve may appear normal with a healthy neuroretinal rim and a small physiologic cup, or it may show extensive central cupping with compression of the peripheral neuroretinal rim. This cupping is often reversible after lowering of the intraocular pressure.

The pathogenesis of the anterior chamber abnormalities in primary congenital-infantile glaucoma is believed to result from a developmental arrest in the angle structure formation (2, 37). Abnormalities of the neurocrest cell migration and subsequent formation of the anterior chamber structures may contribute to this disease. Early descriptions of occlusion of the trabecular meshwork by a membrane (Barkan's membrane) have never been supported by histology of congenital glaucoma eyes (6). The differential diagnosis of congenital glaucoma includes nasolacrimal duct obstruction and epiphora, meglocornea, traumatic ruptures of Descemet's membrane, and other causes of corneal opacification.

Management of primary congenital-infantile glaucoma is almost always surgical (7, 24). Medical therapy may be used as a temporizing measure, but surgical intervention is usually necessary. The principal procedures for control of intraocular pressure in congenital glaucoma are trabeculotomy and goniotomy. These procedures are described further in this text. Postoperative care in patients with congenital-infantile glaucoma includes close observation and repeat examinations under anesthesia at frequent intervals. Corneal edema and opacification may limit the ultimate visual rehabilitation and may contribute to the development of amblyopia. Intraocular pressures below 20mm Hg should be used as a target range in most cases. Multiple procedures are necessary to control the intraocular pressure in approximately 50% of eyes with congenital-infantile glaucoma. Education of the patient's family is critically important in the successful management of infantile glaucoma. Patients with this disease require lifelong follow-up, and frequent physician visits are to be expected.

■ ANIRIDIA

Aniridia is a developmental, usually bilateral, ocular anomaly which includes absence of the normal iris, other ocular abnormalities, and is associated with glaucoma (8, 45, 52). Although the name implies a total absence of the iris, there is always a rudimentary stump of peripheral iris, which may need gonioscopy to be seen. Aniridia is most often an autosomal-dominant inherited disease, but sporadic cases do occur. Approximately 20% of sporadic cases of aniridia will be associated with Wilm's tumor or other genitourinary tract abnormalities. Some of these individuals have a defect on the short arm of the eleventh chromosome. Glaucoma develops in greater than 50% of aniridia patients, although it usually does not present until the second or third decade of life. Some aniridics also exhibit mental retardation.

The clinical presentation of aniridia is variable, and many ocular abnormalities may be associated with aniridia. Progressive corneal pannus and opacification may develop. Early in life, this keratopathy may be limited to the peripheral cornea, but during adolescence and early adulthood, central opacification of the cornea may occur. Congenital cataracts are frequent but are typically not visually significant until later in life. During the third and fourth decades of life, lens opacification may progress rapidly, requiring cataract extraction. However, the primary etiology of decreased visual acuity in aniridic patients is foveal hypoplasia. The abnormal foveal development results in significant decrease in the visual acuity (usually 20/100 to 20/200) and concomitant nystagmus (87). Some families have been described with aniridia and normal foveal development. Other ocular abnormalities include microcornea, lens subluxation, choroidal colobomas, and strabismus.

The glaucoma associated with aniridia is often difficult to control. In the aniridic infant, a rudimentary stump of peripheral iris and an open anterior chamber angle are common. There may be areas of peripheral anterior synechiae, fine iris processes extending across the anterior chamber angle, occasional small blood vessels within the chamber angle, or other congenital anomalies of the anterior chamber angle. Elevation of intraocular pressure most commonly occurs in the second to third decade of life. This is associated with progressive contracture of the anterior chamber angle and closure of the trabecular meshwork by the residual iris. Glaucoma may occur at a younger age without angle-closure, secondary to congenital abnormalities of the anterior chamber angle. In older patients, filtration surgery is the procedure of choice. Goniotomy or trabeculotomies frequently do not work in older children because of the extensive angle-closure. In younger children, goniotomy should be attempted, if the anterior chamber angle is open.

■ PHAKOMATOSES

Phakomatoses refer to a group of disorders in which congenital hamartomas occur primarily in the skin, eye, and central nervous system (82). Other systemic anomalies may be associated with these disorders. The most frequent phakomatoses to be associated with glaucoma are Sturge-Weber syndrome (encephalotrigeminal angiomatoses) and von Recklinghausen's disease (neurofibromatosis). von Hippel Lindau disease and tuberosis sclerosis are occasionally associated with glaucoma (also see Chapter 23).

Sturge-Weber Syndrome

Sturge-Weber syndrome is a phakomatosis characterized by hemangiomas of the face and eye (55, 93). The classic presentation includes a "port wine stain" or hemangioma of the facial skin in the distribution of the trigeminal nerve and is virtually diagnostic of this syndrome (Figure 45–7) . These congenitally occurring hemangiomas may be associated with an ipsilateral leptomeningeal angioma, which may result in a seizure disorder. The facial hemangiomas are most typically unilateral but may occur bilaterally. Hemangiomas of the eye may involve both the episclera and the choroid. Approximately 50% of children born with lid and ocular involvement of the hemangiomas will develop glaucoma. The glaucoma may be evident in early childhood or may develop in early adulthood. Sturge-Weber syndrome is nonhereditary.

There are two potential etiologies for elevated intraocular pressure in individuals with Sturge-Weber syndrome. Anterior segment anomalies and faulty development of the aqueous drainage pathways or increased episcleral venous pressure may both contribute to elevated intraocular pressure (93).

Therapy for the glaucoma associated with Sturge-Weber syndrome depends on the age of onset for the elevation of intraocular pressure (33). Patients with childhood onset almost always require surgical intervention, while adult onset may be treated medically. The surgical procedures of choice in children with Sturge-Weber syndrome are goniotomy and trabeculotomy. The rationale for these procedures is threefold. First, filtration surgery during childhood typically has a poor prognosis for success. Second, many children are believed to have developmental anomalies of the anterior chamber angle which contribute to the glaucoma and may be amenable to goniotomy or trabeculotomy. Finally, associated choroidal hemangiomas found in Sturge-Weber syndrome may cause rapid expansion of choroidal effusions or suprachoroidal expulsive hemorrhages during or shortly after glaucoma filtration surgery in these patients. A decreased intraocular pressure after filtration surgery increases the risk of these complications. Goniotomy and trabeculotomy result in less profound lowering of the intraocular pressure in the immediate postoperative period and may decrease the incidence of these problems. In adults, filtration surgery may be necessary if medical therapy is inadequate. Prophylactic sclerotomies placed before filtration surgery is recommended in these cases.

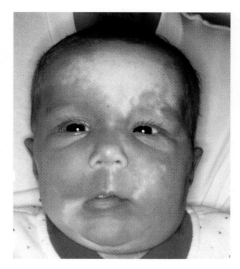

Figure 45–7.
Sturge-Weber Syndrome: A child with a facial hemangioma (port wine stain) in the trigeminal distribution. This child also had glaucoma and a large choroidal hemangioma in the left eye.

Von Recklinghausen's Disease

Neurofibromatosis 1 or von Recklinghausen's disease is an autosomally dominant inherited phakomatoses which may be associated with glaucoma (31, 53). The classic findings of von Recklinghausen's disease include pigmented skin lesions (café au lait spots), central nervous system and skin neurofibromas, acoustic neuromas, and schwanomas. Glaucoma is more frequent in eyes in which neurofibromas involve the ipsilateral upper eye lid. Anterior chamber angle dysgenesis and neurofibromatous tissue in the anterior chamber angle have been reported. Another common ocular finding with neurofibromatosis is the presence of Lisch nodules (40). These are yellow-pigmented nodules on the iris stroma which occur in almost all children with neurofibromatosis by late childhood. Management of elevated intraocular pressure in neurofibromatosis is difficult. Medical therapy should be attempted primarily, with surgical intervention used only if medical therapy failures.

■ AXENFELD-RIEGER SYNDROME (ANTERIOR SEGMENT DYSGENESIS)

Axenfeld-Rieger Syndrome includes a spectrum of developmental disorders which are present at birth and may be associated with glaucoma (69). In 1920, Axenfeld described a patient with strands of iris tissue extending from the peripheral iris to an anteriorly displaced Schwalbe's line (4). Later, Rieger described a similar case in which iris atrophy was also evident (62). The anteriorly displaced Schwalbe's line was later given the name "posterior embryotoxon" of the cornea, and these disorders were included under the category of "mesodermal dysgenesis (69)." Mesodermal dysgenesis is a misnomer as the embryonic cause is most likely a defect of the neuralcrest cell migration. The term anterior segment dysgenesis is more appropriate. Posterior embryotoxon occurs in up to 15% of normal eyes.

Today, Axenfeld-Rieger syndrome defines a spectrum of anomalous conditions of the cornea, iris, anterior chamber angle, and lens (69, 90). Axenfeld's anomaly is defined as a developmental disorder with peripheral iris strands attaching to an anteriorly displaced Schwalbe's line, while Rieger's anomaly denotes the additional central iris findings of corectopia and atrophy. Axenfeld's syndrome includes the development of glaucoma, and Rieger's syndrome may have a multiple of other anomalies including glaucoma and nonocular developmental defects. These disorders are almost always bilateral and often there is a family history with an autosomal-dominant inheritance pattern. There is no sex predilection for these disorders.

On examination, individuals with Axenfeld's anomaly characteristically show a prominent and anteriorly displaced Schwalbe's line, which may be seen without gonioscopy. Strands of peripheral iris stroma extend up to Schwalbe's line and occur throughout the entire chamber angle (Figure 45–8). The cornea is usually normal although both microcornea and megalo-

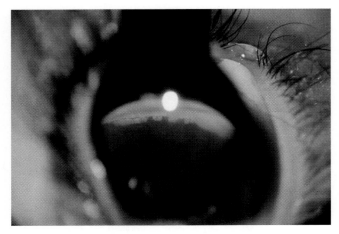

Figure 45–8.
Axenfeld-Rieger's Syndrome: Gonioscopic view of a child's eye with strands of tissue extending from the peripheral iris to a prominent, anteriorly-displaced Schwalbe's line.

cornea have been described. Strabismus is more common in patients with Axenfeld-Rieger's syndrome than in the general pediatric population. Other associated ocular abnormalities include limbal dermoids, congenital cataracts, chorioretinal colobomas, macular degeneration, retinal detachments, and hypoplasia of the optic nerves.

Nonocular findings associated with Rieger's syndrome include small, displaced teeth and occasional absence of teeth (69). Maxillary hypoplasia, hypertelorism, and midfacial and midline central nervous system anomalies have been reported. Pituitary deficiencies with growth hormone insufficiency may occur, and children should be monitored for normal developmental milestones. Genitourinary abnormalities have also been described with this syndrome.

More than 50% of individuals with Axenfeld-Rieger's syndrome will develop glaucoma. This may present as an infantile glaucoma but more commonly appears in later childhood or even early adulthood. Glaucoma associated with this syndrome may be difficult to control, requiring multiple surgical procedures. Intraocular pressure is infrequently controlled with medical therapy, and goniotomy or trabeculotomy is the primary surgical option. With glaucoma presenting later in life, trabeculectomy may also be considered. Irido-corneal adhesions may make goniotomy difficult to complete and trabeculotomy is preferred by some clinicians (also see Chapter 51).

■ PETER'S ANOMALY

Peter's anomaly is a bilateral congenital disorder which can be associated with infantile glaucoma (5, 45). This anomaly is characterized by central defects in Descemet's membrane and the corneal endothelium, with thinning of the central corneal stroma. Adhesions extend from the borders of the corneal defect to the central iris in most cases. Apposition of the lens to the central corneal defect may also occur. Most cases are nonhereditary, although autosomal-recessive and autosomal-dominant cases have been reported. Chromosomal abnormalities have also been described. Approximately 50% of patients with Peter's anomaly will develop glaucoma, usually at birth or during early childhood. Structural abnormalities of the anterior chamber angle are usually present, and the glaucoma is frequently difficult to control. Central corneal abnormalities often require penetrating keratoplasty and removal of the lens. Trabeculotomy or trabeculectomy are the surgical procedures done most frequently for control of the glaucoma (also see Chapter 51).

■ RETINOPATHY OF PREMATURITY

Retinopathy of prematurity, or retrolental fibroplasia, is a bilateral disease occurring in prematurely born children, especially those who received oxygen therapy (25, 27, 39). At the time of the premature birth, the retinal vascularization is incomplete and subsequent vascularization develops abnormally. This may lead to a variety of sequelae, including vitreous hemorrhage, retinal detachment, and retrolental fibrotic membrane formation. With the development of fibrotic tissue posterior to the lens, a secondary angle-closure glaucoma may develop. This occurs as the lens-iris diaphragm is shifted anteriorly by the retrolental mass. When glaucoma occurs in infancy or early childhood, lens removal with a concurrent vitrectomy and removal of the retrolental fibrotic mass is usually required. Such eyes have a guarded visual prognosis, despite surgical intervention. Angle-closure glaucoma has also been reported in early adulthood, during the second to fourth decades of life, in eyes with a history of retinopathy of prematurity. These individuals are more amenable to medical therapy, as well as laser iridotomy treatments if there is a pupillary block component (also see chapter on Pediatric Retinal).

PERSISTENT HYPERPLASTIC PRIMARY VITREOUS

Persistent hyperplastic primary vitreous, or PHPV, is almost always unilateral and occurs most often in microphthalmic eyes (61). Failure of the regression of the primary vitreous results in a contractile retrolental fibrous mass which may be attached to the posterior surface of the lens. Classically, the ciliary processes are drawn centrally and elongated. PHPV is part of the differential diagnosis of leukocoria and must be differentiated from intraocular tumor. Microphthalmia frequently occurs with PHPV but rarely occurs with retinoblastoma. Progressive cataract formation and in-

creased posterior pressure shifting the lens-iris diaphragm forward results in a secondary angle-closure glaucoma. Intraocular hemorrhages may result in aqueous humor outflow obstruction. Therapy for PHPV and the associated glaucoma includes removal of the cataract and retrolental mass. The visual prognosis is poor in eyes with glaucoma. Early surgery to remove the lens and retinolental mass in PHPV results in more favorable visual outcomes and decreases the likelihood of secondary glaucoma (also see Chapter 21).

RUBENSTEIN-TAYBI SYNDROME

Rubenstein-Taybi syndrome is a rare disorder which includes mental retardation, congenital cataracts, and congenital glaucoma (92). These children frequently have large thumbs and great toes, which has resulted in the name "broad thumb syndrome." Large physiologic

cups, as well as posterior segment colobomas, are seen in these children. Traditional goniotomy or trabeculotomy surgery for this form of infantile glaucoma is recommended (also see Chapter 23).

RUBELLA

Congenital rubella syndrome is seen in newborns in whom there was maternal exposure to rubella during pregnancy (10). The syndrome includes congenital glaucoma, congenital cataracts, microcornea, and pigmented retinopathy. These children may also have cataracts and central nervous system abnormalities.

Rubella keratitis may develop and result in central corneal opacification. Management of glaucoma in these individuals usually calls for surgery. Goniotomy or trabeculotomy is recommended as the primary therapy, but frequently, multiple surgeries are needed. Postoperative uveitis is common (also see Chapter 21).

LOWE'S SYNDROME

Lowe's syndrome, or oculocerebrorenal syndrome, is characterized as a sex-linked recessive anomaly which includes aminoaciduria, renal failure, and mental retardation (86). This is seen in male infants, and congenital

glaucoma and cataracts are the most frequent ocular abnormalities. Goniotomy or trabeculotomy is recommended as the primary procedure, although the prognosis is guarded (also see Chapter 21).

REFERENCES

1. Abedin, S, Simmons, RJ, Grant, WM: Progressive low-tension glaucoma. Treatment to stop glaucomatous cupping and field loss when these progress despite normal intraocular pressure, Ophthalmology 1982, 89:1.
2. Anderson DR: The development of the trabecular mesh-

work and its abnormality in primary infantile glaucoma. Trans Am Ophthal Soc 1981, 79:458.
3. Armaly, MF, Wang, Y: Demonstration of acid mucopolysaccharides in the trabecular meshwork of the Rhesus monkey. Invest Ophthal 1975, 14:507.

4. Axenfeld TH: Embryotoxon cornae posterious. Der Deutsch Ophtla Ges 1920, 42:301

5. Azuma I: Peters' anomaly associated with glaucoma and chromosomal abnormality. Folia Ophthal Jap 1984, 35:1869.

6. Barkan O: Pathogenesis of congenital glaucoma. Gonioscopic and anatomic observation of the angle of the anterior chamber in the normal eye and in congenital glaucoma. Am J Ophthal 1955, 40:1.

7. Barkan O: Goniotomy for the relief of congenital glaucoma. Br J Ophthal 1948, 32:701.

8. Beauchamp GR: Anterior segment dysgenesis, keratolenticular adhesion and aniridia. J Ped Ophthal Strab 1980, 17:55.

9. Becker, B, Unger, HH, Coleman, SL, Keates, EU: Plasma cells and gamma-globulin in trabecular meshwork of eyes with primary open-angle glaucoma. Arch Ophthal 1963, 70:38.

10. Boniuk M: Glaucoma in the congenital rubella syndrome. Int Ophthal Clin 1972, 12:121.

11. Brown, GC, Magargal, LE, Schachat, A, Shah, H: Neovascular glaucoma: etiologic considerations. Ophthalmology 1984, 91:315.

12. Campbell, DG: Pigmentary dispersion and glaucoma. A new theory. Arch Ophthal 1979, 97:1667.

13. Campbell, DG, Essigmann, EM: Hemolytic ghost cell glaucoma. Further studies. Arch Ophthal 1979, 97:2141.

14. Campbell, DG, Simmons, RJ, Grant, WM: Ghost cells as a cause of glaucoma. Am J Ophthal 1976, 81:441.

15. Canavan, YM, Archer, DB: Anterior segment consequences of blunt ocular injury. Br J Ophthal 1982, 66;549.

16. Chandler, PA: Narrow-angle glaucoma. Arch Ophthal 1952, 47:695.

17. Chandler, PA, Simmons, RJ, Grant, WM: Malignant glaucoma. Medical and surgical treatment. AM J Ophthal 1968, 66:495.

18. Deutsch, TA: Indications for Surgical Management of Hyphema in Patients with Sickle Cell Trait. Arch Ophthal 1984, 102:566–569.

19. Drance, SM, Morgan RW, Bryett, J, et al: Anterior chamber depth and gonioscopic findings among the Eskimos and Indians of the Canadian arctic. Can J Ophthal 1973, 8:255.

20. Dvorak, Theobald, G: Pseudo-exfoliation of the lens capsule. Relation to "true" exfoliation of the lens capsule as reported in the literature and role in the production of glaucoma capsulocuticulare. Am J Ophthal 1954, 37:1.

21. Epstein, DL: Diagnosis and management of lens-induced glaucoma. Ophthalmology 1982, 89:227.

22. Farrar, SM, Shields, MB: Current concepts in pigmentary glaucoma, Surv Ophthalmol 1993, 37(4)233.

23. Fritch CD: Traumatic hyphema. Ann Ophthalmol 1976, 8:1223.

24. Harms H, Dannheim R: Trabeculotomy results and problems. In: Microsurgery in Glaucoma, (ed. Mackenson G). Basel, S. Karger, 1970, -g. 121.

25. Hartnett ME, Gilbert MM, Richardson TM, et al: Anterior segment evaluation of infants with retinopathy of prematurity. Ophthalmology 1990, 97:122.

26. Hayreh, SS, Podhajsky, P: Ocular neovascularization with retinal vascular occlusion. II. Occurrence in central and branch retinal artery occlusion. Arch Ophthal 1982, 100;1585.

27. Hittner HM, Rhodes LM, McPherson AR: Anterior segment abnormalities in cicatricial retinopathy of prematurity. Ophthalmolol 86:803, 1979.

28. Hollows, FC, Graham, PA: Intra-ocular pressure, glaucoma, and glaucoma suspects in a defined population, Br J Ophthal 1966, 50:570.

29. Hoskins, HD Jr.: Neovascular glaucoma: current concepts. Trans Am Acad Ophthal Otol 1974, 78:330.

30. Huang SCM, Soong HK, Benz RM, et al: Problems associated with penetrating keratoplasty for corneal edema in congenital glaucoma. Ophthal Surg 1989, 20:399.

31. Huson S, Jones D, Beck L: Ophthalmic manifestations of neurofibromatosis. Br J Ophthal 1987, 71:235.

32. Hwang, DG, Smith, RE: Corneal complications of cataract surgery. Refract Corneal Surg 1991, 7(1) 77.

33. Iwach AG, Hoskins HD Jr, Hetherington J Jr, Shaffer RN: Analysis of surgical and medical management of glaucoma in Sturge-Weber syndrome. Ophthalmology 1990, 97:904.

34. Karbassi, M, Raizman, MB, Schuman JS: Herpes Zoster Ophthamicas. Surv Ophthalmol 1992, 36(6): 395.

35. Keates RH, Ehrlich DR: Lenses of chance. Complications of anterior chamber implants. Ophthalmology 1978, 85:408.

36. Krachmer, JH: Posterior polymorphous corneal dystrophy: a disease characterized by epithelial-like endothelial cells which influence management and prognosis. Trans Am Ophthal Soc 1985, 83:413.

37. Kupfer C, Kaiser-Kuper MI: Observations on the development of the anterior chamber angle with reference to the pathogenesis of congenital glaucomas. Am J Ophth 1979, 88:424.

38. Kushner, BJ: Ciliary block glaucoma in retinopathy of prematurity. Arch Ophthalmol 1982, 100:1078.

39. Kushner BJ, Sondheimer S: Medical treatment of glaucoma associated with cicatricial retinopathy of prematurity. Am J Ophthal 1982, 94:313.

40. Lewis RA, Riccardi VM: von Recklinghausen neurofibromatosis. Incidence of iris hamartomata. Ophthalmology 1981, 88:348.

41. Li, Y, Yi, Y: Histochemical and electron microscopic studies of the trabecular meshwork in primary open-angle glaucoma. Eye Science 1985, 1:17.

42. Liesgang, TJ: Clinical features and prognosis in Fuch's uveitis syndrome. Arch Ophthal 1982, 100;1622.

43. Lindberg, JG: Clinical investigations on depigmentation of the pupillary border and translucency of the iris. In cases of senile cataract and in normal eyes in elderly persons. Academic Dissertation, Helsinki, 1917. English translation by Tarkkanen, A, Forsius, H, Acta Ophthal Suppl 190, Vol. 66, University Press, Helsinki, 1989.

44. Lowe, RF: Malignant glaucoma related to primary angle-closure glaucoma. Aust NZ J Ophthalmol 1979, 7:11.

45. Margo CE: Congenital aniridia: a histopathologic study of the anterior segment in children. J Ped Ophthal Strab 1983, 20:192.

46. Martin, MJ, Sommer, A, Gold, EB, Diamond, EL: Race and primary open-angle glaucoma. Am J Ophthal 1985, 99:383.

47. McLean, JM: Use of ACTH and cortisone. Discussion of paper of Woods, AC. Trans Am Ophthal Soc 1950, 48:293.

48. Minas, TF, Podos, SM: Familial glaucoma associated with elevated episcleral venous pressure. Arch Ophthal 1968, 80:202.

49. Muller, H: Phacolytic glaucoma and phacogenic ophthalmia. (Lens induced uveitis). Trans Ophthal Soc UK 1963, 83:689.

50. Omerod LD, Baerveldt G, Sunalp MA, Riekhof FT: Management of they hypotonus cyclodialysis cleft. Ophthalmol 1991, 98(9) 1284.

51. Panek, WC, Hololand, GN, Lee, DA, Christensen, RE: Glaucoma in patients with uveitis. Br J. Ophthal 1990, 74:223.

52. Pavlick MA, Walton DS: Genetics of Aniridia: The Aniridia: Wilm's Tumor Association. Int Ophthalmol Clin 1993 33(2) 77.

53. Pearson-Webb MA, Kaiser-Kupfer MI, Eldridge R: Eye findings in bilateral acoustic (central) neurofibromatosis: association with presenile lens opacities and cataracts but absence of Lisch nodules. N Engl J Med 1986, 315:1553.

54. Peters A: Ueber angeborene Defektbildung der Descemetschen Membran. Klin Monatsbl Augenheilkd 1906, 44:27.

55. Phelps, CD: The pathogenesis of glaucoma in Sturge-Weber syndrome. Ophthalmology 1978, 85:276.

56. Pohjanpelto, PEJ, Plava, J: Ocular hypertension and glaucomatous optic nerve damage. Acta Ophthal 1974, 52:194.

57. Pollack, IP: Chronic angle-closure glaucoma. Diagnosis and treatment in patients with angles that appear open. Arch Ophthal 1971, 85:676.

58. Posner, A, Schlossman, A: Syndrome of unilateral recurrent attacks of glaucoma with cyclitic symptoms. Arch Ophthal 1948, 39:517.

59. Prince, AM, Ritch, R: Clinical signs of the pseudoexfoliation syndrome. Ophthalmology 1986, 93:803.

60. Radius, RL, Maumenee, AE: Dilated episcleral vessels and open-angle glaucoma. Am J Ophthal 1978, 86:31.

61. Reese AB: Persistent hyperplastic primary vitreous. Am J Ophthal 1955, 40:317.

62. Rieger H: Dysgenesis mesodermalis Cornae et Iridis. Z Augenheilkd 1935, 86:333.

63. Riesler, JC and Schwartz, B: Miotic-induced malignant glaucoma. Arch Ophthalmol 1972, 87:706.

64. Rodrigues MM, Spaeth GL, Krachmer JH,Laibson PR: Iridochisis associated with glaucoma and bullous keratopathy. Am J Ophthal 1983, 95:73

65. Rodrigues, MM, Spaeth, GL, Weinreb, S, Sivalingam, E: Spectrum of trabecular pigmentation in open-angle glaucoma: a clinicopathologic study. Trans Am Acad Ophthal Otol 1976, 81:258.

66. Roth, M, Epstein, DL: Exfoliation syndrome. Am J Ophthal 1980, 89:477.

67. Rothova, A, van Veenendaal, WG, Linssen, A, et al: Clinical features of acute anterior uveitis, Am J Ophthal 1987, 103:137.

68. Shaffer RN, Weiss DI: Congenital and pediatric glaucomas. CV Mosby, St. Louis, 1970, p. 37.

69. Shields MB, Buckley E, Lintworth GK, Thresher R: Axenfeld-Rieger syndrome. A spectrum of developmental disorders. Surv Ophthal 1985, 29:387.

70. Shields, MB: Progressive essential iris atrophy, Chandler's syndrome, and the iris nevus (Cogen Reese) syndrome: a spectrum of disease. Surv Ophthal 197, 24:3.

71. Shields CL, Shields JA, Shields MB, Augsburger JJ: Prevalence and mechanisms of secondary intraocular pressure elevation in eyes with intraocular tumors. Ophthalmology 1987. 94:839.

72. Simmons, RJ: Malignant glaucoma, Br J Ophthalmol 1972, 56:263.

73. Simmons, RJ: Malignant glaucoma. In: Ritch R, and Shields MB, editors: The secondary glaucomas, St. Louis, 1982, CV Mosby

74. Singh, OS, Simmons, RJ, Brockhurst, RJ, Trempe, CL: Nanophthalmos: a perspective on identification and therapy. Ophthalmology 1982, 89:1006.

75. Smith, RJH: Rubeotic glaucoma. Br J Ophthal 1981, 65:606.

76. Sommer, A, Tielsch, JM, Katz, J, Quigley, HA, Gottsch, JD, Javitt, J, Singh, K and Baltimore Eye Survey Research Group: Relationship between intraocular pressure and primary open angle glaucoma among white and black Americans. Arch Ophthalmol 1991, 109:1090.

77. Sugar, HS: Pigmentary glaucoma. A 25 year review. Am J Ophthal 1966, 62:499.

78. Tomey KF, Traverso CE: The glaucomas in aphakia and pseudophakia. Surv Ophthal 36(2) 1991, 79–112.

79. Urban, RC, Dreger EB: Corticosteroid-induces glaucoma. Int. Ophthalmol Clin, 1993, 33(2) 135.

80. Van Buskirk EM, Leure-duPree AE: Pathophysiology and electron microscopy of melanomalytic glaucoma. Am J Ophthal 1978, 85:160.

81. Van Buskirk EM, Palmer EA: Office assessment of young children for glaucoma. Ann Ophthal 1979, 11:1749.

82. Van der Hoeve, J: Eye symptoms in phakomatoses. Trans Ophthal Soc UK 1932, 42:380.

83. Vogt, A: Vergleichende Uebersicht uber Klinik und Histologie der Alters—und Feuerlamelle der Linsenvorderkapsel. Klin Monatsbl Augenheilkd 1925, 75:1.

84. von Graefe, A: Beitrage zur pathologie und therapie des glaucoms, Arc Fur Ophthalmol 1869, 15:108.

85. von Graefe A: Uber die iridectomie bei glaukom und uber den glaucomatosen process. Graefes Arch Clin Exp Ophthalmol 1857, 3:456.

86. Wadelius C, Fagerholm P, Pettersson U, Anneren G: Lowe oculocerbrorenal syndrome. DNA-based linkage of the gene to Xq24-q26, using tightly linked flanking markers and the correlation to lens examination in carrier diagnosis. Am J Hum Genet 1989, 44:241.

87. Walton, DS: Aniridic glaucoma: the results of goniosurgery to prevent and treat this problem. Trans Am Ophthal Soc 1986, 84:59.

88. Walton DS: Primary congenital open-angle glaucoma. In: Glaucoma, Chandler PA, Grant WM. Lea and Febiger, Philadelphia, 1979, p. 329.

89. Wand, M, Grant WM, Simmons, RJ, Hutchinson, BT: Plateau iris syndrome. Trans Am Acad Ophthal Otol 1977, 83:122.

90. Waring GO III, Rodrigues MM, Laibson PR: Anterior chamber cleavage syndrome. A stepladder classification. Surv Ophthal 1975, 20:3.

91. Watson, PG, Hayreh, SS: Scleritis and episcleritis. Br J Ophthal 1976, 60:163.

92. Weber U, Bernsmeier H: Rubinstein-Taybi syndrome and juvenile glaucoma. Klin Monatsbl Augenheilkd 1983, 183:47.

93. Weiss DI: Dual origin of glaucoma in encephalotrigeminal haemangiomatosis. Trans Ophthal Soc UK, 1973, 93:477.

94. Wesely, P, Liebmann, J, Walsh, JB, Ritch, R: Lttice degeneration of the retina and pigment dispersion syndrome. Am J Ophthal 1993 114(5):539.

95. Wilensky, J: Racial influences in glaucoma. Ann Ophthal 1977, 9:1545.

96. Weiner, MJ, Trentacosts, J, Pon, DM, Albert, DM: Epithelial downgrowth: a 30-year clinico-pathological review. Br J Ophthal 1989, 73:6.

97. Wilson, MC, Shields, MB: A comparison of the clinical variations of the iridocorneal endothelial syndrome. Arch Ophthal 1989, 107:1465.

98. Yanoff M: Glaucoma mechanisms in ocular malignant melanomas. Am J Ophthal 1970, 70:898.

99. Yanoff, M: Iridocorneal endothelial syndrome. Unification of a disease spectrum. Surv Ophthal 1979, 24:1.

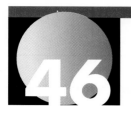

46 Ocular Hypotony

G. A. Cioffi, E. M. Van Buskirk

Clinically significant, ocular hypotony occurs when the intraocular pressure becomes sufficiently decreased to compromise function of the eye, usually below 6mm Hg. Hypotony may be associated with systemic conditions such as severe dehydration or myotonic dystrophy, but more often derives from some ocular abnormality (1, 2, 3, 4, 5). Hypotony may accompany severe uveitis, in which case the intraocular pressure normalizes as the inflammation resolves. More commonly, hypotony comes after intraocular surgery, especially glaucoma filtration surgery, as well as cataract extractions or other procedures. Profound causes of ocular hypotony require an alteration in the physiologic and/or structural integrity of the eye. Since normal aqueous humor formation is relatively stable and episcleral venous pressure ranges from 8 to 12mm Hg, either near-total or total suppression of aqueous humor formation, or an alternative pathway of aqueous humor outflow, must be present to cause profound ocular hypotony. After filtration surgery, excess aqueous humor runoff, uveal effusion with cilio-choroidal detachment, conjunctival leak, or cyclodialysis cleft may all lead to hypotony. The etiology of the ocular hypotony in eyes with decreased visual function should be sought and corrected in a timely fashion, since prolonged hypotony may result in permanent loss of visual function.

Ocular hypotony after filtration surgery may be associated with overfiltration through an exuberant 360° bleb or a thin-wall leaking bleb. These blebs occur more commonly with the use of adjunctive antimetabolite agents with filtration surgery, especially in myopic eyes. Rhegmaogenous retinal detachment may result in mild or profound ocular hypotony. Mild decreases in the aqueous humor production have been observed in eyes with retinal detachments. Aqueous humor may leave the eye via the retinal tear and ultimately be absorbed by the choroid, resulting in hypotony.

Cyclodialysis should always be considered a possible cause of hypotony, either after intraocular surgery or ocular contusion. Cyclodialysis clefts appear in the angle as a white "bared" scleral spur, from which the ciliary body has been detached, with an obvious gap or space between the ciliary body and the sclera. This creates a direct communication between the anterior chamber and the suprachoroidal space, resulting in increased aqueous egress from the anterior chamber.

Many eyes will tolerate relatively decreased, even hypotonus, intraocular pressures indefinitely with no apparent sequelae. Myotonic dystrophy results in bilateral ocular hypotony, which is usually mild and without visual sequelae. The etiology of hypotony in these patients remains unclear.

Other eyes, however, become soft enough to develop intermittent shallowing of the anterior chamber, blurring of vision, intraocular inflammation, cataract formation, uveal effusion, macular edema, disc edema, and choroidal folds. These clinical findings usually mandate intervention. Wound leaks or leaking blebs should be repaired. Chronic uveal effusions will nearly always spontaneously reabsorb. If they do not spontaneously resolve after 3 to 4 months, consideration should be given toward drainage of suprachoroidal fluid.

Sometimes, cyclodialysis clefts will close after administration of parasympatholytic agents, such as atropine, which paralyze the iris sphincter muscle and relax the lens-iris diaphragm. Pure sympathomimetic mydriatic agents, such as phenylephrine, may actually exacerbate the cleft by pulling the iris root toward the pupil. The variety of surgical techniques devised to close cyclodialysis clefts attests to the difficulty of the task. Small clefts can sometimes be closed by applying laser photocoagulation to create adhesion between the detached ciliary body and the overlying sclera. Larger clefts will often respond to penetrating diathermy. Diathermy should be applied using a 1 mm penetrating needle along the limbal extent of the cleft, as determined by gonioscopy. If more conservative therapies fail, surgical closure of the cleft is required.

The workup for ocular hypotony includes a careful history to elicit a previous ocular trauma or surgery. Examination of any surgical or filtration site is crucial in these cases. Even after uncomplicated cataract surgery, inadvertent filtration blebs may occur. A Seidel test should be done in all eyes with previous trauma or surgery, to look for a wound leak, bleb leak, or site of perforation. Gonioscopy should be done to evaluate patients for possible cyclodialysis clefts.

■ REFERENCES

1. Aaberg TM: Experimental serous and hemorrhagic uveal edema associated with retinal detachment surgery. Invest Ophthalmol 1975, 14:243.
2. Brubaker RF, and Pederson JE: Ciliochoroidal detachment. Surv Ophthalmol 1983, 27:281.
3. Dreyer RF: Ocular hypotony in myotonic dystrophy. Int Ophthalmol 1983, 6:221.
4. Meislik J, and Herschler J: Hypotony due to inadvertent cyclodialysis after intraocular lens implantation. Arch Ophthalmol 1979, 97:1297.
5. Ormerod LD, Baerveldt G, and Green RL: Cyclodialysis clefts: natural history, assessment and management. In: Weinstein GW, (ed): Open-angle Glaucoma: Contemporary Issues in Ophthalmology, vol. 3, New York, 1986, Churchill Livingstone.

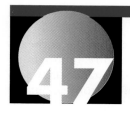# Glaucoma Therapy

G. A. Cioffi, E. M. Van Buskirk

■ GENERAL CONSIDERATIONS FOR GLAUCOMA THERAPY

Currently, almost all therapeutic modalities for the treatment of glaucoma are designed to lower the intraocular pressure. These modalities include medical antihypertensives, laser therapy, and incisional surgery. In clinical practice, individuals with newly diagnosed open-angle glaucoma initially have been treated with medical pressure-lowering agents, followed by argon laser trabeculoplasty, and finally, by surgical filtration procedures, if medical and laser therapies fail. Recently, this step-wise therapeutic approach has been questioned, and the efficacy of initial surgical therapy for glaucoma is being examined (56, 58, 59). With the advent of guarded filtration procedures, the surgical complication rates have been reduced. In addition, proponents of early surgical intervention believe that prolonged use of topical medications adversely affect surgical success rates. Many factors should be considered while individualizing each patient's care. These factors include the patient's diagnosis, the possible side effects of therapy, the cost of therapy, the predicted quality of life of the patient after therapy, and the long-term efficacy of the therapy.

Medical therapy for glaucoma has been greatly expanded during the past several decades. Currently, the clinician has a variety of topical and systemic agents with which to lower intraocular pressure. These agents include drugs which enhance aqueous humor outflow from the eye and drugs which suppress aqueous humor formation. All currently available topical medications exert their effect by changes in the autonomic nervous system. These drugs are subcategorized as cholingeric

agonists, adrenergic agonists, and adrenergic antagonists. Many ocular topical medications were originally derived from systemic cardiovascular medications.

Systemic antiglaucomatous medications are also available. Oral carbonic anhydrase inhibitors form the mainstay of systemic therapy for the control of intraocular pressure. Currently, topical carbonic anhydrase inhibitors are under investigation. Systemic hyperosmotic agents are also used for acute reduction of intraocular pressure, but their use is often limited by their systemic side effects and short duration of action.

New classifications of topical and intracameral glaucoma medications which enhance aqueous outflow through conventional and unconventional pathways, without altering the autonomic nervous system, are under investigation. These include intracameral ethacrynic acid and topical prostaglandins (11, 13, 20).

Many factors contribute to the success of medical therapy. The effectiveness of therapy depends on patient compliance with the medical regimen. With glaucoma, as with any chronic disease, long-term medical therapy is difficult to comply with. Because of the minimal symptoms associated with early glaucomatous optic nerve damage, many patients do not realize the importance of consistent medication application. It is critically important to educate the patient about the disease, glaucoma, and the potential for devastating visual loss. This may enhance the patient's compliance and aid in the tolerance of the prescribed medical regimen.

Side effects resulting from the various medications play an important role in the success of therapy but may be counter-productive to compliance. Side effects range from mild, local irritation to serious life-threatening disorders. Because of the nasolacrimal drainage system, medications applied topically in the eye have ready access to the nasal mucosa. Rapid absorption by the highly vascular tissues of the nasal passages results in a variety of systemic side effects after administration of topical medications. Eyelid closure immediately after the instillation of topical medications and digital-punctal occlusion may decrease the amount of medication flowing into the lacrimal system (81). These two techniques should be taught to every patient and continued for at least 3 minutes after the instillation of topical medications. Allowing 3 minutes between successive medications also ensures absorption of the first topically applied medication and prevents washout by subsequent medications.

The pharmacokinetics of topical medications are important, as well, in determining the effectiveness of these medications for controlling intraocular pressure. The ability to penetrate the cornea and the rate of drug metabolism influence the efficacy and duration of ac-

tion of the various medications. Because the cornea is an alternating lipid-water-lipid structure (epithelium-stroma-endothelium), lipid-soluble substances may penetrate the inner and outer layers of the cornea, but the hydrophilic stroma may remain impermeable (1). Drugs that exist in both an ionized and a nonionized state penetrate best through all the corneal layers.

In recent years, increasing interest in glaucoma therapy not related to control of intraocular pressure has emerged. With the recognition of patients in whom intraocular pressure is never elevated, but glaucomatous optic nerve damage continues, attention has turned to direct preservation of the optic nerve. Various medications have been used to enhance the blood flow to the optic nerve, possibly protecting it from localized ischemic damage. Calcium channel blockers, because of their vasodilative effects, as well as other vaso-modulators, have been investigated for this purpose (46,48). Excitatory neurotransmitters, free radical scavengers, antioxidants, and growth factors are all being investigated for possible direct neural protection abilities (57).

■ TOPICAL MEDICATIONS

Cholinergic Agonists

Cholinergic agonists (parasympathomimetic agents) were the first class of drugs used in the therapy of glaucoma (19, 43, 45). These medications, called "miotics" for their pupillary action, may be either direct-acting or indirect-acting agents. Direct-acting cholingeric agonists stimulate the motor endplates in a similar fashion to acetylcholine, while indirect agents inhibit acetylcholinesterase and potentiate the effects of acetylcholine by preventing its degradation. Pilocarpine is a direct-acting agent. Carbachol has both direct and indirect cholinergic actions. Echothiophate iodide is a pure indirect-acting agent (27,80). Physostigmine sulfate and demecarium bromide are also indirect-acting agents but are rarely used in the therapy of glaucoma. All miotics lower intraocular pressure by enhancing aqueous humor outflow from the anterior chamber. Increased tension on the scleral spur, secondary to contraction of the longitudinal ciliary muscles, is believed to cause alterations in configuration of the trabecular meshwork and Schlemm's canal, resulting in enhanced outflow.

The most frequent side effects resulting from the use of cholinergic agonists are limited to the eyes and ocular adnexa. Concomitant with contraction of the ciliary body muscles, miotics also stimulate the iris sphincter muscle to contract, causing miosis. Miosis dims vision by limiting the amount of light entering the eye

and may be particularly disabling in dim lighting. Miosis also decreases the perceived field of vision. Contraction of the ciliary muscle shifts the lens-iris diaphragm forward and thickens the lens, inducing myopia (49). Fluctuations in vision, secondary to changes in the position of the lens-iris diaphragm between doses, are poorly tolerated in younger patients. Ciliary spasm can occur and may be painful, creating a brow ache, especially at the initiation of therapy. Patients should be warned in advance of this side effect and encouraged to continue the medication since this side effect typically resolves within 1 to 2 weeks. Sustained brow ache is more often seen with carbachol than with pilocarpine. Retinal detachments resulting from contraction of the ciliary muscles and vitreoretinal traction have been reported with all miotics. Patients should undergo a dilated funduscopic examination to rule out asymptomatic peripheral retinal tears or holes before initiating miotic therapy. Cataract development has been associated with miotics, particularly echothiophate iodide. Echothiophate has also been associated with the development of iris cysts.

Systemic toxicosis is rare with pilocarpine and carbachol but may result from cholinergic stimulation. Systemic side effects include diarrhea, nausea, vomiting, increased pulmonary secretions, and diaphoresis. With indirect-acting agents, systemic side effects are much more common and potentially serious. Echothiophate iodide inhibits pseudocholinesterase, as well as cholinesterase, which may potentiate respiratory paralysis after general anesthesia with succinylcholine.

In animal models, pilocarpine decreases unconventional uveoscleral aqueous humor outflow (10). It is unknown if this effect occurs in the human eye, but eyes with limited conventional outflow should not be placed on miotics since elevation of intraocular pressure may result.

Because of the relatively short duration of action of the commonly used miotics, administration 3 or 4 times a day is required. Pilocarpine is available in a variety of concentrations (1 to 10%) and the intraocular pressure-lowering effect to pilocarpine is dose-related up to 4% (up to 6% in darkly pigmented eyes). A variety of sustained-release pilocarpine delivery systems has been developed, as well as long-acting gel preparations. Sustained-release pilocarpine membranes may be preferred by younger individuals since they have a more steady-state delivery and produce less fluctuation in vision. Pilocarpine gel is administered once a day at bedtime and lasts for 20 to 24 hours. With the gel preparations, the maximally induced myopia and miosis occur during sleep and are less bothersome to the patient. Carbachol is available in 0.75 to 3% preparations and is administered 3 times daily. Echothiophate iodide is available in 0.03 to 0.25% concentrations and is administered twice daily.

Adrenergic Agonists

There are two groups of adrenergic agonists used in the therapy of glaucoma: epinephrine compounds and alpha$_2$-adrenergic agonists (4, 5, 18, 29, 35). Epinephrine is a direct-acting sympathomimetic stimulator, believed to enhance both conventional and uveo-scleral aqueous humor outflow. Epinephrine compounds also decrease aqueous humor production.

Local and systemic side effects may limit the usefulness of epinephrine compounds (74). Epinephrine may create local irritation and allergic conjunctivitis, as well as profound rebound hyperemia of the conjunctiva. Conjunctival hyperemia from vessel dilation often causes concern for many patients. The cosmetic appearance of a continual red eye is usually poorly tolerated, although generally harmless. Mild pupillary dilation may occur with adrenergic agonists. One of the most peculiar ocular side effects of these medications is the development of adrenochrome deposits, especially in the inferior fornix conjunctiva. Oxidation of epinephrine compounds results in a conversion to adrenochrome pigment, which is deposited in the conjunctiva. This is a frequent side effect of epinephrine but is infrequent with dipivefrin (dipivalyl epinephrine). Cystoid macular edema has been reported in pseudophakic and aphakic patients using epinephrine compounds. Systemic side effects include elevation of blood pressure, tachycardia, arrhythmias, nervousness, and headaches.

A variety of epinephrine salts are available in concentrations from 0.5 to 2%. Combination medications of epinephrine and pilocarpine are also available. Dipivifrin is a prodrug epinephrine compound that must be chemically cleaved into epinephrine by the corneal esterases as it penetrates the eye. Because of the enhanced corneal penetration of dipivifrin, a lower concentration (0.1%) may achieve the same pressure-lowering effects as higher concentrations of epinephrine. This results in less systemic and extraocular side effects. Both of these medications are administered twice daily. They both show significant intraocular pressure reduction when used in combination with miotics and carbonic anhydrase inhibitors but are minimally additive to beta-adrenergic blockers.

Apraclonidine hydrochloride is the prototype alpha$_2$-adrenergic agonist used in the therapy of glaucoma (24, 35). Apraclonidine hydrochloride is a derivative of clonidine hydrochloride, a potent systemic antihypertensive (35). Topical preparations of clonidine showed promise as intraocular pressure-lowering agents without cardiovascular side effects, but cardiovascular side effects have limited their ultimate usefulness. Side effects associated with apraclonidine include drying of the nasal and buccal mucosa, lightheadedness, lid retraction, mydriasis, and localized allergic reaction. Apraclonidine lowers the intraocular pressure by reducing aqueous humor production.

Apraclonidine is used to diminish the acute intraocular pressure elevations which may occur after laser iridotomies, capsulotomies, and trabeculoplasties. Instillation of a drop of apraclonidine 1% is recommended 1 hour before and immediately after these laser procedures. Apraclonidine 0.5%, administered 3 times a day, has been approved for intraocular pressure control in patients on maximally tolerated medical therapy awaiting surgery.

Adrenergic Antagonists

Beta-adrenergic inhibitors are the most commonly prescribed medications in the treatment of glaucoma (7, 8, 9, 30, 31, 34, 38, 64, 82). Beta-adrenergic antagonists, or "beta blockers," were originally used as a systemic treatment of cardiac arrhythmias and systemic hypertension. Most of these medications nonselectively block both beta$_1$ (heart) and beta$_2$ (pulmonary smooth muscle) adrenergic receptors (timolol maleate, metipranolol hydrochloride, carteolol, and levobunolol hydrochloride). A relatively cardioselective, beta$_1$-adrenergic antagonist is also available (betaxolol hydrochloride) which has less effect on pulmonary smooth muscle. All beta blockers reduce intraocular pressure by decreasing the aqueous humor production. Intraocular pressure reduction of up to 50% is seen with these agents.

Side effects with beta-adrenergic antagonists are numerous, but serious side effects which prevent continued use are rare (55, 68, 72, 76). Ocular allergic reactions have been reported with all of the available beta blockers. Systemic toxicosis, a more serious matter, must be monitored in patients on topical beta blockers. Beta$_1$-adrenergic receptor blockade decreases the pulse rate and reduces myocardial contractility. In susceptible individuals, this cardiovascular depression may be intolerable. Beta$_2$-adrenergic receptor blockade results in smooth muscle contraction of the bronchial airways. This may cause severe bronchospasm and is a major concern in individuals with obstructive or reactive airway disease. Cardioselective beta blockers may be better tolerated in individuals with marginal respiratory status because they produce less bronchoconstriction. A nonselective, beta-adrenergic blocker with intrinsic sympathomimetic (carteolol) activity is also available. Intrinsic sympathomimetic activity does not interfere with the beta-blocking activity of this medication. However, hopes that the intrinsic sympathomimetic activity would limit systemic side effects associated with beta blockers have not been shown. Other side effects of the beta blockers include reduced tolerance of exercise, fatigue, depression, lethargy, syncope, impotence, and reduced libido. Myasthenia gravis may also be aggravated by all the beta blockers.

Timolol maleate, betaxolol hydrochloride, and levobunolol hydrochloride are all prepared in a 0.25 and 0.5% concentration. Betaxolol is additionally provided in a 0.25% suspension. Metipranolol hydrochloride is provided in a 0.3% concentration, and carteolol in a 1% solution. Once a day administration in the morning or twice a day administration is recommended with all beta blocker preparations. Maximum intraocular pressure-lowering effects may often be achieved with once-daily dosing. The higher drug concentrations are usually required to sustain the longer duration of action and allow once-a-day dosing. The maximal intraocular pressure-lowering effect from a single dose is seen within 2 hours of administration, but 2 to 4 weeks of continuous administration may be required to achieve maximal intraocular pressure lowering. The effects of beta blockers on intraocular pressure may be sustained for 2 to 4 days after discontinuation, and some intraocular pressure-lowering effect may be seen for 2 to 3 weeks.

■ SYSTEMIC MEDICATIONS

Carbonic Anhydrase Inhibitors

Carbonic anhydrase inhibitors are systemically administered medications which reduce aqueous humor formation to decrease the intraocular pressure (3). These medications directly inhibit the carbonic anhydrase activity within the ciliary body. Acetazolamide and methazolomide are the most commonly used carbonic anhydrase inhibitors. Other systemic carbonic anhydrase inhibitors include dichlorphenamide and ethoxzolamide. Carbonic anhydrase inhibitors may be administered orally or intravenously. Acetazolamide has a shorter duration of action than methazolomide and must be administered 4 times daily (125 to 250 mg). Sustained-release acetazolamide capsules (500 mg) are available for twice-a-day dosing. Methazolomide (25 to 50mg) is administered 3 times a day.

These agents produce a systemic metabolic acidosis and their use is often limited by their side effects (21, 23, 36). Prolonged use of carbonic anhydrase inhibitors is typically reserved for individuals in whom topical therapy is insufficient or not tolerated. Many clinicians will proceed to laser surgery or filtration surgery before administering continual anhydrase inhibitor therapy. Side effects of carbonic anhydrase inhibitor therapy are typically dose-related. Almost all patients develop paresthesias in their fingers and toes. Loss of appetite, fatigue, gastrointestinal upset, and weight loss are all common complaints associated with carbonic anhydrase inhibitor therapy. Severe depression and decreased libido are less common side effects. All carbonic anhydrase inhibitors increase urinary excretion. Carbonic anhydrase inhibitors may exacerbate potassium depletion, especially in individuals on other diuretics. Calcium oxalate and calcium phosphate renal calculi may result from carbonic anhydrase inhibitor use. Blood dyscrasias and even aplastic anemia may result from these medications, but rarely. Finally, because of the chemical derivation of carbonic anhydrase inhibitors from sulfonamide drugs, there can be allergic cross-reactivity between these classes of drugs. Topical carbonic anhydrase inhibitors are in the final stages of clinical research trials and are likely to soon find their way to the commercial market. These medications may minimize systemic side effects and offer a new pressure-lowering modality for glaucoma therapy.

Hyperosmotic Agents

Hyperosmotic agents are systemically administered medications which lower intraocular pressure by increasing the plasma osmolality, resulting in vitreous dehydration (40, 54, 78). Fluid is osmotically drawn from the vitreous cavity into the circulation. These agents rapidly reduce intraocular pressure. Mannitol, glycerin, and isosorbide are the most frequently used hyperosmotic agents. Hyperosmotic agents are only used as a short-term therapy. Glycerin and isosorbide are administered orally, while mannitol is administered intravenously.

The potential side effects from hyperosmotics include headache, mental disorientation, gastrointestinal upset, and diuresis. Intracranial hemorrhages and congestive heart failure have also been reported. Glycerin may result in hyperglycemia in diabetic patients because it is metabolized. Isosorbide can be used safely in diabetics since it cannot be metabolized. In acute angle-closure glaucoma, intervenous mannitol may be used to rapidly reduce the intraocular pressure and avoid oral intake in patients with nausea. The dose for IV mannitol is 1 to 2 g per kg every 6 to 8 hours.

Laser Surgical Procedures

■ ARGON LASER TRABECULOPLASTY

During the early 1970s, attempts were made with a variety of lasers to enhance aqueous humor outflow through the trabecular meshwork in open-angle glaucoma, by puncturing the trabecular meshwork with laser energy (32, 79). Despite the failure of these procedures to create actual holes in the trabecular meshwork, a decrease in the intraocular pressure was observed in some eyes several days to weeks after the procedure. In 1979, Wise and Witter published a pilot study describing an argon laser procedure for the control of intraocular pressure (77). The authors placed evenly spaced argon laser burns for the entire circumference of the trabecular meshwork. Approximately three-quarters of their patients experienced significant lowering of the intraocular pressure, some lasting for several years. This technique, known as argon laser trabeculoplasty, has changed little since its original description. Many theories attempting to explain the effect of the trabeculoplasty laser burns have emerged. Initial impressions that laser trabeculoplasty mechanically altered the trabecular meshwork have largely been dispelled. It is now thought that a cascade of biologic events is initiated by the argon laser burns (73, 71). An alteration in the production of glycosaminoglycans by the trabecular meshwork cells and accelerated turnover of the extracellular matrix, enhances outflow through the trabecular meshwork after laser treatment. Argon laser trabeculoplasty has gained wide acceptance in the treatment of open-angle glaucoma.

Most clinicians use some modification of the following technique, when using argon laser trabeculoplasty. An alpha$_2$-adrenergic receptor agonist is instilled in the eye 30 to 60 minutes before the procedure. The initial treatment may extend for a 180° or 360° of the trabecular meshwork. An indirect gonioscopy lens, such as the Goldmann three-mirrored lens with antireflective laser coating, is used for the procedure. Laser burns are evenly spaced and applied to the anterior portion of the trabecular meshwork. Twenty to twenty-five laser burns are placed in each quadrant. Laser spot size of 50 microns burn duration of 0.1 seconds, and laser energy of 800 to 1200 mV are recommended, using an argon blue-green laser (488 nm). After the procedure, a second drop of the alpha$_2$-adrenergic agonist is instilled, and the intraocular pressure is monitored for 1 to 3 hours after the procedure. Topical corticosteroid therapy is used for the first week after the procedure to minimize postoperative inflammation. Patients are reexamined at 1 week and 6 weeks after the procedure.

The pressure-lowering effects of argon laser trabeculoplasty often are not evident until 4 to 6 weeks after the procedure. Short-term success rates range between 65 to 97% (52). Each year, approximately 10% of eyes, which initially respond favorably, will lose intraocular pressure control. Many factors such as patient age, phakic status of the eye, and preoperative glaucoma diagnosis, influence the success rates. Several authors have reported better-than-average success with argon laser trabeculoplasty in pseudoexfoliation and pigmentary glaucoma. Some reports suggest better results in phakic eyes as compared with aphakic or pseudophakic eyes. Poor results are typically reported in congenital, uveitic, and post-traumatic glaucomas. Argon laser trabeculoplasty may be repeated or the remaining 180° may be treated, if the initial treatment was efficacious.

Complications after argon laser trabeculoplasty are relatively rare. Initial studies reported up to 50% of treated eyes had significant postoperative pressure elevations. With the standardization of the laser treatment parameters and the emergence of alpha$_2$-adrenergic agonists, this complication has been minimized. However, patients should be monitored for 1 to 3 hours after the procedure, since most pressure elevations will occur during this time period. Intraocular hemorrhage, peripheral anterior synechiae, corneal burns, and postoperative intraocular inflammation have all been reported.

■ OTHER LASER PROCEDURES

Laser Iridotomy

With the advancements in lasers during the 1950s and 1960s, the treatment of angle-closure glaucoma was greatly altered (42). Laser iridotomy became the preferred form of treatment for angle-closure glaucoma associated with pupillary block. The complications associated with surgical iridectomies are almost entirely eliminated by this therapy. In addition, prophylactic laser iridotomies may be placed in eyes with appositionally closed anterior chamber angles which may be predisposed to either acute episodes of angle closure or chronic angle-closure glaucoma. Surgical iridectomies still are rarely done when extensive corneal edema or corneal opacification prevent adequate visualization of the iris and the placement of laser iridotomy.

A variety of techniques have been described to create a laser iridotomy. The argon laser and the neodymium:YAG (Nd:YAG) lasers are both currently used to create laser iridotomies. Thick irides may be difficult to penetrate with argon laser, and the neodymium:YAG laser is useful in these eyes. It is preferable for lightly colored irides, as well, since with little iris pigmentation, they absorb the argon laser energy poorly. The iridotomy is usually placed in the superior iris, under the superior eyelid. The iridotomy is placed peripherally, approximately two-thirds the distance from the pupil to the iris root. If possible, the iridotomy is placed within an iris crypt, to enhance penetration of the iris by the laser energy.

When using the argon laser to do an iridotomy, a two-step procedure is often most efficacious. Initially, burns are used to stretch the iris and create a taut surface. These burns are created with decreased power, large spot size, and long durations (200 to 400 mW, 200 to 500 μm and 0.2 to 0.5 seconds). Burns of higher power, shorter duration, and smaller spot size are then used to penetrate the iris at the center of the stretch burns (600 to 1200 mW, 0.1 seconds, and 50 μm).

The neodymium:YAG laser may also be used to do an iridotomy. Typical parameters used with the neodymium:YAG laser are 1 or 2 bursts per application and an energy setting of 1 to 5 millijoules per burst. Because of the posterior shock waves initiated by the photo-disruption nd:YAG laser, lens injury has been a concern. Peripheral placement of the iridotomy and careful aiming on the surface of the iris can prevent this complication.

Complications with either argon laser or Nd:YAG laser iridotomies may occur. Corneal edema may result from burns placed superficially in the iris (argon laser) or anteriorly aimed (Nd:YAG laser), especially in the setting of a shallow anterior chamber. Mild postoperative, anterior uveitis is frequent and may be controlled with topical corticosteroids prescribed for 4 to 7 days after the procedure. Hemorrhage from the site of iridotomy is reported more frequently after the Nd:YAG iridotomies. The argon laser cauterizes the site of the iridotomy, thus preventing this complication. If postoperative hemorrhage is a concern, the argon laser may be used initially to cauterize the site of the iridotomy and the Nd:YAG can be used to penetrate the iris. Postoperative elevation of intraocular pressure may occur either transiently or permanently. Perioperative treatments with pilocarpine and alpha$_2$-adrenergic agonists have almost eliminated this complication. Late closure of the iridotomy site by migration of pigment epithelial cells may occur. Usually, this is easily remedied by repeating the laser iridotomy.

■ LASER IRIDOPLASTY

Argon laser peripheral iridoplasty is useful in certain situations to enhance opening of the anterior chamber angle (53). With laser iridoplasty, circumferential argon laser burns are placed on the peripheral iris to contract the iris, thereby pulling it out of the angle. This is most effective in angle-closure glaucoma resistant to opening after placement of an iridotomy, plateau iris syndrome, and nanophthalmos. Large burns (300 to 500 μm) of long duration (0.2 to 0.5 seconds) and moderate power (200 to 400 mW) are typically used. The laser burns are placed for 360° around the peripheral iris. An indirect gonioscopy lens may be used to place the burns on the peripheral iris. Twenty-five to thirty burns are placed around the circumference of the iris. Complications after this therapy are rare. However, successful anatomic opening of the anterior chamber angle occurs in only approximately 50% of patients.

Other laser therapies for glaucoma have been described. These include laser pupilloplasty, internal openings of filtering fistulas, and goniophotocoagulation, among others. The application of these techniques is rare and outside the scope of this text.

Incisional Surgical Procedures

■ TRABECULECTOMY

Trabeculectomy is the most frequently performed incisional operation for the control of elevated intraocular pressure in adult glaucoma (14, 66). Various filtering procedures have been developed to shunt the aqueous humor from the anterior chamber to a subconjunctival reservoir. These procedures provide an alternative pathway of less resistance for aqueous humor egress from the eye. It is believed that the aqueous humor either filters through the conjunctiva from the reservoir mixing with the tears, or it is absorbed by the vascular tissue of the episclera and conjunctiva.

Surgical Technique

A complete description of all surgical procedures done for the control of intraocular pressure is outside the scope of this text. Trabeculectomy, or guarded filtration surgery, is now the most common filtering procedure used in glaucoma (Figure 47–1) Typically, a trabeculectomy is done in the superior nasal or superior temporal quadrant. A conjunctival incision is made approximately 10 mm posterior to the limbus. This incision extends through the conjunctiva, Tenon's capsule and episcleral tissues, to the level of bare sclera. The incision is extended circumferentially for approximately 8 to 12 mm. With both blunt and sharp dissection, a limbal-based conjunctival-Tenon's flap is elevated. This dissection extends to the superior limbus and electrocautery can be used to obtain hemostasis. A paracentesis is done, usually in the temporal quadrant away from the site of the trabeculectomy. At the trabeculectomy site, a limbal-based, scleral flap is developed. The scleral flap may be any shape, usually measures approximately 4 mm across the base, and extends 2 to 3 mm from the limbus. The scleral flap is developed with a spatulated blade and is approximately 0.5 millimeter in thickness. The flap is advanced anteriorly until the surgical limbus is identified. While reflecting the scleral flap inferiorly,

an incision is made into the anterior chamber. The incision should enter the anterior chamber, slightly anterior to the trabecular meshwork. A block of trabecular meshwork is excised with a scalpel blade or a membrane punch. The base of the iris typically presents itself into the translimbal fistula. A surgical iridectomy is done, and the iris is redeposited into the anterior chamber. The scleral flap is loosely reapproximated into its original position with a suture. A variety of techniques have been developed for reapproximating the scleral flap. These include a single suture, multiple sutures, and releasable sutures. Flow through the trabeculectomy site may be assessed by infusing saline solution into the anterior chamber through the previously placed paracentesis. The scleral flap should be reapproximated so that flow easily egresses from the anterior chamber, but the anterior chamber should remain formed when infusion is discontinued. The conjunctival wound is closed with a running, horizontal mattress suture. A variety of locking or interrupted suture closures have also been described. A two-layer closure, which first reapproximates Tenon's capsule, followed by an overlying closure of conjunctiva, may also be used. Infusion into the anterior chamber will reestablish the chamber and inflate the filtering reservoir.

Postoperative management includes topical cycloplegics and antibiotics for the first 1 to 2 weeks after surgery. Topical corticosteroids are also used to suppress intraocular, conjunctival, and episcleral inflammation. The corticosteroid therapy is thought to reduce scar formation and failure of the filtering bleb (see Modulation of Wound Healing After Glaucoma Filtration Surgery).

Clinical Appearance of the Filtration Bleb

A properly functioning filtering reservoir or "bleb" has several important clinical characteristics which can be

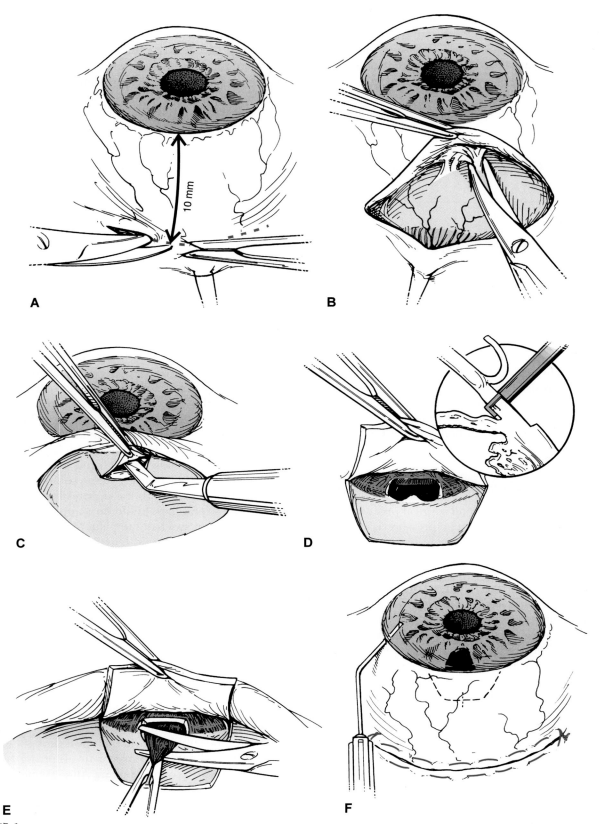

Figure 47–1.
Trabeculectomy, basic surgical steps: A) superior conjunctival/Tenon's capsule incision, approximately 10 mm from limbus, B) dissection of limbus-based, conjunctival flap, C) dissection of scleral flap, D) excision of limbal tissue, E) surgical iridectomy, and F) reconstitution of anterior chamber and inflation of filtration bleb after conjunctival closure.

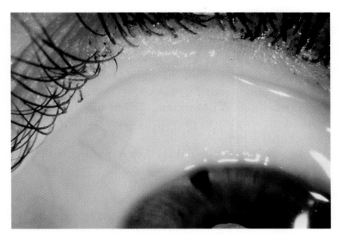

Figure 47–2.
Filtration Bleb: Minimally elevated, diffuse, avascular filtration bleb. Note peripheral iridectomy.

seen on biomicroscopic examination. These favorable characteristics include microcysts of fluid within the conjunctival epithelium overlying the bleb, a decreased diffuse bleb profile, and minimal vascularization of the conjunctiva (Figure 47–2). Although the appearance of a functioning bleb may vary greatly, these characteristics are most often found in blebs exhibiting adequate intraocular pressure control. Failing filtering blebs are more often associated with increased vascular injection of the conjunctiva over the filtration bleb, a thickened appearance of the epithelium which is devoid of microcysts, and a circumscribed, elevated, or "domed" bleb. A failed bleb eventually flattens and may become indistinguishable from the surrounding tissue. Although these characteristics are good clinical guidelines for the assessment of filtration blebs, many eyes exhibit multiple poor prognostic clinical signs but maintain adequate pressure control.

■ FULL-THICKNESS FILTRATION PROCEDURES

Other fistulizing filtration procedures were successfully used in the past. Full-thickness procedures, which lack the guarded outflow provided by the trabeculectomy flap, were popular between the 1940s to 1970s. These included posterior lip sclerectomy, trephinating procedures, and thermosclerostomy (Scheie procedures). More recently laser sclerostomies, both Ab Externo and Ab Interno, have become popular. These procedures typically share the same complications and problems of older full-thickness procedures: principally postoperative flat anterior chambers, choroidal detachment and hemorrhages, and cataract formation. Limited success has been achieved with these laser procedures because of these postoperative complications. In addition, most studies agree that the complication rate with trabeculectomy surgery is lower than with full-thickness procedures, and the success rate is higher, although lower ultimate intraocular pressures may be achieved after full-thickness procedures.

■ MODULATION OF WOUND HEALING AFTER GLAUCOMA FILTRATION SURGERY

The most common cause of filtration failure is excessive scarring at the fistula site and within the subconjunctival space. Many factors increase the risk of filtration surgery failure, including history of previous ocular surgery, ocular inflammation, anterior segment neovascularization, black heritage, and youth. Fibroproliferation and vascular ingrowth result in scar tissue formation that leads to filtration failure. Modulation of the normal wound healing response and minimization of subconjunctival scarring is desirable to maintain the translimbal fistula and the subconjunctival filtration reservoir (17, 28, 61, 63, 67). Inhibition of fibroblast activity has been attempted with a variety of adjunctive therapies at the time of glaucoma surgery or during the perioperative period.

Two primary modalities are currently used in clinical practice: antiinflammatory and antimetabolite medications. Antiinflammatory medications such as corticosteroids (topical, local injections, and systemic), act by suppressing the inflammatory response after filtration surgery. By decreasing the inflammatory cell (macrophages and neutrophils) infiltration at the wound site, there is less stimulus for fibroblast activity and scar tissue formation. Corticosteroids are generally administered immediately after surgery and during the first 4 to 8 postoperative weeks. Corticosteroids may be given as a subconjunctival injection at the conclusion of the filtration surgery and in a short burst of orally administered medication after surgery, as well. Orally administered corticosteroids should be tapered quickly over the first 2 postoperative weeks. Topical steroids are strongly recommended after all filtration surgeries. Topical prednisolone acetate, 4 to 6 times each day, should be administered for several weeks. This topical treatment can be weaned, based on the amount of intraocular and conjunctival inflammation. Both intraocular and conjunctival inflammation should subside before withdrawal of steroid therapy. It should be remembered that intraocular inflammation may resolve first; conjunctival and subconjunctival inflammation may be longer lasting. Left untreated, conjunctival inflammation may result in filtration failure.

Antimetabolite therapy inhibits cellular fibroproliferation after filtration surgery. Currrently, two antimetabolites are used in clinical practice, 5-fluorouracil and mitomycin C (17, 67). Both are applied to the subconjunctival and scleral tissues at the time of filtration surgery, and 5-fluorouracil may also be administered postoperatively as a series of subconjunctival injections. 5-fluorouracil is a chemotherapeutic agent which inhibits DNA and RNA synthesis, thereby preventing cellular proliferation. The Fluorouracil Filtering Surgery Study was a multi-center investigation which showed the usefulness of 5-fluorouracil in enhancing filtration surgery success. The Fluorouracil Filtering Surgery Study used 5-fluorouracil subconjunctival injections (5 mg), twice a day for the first week after surgery and once a day for the second week after surgery (67). Less frequent dosing is equally effective and minimizes complications (75). An average of five to ten injections is now recommended during the first 2 postoperative weeks. The frequency of postoperative injections is judged by the amount of conjunctival inflammation and the appearance of the filtration bleb. 5-fluorouracil is withheld in patients with corneal epithelial defects or severe epitheliopathy in whom defects may occur. Normal corneal epithelial turnover is inhibited by 5-fluorouracil, and corneal erosions may result from minor trauma or abrasions. Reports of conjunctival melts and prolonged hypotony after 5-fluorouracil treatment have been described. Initially, 5-fluorouracil was recommended only for patients at increased risk of filtration failure (anterior segment neovascularization, ocular inflammation, and youth). Antimetabolite therapy should now be considered in every filtration surgery.

Mitomycin-C is another antimetabolite which is administered at the time of filtration surgery (17). Because of the repeated postoperative injections typically involved in 5-fluorouracil administration, clinicians have looked for a more convenient and patient-friendly method of antimetabolite administration. Mitomycin C is an alkylating agent that prevents DNA synthesis and inhibits cellular proliferation. It was initially used in ophthalmic surgery to prevent recurrence of surgically excised pterygium.

Mitomycin C is applied for 1 to 5 minutes with a gel foam sponge, soaked in the solution (0.1 to 0.5 mg/ml) at the time of filtration surgery. After dissection of the conjunctival flap, the sponge is placed in the subconjunctival space. Extensive irrigation with saline solution immediately after mitomycin C application minimizes prolonged tissue exposure and intraocular toxicosis. Limbus-based conjunctival flaps are preferred for filtration procedures with mitomycin C to decrease the possibility of postoperative wound leaks at the limbus, which may occur with fornix-based surgery. Currently, the use of mitomycin C is reserved for patients at an increased risk of filtration failure, although some clinicians advocate its routine use.

Mitomycin C induces some specific and serious complications. These include wound and bleb leaks, conjunctival melts, prolonged hypotony, postoperative infections, and choroidal detachments. Wound or bleb leaks are more likely to occur after mitomycin C therapy because of the extreme inhibition of the normal healing response of the incision site or at bleb perforation sites. Ocular hypotony occurs more frequently after mitomycin C filtration surgery, from overfiltration and transconjunctival bleb leaks. Perhaps, the most worrisome aspect of mitomycin C administration is its unpredictability from individual to individual. Both the imprecision of the drug delivery and the variability of response to the drug among different individuals, results in great variations in surgical outcomes after mitomycin C administration. Further studies are currently underway to standardize administration and investigate the risks and benefits of mitomycin C adjunctive antimetabolite therapy.

■ TRABECULOTOMY AND GONIOTOMY

The mainstay of therapy for congenital or infantile glaucoma is surgical. Medical therapy may occasionally be used but usually is unsuccessful as long-term therapy. Trabeculotomy and goniotomy are the principal procedures used to enhance aqueous outflow, by eliminating the resistance produced by the developmentally abnormal anterior chamber angle and establishing patency to Schlemm's canal (2, 41). The choice between these procedures remains primarily a personal preference, but, in some cases, the choice may be determined by the presence or absence of corneal edema. Goniotomy requires clear visualization of the anterior chamber angle. Trabeculotomy uses an external approach to the anterior chamber angle and, therefore, is less dependent on visualization of the anterior chamber.

Trabeculotomy involves an external dissection, similar to that used in trabeculectomy. After dissection of a fornix-based conjunctival flap, a partial-thickness limbal-based scleral flap is developed, extending 4 mm posterior to the limbus with a 4-mm width. A radial incision is made underneath the scleral flap, down to the level of Schlemm's canal. In the buphthalmic eye, limbal structures may be stretched and identification of Schlemm's canal can be difficult. Once Schlemm's canal is identified, a monofilament nylon suture is passed into the canal in either direction to establish its patency and assure correct identification of the canal. After this, a forked probe, or "trabeculotome," is passed into the canal and rotated into the anterior chamber. The trabeculotome is angled to conform to the curved pattern of the canal. A second trabeculotome is passed in the opposite direction and rotated into the anterior chamber. This procedure requires little or minimal visualization of the anterior chamber, but the trabeculotome should be rotated parallel to and above the plane of the iris, to prevent peripheral lens or iris damage. Trabeculotomy establishes aqueous outflow directly from the anterior chamber and into Schlemm's canal. Postoperative miotics are used to constrict the pupil and keep the peripheral iris from occluding the incision site.

Goniotomy was first described by Barkan in 1942 (2). He thought that with direct visualization of the anterior chamber angle, congenital glaucoma could be treated by incising the membrane that was present over the trabecular meshwork ("Barkan's membrane"). To perform a goniotomy, a direct gonioscopy lens is used to visualize the anterior chamber angle structures. A goniotomy knife is passed from a paracentesis opposite to the visualized anterior chamber angle, across the anterior chamber. If the anterior chamber is shallow before or during this procedure, a visco-elastic substance or saline infusion may be used to maintain the depth of the chamber. The knife is used to incise the inner layers of the trabecular meshwork. This eliminates the resistance from the abnormally developed chamber angle, enhancing outflow facility in these eyes. The original membrane described by Barkan has never been identified histologically, yet this procedure remains a successful treatment for congenital-infantile glaucoma.

Both trabeculotomy and goniotomy are successful in the control of infantile or congenital glaucoma. Most surgeons report 75 to 90% success rates with either procedure, although repeat operations are common, occurring in as many as 50% of eyes. Children in whom glaucoma is detected immediately after birth or late in childhood have a less favorable prognosis than those detected during early childhood. Severe buphthalmos increases the surgical difficulty of both surgical procedures and results in a less favorable response to surgery. There are many advocates for each of these surgical procedures and each has a place in the management of congenital-infantile glaucoma.

■ SETON PROCEDURES

Postoperative scarring and closure of the filtration fistula is the most common cause of failure in both full-thickness and partial-thickness filtering procedures (62). In eyes prone to extensive postoperative inflammation, postoperative intraocular bleeding, or scar tissue proliferation, placement of a seton or glaucoma tube shunt may be advisable for intraocular pressure control. Implantation of a seton should be considered in a variety of situations, including eyes with active neovascular glaucoma in which a surgical iridectomy is not possible, eyes with multiple filtration failures especially if associated with prolonged inflammation, eyes with multiple previous surgeries in which conjunctival dissection and development of a filtration bleb is impossible, and in childhood glaucomas in which primary procedures have failed. It is hypothesized that setons control intraocular pressure in a similar fashion to traditional filtration surgery. Setons provide a translimbal tube which enters the anterior chamber and drains aqueous humor to a posterior subconjunctival reservoir (33, 44, 60). The translimbal tube prevents scar tissue closure of the fistula. A variety of implants have been developed. The main difference among these implants is the design of the plate attached to the posterior aspect of the tube. The plate mechanically maintains the subconjunctival drainage reservoir. Most setons are made with a silicon or silastic anterior chamber tube, and a variety of plastics and silicones have been used for the posterior drainage plates. Many modifications have been made within the plates and within the tubes to prevent excessive drainage, especially during the early postoperative period. Because of the consequences of postoperative hypotony, setons have been developed with intraluminal pressure-dependent valves which prevent excessive aqueous outflow. A variety of surgical techniques, including intraluminal stents or extraluminal phimosis sutures, have also been developed to prevent excess aqueous outflow.

■ CYCLODESTRUCTIVE SURGICAL PROCEDURES

Just as medical therapy may either increase aqueous humor outflow from the eye or decrease aqueous production, so may surgical procedures. Filtration operations increase aqueous humor outflow from the eye, while cyclodestructive procedures reduce the aqueous production. The two most common cyclodestructive procedures are cyclocryotherapy and trans-scleral cyclophotocoagulation (6, 50). In cyclocryotherapy, a nitrous oxide or carbon dioxide gas cryotherapy probe is used. These probes can be cooled −60° to −70° celsius and produce trans-scleral freezing of the ciliary processes. Freezing applications in this temperature range result in either direct cell death of the ciliary epithelium or infarction with secondary cell death and ischemic necrosis. The most common technique used for cyclocryotherapy involves placement of the cryoprobe directly on the perilimbal conjunctiva. The cryoprobe is placed approximately 1 mm posterior to the cornealscleral limbus. One or two quadrants are treated in a single session, and three to four applications are applied in each quadrant. More extensive applications or repeat applications can be done at a later time.

Trans-scleral cyclophotocoagulation is also used to suppress aqueous formation by destroying the ciliary epithelium. A variety of lasers are now used for this procedure, including neodymium:YAG lasers, argon lasers, krypton lasers, and semiconductor diode lasers. Neodymium:YAG lasers use both noncontact slit lamp delivery systems and contact fiberoptic probe systems. Retrofocusing of the laser energy allows the maximal laser energy to be delivered internally, within the eye, at the level of the ciliary body. These lasers destroy the ciliary body epithelium by inducing ischemic necrosis, resulting in marked atrophy of the ciliary processes. Noncontact neodymium:YAG lasers deliver energy levels up to 9j while contact laser cyclophotocoagulation units deliver maximum powers of approximately 10W. A variety of techniques are used with the various contact and noncontact units. Treatment may vary from 1 to 4 quadrants, depending on the pressure-lowering needs and the glaucoma diagnosis. In general, cyclodestruction with photocoagulation is thought to be more controlled and predictable than with cryotherapy. Preoperative retrobulbar anesthesia is needed for both cyclocryotherapy and trans-scleral cyclophotocoagulation. Postoperative complications include both transient and permanent intraocular pressure elevations, intraocular inflammation, and hypotony. Pain is the most frequent postoperative complaint and is the result of intraocular inflammation. Suppression of the postoperative inflammation and control of pain with corticosteroid therapy and oral analgesics are almost always necessary. Cycloplegics also help control postoperative pain after these procedures.

Other forms of cyclodestructive procedures have been described. These include transpupillary-intraocular cyclophotocoagulation, ultrasonic cyclodestruction, and endoscopic cyclophotocoagulation. These techniques have limited usefulness in the clinical setting.

■ MANAGEMENT OF COEXISTING GLAUCOMA AND CATARACT

The management of the patient with coexisting visually significant cataracts and glaucoma includes at least four options: (a) cataract surgery alone; (b) glaucoma filtration surgery followed by cataract extraction at a later time; (c) cataract extraction followed by glaucoma filtration surgery; and (d) combined cataract and glaucoma surgery in a single setting. Removal of the cataract in either angle-closure or open-angle glaucoma may, in itself, result in a lower intraocular pressure. However, many eyes with glaucoma exhibit pressure elevations after cataract extraction. Indications for cataract extraction in eyes with glaucoma follow typical guidelines for removal of cataracts. However, some clinicians prefer a more conservative approach, allowing a greater decrease in visual acuity before cataract extraction is considered, because of possible postoperative complications and lack of intraocular pressure control.

A filtration procedure alone should be considered in glaucoma patients with uncontrolled intraocular pressures, despite maximal tolerated medical therapy. Filtration procedures, when completed without concomitant cataract extraction, are more successful in long-term pressure management. As with any intraocular surgery, filtration surgery increases the progression of cataracts, especially in eyes with postoperative shallow or flat anterior chambers. For eyes in which filtration surgery is done alone, cataract extraction should be postponed at least 6 months to allow the filtering bleb to become well established. Subsequent cataract extraction may be done through an inferior temporal scleral incision or a clear corneal incision, to avoid the superior filtration bleb. No matter how distant and atraumatic the subsequent cataract extraction, the associated inflammation and wound healing response can stimulate fibrosis in the bleb and filtration failure.

In eyes with well-controlled intraocular pressures on tolerated medical therapy, cataract extraction without filtration surgery is the best alternative. Postoperative intraocular pressure elevations, secondary to intraocular inflammation or incomplete removal of visco-elastic aqueous substitutes, are a concern. Careful attention to minimizing operative intraocular manipulation, removal of all visco-elastic substances, and the possible use of additional pressure-lowering agents during the early postoperative period may avert this problem. Placement of anterior chamber lenses in eyes with preexisting glaucoma poses a significant risk for postoperative uncontrolled glaucoma. Performance of the cataract extraction in either the superior nasal or superior temporal quadrant, instead of directly at the vertical meridian, preserves the adjacent quadrant for later filtration surgery, should it become necessary. Filtration surgery with adjunctive antimetabolites in pseudophakic eyes, especially with posterior chamber intraocular lenses, has a good success rate. Therefore, initial cataract surgery, followed by filtration surgery if needed at a later time, is often the best surgical sequence.

Cataract surgery in combination with glaucoma filtering surgery may be considered for eyes in which the intraocular pressure is uncontrolled, and there is a significant decrease in visual acuity secondary to cataract formation. Many combined filtration and cataract procedures have been described, and a complete description of these procedures is outside the scope of this text. It is generally believed that postoperative visual acuity recovery is delayed and filtration surgery success is slightly decreased, in eyes undergoing combined procedures, as opposed to separate procedures. However, many surgeons report excellent results, both in terms of visual acuity and pressure control, after these combined procedures.

■ COMPLICATIONS OF FILTRATION SURGERY

Flat Anterior Chamber

After any type of anterior segment surgery, the anterior chamber may become shallow or flat. A flat chamber refers to corneal endothelial contact with an underlying structure, such as the iris, lens, or vitreous humor. Lenticular-corneal touch or vitreal-corneal touch are particularly a matter of concern, because of the possibility of cataract formation, corneal decompensation, and filtration surgery failure. Peripheral iris-corneal touch is frequently seen after filtration surgery and usually resolves spontaneously. The level of intraocular pressure is important in the assessment of the postoperative shallow or flat anterior chamber. If the eye is hypotonous, excess aqueous humor runoff is the most frequent cause of a flat anterior chamber, and the clinician should examine the eye for the possibility of a wound/bleb leak or overfiltration of the glaucoma filtering procedure (22, 26). In addition, choroidal detachments may result from the hypotony or may perpetuate the hypotony if a concurrent ciliary body detachment occurs (7). If the intraocular pressure is normotensive or hypertensive, a flat chamber typically derives from increased pressure behind the iris: pupillary block glaucoma, acute expansion of the suprachoroidal space (either serous or hemorrhagic), aqueous humor misdirection, or diversion and accumulation in the vitreous cavity (malignant glaucoma) (15).

Assessment and management of a wound/bleb leak is described later in this text. Hypotony secondary to overfiltration is usually accompanied by a large filtration bleb with excessive aqueous humor egress. This may be decreased by placement of an oversized soft contact lens, a shell tamponade, or by patching the eye. These techniques are intended to compress the filtration bleb and limit the egress of aqueous from the anterior chamber. Overfiltration may also be seen after placement of a glaucoma seton. Choroidal detachments frequently occur after filtration surgery. These appear as bullous elevations of the peripheral fundus and are seen in almost all eyes with a pressure below 4mm Hg. Hemorrhagic choroidal detachments are typically darker and less mobile than serous detachments. Hemorrhagic detachments are associated with rapid expansion, intense pain, and loss of vision. Choroidal detachments may be the result of prolonged hypotony or may themselves contribute to the hypotony because of a secondary ciliary body detachment and hyposecretion of aqueous humor. If direct visualization of the posterior segment is not possible, ultrasonography may assist in assessing these postoperative problems (Figure 47–3).

In the absence of a patent iridectomy, pupillary block glaucoma may result in a postoperative flat anterior chamber after any intraocular surgery. Establishing an iridectomy, either with laser or surgically, is both diagnostic and therapeutic. If a patent iridectomy is present, the anterior chamber is flat, and the eye has a normal or elevated intraocular pressure, the possibility of suprachoroidal hemorrhage or malignant glaucoma should be investigated.

Malignant glaucoma (aqueous misdirection syndrome or ciliary block glaucoma) may be difficult to both diagnose and manage. Misdirection of the aqueous humor into the vitreous cavity expands the vitreous, shifts the lens-iris diaphragm anteriorly, and rotates the ciliary body forward. Even in the presence of a patent iridectomy, the diversion of aqueous humor into the posterior cavity persists and results in shallowing or flattening of the anterior chamber. This syndrome is most often seen in eyes with a history of angle-closure glaucoma and in hyperopic eyes. Medical therapy should be tried first with malignant glaucoma. Maximal cycloplegia and aqueous humor suppression are the first line of therapy. If medical therapy is unsuccessful, laser therapy

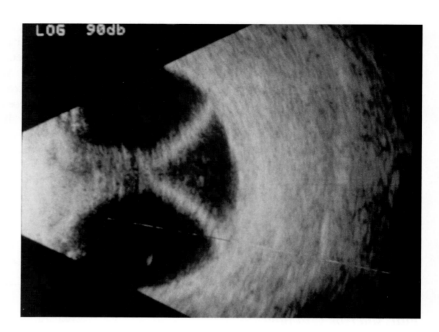

Figure 47–3.
Ultrasonography of Choroidal Detachment (B-Scan): Large, centrally touching ("kissing") choroidals in a hypotonus eye after filtration surgery.

may be tried in the pseudophakic eye. Disruption of the anterior hyaloid face (vitrotomy) and the posterior lens capsule with a neodymium:YAG laser may allow the entrapped aqueous humor to flow into the anterior chamber. If this is unsuccessful, a more complete posterior vitrectomy may be needed to alleviate this complication.

Prolonged irido-corneal touch from peripheral shallowing of the anterior chamber may result in the formation of peripheral anterior synechiae. This problem is best treated by conservative medical management, with topical suppression of intraocular inflammation and maximal cycloplegia. Lenticular-corneal touch is more worrisome because of the possible rapid formation of a cataract and corneal decompensation. Conservative medical therapy (maximal cycloplegia) may be tried in this situation, but surgical intervention should not be delayed if immediate results within 24 hours are not seen. When conservative therapies do not result in reformation and maintenance of the anterior chamber, surgical intervention is required. The management of choroidal detachments, either hemorrhagic or serous, is controversial. Most surgeons will observe choroidal detachments for long periods of time (several weeks to months) if the anterior chamber remains formed. If the anterior chamber is flat and an associated choroidal detachment is present, reformation of the anterior chamber and drainage of the choroidal detachments is recommended, 1 to 2 weeks after the initial surgery. Centrally touching choroidal detachments (kissing choroidals) may require drainage at an earlier time to prevent adhesions between the retinal surfaces.

Bleb Failure and Management

Encapsulated Bleb

Encapsulation of the filtration bleb is the most common cause of failure during the first 3 months after surgery (69, 70). The encapsulated bleb clinically appears as an elevated, domelike filtration bleb that extends several millimeters above the surface of the globe. Filtration bleb encapsulation may occur after any type of filtration surgery, including trabeculectomy, full-thickness procedures, and even seton glaucoma shunts. The bleb becomes sharply demarcated with marked vascular injection, especially surrounding the bleb. The conjunctiva is distended and tightly stretched over the dome of an impermeable, subconjunctival, fibrotic wall. The fibrosis and thickening of the subconjunctival tissue, which becomes impermeable to filtration of aqueous humor, is responsible for the loss of pressure control in the encapsulated bleb.

A patent translimbal fistula from the anterior chamber to the encapsulated bleb is maintained. The vast majority of encapsulated blebs will spontaneously regain function without any surgical intervention. However, many weeks may be required for spontaneous resolution, and medical control of intraocular pressure may be required during this period. Topical beta-adrenergic blockers to suppress aqueous humor production, in conjunction with topical corticosteroids to inhibit further subconjunctival fibrosis, comprise the mainstay of medical management. Direct manual compression over the surface of the encapsulated bleb may promote thinning of the thickened fibrotic wall and enhance permeability, thereby leading to better aqueous filtration. This may be accomplished by direct compression with a moistened cotton-tipped applicator on the surface of the domed, encapsulated bleb.

At least 80 to 90% of encapsulated filtration blebs will regain adequate filtration over a 4- to 12-week period. During this time, the bleb wall thins and microcystic changes of the conjunctival epithelium increase in the area surrounding the encapsulated bleb. The bleb also becomes less vascular, less elevated, and the conjunctiva loosens over the surface of the encapsulation.

If spontaneous resolution of filtration and control of intraocular pressure are not achieved within 60 to 90 days, surgical revision of the encapsulation may be required. This involves incisional revision by needling of the filtration bleb, or complete excisional revision by reopening of the original conjunctival incision and excising of the thickened encapsulated wall. Needling can be done in the office by incising the fibrotic wall of the encapsulated bleb with a subconjunctival needle. This procedure, by far the simplest, is successful in approximately 50% of nonresolving bleb encapsulations and should be attempted before excisional revision.

The Episcleral Membrane

Proliferation of episcleral membranes, with overgrowth of the external opening of the filtration fistula, is a common cause of late filtration failure. Clinically, the filtration bleb becomes small and contracted, with minimal elevation over the surface of the globe. Microcystic changes of the conjunctiva decrease with the progression of the episcleral membrane and blockage of flow of aqueous humor into the subconjunctival space. The overlying conjunctiva is usually mobile and can be slid over a grayish, glistening fibrotic membrane which appears over the site of the external scleral, filtration opening. Adjunctive antimetabolite therapy at the time of surgery decreases the proliferation of these episcleral membranes. Episcleral membranes rarely respond to digital massage, direct compression, or incisional needling. Most frequently, bleb failure which results from episcleral membrane proliferation requires surgical revision and removal of the membrane.

Fistula Obstruction

The internal opening of the fistula may also become obstructed, preventing egress of the aqueous humor from the anterior chamber. The etiology of obstruction of the internal fistular opening can often be visualized with gonioscopy. The most common sources of the obstruction of the fistula are corneoscleral tissue, iris, ciliary body processes, lens material, or vitreous humor.

Any of these structures may also provide a template for fibrous scar tissue growth and obstruction of the fistula. Just as migrating iris epithelium may obstruct a peripheral iridotomy, proliferation of this tissue may also obstruct the internal fistular opening.

Depending on the source of obstruction, nd:YAG laser may be used to reopen the fistula. With fibrotic membrane proliferation, nd:YAG laser may be used to perforate the membrane, allowing aqueous humor egress. With obstruction secondary to vitreous herniation into the anterior chamber, vitreous bands may sometimes be cut with the nd:YAG laser. However, vitreous herniation and fistular obstruction most often requires a second operation and vitrectomy.

Tight Scleral Flap

After guarded partial-thickness filtration surgery (trabeculectomy), overly tight closure of the scleral flap may prevent filtration. In the early postoperative period, a tight scleral flap may become adherent to the underlying scleral bed with fibrin and other blood products acting to "glue" the flap in place. Sutures placed at the time of surgery which are too tight may also prevent filtration. In either case, no bleb elevation is seen clinically. Frequently, the flap may be loosened with gentle manipulation at the filtration site with a cotton-tipped applicator. If a tight suture is evident, transconjunctival laser suture lysis is completed with an argon laser. Some clinicians purposely place multiple tight sutures at the time of filtration followed by sequential laser lysis, in an attempt to titrate filtration outflow after surgery. In addition, a variety of releasable sutures, which can be removed during the first 2 postoperative weeks, have been devised.

Late closure of the scleral flap may occur months to years after the initial surgery and is most often the result of gradual fibrosis of the flap with progressive adhesion to the underlying sclera. As the flap becomes adherent to the underlying scleral bed, the overlying filtration bleb gradually contracts and collapses. In almost all of these cases, surgical revision at the same site or a second trabeculectomy at a distant site must be completed.

Wound and Bleb Leaks

A leak of aqueous humor after filtration surgery may occur either at the original conjunctival incision or at a separate conjunctival site. Incision or wound leaks are most commonly the result of inadequate closure of the conjunctival and Tenon's capsule incision. Laxity in the suture of a running conjunctival closure will result in an aqueous humor leak at the wound site. Although antimetabolites are frequently cited as the etiology of wound leaks, careful attention to the wound closure at the time of filtration surgery will result in almost total elimination of this postoperative complication. Wound leaks occur slightly more frequently after fornix-based incisions, in which the wound is placed at the corneal limbus.

Conjunctival bleb leaks, "button holes," may occur at the time of surgery or shortly postoperatively. Conjunctival button holes most often occur during the dissection and elevation of the conjunctival flap, especially in eyes with a history of previous surgery and subconjunctival adhesions. Infrequently, these bleb leaks may close spontaneously. More often, the aqueous humor will leak through the perforation site and the bleb will collapse. Closure of bleb leaks is most successful with a tapered microvascular needle. Large bleb leaks may be closed in a running horizontal mattress fashion, while smaller bleb leaks can be closed either with a purse-string suture or interrupted sutures.

Conjunctival bleb leaks may also occur many months to years after the original filtration surgery. These are associated with thin, transparent, cystic filtration blebs and are more often seen after full-thickness filtration procedures or filtration surgery done with adjunctiva antimetabolites. Frequently, a small hole in the surface of the bleb will be seen, creating a positive Seidel test (Figure 47–4). With thin-walled conjunctival blebs, the conjunctival wall is diaphanous and a single site of leakage may not be ascertained. Extensive tissue necrosis associated with antimetabolite therapy may result in progressive thinning of the bleb wall and the development of so-called "melt holes." The intraocular pressure is typically decreased with bleb leaks, although the bleb and anterior chamber may remain formed. In some cases, topical aqueous suppressants, in combination with topical antibiotic therapy, will result in closure of filtration bleb leaks. Aqueous suppression is used to slow the flow

of aqueous humor through the bleb leak, while antibiotic therapy is used to stimulate low-grade inflammation of the conjunctiva to promote wound healing and to protect against intraocular infection. In addition, application of a large diameter soft contact lens or patching the eye may help in resolution of the bleb leak. If conservative medical therapy is unsuccessful, surgical closure of the leak with excision of the portion of leaking conjunctiva may be required.

Cataract Formation

Formation of cataracts may occur after any form of intraocular surgery. It is estimated that 25 to 30% of eyes after filtering surgery will develop cataracts (16, 39, 47, 65). There are many proposed mechanisms for this complication. Violation of the lens capsule at the time of surgery may result in an instantaneous cataract or development of a cataract at a later date. Caution must be used when completing surgical iridectomies, either in combination with trabeculectomy or as a surgical procedure for angle-closure glaucoma, because the lens periphery may be damaged. Postoperative flat anterior chambers, especially with lenticular corneal touch, greatly increases the chance of postoperative cataract formation. Extended postoperative inflammation may also lead to cataract formation.

Infection

Intraocular infection after filtration surgery is an uncommon, but potentially devastating, complication (12, 25, 37). Thin-walled filtering blebs, blebs after full-thickness procedures, and filtration procedures completed with adjunctive antimetabolite therapy are all at a higher risk of developing postoperative endophthalmi-

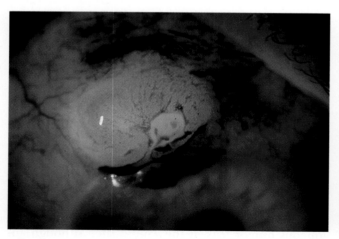

Figure 47–4.
Filtration Bleb Leak: Thin-walled, elevated filtration bleb with aqueous humor leak identified using fluoresceing and cobalt blue illumination (positive Seidel test).

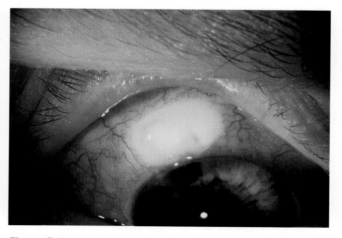

Figure 47–5.
Filtration Bleb Infection: Extensive conjunctival inflammation with well-demarcated, milky-white, thin-walled bleb.

tis. After any form of filtration surgery, the possibility of endophthalmitis is increased, because of the permanent fistulization through one of the layers of the eye and increased intraocular access by pathogens. For these reasons, any external infection or conjunctivitis should be treated aggressively in eyes after filtration surgery.

Postoperative infection in an eye with a filtering procedure may stay localized to the filtration bleb. Clinically, the episcleral and conjunctival vasculature becomes significantly injected, but the filtration bleb is typically thin-walled, avascular, and milky-white in appearance (Figure 47–5). These filtration blebs may develop spontaneous leaks of aqueous humor through the wall of the conjunctiva or a frank hole through the conjunctiva may be seen. White cells may be seen circulating in the anterior chamber and may be layered in the bleb itself. Fulminant endophthalmitis may occur within hours to days after the onset of a localized bleb infection. Gram stain of the surrounding conjunctiva is always recommended. An anterior chamber tap, with Gram stains and cultures, should be done in eyes with significant anterior chamber inflammation. Management includes immediate initiation of broad spectrum antibiotics. A vitreous tap should also be considered in more extensive infections. Streptococci and *Hemophilus influenza* are the two most frequently reported bacterial pathogens associated with filtering bleb infections. Treatment of the infection and preservation of the eye should be the first priority, but maintenance of the filtration bleb should also be considered. Periocular corticosteroids may be used to minimize the secondary inflammatory response and prevent filtration failure.

■ REFERENCES

1. Akers MJ: Ocular bioavailability of topically applied ophthalmic drugs. Am Pharm 1983, NS23:33.
2. Barkan O: Operation for congenital glaucoma. Am J Ophthalmol 1942, 25:552.
3. Becker B: Decrease in intraocular pressure in man by a carbonic anhydrase inhibitor, Diamox. Am J Ophthal 1954, 37:13.
4. Becker B, Ley AP: Epinephrine and acetazolamide in the therapy of the chronic glaucomas. Am J Ophthal 1958, 45:639.
5. Becker B, Pettit TH, Gay AJ: Topical epinephrine therapy of open-angle glaucoma. Arch Opthal 1961, 66:219.
6. Beckman H, Sugar HS: Neodymium laser cyclocoagulation. Arch Ophthalmol 1973, 90:27.
7. Bellows AR, Chylack LT, Hutchinson BT: Choroidal detachment: Clinical manifestation, therapy and mechanism of formation. Ophthalmol 1981, 88:1107.
8. Berry DP, Van Buskirk EM, Shields MB: Betaxolol and timolol. A comparison of efficacy and side effects. Arch Ophthal 1984, 102:42.
9. Berson FG, Cinotti A, Cohen H, et al: Levobunolol. A beta-adrenoceptor antagonist effective in the long-term treatment of glaucoma. Ophthalmology 1985, 92:1271.
10. Bill A, Phillips CI: Uveoscleral drainage of aqueous humor in human eyes. Exp Eye Res 1971, 12:275.
11. Bito LZ, Baroody RA: The ocular pharmacokinetics of eicosanoids and their derivatives. I. Comparison of ocular eicosanoid penetration and distribution following the topical application of PGF$_{2a}$ PGF$_{2a}$-1-methyl ester, and PGF$_{2a}$-1-isopropyl ester. Exp Eye Res 1987, 44:217.
12. Brown RH, Yang LH, Walker SD, Lynch MG, Martinez LA, Wilson LA: Treatment of bleb infection after glaucoma surgery. Arch Ophthalmol 1994, 112:57.
13. Camras CB, Bito LZ, Eakins KE: Reduction of intraocular pressure by prostaglandins applied topically to the eyes of conscious rabbits. Invest Ophthal Vis Sci 1977,16:1125.
14. Cairns JE: Trabeculectomy. Preliminary report of a new method. Am J Ophthal 1968, 5:573.
15. Chandler PA, Simmons RJ, Grant WM: Malignant glaucoma. Am J Ophthalmol 1968, 66:(3): 495.
16. Chauvaud D, Clay-Fressinet C, Pouliquen Y, Offret G: Opacification of the lens after trabeculectomy. Arch Ophthal (Paris) 1976, 36:379.
17. Chen CW, Huang HT,Bair JS, Lee CC: Trabeculectomy with simultaneous topical application of mitomycin-C in refractory glaucoma. J Ocul Pharmacol 1990, 61-75.
18. Coleman AL, Robin AL, Pollack IP, et al: Cardiovascular and intraocular pressure effects and plasma concentrations of apraclonidine. Arch Ophthal 1990, 108:1264.
19. Drance SM, Nash PA: The dose response of human intraocular pressure to pilocarpine. Can J Ophthal 1971, 6:9.
20. Epstein DL, Freddo TF, Bassett-Chu S, et al: Influence of ethacrynic acid on outflow facility in the monkey and calf eye. Invest Ophthal Vis Sci 1987, 28:2067.
21. Epstein DL, Grant WM: Carbonic anhydrase inhibitor side effects. Serum chemical analysis. Arch Ophthal 1977, 95:1378.
22. Fourman, S: Management of cornea-lens touch after filtering surgery for glaucoma. Ophthalmol, 1990, 97:424.
23. Fraunfelder FT, Meyer SM, Bagby GC Jr, Dreis MW: Hematologic reactions to carbonic anhydrase inhibitors. Am J Ophthal 1985, 100:79.
24. Gharagozloo NZ, Relf SJ, Brubaker RF: Aqueous flow is reduced by the alpha-adrenergic agonist, apraclonidine hydrochloride (ALO 2145) Ophthalmology 1988, 95:1217.
25. Hattenhauer JM, Lipsich MP: Late endophthalmitis after filtering surgery. Am J Ophthalmol 1971, 72:1097.
26. Hoskins HD, Kass M: Complications and failure of filtering surgery. In: Hoskins HD, Kass M (eds): Becker-Schaffer's Diagnosis and Therapy of the Glaucomas. CV Mosby, St. Louis, 1989, 583.

27. Hung PT, Hsieh JW, Chiou GCY: Ocular hypotensive effects of N-demethylated carbachol on open angle glaucoma. Arch Ophthal 1982, 100:262.

28. Jampel HD, McGuigan LJ, Dunkelberger GR, et al: Cell proliferation after experimental glaucoma filtration surgery. Arch Ophthalmol 1988, 106:89.

29. Kaback MD, Podos SM, Hargin TS Jr., et al: The effects of dipivalyl epinephrine on the eye. Am J Ophthal 1976, 81:768.

30. Katz IM, Hubbard WA, Getson AJ, Gould AL: Intraocular pressure decrease in normal volunteers following timolol ophthalmic solution. Invest Ophthal 1976, 15:489.

31. Kitazawa Y, Axuma I, Takase M: Evaluation of the effect of carteolol eyedrops for primary open-angle glaucoma and ocular hypertension. Igaku No Ayumi 1983, 127:859.

32. Krasnov MM: Laser puncture of the anterior chamber angle in glaucoma. Vestn Oftal 1972, 3:37.

33. Krupin T, Podos SM, Becker B: Valve implants in filtering surgery. Am J Ophthalmol 1976, 81:232.

34. Kruse W: Metipranolol—a new beta receptor blocking agent. Klin Monatsbl Augenheilhd 1983, 182:582.

35. Lee DA, Topper JE, Brubaker RF: Effect of clonidine on aqueous humor flow in normal human eyes. Exp Eye Res 1984, 38;239.

36. Lichter PR: Reducing side effects of carbonic anhydrase inhibitors. Ophthalmology 1981, 88:266.

37. Mandelbaum S, Forster RK, Gelender H, Culbertson W: Late onset endophthalmitis associated with filtering blebs. Ophthalmology 1985, 92:964.

38. Maerte HJ, Merkle W: Long-term treatment of glaucoma with propranolol ophthalmic solution. Klin Monatsble Augenheilkd 1980, 177:437.

39. Marion JR, Shields MB: Thermal sclerostomy and posterior lip sclerectomy: a comparative study. Ophthal Surg 1978, 9:67.

40. Masiakowski J, Warchalowska D, Orlowski WJ: Effect of osmotic agents on intraocular pressure. I. Survey of pharmacological possibilities. Klin Oczna 1973, 43:365.

41. McPherson SD, Berry DP: Goniotomy vs. external trabeculotomy for developmental glaucoma. Am J Ophthalmol 1983, 3:95.

42. Meyer-Schwickerath G: Erfahrungen mit der Lichtokoagulation der Netzhaut under der Iris. Ophthal 1956, 10:91.

43. Mindel JS, Kharlamb AB: Alteration of acetylcholine synthesis by pilocarpine. Arch Ophthal 1984, 102:1546.

44. Molteno ACB: New implants for drainage in glaucoma. Br J Ophthalmol 1969, 43:606.

45. Nagataki S, Brubaker RF: Effect of pilocarpine on aqueous humor formation in human beings. Arch Ophthamol 1982, 100:818.

46. Netland PA, Chaturvedi N, Dreyer EB: Calcium channel blockers in the management of low tension and open-angle glaucoma. Am J Ophthal 1993, 15:608.

47. O'Connell EJ, Karseras AG: Intraocular surgery in advanced glaucoma. Br J Ophthal 1976, 60:124.

48. Piltz JR, Bose S, Grunwald JE, Petrig BL, Riva ED: Effect of nimodipine on automated threshold perimetry, spatial contrast sensitivity and macular blood flow in normal tension glaucoma and controls. Invest Ophthal Vis Sci 1993, 34(S):1287.

49. Pooinoosawmy D, Nagasubramanian S, Brown NAP: Effect of pilocarpine on visual acuity on the dimensions of the cornea and anterior chamber. Br J Ophthal 1976, 60:676.

50. Prost M: Cyclocryotherapy for glaucoma. Evaluation of techniques. Surv Ophthal 1983, 28:93.

51. Radius RL, Diamond GR, Pollack IP, Langham ME: Timolol. A new drug for management of chronic simple glaucoma. Arch Ophthal 1978, 96:1003

52. Reiss GR, Wilensky JT, Higginbotham EJ: Laser trabeculoplasty. Surv Ophthal 1991, 35(6):407.

53. Ritch R: Argon laser treatment for medically unresponsive attacks of angle-closure glaucoma. Am J Ophthal 1982, 94:197.

54. Robbins R, Galin MA: Effect of osmotic agents on the vitreous body. Arch Ophthal 1969, 82:694.

55. Schoene RB, Martin TR, Charan NB, French CL: Timolol-induced bronchospasm in asthmatic bronchitis. JAMA 1981, 245:1460.

56. Schultz JS: Initial Treatment of Glaucoma: Surgery or Medications. III. Editorial. Chop or Drop? Surv Ophthalmol 37:4, 293.

57. Schumer RA, Podos SM: The Nerve of Glaucoma! Arch Ophthalmol 1994, 112(1):37.

58. Sharir M, Zimmerman TJ: Initial Treatment of Glaucoma: Surgery or Medications. II. Medical Therapy. Surv Ophthalmol 1993, 37:4, 293.

59. Sherwood MB, Migdal CS, Hitchings RA: Initial Treatment of Glaucoma: Surgery or Medications. I. Filtration Surgery. Surv Ophthalmol 1993, 37:4, 293.

60. Shocket SS: Investigation of the reasons for success and failure in the anterior shunt to the encircling band procedure in the treatment of refractory glaucoma. Trans Am Ophthalmol Soc 1986, 84:743.

61. Skuta GL, Parrish RK Jr: Wound healing in glaucoma filtering surgery. Surv Ophthalmol 1987, 32:149.

62. Skuta LG, Parrish RK: Wound healing in glaucoma filtering surgery. Surv Ophthalmol 1987, 32:149.

63. Starita RJ, Fellman RL, Spaeth GL, et al. Short and long-term effects of postoperative corticosteroids on trabeculectomy. Ophthalmology 1985, 92:938.

64. Stewart RH, Kimbrough RL, Ward RL: Betaxolol vs timolol. A six month double blind comparison. Arch Ophthal 1986, 104:46.

65. Sugar HS: Cataract and filtering surgery. Am J Ophthal 1970, 69:740.

66. Sugar HS: Experimental trabeculectomy in glaucoma. Am J Ophthal 1961, 51:623.

67. The Fluorouracil Filtering Surgery Study Group. Fluorouracil filtering surgery study one-year follow-up. Am J Ophthalmol 1989, 108:625.

68. Van Buskirk EM: Adverse reactions from timolol administration. Ophthalmology 1980, 87:447.

69. Van Buskirk EM: Filtration Blebs: Clinical Variations in Wound Healing. In: Drance S, Van Buskirk EM, Neufeld AH (eds), Pharmacology of Glaucoma. Williams & Wilkins, Baltimore, 1992, 1.

70. Van Buskirk EM: The failing filter. In: Wright KW (ed) Color Atlas of Ophthalmic Surgery: Glaucoma, Lippincott-Raven, Philadelphia, 1992, 105.

71. Van Buskirk EM: Pathophysiology of laser trabeculoplasty. Surv Ophthal 1989, 33:264.

72. Van Buskirk EM, Fraunfelder FT: Ocular beta blockers and systemic effects. Am J Ophthalmol 1984, 98;623.

73. Van Buskirk EM, Pond V, Rosenquist RC, Acott TS: Argon

laser trabeculoplasty. Studies of mechanism of action. Ophthalmology 1984, 91:1005.

74. Wandel T, Spinak M: Toxicity of dipivalyl epinephrine. Ophthalmology 1981, 88:259.

75. Weinreb RN: Adjusting the dose of 5-fluorouracil after filtration surgery to minimize side effects. Ophthalmology 1987, 94:564.

76. Weinreb RN, Van Buskirk EM, Cherniack R, Drake MM: Long-term betaxolol therapy in glaucoma patients with pulmonary disease. Am J Ophthal 1988, 106:162.

77. Wise JB, Witter SL: Argon laser therapy for open-angle glaucoma. A pilot study. Arch Ophthal 1979, 97:319.

78. Wisznia KI, Lazar M, Leopold IH: Oral isosorbide and intraocular pressure. Am J Ophthal 1970, 70:630.

79. Worthen DM, Wickham MG: Argon laser trabeculotomy. Trans Am Acad Ophthal Otol 1974, 78:371.

80. Zimmerman TJ, Dukar U, Nardin GF, et al: Carbachol dose response. Am J Ophthal 1989, 108:456.

81. Zimmerman TJ, Kooner KS, Kandarakis AS, Ziegler LP: Improving the therapeutic index of topically applied ocular drugs. Arch Ophthal 1984, 102:551.

82. Zimmerman TJ, Kaufman HE: Timolol. A beta-adrenergic blocking agent for the treatment of glaucoma. Arch Ophthal 1977, 95:601.

IX Anterior Segment and External Diseases

Section Editor: Thomas J. Liesegang

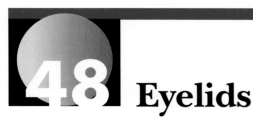

48 Eyelids

Diseases of the Eyelid Margin

Thomas J. Liesegang

Eyelid margin inflammation (blepharitis) is one of the most common problems in ophthalmology. Lid inflammation affects patients of all ages with either an acute or prolonged inflammatory reaction. Despite its frequency, our knowledge of the pathophysiology and treatment are rudimentary. Treatment is time-consuming and frequently, not completely effective. There are recognized distinctive forms of blepharitis which will be described. Several of these are frequently present together with multiple approaches required (15). Clinically, these diseases have been divided into those which involve mainly the base of the eyelashes (seborrheic blepharitis, staphylococcal blepharitis) and those which involve the meibomian glands (meibomian gland dysfunction). (For anatomic description, see Chapter 1, Figure 1–7A) (Table 48–1).

■ SEBORRHEIC BLEPHARITIS

Patients with seborrheic blepharitis complain of continuous burning, itching, light sensitivity, and heaviness of the lids. Although it can occur at any age, it is frequently found in the elderly, especially those of Anglican descent. It is often associated with seborrhea of the scalp, brow, and facial area or of the ears or sternal skin. Significant findings include eyelid inflammation and dry flakes (dandruff) on the lids (dry seborrheic blepharitis). A variant of this consists of oily secretions and greasy deposits on the eye lashes (wet seborrheic blepharitis) which may dry to form crusts (scurf). This greasy form may be associated with meibomian gland dysfunc-tion (14) (Figure 48–1). With chronicity, some patients develop corneal involvement with a punctate keratopathy in the interpalpebral space. *Pityrosporum ovale* and *orbiculare* are budding yeasts plentiful in the scrapings from seborrhea, but their significance remains debatable. This disease is chronic and incurable. Mild forms can respond to lid hygiene (hot compresses and lid massage with removal of the lid flakes with mild soaps or commercially prepared eye pads). Seborrheic blepharitis may be florid in patients with AIDS with a response to 2% ketoconazole cream (18).

■ STAPHYLOCOCCAL BLEPHARITIS

Patients with *Staphylococcal blepharitis* often complain of burning, itching, and irritation, especially in the morning (22). They may report difficulty opening their eyes in the morning with their lids matted or stuck together. Compared with seborrheic blepharitis patients, patients with *S. blepharitis* are younger and more frequently female. During acute *S. blephararitis*, perifolliculitis can lead to ulceration and fibrinous exudates on the lid

TABLE 48–1
Classification of Blepharitis

Anterior Lid Margin
  Seborrheic blepharitis
    Dry seborrhea
    Wet seborrhea (associated with meibomian gland dysfunction)
  Staphylococcal blepharitis
  Mixed seborrheic and staphylococcal blepharitis
Posterior Lid Margin
  Meibomian gland dysfunction
    With rosacea dermatitis
    Without rosacea dermatitis
Localized lid margin disease
  External hordeolum
    Infection of Zeis gland
  Internal hordeolum
    Infection of meibomian gland
  Chalazion
    Lipogranulomatous reaction in meibomian gland

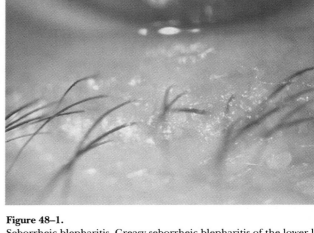

Figure 48–1.
Seborrheic blepharitis. Greasy seborrheic blepharitis of the lower lid. The patient also had rosacea of the facial area but without significant meibomian gland dysfunction.

margin. Typical changes of chronic blepharitis include crusting and hard brittle scales on the base of the lashes. When these scales encircle the lash they are known as collarettes. The eyelid margins are typically dry, thickened, and hyperemic (rosettes) and the eye lashes may be matted together in tufts. Structural alterations with chronicity include telangiectasia, hypertrophy, and notching or irregularity (tylosis). Lashes are frequently short, misdirected, broken, or absent (madarosis) from hair follicle damage. Localized poliosis (whitening) of individual eye lashes occurs from damage to the pilosebaceous unit by staphylococcus. External and internal hordeola are common during the lifetime of the individual. An external hordeolum (sty) is an abscess of the gland of Zeis on the anterior lid margin and is associated with pain, redness, and swelling. An internal hordeolum is an infection within the meibomian gland of the posterior lid margin. It causes intense pain and swelling and may point to either the conjunctival or the skin side.

S. blepharitis is frequently associated with corneal changes either in the form of a fine epithelial keratitis of the lower half of the cornea (especially common in the morning) or with catarrhal corneal infiltrates or ulcers, usually at the 2 to 4-o'clock or 8 to 10-o'clock area of the peripheral cornea. These catarrhal lesions are separated from the limbus by a lucid interval; they are sterile and represent immunologic response to bacterial antigen. Neovascularization of the cornea sometimes occurs.

Staphylococcus aureus has traditionally been the cause of this condition, although it can also be associated with colonization of the lids with *Staphylococcal epidermidis*, *Propionibacterium acnes*, and *Corynebacterium species* (23). From a rabbit model of *S. blepharitis*, it was postulated that the pathogenesis of *S. blepharitis* relates to a hypersensitivity reaction to the *S. aureus* cell wall, particularly to ribitol teichoic acid (9,16). Alternatively, the many toxins from staphylococcus may play a role (20, 25). Therapy of *S. blepharitis* involves lid hygiene with the addition of a suitable topical antibiotic ointment to the base of the eyelashes for a period of several weeks. In some patients, systemic antibiotics are indicated. Lid cultures are done in cases resistant to therapy. Prophylactic lid hygiene is done to reduce recurrences. Angular blepharitis is a maceration, fissuring, scaling, lichenification, and redness usually at the external canthus associated with a conjunctivitis and frequently with *S. blepharitis*. A redundant dermatochalasis may contribute to the pathogenesis in some patients. *Moraxella lacunata* or *S. aureus* are usually implicated. Therapy is the same as for *S. blepharitis*.

The skin of the eyelid can also be affected secondarily from impetigo or infectious eczematoid dermatitis.

■ MEIBOMIAN GLAND DYSFUNCTION

The meibomian glands are tubuloalveolar sebaceous glands of the eyelid margin that resemble cutaneous holocrine glands. The meibomian gland secretions consist of sterol esters and waxes, but lack the high triglyceride levels found in sebum. Initial changes in meibomian gland dysfunction consist of keratinization of the ductal epithelium and the meibomian gland orifices, leading to plugging of the ducts with desquamated epithelial cells. The glands become dilated and cystic with changes in the lipid composition because of this stagnation (25). Microbial lipases from *P. acnes* and other bacteria contribute to producing irritating fatty acids which may alter tear film stability (13).

Meibomian gland dysfunction is characterized by bilateral, prolonged, posterior eyelid margin inflammation. Patients complain of redness and burning, presumably from the free fatty acid irritation. Meibomian gland inspissation and occlusion with pouting of the orifices is typical. A thick, yellowish oil can be expressed from individual meibomian glands unless the secretions are inspissated in the orifice (Figure 48–2). Spotty hyperemic areas of telangiectatic blood vessels fan across the eyelid margin. An oily sheen with mucin particles appear in the tear film and lipid residues with foamy tears may collect on the lid margin. Redundant conjunctiva may be seen. Conjunctival hyperemia is seen in prolonged cases. The cornea may manifest diffuse epithelial erosions; with chronicity, superficial stromal vascularization with pannus formation is seen.

Patients may develop an acute infection of an occluded meibomian gland (internal hordeolum) or a prolonged obstruction with lipogranulomatous formation (chalazia) (17). Chalazia typically erupt under the conjunctival surface, but can also erupt through the tarsus and into the subcutaneous tissue. They may resolve on their own. Occasionally, an incision and drainage or intralesional steroid injections are necessary (19). With resolution, chalazions frequently result in permanent stellate conjunctival scarring and distortion of the eyelid margin.

Eyelid margin cultures are not indicated but will reveal lipophilic organisms such as *P. acnes* and *Corynebac-*

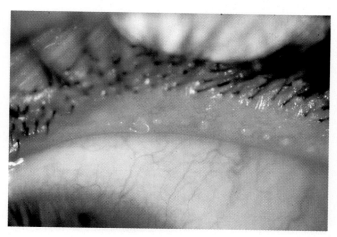

Figure 48–2.
Meibomian gland dysfunction. Oily secretions extruding from the meibomian gland orifices in a patient with meibomian gland dysfunction.

terium species (11). Chromatographic analysis of meibomian gland lipids is a complex research tool at present. Eyelid hygiene with eyelid massage and expression of meibomian glands should be taught. Ointments should be avoided. Topical corticosteroids are helpful in some of the corneal complications but should generally be avoided. Oral tetracycline or doxycycline are effective in reducing the symptoms associated with meibomian gland dysfunction by an effect on altering the oily products of the meibomian gland (21) perhaps because of its ability to bind zinc.

■ ROSACEA BLEPHAROCONJUNCTIVITIS

Rosacea is a common inflammatory disorder of the facial skin and chest with an onset primarily between ages 30 and 50. Although more common in females, it is frequently more severe in males. The early stages consist of facial erythema or a "ruddy" complexion. Fine telangiectasia of the skin occur with inflammatory papules and pustules. Severe involvement leads to dilated nodules on the face and rhinophyma. Ocular symptoms and signs are common and may precede the significant skin changes (3); there may be poor correlation with the ocular findings and the degree of skin involvement (Figure 48–3). There is a genetic predisposition in patients of Celtic-born northern European ancestry.

The ocular findings are the same as found with meibomian gland dysfunction and the ocular treatment is the same (4). Topical metronidazole is effective in rosacea dermatitis. It is not available in an ocular preparation. There are no studies available to indicate

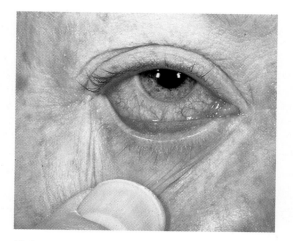

Figure 48–3.
Rosacea. Rosacea of the facial area and an associated meibomian gland dysfunction and rosacea conjunctivitis characterized by hyperemia and irritation.

whether controlling the dermal component may have an effect on ocular manifestations. The etiology of rosacea (and the related meibomian gland dysfunction) may be a dermal dystrophy with changes in the perivascular collagen leading to small vessel dilation and incompetence. Leakage of inflammatory substances into the perivascular space may lead to lymphedema with the formation of papules, pustules, and lupoid nodules. There may be widespread lability of vascular regulatory mechanisms, accounting for increased tendency to flush and for migraine (1).

■ OTHER CAUSES OF EYELID MARGIN INFLAMMATION

Demodex foliculorum is a hair follicle mite found in a high percentage of eye lash follicles with or without blepharitis. Their role in blepharitis remains unclear (5). Symptoms may include itching and pain with significant infestations. Diagnosis is established by finding semitransparent, almost plastic, thin, tubelike crusting of the skin around the lashes. This excess keratin may be a result of abrasive action of the mites' sharp claws. Examination of the epilated lashes by light microscopy will confirm the mites. Treatment is with lid scrubs and antibiotic ointments (8).

The *crab louse, Phthirus pubis,* is usually found in the hairs of the genital region; occasionally infestation of the beard, eye brows, axilla, and eye lashes may occur (Figure 48–4). Transmission is by direct contact with an infested individual or with use of infested personal articles. Involvement of the eyelids causes itching and burning. The eyelids show tiny pearly white nits (eggs or egg cases) attached to the lashes. The transparent adult lice are difficult to see without a slit lamp magnification. After attaching to the base of the lashes, the louse feeds every few hours on the eyelid skin. The female may lay several eggs per day. The eggs hatch in about 8 days into nymphs which mature over 2 weeks. The conjunctiva may have an irritative conjunctivitis. The ideal therapy has yet to be established. Mechanical removal of nits and lice is time-consuming. A thick occlusive application of ophthalmic ointment (Eucerin ointment or Lacri-Lube) may smother the adult. Topical application of fluorescein 20% with a swab can dislodge the parasites. Application of lindane 1% (Kwell) lotion or malathion 0.5% (Ovide) can be effective. Cryotherapy and argon laser phototherapy are alternative treatments. All contacts need to be treated with delousing of all personal items and clothing. The remainder of the body needs treatment with delousing shampoos. Retreatment may be necessary (6,25).

Molluscum contagiosum is caused by a pox virus resulting in multiple waxy, umbilicated wartlike growths along the lid margins and can also be found on the eyelids and face (also see plastic section). It is associated with a serous follicular conjunctivitis and punctate keratitis as a result of the virus being shed into the tear film (Figure 48–5). Severe disseminated disease with this double-stranded DNA virus may occur in patients with AIDS. The diagnosis is based on the characteristic appearance. Therapy is surgical with removal of the growths by excision, chemical cauterization, or cryotherapy.

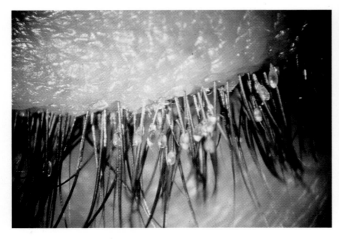

Figure 48–4.
Parasitic blepharitis. Phthirus pubis crab louse nits on the lid margin. The patient had concomitant pubic lice.

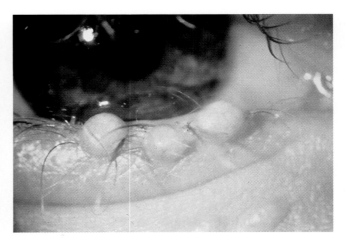

Figure 48–5.
Molluscum contagiosum. The viral legions of molluscum contagiosum on the lower lid in a patient with a follicular conjunctivitis. The patient responded to cryotherapy of the lesions.

Verruca vulgaris is caused by the same papovavirus causing the common wart. It frequently appears on the eyelid margin. It may be pedunculated or broad-based and multilobulated. A secondary mild papillary conjunctivitis and epithelial keratitis may be present. Excision with cauterization or cryotherapy may be curative, although recurrences are possible.

Infection of the Eyelid Skin

■ IMPETIGO

Impetigo of the eyelids is usually associated with infection of the face (7). This superficial skin infection is caused by Group A streptococcus or *S. aureus*. The infection begins as a small macule that enlarges, vesiculates, and then pustulates. Bullae can form and become crusted. The crusts are usually thin and varnishlike in *staphylococcal impetigo* and are thick and honey-colored in *streptococcal impetigo*. The infection can spread by finger or towels and satellite lesions can be found in other skin locations. It is most common in children. The streptococcal skin infection can be associated with glomerulonephritis. The disease is diagnosed by its characteristic clinical appearance. Culture should be taken to guide antimicrobial therapy. Treatment consists of gentle washing of the affected areas, followed by application of bacitracin or erythromycin ointment. Oral administration of erythromycin in effective for bullous impetigo caused by *S. aureus* and oral penicillin is the best initial therapy for group A streptococcal infections.

■ INFECTIOUS ECZEMATOID DERMATITIS

Infectious eczematoid dermatitis is a vesiculated, pustular, crusting, or lichenified change of the eyelid skin seen in association with *staphylococcal blepharitis*. It is caused by a sensitization to staphylococcal products, which serve as haptens. The *staphylococcal blepharitis* needs to be treated with topical and sometimes systemic antibiotics. Topical corticosteroids creams help control the eczematoid lid reaction.

■ ERYSIPELAS

Erysipelas is a deeper skin infection caused by *Streptococcus pyogenes* (2, 12). It is characterized by warm, red, swollen lesions with sharply raised, violaceous, readily outlined borders. Vesicles or bulla are often present. Systemic symptoms of headache, joint pain, chills, and fever may occur. Systemic penicillin is indicated.

There are multiple other infectious diseases which can involve the lids, including bacterial (anthrax, syphilis), viral (HSV, VZV, varicella, vaccinia), fungal (blastomycosis, coccidioidomycoses, cryptomycosis, sporotrichosis, mycetoma, aspergillosis, candidiasis), mycobacterial (tuberculosis, atypical mycobacterial, leprosy), and parasitic (myiasis, leishmaniasis, onchocerciasis, dirofilariasis, cysticercosis) (10, 24). Some are discussed in different sections and some are rare.

■ REFERENCES

1. Bajart AM: Lid inflammation. In: Albert, DM, Jakobiec, FA (eds). Principles and practice of ophthalmology. Philadelphia: WB Saunders, 1994: Volume 1:101–116.
2. Bernard, P, Bedane, C, Mournier, M, et al: Streptococcal cause of erysipelas and cellulitis in adults. Arch Dermatol, 1989: 125:779.
3. Browning, DJ, Proia, AD: Ocular rosacea. Surv Ophthalmol, 1986: 31:145.

4. Cory, CC, Hinks, W, Burton, JL, Shuster, S: Meibomian gland secretions in the red eyes of rosacea. Br J Dermatol, 1973: 88:25–27.

5. Coston, TO: Demodex folliculorum blepharitis. Trans Am Ophthalmol Soc, 1967: 65:361.

6. Couch, JM, Green, WR, Hirst, LW et al: Diagnosing and treating phthirus pubis palpebrarum. Surv Ophthalmol, 1982: 26:219–225.

7. Demidovich, CW, Wittler, RR, Ruff, ME, et al: Impetigo. Am J Dis Child, 1990: 144:1313.

8. English, FP, Nutting, WB: Demodicosis of ophthalmic concern. Am J Ophthalmol, 1981: 91:362–372.

9. Ficker, L, Ramakrishnan, M, Seal, D, et al: Role of cell-mediated immunity to staphylococci in blepharitis. Am J Ophthalmol, 1988: 106:514.

10. Glover AT: Eyelid infection. In: Albert DM, Jakobiec FA (eds). Principles and practice of ophthalmology. Philadelphia: WB Saunders, 1994: Volume 3:1702–1712.

11. Groden, LR, Murphy, B, Rodnite, J, et al: Lid flora in blepharitis. Cornea, 1991: 10:50.

12. Matoba, AY: Acute bacterial infections of eyelids and tarsal plate. Ophthalmol Clin North Am, 1992: 5:169.

13. McCulley JP: Meibomitis. In: Kaufman, HE, Barrou, BA, McDonald, MB, Waltman, SR. The Cornea. New York: Churchill Livingstone, 1988: 125–138.

14. McCulley, JP, Dougherty, JM: Blepharitis associated with acne rosacea and seborrheic dermatitis. Int Ophthalmol Clin, 1985: 25:159.

15. McCulley, JP, Dougherty, JM, Deneau, DG: Classification of chronic blepharitis. Ophthalmology, 1982: 89:1173.

16. Mondino, BJ, Caster, AI, Dethlefs, B: A rabbit model of staphylococcal blepharitis. Arch Ophthalmol, 1987: 105:409–

17. Nicolaides, N, Flores, A, Santos, EC, et al: The lipids of chalazia. Invest Ophthalmol Vis Sci, 1988: 29:482.

18. Ostler HB: Blepharitis. In: Tasman, W, Jaeger, EA (eds): Duane's Clinical Ophthalmology. Philadelphia: Lippincott-Raven, 1989: Volume 4: Chapter 22.

19. Pizzarello, LD, Jakobiec, FA, Hofeldt, AJ, et al: Intralesional corticosteroid therapy of chalazia. Am J Ophthalmol, 1978: 85:818–821.

20. Raskin, EM, Speaker, MG, Laibson, PR: Blepharitis. Inf Dis Clin North Am, 1992: 6:777–787.

21. Salamon, SM: Tetracyclines in ophthalmology. Surv Ophthalmol, 1985: 29:265–275.

22. Smolin, G, Okumoto, M: Staphylococcal blepharitis. Arch Ophthalmol, 1977: 95:812.

23. Valenton, M, Okumoto, M: Toxin producing strains of Staphylococcus epidermidis. Arch Ophthalmol, 1973: 89:186.

24. Weinberg, RS: Selected inflammatory diseases of the skin and eye. Ophthalmol Clin of North Am, 1992: 5:215.

25. Wilhelmus, KR: Inflammatory disorders of the eyelid margins and eyelashes. Ophthalmol Clin North Am, 1992: 5:187–194.

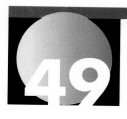

49 Tear Dysfunction

Thomas J. Liesegang

◼ ANATOMY AND PHYSIOLOGY OF THE TEAR FILM (ALSO SEE PLASTIC SECTION LACRIMAL SYSTEM)

The precorneal tear film handles several important functions in maintaining the metabolic, protective, and physiologic health of the corneal epithelium. It provides a moist environment for the surface epithelial cells of the conjunctiva and the cornea. Along with the lids, it washes away noxious stimuli. Tears contain antimicrobial products and can carry antiinflammatory products of the body to a site of injury. The tear film transports metabolic products (oxygen, CO_2) to and from the surface cells. It provides a smooth refracting surface over the cornea for precise vision.

The precorneal tear film is composed of three layers: the outer layer (a thin oily or lipid layer), the middle layer (a thick aqueous layer), and the inner layer (a thin mucin layer) (Figure 49–1) (Table 49–1). The mucin layer is firmly attached to the conjunctiva and corneal epithelium; the aqueous and mucous layers are partially mixed and are held together as an aggregate of colloidal droplets through electrostatic attractive forces. The entire tear film is approximately 7 μm thick. The tear film is thickest immediately after a blink and thins progressively until the next blink, or until the tear film breaks up. The average tear film production in humans is approximately 1.2 μm per minute and the tear fluid averages 7 μm. Approximately 1.1 μm of this total volume lies in the preocular tear film within the palpebral fissure. Approximately 2.9 μm is within the marginal strip, and approximately 4.5 μm is within the fornices (6).

Lipid Layer

The lipid layer is approximately 0.1 to 0.5 μm thick. It is derived from the meibomian gland in the upper and lower lids and consists of esters, triacylglycerols, free sterols, sterol esters, and fatty acids. The lipid layer behaves as a film, independent of the aqueous layer beneath it, and is firmly anchored at the orifices of the meibomian glands with debris in the tear film floating in the underlying aqueous portion. During lid closure, the lipid layer thickens and during lid opening the layer thins, remaining continually intact. The function of this lipid layer is to inhibit the evaporation of the tears, especially under conditions of decreased humidity or wind. It also acts as a hydrophobic barrier to prevent overflow of tears and protects the aqueous layer from polar lipid contamination that could rupture the tear film prematurely (13).

Aqueous Layer

The major portion of the tear film is the aqueous layer which is almost 7 μl thick. The aqueous portion is formed primarily by the lacrimal gland and the accessory lacrimal glands of Krause and Wolfring. The main lacrimal gland is divided into an orbital and palpebral portion by the levator aponeurosis and lies deep in the superior temporal fornix. The majority of the accessory

TABLE 49-1
The Precorneal Tear Film

Layer	Source	Function
Superficial Layer: Lipid (~0.5 μm)	Meibomian glands Glands of Zeis Glands of Moll	Lubrication Retards evaporation Keeps layers thick
Middle Layer: Aqueous (~7.0 μm)	Lacrimal gland Glands of Krause Glands of Wolfring	Hydration Lubrication Antimicrobial agent Removes debris Brings nutrients Basic and reflex secretion
Inner Layer: Mucin (~0.1 μm)	Conjunctival goblet cells	Reduces surface tension Lubrication

glands of Krause lie in the superior temporal fornix, with a few lying in the inferior temporal fornix. The glands of Wolfring are larger, but fewer in number than the glands of Krause and lie in the conjunctiva near the forniceal side of the tarsal plates. Most of the aqueous fluids arrive from the superior temporal fornix, travel into the marginal tear strip, and then into the lacrimal puncta.

There has been a classic interpretation of lacrimal secretory system that divides the system anatomically into two parts: the basic secreters (goblet cells and ac-

cessary lacrimal gland) which provide the normal tear film, and the reflux secreters (the main lacrimal gland) which provide excess tears during irritation or crying. Both probably work simultaneously instead of with this clear-cut distinction.

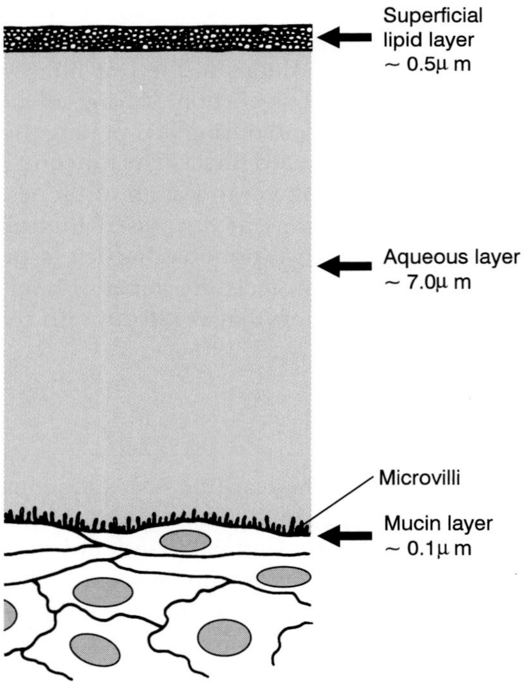

The lacrimal gland is innervated by both sympathetic and parasympathetic nerves. Parasympathetic stimulation causes lacrimal gland secretion as do beta adrenergic agonists. Parasympathetic blockers and beta adrenergic blockers can diminish lacrimal gland secretion clinically (6). The relationship between sympathetic fibers to the lacrimal gland remains unresolved. The main and accessory lacrimal gland secretion is regulated both centrally and peripherally. Centrally, parasympathetic nerves innervate the lacrimal gland tissue; this activity is modulated by sensory reflex arcs and emotion. The lacrimal gland cells might also be stimulated directly by neurohumoral agents.

Mucin Layer

The inner mucin layer of the tear film is thin and produced by the conjunctival goblet cells and the mucous secretory cells of the lacrimal gland. The mucin layer is made up of glycoprotein and mucopolysaccharide. This layer is essential for spreading the aqueous layer of the tears and maintaining contact between the aqueous layer and the corneal epithelium by rendering the corneal epithelium wettable. The mucin in the tear film dissolves in the aqueous layer. This helps lower the surface tension with the aqueous layer and enables it to wet more readily. Mucin then has three roles in maintaining a stable tear film (13); 1) mucin dissolved in the aqueous component increases the film pressure of the superficial lipid layer and renders it more stable; 2) the absorbed mucin renders the surface of the cornea wettable; 3) an adequate layer of mucin masks lipid molecules arriving at the corneal surface and thereby, maintains its hy-

Superficial lipid layer ~ 0.5μ m

Aqueous layer ~ 7.0μ m

Microvilli

Mucin layer ~ 0.1μ m

Figure 49–1.
The structure of the precorneal tear. Film drawn to scale.

drophilic character. An estimate of the effectiveness of the mucin layer can be made by measuring the tear breakup time or by performing a goblet cell count.

Tear Film Composition

The aqueous layer contains water-soluble contents including inorganic salts, glucose, urea, protein, and trace elements (9) (Table 49–2). The tear film has a unique electrolyte composition which is increased especially in potassium. The osmolality of the normal human tear averages 302 mOsm/l. Lowest in the morning after prolonged lid closure, it increases as the day progresses, primarily because of evaporation. Although glucose is present in the tear film, it is too decreased to supply the needs of the corneal epithelium. The cornea obtains its glucose from the aqueous humor. Oxygen in the tear film is probably the only metabolite the cornea obtains from the tear film. With the eyes open, a partial pressure of 155mm Hg of oxygen is maintained; with the lids closed, an oxygen partial pressure of 55mm Hg is maintained from diffusion of oxygen through the conjunctival capillary bed (6).

There are many different types of protein in the tear fluid, some of which come from the lacrimal gland and others from the serum. Proteins contained in the tear film include tear specific prealbumin, beta-lysine, lactoferrin, lysozyme, nonlysosomal antibacterial factor, immunoglobulin, and complement (10). These proteins help to lower the surface tension of the tears, which in turn helps to maintain a continuous tear film over the cornea (18). Lysozyme (muramidase) destroys bacterial cell membranes by disrupting the N-acetylglucosamine-N-acetylneuraminic acid polymers; this plays a role in maintaining the sterility of the tear film. Lysozyme is probably secreted by the lacrimal gland and decreased levels have been correlated with keratoconjunctivitis sicca. Numerous methods to measure tear lysozyme are available but are hampered by procedural details and interpretation. Beta-lysine ruptures cell membranes by unknown mechanisms and is also antibacterial. Lactoferrin is bactericidal, probably by virtue of its ion-binding capacity and also by the interaction with complement. Lactoferrin is probably secreted by the lacrimal and accessory lacrimal glands.

Although all the immunoglobulins are found in normal human tears, only IgA is found in significant quantities. Tears may contain specific antibodies to a number of viruses (for example HSV), although the presence of antibodies does not influence the disease. The role of IgA is unclear but may act to inhibit adherence of bacteria to mucous membranes (13). The entire complement pathway (both classic and alternate) is present in normal human tears. The complement system builds a cell membrane-bound protein chain that eventually lyses the bacterial cells. Epidermal growth factor is syn-

TABLE 49–2
Tear Fluid

Physical Properties	Value (approximate)
pH	6.5–7.6
Osmolarity	302 mOsm/L
Volume	6.5 μl
Flow rate	1.2 μl/min
Evaporation rate	10.1×10^{-7} g/cm/sec
Refractive index	1.336
Surface tension	40.1 dyne/cm

Composition of Tears	Concentration (approximate)
Water	98.2%
Electrolytes	
Sodium	145 mEq/L
Potassium	20 mEq/L
Chloride	128 mEq/L
Bicarbonate	26 mEq/L
Calcium	2.11 mg/dl
Magnesium	trace
Zinc	trace
Metabolites	
Glucose	3 mg/dl
Lactate/pyruvate	present
Urea	7–20 mg/dl
Protein	
Prealbumin	trace
Lysozyme	1–2 g/l
Lactoferrin	trace
Immunoglobin A	10–100 mg %
Immunoglobin G	trace
Immunoglobin E	26–144 mg/ml
Complement	1:4
Glycoproteins (hexosamine)	trace
Enzymes	
Lysosomal enzymes	$2–10 \times$ serum
Lactate dehydrogenase	high levels
Amylase	similar to urine
Peroxidase	10^3 U/I
Lipids	
Cholesterol	200 mg %
Meibomian lipids (hydrocarbons, wax esters, cholesterol esters, triglycerides, diglycerides, free fatty acids, free cholesterol, phospholipids)	trace

Modified from: Farris RL: Abnormalities of the tears and treatment of dry eyes. In: Kaufman, NE, Barron, BA, McDonald, MB, Waltman, SR (eds). The cornea. New York: Churchill Livingstone, 1988: 139–159. **and** Lamberts, DW: Physiology of the tear film. In: Smolin, G, Thoft, FA (eds). The cornea. Third edition. Boston: Little, Brown and Co., 1994:439–455.

thesized in the lacrimal gland and identified in the tear film; it may play a role in corneal epithelial repair from constant microtrauma.

Tear Dynamics

The tear film is inherently unstable with complex features permitting the intact tear film (15). The human tear film is a constantly changing fluid membrane with flow occurring only in the aqueous layer (13). The lipid layer remains intact between blinks and the mucin layer remains adherent to the epithelium. After a blink, the three layers of the tear film are intact and relatively distinct. As the eye remains open, the aqueous layer begins to evaporate and thin: in effect, bringing the lipid layer closer to the mucin layer. The tear film will break up eventually if the eye is held open long enough (13). During the blink, the lipid layer is compressed between the closing lids. Through shear forces across the aqueous layer, conjunctival mucin is spread over the epithelium, providing it with a fresh surface (3). Other debris is washed through the lacrimal aqueous portion to the upper and lower puncta (13). (See Plastics Section, Chapter 24 Lacrimal System for further discussion of tear drainage.)

Effect of Drugs on Tear Flow

Autonomic drugs have an inherent effect on tear flow. Parasympathetic stimulation produces depolarization of secretory cell membranes and constriction of the excretory ducts of the lacrimal gland. Sympathetic stimulation does not produce changes in the secretory cells or in the tear outflow of the lacrimal gland directly. Various drugs, such as the muscarinic, sympathomimetic, antihypertensive, and miscellaneous drugs will stimu-

TABLE 49–3
Effect of Drugs on Tear Flow

Drugs That Decrease Tear Flow
Antimuscarinic drugs (atropine, scopolamine and similar drugs)
Antihistamines
General anesthetics
Beta adrenergic blockers (systemic and topical)
Some antihypertensives (hydrochlorothiazide)
Antidepressants
Beta adrenergic blockers

Drugs That Increase Tear Flow
Muscarinics (pilocarpine, methacholine, carbachol, neostigmine, bethanechol)
Sympathomimetic (epinephrine, ephedrine)
Antihypertensive (reserpine, hydralazine)
Some general anesthetics (ketamine)
Fluorouracil
Marijuana
Bromhexine

late lacrimation (2) (Table 49–3). Several drugs, such as the antimuscarinics, will decrease tear flow. Many over-the-counter sedatives, nasal decongestants, antitussives, or antidiarrheal medications may have antimuscarinic components. Antihistamines and beta-adrenergic blockers (topical or systemic) decrease the tear flow. Most general anesthetics produce a marked decrease in tear production.

■ CLASSIFICATION OF DISEASES OF TEAR DYSFUNCTION

All diseases of tear dysfunction cause a detrimental effect on the ocular surface, leading to corneal and conjunctival epithelial disruption. Based on the research of Holly and Lemp, it is reasonable to consider five pathogenic pathways to tear dysfunction with an overlap of many of the mechanisms of disease. These five pathways include aqueous tear deficiency, mucin deficiency, lipid abnormalities, lid surfacing abnormalities, and epitheliopathies (4, 9, 13, 14) (Table 49–4).

Aqueous Tear Deficiency

The aqueous components constitute the bulk of the precorneal tear film and aqueous deficiency is by far, the most common cause of tear dysfunction states and dry eyes. Deficiency of aqueous tear production can occur in rare conditions such as the congenital abnormal-

ities of alacrima, hypoplasia of the lacrimal glands, or congenital paresis of the seventh cranial nerve, or as part of the Riley-Day syndrome, a generalized dysfunction of the autonomic nervous system.

Acquired causes of aqueous tear deficiency include trauma to the lacrimal gland (surgical, radiation), inflammation of the lacrimal gland (Sjogren's syndrome, mumps, trachoma), infiltration of the lacrimal gland (amyloid, sarcoid, lymphoma), drug effects (antihistamines, antimuscarines, general anesthetics), and neuroparalytic hyposecretion (brain stem lesion) (Table 49–4). Aqueous tear production normally decreases with age without causing symptoms in most patients. In some patients, the deficiency can be severe enough to lead to the development of ocular surface disease (keratoconjunctivitis sicca). Symptoms range from foreign body sensation, irritation, grittiness, redness of the eyes,

TABLE 49–4
Classification of Ocular Surface Disorders

Aqueous Tear Deficiency

Congenital
  Riley-Day syndrome
  Ectodermal dysplasia
  Absent lacrimal gland
Acquired Age-Related Lacrimal Gland Atrophy
  Trauma to Lacrimal Gland
    Injury
    Removal of lacrimal gland
    Radiation
  Inflammation of Lacrimal Gland
    Sjögren syndrome (1° or 2°)
    Mumps
    Trachoma
  Infiltrations of the Lacrimal Gland
    Sarcoid
    Lymphoma
    Amyloid
  Drug Effects
    Antihistamines
    Antimuscarinics
    General anesthetics
    Beta blockers
  Neuroparalytic hyposecretion
    Brainstem lesions
  Postsurgical
    Blepharoplasty

Mucin Deficiency

Vitamin A Deficiency
Goblet Cell Destruction
  Chemical burn
  Cicatricial pemphigoid
  Erythema multiforme
  Trachoma
Drug-Induced Pseudopemphigoid

Lipid Abnormalities

Absent meibomian glands
Destruction of meibomian glands
Meibomian gland dysfunction

Lid Surfacing Abnormalities

Lid malpositions
Exposure keratitis
Entropion
Ectropion
Symblepharon
Lagophthalmos
Keratinized lid margins

Corneal Epitheliopathies

Corneal scars
Corneal ulcer, erosions, dellen
Corneal elevations
Neurotrophic changes

and burning, to a severe, debilitating surface pain. The symptoms typically get worse throughout the day as evaporation from the tear film increases.

Clinical signs of aqueous deficiency include a scanty tear film meniscus over the inferior lid margin, increased debris in the tear film, and an increase in mucous strands in the inferior fornix (Table 49–5). The more severe forms may show a *filamentary keratitis* consisting of dry sheets of desquamated epithelial cells mixed with desiccated mucin. Shearing action on these filaments can cause a great deal of surface pain. Diminished antibacterial components in the tear film increase the risk of surface infection.

Keratoconjunctivitis sicca is usually bilateral and symmetric, although occasionally it is asymmetric. Keratoconjunctivitis sicca most commonly develops in the absence of other systemic disease. Women in the menopausal and postmenopausal age group are the most common victims, although no well-controlled studies have documented a hormonal association. A host of autoimmune diseases can be associated with keratoconjunctivitis sicca. Approximately 10 to 20% of patients with rheumatoid arthritis have keratoconjunctivitis sicca. The histologic changes in keratoconjunctivitis sicca are those of generalized atrophy of the acinar and interstitial tissue of the lacrimal glands.

Sjögren syndrome is a distinct subset of patients with severe aqueous deficiency. It is a chronic autoimmune disorder with multisystem abnormalities including dry eyes (keratoconjunctivitis sicca), dry mouth, and xerostomia (1, 12, 20). It may occur in isolation (primary Sjögren's syndrome) or in association with other autoimmune diseases (secondary Sjögren's syndrome). Clinical studies suggest that there are definite genetic, immunopatho-

TABLE 49–5
Clinical Signs of Tear Dysfunction

        Conjunctival hyperemia
        Conjunctival redundancy
        Decreased tear break up time
        Debris in tear film
        Tear film meniscus decreased
        Rose bengal staining
        Fluorescein staining
        Corneal surface reflexes irregular
        Punctate epithelial keratitis
        Filaments or mucous plaques
        Poor or incomplete blinking
        Corneal thinning/perforation

logic, serologic, and clinical differences between primary and secondary Sjögren's syndrome. The autoimmune diseases associated with keratoconjunctivitis sicca and xerostomia include rheumatoid arthritis, systemic lupus erythematosus, progressive systemic sclerosis, Hashimoto's thyroiditis, polymyositis, polyarteritis nodosa, and Waldenstrom's macroglobulinemia. Patients with primary or secondary Sjögren's have a higher risk of developing lymphoma or lymphoproliferative disease, possibly related to a reduction in natural killer cell activity. Females are more frequently affected by primary Sjögren's syndrome in a ratio of 9 to 1. Onset of disease is between the ages of 40 and 60.

Developments in immunology, molecular biology, and virology have influenced our understanding of Sjögren's syndrome. The disease is characterized by mononuclear infiltration of the lacrimal and salivary glands, leading to destruction of the ductal and acinar structures, resulting in deficiency of tears in saliva. The predominant lymphocytic infiltration consists of helper T cells. A genetic inborn abnormality of the lymphocytes may allow them to home to exocrine glands. Alternatively, the Epstein-Barr virus may play a role in the pathogenesis of Sjögren's syndrome. Pflugfelder et al have reported the detection of Epstein-Barr virus genomic sequences in peripheral blood mononuclear cells, lacrimal glands, and tears of the Sjögren's patients, although the significance remains unknown (19).

Mucin Deficiency

Since mucin is produced predominately by the goblet cells of the conjunctiva and possibly a small amount by the main lacrimal gland, those diseases which damage the conjunctiva are candidates to cause a mucin deficiency. These mucin deficient conditions affect the stability of the tear film, leading to drying and nonwettability of the ocular surface and ultimately to keratinization (17). These diseases include vitamin A deficiency, ocular pemphigoid, drug-induced pemphigoid, erythema multiforme (Stevens-Johnson syndrome), trachoma, chemical burns, and irradiation. Vitamin A deficiency selectively affects conjunctival goblet cells. Vitamin A also plays a part in controlling the differentiation of epithelial cells; vitamin A deprivation favors the production of keratinized epithelial cells, whereas the presence of vitamin A shifts the differentiation to mucin-producing cells. Treatment with vitamin A can reverse these conjunctival changes. The other conditions enumerated destroy the conjunctiva with inflammation in a nondiscriminatory way. The hallmark of a mucin-deficient dry eye is the unstable tear film manifested with a rapid tear film breakup.

Lipid Abnormalities

True lipid deficiencies are rare, as in congenital anhidrotic ectodermal dysplasia and in extensive injuries to the lid margin. More frequently, there are qualitative changes in lipid secretion associated with meibomian gland dysfunction. Meibomian gland products are important in stabilizing the tear film. Abnormalities of meibomian gland secretion cause a change in lipid viscosity, a change in the melting point, and an obstruction of the meibomian orifices. Excessive oil in the tear film can cause foamy tears. Bacteria can invade meibomian glands and secrete lipases that hydrolyze lipids to produce various types of fatty acids which can rupture the tear film and are toxic to the corneal epithelium. Obstruction of the meibomian gland from thick secretions may result in decreased oils, with an increase in tear film osmolality with accelerated evaporation from the surface. Obstruction of the meibomian glands has been correlated with morphologic changes in the glandular structure, showing dropout of glands and involution and atresia of ductules. Systemic isoretinoin (Accutane) can cause similar temporary involutional changes (14).

Lid Surface Abnormalities

The blink function of the lid serves to resurface the eye with tears. Fresh mucin is distributed, debris is washed away, and a new surface is created. When the normal lid movement is impeded, the cornea develops an area on nonwetting and subsequent desiccation. A dry area may dehydrate to the extent that a shallow crater, called a dellen, may appear. The epithelium may remain intact and most dellen will disappear with patching or with frequent use of artificial tears. Secondary keratinization may occur with even poorer wettability.

Any malposition of the lid or restriction in lid movement can cause these lid surfacing abnormalities. The normal Bell's phenomena (upward rotation of the globe when the eye is closed) is a normal protective mechanism, but is absent in approximately 5% of individuals.

Epitheliopathy

The intact tear film is dependent on a smooth uninterrupted epithelial surface. Any abnormality of the surface can affect the stability of the overlying tear film. Corneal surface irregularities can occur with corneal scars, elevations, erosions, and corneal dystrophies. Corneal anesthesia, as in fifth nerve damage, and after herpes zoster ophthalmicus, can lead to neurotrophic changes affecting epithelial turnover and production of a smooth corneal surface.

■ TEAR DYSFUNCTION SYNDROMES

Manifestations of Tear Dysfunction

Mild cases of tear dysfunction syndrome cause a foreign body sensation, itching, burning, and moderate conjunctival injection. Symptoms are worse in the afternoon and exacerbated by wind, air conditioning, heating, smoke, or prolonged reading. In severe keratitis, there may be blurred vision, photophobia, or pain. Patients may be unable to produce tears during crying. Some patients state that their eyes are dry but may have paradoxical watering from reflex tear production and excess mucous precipitation.

The signs of tear dysfunction syndrome include an absent or scanty tear meniscus, increase of debris in the precorneal tear film, and conjunctival injection (Table 49–5). The palpebral conjunctiva may be edematous, hyperemic, and thrown into folds; in addition, a variable fine, medium, or coarse epithelial keratitis occurs. Epithelial or mucoid filaments are often formed in the interpalpebral area. In severe cases, recurrent *staphylococcal blepharoconjunctivitis* may occur. Use of the slit lamp with the broad beam, as well as the slit beam is required to detect most of these clinical findings.

Clinical and Laboratory Diagnostic Tests

There is no one reliable objective test to establish the diagnosis of tear dysfunction syndrome. The clinical picture, with the addition of either diagnostic or laboratory tests, suggests the diagnosis. The best clinical tests are the rose bengal dye test, the measurement of the tear breakup time, and the Schirmer test.

Rose bengal is a water soluble vital stain, specific for altered conjunctival and corneal epithelium and mucous filaments. Unlike fluorescein, it does not stain the precorneal tear film. A 1% solution of rose bengal dye can be placed on an applicator stick and touched to the bulbar conjunctiva. Alternatively, rose bengal strips can be moistened with irrigating solution and touched against the bulbar conjunctiva. VanBijsterveld developed a scoring system for staining shown in three zones: nasal bulbar conjunctiva, cornea, and temporal bulbar conjunctiva. This test has been used in studies and for monitoring patients (22). The pattern of staining can also be used to differentiate keratoconjunctivitis sicca, meibomian gland dysfunction, nocturnal lagophthalmos, and superior limbic keratoconjunctivitis (6).

The tear breakup time is defined as the interval between a complete blink and the development of the first randomly distributed dry spot on the tear film. A drop of fluorescein instilled in the eye allows the tear film to be observed using the cobalt blue light of the slit lamp.

The normal breakup time is greater than 10 seconds. Less than 10 seconds suggests an unstable tear film and is most consistently found in mucin deficient states.

Schirmer's test is a measure of tear secretion during a specified time (11). The test is done with a standardized strip of filter paper that is rested over the lower lid and extended onto the forniceal conjunctiva. The test can be done without topical anesthesia (reflex secretion) or with topical anesthesia (basic secretion). The test is usually measured after 5 minutes. The patient can have the eyes either closed or open. Less than 8mm of wetting indicates probable hyposecretion. The test has poor specificity and sensitivity, but nonetheless is widely practiced (also see Chapter 24, The Lacrimal System for Schirmer tests).

There are a number of laboratory tests used for diagnosing tear dysfunction states but they are not readily available in the clinical setting. These tests include tear osmolality, tear lysozyme measurement, lactoferrin content, fluorescein dilution tests, tear mucin measurement, and impression cytology. Tear osmolality is significantly increased in patients with keratoconjunctivitis sicca and usually measures above 310 milliosmols/liter (5,7,8). A micropipette is used to collect a small sample of tears minimizing reflex secretion. The expense of the instrumentation limits the usefulness of this test. The tear lysozyme is decreased in a number of dry eye disorders. There are several ways to measure tear lysozyme with the agar diffusion method being the most popular. A uniform suspension of Micrococcus lysodeikticus, an organism whose cell wall is destroyed by lysozyme, is placed on an agarose gel slab. A tear sample is placed in a small hole cut into the gel and then incubated at room temperature or 37° centigrade. The zone of clearing around the well corresponds to the concentration of lysozyme in the sample. Radial immunodiffusion is an alternative test.

Tear lactoferrin can be measured with radial immunodiffusion techniques with a commercially available plate, the lactoplate. The lactoplate contains antibodies to human lactoferrin; a 4mm filter paper disc with tear lactoferrin results in an antigen antibody precipitation ring within the agarose gel.

Fluorescein dilution tests are done in different ways, employing similar basic fundamentals. A small, nonirritating fluorescein drop of known volume is placed on the eye and mixed with tears. Subsequent levels of fluorescence are measured with a fluorophotometer, or visual inspection is used to calculate the tear volume.

Tear mucin measurement can be approximated from tear hexosamine. Hexosamine levels are decreased in mucin deficient disorders and normal in keratoconjunctivitis sicca.

Impression cytology is a noninvasive diagnostic test with cellulose acetate filter disks pressed onto the conjunctival surface and then removed (16). The disks pull off loosely attached conjunctival surface cells. The specimen is fixed, stained, and examined for morphologic abnormalities such as determination of goblet cell density, squamous metaplasia, and keratinization. This test is limited by the experience of the microscopic interpretation.

Treatment of Tear Dysfunction Syndromes

There are a number of management options which should be tailored to the individual patient depending on the severity of the disease. Supplementation of tears is the most common form of therapy with either drops, ointments, or inserts. A proliferation of tear substitutes are commercially available over the counter. There are newer products with adsorptive polymers to help increase contact time and newer products based on lower osmolality. Choosing an artificial tear is arbitrary at present with a trial approach generally recommended. Most artificial tears are combinations of methylcellulose, hydroxyethyl cellulose, polyvinyl alcohol, polyvinylpyrrolidone, dextran, or hydroxypropyl methylcellulose. Most commercially available tears contain preservatives which can damage the conjunctiva and cornea and also cause hypersensitivity. Artificial tears without preservative are now available but costly, since they are made for single use (Refresh, Celluvisc, Tears Naturale-Free, Bion). Bland ophthalmic ointments are helpful at night, although difficult to use during the day because of visual blurring (Hypotears, Refresh, Lacri-Lube). Sustained-release inserts and gels may help a selected subset of patients with moderate to severe keratoconjunctivitis sicca. They are expensive, tend to extrude, and are more difficult for some patients to handle. Other attempts at producing artificial tears include solutions made from diluted Healon, autologous serum, and vitamin A ointment. There are no good (reliable?) controlled studies showing improved effect of these latter techniques.

Patients should receive instructions on techniques to preserve existing tears. Glasses should be worn at all times to retard evaporation. Swimmers' goggles, moist chamber spectacles, lid taping, bandage contact lenses, and punctal occlusion are other alternatives to make a moist chamber around the eye. Bandage soft contact lenses are helpful in selective circumstances, but carry significant risk. They may be especially helpful in filamentary keratitis, mucin deficient dry eyes, and exposure keratitis. Concomitant use of artificial tears is recommended and vigilance for complications of contact lenses.

Punctal occlusion can be accomplished by solid gelatin rods, cyanoacrylate adhesives, silicone plugs, cautery, or laser (21). There is a trend to move to these surgical techniques earlier in treatment. The stimulation of the lacrimal gland to produce tears has been tried in Europe with Bromhexine but is rarely used in the United States, because of diminishing effectiveness with prolonged use.

In patients with mucous plaques or filaments, the use of 10 to 20% acetylcysteine 4 to 5 times a day can decrease the viscosity of the surface mucin. Parotid duct implantation has been largely abandoned. A lateral tarsorrhaphy can help in maintaining structural integrity and decreasing the exposed ocular surface, especially in patients with lagophthalmos, persistent epithelial defects, and noninfectious ulcers. In the early stages of Sjögren's syndrome, and specifically in young patients, systemic steroids may modulate the immunologic reaction before the irreversible destruction of glandular tissue and before the onset of permanent scarring and fibrosis. Otherwise, systemic immunosuppressive agents have not been effective in alleviating tear dysfunction. Therapy should be directed at the other autoimmune components of secondary Sjögren's syndrome as appropriate.

■ REFERENCES

1. Bloch K, Buchanan W, Wohl M, et al: Sjogren's syndrome. A clinical, pathological and serological study of 62 cases. Medicine 1965:44:187.
2. Crandall, DC, Leopold, IH: The influence of systemic drugs on tear constituents. Ophthalmology, 1979: 86:115.
3. Doane, MB: Blinking and the mechanics of the lacrimal drainage system. Ophthalmology, 1981: 88:844.
4. Farris, RL: Abnormalities of the tears and treatment of dry eyes. In: Kaufman, HE, Barron, BA, McDonald MB, Waltman, SR: The cornea. New York: Churchill Livingstone, 1988: 139–159.
5. Farris RL, Stuchell RN, Mandell ID: Tear osmolarity variation in the dry eye. Trans Am Ophthalmol Soc, 1986: 84:250.
6. Gilbard, JP: Dry eye disorders. In: Albert, DM, Jakobiec FA (eds): Principles and practice of ophthalmology. Philadelphia: W. B. Saunders, 1994: 257–276.
7. Gilbard JP, Farris RL: Tear osmolarity and ocular surface disease in keratoconjunctivitis sicca. Arch Ophthalmol 1979: 97:1642.
8. Gilbard JP, Rossi SR, Gray KL, et al: Tear film osmolarity and ocular surface disease in two rabbit models for keratoconjunctivitis sicca. Invest Ophthalmol Vis Sci 1988: 29:374.

9. Holly, FJ, Lemp, MA: Tear physiology and dry eyes. Surv Ophthalmol 1977: 22:69.

10. Janssen, PT, van Bijsterveld, OP: Origin and biosynthesis of human tear proteins. Invest Ophthalmol Vis Sci, 1983: 24:623.

11. Jordan A, Baum J: Basic tear flow. Does it exist: Ophthalmology, 1980: 87:920.

12. Kassan SS, Gardy M: Sjögren's syndrome: An update and overview. Am J Med 1978: 64:1037.

13. Lamberts, DW: Physiology of the tear film. In: Smolin G, Thoft RA (eds): The Cornea. Third edition. Boston: Little, Brown and Company, 1994: 439–455.

14. Lemp, MA, Chacko, B: Diagnoses and treatment of tear deficiencies. In: Clinical Ophthalmology. Tasman, W, Jaeger, EA (eds): Philadelphia: JB Lippincott Co., 1994: Volume 4, Chapter 14.

15. Mishima S: Some physiological aspects of the precorneal tear film. Arch Ophthalmol, 1965: 73:233.

16. Nelson JD, Havener VR, Cameron JD: Cellulose acetate impressions of the ocular surface. Dry eye states. Arch Ophthalmol 1983: 101:1869.

17. Nichols, BA, Chiappino, ML, Dawson, CR: Demonstration of the mucous layer of the tear film by electron microscopy. Invest Ophthalmol Vis Sci, 1985: 26:464.

18. Ostler, HB: Diseases of the external eye and adnexa. Baltimore: Williams and Wilkins, 1993: 361–364.

19. Pflugfelder, SC, Crouse, C, Pereira, I, Atherton, S: Amplification of Epstein-Barr genome sequences in blood cells, lacrimal glands, and tears from primary Sjögren's syndrome patients. Ophthalmology 1990: 97:976–984.

20. Sjögren H, Bloch KJ: Keratoconjunctivitis sicca and the Sjögren syndrome. Surv Ophthalmol 1971: 16:145.

21. Tuberville AW, Frederick WR, Wood TO: Punctal occlusion in tear deficiency syndromes. Ophthalmology 1982: 89:1170.

22. Van Bijsterveld, OP: Diagnostic tests in the sicca syndrome. Arch Ophthalmol 1985: 82:10.

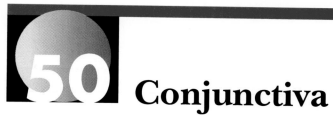

50 Conjunctiva

Thomas J. Liesegang

■ BASIC CONJUNCTIVAL REACTIONS

The conjunctiva is a mucous membrane that covers the inner surface of the upper and lower lids and extends to the limbus on the surface of the globe. Major functions of the conjunctiva are to provide the tear film mucous layer and to provide immune tissue and antimicrobial agents to protect the ocular surface. All ducts associated with the aqueous, lipid, and mucin components of the tear film enter the conjunctival epithelium. The surface epithelium is a unique nonkeratinized squamous type with goblet cells intercalated within. A highly vascularized substantia propria provides connective tissue support, sensory innervation, and immune capabilities. Three regions of the conjunctiva are recognized: palpebral conjunctiva, bulbar conjunctiva, and forniceal conjunctiva.

The conjunctiva has limited ways of responding to disease processes. Many of these responses are nonspecific, but others can be characteristic with a limited differential diagnosis. The following is a description of these responses (63).

A local or diffuse vascular dilatation is invariably present in most conjunctival inflammatory processes. This conjunctival hyperemia must be distinguished from scleritis, episcleritis, and ciliary injection. The blood vessels of the palpebral conjunctiva derive from the superior and inferior tarsal arcades. Three layers of vascular network can be discerned on the surface of the eye; the bulbar conjunctival plexus of subepithelial vessels, the capillary meshwork of Tenon's capsule, and the deep episcleral network composed of large and small vessels. The bulbar conjunctival vessels are branches of the ophthalmic artery and the episcleral network comes from the ciliary artery. There are some anastomoses between these vessels, but careful direct observation with white or green light of the slit lamp can distinguish the predominant cause of the hyperemia on the basis of the depth, distribution, pattern, moveability, and color of the vascular dilatation.

Conjunctival edema (chemosis) occurs from increased capillary permeability, vascular endothelial damage, vasomotor instability, blockage or congestion of orbital lymphatics, obstruction of venous drainage, reduced osmotic pressure (nephrotic syndrome), or myxedema. It is characterized by a translucent swelling of the bulbar conjunctiva, folds or rugae of the cul-de-sac, and tarsal papillae. The swelling may protrude through the interpalpebral fissure.

Conjunctival discharge may be watery, mucoid, mucopurulent, or purulent. It is a composite of tears, mucin, fibrin, epithelial debris, inflammatory cells, and serum products. A serous (watery) discharge occurs in the early stages of any conjunctival infection or inflammation and continues during toxic or viral infections. A mucoid discharge of fibrin and mucin is characteristic of persistent allergic conjunctival inflammation. Purulent discharge typifies bacterial infections.

Conjunctival papillae are dotlike telangiectatic vascular changes most easily visible in the tarsal conjunctiva. With progression, these dilated vessels sprout capillaries which become surrounded by edema and a mixed inflammatory cell infiltrate, producing raised elevations under the conjunctival epithelium (Figure 50–1). Papillae develop only in areas where the conjunctiva is firmly attached to the underlying tissue (e.g., tarsus, semilunar fold, limbus). A mild papillary reaction produces a smooth, velvety appearance. With pro-

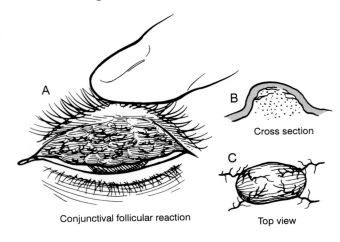

Conjunctival follicular reaction

B — Cross section

C — Top view

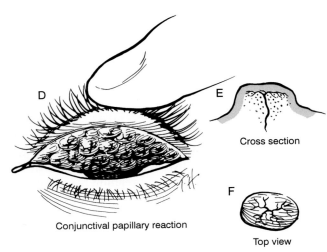

Conjunctival papillary reaction

E — Cross section

F — Top view

Figure 50–1.
Papillary and follicular response. Illustration of the morphologic and cellular composition of a conjunctival papillary and follicular response. Papillae tend to have a central vascular core with chronic inflammatory cells. Follicles are avascular with blood vessels at the base. Follicles are collections of lymphocytes.

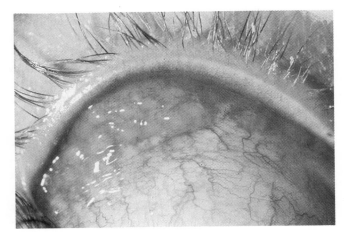

Figure 50–2.
Follicular conjunctivitis. A conjunctival follicular response in a patient with chlamydial conjunctivitis. The follicles are small, round, slightly elevated avascular structures with clusters of lymphocytes.

TABLE 50–1
Causes of a Follicular Conjunctivitis

Acute Follicular Response
Adenovirus
Pharyngoconjunctival fever (Adeno type 3, 4, 7)
Epidemic keratoconjunctivitis (Adeno type 8, 19)
Herpes simplex virus conjunctivitis
Chlamydial conjunctivitis
Inclusion conjunctivitis
Acute trachoma
Acute hemorrhagic conjunctivitis (picornavirus)
Rubella conjunctivitis
Newcastle virus conjunctivitis

Chronic Follicular Response
Chlamydia
Inclusion conjunctivitis
Trachoma
Chronic blepharitis
Moraxella
Molluscum contagiosum
Drug-induced toxic reaction
Glaucoma medications
Antiviral medications
Antibiotic medications
Preservatives
Eye cosmetics
Axenfeld follicles of childhood (folliculosis)
Rosacea conjunctivitis

longed, recurrent, or severe conjunctival inflammation, the anchoring fibers weaken, leading to confluent papillae hypertrophy. There are many causes of acute and long-term conjunctival inflammations which produce a papillary response. In giant papillae, several cores of ves-

TABLE 50–2
Causes of Inflammatory Conjunctival Membranes

True Membranes (Associated With Ulceration and Hemorrhage)
Corynebacterium diphtheriae
Neisseria gonorrhoeae
Beta hemolytic streptococcus
Erythema multiforme major

Pseudomembranes (Not Associated With Hemorrhage)
Viral
Adenovirus (especially epidemic keratoconjunctivitis)
Herpes virus
Bacterial
Staphylococcus, pneumococcus
Pseudomonas aeruginosa
Chemical burns
Ocular pemphigoid
Ligneous conjunctivitis

TABLE 50–3
Causes of Cicatrizing Conjunctivitis

Ocular cicatricial pemphigoid
Atopic keratoconjunctivitis
Erythema multiforme major (Stevens-Johnson Syndrome)
Chemical burns
Diphtheria conjunctivitis
Rosacea keratoconjunctivitis
Epidemic keratoconjunctivitis
Carcinoma (squamous cell, sebaceous cell)
Trachoma
Sarcoidosis
Traumatic scars

sels can be seen to penetrate the papillae at different areas and then branch. Giant papillae develop in vernal, atopic, and giant papillary conjunctivitis.

Conjunctival follicles are small, round, slightly elevated avascular structures which are clusters of lymphocytes with an active germinal center, surrounded by plasma cells and some mast cells. Vessels are not visible within the follicle. Follicles may develop at the edge of the tarsus and in the cul-de-sac as a nonspecific response to inflammation. Tarsal and bulbar follicles are more specific and suggestive of viral, chlamydial, or toxic conjunctivitis (Figures 50–1 and 50–2); (Table 50–1). A benign follicular reaction *(folliculosis)* represents a propensity of young patients to develop follicles from antigenic stimulation. These are characterized by insidious onset and absence of symptoms or other signs.

A *membranous conjunctival* reaction is composed of fibrin, fibrinous byproducts, leukocytes, and necrotic material deposited within and on the surface of the conjunctiva from inflamed, leaking blood vessels. Stripping of the membrane from the conjunctiva exposes a raw bleeding surface and granulation tissue. Healing takes place with considerable subepithelial scarring. Diphtheritic conjunctivitis is the prototypic cause. A pseudomembranous conjunctivitis is composed of the same transudate products, but when the pseudomembrane is stripped away, the underlying conjunctival surface is relatively intact and only minimal bleeding occurs. The pseudomembrane is characteristic of viral epidemic keratoconjunctivitis. Scars, symblepharon, entropion, and trichiasis are potential sequelae to membranous or pseudomembranous conjunctivitis. (Tables 50–2 and 50–3).

Conjunctival ulcerations are frequently overlooked because of other intense conjunctival responses. These ulcers can be caused by trauma or any severe conjunctival inflammatory reaction which causes the normal cell junctions to lose their integrity. They occur in herpes simplex viral infection, factitious injuries, primary syphilis, pemphigoid, toxic epidermal necrolysis, erythema multiforme major, membranous conjunctivitis, pseudomembranous conjunctivitis, and granulomatous conjunctivitis. A symblepharon may result.

Chronic granulomas appear as nodules of variable size (up to 6 mm). They are commonly elevated, highly vascularized, and appear as sessile or polypoid masses. They are often associated with necrosis. Conjunctival granulomas can develop in response to foreign bodies, sarcoid, tuberculosis, or as Parinaud's oculoglandular syndrome in which there is a grossly visible preauricular lymph node.

Conjunctival cytology with Giemsa stain may be helpful in determining the etiology of the conjunctivitis. Table 50–4 lists the differential diagnosis depending on the predominant cytologic pattern.

TABLE 50–4
Cytology of Conjunctival Scrapings

Predominant polymorphonuclear response
  Bacterial conjunctivitis
  Severe viral or chlamydial conjunctivitis
  Allergic conjunctivitis
  Chemical or irritative conjunctivitis
  Any severe or membranous conjunctivitis
  Erythema multiforme major
  Giant papillary conjunctivitis
Predominant lymphocytic and mononuclear response
  Adenoviral conjunctivitis
  Herpes simplex conjunctivitis
  Chronic drug induced
  Molluscum contagiosum conjunctivitis
Predominant eosinophilic response
  Vernal conjunctivitis
  Atopic conjunctivitis
  Hay fever conjunctivitis
  Drug allergy
Mixed polymorphonuclear and mononuclear response
  Chlamydia conjunctivitis
  Adenoviral conjunctivitis
  Any severe acute or chronic conjunctivitis
Large macrophages, plasma cells
  Chlamydia conjunctivitis
Keratinized epithelial cells
  Tear dysfunction states
  Pemphigoid
  Superior limbic keratoconjunctivitis
  Vitamin A deficiency
  Radiation conjunctivitis
  Chemical burns
  Erythema multiforme major
  Trachoma
  After any severe conjunctivitis
Multinucleated epithelial cells
  Herpes simplex conjunctivitis
  Varicella zoster conjunctivitis
  Radiation
Neoplastic cells
  Cornea dysplasia
  Squamous cell carcinoma
  Sebaceous cell carcinoma
  Conjunctival melanoma

■ CONJUNCTIVAL INFECTIONS

Bacterial

Although the outer eye is constantly exposed to microorganisms, infection of the conjunctiva is relatively rare. There are multiple host defense mechanisms which work in concert to prevent infection. Bacterial conjunctivitis is an inflammatory reaction of the conjunctiva after exposure to certain pathogenic bacteria. It is usually self-limited in its course. The frequency and cause are influenced by age, climate, and the social and hygienic conditions. The severity of the infection depends on the inoculum size, pathogenicity and virulence of the organism, as well as the mechanical, humoral, and cellular host defense mechanisms.

Bacterial conjunctivitis is frequently divided into acute, hyperacute, and chronic forms based on the clinical course (25, 49, 80). This classification is helpful in assessing the potential causes and starting therapy. The common potential responsible organisms are listed in Table 50–5.

The patient with acute bacterial conjunctivitis usually develops watering and irritation of the eyes followed by mucopurulent discharge and sticking of the lids together in the morning. One eye is usually involved, followed quickly by involvement of the second eye. On examination, the conjunctiva is diffusely injected, a mucopurulent exudate is present in the inferior fornix, and there is usually no preauricular lymph node. The most common bacteria isolated include *Staphylococcus aureus*, *Haemophilus aegyptius*, *Haemophilus influenze* and *Streptococcus pneumoniae*. There are some distinguishing features about the clinical picture of these infections which might suggest the specific organism. Petechial conjunctival hemorrhages are common with *S. pneumoniae* and Haemophilus infections. Marginal corneal infiltrates are more common with Haemophilus. *S. pneumoniae* is more common in children and in cooler climates. Haemophilus is more common in young children, especially in warmer climates, and may be associated with a bluish, discolored preseptal cellulitis or systemic symptoms. *Haemophilus cellulitis* needs to be recognized because of potential septicemia, meningitis, septic arthritis, and endogenous endophthalmitis. *Streptococcus pyogenes* and *Corynebacterium diphtheriae* can produce a conjunctivitis with membrane formation.

The responsible organism can usually be identified on the Gram stain or with culture. These laboratory studies are not usually done except in situations of severe or prolonged infection or in situations of localized and systemic infection. The treatment of bacterial conjunctivitis consists of topical antibiotic drops or ointments based on the clinical appearance and likely responsible organisms. Cultures can guide therapy in selected circumstances. Sulfacetamide, trimethoprim sulfate, polymyxin B sulfate, erythromycin, and chloramphenicol are commonly used.

Hyperacute bacterial conjunctivitis is typically caused by *Neisseria gonorrhea* or *Neisseria meningitides* acquired by autoinoculation from infected genitalia

TABLE 50–5
Causes of Bacterial Conjunctivitis

Acute
Staphylococcus aureus
Haemophilus aegyptius
Haemophilus influenzae
Streptococcus pneumoniae
Streptococcus pyogenes
Pseudomonas aeruginosa
Corynebacteria diphtheriae

Hyperacute
Neisseria gonorrhoeae
Neisseria meningitides
Corynebacteria diphtheriae
Haemophilus influenzae
Beta streptococcus

Chronic
Staphylococcus aureus
Moraxella lacunata
Proteus
Klebsiella
Serratia
Beta streptococcus

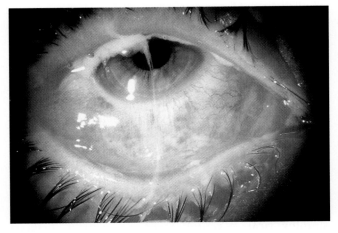

Figure 50–3.
Hyperacute bacterial conjunctivitis. Hyperacute bacterial conjunctivitis with marked conjunctival hyperemia, purulent discharge, and chemosis of the conjunctiva in a sexually active male. Gram stain and culture confirmed *Neisseria gonorrhea*.

(Figure 50–3). It is most commonly seen in adolescents and young adults, especially in the warmer months. There is a unilateral or bilateral conjunctival hyperemia which rapidly progresses to copious purulent discharge, swelling of the lids, chemosis of the conjunctiva, and frequently conjunctival membrane formation. There may be a tender preauricular lymph node. Corneal involvement may occur with punctate epithelial keratitis or peripheral stromal infiltration and ulceration. This corneal ulceration can rapidly progress to corneal perforation as a result of bacterial toxins or the production of conjunctival inflammatory products. The findings in *Neisseria gonorrhoeae* conjunctivitis are usually more prominent than in *Neisseria meningitides* conjunctivitis. Rarely other organisms such as *S. aureus*, Streptococcus, *Haemophilus influenza* or Pseudomonas can cause an explosive conjunctivitis.

Gram stain and culture are recommended in all cases of hyperacute conjunctivitis because of the need to confirm the specific initiating bacteria. The Gram stain will show exuberant polymorphonuclear cells. The treatment is based on the specific causative pathogen. Gonococcal conjunctivitis should be treated with both topical and full doses of systemic antibiotics. Parenteral therapy includes ceftriaxone or penicillin. Therapy should be accompanied by frequent saline conjunctival irrigation. Topical therapy includes bacitracin, gentamycin, or tetracycline ointment. Patients and their companions should be further evaluated for other venereal disease. Severe streptococcal conjunctivitis should be treated with systemic penicillin and topical erythromycin. If *C. diphtheria* is identified, systemic penicillin or erythromycin should be used along with diphtheria antitoxin. Conjunctival scarring can result from any severe bacterial conjunctivitis.

In chronic bacterial conjunctivitis, the findings are variable and usually related to a source of organisms in the ocular adnexal tissues. *S. aureus* and *Moraxella lacunata* are frequently implicated in association with Staphylococcal blepharitis or angular blepharitis, respectively. Other organisms such as Proteus, Klebsiella, and Serratia are inhabitants of the respiratory or GI tract and can be carried to the conjunctival sac in patients with chronic disease. The production of toxins is common with *S. aureus* and Moraxella and the conjunctival reaction may be a combination of responses to bacteria and to toxin. Corneal findings are common in chronic bacterial conjunctivitis especially involving the inferior cornea in the form on punctate epithelial erosions, marginal corneal ulcerations, or phlyctenular keratitis.

Patients with chronic conjunctivitis need a careful assessment of the ocular adnexa (lids, nasolacrimal drainage), as well as the respiratory, gastrointestinal and genitourinary system. There should be a review of hygienic practices (e.g., contact lens, cosmetic products,

the use of topical eye drops) to evaluate all potential sources of bacteria.

Therapy of chronic bacterial conjunctivitis is based on finding a causative organism and finding the route of entry. Cultures may help suggest a potential source. Altering the route of infection and good ocular hygiene are essential. Topical broad-spectrum antibiotics such as bacitracin, erythromycin and rarely systemic antibiotics (tetracycline, doxycycline) may be indicated based on the specific organism. Prolonged use of any antibiotic is discouraged.

Viral

Various viruses are a common cause of conjunctivitis in patients of all ages (66). (Table 50–6). The adenovirus is by far the most common cause, with various serotypes responsible. Less common causes include picornaviruses, herpes simplex virus, varicella zoster virus, vaccinia virus, and the virus of molluscum contagiosum. Rare conjunctivitis is seen during systemic infection with influenza virus, Epstein-Barr virus (infectious mononucleosis), and paramyxovirus (mumps, rubeola). Viral conjunctivitis, although usually benign and self-limited, tends to last longer than bacterial conjunctivitis and is more symptomatic. Almost all are associated with an acute follicular conjunctival reaction with a preauricular lymph node.

Adenoviral infections of the conjunctiva cause extreme tearing, redness, and foreign body sensation. This complex is called a catarrhal conjunctivitis. When the cornea is involved, there is intense photophobia. There may a history of exposure to another individual with a red eye and frequently, there are symptoms of an upper respiratory infection. The infection may be unilateral or bilateral. On examination there is lid edema, ptosis, conjunctival hyperemia and watering, conjunctival follicles, and fine papilla (especially in the lower lid). Occasionally there is pseudomembrane formation and preauricular lymph node involvement. There are particular subtypes of adenovirus which cause two distinct syndromes: pharyngoconjunctival fever and epidemic keratoconjunctivitis. Both these viruses tend to occur in epidemics in the Western world because of decreased levels of natural immunity. There is no animal reservoir.

Pharyngoconjunctival fever is most commonly associated with adenovirus 3 and 7 and usually occurs in children. Patients have symptoms of an upper respiratory infection (pharyngitis and fever), along with bilateral watery conjunctival discharge, hyperemia, chemosis, foreign body sensation, and preauricular lymph nodes. This disease is self-limited over 2 to 3 weeks and is highly contagious.

Epidemic keratoconjunctivitis (EKC) is most commonly associated with adenovirus 8, 19, and 37, and usually occurs in adults between the ages of 20 and 40. The symptoms and signs are usually isolated to the eye with severe lid and conjunctival edema, conjunctival hyperemia,

TABLE 50–6
Viral Infections of the External Eye

DNA Viruses	
Herpes virus	
Herpes Simplex I & II	Blepharitis, conjunctivitis, keratitis
Varicella zoster	Blepharitis, conjunctivitis, keratitis
Epstein-Barr	Keratitis
Adenovirus	Conjunctivitis, keratitis
Papovavirus	
Papilloma	Conjunctival warts
Poxvirus	
Vaccinia	Blepharitis, conjunctivitis, keratitis
Variola	Conjunctivitis, keratitis
Molluscum contagiosum	Blepharitis, follicular conjunctivitis, keratitis
RNA Viruses	
Picornavirus	
Enterovirus	Acute hemorrhagic conjunctivitis
Coxsackie	Acute hemorrhagic conjunctivitis
Paramyxovirus	
Measles	Follicular conjunctivitis, keratitis
Mumps	Follicular conjunctivitis, keratitis
Newcastle	Follicular conjunctivitis, keratitis
Retrovirus	
Human immunodeficiency virus	
Togavirus	
Rubella	Catarrhal or follicular conjunctivitis
Orthomyxovirus	
Influenza	Conjunctivitis

and watery discharge, and a marked follicular and papillary reaction, occasionally associated with petechial conjunctival hemorrhages. There may be swelling of the plica and occasionally, the presence of a pseudomembrane and tender preauricular lymph node. One eye is usually involved and the second eye becomes involved within 7 days (usually with a milder coarse). Occasionally, there are symptoms of a mild upper respiratory infection. This syndrome is associated with characteristic evolving corneal lesions which initially present with small punctate keratitis associated with photophobia. Over several days, these lesions coalesce and they become deeper, subepithelial nummular lesions which can decrease vision if located centrally. The early corneal lesions are associated with virus in the epithelial cells; the later subepithelial infiltrates appear to be hypersensitive reactions at the level of Bowman's membrane (12) (Figures 50–4 and 50–5). Untreated, the subepithelial infiltrates resolve over weeks or months. EKC, as the name implies, is contagious and spread among household members and school children. It is frequently spread by health care givers. Seasonal epidemics have been associated with swimming pools. There may be an incubation period of 1 week and the

individual may be contagious for several weeks after the onset of the conjunctivitis. The virus may be recovered from nonporous surfaces weeks later.

The diagnosis is usually made on the clinical features alone. Other causes of follicular conjunctivitis must be considered (for example HSV, chlamydia). Cytology of the conjunctival scrapings reveal lymphocytes with intranuclear inclusions. A cotton swab of the conjunctiva placed into chlamydial transport media can be used to transport the culture to the lab for viral culture, usually available with results in 2 to 7 days. There are adenoviral enzyme immunoassays with good specificity for adenoviral antigen. Immunofluorescence, immunoperoxidase, electron microscopy, and polymerase chain reaction are alternative detection techniques (29).

The most important aspect of therapy for adenoviral conjunctivitis is to prevent transmission, especially in the health care facility. Careful hand washing before seeing each patient, proper cleansing of instruments that touch a patient's eye, and frequent changing of multiuse ophthalmic drops is vital. Using a single infection examination room, along with educating the staff and patient are essential in each ophthalmologist's of-

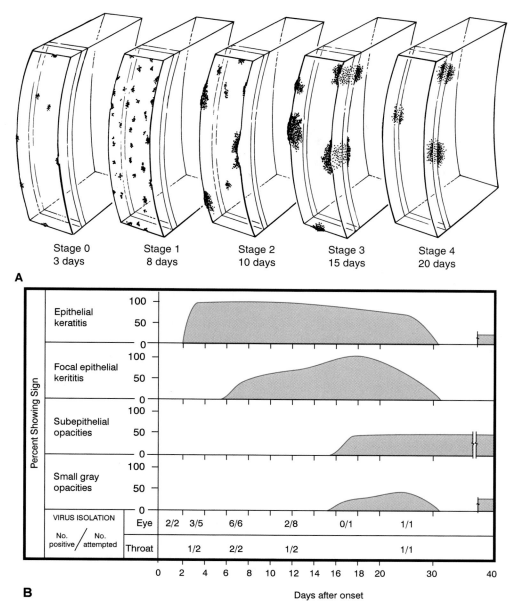

Figure 50–4.
Epidemic keratoconjunctivitis keratitis. The time course and schematic drawings of the different types of keratitis seen with adenovirus Type 8 infection causing epidemic gonorrhea. Modified from Jones DB, Viral and Chlamydia Keratoconjunctivitis. *In* Symposium on medical and surgical diseases of the Cornea. St. Louis. CV Mosby 1980. p. 497-523.

fice, especially in the setting of an epidemic. The individual patient should use contagion and isolation precautions for at least 2 weeks. Currently, there is no effective antiviral therapy, although limited research is promising (29). Compresses, vasoconstriction, and topical nonsteroidal antiinflammatory drugs may reduce some symptoms. Secondary bacterial conjunctivitis is rare. Use of topical corticosteroids is discouraged but occasionally used in situations such as severe pseudomembranes and severe subepithelial infiltrates in the visual axis. The subepithelial infiltrates usually return when the topical corticosteroid is withdrawn and many

believe the steroid simply prolongs the disease process.

Acute hemorrhagic conjunctivitis has been reported in epidemics in various locations throughout the world and in the southern United States in association with two major picornavirus: enterovirus 70 and Coxsackie virus A24. Children and young adults in the lower socioeconomic classes are most susceptible. There is a rapid onset of watery discharge, foreign body sensation, burning, and photophobia within 24 hours of exposure. Ocular signs include bilateral follicular conjunctivitis, lid edema, bulbar hemorrhages, and preauricular lymph nodes. The disease resolves over 1 week with oc-

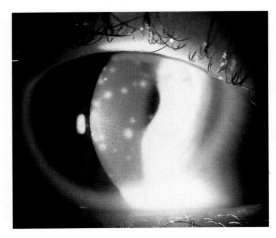

Figure 50–5.
Epidemic keratoconjunctivitis. Persisting subepithelial infiltrates in the cornea of a patient with acute epidemic keratoconjunctivitis 1 month before. These infiltrates are an immune response and will resolve on their own.

casional neurologic symptoms (radiculomyelitis). There is no effective therapy. Contagion and isolation precautions should be used.

Chlamydial

The genus chlamydia comprise a group of eubacteria with the species Chlamydia trachomatis associated with human disease. Chlamydia are only capable of growth within eukaryotic host cells. Strains of C. trachomatis are associated with trachoma, adult inclusion conjunctivitis, neonatal conjunctivitis, urethritis, and cervicitis. The biologic hallmark that separates chlamydia from all other bacteria is its developmental cycle, initiated by attachment and invasion of host cells with elementary bodies, the extracellular and infectious form of the organism. Once the elementary body enters a host cell, it initiates changes in the macromolecular structure of the outer membrane and its chromosome to become the vegetative and noninfective form called the reticulate body. The chlamydia growth cycle produces hundreds of progeny per cell which escape as elementary bodies.

Trachoma is a chronic follicular conjunctivitis invariably caused by C. *trachomatis* serotypes A, B, Ba, or C. It is the leading cause of preventable blindness in the world, although it is sporadic in the United States. Epidemics of bacterial conjunctivitis, often spread by flies, complicate the epidemiology of trachoma in hyperendemic areas. Common bacterial pathogens associated with trachoma include H. aegyptius, S. pneumoniae, and Moraxella. Patients in hot, dry, dusty climates are at greater risk, especially those in a lower socioeconomic class (77).

Clinically, trachoma is a chronic follicular conjunctivitis that leads to conjunctival and corneal scarring

(88). There are four stages of the disease based on the developmental changes in the conjunctival follicles, papillary hypertrophy, and scar formation. Initially, after a 5-day incubation period, the eye becomes red and inflamed. There may be a purulent discharge and a tender preauricular lymph node. Stage 1 follicles appear by 3 weeks, consisting of immature follicles on the upper tarsus, minimal papillary hypertrophy, and faint subepithelial opacities and punctate epithelial keratitis. Stage 2 has well-developed mature follicles on the upper tarsal conjunctiva with punctate keratitis, limbal follicles, and a corneal pannus. In Stage 2A, there is acute inflammation with papillary hypertrophy obliterating the follicles, intense cellular infiltration, pannus, and infiltration extending from the upper limbus. In Stage 3, the follicles have undergone necrosis and scarring with papillary hypertrophy and islands of cellular infiltration between scars. Trichiasis and entropion begin to develop. Stage 4 is a completely cicatrized and scarred smooth conjunctiva with absent follicles and papillary reaction with no inflammatory reaction. There is no punctate keratitis but variable trichiasis, entropion, and corneal scarring. The findings, which help confirm the clinical diagnosis at any time during the disease, consist of a micropannus located superiorly, epithelial keratitis, subepithelial infiltrates, limbal follicles, and limbal depressions (called Herbert's pits). Herbert's pits are residual scars from prior limbal follicles. When superimposed infection with Haemophilus or other bacteria occur, the keratitis is particularly severe, leading to ulceration with perforation or scarring.

In endemic areas, the diagnosis is made on clinical criteria. Laboratory studies are helpful, especially in the Western world, to help confirm the diagnosis. The histologic section of the tarsus and subepithelial tissue of patients with active trachoma reveals papillary hypertrophy of the epithelium and diffuse infiltration of the subepithelial tissues with lymphocytes and plasma cells. The large number of suppressor/cytotoxic and helper T cells, supports a role for cell-mediated immunity and the local response to Chlamydia trachomatis, ocular infection of the conjunctiva, and corneal epithelial cells. As follicles develop in the conjunctiva or limbus, extensive necrosis occurs leading to scar formation in the conjunctiva and small ulcers (Herbert's pits) in the limbus which ultimately fill in. The corneal scarring is a result of corneal complications of disease but also a result of secondary complications such as keratitis sicca, entropion, trichiasis, and repeated corneal erosions.

Adult inclusion conjunctivitis is an oculogenital disease produced by C. *trachomatis* serotypes D, E, F, G, H, I, J, K. Unlike trachoma, it is common in urban and industrialized areas. It is frequently found in patients with other venereal diseases and has been associated with urethritis in men and cervicitis in women. These genital diseases may be relatively asymptomatic. In contrast to the eye-to-eye transmission of trachoma, adult inclusion disease is transmitted from hand to eye or from genitalia to eye. After an incubation period of 2 days to 2 weeks, the symptoms usually begin with a unilateral red irritated eye with a mucopurulent discharge, and the lids matted together upon awakening. The disease later becomes bilateral with a tender preauricular lymph node. There are usually no other constitutional symptoms. The conjunctiva is hyperemic with follicles usually not developing for several weeks and then are relatively large. The follicles are usually on both the upper and lower conjunctiva but more marked in the inferior conjunctival fornix. Follicles may develop in the limbal areas or bulbar conjunctiva. The conjunctival discharge is usually persistently mucopurulent.

Corneal involvement occurs in some patients, usually as a superficial epithelial keratitis. Occasionally, there are large, coarse punctate epithelial lesions distributed randomly over the cornea. In severe cases, macroulcerations, peripheral corneal infiltrates, or corneal edema may develop. A micropannus frequently develops at the superior limbus, but rarely leads to a significant visual problem.

Untreated, adult inclusion conjunctivitis persists for months, usually in the form of a marked follicular reaction, or as subepithelial infiltration, or with a low-grade mucopurulent discharge. There is usually no conjunctival scarring as there is with trachoma. The differential diagnosis is that of an acute or chronic follicular conjunctivitis. Adult chlamydial conjunctivitis is usually delayed in its diagnosis because of the absence of distinct signs in the early course. In distinction to trachoma, the disease may resolve without telltale signs if effectively treated.

Neonatal inclusion conjunctivitis (blennorrhea) is a chlamydial infection of newborns acquired during passage through the infected birth canal of the mother. It is increasing in industrialized countries with an incidence of 2 to 6% of births. The incidence of chlamydial infection of the cervix may be as increased as 11% in sexually active women with a 20% risk of transmission at birth (88). Systemic infection of newborns results in the distinctive chlamydial pneumonia syndrome and a gastrointestinal syndrome (88). Because of the neonates immature immune system, follicles cannot usually develop. Signs of infection occur 5 to 14 days postpartum with unilateral or bilateral papillary conjunctivitis. Occasionally, a mucopurulent discharge or inflammatory membranes may form. The cornea may exhibit a fine or coarse diffuse superficial punctate keratitis with peripheral subepithelial infiltrates and a pannus. The conjunctival disease is self-limited, but may last up to a year (1).

Conjunctival cytology will reveal cytoplasmic inclusions in Giemsa stain along with polymorphonuclear cells and lymphocytes. Chlamydia culture on McCoy cells are more frequently positive in neonates than in adults. Other laboratory tests include microtiter indirect immunofluorescence, fluorescein-conjugated monoclonal antibodies, complement fixation, and polymerase chain reaction-enzyme immunoassay.

Therapy of neonatal chlamydial infection requires systemic antibiotics. Oral erythromycin is administered for 14 days. Maternal screening has decreased the incidence of neonatal inclusion conjunctivitis.

Neonatal Conjunctivitis (Ophthalmia Neonatorum)

Conjunctivitis in the newborn is a distinct entity during the first 28 days of life with multiple different causes (Table 50–7). An infection can be acquired from the birth canal, from hospital workers, or the conjunctivitis may represent a clinical reaction to the Credé prophylaxis with silver nitrate 1% drops. Credé prophylaxis in newborns was introduced years ago to prevent Neisseria gonorrhoeae conjunctivitis (Figure 50–6). It has been replaced in many states with erythromycin or tetracycline ophthalmic ointment because these are effective against both Neisseria and chlamydia. Erythromycin and tetracycline ointment do not usually cause a conjunctival reaction. Povidone-iodine has been recently reported to be highly effective and safe (34A,34B).

Specific Causes

Chemical reaction to silver nitrate (Credé) usually occurs within 24 hours. It is associated with an injection and rarely a purulent reaction with polymorphonuclear cells. No specific therapy is required.

Neonatal chlamydial infection has been discussed in the prior section.

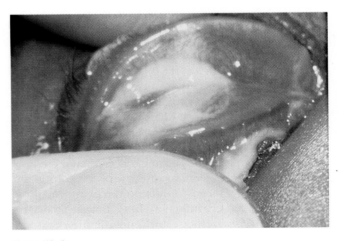

Figure 50–6.
Neonatal conjunctivitis. An acute purulent conjunctivitis within the first few days of life in this newborn. Giemsa stain and culture confirmed chlamydia,

TABLE 50–7
Diagnosis and Treatment of Neonatal Conjunctivitis

Agent	Day of Onset	Discharge	Corneal Involvement	Lab Findings	Therapy
1. Silver nitrate irritation	1 d	Hyperemia Rare purulent	Rare keratitis or scarring	PMN on Giemsa	None necessary
2. Neisseria gonorrhea	3–5 d	Mucopurulent	Corneal abscess, perforation	Gram (−) cocci and PMN on Gram stain Positive culture	Systemic penicillin or cephtiaxone Saline lavage Topical erythromycin ointment
3. Neonatal chlamydia	5–10 d	Purulent	Epithelial keratitis Superior micropannus	PMN with inclusions on Giemsa Positive culture Immunofluorescent tests +	Topical erythromycin Oral erythromycin Treat parents
4. Staphylococcus aureus, Streptococcus pneumoniae	5–10 d	Catarrhal or mucopurulent	Punctate keratopathy	Gram (+) cocci and PMN on Gram stain Positive culture	Topical erythromycin
5. HSV Type II	3–15 d	Catarrhal	Epithelial or stromal disease	Multinucleated giant cells on Giemsa Positive culture Immunofluorescent tests +	Topical trifluorothymidine Systemic acyclovir
6. Haemophilus	5–10 d	Catarrhal or mucopurulent	Rare punctate keratopathy	Gram (−) coccobacillus on Gram stain	Topical erythromycin ointment Systemic cephalosporin

Gonococcal conjunctivitis occurs at approximately 48 hours after birth; however, it may occur earlier if there was rupture of amniotic membranes several hours before delivery. Typically, gonococcal conjunctivitis presents with severe purulent discharge and conjunctival and lid edema often associated with a keratitis. N. gonorrhoeae bacteria can penetrate intact corneal epithelium and can cause corneal ulcer and even corneal perforation if left untreated. A diagnosis is made by identifying gram negative intracellular diplococci on conjunctival scrapings. The treatment for gonococcal conjunctivitis is topic erythromycin ointment with systemic third-generation cephalosporin (Ceftriaxone I.V. 30 −50 mg/kg per day in divided doses). Alternatively, 1 g Ceftriaxone I.M. has been reported to be effective (29A).

Herpes Simplex type II can cause neonatal conjunctivitis which is usually associated with a keratitis and corneal staining. Herpes keratoconjunctivitis usually occurs as an isolated eye infection, but it may be associated with systemic invovement and encephalitis. Systemic herpes infection in a neonate is a devastating disease with an increased morbidity and mortality. The onset of herpes keratoconjunctivitis is usually between 1 and 2 weeks postpartum, presenting as a serous discharge with moderate conjunctival injection. In contrast to other infectious causes for neonatal conjunctivitis, herpes almost always presents as a unilateral infection. The keratitis results in positive fluorescein staining, most often in a geographic or dendritic pattern. The diagnosis is confirmed by obtaining viral cultures. However, the virus may take up to 7 to 10 days to become positive. When herpes neonatal conjunctival is suspected, immediately start topical trifluorothymidine (viroptic) every 2 hours and consider systemic acyclovir if there is a question about systemic involvement (also see Neonatal herpes simplex; cornea section).

S. aureus or other gram-positive organisms can cause a conjunctivitis in newborns arising from either the mother or the hospital personnel. There is usually a catarrhal to mucopurulent discharge with gram-positive cocci seen on Gram stain. It responds to topical erythromycin ointment. Systemic therapy is usually not necessary.

Evaluation and Treatment of Newborn with Conjunctivitis

Because of the potential visual loss, neonatal conjunctivitis requires a systematic approach to provide appropriate therapy as soon as possible (13). A detailed maternal history should discuss venereal disease, and documentation of how long the placental membranes were ruptured. The type of ocular prophylaxis and the time of onset of the conjunctivitis should be documented. Examination should evaluate for lid edema, skin findings, type of discharge, and corneal involvement. Systemic examination should search for other signs of chlamydial or gonococcal infection. Conjunctival scraping should be done with a metal spatula and examined with Gram, Giemsa, and Papanicolaou immunofluorescent stains or other specialized techniques. Cultures for a virus, chlamydia, and bacteria are appropriate. Specific treatment is directed by the results of the laboratory evaluation.

The initial treatment of a neonate with conjunctivitis is to start topical erythromycin ointment and systemic ceftrioxone. This treatment should be given immediately, as soon as cultures have been taken. Once the laboratory results are known, then therapy can be altered to specifically treat the offending organism.

Prevention is an important aspect and can be accomplished by surveillance of women during the third trimester of pregnancy and postnatal administration of topical antimicrobial agents. The Centers for Disease Control and Prevention and the American Academy of Pediatrics have recommended either 1% tetracycline ointment or .5% erythromycin as alternative therapies to 1% silver nitrate drops. The use of povidone-iodine is being evaluated (34A,34B).

■ IMMUNOLOGIC CONJUNCTIVAL INFLAMMATION

Some immunologic diseases which can affect the conjunctiva correlate with one of the four types of hypersensitive reactions of Gell and Coombs. In most, the entire immunologic components are not clearly defined (Table 50–8) (22).

Seasonal Allergic Conjunctivitis

Seasonal allergic conjunctivitis (hay fever) along with seasonal allergic rhinitis is an example of a pure Type 1 hypersensitivity reaction. The ragweed pollen causes IgE antiragweed antibody production and adoptive transfer has been shown with the experimental disease in animals. Along with asthma and atopic dermatitis, allergic conjunctivitis is one of the major atopic diseases which affect up to 10% of the general population. The typical symptoms of seasonal allergic conjunctivitis consists of ocular tearing and itching, often in association with the nasal congestion and sneezing of seasonal allergic rhinitis. There is usually a positive family history of some atopic disease. Examination reveals mild bulbar conjunctival edema with occasional slight mucous in the tear film and the inferior cul-de-sac. Laboratory tests are usually not indicated to confirm the diagnosis. Conjunctival scrapings or biopsy will reveal mast cells and eosinophils and quantitative serum IgE levels will be increased. Skin tests may reveal multiple environmental allergens.

Therapy is directed at multiple components in the reaction scheme: avoidance of environmental allergens, mast cell stabilizing agents during the allergy season (cromolyn, nedocromil, lodoxamide), systemic antihistamines after exposure, topical ocular antihistamines, and topical corticosteroids. Desensitization immunotherapy directed by an allergist is indicated in severe cases.

Vernal Keratoconjunctivitis

Vernal keratoconjunctivitis is an allergic inflammatory condition with characteristic giant papillae, usually on the upper tarsal conjunctiva and less commonly on the limbus (Figure 50–7). It is probably a combination of Type 1 and Type 4 Gell and Coombs hypersensitivity reaction. It most commonly occurs in the spring (hence vernal) although perennial forms also occur. It affects predominately young men but resolves in most patients over time. There is usually a personal or family history of other atopic reactions. Although worldwide in distribution, it is most common in the Mediterranean region and Central and South America.

The predominant symptoms are ocular itching with associated tearing, burning, mucous production, and

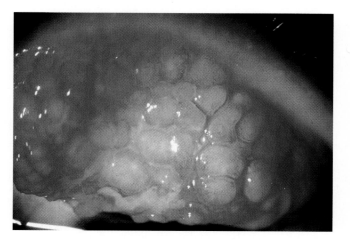

Figure 50–7.
Vernal conjunctivitis. A marked giant papillary conjunctival reaction of the upper lid in a 13-year-old boy with severe palpebral vernal conjunctivitis.

TABLE 50–8
Immunologic Diseases of the Conjunctiva With the Most
Likely Type of Hypersensitivity

Type I (Anaphylactoid)
Seasonal allergic conjunctivitis
Vernal keratoconjunctivitis (probably also Type IV)
Atopic keratoconjunctivitis (probably several types)
Giant papillary conjunctivitis (probably several types)
Acute and chronic allergic reaction

Type II (Cytotoxic)
Ocular cicatricial pemphigoid
Pemphigus vulgaris
Dermatitis herpetiformis
Pseudopemphigoid

Type III (Immune complex)
Erythema multiforme (Stevens-Johnson syndrome)
Toxic epidermal necrolysis
Keratoconjunctivitis sicca
Rheumatoid arthritis
Various collagen vascular diseases
Wegener granulomatosis
Relapsing polychondritis
Reiter syndrome

Type IV (Cell–Mediated)
Phlyctenulosis
Contact dermatoconjunctivitis
Graft versus host disease
Giant papillary conjunctivitis

light sensitivity. The giant papillae on the upper tarsal conjunctiva may have the appearance of cobblestones and are the probable cause of a diffuse superficial punctate keratitis or ulceration. A morphologic shield ulcer may develop which is persistent and can lead to microbial infection or corneal scarring. A limbal form of vernal with large papillae at the corneoscleral limbus is more common in blacks. There may be accumulation of inflammatory cells (mainly eosinophils) near the limbus within papillae called Horner-Trantas' dots. Up to 27% of patients may have permanent visual loss as a result of vernal keratoconjunctivitis (11).

The mainstay of therapy is allergen avoidance which is best evaluated by an allergy specialist. Systemic antihistamines (terfenadine, astemizole, hydroxyzine) can be effective in relieving many symptoms. Topical ocular mast cell stabilizing agents are essential agents. Cromolyn has shown to be effective; nedocromil and lodoxamide may be equally efficacious. Topical corticosteroids are used at strategic intervals for pulse therapy with taper and discontinuance as soon as possible. Long-term corticosteroid use should be discouraged.

The shield ulcers are notoriously resistant to therapy with options including topical N-acetylcysteine, bandage contact lens therapy, lubricants, and the investigational use of fibronectin and epidermal growth factor.

Giant Papillary Conjunctivitis

Giant papillary conjunctivitis is a papillary conjunctival reaction of the upper tarsal conjunctiva originally described in patients with contact lens intolerance, itching, and excessive mucous production. The reaction is a result of sensitization to allergic material present on the surface of the contact lens, coupled to the trauma that occurs with each blink over the contact lens. It affects at least 10% of the 24 million patients who wear contact lenses in the United States. Biopsy of the conjunctival papillae reveal mast cells and eosinophils and occasionally basophils. Therapy consists of discontinuing contact lenses, although most patients will resist this option. Proper lens hygiene, limitation of contact lens wear, and modification of contact lens design or wearing pattern may lessen the symptoms. The disease is most common with soft contact lenses but can be seen with all types of contact lenses, as well as ocular cosmetic shells. The use of daily disposable lenses, or at least frequent replacement, is the most appropriate alternative for these patients. Topical lubrication may also help. Topical corticosteroids should be avoided. The mast cell stabilizers (cromolyn, nedocromil, lodoxamide) may be helpful in some patients (4).

Atopic Keratoconjunctivitis

Atopic keratoconjunctivitis is an allergic keratoconjunctivitis seen in association with atopic dermatitis (eczema). Atopic dermatitis often occurs in childhood but can also be seen in adolescents and adults. Three percent of children under age three have atopic dermatitis. In addition to immunologic abnormalities, patients also have abnormal reactivity of the skin to various stimuli. This reactivity may represent a metabolic or biochemical defect which is genetically determined. The relationship of the disease to specific allergens is usually difficult to establish. Serum IgE concentrations are usually elevated in patients with atopic dermatitis and defects in cellular immunity are also evident. The disease may be related to a deficiency of T-suppressor cells in terminating IgE antibody response to certain allergens. IgE binds to mast cells in the skin, causing release of histamine and other chemical mediators. Skin in patients with atopic dermatitis has an excessive response to these mediators.

Conjunctival involvement is common in atopic dermatitis associated with symptoms of itching, burning, and mucoid discharge. The conjunctiva can appear hyperemic and chemotic during active disease and with chronicity become pale and congested with a papillary reaction. The papillae are usually in the inferior palpebral conjunctiva without formation of large papillae. Trantas' dots of eosinophils can be seen at the limbus. Scarring of the conjunctiva can result in symblepharon, entropion, and trichiasis (23, 28, 34). Corneal findings include a punctate keratitis, most common inferiorly. Marginal ulcers, vascularization, and corneal opacification occur. Keratoconus and herpes simplex virus infections are more common in atopic patients. Anterior and posterior subcapsular cataracts occur in approximately 10% of patients at a relatively young age and may progress rapidly.

The diagnosis is based on a constellation of clinical signs. There is no one laboratory test to confirm the diagnosis. Identification and avoidance of allergens is a primary focus of prevention. A fluorinated corticosteroid in a water-soluble base is used for skin lesions. Multiple other dermatologic regimens are available in the dermatologic armamentarium. Oral antihistamines are frequently beneficial; oral corticosteroids are reserved for short-term pulsed therapy. Symptomatic treatment of eye symptoms include cold compresses, topical vasoconstrictors, and mast cell stabilizers (cromolyn, nedocromil, lodoxamide). Topical corticosteroids may be used for short periods when there is increased inflammation, but long-term use should be avoided. Some patients with atopic dermatitis have the hyper-IgE syndrome. These patients have recurrent pyogenic skin and lung infections, significantly elevated serum IgE, and defective neutrophils. These patients may be improved by plasmapheresis (5).

Ocular Cicatricial Pemphigoid

Evidence is accumulating that the disease of ocular cicatricial pemphigoid, pemphigus vulgaris, and dermatitis herpetiform are possible examples of a Type 2 Gell and Coombs hypersensitivity phenomena. Autoantibodies are detected at the ocular and dermatologic sites and the autoantibodies are pathogenic (21,22).

Ocular cicatricial pemphigoid is a systemic autoimmune disease of the eye and the skin. Unlike bullous pemphigoid, cicatricial pemphigoid does not produce scarring of the skin; cicatricial pemphigoid is associated with conjunctival and other mucous membrane scarring, especially in the esophagus, trachea, pharynx, mouth, nose, anus, urethra, and vagina. The disease is rare but frequently not recognized in its early stages. It affects all races across the world but is slightly more common in females in their 60s and 70s. There may be a genetic predisposition linked to the HLA-DQw7 gene (2). There may be specific exciting agents that cause the disease. There is a drug-induced form of the disease originally associated with the systemic drug practolol. A localized ocular disease (pseudopemphigoid) has been

seen in association with the use of topical glaucoma medications including pilocarpine, epinephrine, timolol, and echothiophate (33).

Autoantibodies to a component of conjunctival basement membrane zone is the hallmark of ocular pemphigoid. Traditional techniques cannot usually detect circulating autoantibodies and more sensitive techniques may be required (3). The antigen in the basement membrane appears to be a 205 kilodalton protein (22). The antibody deposition appears to result in complement activation with a cascade of events, including mast cell degranulation, liberation of vasoactive amines, recruitment of macrophages and lymphocytes, liberation of cytokines, vascular damage, and up regulation of fibroblasts (22). The predominant immunologic cell is the helper T lymphocyte and macrophages, both in the ocular tissue and the circulation, emphasizing that it is a systemic autoimmune disease.

Foster has described four clinical stages of ocular cicatricial pemphigoid (21). Stage 1 has mild conjunctival changes and keratitis with subtle subepithelial fibrosis of the conjunctiva. Stage 2 has further cicatrization with foreshortening of the inferior fornix (Figure 50–8). Stage 3 has obvious symblepharon, and Stage 4 is advanced disease with ankyloblepharon and keratinization of the cornea. A dry eye generally does not occur until the more advanced stages. There is a relative decrease in goblet cells and later deformation of lash follicles, trichiasis, compromise in the meibomian gland ductules leading to corneal epithelial defects, secondary infection, and corneal neovascularization.

The definitive diagnosis requires the demonstration of immunoglobin or complement deposition at the epithelial basement membrane zone by immunologic techniques from active inflamed conjunctiva. This is

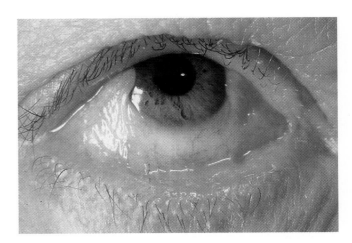

Figure 50–8.
Ocular pemphigoid. Severe conjunctival foreshortening and symblepharon in a patient with moderately advanced ocular cicatricial pemphigoid. There was also mucous membrane involvement of the mouth and nose.

best done in a skilled immunopathology laboratory. Because it is a systemic disease, ocular cicatricial pemphigoid is best managed by the ophthalmologist in conjunction with a chemotherapist or dermatologist. The therapy is then modified based on the therapeutic response and the tolerance of the systemic medications. If the ocular cicatricial pemphigoid is active, the initial therapy recommended is dapsone (provided the patient is not allergic to sulfa and is not glucose-6-phosphate dehydrogenase deficient). If the response to dapsone is incomplete, alternate medications may be added, including methotrexate, azathioprine, corticosteroids, or cyclophosphamide. Steroids are usually used only for the short-term, whereas the other agents are used for longer periods, if not indefinitely (59). Cyclosporin has not proven to be effective (22).

Attention to other details of the ocular condition is essential. Abnormal or aberrant lashes need to be removed with epilation or permanent destruction with electrolysis, cryoablation, or marginal lid rotation and follicle extirpation. Mucous membrane grafting may be required for extensive keratinized conjunctiva. Tear dysfunction states require lubrication and punctal occlusion. Corneal exposure and lagophthalmos may require tarsorrhaphy. Corneal transplant surgery is fraught with postoperative problems and is only recommended in rare circumstances; a keratoprosthesis is a better surgical alternative for many of the advanced patients.

Pemphigus Vulgaris

Pemphigus vulgaris is a fatal autoimmune skin disease affecting all ages with a widespread distribution but especially common among Ashkenazi Jews. Susceptibility to the disease is carried on the HLA-DQ3 gene (Foster 94). The antigen is a 130 kilodalton glycoprotein in the intercellular cement of epithelial cells; circulating autoantibodies activate complement and dissolve the bonds between the adjacent epithelial cells resulting in blisters under the surface epithelium which may rupture. There are occasional lid manifestations of pemphigus, but ocular manifestations are rare. Conjunctival bulla may occasionally rupture. Therapy is directed at hydration, control of sepsis, and the use of increased dose systemic corticosteroids and cytoxan immunosuppressive treatment.

Dermatitis Herpetiformis

Dermatitis herpetiformis is an autoimmune blistering dermatosis characterized by a pruritic eruption of the skin. Ocular (cicatrizing conjunctivitis) and other mucous membrane involvement is rare. The autoantibody is in the IgA class and biopsy of affected skin shows deposition of IgA and complement in a granular pattern at the dermal-epidermal junction. There is an HLA-DR3/HLA-B8 gene association. Dapsone therapy with systemic corticosteroids is usually effective.

Erythema Multiforme Major (Stevens-Johnson Syndrome)

Erythema multiforme major is a systemic disease, probably precipitated by a Type 3 hypersensitivity reaction to a microbe. Mycoplasma pneumonia is a common cause in children; herpes simplex virus and other viral diseases including polio, vaccinia, variola, and mumps have been associated with Stevens-Johnson syndrome (22). Other microbial agents have also been implicated. Although some drugs have been clearly implicated in cases of Stevens-Johnson syndrome (sulfonamides, tetracycline, penicillin, and so forth), in most instances the hypersensitivity reaction is probably a reaction to the microbe for which the patient was prescribed the medication.

Systemic manifestations include fever, malaise, headache, loss of appetite, and nausea. A generalized erythematous papular eruption later emerges to a bull's-eye lesion with an erythematous center surrounded by a zone of normal skin and then a zone of erythematous skin. The soles and palms are typically involved. Mucous membranes are involved especially the nose, mouth, vagina, anus, and conjunctiva.

The conjunctiva may have bulla which rupture leading to symblepharon, infection, or keratopathy. Subepithelial fibrosis causes conjunctival foreshortening, symblepharon formation, distorted lids, lashes and meibomian glands, and chronic keratopathy secondary to the abnormal lids, lashes, meibomian gland, and tear dysfunction. This can lead to corneal ulceration, neovascularization, or stromal ulceration. In some patients there are periodic recurrences and recrudescences of the disease (24).

The immunopathology suggests that the disease results from a combined mechanism involving circulating IgA immune complexes and a lymphocytic vasculitis in the areas where the complexes lodge. Therapy is directed at general support during the acute phase with hydration and surveillance for infection. The use of systemic corticosteroids remains controversial. Acute care of the ocular symptoms includes ocular hygiene to remove any discharges, the gentle separation of conjunctival adhesions, and the use of topical antibiotics and topical corticosteroids. There are no controlled studies to establish the correct protocol of therapy. Immunosuppressive therapy does not seem to be indicated except in the rare patient in whom an immunologically driven recurrent Stevens-Johnson syndrome has been shown (24). In these patients, immunohistochemistry of the conjunctiva shows IgA deposition in vessel walls with lymphocytic microvasculitis.

The chronic ocular disease requires attention to trichiasis and dystrichiasis (preferably through permanent destruction of the hair follicles), attention to meibomian gland dysfunction (lid hygiene), and treatment of keratopathy secondary to the abnormal lid, lashes, and tear dysfunction. Mucus membrane grafting is occasionally necessary for severely keratinized tissue.

Kawasaki Syndrome

This is an acute mucocutaneous inflammatory disease with systemic vasculitis usually occurring in children under 5 years of age. It is associated with fever of unknown origin (greater than 5 days), bilateral conjunctivitis, oral mucous membrane "injection, strawberry tongue," erythema of palms and soles with edema of the hands and feet, polymorphous exanthem, and cervical lymphadenopathy. The conjunctiva injection, typically spares the limbal area, and a mild iritis may occur. The most important complication is a systemic vasculitis that can cause coronary aneurysm and thrombosis, leading to sudden death in approximately 1% of cases. The etiology is unknown and treatment is supportive.

Toxic Epidermal Necrolysis

Lyell's syndrome, or toxic epidermal necrolysis, occurs in children as a result of staphylococcal toxin products causing a generalized peeling of the epidermis in large geographic areas of the skin and mucus membranes (48). A form of toxic epidermal necrolysis in adults may be caused by other microbes. As in Stevens-Johnson syndrome, medications (usually taken because of the systemic infection) are implicated in the disease but their role remains uncertain. The ocular manifestations are similar to Stevens-Johnson syndrome and the therapy is the same. Children with Staphylococcus aureus as the inciting agent require systemic antibiotics.

Phlyctenulosis

Phlyctenulosis is a granulomatous disease occurring in the conjunctiva, the limbus, or the cornea (81). It appears to be a Gell and Coombs Type 4 delayed hypersensitivity reaction to bacterial protein. It was common when tuberculosis was prevalent, but more recently has been seen in association with staphylococcal proteins. Candida, coccidioides, and lymphogranuloma vener-eum have also been associated with phlyctenulosis.

The inflammatory lesion initially has an intact epithelium which later ulcerates at the apex and resolves over a period of time. A corneal or limbal scar may result. Topical corticosteroids are effective in resolving the disease. Systemic tetracycline has also been effective.

Attention to the staphylococcal blepharitis is important to prevent recurrences. High-risk groups may require screening for tuberculosis.

Contact Dermatoconjunctivitis

Contact dermatoconjunctivitis is a Type 4 hypersensitive reaction of the skin and conjunctiva most frequently associated with atropine, neomycin, penicillin, or antazoline. Typical findings include an erythematous scaling dermatitis affecting the upper and lower lids with an erythematous conjunctiva (Figure 50–9). Patch skin tests can confirm the allergen with a classic delayed type hypersensitivity reaction occurring at 48 to 72 hours. Therapy involves withdrawal of the medication along with cool compresses and occasionally hydrocortisone skin cream to the affected area.

Graft versus Host Disease

Graft versus host disease occurs in approximately 40% of patients after bone marrow transplantation and is related to donor T lymphocytes attacking the recipient cells. The primary targets of attack are the skin, liver, intestine, oral mucosa, conjunctiva, lacrimal gland, vaginal mucosa, and esophageal mucosa. Only 45% of patients with moderate or severe acute graft versus host disease survive long-term (78).

Immunosuppressive therapy has been used to prevent acute graft versus host disease, usually using methotrexate and cyclosporine. Chronic graft versus host disease develops 3 to 15 months after bone marrow transplantation with T-cell infiltration in target tissues with complement and autoantibodies deposited at the dermal-epidermal graft junction. The most effective prevention of chronic graft versus host disease is to pre-

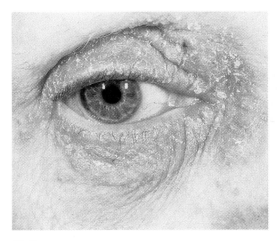

Figure 50–9.
Contact dermatitis. A contact dermatitis of the periocular skin in an older woman treated 3 days previously for a bacterial conjunctivitis with neosporin polymyxin B ophthalmic solution.

vent acute graft versus host disease. Therapy of chronic graft versus host disease is with multiple immunosuppressive therapy, especially azathioprine and cyclosporine.

The ocular effects of graft versus host disease can be devastating. Severe keratoconjunctivitis sicca can occur with epithelial erosions and stromal ulceration. Perma- nent punctal occlusion and tarsorrhaphy should be considered early in the course. A chronic conjunctivitis is seen in graft versus host disease which is immunologically driven and requires systemic immunosuppression. Topical 2% cyclosporine may have a limited effect (22). Cataract, uveitis, and retinitis may be part of this syndrome.

■ OTHER CONJUNCTIVAL INFLAMMATIONS

Superior Limbic Keratoconjunctivitis

Superior limbic keratoconjunctivitis is a cause of chronic and recurrent bilateral keratoconjunctivitis. It occurs most commonly between ages 20 and 60, primarily in females. There is no geographic or racial predilection, but abnormal thyroid function is present in up to 50% of patients. The disease has a characteristic course of remissions and exacerbations with usually no visual sequela.

The symptoms consist of burning, foreign body sensation, photophobia, and tearing. The inferior conjunctiva is usually normal, but the upper tarsal conjunctiva has a papillary reaction. The upper bulbar conjunctiva is thickened, edematous, and injected, and can override the peripheral limbus. The involved bulbar conjunctiva and superior limbus stain intensely with rose bengal. Occasionally, coarse and long filaments are attached to the involved bulbar conjunctiva and limbus. A fine epithelial keratitis occurs in association with a micropannus.

Giemsa-stained scrapings from the superior bulbar conjunctiva show keratinization of the epithelial cells. Papanicolaou-stain scrapings of the superior bulbar conjunctiva show nuclear chromatin condensed into unusual figures (85). Biopsy of the bulbar conjunctiva reveals acanthosis, keratinization, and dyskeratosis. The cause of the disease is unknown but may relate to an increased tension of the upper lid against the globe and increased mobility of the upper bulbar conjunctiva.

There have been multiple therapies directed at superior limbic keratoconjunctivitis. Dilute liquid silver nitrate applied to the conjunctiva can relieve some symptoms. Simple mechanical scraping, bandage soft contact lenses, and thermal cautery of the superior bulbar conjunctiva can also be effective. Resection of superior bulbar conjunctiva is indicated in the cases that do not respond to other therapy (64).

Contact Lens Induced Keratoconjunctivitis

Contact lens induced keratoconjunctivitis can simulate superior limbic keratoconjunctivitis (76). Symptoms include redness, irritation, itching, and photophobia with slightly reduced vision. The superior corneal epithelium is irregular, thickened, and gray. Subepithelial opacities may be present. A pannus may extend several millimeters onto the cornea. The superior tarsal conjunctiva may display mild papillary response. Filaments are usually present. The condition may progress if the contact lenses are not discontinued and cause significant corneal scarring and vascularization. The conjunctival scrapings reveal early keratinization with moderate polymorphonuclears and lymphocytes. The biopsy is similar to superior limbic keratoconjunctivitis. The disease is probably caused by mechanical factors but may be specifically related to the thimerosal in the lens care solution. Cessation of the soft contact lens wear is essential. I have not seen it in association with rigid contact lenses. Symptoms and signs may take years to resolve. When quiescent, a rigid gas permeable contact lens with avoidance of thimerosal containing solutions is appropriate.

Floppy Eyelid Syndrome

The floppy eyelid syndrome is a cause of chronic papillary conjunctivitis probably related to a lax easily everted upper lid (10). Patients complain of irritation, redness, and mucous discharge. The symptoms are usually worse in the morning and get better during the day. Most patients with the disorder are obese with the most prominent ocular feature being a loose upper lid which may spontaneously evert. The superior tarsal conjunctiva has a papillary response with some mucous strands. A coarse punctate keratopathy, a superior corneal pannus, filaments, and a mild ptosis may be present.

The pathogenesis of the loose upper lid is unknown, but it has been proposed that lid eversion occurs during sleep, resulting in contact of the upper lid and cornea with the pillow. Treatment is aimed at eliminating the eversion of the upper lid. Taping the lids shut may help. Permanent relief can be obtained with a horizontal lid shortening procedure (56).

Mucus Fishing Syndrome

The mucus fishing syndrome is a self-induced mechanical trauma to the conjunctiva during the course of removing mucus filaments from the eye. The mucus filaments are caused by a number of mechanisms, most commonly being keratoconjunctivitis sicca. The patient exacerbates the symptoms by removing mucus with cotton balls, the finger, or other instruments. The conjunctival trauma is evident when the patient shows the technique of removal. Rose bengal staining is usually positive. Treatment involves the cessation of touching the eye and the institution of treatment for the underlying condition (51).

Ligneous Conjunctivitis

Ligneous conjunctivitis is a chronic bilateral conjunctivitis of unknown etiology seen in childhood. Patients may have acute systemic symptoms at the time of development. The eyes are injected with mucoid discharge. There are thick conjunctival membranes which exhibit a hard boardlike appearance. The membranes may be sessile or pedunculated on the bulbar or tarsal conjunctiva. If the membranes are removed, bleeding occurs and the membranes will reform in several days. The disease may persist for months or years. The white or yellowish ligneous growth appears to mold and conform to the tarsal and bulbar conjunctiva (32).

Conjunctival scrapings reveal degenerated inflammatory cells. Histochemically, the lesion is composed of mucopolysaccharides. The pathogenesis is poorly defined, but immunologic studies suggest an association with streptococcal infection. Currently, there is no satisfactory treatment, although hyaluronidase, fibrinolysin, alpha chymotrypsin, cryotherapy, cromolyn, cyclosporine, and azathioprine have all been tried in patients with variable results. It may be an autosomal recessive disorder. Spontaneous resolution usually takes place over time (55).

Masquerade Syndrome

Most conjunctival tumors grow in an exophytic pattern and are easily recognized. Occasionally, conjunctival tumors such as squamous cell carcinoma or a meibomian gland carcinoma may grow in a diffuse minimally elevated pattern and appear as a chronic conjunctivitis. This is a unilateral conjunctivitis with a diffusely inflamed, moderately thickened conjunctiva, with vascular tufts or subepithelial scarring. The cornea may display a diffuse nonspecific punctate keratitis (8). A biopsy or a conjunctival scraping will reveal the atypical tumor cells. Specimens may be necessary from multiple areas to confirm the diagnosis. Treatment is based on the specific tumor type.

Toxic Conjunctival Reactions

Toxic conjunctival reactions are much more common than allergic reactions and can have different manifestations (89–91). Toxic papillary keratoconjunctivitis is a direct chemical irritation from the drug or the preservative. These toxic reactions usually take several weeks to develop. Symptoms include irritation, usually without itching. There is hyperemia, nonspecific papillary conjunctivitis, and scant discharge. Punctate staining of the cornea and conjunctiva are usually most prominent in the inferior nasal conjunctiva and cornea. Significant toxicosis can lead to chronic epithelial defects. The most common causative agents of toxic papillary conjunctivitis are the aminoglycoside antibiotics, antiviral agents, and the preservative benzalkonium chloride. A dry eye, prolonged use of medications, and use of multiple medications contribute to this reaction. Treatment is to withdraw the medication and/or preservative. Topical corticosteroids are usually of no value (and usually contain benzalkonium). Preservative-free artificial tears or ointments may relieve symptoms. Prolonged reactions may lead to pseudopemphigoid discussed previously in association mainly with glaucoma medications. Alternate glaucoma therapy should be selected.

A toxic follicular conjunctivitis can occur in association with certain drugs. Symptoms of allergy are usually absent. The toxic follicular reaction results from the ability of certain drugs to act as nonantigenic mitogens which induce mitoses and lymphoblastic transformation of lymphocytes by nonimmunologic means (89). Toxic follicular reactions take weeks to develop (approximately 15 months in the case of dipivalyl epinephrine). Follicular conjunctivitis is the main finding with unimpressive conjunctival hyperemia. There is a proliferation of subepithelial conjunctival lymphocytes with true lymphoid follicles in both the palpebral and bulbar surface. There is usually no conjunctival discharge. Only a few specific drugs (and not preservatives) elicit a toxic follicular reaction. These include all the topical antiviral agents (idoxuridine, vidarabine, triflurothymidine), glaucoma medications (dipivalyl epinephrine, echothiophate, pilocarpine), and cycloplegic agents (atropine, homatropine). Therapy involves withdrawal of the drug. In some instances, replacement of drug with a fresh drug may be helpful.

■ CONJUNCTIVAL DEGENERATIONS

Pingueculae are triangular, yellow-white elevated conjunctival nodules adjacent to the 3- and 9-o'clock limbus. They occur more commonly on the nasal side and are bilateral. They are related to the combined effect of

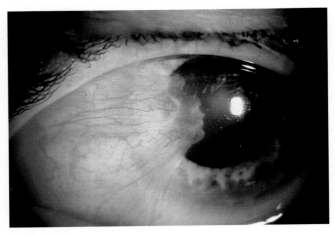

Figure 50–10.
Pterygium. A fleshy injected vascular pterygium almost to the visual axis on the nasal aspect of a farmer who spends a great deal of time outdoors. There is slight regular astigmatism in this eye.

age and exposure to ultraviolet light. Histopathologically, a pinguecula consists of abnormal subepithelial collagen which is hyalinized and has increased curling and basophilia characteristic of elastotic degeneration (6). The overlying epithelium is slightly thinned but may be thickened or even dysplastic. Pingueculae usually are asymptomatic but can grow into pteryia. They rarely become inflamed and symptomatic (pingueculitis) (79). Pingueculitis can be treated with observation, topical corticosteroids, and rarely excision.

Pterygia are fibrovascular overgrowths of the bulbar conjunctiva onto the cornea. They are located in the palpebral fissure most commonly on the nasal side with a triangular configuration with the base peripheral and the apex central over the cornea. A pigmented iron line, the Stocker line, may be seen on the corneal edge of the pterygium head. The body of the pterygium varies in thickness and injection; budding blood vessels

and active vascularization are signs of progressive growth. The head of the pterygium is firmly adherent to the cornea and may destroy Bowman's membrane, but otherwise the pterygium can usually be lifted up (Figure 50–10). Pterygia, similar to pinguecula, are related to climatic factors, especially ultraviolet radiation and a windy atmosphere (57). They are most common in central American, the Caribbean, and the southern United States, especially in outdoor laborers. Patients are usually young. The disease may progress to the central area or growth may cease at any time. Histologically, the changes are similar to pinguecula with thickening and elastotic degeneration of the subepithelial connective tissue. The overlying corneal epithelium may be dysplastic.

Although a pterygium is usually asymptomatic, it can cause tearing, foreign body sensation, and may induce with the rule or irregular astigmatism by tension on the cornea in the visual axis. Limitations of eye movement can occur, especially with recurrences when the horizontal recti muscles are involved. A pterygium may occasionally be removed because of astigmatism, involvement of the visual axis, or because of cosmetic problems. The recurrence rate is increased, although much lower with recent approaches. Some techniques have been tried for pterygium removal including bare sclera technique, beta irradiation, conjunctival grafts, lamellar corneal grafts, and the use of thio-tepa or mitomycin postoperatively (68, 82). For primary or recurrent pterygia, many prefer a conjunctival autograft after simple excision and smoothing of the corneal surface with a diamond corneal burr (41). Topical mitomycin is an alternative but is associated with significant risk of ischemic ocular damage (31, 74). Rarely, a peripheral lamellar corneal graft is required to free up scarred tissue. Recurrences can occur as early as a few weeks after removal of the pterygium.

■ CONJUNCTIVAL TUMORS

Tumors affect the conjunctiva and the cornea in an inseparable fashion since the corneal epithelium is continuous with the conjunctival epithelium. The most common neoplasias which arise from the conjunctiva and cornea are from disturbances of the squamous cells or from proliferation of the intraepithelial dendritic melanocytes. There are also congenital abnormalities which may simulate a neoplasm and there are also less common neoplasms arising from the underlying mesenchymal tissues.

Congenital Lesions

Choristomas are tumorlike growths which contain epithelial and dermal elements not normally indigenous

to the site in which it is found (75). The dermoid and dermolipoma are examples of choristomas. The dermoid is a small circumscribed solid tumor usually found in the inferior temporal portion of the cornea although occasionally isolated on the cornea. It can be from a few millimeters in size up to 10 millimeters in size and is usually tan or white (Figure 50–11). Although most are asymptomatic, they can be associated with astigmatism, irritation, and disturbances of the tear film. Histopathologically, they are composed of collagenous tissue embedded with dermal elements of sweat glands, fat, and pilosebaceous units. Dermolipomas are similar to dermoids but have a more yellowish color and a location in the conjunctiva near the insertion of the lateral rectus muscle and the superior fornix. They are composed pri-

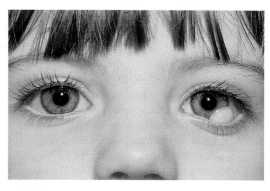

Figure 50–11.
Limbal dermoid. A young child with a dermoid tumor at the corneal limbus. It was removed with a shave keratectomy.

marily of fat without pilosebaceous units. No treatment is usually required for either condition; the dermoid may be removed with a shave or lamellar dissection because of cosmesis, irritation, or astigmatism. Caution is required in removal of the dermolipoma to investigate the posterior extent of involvement and the potential damage to the lacrimal gland. Dermoids and dermolipomas can grow during youth but do not undergo neoplastic transformation. A rare form of a choristoma is an ectopic lacrimal gland which is highly vascularized and fleshy and may extend onto the cornea (69).

Epithelial Tumors

Papillomas

There are two types of papillomas of the conjunctiva: infectious and noninfectious. The infectious conjunctival papilloma is a benign tumor usually asymptomatic in children or young adults, occurring most commonly in

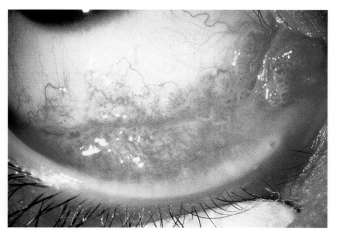

Figure 50–12.
Conjunctival papilloma. A recurrent conjunctival papillomatous growth in the inferior conjunctiva and caruncle area. It had previously been treated with cryotherapy.

the inferior fornix, especially near the caruncle (Figure 50–12). The tumors may be multiple or bilateral in distribution. They tend to be pedunculated fleshy growths with little associated inflammatory reaction. The papovavirus has been implicated in the etiology of these lesions with hand-to-eye transmission (44, 53). They rarely undergo malignant transformation and resolve within a 2-year period (92). Treatment is usually conservative; surgical excision combined with cryotherapy is the procedure of choice (26). Recurrences are frequent and the treatment can be instrumental in spreading this viral infection.

The noninfectious papilloma occurs in older individuals at a single site, usually at the limbus. It tends to be sessile with large feeder vessels. The translucency of the conjunctiva permits visualization of the central vascular core. It may be difficult to distinguish from a premalignant squamous neoplasia. It is treated as other squamous cell neoplasias with excision and cryotherapy.

The inverted conjunctival papilloma, also as known as benign mucoepidermoid carcinoma of the conjunctiva, is a variant of squamous cell papilloma. It shows an endophytic growth pattern, rather than the usual exophytic pattern. It can have an indolent course. Histopathologically, there is invasion of benign epithelial cells into underlying connective tissue (38).

Inflammatory Epithelial Tumors

Benign hereditary intraepithelial dyskeratosis is a bilaterally inherited disorder (autosomal dominant) with an increased degree of penetrance. It usually appears in the first decade of life and affects primarily the Haliwa Indians who come from sections of North Carolina. It has also been reported elsewhere. Bilateral elevated hyperplastic lesions with foci of white keratin or dilated vessels are seen. They are usually nonprogressive although occasionally can cause loss of vision. Associated lesions are rarely seen in the oral pharynx or buccal mucosa. On histopathologic assessment, the conjunctival epithelium is acanthotic and exhibits premature keratinization of cells (dyskeratosis) with a surface layer of keratin. There is no malignant change. Local excision is the treatment of choice but recurrences occur (71, 83).

Pseudoepitheliomatous hyperplasia is a benign reactive proliferation of the conjunctiva or corneal epithelium that typically develops rapidly over weeks or months (84). It is frequently seen in association with a preexisting inflammatory lesion such as a pingueculum or pterygium. The lesion has a white, hyperkeratotic surface with a central umbilication, like a keratoacanthoma. On histopathologic assessment, the conjunctival epithelium shows acanthosis, parakeratosis, and hyperkeratosis with long-term inflammatory cells. There is no conversion to malignancy. A keratoacanthoma, probably a variant of the pseudoepitheliomatous hyperplasia, can rarely occur on the conjunctiva (72). The pyogenic granuloma ("proud flesh") is an inflammatory vascular response to an insult to the conjunctiva. It is seen most frequently after strabismus or pterygium surgery, or after chemical burns. It rarely arises de novo. It is a red vascular mass which develops rapidly. The pathologic assessment shows dilated capillaries and a cellular infiltrate of lymphocytes, plasma cells, and scattered polymorphonuclear cells (it is not a granuloma). It can be treated with excision, with cauterization to the base of the lesion (65).

Conjunctival Intraepithelial Neoplasia

Conjunctival and corneal neoplasia have stimulated considerable debate about their classification, natural history, and subsequent treatment options (17). There have been multiple terms used to describe what is now termed conjunctival (or corneal) intraepithelial neoplasia. It is usually seen as a unilateral condition in fair-skinned men in middle or late age with a history of ultraviolet exposure and perhaps additional risk factors associated with smoking, petroleum derivatives, and contact with the human papillomavirus (58). The human papillomavirus was detected by polymerase chain reaction in 88% of tissue samples, although the clinical significance still remains unclear (45, 52, 62).

Conjunctival intraepithelial neoplasia has the clinical appearance of a translucent or gelatinous thickening of the conjunctiva with a variable degree of keratinization (Figure 50–13). Occasionally, a papillomatous-like lesion is present. Almost all arise at the limbus and can spread either onto the conjunctiva or the cornea. When it is present on the cornea, there is frequently a frosted glass appearance with a fimbriated margin and clusters of gray spots. It is rarely confined to the cornea and may have a migrating pattern (86). The term connotes a neoplasm confined to the epithelium. There is an abnormality in the maturation of epithelial cells with gradation from subtle alterations to frank anaplasia probably in a continual spectrum. Most lesions do not progress to invasive squamous cell carcinoma but they have the propensity to do so. As long as the disease remains confined to the intact basement membrane, metastasis does not occur. It can become an invasive squamous cell carcinoma with risk of intraocular extension and metastasis. The clinical appearance, and the degree of dysplasia does not affect the prognosis. The treatment of conjunctival intraepithelial neoplasia is primarily with wide local excision with the addition of cryotherapy. When the lesion is large, this may mean significant loss of epithelium and the need for conjunctival autografts. Recurrences still occur but in only approximately 5% if the initial pathologic specimen shows clear margins.

Invasive Squamous Cell Carcinoma

Invasive squamous cell carcinoma is a rare extension of conjunctival intraepithelial neoplasia with invasion through the basement membrane in either a microinvasive or macroinvasive pattern. The lesion tends to be clinically larger than conjunctival intraepithelial neoplasia and may have a feeder vessel or be seen as a recurrence of prior conjunctival intraepithelial neoplasia. The adherence of the lesion to the underlying sclera is a marker for possible invasion. On histopathologic examination, these lesions show a bizarre pleomorphic change of the epithelium with epidermoid and spindle cells showing acanthosis, dyskeratosis, and anaplasia. A majority of the lesions are just locally invasive and can be treated with surgical excision with a keratectomy or sclerectomy combined with cryotherapy (67). Intraocular, orbital, and distant metastases can occur, and require individual approaches to therapy (27, 61).

Mucoepidermoid carcinoma and spindle cell carcinoma are variants of squamous cell carcinoma which tend to be more locally aggressive. Mucoepidermoid carcinoma can arise anywhere on the conjunctiva and tends to invade tissues early in the course, although they do not usually metastasize (7). Spindle cell carcinoma is a rare, aggressive variant with propensity for rapid invasion resulting in corneal perforation (9). Both variants require a more aggressive surgical approach.

Sebaceous Carcinoma

Sebaceous carcinoma most commonly arises from the sebaceous glands of the eyelid and presents in the eyelid as a mass. There are variants, however, which may affect the conjunctiva, such as an intraepithelial (pagetoid) spread to the conjunctiva but may also arise de

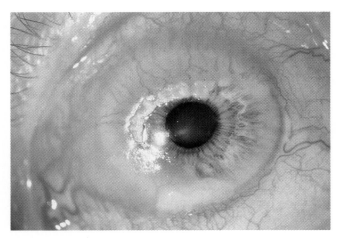

Figure 50–13.
Conjunctival intraepithelial neoplasia. A diffuse conjunctival intraepithelial neoplasia rising in the limbal area and spreading circumferentially around the cornea. It was removed with excision leaving Bowman's membrane intact.

novo in the conjunctiva (50). Pagetoid spread onto the conjunctiva causes an inflammatory reaction, perhaps related to sebaceous material secreted by the tumor cells. The primary tumor is most frequently on the upper lid (50%), and less commonly in the lower lid (20%) or diffuse (15%), or at the caruncle. It is more common in females in their 50s and 60s with Asians being more frequently affected (60). There is often a delay in making the diagnosis in the absence of a distinct palpable lid mass. A frequent scenario is the presence of a prolonged unresponsive conjunctivitis with the diagnosis finally being established after a conjunctival biopsy. Pathologically, sebaceous elements are found within the tumor, best shown by fat stain or ultramicroscopic studies. The pagetoid spread may involve only the superficial epithelial layers and spare the basilar layers.

The treatment is primarily surgical with a wide surgical margin. The conjunctival involvement is best mapped before surgery to plan the surgical approach. Conjunctival involvement of less than 50% can sometimes be managed with excision and cryotherapy to the involved conjunctiva. If orbital invasion is found, then exenteration is advocated. Lymph node involvement requires aggressive therapy; some of these patients have survived long-term. Close followup of all patients is necessary because of a increased recurrence rate and mortality rate (14). Factors associated with a poor prognosis include invasion of vascular or lymphatic tissue, diffuse involvement of both lids, multicentric origin, tumor diameter greater than 10 mm, and symptoms for greater than 6 months (70).

Pigmented Conjunctival Lesions

Pigmented lesions of the conjunctiva or sclera arise from melanocytes capable of producing pigment granules of melanin within melanosomes. They are derived from dendritic, nevus, or fusiform melanocytes (35). Table 50–9 lists the types of melanocytes and the associated lesions they produce (46). Since clinicians encounter melanocytic lesions in various clinical settings, it is easier to classify melanocytic lesions into congenital melanosis, nevi, acquired melanosis, and conjunctival melanoma. The differential diagnosis of these classes of melanocytic conjunctival lesions is shown in Table 50–10 (18, 19, 37, 46).

Congenital melanosis can consist of benign epithelial melanosis, or the subepithelial lesions of melanosis oculi, oculodermal melanosis, and pigmented episcleral spot. Benign epithelial melanosis is a common, flat, patchy, brown pigmentation of the conjunctival epithelium most frequently seen in blacks and darkly complexioned patients. It can occur in whites. It is bilateral, and usually asymmetric. Melanosis oculi is a diffuse or localized unilateral irregular-bordered pigmentation of

TABLE 50–9
Types of Melanocytes and Associated Lesions

Dendritic
   Benign epithelial melanosis of conjunctiva
   Primary acquired melanosis of conjunctiva*
   Secondary acquired melanosis of conjunctiva
Nevus
   Junctional conjunctival nevus*
   Subepithelial conjunctival nevus
   Compound conjunctival nevus*
Fusiform
   Nevus of Ota* (involving skin, conjunctiva, episclera, and sclera)
   Melanosis oculi* (involving conjunctiva, episclera, and sclera)
   Blue nevus of sclera
   Cellular blue nevus of sclera
   Pigmented episcleral spots

* Malignant potential

the episclera often associated with a unilateral increase in ocular pigment in the iris or choroid. It does not affect the conjunctiva. There is a decreased risk of developing uveal (but not conjunctival) melanoma. Oculodermal melanosis (the nevis of Ota) is an ipsilateral pigmentation of the periocular skin in addition to the findings of melanosis oculi and with no risk of developing conjunctival melanoma. The pigmented episcleral spot of Axenfeld is a loop from an intrascleral nerve that has perforated through the sclera.

TABLE 50–10
Melanocytic Conjunctival Lesions

Congenital melanosis
   Benign epithelial melanosis of conjunctiva
   Subepithelial lesions
      Melanosis oculi*
      Oculodermal melanosis (nevus of Ota*)
      Pigmented episcleral spot
Nevi
   Intraepithelial (junctional)*
   Subepithelial
   Compound*
   Spindle epithelioid ("juvenile melanoma")
   Blue nevus
   Cellular blue nevus
Acquired epithelial melanosis
   Primary acquired melanosis*
   Secondary acquired melanosis (bilateral)
Melanoma of conjunctiva*
   From nevi, from acquired melanosis, or de novo
   From metastatic or intraocular extension

* Malignant potential

Melanocytic nevi are common hamartomatous lesions of the conjunctiva. They usually appear within the first two decades of life and may grow with puberty, hormones, or solar exposure. They are rarely malignant, with malignancy related primarily to the junctional activity at the epithelial-subepithelial layer. They have variable pigment and frequent epithelial inclusion cysts and mucous-producing goblet cells.

Acquired melanosis may be secondary to a variety of conjunctival irritants such as disease (chronic conjunctival disorders or because of chemicals, hormones or radiation) (Figure 50–14). Primary acquired is a poorly circumscribed diffuse irregular hyperpigmentation of the bulbar conjunctiva, usually near the limbus. It can be multifocal and is seen almost exclusively in whites, where it has the propensity to become malignant. The present approach to the diagnosis of these disorders is with the conjunctival biopsies to stage the lesion. Stage 1A shows no atypia and rarely converts to melanoma. Stage 1B has atypia which can have either a decreased risk of progression to melanoma (if the growth pattern confined to the basilar epithelium) or a increased risk of progression to melanoma (if the growth pattern is not confined to the basilar epithelium). Stage 2 implies invasion and requires aggressive surgical approach with excision of nodules of melanoma and extensive cryotherapy to the remaining pigmentation.

Melanoma of the conjunctiva can arise de novo, from nevi, or from acquired melanosis with the latter probably being the most common source (Figure 50–15). They are rare tumors but need aggressive therapy because of a mortality rate of approximately 26% (20, 46). Extensive surgical removal should be done followed by extensive cryotherapy to the base and margins (36, 46). Recurrences are frequent but may respond to further excision. Local intralymphatic spread may oc-

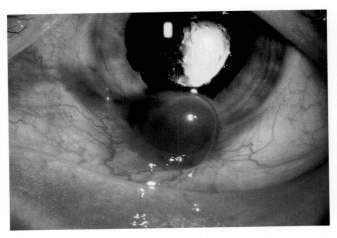

Figure 50–15.
Conjunctival melanoma. A conjunctival melanoma arising de novo in a 50-year-old white male.

cur. Extensive lymph node dissection may be curative in some patients. Any organ can be the site of metastatic involvement with only palliative treatment available.

Soft Tissue Tumors

Lymphoproliferative Lesions

Ocular adnexal lymphoproliferative lesions consist of a spectrum of entities including reactive lymphoid hyperplasia, atypical lymphoid hyperplasia, and lymphoma (16, 47). There are no clinical or radiologic signs which can clearly distinguish the reactive processes from a true lymphoma. A similar pattern is evident in other mucosa-associated lymphoid tumors elsewhere in the body. Lymphocytes normally reside in the substantia propria of the conjunctiva and can undergo hyperplasia in response to a stimulant (42, 43).

Reactive lymphoid hyperplasia is a hypercellular lesion of mature lymphocytes and scattered plasma cells and histiocytes. They are T-cell rich polyclonal lesions and have a counterpart in mucosa-associated lymphoid tissues in other sites. Up to 20% may be capable of transformation to a lymphoma. Atypical lymphoid hyperplasia is a monotonous and monomorphous sheet of diffuse or follicular lymphoid proliferating cells with a subpopulation of atypical cells suggestive of lymphoma. They are usually polyclonal on immunologic testing.

The diagnosis of lymphoma in the ocular adnexa is difficult because criteria such as effacement of preexisting architecture or invasion of the capsule cannot be applied. In distinction to lymphoma elsewhere, most ocular adnexal lymphomas are well differentiated low-grade small lymphocytic lymphomas which have a biologic resemblance to extranodal lesions in the lung, gut, and parotid gland known as mucosa-associated lymphoid tumors (30, 39).

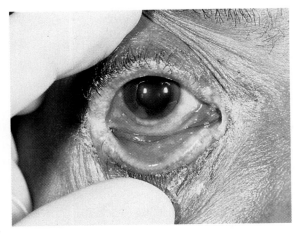

Figure 50–14.
Secondary acquired melanosis. A 30-year-old black male with recurrent atopic keratoconjunctivitis resulting in stimulation of the conjunctival melanocytes.

Even if the lymphoma becomes widespread, the small well-differentiated lymphocytic lymphoma is associated with long survival. Twenty-five percent of these small cell lymphomas will develop a systemic lymphoma whereas 68% of the less well-differentiated lymphomas may develop systemic lymphoma. The 5-year survival for patients with low-grade ocular adnexal lymphoma is better than that associated with a low-grade lymphoma in other sites and may not be much different than that expected in the general population.

Immunologic and molecular genetic studies have enhanced our knowledge but not necessarily clarified the issue. The evolution from polyclonal to monoclonal has been substantiated in some lesions and lymphoma can evolve in its differentiation. The ocular lymphoproliferative lesions probably represent a spectrum of changes from polyclonal to monoclonal and then further capacity for malignant transformation because of a metastable condition.

There are no good clinical signs to confirm the stage in the spectrum of the lymphoproliferative lesion. Patients are usually in their seventh decade with no acute conjunctival or orbital inflammatory changes. The lymphoid lesions are frequently salmon-colored patches and can be pebbly or firm rubbery nodules (Figure 50–16). CT scanning will reveal the lesions with distinctive molding to the globe to surrounding structures. A biopsy of the conjunctival or orbital lesion is necessary with fresh tissue submitted for immunologic studies and histopathologic examination. (54). Appropriate staging is done to find other possible sites of disease. Low-grade lymphomas have a long clinical evolution and current modes of therapy usually cannot eradicate the disease process. Treatment then is complex with consideration given to withholding any therapy based on the features of the lesion, the extent and site and size of involvement, the age of the patient and symptoms, the bone marrow function, and the threat to vital organs. Therapy for the mid and increased grade lymphomas is recommended with radiation locally (if the disease is confined to the ocular adnexal area) and chemotherapy (if the disease is beyond the orbit). Patients need to be continually monitored for additional evidence for lymphoma elsewhere.

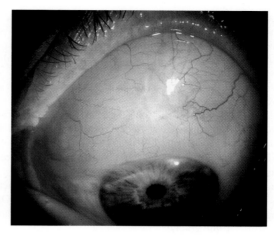

Figure 50–16.
Conjunctival lymphoma. A fleshy growth arising in the superior cul-de-sac. Histopathologic assessment and immunocytochemistry studies confirmed a low-grade lymphoma.

Kaposi Sarcoma

Ocular adnexal Kaposi sarcoma has been increasingly common in association with immunosuppression especially in patients with AIDS (23, 87). It presents with a characteristic reddish or bluish vascular conjunctival lesion which may be nodular or diffuse. There are perhaps three histologic types: Type 1 with dilated vascular channels lined by flat endothelial cells; Type 2 with fusiform endothelial cells with patches of spindle cells; Type 3 with spindle cells (15). Most lesions progress slowly and rarely invade although they may cause symptoms because of their bulk. Kaposi sarcomas usually respond to radiation, but occasionally excision can be done.

Mesenchymal Tumors

There are a variety of tumors which contain tissue elements from the substantia propria. These include the lymphoma discussed previously and the much rarer lesions such as neurofibroma, schwannoma, rhabdomyosarcoma, myxoma, metastatic lesions, hemangiopericytoma, lymphangioma, xanthomatous lesions, leukemia, and pseudotumor.

■ REFERENCES

1. Adamis AP, Schein OD: Chlamydia and acanthamoeba infections of the eye. In: Albert, DM, Jakobiec, FA (eds): Principles and Practice of Ophthalmology. Philadelphia: WB Saunders: 1994: Volume 1, Chapter 9.
2. Ahmed, AR, Foster, CS, Zaltas, M, et al: Association of DQW 7 with ocular cicatricial pemphigoid. Proc Natl Acad Sci, 1991: 88:11579–11582.
3. Ahmed, AR, Kahn, KNA, Wells, P, et al: Preliminary serological studies comparing immunofluorescence assay with radioimmunoassay. Curr Eye Res, 1989: 8:1011–1019.
4. Allansmith, MR, Ross, RN: Ocular allergy and mast cell stabilizer. Surv Ophthalmol, 1986: 30:229–244.
5. Aswad MI, Tauber J, Baum J.: Plasmapheresis treatment in patients with severe atopic keratoconjunctivitis. Ophthalmology 1988: 95:444.
6. Austin P, Jakobiec HA, Iwamoto T: Elastodysplasia and

elastodystrophy as pathologic bases of ocular pterygium and pingueculum. Ophthalmology 1983; 90:96.

7. Brownstein S: Mucoepidermoid carcinoma of the conjunctiva with intraocular invasion. Ophthalmology 88:1226, 1981.

8. Brownstein, S, Codere, F, Jackson, WB: Masquerade syndrome. Ophthalmology, 1980: 87:259.

9. Cohen B, Green W, Nicholas T, et al: Spindle cell carcinoma of the conjunctiva. Arch Ophthalmology 98:1809, 1980.

10. Culbertson, WW, Ostler, HB: The floppy lid syndrome. Am J Ophthalmol, 1981: 92:568.

11. Dart JKG: The epidemiology of vernal keratoconjunctivitis. Proceedings of the Second Fisons International Ophthalmology Workshop. Bollington, Cheshire England. Pennine, 1989: 26–37.

12. Dawson, C, Hanna, L, Togni, B: Adenovirus type 8 infections in the United States. IV. Observations on the pathogenesis of lesions in severe eye disease. Arch Ophthalmol, 1972: 87:258.

13. deToledo, AR, Chandler, JW: Conjunctivitis in the newborn. Infect Dis Clin North Am, 1992: 6:807–813.

14. Doxanas M, Green W: Sebaceous gland carcinoma. Arch Ophthalmol 102:245, 1984.

15. Dugel PU, Gill PS, Frangieh GT, et al: Ocular adnexal Kaposi's sarcoma in acquired immunodeficiency syndrome. Am J Ophthalmol 110:500, 1990.

16. Ellis J, Banks P, Campbell J, Liesegang T.: Lymphoid tumors of the ocular adnexa. Ophthalmology 1985;92:1311–1323.

17. Erie JC, Campbell RJ, Liesegang TJ: Conjunctival and corneal intraepithelial and invasive neoplasia. Ophthalmology 93:176, 1986.

18. Folberg R, Jakobiec FA, Bernardino VB, Iwamoto T. Benign conjunctival melanocytic lesions: clinicopathologic features. Ophthalmology 1989;96:436–461.

19. Folberg R, McLean IW. Primary acquired melanosis and melanoma of the conjunctiva: terminology, classification, and biologic behavior. Hum Pathol 1986;17:652–654.

20. Folberg R, McLean IW, Zimmerman LE. Conjunctival melanosis and melanoma. Ophthalmology 1984;91:673–677.

21. Foster, CS: Cicatricial pemphigoid. Trans Am Ophthalmol Soc, 1986: 84:527–663.

22. Foster CS: Immunologic disorders of the conjunctiva, cornea, and sclera. In: Albert, DM, Jakobiec, FA (eds): Principles and Practice of Ophthalmology. Philadelphia: WB Saunders: 1994: Vol 1, Chapter 10.

23. Foster, CS, Calonge M. Atopic keratoconjunctivitis. Ophthalmology 1990: 97:992–1000.

24. Foster, CS, Fong, LP, Azar, D, Kenyon, KR: Episodic conjunctival inflammation after Stevens-Johnson syndrome. Ophthalmology, 1988: 95:453–462.

25. Foulks GN: Bacterial infectious of the conjunctiva and cornea. In: Albert, DM, Jakobiec, FA. Principles and Practice of Ophthalmology. Philadelphia: WB Saunders, 1994: V. 1, Chapter 7:162–171.

26. Fraunfelder FT, Wallace TR, Farris HE, et al: The role of cryosurgery in external ocular and periocular disease. Trans Am Acad Ophthalmol Otolaryngol 83:713–724, 1977.

27. Freedman J, Rohm G: Surgical management and histopathology of invasive tumors of the cornea. Br J Ophthalmol 63:632, 1979.

28. Garrity, JA, Liesegang, TJ: Ocular complications of atopic dermatitis. Can J Ophthalmol, 1984: 19:21.

29. Gordon JS: Adenovirus and other nonherpetic viral diseases. In: Smolin, G, Thoft, RA (eds): The Cornea. Third Edition. Boston: Little, Brown & Co., 1994: 215–227.

29a. Haimovici, R., Roussel T. J., Treatment of gonococcal conjunctivitis with single dose intermuscular Ceftriaxone. Am J Ophthalmol 1989; 107: 511–514.

30. Hardman-Lea S, Kerr-Muir M, Wotherspoon AC, et al: Mucosal-associated lymphoid tissue lymphoma of the conjunctiva. Arch Ophthalmol 112:1207–1212, 1994.

31. Hayasaka S, Noda S, Yamamoto Y, Setogawa T: Postoperative instillation of low-dose mitomycin C in the treatment of primary pterygium. Am J Ophthalmol 1988; 106:715–718.

32. Hidayat, AA, Riddle, PJ: Ligneous conjunctivitis: a clinicopathologic study of 17 cases. Ophthalmology, 1927: 94:947.

33. Hirst, LW, Werblin, T, Novak, M et al: Drug-induced cicatrizing conjunctivitis simulating ocular pemphigoid. Cornea, 1982: 1:121.

34. Hogan, MJ: Atopic keratoconjunctivitis. Trans Am Ophthalmol Soc, 1952: 50:265.

34a. Isenberg, SJ, Apt, L, Wood, M: A controlled trial of povidone-iodine as prophylasis against ophthalmia neonatorum. New Engl J Med 1995; 332(9):562–566.

34b. Isenberg et al: Povidone-iodine for ophthalmia neonatorum prophylaxis. Am J Ophthalmol 1994;118 (6): 701–706.

35. Jakobiec FA. The ultrastructure of conjunctival melanocytic tumors. Trans Am Ophthalmol Soc 1984;82:599–752.

36. Jakobiec FA, Brownstein S, Albert W, et al: The role of cryotherapy in the management of conjunctival melanoma. Ophthalmology 89:502, 1982.

37. Jakobiec FA, Folberg R, Iwamoto T. Clinicopathologic characteristics of premalignant and malignant melanocytic lesions of the conjunctiva. Ophthalmology 1989;95:147–166.

38. Jakobiec FA, Harrison W, Aronian D: Inverted mucoepidermoid papillomas of the epibulbar conjunctiva. Ophthalmology 94:283, 1987.

39. Jakobiec FA, Iwamoto T, Patell M, Knowles DM: Ocular adnexal monoclonal tumors with a favorable prognosis. Ophthalmology 1986;93:1547–1557.

40. Jakobiec FA, Rini FJ, Fraunfelder FT, Brownstein S. Cryotherapy for conjunctival primary acquired melanosis and malignant melanoma: experience with 62 cases. Ophthalmology 1988;95:1058–1069.

41. Kenyon KR, Wagoner MD, Hettinger ME: Conjunctival autograft transplantation for advanced and recurrent pterygium. Ophthalmol 1985;92:1461.

42. Knowles DM, Jakobiec FA: Ocular adnexal lymphoid neoplasm: clinical, histopathologic and electron microscopic and immunologic characteristics. Hum Pathol 1982;13:148–162.

43. Knowles DM, Jakobiec FA, McNally L, Burke JS: Lymphoid hyperplasia and malignant lymphoma occurring in

the ocular adnexa (orbit, conjunctiva and eyelids). Hum Pathol 1990;21:959–973.

44. Lass JH, Grove AS, Paple JJ, et al: Papillomavirus in human conjunctival papillomas. Am J Ophthalmol 95:364–368, 1983.

45. Lauer SA, Malter JS, Meier AJ: Human papillomavirus type 18 in conjunctival intraepithelial neoplasia. Am J Ophthalmol 110:23, 1990.

46. Liesegang TJ: Pigmented conjunctival and scleral lesions. Mayo Clin Proc 1994;69:151–161.

47. Liesegang TJ: Ocular adnexal lymphoproliferative lesions. Mayo Clin Proc 1993:68:1003–1010.

48. Lyell A: Toxic epidermal necrolyses: A reappraisal. Br J Ophthalmol, 1979: 100:69.

49. Mannis MJ: Bacterial conjunctivitis. In: Tasman, W, Jaeger, EA (eds): Duane's Clinical Ophthalmology. Philadelphia: Lippincott-Raven, 1990: Volume 4, Chapter 5.

50. Margo C, Lessner A, Stern A: Intraepithelial sebaceous cell carcinoma of the conjunctiva and the skin of the eyelid. Ophthalmology 99:227, 1992.

51. McCulley, JP, Moore, MB, Matoba AY: Mucus fishing syndrome. Ophthalmology, 1985: 92:1262.

52. McDonnell JM, Mayr AJ, Martin WJ: DNA of human papillomavirus type 16 is dysplastic and malignant lesions of the conjunctiva and cornea. New Engl J Med 320:1442, 1989.

53. McDonnell PJ, McDonnell JM, Kessis T, et al: Detection of human papillomavirus type 6/11 DNA in conjunctival papillomas by insitu hybridization with radioactive probes. Hum Pathol 18:1115, 1987.

54. Medeiros LJ, Harmon DC, Lingood RM, Harris NL: Immunohistologic features predict clinical behavior of orbital and conjunctival lymphoid infiltrates. Blood. 74:2121–2129,1989.

55. Melikian, HE: Treatment of ligneous conjunctivitis. Ann Ophthalmol, 1985: 17:763.

56. Moore, MB, Harrington, J, McCulley, JP: Floppy eyelid syndrome: Management including surgery. Ophthalmology, 1986: 93:184.

57. Moran DJ, Hollows FC: Pterygium and ultraviolet radiation: a positive correlation. Br J Ophthalmol 1984; 68:343.

58. Napora C, Cohen EJ, Genvert GL, et al: Factors associated with conjunctival intraepithelial neoplasia: A case control study. Ophthalmic Surg 21:27, 1990.

59. Neumann, R, Tauber, J, Foster, CS: Remission and recurrence after withdrawal of therapy for ocular cicatricial pemphigoid. Ophthalmology, 1991: 98:383–395.

60. Ni C, Searl SS, Kuo PK, et al: Sebaceous cell carcinomas of the ocular adnexa. Int Ophthalmol Clin 22:23, 1981.

61. Nicholson DH, Herscheler J: Intraocular extension of squamous cell carcinoma of the conjunctiva. Arch Ophthalmol 95:843, 1977.

62. Odrich MG, Jakobiec FA, Lancaster WD, et al: A spectrum of bilateral squamous conjunctival tumors associated with human papillomavirus type 16. Ophthalmology 98:626, 1991.

63. Ostler HB: Diseases of the External Eye and Adnexa. Baltimore: Williams & Wilkins, 1993: 67–74.

64. Passons, GA, Wood, TO: Conjunctival resection for superior limbic keratoconjunctivitis. Ophthalmology, 1984: 91:966.

65. Patten JT, Hyndiuk RA: Granuloma pyogenicum of the conjunctiva. Ann Ophthalmol 7:1588, 1975.

66. Pavan-Langston D: Viral diseases of the cornea and external eye. In: Albert, DM, Jakobiec FA (eds): Principles and Practice of Ophthalmology. Philadelphia: WB Saunders: 1994: Vol 1, Chapter 6.

67. Peksayar G, Soyturk MK, Demiyont M: Long-term results of cryotherapy on malignant epithelial tumors of the conjunctiva. Am J Ophthalmol 107:337, 1989.

68. Poirer RH, Fish JR: Lamellar kertoplasty for recurrent pterygium. Opthalmic Surg 1976; 7:38.

69. Pokorny KS, Hyman BM, Jakobiec FA, et al: Epibulbar choristomas containing lacrimal tissue. Clinical distinction from dermoids and histologic evidence of an origin from the palpebral lobe. Ophthalmology 94:1249, 1987.

70. Rao NA, Hidayat AA, McLean IW, et al: Sebaceous carcinomas of the ocular adnexa: A clinicopathologic study of 104 cases, with five-year follow-up data. Hum Pathol 13:113, 1982.

71. Reed JW, Cashwell LF, Kintworth GK: Corneal manifestations of hereditary benign intraepithelial dyskeratosis. Arch Ophthalmol 97:297, 1979.

72. Roth AM: Solitary keratoacanthoma of the conjunctiva. Am J Ophthalmol 85:647, 1978.

73. Shuler JD, Holland GN, Miles SA, et al: Kaposi sarcoma of the conjunctiva and eyelids associated with the acquired immunodeficiency syndrome. Arch Ophthalmol 107:858, 1989.

74. Singh G, Wilson MR, Foster CS: Mitomycin eye drops as treatment for pterygium. Ophthalmol 1988;95:813.

75. Spencer WH, Zimmerman LE: Conjunctiva. In Spencer WH (ed): Ophthalmic Pathology: An Atlas and Textbook. Philadelphia, WB Saunders, 1985, 109.

76. Stenson, S: Superior limbic keratoconjunctivitis associated with soft contact lens wear. Arch Ophthalmol, 1983: 101:402.

77. Stephens RS: Chlamydial keratitis and conjunctivitis. Chlamydiology. In: Smolin, G, Thoft, RA (eds): The Cornea. Third edition. Boston: Little, Brown & Co., 1994: 227–282.

78. Storb, R, Prentice, RL, Buchner, CD, et al. Graft-versus-host disease and survival in patients with aplastic anemia treated by marrow grafts from HLA-identical siblings: Beneficial effect of a protective environment. N Engl J Med, 1983: 30:302–307.

79. Sugar S, Koebernick S: Localized irritative lesions involving pingueculae. Am J Ophthalmol 1964; 57:94.

80. Syed, NA, Hyndiuk, RA: Infectious conjunctivitis. Inf Dis Clin No Am, 1992: 6:789–805.

81. Thygeson, P: Observations on non-tuberculosis phlyctenular keratoconjunctivitis. Trans Am Acad Ophthalmol Otolaryngol, 1954, 58:128.

82. Townsend WM: Pterygium. In Kaufman HE, editors: The Cornea. New York 1988, Churchill Livingstone.

83. Von Sallman L, Pataton D: Hereditary benign intraepithelial dyskeratosis: I. Ocular manifestations. Arch Ophthalmol 63:421, 1960.

84. Walter WL: Pseudo-epitheliomatous hyperplasia of the conjunctiva. Am J Ophthalmol 53:999, 1962.

85. Wander, AH, Musukawa, T: Unusual appearance of condensed chromatin in conjunctival cells in superior limbic keratoconjunctivitis. Lancet, 1981: 2:42.

86. Waring GOI, Roth AM, Ekins MB: Clinical and pathological descriptions of 17 cases of corneal intraepithelial neoplasia. Am J Ophthalmol 97:547, 1984.

87. Weiter JJ, Jakobiec FA, Iwamoto T: The clinical and morphologic characteristics of Kaposi's sarcoma of the conjunctiva. Am J Ophthalmol 89:546, 1980.

88. Whitcher JP: Chlamydial keratitis and conjunctivitis. Chlamydiology. In: Smolin, G, Thoft, RA (eds): The cornea. Third edition. Boston: Little, Brown & Co., 1994: 282–293.

89. Wilson FM: Toxic and allergic reactions to topical ophthalmic medications. In: Grayson's Diseases of the Cornea. Robert C. Arffa (ed) Mosby Year Book, Baltimore: 1991, Chapter 28.

90. Wilson, FM, II. Adverse external ocular side effects of topical ophthalmic medications. Surv Ophthalmol, 1979: 24:57.

91. Wilson FM, II. Adverse external ocular effects of topical ophthalmic therapy: An epidemiologic, laboratory, and clinical study. Trans Am Ophthalmol Soc, 1983: 81:854.

92. Wilson FM, Ostler HB: Conjunctival papilloma in siblings. Am J Ophthalmol 77:103–107, 1974.

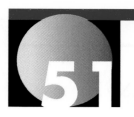

51 Cornea

Thomas J. Liesegang

■ EXAMINATION OF THE CORNEA

Symptoms of corneal disease can include injection of the eye, blurred vision, pain, photophobia, tearing, discharge, swelling of the lids, swelling of the conjunctiva, or blepharospasm. The external examination of the outer eye should be done before using a slit lamp biomicroscope. Daylight is best for detecting true color changes in the conjunctiva and sclera as well as the limbal tissue. The blink rate and amplitude should be observed to detect frequent blinking as in photophobia, incomplete blinking, or blepharospasm. Photophobia can result from several corneal inflammatory conditions. A penlight examination should include anterior segment structures which could influence the cornea (e.g., inflammation of the eyelids, scleritis, conjunctival abnormalities). An area of localized perilimbal injection suggests a peripheral lesion of the cornea.

Slit Lamp Techniques

The slit lamp biomicroscope has two rotating arms, one for the slit lamp illumination unit and the other for the corneal biomicroscope. The adjustable eye pieces allow for a stereoscopic image. The slit lamp has an adjustable light beam with multiple magnifications. The illumination and microscope arm can be focused onto the same spot (direct illumination) or at different locations (indirect illumination). There are several variations of these illumination techniques which allow identification and resolution of corneal and limbal disease (Figure 51–1).

Diffuse illumination with the slit lamp can be done by placing a ground glass diffuser over the light source or by rotating the ocular out of focus in relationship to the light. Most examiners will use a broad light beam of reduced intensity and illuminate the eye from an oblique angle.

With slit or narrow illumination, the light and microscope are focused on the same spot and the slit aperture is narrowed. This direct focal technique allows precise localization of lesions in the cornea and anterior segment with the highest detail. When focused into the anterior chamber, an inflammatory reaction can also be determined.

With indirect illumination, the light beam and microscope are focused at different adjacent spots and this allows the resolution of tiny opacities with three-dimensional images.

With limbal or scleral scatter, the light is directed at the limbus and the cornea is viewed with the microscope. This gives a backscattered light by total internal reflection. This allows better visualization of corneal edema or corneal infiltration.

With the retroillumination technique, light is projected through the edge of the pupil with any abnormality of the iris or cornea seen highlighted through the microscope against a red fundus reflex.

Specular reflection is a technique which sets the slit beam at 60 to 80 degrees from the viewing arm with a narrow slit. The angle of observation is equal to the angle of illumination and this allows structures on the front or back surface of the eye to be assessed.

A combination of these slit lamp techniques allows observation of lesions in the cornea and accentuates the abnormalities. The slit can be used to approximate corneal thickness, anterior chamber depth, and a short beam is used to detect anterior chamber reaction. Spec-

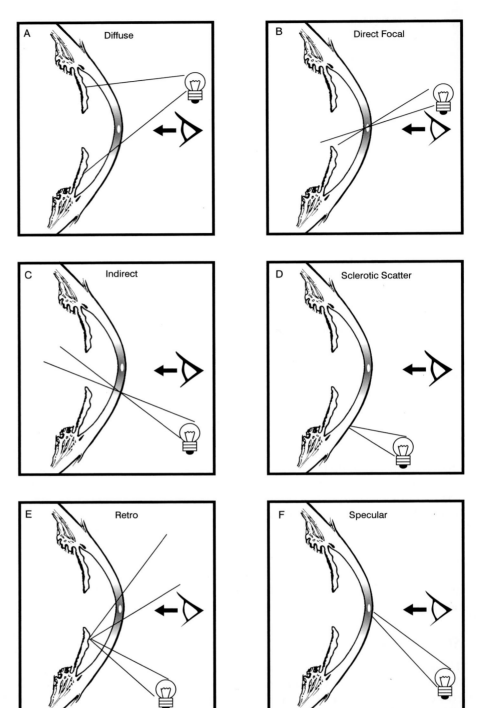

Figure 51–1.
Slit lamp illumination techniques. Different examining techniques used in the slit lamp biomicroscope which are useful in detecting and diagnosing corneal and anterior segment disease. A combination of techniques is necessary to determine the location and surrounding findings in a specific corneal disorder. Modified from Peyman, Sanders, Goldberg (eds): Sugar J. Corneal Examination. In: Principles and Practice of Ophthalmology. Philadelphia: WB Saunders, 1980, p. 392.

ular reflection outlines the endothelial cells. Direct, slit, and retroillumination technique can identify abnormalities of the iris or lens. The anterior vitreous can be viewed with a slit lamp biomicroscope, but special lenses are needed to view the posterior vitreous and retina.

External and slit lamp photography is important in following the course of corneal disease processes and/or surgery. Anterior segment fluorescein angiography has been used to study the circulation of the conjunctiva, episclera, sclera, as well as the vessels in the corneal limbus. It is especially helpful in patients suspected of having vasculitis or vascular nonperfusion.

Corneal Surface and Curvature

The corneal surface and curvature can be evaluated by a number of instruments. Keratometry determines the central corneal curvature by use of an image-doubling device which measures the greater and lesser radii of the oval image of a circle reflected from the corneal surface. Results can be reported as radius of curvature in millimeters or in refracting power in diopters. This keratometer can only measure the central curvature and has limited usefulness in irregular astigmatism or in instances where more information is needed about the peripheral cornea.

More qualitative information about the corneal curvature can be obtained from instruments that reflect the images of multiple concentric circles from the corneal surface. These keratoscopes allow analysis of corneal curvature in both central and peripheral zones. Examples of these are the hand-held Klein keratoscope and Placido disk. Photokeratoscopy can record the image on film. The steepness and flatness of the cornea as well as areas of astigmatism can be discerned. Video keratoscopes are computer assisted machines which capture a topographic map of the cornea and analyze the corneal contour. Since a large number of rings are produced, both the central and peripheral cornea can be measured producing dioptric maps in color-coded patterns which allow interpretation of subtle power distribution on the anterior surface of the cornea (444).

Retinoscopy is valuable in examining the cornea since it can detect subtle changes in the corneal reflex from disturbances of the surface and can be used to detect regular and irregular astigmatism.

Specular Photomicroscopy

Specular photomicroscopy uses the principal of specular reflection to permit visualization and photography of the corneal endothelial mosaic on the back of the cornea. Initial specular microscopic techniques involved the use of a photomicroscope attached to an applanating cone. Wide-field specular photomicroscopes are now available and regional corneal anatomy can be compared. The cornea has to be reasonably clear to allow visualization of the specular reflex. The normal corneal endothelial cell density decreases with age but is normally approximately 2400 cells per square millimeter in middle and older age (Figure 51–2). The coefficient of variation in mean cell area is defined as the mean cell area divided by the standard deviation of the mean cell area; an increased coefficient of variation is a sensitive indicator of endothelial instability. Pleomorphism is a measure of the increased variability in cell shape, usually recorded as the percentage of cells deviating from the normal hexagonal shape. Hexagonal cell percentage greater than 50% generally reflects a healthy endothelium. Polymegathism is a variation in cell size and has been correlated with endothelial dysfunction and with the risk of developing future corneal decompensation. Endothelial cell counts and endothelial cell morphology reflect endothelial physiologic function, although not necessarily in a linear relation. The main value of the technique is in screening patients with suspected endothelial disease or in following patients with serial progressive changes in the endothelium as a result of some insults such as increased intraocular pressure, uveitis, intraocular lenses or other form of surgery, contact lenses, or monitoring the effects of pharmaceutical agents (10).

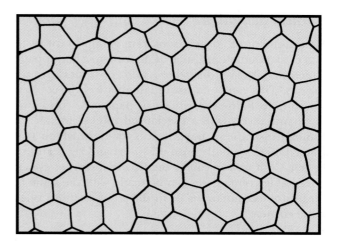

Figure 51–2.
Corneal endothelial pattern. A schematic drawing of the endothelial layer of the cornea demonstrating the hexagonal pattern of the cells, the slight difference in cell shape and size, and the continuous pattern of coverage.

Pachometry

Corneal thickness is a sensitive indicator of endothelial physiology and correlates well with other measures of corneal function. The pachometer is an instrument which measures corneal thickness. Optical pachometers attach to the slit lamp and, although they can be accurate, they are associated with significant interobserver variability. Ultrasonic pachometers are available which are highly accurate and used reliably in refractory surgery. Specular microscopes that applanate the cornea have a pachometer attached to the focusing apparatus so that the corneal thickness can be measured simultaneously.

Tandem Scanning Confocal Microscope

The tandem scanning confocal microscope has the ability to study all cell layers of the cornea, even in the presence of inflammation, edema, or scarring. An applanating cone attached to a microscope enables scanning the cornea through a fixed point of illumination. Images are captured on videotape with enhancement and analysis through a computer system. Morphologic evaluation of organisms and other cells are possible in the epithelium and endothelium as well as within the stroma because of the lateral and axial resolution and serial optical sectioning capabilities (69).

Corneal Sensation

Measurement of corneal sensation is important in several clinical situations, such as neurotropic keratopathy, trigeminal nerve disorders, and postoperative eye surgery. This can be measured qualitatively by comparison with the fellow eye with tissue paper or a cotton wisp or quantitatively with a specialized esthesiometer. The Luneau instrument has a nylon filament which is retracted incrementally until it is short and rigid and can be felt. Comparison can be made with the other eye and reasonable comparison can be made with the same eye on future examinations or in different portions of the same cornea.

Anterior Segment Echography

Anterior segment echography is occasionally used to detect foreign bodies, evaluate ciliary body or iris cysts, to evaluate for tumors, or to evaluate the extent of trauma as well as to measure the eye for placement of an im-

plant. Newer B-scan methods are available for increased resolution evaluation of the anterior segment (ultrasonic biomicroscopy).

Special Stains

Special stains are useful in evaluating the corneal surface and can also be used to evaluate tear function and lacrimal drainage. Topical fluorescein is used to evaluate the tear film, to detect punctate and ulcerative epithelial defects, and to detect leakage from the anterior chamber (Seidel test). Fluorescein is detected with a cobalt blue light filter. It is a nontoxic water soluble dye which can enter the corneal stroma and the anterior chamber, especially in the presence of an epithelial defect. Rose bengal is a derivative of fluorescein which stains devitalized cells or cells which lack a mucin layer. It is especially useful in detecting the epithelial defects in keratoconjunctivitis sicca. Rose bengal can also be used as a photosensitizer and may have an antiviral effect (112).

■ CORNEAL RESPONSE TO DISEASE AND INSULTS

The cornea has a limited number of responses to a wide variety of insults or diseases. There are ways of classify-

ing the major corneal responses which may offer a clue to a diagnostic problem. In most of these conditions, it

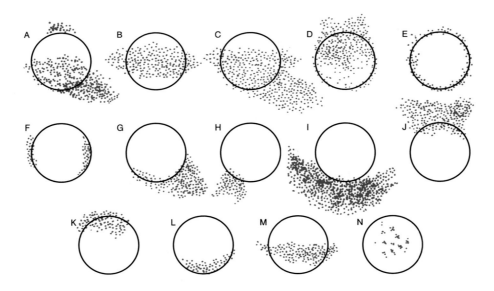

Figure 51–3.
Corneal staining patterns. Staining patterns of various conditions are shown. A. Drug-induced toxicosis or allergy; B. Keratoconjunctivitis sicca; C. Keratoconjunctivitis sicca with superimposed drug toxicosis or allergy; D. Contact lens induced keratoconjunctivitis; E. Limbal staining and soft contact lens wear without papillary keratoconjunctival reaction; F. Typical hard contact lens–induced staining; G. Staining caused by inferior nasal gravitation of increased amounts of conjunctival mucous, especially in patients who rub their eyes; H. Staining from recent insertion of Schirmer strip; I. Factitious (self-induced) conjunctivitis from rubbing or scraping of inferior conjunctiva or from installation of irritating substance into lower cul-de-sac; J. Superior limbic keratoconjunctivitis. K. Fine punctate epithelial keratopathy of vernal catarrh, floppy eyelid syndrome, or early contact lens induced keratoconjunctivitis; L. Staphylococcal blepharoconjunctivitis; M. Lagophthalmos; N. Focal epithelial keratitis caused by adenovirus, molluscum contagiosum, inclusion conjunctivitis, or Thygeson's superficial punctate keratitis.
Modified from Wilson: Trans Am Ophthalmol Soc 1983;81:854.

TABLE 51–1
Differential Diagnosis of Pathologic Corneal Responses

Punctate epithelial keratitis (fine, slightly depressed epithelial lesions)
  Systemic disease (keratitis sicca)
  Viral disease (herpes simplex, herpes zoster, adenovirus, molluscum contagiosum)
  Bacterial disease (Staphylococcal blepharitis)
  Chlamydial disease (inclusion conjunctivitis, trachoma)
  Trauma (trichiasis, recurrent erosion, exposure)
  Toxic (drug or preservative induced)
  Neurologic (neurotrophic keratitis)
  Allergic (vernal conjunctivitis, atopic)
  Unknown (superior limbic keratoconjunctivitis, Thygeson's superficial punctate keratitis)
Superficial epithelial keratopathy (round, small or large accumulations of epithelial cells)
  Blepharitis
  Meibomian gland dysfunction
  Lid position abnormalities (trichiasis, entropion, ectropion, lagophthalmos)
  Viral lid disease (HSV, VZV, molluscum contagiosum)
  Viral conjunctival disease (adenovirus, chlamydial disease)
  Drug toxicosis
  Dermatoses (psoriasis, ichthyosis, mycosis fungoides)
  Conjunctival scarring (pemphigoid, Stevens-Johnson)
  Allergic disease (vernal, atopic)
Focal epithelial keratitis (coarse grouped epithelial lesions)
  Thygeson superficial punctate keratitis
  Herpes simplex
  Herpes zoster
  Adenovirus
  Adult inclusion conjunctivitis
  Drug toxicosis
  Measles
Dendritic keratopathy (epithelial elevations in a dendritic pattern)
  Herpes simplex
  Herpes zoster
  Contact lens induced
  Mucoid plaque
  Healing epithelial defect (e.g., recurrent erosion)
Subepithelial nummular opacities
  Viral (HSV, VZV, EKC)
  Unknown (Nummular keratitis)
  Leprosy
  Chlamydia (trachoma, adult inclusion conjunctivitis)
Filamentary keratitis (small mucoid deposits adherent to the corneal surface)
  Viral (HSV)
  Mechanical (after patching)
  Traumatic (after corneal abrasions)

  Keratoconjunctivitis sicca
  Superior limbic keratoconjunctivitis
  Neurotrophic keratopathy
  Drug toxicosis
Superficial corneal vascularization (micropannus <2 mm beyond limbus)
  Contact lens wear
  Superior limbic keratoconjunctivitis
  Vernal conjunctivitis
  Inclusion conjunctivitis
  Staphylococcal blepharitis
Superficial corneal neovascularization (gross pannus >2 mm beyond limbus)
  Contact lens wear
  Acne rosacea
  Atopic keratoconjunctivitis
  Phlyctenulosis
  Trachoma
  Staphylococcal blepharitis
  Herpes simplex keratitis
Increased visibility of corneal nerves
  Keratoconus
  Neurofibromatosis
  Multiple endocrine neoplasia type 1
  Fuchs corneal dystrophy
  Ichthyoses
  Aging
  Primary amyloidosis
  Refsum's syndrome
Corneal pigment whorls
  Amiodarone
  Fabry's disease
  Iron
  Chloroquine
  Chlorpromazine
  Indomethacin
  Tamoxifen
  Tilerone
  Quinacrine
Corneal Crystals
  Schnyder crystalline dystrophy
  Tangier disease
  Lecithin cholesterol–acyltransferase deficiency
  Band keratopathy
  Cystinosis
  Tyrosinosis
  Hyperuricemia
  Multiple myeloma
  Porphyria
  Secondary lipid keratopathy

Modified from Arffa RC. Grayson's Diseases of the Cornea. Mosby Year Book. St. Louis, 1991, p 47–55.

is pattern recognition which permits a diagnosis (1, 42). Among the important clinical findings are the pattern of epithelial staining (punctate epithelial keratitis, superficial epithelial keratopathy, focal epithelial keratitis), presence of corneal filaments or subepithelial nummular opacities, increased visibility of corneal nerves, decreased corneal sensation, corneal deposits or crystals, immune corneal rings, and the location and depth of corneal vascularization. Diseases to be considered in the presence of these responses are tabulated in Tables 51–1 and 51–2 modified from the work of many (17, 303). The pattern of staining on the cornea or conjunctiva with rose bengal or fluorescein is also suggestive of a specific etiology as shown in Figure 51–3.

The vast collection of diseases of the cornea will be divided for purposes of presentation into the following sections which will discuss specific entities: 1) corneal dysgenesis, degenerations and dystrophies; 2) corneal infections; 3) surface diseases of the anterior segment; and 4) peripheral corneal inflammatory disease.

■ CORNEAL DYSGENESIS

The corneal structural alterations caused by abnormalities in development present at birth and can be caused by genetic, traumatic, toxic, or infectious problems during gestation. They are usually attributable to problems in development occurring between the sixth and sixteenth week of gestation. They may be inherited, are nonprogressive, and can be unilateral or bilateral. They can be central, peripheral, or the entire cornea can be involved; sometimes associated systemic abnormalities are present. They can be divided into abnormalities of corneal size, shape and curvature, or diseases of anterior segment dysgenesis (mesodermal dysgenesis).

TABLE 51–2
Principal Etiologic Agents in Epithelial Keratitis

Infections
Herpes simplex virus
Herpes zoster virus
Molluscum contagiosum
Measles
Mumps
Adenoviral disease
Infectious mononucleosis
Chlamydia inclusion
Trachoma
Staphylococcal blepharitis

Mechanical
Exposure, poor blink
Keratitis sicca
Trichiasis
Entropion
Occlusion
Spray keratitis (aerosols)
Posttraumatic erosion
Overuse of contact lenses

Toxic
Medication (neomycin, gentamycin, timolol, topical anesthetics)
Radiation
Chemicals or toxins
Ultraviolet light
Arc welding
Acne rosacea

Others
Neurotrophic
Anterior membrane dystrophy
Recurrent erosion

Unknown Cause
Superficial punctate keratitis of Thygeson
Superior limbic keratitis of Theodore

Abnormalities of Corneal Size, Shape, or Curvature

Microcornea

A corneal diameter less than 10 mm is termed microcornea. If the entire eye is small but otherwise normal, the condition is called nanophthalmos. Microcornea can be unilateral or bilateral and transmitted as an autosomal dominant or recessive trait. The corneal curvature can be flat or steep. The visual acuity can be normal in the absence of other accompanying ocular abnormalities. Microcornea, however, can be associated with a wide variety of ocular conditions (congenital glaucoma, angle closure glaucoma, persistent hyperplastic vitreous, cataract, coloboma, corneal leukoma, iris coloboma) or systemic syndromes (Ehlers-Danlos, Weill-Marchesani, Rieger syndrome, fetal alcohol syndrome, rubella, trisomy 13–15).

Megalocornea

A cornea that measures 13 mm or more in the horizontal diameter is known as megalocornea. It is usually bilateral and symmetric and an x-linked recessive trait probably linked to the Xq12-q26 region; 90% of patients are males. Occasionally this is transmitted as an autosomal dominant trait and rarely autosomal recessive. The cornea is otherwise normal and the condition is nonprogressive. Other ocular abnormalities may be present including a deep anterior chamber, ectopic lentis, anterior embryotoxon, Krukenberg spindle, heavy pigmentation of trabecular meshwork, arcus senilis, and iris transillumination defects. Megalocornea can be associated with the systemic syndromes of Down, Marfan, and Apert.

Cornea Plana

In cornea plana, the corneal curvature measures 20 to 30 diopters (normal 42 to 46). This corresponds to the normal curvature of the sclera. Some scleralization of the cornea occurs and this may be a form of sclerocornea. Rarely diffuse opacification of the central cornea can be seen. There is usually a hyperopic refractive error in this dominant or recessive condition. There may be concurrent anterior segment abnormalities (iris coloboma, congenital cataract, glaucoma) or systemic conditions (osteogenesis imperfecta, Hurler syndrome, Trisomy 13).

Anterior Segment Dysgenesis

Anterior segment dysgenesis (also called mesenchymal dysgenesis) is a spectrum of corneal, iris, angle, and lens abnormalities that appear to be related to abnormal development of mesenchyme-derived neural crest forming the anterior segment of the eye (16, 441, 442) (Figure 51–4). It includes the disorders posterior embryotoxon, Axenfeld anomaly, Reiger anomaly, Peters anomaly, and circumscribed posterior keratoconus. During early development, mesenchyme migrates centrally across the opening of the optic cup in waves: the first wave gives rise to the corneal endothelium, the second to the corneal stroma, and the third to the iris stroma. As the tissue organizes and recedes, the anterior segment structures are developed. Incomplete migration and differentiation, or incomplete recession of the mesenchyme, causes these congenital abnormalities. Waring et al have suggested a stepladder classification, which although not pure, is helpful in understanding these conditions and making a specific diagnosis in many patients (424).

Posterior Embryotoxon

Posterior embryotoxon is a thickened and more centrally displaced anterior border ring of Schwalbe. This is a normal circumferential collagenous band at the junction of Descemet's membrane and the trabecular meshwork. It is usually visible only by gonioscopy, but in patients with posterior embryotoxon it is visible at the slit lamp. Posterior embryotoxon is often inherited as an autosomal dominant trait. In itself, it does not cause any visual problems.

Axenfeld Anomaly and Syndrome

In Axenfeld anomaly, posterior embryotoxon is accompanied by iris strands extending across the anterior chamber to attach to a prominent Schwalbe's line. When glaucoma occurs because of secondary angle anomalies, the condition is called Axenfeld syndrome. Both conditions are dominantly inherited and rarely can be associated with systemic disease.

Rieger Anomaly and Syndrome

In Rieger anomaly there is posterior embryotoxon, prominent iris processes, and atrophy of the iris stroma. Iris abnormalities may consist of peripheral anterior synechia, corectopia, ectropion uvea, and pseudopolycoria. Glaucoma occurs in 50 to 60%. Rieger syndrome consists of Rieger anomaly plus other skeletal, facial, cranial, or dental anomalies. Transmission is usually autosomal dominant.

Circumscribed Posterior Keratoconus

This is a rare disorder characterized by one or more localized crater defects on the posterior corneal surface with the concavity facing towards the anterior chamber. It is usually unilateral and central with a mild stromal haze overlying. The anterior corneal surface is normal and progression does not occur. Both Descemet's membrane and endothelium are present but show distinct abnormalities. There may be other associated anomalies of anterior segment dysgenesis. It has no relationship to anterior keratoconus.

Peters Anomaly

Peters anomaly is a central corneal opacity, usually bilateral, corresponding to defects in the posterior stroma, Descemet's membrane and endothelium. Most cases are sporadic, although inheritance patterns are recognized in some. There are two variants. Peters anomaly Type 1 shows typical nebular opacities in the pupillary access, bordered by iris strands that cross the anterior chamber from the iris collarette. The lens is clear. Peters anomaly Type 2 has the same corneal findings but the lens has a cataract or is dislocated. This latter type is associated with more severe ocular and systemic malformations. This congenital anomaly is probably caused by incomplete central migration of mesenchyme (384). When systemic anomalies such as cardiac defects, cleft lip, cleft palate, craniofacial dysplasia, or skeletal changes occur, it is called Peters-plus syndrome.

Sclerocornea

In sclerocornea, the scleral opaque tissues extend onto the peripheral cornea and sometimes onto the central cornea (Figure 51–5). Most cases are bilateral, although asymmetric and stationary. There is no evident hereditary pattern. Many cases are associated with cornea

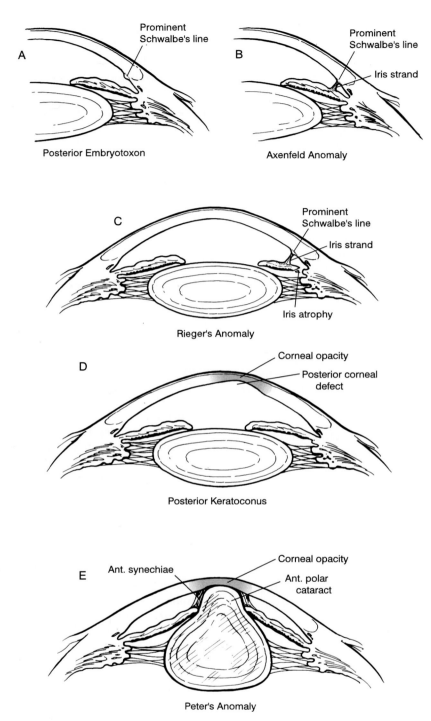

Figure 51–4.
Corneal dysgeneses syndromes. A. Posterior embryotoxon is a prominent ring of Schwalbe; B. Axenfeld anomaly is a prominent ring of Schwalbe with iris strands to the ring; C. Rieger anomaly is a prominent ring of Schwalbe, prominent iris strands, and iris atrophy with corectopia. D. Posterior keratoconus is a defect in the posterior cornea with overlying corneal scarring. E. Peters anomaly comes in various forms all having a central corneal scar with a posterior defect and central iris adhesions.

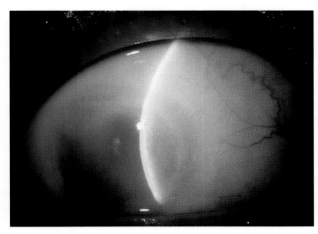

Figure 51–5.
Sclerocornea. A 20-year-old boy born with sclerocornea with extension of the opaque scleral tissues onto the cornea and absence of the usual limbal change in contour. The other eye had minimal sclerocornea with good visual acuity.

plana discussed above. Other ocular or somatic abnormalities can be associated. Ultrastructural studies show that the abnormal tissue has features of the sclera. Sclerocornea probably results from developmental arrest of limbal differentiation.

Congenital Hereditary Endothelial Dystrophy

Congenital hereditary endothelial dystrophy (CHED) is now more appropriately classified as an anterior segment dysgenesis. At birth, or shortly after, there is bilateral corneal edema not associated with vascularization or inflammation. The stroma is significantly swollen with slight epithelial edema and thickening of Descemet's membrane (see Posterior Corneal Dystrophies for further discussion).

■ CORNEAL DEGENERATIONS

Corneal degenerations are usually unilateral or at least asymmetric, located peripherally and frequently accompanied by vascularization. They occur usually in middle life without an inheritance pattern and may be progressive. They may be caused or exacerbated by aging, trauma, or other ocular inflammations (15, 378, 384).

Corneal Aging Changes

Corneal aging is associated with biometric and clinical changes which are summarized by Greiner and Kenyon (151). The cornea is relatively large at birth (9.5 mm) and reaches full size of approximately 11.7 mm by age 1 or 2. Thus, although the eye volume increases nearly threefold, the cornea changes little between birth and full maturity. The central corneal thickness of 0.520 mm is approximately the same in newborn and the aged with no evident significant variation. The corneal curvature is steep at birth (7.11 mm) but becomes flatter until adulthood (7.80 mm). With age, the cornea has a tendency to become steeper, perhaps related to changes in astigmatism. During aging, astigmatism changes from primarily with the rule to against the rule, probably associated with a decrease in eyelid tension (13,418). The corneal asphericity changes with age from a flat cornea centrally (compared with the periphery) to the opposite in adults where the central cornea is steeper than the periphery (427). With age, the cornea has a decrease in refractive index as well as becoming overall flatter. Astigmatism in the eye is influenced most by the cornea, although the lens can affect the total astigmatism. Infants have little astigmatism, but it increases during childhood, especially in those patients with increased spherical refractive errors (166). If astigmatism is marked, it usually changes little in young adults. With the rule astigmatism is present in 92% of children age 10 but only 14% of patients at age 80 (151). Astigmatism can vary perhaps related to the effects of corneal hydration and eyelid pressure on the aging cornea (406).

Clinical signs of aging affect most layers of the cornea (151). The corneal epithelium has a decrease in luster and a decrease in the refractive index probably associated with changes in hydration or with decline in lubricating properties of the tear film. There is a decline in corneal sensation beginning after age 40, possibly related to decrease in water content, nerve atrophy, or thickening of the fibrous structure of the cornea (273). There is a significant increase in measured corneal fragility although the reason it is clinically significant is unknown (274).

There is increase in corneal stromal relucency and increase in light scattering in the cornea with age correlating with a decrease in the distance between the collagen fibers and a breakdown of collagen fibers. The Hudson-Stahli line is a thin pigment line in the central lower cornea composed of iron deposition in the cytoplasm of epithelial cells. It occurs in most patients over age 50, especially males. It does not disturb the vision (141).

Aging changes in Bowman's layer can be manifested as a crocodile shagreen (mosaic shagreen of Vogt) which are grayish white polygonal opacities most prominent centrally. It is usually bilateral and does not affect vision. A similar morphologic change can also been seen in association with hypotony.

Descemet's membrane is the basement membrane secreted by the corneal endothelium. It has an anterior vertical banded pattern of collagen and a posterior nonbanded pattern of collagen. It doubles in thickness every 40 years although it is not necessarily uniform throughout age and cannot be used to predict age. Hassall-Henle warts are localized thickenings in the periphery of the endothelium which are excrescences of Descemet's that project toward the anterior chamber. They are round, small, and break up the endothelial mosaic. They are similar to corneal gutatta except that they occur in the periphery. Gutatta are located centrally and occur more commonly with age, especially with females. They may be an indication of future endothelial degeneration. They are a prominent part of Fuchs' endothelial dystrophy and also occur in association with trauma or inflammation, where they may be transient. The endothelial cell density on the back of the cornea is important in maintaining corneal deturgescence. At birth approximately 3000 cells per square millimeter are present, and they decrease to approximately 2000 cells per square millimeter in later life with progressive enlargement of the original endothelial cells to fill in the gap. The source of the cell loss is unknown but is hastened with intraocular surgery and corneal inflammation. The endothelial mosaic is hexagonal in childhood. With the decrease in cell density, the cells enlarge, migrate, and reorganize to maintain an intact layer. The decrease of hexagonal cells with age is a faithful marker of the health of the cornea. The mean cell size and degree of variation of cells increases with age as the number of hexagonal cells decrease (169, 222, 394, 423).

It is difficult to separate the normal aging changes discussed here from the corneal degenerations, in that the latter are frequently an extension of the former. Listed below are some of the more common degenerative changes.

Epithelial Basement Membrane Dystrophy

The epithelial basement membrane dystrophy (discussed under dystrophies) may be more appropriately termed a degenerative condition.

Limbal Girdle of Vogt

The limbal girdle of Vogt is a symmetric arcuate yellowish-white opacity in the peripheral cornea which is a degeneration of Bowman's layer. It is seen at the 3- and 9-o'clock positions in patients over age 40. It does not encircle the cornea. It may be separated from the limbus by a transparent interval. Histologically, there is destruction of Bowman's layer with deposition of calcium in areas of elastotic and hyalin degeneration with hypertrophy of the overlying epithelium. It resembles early band degeneration (395).

Corneal Farinata

Corneal farinata is a bilateral speckling of small grayish-white opacities in the deep corneal stroma best seen with retroillumination. It does not affect vision and can be a familial trait.

Corneal Arcus

Corneal arcus is an asymmetric bilateral infiltration of white-yellowish deposits in the peripheral cornea characterized by a narrow band of clear peripheral cornea. It begins in the inferior and then superior cornea but can extend to encircle the cornea. The deposits of cholesterol, cholesterol esters, and neutral glycerides are located in the extracellular corneal stroma. It is associated with age but also with elevated cholesterol and low density lipoprotein. It is seen in nearly all patients over age 80 but occurs earlier in blacks. Evaluation for hyperlipidemia should be done in patients under age 40 (12, 81). Unilateral or asymmetric arcus may indicate carotid vascular disease on the less affected side.

Senile Marginal Furrow

Senile marginal furrow degeneration is a noninflammatory corneal thinning which develops in the periphery usually in association with arcus senilis. The inner margin is steeper than the outer margin. It begins in the inferior cornea and can extend 360° around the cornea. Histologically, there is fragmentation of corneal collagen.

Terrien Marginal Degeneration

Terrien marginal degeneration is a distinct variant of marginal corneal thinning seen in young males, often bilateral but asymmetric. It generally starts superiorly as an opacification and slowly progresses over years with stromal thinning and ectasia with an intact epithelium. A yellow border of lipid is characteristically present at the advancing edge with vessels traversing. The astigmatism is usually against the rule and marked; corneal perforation can occur with minor trauma. There is a form associated with inflammation, necrosis, and neovascularization of the peripheral cornea (20). Electron microscopy has shown increased lysosomal activity in histiocytic cells with active phagocytosis of collagen and ground substance (400). When extreme corneal thinning develops, a lamellar or full thickness corneoscleral graft may be necessary, although gradual thinning of the graft may also occur (53).

Band Keratopathy

Band keratopathy is a deposition of hydroxyapatite deposits of calcium carbonate in the epithelial basement

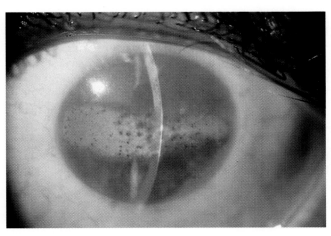

Figure 51–6.
Band keratopathy. A deposition of calcium carbonate in the epithelial basement membrane of a 20-year-old man with long-standing juvenile rheumatoid arthritis. This band keratopathy is periodically removed with chelation with EDTA.

membrane, Bowman's layer, and a superficial stroma (Figure 51–6). It is seen in association with localized ocular inflammatory diseases or systemic diseases. It is more commonly seen in conditions where calcium or bone is deposited in other portions of the eye (294). In calcific band shaped keratopathy, the band is largely in the palpebral fissure and has a Swiss cheese appearance with holes where corneal nerves penetrate. Histopathologically, the earliest changes consist of basophilic staining of the basement membrane followed by involvement of Bowman's membrane. The cause of the gray-white calcium precipitation may involve gaseous exchanges at the corneal surface leading to decreased carbon dioxide and elevated pH (294). Alternatively, precipitation of calcium may be triggered by elevation

TABLE 51–3
Causes of Band Keratopathy

Ocular Disease	Systemic Conditions
Chronic uveitis (esp. JRA)	Hypercalcemia
Long standing glaucoma	Renal failure
Long standing corneal edema	Hyperparathyroidism
Ph thisis bulbi	Sarcoidosis
Spheroidal degeneration	Multiple myeloma
Intracorneal viscoat	Vitamin D excess
Interstitial keratitis	Milk alkali syndrome
Exposure keratopathy	Paget disease
	Bone metastates
	Ichthyosis
	Gout (urate)
	Discoid lupus erythematosus

of pH, evaporation, or an increase in calcium or phosphate locally. The calcific deposits owing to local ocular disease are usually extracellular, whereas the deposits are intracellular with systemic disease. Band keratopathy can also occur from deposition of urates in the cornea; these are usually brown (115). Mercury-containing eye drops (previously used in preservatives) can cause band keratopathy (198). Severe dry eye, probably because of the concentration of tear calcium, can be associated with band keratopathy (231). Some of the local and systemic causes of band keratopathy are shown in Table 51–3. Many situations are idiopathic.

Band keratopathy can be treated with the application of calcium-binding agents such as 0.4% ethylenediaminotetra-acetic acid (EDTA) or by superficial keratectomy (452).

Corneal Amyloidosis

Corneal deposits of amyloid can be seen in localized amyloidosis (primary or secondary) and in primary systemic disease. It is not seen in secondary systemic amyloidosis. These deposits are not associated with inflammation. Clinically, the corneal amyloid lesions are salmon pink or yellow raised fleshy masses which create a nodular corneal or conjunctival surface (139). Primary localized amyloidosis occurs in lattice corneal dystrophy, gelatinous droplike dystrophy, and polymorphic stromal dystrophy. These are discussed under stromal corneal dystrophies. Secondary localized amyloidosis is seen in corneal trauma and other anterior corneal disorders (neoplasms, trachoma, glaucoma, lipoidal degeneration, climatic droplet keratopathy) and may be present in up to 35% of corneal pathologic assessment specimens (267). There are three kinds of secondary amyloid deposits: subepithelial masses resembling degenerative pannus, lamellar deposits in the deep stroma, and perivascular deposits associated with corneal neovascularization. In primary systemic amyloidosis, purpuric and papillary lesions of the eyelid and conjunctiva occur with occasional skin changes, cranial nerve palsies, visceral symptoms, ophthalmoplegia, and ptosis. In a familial form, veil-like vitreous opacities or glaucoma occurs (194).

The amyloid protein is identical to amyloid elsewhere. Histopathologically, the deposits are amorphous, eosinophilic, hyalin-like without inflammatory reaction. Amyloid stains metachromatically with crystal violet or methyl violet, produces secondary fluorescence with thioflavine, and shows unique red-green birefringence after Congo red staining. There are several amyloid types probably produced as defective immunoglobins from tissue or from serum (83). Therapy of secondary localized corneal amyloidosis is usually surgical removal either by scraping or deep lamellar or penetrating keratoplasty.

Spheroidal Degeneration

Several names have been applied to the golden brown, spherical, translucent, droplike deposits seen in the subepithelial layers of the conjunctiva and cornea. It has been variously termed in different parts of the world as spheroidal degeneration, climatic droplet keratopathy, elastoid degeneration, proteinaceous degeneration, Labrador keratopathy, and chronic actinic keratopathy. These nonhereditary, climate-related deposits begin peripherally at 3- and 9-o'clock and remain in the interpalpebral zone as they advance centrally. The deposits may opacify, coalesce, darken, and autofluoresce. Spheroidal degeneration has been divided into three types: primary corneal, secondary corneal, and conjunctival (127, 128, 129, 158). Primary corneal spheroidal degeneration is related to age and is usually bilateral without association with ocular disease. Patients complain of intermittent pain, deterioration of vision, and photophobia. The second corneal type is seen in association with long-standing ocular disease (Fuchs' corneal dystrophy, lattice dystrophy, chronic herpes infection) or in adverse climatic conditions. This may be unilateral or bilateral, and either central or peripheral. The conjunctival form can occur in isolation, or in association with either of the corneal types; it is seen in association with pterygium and pingueculum (21, 293, 401). Actinic exposure is probably the initiator of all types of spheroid degeneration since it is more common in areas of the world with greater amounts of sunlight, extremes of temperature, and patients with outdoor occupations (138, 402). On histopathologic examination, the spheroidal material in the epithelium and superficial stroma is an acidophilic, Periodic acid-Schiff negative, amorphous mass. By electron microscopy, it is proteinaceous and extracellular. Spheroidal degeneration is of unknown cause but most likely represents an elastotic degeneration of stromal collagen. It may result from an interaction of ultraviolet light and plasma proteins within the corneal stroma (186). The disease usually requires no treatment although rarely superficial keratectomy, or lamellar or penetrating keratoplasty is required.

Salzmann Degeneration

Salzmann degeneration is a noninflammatory condition with multiple, superficial, bluish-white nodules in the midperiphery sometimes arranged in a circular fashion around the pupil. They usually develop slowly and are asymptomatic unless they affect visual axis. Rarely they can erode the epithelial surface. This degeneration occurs in adults and is usually asymmetrically bilateral and more common in females. It is seen in association with prior corneal inflammation from phlyctenular disease, trachoma, vernal keratoconjunc-

tivitis, interstitial keratitis, epithelial basement membrane disease, and contact lens wear (453).

Histopathologic examination shows degenerative changes in the corneal epithelium with variable thinness. There is excessive secretion of basement membrane-like material with a break in Bowman's layer (414). There is degeneration of collagen perhaps with an active immune process. Treatment is usually not necessary. Simple excision or stripping can be sufficient; rarely, lamellar or penetrating keratoplasty is necessary. Recurrence can occur (371).

Corneal Keloids

Corneal keloids are rare, hypertrophic scars after corneal injury, inflammation, or trauma. They have a higher incidence in blacks. They are a result of exuberant myofibroblasts originating from stromal cells (173). Therapy is surgical but can result in a recurrence of the same problem (297).

Lipid Degeneration

Lipid degeneration of the cornea can occur in primary or secondary form. Rare primary lipid degeneration occurs with no prior history of ocular disease (8, 130, 357). Consideration should be given to rare causes of serum lipoprotein abnormalities such as Tangier disease and lecithin-cholesterol acyltransferase (LCAT) deficiency (144) although serum lipids are usually normal. Secondary lipid degeneration is more common and is a result of corneal vascularization from trauma, interstitial keratitis, and especially herpes zoster keratitis. The lipid is a dense, yellow-white opacification or cholesterol crystals that may fan out with feathery edges from leaking blood vessels. The material consists of neutral fats, phospholipids, and cholesterol in both the primary and secondary lipid degenerations. The specific pathogenesis is unknown.

Argon laser treatment of corneal vessels can reduce the extent or density of the lipid opacities. Rarely, surgical penetrating keratoplasty is required with possible recurrences in the graft (130).

Coat's White Ring

Coat's white ring is a small white corneal semicircular ring usually located in an area of prior corneal injury from a foreign body. It represents iron deposits at the level of Bowman's layer or the anterior stroma (290).

Iron Deposition

Iron deposition of the cornea is seen secondarily in clinical settings (Figure 51–7). Hudson-Stahli line is seen in the lower central cornea as a normal aging change.

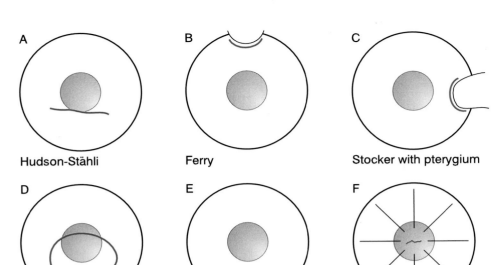

A. Hudson-Stähli

B. Ferry

C. Stocker with pterygium

D. Fleisher (keratoconus)

E. Pigment around Coats ring

F. Pigment with radial keratotomy

Figure 51–7.
Corneal iron lines. Pattern of pigment iron lines as seen with A. Hudson Stähli line which is a physiologic variant; B. Ferry line in front of a bleb; C. Stocker line in front of a pterygium; D. A Fleischer line at the base of a keratoconus ring; E. Pigment around a Coats' ring; F. Pigment near incisions of radial keratotomy.

Ferry's line is seen in advance of a filtering bleb. Stocker's line is seen adjacent to the head of a pterygium. Fleischer's ring is seen at the base of a keratoconus cone. Histologic examination all reveals hemosiderin deposits in the basal corneal epithelial cells and the condition is probably related to poor tear flow or surface wetting (27,141,181). The source of the iron may be perilimbal blood vessels (49). Metallic foreign bodies and therapeutically used metals (copper, gold, silver, iron) can also be deposited in the cornea (49).

■ CORNEAL DYSTROPHIES

Corneal dystrophies usually appear in the first or second decade of life and show a hereditary pattern (usually autosomal dominant), and are symmetric, bilateral and may be progressive. There is generally no systemic disease. They also tend to affect the central cornea without signs of local inflammation. Exceptions to each of these generalizations occur (Table 51–4). The corneal dystrophies have been classified anatomically since only a few of them have a unifying pathogenic mechanism (Table 51–5), (Figure 51–8). There is some overlap of the degenerative disorders and the dystrophies as well as the ectatic corneal changes.

TABLE 51–4
Characteristics and Exceptions of Corneal Dystrophies

Characteristic	Exceptions
Autosomal dominant heredity	Autosomal recessive
	Macular dystrophy
	May be autosomal recessive
	Congenital hereditary endothelial dystrophy
	Posterior polymorphous dystrophy
Bilateral involvement	Rare unilateral cases
Central involvement	—
Onset early in life	Fuchs dystrophy in later life
	Epithelial basement membrane dystrophy in mid-life
Slowly progressive	Some relatively stable
One layer of corneal involved	Macular dystrophy involves stroma and endothelium
No associated systemic disease	Central crystalline dystrophy may have high cholesterol

TABLE 51–5
Principal Corneal Dystrophies

Anterior Corneal Dystrophies

Epithelial basement membrane (map–dot–fingerprint)
Meesmann
Reis Bückler
Gelatinous droplike

Stromal Dystrophies

Macular
Granular
Lattice
  Type I
  Type II
  Type III
Schnyder crystalline
Fleck
Central cloudy

PreDescemet's Dystrophies

(Multiple variants)

Posterior Corneal Dystrophies

Congenital hereditary endothelial
Corneal guttata
Fuchs endothelial
Posterior polymorphous

Anterior Corneal Dystrophies

Dystrophies of the anterior cornea can involve the epithelium, basement membrane, and Bowman's membrane. The major ones are the epithelial basement membrane dystrophy, Meesmann dystrophy and Reis-Bückler dystrophy (Figure 51–9).

Epithelial Basement Membrane Dystrophy

The epithelial basement membrane (also called Cogan microcystic epithelial dystrophy or map-dot-fingerprint dystrophy) is a common bilateral epithelial dystrophy with occasional autosomal dominant inheritance (220, 422). In one study, as many as 75% of patients over age 50 may have one of these abnormalities (430). This frequency suggests more of a corneal degeneration. It is more common in women, usually in the 40 to 70 age range (221). The pattern of epithelial and basement membrane abnormalities varies considerably as do the symptoms. Maps, fingerprints, dots, blebs, and nets may be seen; they vary in location and presence from time to time (Figure 51–10). The dots are intraepithelial white opacities of varying size which look like putty. Occasionally they are clustered with slight elevation of the epithelium over the dots. Fingerprint lines are groups of concentric contoured lines, some long and thick in various areas of the cornea best seen in retroillumination. Maps are geographic shaped irregular circumscribed areas which vary in size and have a ground glass appearance. They are best seen with broad oblique illumination. Blebs are clear, round, bubblelike areas best seen with retroillumination (previously bleb-like dystrophy). Nets are rows of blebs or refractile lines that follow the normal anterior corneal mosaic.

Although most patients are asymptomatic, many patients have decreased vision from surface irregularities or they may get recurrent epithelial erosions. Irregular astigmatism can result in variable vision. Symptoms of recurrent erosions include pain, tearing, foreign body sensation, and photophobia. Characteristically, the

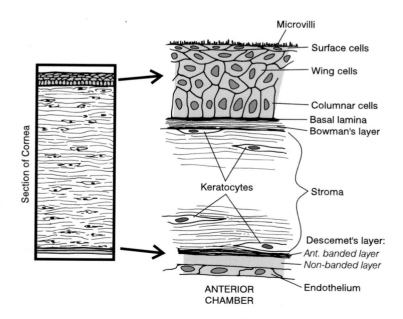

Figure 51–8.
Layers of the cornea. A schematic drawing emphasizing the different layers of the cornea with corneal dystrophies affecting predominantly one of the layers.

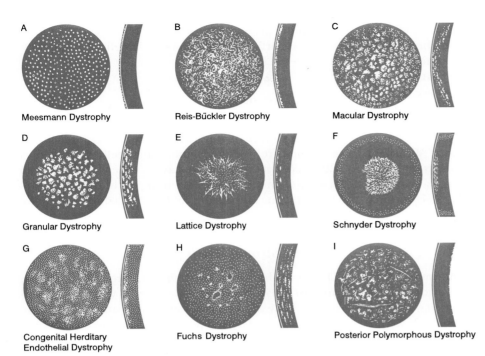

Figure 51–9.
Corneal dystrophy patterns. A. Meesmann dystrophy; B. Reis Bückler dystrophy; C. Macular dystrophy; D. Granular dystrophy; E. Lattice dystrophy; F. Schnyder's dystrophy; G. Congenital hereditary endothelial dystrophy; H. Fuchs dystrophy; I. Posterior polymorphous dystrophy. Modified from Goldberg (ed): Bron AJ, Tripathi RC. Corneal Disorders. In: Genetic and Metabolic Eye Disease. Boston: Little Brown, 1974, p. 283.

symptoms develop upon awakening in the morning and many individuals can anticipate an erosion before opening their eyes (118). Similar symptoms of recurrent corneal erosion can also be associated with trauma, but these erosions are localized to the area of prior corneal injury. The symptoms of anterior membrane corneal dystrophy tend to decrease over time (usually years). The histopathologic assessment shows epithelial basement abnormalities with intraepithelial extensions. The dot opacities are intraepithelial microcysts filled with nuclear and cytoplasmic debris representing liquified epithelial cells beneath aberrant epithelial basement membrane. The maplike changes are multilaminar thickenings of the basement membrane into the overlying epithelium which usually lacks hemidesmosomes. Fingerprint lines are linear projections of fibrogranular material into the epithelial layer with a thickened basement membrane. Blebs are localized mounds of fibrogranular protein between Bowman's layer and epithelial basement membrane (325, 350).

Epithelial basement dystrophy is common with symptoms overall rare. Recurrent corneal erosions are treated with hypertonic solutions or ointments, patching, or bandage soft contact lens therapy. In severe cases, scraping of the redundant epithelial basement membrane, superficial keratectomy, or excimer phototherapeutic keratectomy is helpful (60, 61, 454). Anterior stomal puncture with a needle tip or laser may result in production of a new basement membrane with a fibrocytic reaction (193, 266). This is usually only indicated if the area of recurrent erosion can be identified. Irregular astigmatism from the dystrophy is frequently improved with a rigid gas permeable contact lens.

Meesmann Dystrophy

Meesmann corneal dystrophy (hereditary epithelial dystrophy) is a rare dominantly inherited symmetric disorder of the corneal epithelium evident early in life without symptoms. Patients may later complain of foreign

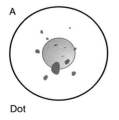

Dot

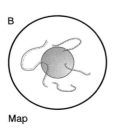

Map

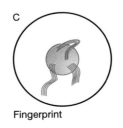

Fingerprint

Figure 51–10.
Anterior membrane corneal dystrophy. The map-dot-fingerprint patterns of anterior membrane corneal dystrophy.

body sensation and slightly decreased vision (51, 114). Intraepithelial cysts are seen as myriad small clear or opaque punctate opacities in the interpalpebral zone of the cornea seen best with direct focal illumination. By retroillumination, the cysts are uniform in size and some may stain with fluorescein. The cysts are accumulations of PAS positive degenerative cellular material and basement membrane-like debris (407). Stocker and Holt described a similar condition in several patients (389). Treatment is usually not necessary. Wearing a soft contact lens may reduce the symptoms as well as decrease the number of cysts (43). With surgical scraping, the disease tends to recur. Superficial keratectomy may result in disappearance of the disease (80).

Reis-Bückler Dystrophy

Reis-Bückler is a dystrophy affecting Bowman's layer which is usually bilateral, symmetric, and evident in the first and second decade of life. It is associated with symptoms of painful recurrent corneal erosions (57, 334). It is an autosomal dominant trait with a strong penetrance pattern (157). Over time, patients develop surface scarring and an irregular corneal epithelium with astigmatism. On biomicroscopy, there is an irregular epithelium with patchy gray opacities at Bowman's layer with a reticulated pattern and a diffuse superficial stromal haze. The primary pathogenesis may be because of fragmentation of the collagen fibrils of Bowman's layer with the epithelial lesions as a secondary change (5, 152, 170, 191, 315, 335, 455, 456). Immunofluorescent staining, however, shows localization of laminin and antigen (45).

The irregular surface produces irregular astigmatism which is best treated with a hard contact lens. The recurrent corneal erosions become less common with time as Bowman's membrane is replaced by scar tissue. Medical therapy may be used to treat these symptoms. Superficial keratectomy is helpful in many, but the disease may recur (51). Lamellar keratoplasty is indicated in a few patients but it also may recur (4,299).

The Grayson-Wilbrandt dystrophy (49), honeycomb dystrophy (403, 456), and Waardenberg and Jonkers dystrophy (445) are probably clinical variants of the Reis-Bückler dystrophy.

Gelatinous Droplike Dystrophy

Gelatinous droplike dystrophy is a clinical manifestation of primary localized corneal amyloidosis (206, 280, 428). It is bilateral with an autosomal recessive inheritance pattern. It may be more common in Japan. It presents early in life with gelatinous mulberry-like elevated corneal lesions. Symptoms of decreased visual acuity, lacrimation, and photophobia occur. The lesions predominantly involve the epithelium and anterior stroma.

Histopathologic studies have shown corneal amyloid containing protein AP but not protein AA (6). Therapy is with superficial keratectomy or lamellar keratoplasty. It can recur in the graft.

Vortex Dystrophy

Vortex dystrophy is a toxic keratopathy, not a dystrophy. A vortex pattern of abnormal pigmented epithelial cells is formed from altered limbal stem cells. It is seen in Fabry's disease (125) as well as in corneal deposits from systemic medications including chloroquine, indomethacin, quinacrine, chlorpromazine, and amiodarone.

Corneal Stromal Dystrophies

The corneal stromal dystrophies are noninflammatory, nonvascularized stromal opacities of varying size and shape. They are bilateral and fairly symmetric hereditary disorders. There is no medical therapy so occasionally penetrating keratoplasty is necessary. The distinctive features of the conditions are shown in Table 51–6.

Macular Dystrophy

Macular dystrophy is inherited as an autosomal recessive disease, so asymptomatic carriers are not aware that they carry the gene. It is bilateral, asymmetric, and affects the anterior layers of the stroma with indistinct diffuse grayish-white spots in the first decade of life. The opacities become deeper over time as well as spread peripherally (Figure 51–11). Descemet's membrane may opacify later in the disease although the epithelium remains smooth until the later stages of the disease. Endothelial involvement can occur. Patients may have a history of recurrent corneal erosions and decreased corneal sensation.

Macular dystrophy may result from a deficiency of a hydrolytic enzyme and may be a localized mucopolysaccharidosis (212). On histopathologic examination, the lesions stain intensely with Alcian blue and colloidal iron, minimally with periodic acid–Schiff, and not with Masson's trichrome. The abnormal material is keratin sulfate-like glycosaminoglycan (acid mucopolysaccharide) that accumulates intracellularly within keratocytes, endothelial cells, as well as extracellularly (136). The cells die as the stored material increases. The accumulation of mucopolysaccharide is within the endoplasmic reticulum and not in the lysosomal vacuoles as seen in systemic mucopolysaccharidoses (179). Two subtypes of macular dystrophy have been immunohistochemically identified. Type 1 is characterized by an absence of antigenic keratin sulfate in the cornea and serum (405). In Type 2, antigenic keratin sulfate is present in the cornea and the serum (99,457).

TABLE 51–6
Corneal Stromal Dystrophies

Dystrophy	Inheritance	Abnormal Substance	Histopathologic Findings	Electron Microscope
Macular	Autosomal Recessive	Glycosaminoglycan	+ PAS + Alcian blue + Colloid iron	Membrane bound vacuoles with fibrillogranular material
Granular	Autosomal Dominant	Hyaline degeneration	+ Masson Trichrome + PAS	Electron dense Rhomboid–shaped rods
Lattice	Autosomal Dominant	Amyloid	+ Masson Trichrome + PAS + Birefringence + Dichroism + Thioflavin T	Nonbranching fibrils of amyloid
Fleck	Autosomal dominant	Glycosaminoglycans & lipids	+ Alcian blue + Colloidal iron + Oil red O	Cytoplasmic Membrane-bound vacuoles with fibrillogranular material
Central Crystalline	Autosomal Dominant	Neutral fats cholesterol	+ Oil red O	Notched rectangular crystals
Gelantinous drop–like	? Autosomal recessive	Amyloid	+ Masson Trichrome + PAS + Birefringence + Dichroism + Thioflavin T	Amyloid fibrils
Central Cloudy	Autosomal dominant	—	—	—

Visual loss may require corneal transplantation by the fourth decade of life. The disease may recur in the donor graft (7, 211, 339). Host keratocytes invade the graft and produce abnormal glycosaminoglycan.

Granular Corneal Dystrophy

Granular corneal dystrophy is an autosomal dominant bilateral and symmetric disease with white opacities ap-

pearing in the first decade of life. Over time, the opacities enlarge, and extend deeper. The lesions are bread crumb-like in pattern and are relatively distinct and demarcated (Figure 51–12) The cornea between the lesions is clear. There are two varieties. In Type 1, the vision deteriorates to approximately 20/200 and there are symptoms of recurrent erosion. In Type 2, the opacities are fewer in number and there are no symptoms of

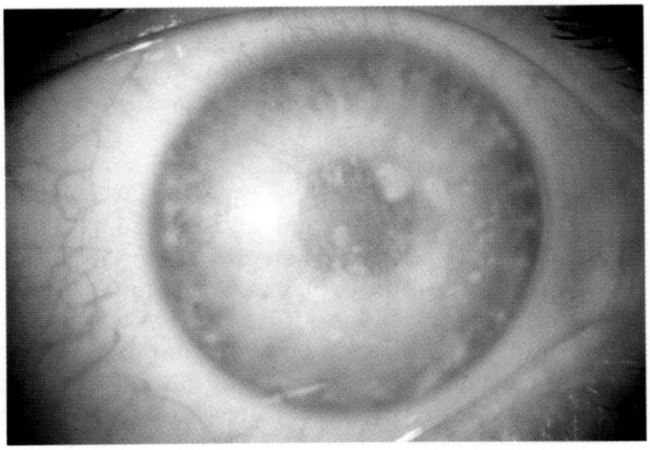

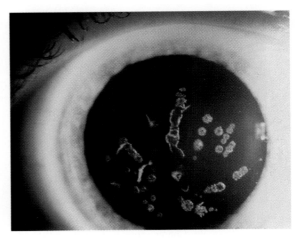

Figure 51–11.
Macular corneal dystrophy. Deposits of glycosaminoglycan in the corneal stroma in a patient with autosomal recessive macular corneal dystrophy. Both eyes were equally involved.

Figure 51–12.
Granular corneal dystrophy. Bread crumb deposits of granular corneal dystrophy in a patient with bilateral disease who maintained good visual acuity without recurrent erosions.

erosion (120, 348). In a third variant, there may be recurrent erosions in infants (50, 355). There are interfamilial and intrafamilial variations in the disease (277).

The opacities consist of areas of hyalin degeneration in which stromal fibers appear "granular" (189). The eosinophilic hyalin is a noncollagenous protein containing tyrosine, tryptophan, arginine, and sulfur-containing amino acids (137, 345). The lesions stain intensely red with Masson trichrome, weakly with PAS, and not with Verhoeff stain. Electron-dense rodlike deposits of amorphous material is seen on electron microscopy. This is probably produced by abnormal keratocytes (156, 446).

No treatment is usually required in granular corneal dystrophy since visual acuity remains good in most patients. Recurrent corneal erosions may cause symptoms. In rare cases, scraping, or lamella or penetrating keratoplasty may be necessary. Recurrence in the graft (usually anterior and peripherally) can take place (55, 341, 408).

Lattice Corneal Dystrophy

Lattice corneal dystrophy is an autosomal dominant disease with characteristic pipestem lattice figures in the corneal stroma (Figure 51–13). Symptoms begin shortly after the first decade and include decreased vision and recurrent erosion. As the disease progresses, it goes deeper and deeper although it leaves the limbus relatively free of disease. As the superficial haze increases, it is more difficult to visualize the typical lattice lesions (examination of a younger relative may help confirm the diagnosis). The dystrophy progresses, and by age 40, frequently corneal transplantation is necessary. Symp-

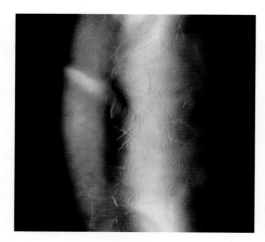

Figure 51–13.
Lattice corneal dystrophy. Characteristic lattice lines in the corneal stroma of a patient with a moderate decrease in visual acuity and recurrent corneal erosions. This autosomal dominant disease was bilateral; the other eye had undergone a penetrating keratoplasty with amyloid showed on histopathologic staining.

toms of recurrent corneal erosions occur because of poor basement membrane adhesion (118); symptoms of decreased visual acuity result from the superficial corneal scars.

Lattice dystrophy Type 1 is a familial form of amyloidosis limited to the cornea (45, 189, 210). This may be secondary to collagen degeneration, perhaps because of lysosomal enzymes elaborated by abnormal keratocytes. Amyloid is an extracellular complex of chondroitin, sulfuric acid and protein. The fibrillar material stains with Congo red, exhibits birefringence, and dichroism. On transmission electron microscopy, the fine electron dense fibrils of 80 to 100 angstroms diameter are present without periodicity. Evaluation of corneas has shown the presence of amyloid P component but staining for amyloid A protein is controversial (146, 279, 280, 431).

Lattice Type 2 is associated with a familial form of systemic amyloidosis. It is associated with progressive cranial and peripheral nerve palsies, protruding lips, blepharochalasis, a masklike facies, and floppy ears (46, 383) (Meretoja Syndrome). The onset of corneal findings is later and ocular symptoms are less severe than in Type 1. The lattice lines are fewer and more radially oriented but thicker than in Type 1. Histologic examination reveals amyloid deposits beneath Bowman's layer as well as in arteries, peripheral nerves, sclera and skin. The amyloid may be slightly different than Type 1 amyloid because it shows loss of Congo red stain after treatment with permanganate (262, 269, 431).

Lattice Type 3 is an autosomal dominant condition with broad lattice-like lines and diffuse subepithelial opacities. The symptoms don't occur until middle age. Recurrent erosions are absent but visual acuity declines in older patients. The stromal deposits of amyloid are larger than in Type 1 or Type 2. There is positive staining for amyloid P protein, but weak staining for amyloid A protein (165). The cornea may develop secondary amyloid deposits associated with several chronic ocular diseases or in patients with apparent granular or Reis-Bücklers dystrophy. Patients from Avellino, Italy, may also have some amyloid deposits in the stroma (Avellino corneal dystrophy) (253).

The amyloid deposits vary among the different amyloidoses. In immunoglobin primary systemic amyloidosis, the amyloid contains fragments of immunoglobin-like chains. In hereditary systemic amyloidosis, the protein is transthyretin, a plasma prealbumin. In secondary systemic amyloidosis, it is protein A which may be a degradation product in the serum unrelated to immunoglobins. Primary and secondary amyloid deposits are associated with structural Protein P present in normal serum. In lattice corneal dystrophy Type 1, immunoglobin light change are not present, but structural Proteins P are present. Protein AA and Protein AP are present in lattice dystrophy in a variable fashion. In

Type 2, Protein AA is present in some patients and Protein AP is present in others. In Type 3, both Protein AP and AA are found (165). Immune types of amyloid are not found in Types 1, 2 or 3 (165, 280, 346, 387).

Polymorphic amyloid degeneration is a common condition in patients over age 40 and is seen as bilateral punctate and filiform stromal deposits at all levels of the cornea, especially deep. There is no progression, no hereditary pattern, and the condition is probably more a corneal degeneration. Amyloid has been confirmed histologically (216, 254).

The treatment of the severe forms of lattice dystrophy (Type 1 and 2) may require penetrating keratoplasty. Patients do well with surgery although recurrences in the graft are frequent (48%) (226, 268). With recurrence, the dystrophy does not usually appear as lattice lines, but as a diffuse anterior stromal haze with diffuse subepithelial opacities.

Schnyder's Crystalline Dystrophy

Schnyder's crystalline dystrophy is an autosomal dominant condition which appears in the first decade of life, progresses for a few decades, and then stabilizes (243, 247). There are round or oval central opacities of fine, needle-shaped polychromatic crystals (Figure 51–14). There have been five morphologic types of these opacities: 1) discoid central opacity, 2) discoid central with indistinct edges, 3) discoid lesions with a garland margin, 4) annular opacities with fine crystals and a clear center, 5) annular opacities with crystalline edges. The opacification is mainly in the anterior stroma although deeper deposits can occur. There is usually a dense corneal arcus. The dystrophy is frequently associated with hyperlipidemia, genu valgum, and xanthelasma.

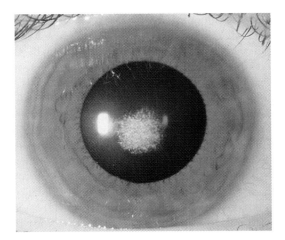

Figure 51–14.
Schnyder's crystalline dystrophy. Needle-shaped polychromatic crystals of cholesterol in the central cornea in a patient with autosomal dominant bilateral Schnyder's crystalline corneal dystrophy.

Histopathologic changes include focal accumulations of glycogen in the basement membrane and Bowman's layer. Rectangular cholesterol crystals are randomly located among the stromal collagen fibrils with widespread neutral lipids throughout the stroma. The cholesterol deposits are both esterified and unesterified (349, 352). There are foci of lipid deposition in deeper corneal layers. The pathologist needs to be contacted since paraffin storage or formation will dissolve the lipids. Special oil red stains are used to confirm the diagnosis.

Therapy is not usually required although penetrating keratoplasty is occasionally required. Recurrences still occur in the graft. Phototherapeutic keratectomy with the excimer laser has been used in a few instances. Serum lipid profiles should be obtained.

Fleck Dystrophy

Fleck (speckled or mouchetee) dystrophy of François-Neetens is an autosomal dominant dystrophy presenting early in life. Subtle grayish specks or punctate opacities which are dandruff-like are present in all layers of the cornea with some rings with centers which are clearer. There is usually no visual disability although photophobia is occasionally present (327, 392).

Histopathologic examination reveals abnormal keratocytes which stain glycosaminoglycans and lipids within intracytoplasmic vacuoles. Transmission electron microscopy shows abnormal keratocytes with fibrogranular substance (291). No treatment is usually necessary.

Central Cloudy Dystrophy

Central cloudy dystrophy of Francois is an autosomal dominant condition which occurs early as a bilateral deep opacification of the central corneal stroma. The lesions are cloudy, grey, polygonal areas without definite structure or distinct margin. This may be a form of posterior crocodile shagreen. No therapy is required (47, 391).

Pre-Descemet's Dystrophies

Pre-Descemet's dystrophies are a variety of posterior stromal opacities seen in patients in the fourth decade and are primarily a form of corneal degeneration. Various patterns of small, deep stromal opacities have been described including shapes of dendritic, circular, comma, linear, filiform, and boomerang. Corneal farinata, consisting of tiny punctate opacities in the deep stroma, may be considered in this group. Histopathologic examination in one case showed cytoplasmic vacuoles within keratocytes with lipid-like material (93). No treatment is required (110, 422).

Posterior Corneal Dystrophies

Posterior corneal dystrophies affect Descemet's membrane and the endothelium. These include congenital hereditary endothelial dystrophy, Fuchs endothelial dystrophy, posterior polymorphous dystrophy, and the iridocorneal endothelial syndrome.

Congenital Hereditary Endothelial Dystrophy

Congenital hereditary endothelial dystrophy (CHED) can be inherited in an autosomal dominant or autosomal recessive form with the latter being more common and more severe (208, 233). The recessive form is present at birth or develops in the neonatal period associated with nystagmus. Patients with dominantly inherited disease develop opacities at a few years of age and do not have nystagmus (192). The clinical picture is that of corneal edema which can vary from a mild haze to severe ground glass appearance (Figure 51–15). The corneal diameter is normal but the corneal thickness is two or three times normal. The intraocular pressure is normal. Relatives of patients with congenital hereditary endothelial dystrophy can manifest abnormalities similar to posterior polymorphous dystrophy (311, 441). Guttate are not present and corneal sensation and intraocular pressure are normal.

The histopathologic assessment shows a degeneration of the endothelium with a normal anterior banded portion of Descemet's membrane, indicating that the endothelium was functionally normal through the fifth month of gestation. The posterior nonbanded portion of Descemet's membrane is variably thickened with a layer of aberrant collagen (199, 205, 343). Guttata do not form but endothelial cells are absent or atrophic.

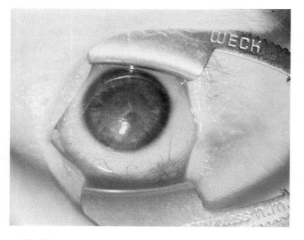

Figure 51–15.
Congenital hereditary endothelial dystrophy. A baby with a cloudy and thickened but normal sized cornea. The patient had a bilateral disease with nystagmus.

Therapy is with corneal transplantation which is more technically difficult in children (393).

Fuchs' Endothelial Dystrophy

Fuchs' endothelial dystrophy is a common corneal dystrophy with an autosomal dominant tendency occurring more frequently in women than in men (92, 218). It was originally described as an epithelial degeneration but is a disease of the posterior cornea (132). It is bilateral, often asymmetric, and affects the central cornea of middle age and older patients. Originally it begins with corneal excrescences (guttata) on Descemet's membrane and occasional pigment dusting of the endothelium. Guttae are wartlike endothelial excrescences which appear as refractile circular excavations on the endothelial surface by direct illumination and as black holes in the endothelial mosaic on specular reflection. They develop centrally and spread peripherally. Over time, a thickening of Descemet's membrane develops with a beaten-metal appearance. In some instances, guttate are not evident but a thickening of Descemet's membrane is evident (3). The merging of the common normal guttata of aging into Fuchs' corneal dystrophy is continuous with no clear distinction among ophthalmologists clinically. Stromal edema from endothelial cell dysfunction causes glare and hazy vision and gradually the epithelium develops small clear cysts and roughening of the corneal epithelium (bedewing). Large epithelial bullae can rupture causing acute pain (443). With continued progression, there is subepithelial connective tissue causing a pannus which may alleviate the corneal edema from ruptured bullae and may help with the pain. Corneal neovascularization, however, may progress, making future corneal transplantation surgery at increased risk. There may be an associated shallow anterior chamber and either angle closure glaucoma or open angle glaucoma (323).

The early stages are characterized by thickened collagenous Descemet's membrane produced by the abnormal endothelial cells. These thickenings present with visible corneal guttata in different patterns (171). Simple corneal guttata may be present in up to 70% of patients over age 40 (246). These excrescences flatten the corneal endothelial cells or push them aside, resulting in abnormal endothelial cell size and loss of the normal hexagonal pattern. The disease is caused by abnormal endothelial cell products in early life although it usually doesn't become manifest until middle age (42). With progressive endothelial thinning and loss of function, stromal edema develops correlating with the decreased density of sodium and potassium ATPase pumps (263). The corneal collagen may be of altered quality (63). Bowman's membrane is disrupted by subepithelial connective tissue of an abnormal basement membrane-like material. Intracellular and intercellular epithelial edema results in bullae which rupture.

Fuchs' corneal dystrophy is diagnosed at the slit lamp with the typical corneal findings. In some cases, corneal guttata are not evident but a thickened Descemet's membrane is found. Looking at the other eye, or other family members, can help establish the diagnosis. Rarely, the disease is so subtle as to be diagnosed only after the onset of corneal edema after uncomplicated cataract surgery. The edema is characteristically worse in the morning (after prolonged lid closure) and gets better during the day associated with evaporation. Epithelial edema first appears as fine clear cysts with nodular elevations of the surface (bedewing) best seen with retroillumination as a fine patina pattern. Fingerprint lines are frequently seen. As the cysts coalesce, large bullae form which can rupture (causing pain), or interfere with vision.

The medical therapy of corneal edema is effective only in the early stages. Hypertonic ointment or drops (5% sodium chloride) can help extract fluid. Warm dry air or a hair dryer held at arms length can help increase surface evaporation. A bandage soft contact lens (fit loose and of increased water content) may reduce the epithelial ruptures. In some instances, increased intraocular pressure may accompany and contribute to the corneal edema; lowering the intraocular pressure may help alleviate some edema. The primary form of therapy in advanced corneal edema (for example, visual acuity less than 20/80) is with a penetrating keratoplasty. Results are best when the edema is limited to the central cornea. Although 80% of grafts remain clear for 2 years, there is a fairly increased recurrence of graft edema (failure), probably related to poor residual endothelial cell function (298, 388). Since many patients may have a narrow angle, consideration should be given to a peripheral iridectomy and the concomitant removal of a cataract which is frequently present. The graft is usually 0.25 to 0.50 mm oversized than the donor hole to allow for a deeper anterior chamber angle. Cystoid macular edema still limits vision in many patients in addition to the risks of graft failure, graft rejection, and glaucoma.

In patients not suitable for penetrating keratoplasty or in whom penetrating keratoplasty has failed, removal of the epithelium and cauterization of Bowman's layer may be advisable to reduce bullae formation. A conjunctival flap is also a good alternative if the conjunctiva has not previously been disturbed.

Corneas which have borderline Fuchs' corneal dystrophy will frequently decompensate with the additional stress of anterior segment surgery or anterior segment inflammation (3). Some of these might be predicted ahead of time on the basis of close clinical observation at the slit lamp or by the use of specular microscopy to evaluate the morphology of the corneal endothelium. There is still, however, no good measure of corneal endothelial function except the use of various stress tests which deprive the eye of oxygen and further stress ATPase pump function. The decision to proceed with cataract surgery alone or to do a combined penetrating keratoplasty and cataract extraction is based on the degree of stromal edema. This is a controversial area, although most corneal surgeons would delay corneal transplantation until epithelial edema develops.

Posterior Polymorphous Dystrophy

Posterior polymorphous dystrophy (PPMD) is a bilateral dominantly inherited dystrophy with strong penetrance which is usually stationary or slowly progressive and usually does not interfere with visual function (159). It may be congenital or develop early in life. There are vesicular or annular polymorphous deposits surrounded by clear halos at the level of Descemet's membrane by slit lamp biomicroscopy (76, 185). In some instances, the entire posterior corneal surface can have a peau d'orange appearance of beaten metal. Another pattern is linear gray thickening of Descemet's membrane. These may appear as irregular scalloped parallel lines with intervening clear bands. They can be oriented vertically or horizontally and can be confused with Descemet's tears (75, 148). In rare instances, specular microscopy is necessary to establish or to suggest the diagnosis or to monitor disease progression (52, 168, 258). Rarely, progression causes endothelial decompensation. Although usually an isolated event, it has been associated with band keratopathy, peripheral anterior synechia, glaucoma, guttata, or other anterior segment dysgenesis (prominent Schwalbe's line, iridocorneal adhesions) (148).

There have been several pathologic studies confirming that the endothelial cells in posterior polymorphous dystrophy morphologically and immunologically resemble epithelial cells. These cells have microvilli by scanning electron microscopy and contain epithelial keratin and have well-developed desmesomes (40, 344, 347). Other studies have shown a similarity of these cells to fibroblasts (148). The abnormal endothelium can extend across the trabecular meshwork and onto the iris (217, 340, 347). Therefore, the disease may represent an aberrant differentiation of neural crest cells similar to the iridocorneal endothelial syndrome (see below) (25). The disease can be confused with the iridocorneal endothelial syndrome except that the iridocorneal endothelial syndrome is unilateral and sporadic. The cause of the embryonal precursors undergoing abnormal differentiation into epithelial-like cells is unknown; because of its appearance, it is thought to develop either late in gestation or shortly after birth. If it presents at birth, it must be distinguished from other causes of a cloudy cornea at birth.

No treatment is usually required for posterior polymorphous dystrophy. Mild epithelial edema is treated as in Fuchs' endothelial dystrophy. Rarely, penetrating keratoplasty may be necessary, but the disease may recur in the graft (41). The associated anterior segment conditions may affect the prognosis. If extensive angle involvement is present, the resultant glaucoma is difficult to manage.

Iridocorneal Endothelial Syndrome

The iridocorneal endothelial (ICE) syndrome is perhaps a single disease with variations previously termed Chandler syndrome, essential iris atrophy, and iris nevus (Cogan-Reese) syndrome (66, 105, 342, 372, 374, 375, 458). This is not really a corneal dystrophy in that it is unilateral, nonfamilial, and more common in women age 30 to 50. It is considered here because of its confusion with and similarity to other corneal dystrophies. The fellow eye is usually normal.

The primary abnormality in the iridocorneal endothelial syndrome is in the abnormal corneal endothelium which has epithelial-like features. The cornea typically exhibits a posterior collagenous layer with an endothelial membrane overgrowth across the cornea, trabecular meshwork, and the iris (203, 351). Iris nodules or iris holes appear later. The endothelial malfunctions cause corneal edema and allow a Descemet's membrane-like tissue to grow over the iris. Contraction of the membrane causes various iris abnormalities and distortions as well as peripheral anterior synechiae. Specular microscopy can help distinguish this condition in several situation revealing pleomorphism, polymegathism, and intracellular dark areas (44, 52, 167, 289, 375).

The relative prominence of the clinical features varies and hence the original three different clinical diseases. In essential iris atrophy, the features of iris atrophy, iris hole formation, and corectopia predominate (372). In Chandler's syndrome, the corneal endothelial changes and stromal edema are most prominent (71, 307). In the iris nevus syndrome, nodular pigmented elevations are present on the iris surface (82). The most prominent finding is usually a beaten-metal appearance to the endothelium with a later development of stromal and epithelial edema. The latter iris changes include an atrophy, peripheral anterior synechia, stretching of the iris with hole formation, and ectropion uvea. The pupil is usually eccentric (the essential iris variation) (66). In others, yellow or brown pedunculated nodules are present on the iris surface (the Cogan-Reese variant) (355, 373). These nodules are not true nevi, but iris tissue prolapsing through a membrane on the surface of iris.

The symptoms of the iridocorneal endothelial syndrome arise from corneal edema, pupillary distortion, and elevated intraocular pressure. Corneal edema can result from only a slight elevation in intraocular pressure and may respond to lowering the intraocular pressure. Patients may require glaucoma filtration surgery, corneal transplantation surgery, or both. The prognosis can be favorable (62, 91).

Ectatic Corneal Dystrophies

Keratoconus

Anterior keratoconus is an axial ectasia or corneal protrusion of the axial cornea (Figure 51–16). It begins as a subtle irregular astigmatism as evidenced by a distorted corneal image on the Placido disk, retinoscope, keratometer, keratoscope, and computerized keratographs. It is usually first detected in adolescence and can progress slowly or rapidly. The inheritance pattern is difficult to define, although a definite familial tendency is present. Form fruste of the disease can be found in a less involved eye or in family members. It is more common in females (2:1).

In its early stages, the corneal cone can be difficult to appreciate. Corneal topography analysis systems have significantly increased our awareness of keratoconus and permit detection in advance of slit lamp findings (250, 329). Retinoscopy reveals a characteristic scissor reflex. There are different forms of keratoconus: the predominant type is the nipple-shaped cone (generally smaller and central) or the larger, oval or sagging cone (317). The apex of the nipple cone is usually directed slightly infero nasally; the apex of the sagging cone is often displaced to the infero temporal quadrant. On downgaze, the lower lid can be distorted by the protrusion causing Munson's sign. Vertical striae (Vogt's striae) or stress lines of Descemet's can be seen by slit lamp. These are characteristically flattened by slight pressure on the globe. There is increased visibility of corneal nerves, a deposit of iron pigment in the epithelium at the base of the cone (Fleischer line), and frequent subepithelial scarring at the apex of the cone. Acute hydrops can occur from stretching of Descemet's membrane beyond its elastic breaking point; the marked local conical edema usually resolves over two months with residual stromal scarring.

Keratoconus has been seen in association with ocular and systemic conditions, most frequently atopic dermatitis (381), vernal keratoconjunctivitis (90), Marfan syndrome, Down syndrome, and retinitis pigmentosa. Frequent rubbing of the eye has long been touted as a potential cause of keratoconus (65) as well as the long-term use of contact lenses (249).

The histopathologic examination of keratoconus shows a focal disruption of Bowman's layer with irregular epithelial thickness and an abnormal basement membrane in areas where Bowman's membrane is ab-

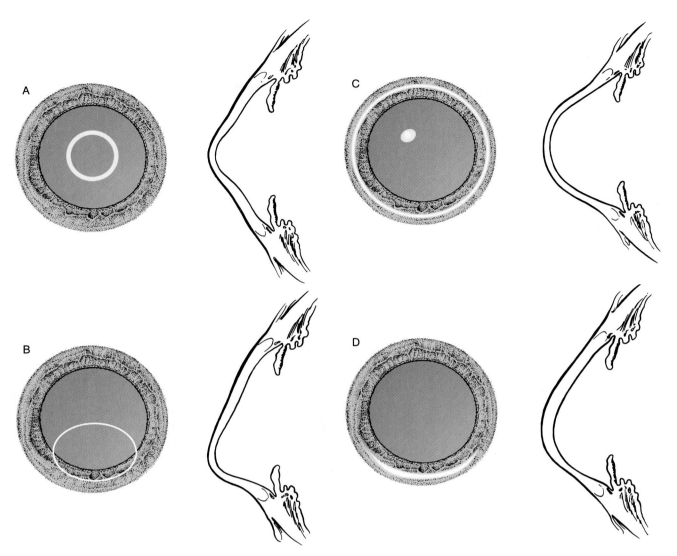

Figure 51–16.
Corneal ectasia. The corneal protrusions seen in A, Keratoconus (round and oval forms); B, Keratoglobus and C, Pellucid marginal degeneration.

sent. With hydrops, torn edges of Descemet's membrane are shown; endothelial cells migrate over the exposed stroma to deposit a new Descemet's membrane (390). The earliest changes can be at the basal cells of the epithelium with perhaps release of proteolytic enzymes. There is decreased sulfated keratan sulfate (134) and protein related abnormalities (305).

Keratoconus is treated with myopic and astigmatic spectacles initially. A rigid contact lens is frequently necessary for the irregular astigmatism which develops. When contact lenses can no longer be worn, occasionally superficial keratectomy, lamellar keratectomy (surgical or laser induced) or an epikeratoplasty may be useful (264). Penetrating keratoplasty is the definitive treatment for advanced cases and is required in approximately 20% of patients and has a fairly good prognosis. In view of the young age of these patients, a re-

jection of tissue is increased over the life of the patient. Recurrences can occur in the graft. Patients still have an increased incidence of astigmatism after penetrating keratoplasty frequently requiring the use of a gas permeable contact lens.

Keratoglobus

Keratoglobus is a rare bilateral corneal ectasia in which the entire cornea is thin. This causes extensive myopia and astigmatism with risk of perforation with minor trauma or risk of acute hydrops.

Keratoconus and keratoglobus have been observed in different members of the same family (70, 150). The pathologic assessment has shown stromal thinning with breaks in Bowman's layer. Contact lenses are a risk because of the thin cornea. Corneal transplantation is technically difficult because of the thin bed. A tectonic lamellar onlay graft is preferable with a full thickness penetrating keratoplasty to follow if necessary.

Pellucid Marginal Degeneration

Pellucid marginal degeneration is a rare form of corneal ectasia with an arcuate band of corneal thinning in the inferior cornea usually between 4- and 8-o'clock. It has no ulceration and the stroma is clear and nonvascularized. The thinning is separated from the limbus by a small amount of clear cornea. The rest of the cornea is of normal thickness and architecture. An against the rule astigmatism is present. The ectasia tends to occur in patients between the ages of 20 and 40 and it may continue to progress over years. It can rarely cause a corneal rupture in association with mild trauma. It has features in common with keratoconus but has a distinct peripheral location and lacks a conical shape. It may be a form fruste of keratoconus since other family members may have increased astigmatism.

The marked astigmatism is usually corrected with glasses. Contact lenses are not a good alternative because of the eccentric location of the thinning. Lamellar tissue grafting with a crescentic donor tissue is technically difficult but may be the best option. It can be followed by penetrating keratoplasty if necessary.

■ CORNEAL INFECTIONS

Viral Infections of the Cornea

Viral infections tend to affect both the conjunctiva and cornea, although in some instances affect only the cornea, especially as a recurrent infection or as a recrudescence or recurrence of an immune reaction triggered by the virus or viral antigen. Infections caused by herpes simplex, varicella zoster virus, Epstein-Barr virus, cytomegalovirus, adenovirus, poxvirus, paramyxovirus, picornavirus, and togavirus will be addressed with a discussion of their widespread ocular and systemic effects.

Herpes Simplex Virus

Epidemiology

Herpes simplex virus is the most common infectious cause of corneal blindness in the Western hemisphere. The epidemiology of ocular herpes simplex virus is much less known compared with the epidemiology of nonocular (mainly genital) herpes simplex virus (235). It has multifaceted presentations and mechanisms of disease which lead to confusion with other clinical entities. The herpes simplex virus is a DNA virus with two antigenically related strains, Type 1 and Type 2. Humans are the only natural reservoir although many animal systems have been developed as research tools to investigate this disease. There is a gradual increase in serum antibody titer to HSV Type 1 throughout life beginning in childhood; herpes simplex virus Type 2 antibodies correlate with the onset and frequency of multiple sexual partners. By age 5 years, 60% of children have been infected with herpes simplex virus Type 1, usually through contact with an infected relative, by the oral or nasal route. This primary episode of herpes simplex virus results in a generalized viral infection which is only occasionally accurately identified as herpes simplex infection. Ocular involvement occurs in only approximately 1% of primary herpes simplex virus, although up to 20% of patients with acute primary ocular herpes simplex virus may be presenting with their first manifestation of any herpes virus infections. During primary infection of the oral or nasal area (or the eye), the virus gains access to nerve endings and ultimately the trigeminal ganglion where the virus establishes an active latency in some of the nuclei. Autopsy studies have confirmed that almost all patients with serum antibodies titers to HSV Type 1 will have a latent HSV identified in the trigeminal ganglion. The vast majority of episodes of ocular herpes simplex virus and episodes of herpes simplex virus on the face or lip represent reactivations of herpes simplex virus from latency by several methods of initiation (for example, stress, fever, etc.) with a final common pathway perhaps being related to prostaglandins. Ongoing studies are trying to define the role of latent virus in the cornea or other local ocular tissues.

Herpes simplex virus Type 2 is much less likely to involve the eye although approximately 5% of cases can be attributed to HSV Type 2 primarily related to neonatal HSV infection caused by passage through an infected birth canal. There are trends indicating a higher incidence of genital HSV caused by Type 1; and subsequently future neonatal HSV may be more frequently caused by Type 1 (23, 310).

An epidemiologic study of ocular herpes simplex virus suggests an incidence of 8.4 new cases per 100,000 person years in the United States, which compares with 11.7 new cases of ocular herpes zoster ophthalmicus per 100,000 persons per year (235). Herpes simplex virus has a much high recurrence rate so most ophthalmologists see more patients with herpes simplex virus than herpes zoster. Recurrences of the ocular disease are far less common than recurrences of either genital or oral herpes simplex virus. The recurrence rate of ocular herpes simplex virus is approximately 40 to 70% over a 5-year period (33, 219, 235, 376, 434). Despite its frequent recurrences, loss of significant vision from herpes simplex virus is relatively uncommon (although most memorable by the ophthalmologists who deal with this frustrating recurrent disease).

Initial episodes of ocular herpes simplex virus are characterized by blepharitis or conjunctivitis in 54%, epithelial keratitis in 63%, stromal keratitis in 6%, and uveitis in 4%. With recurrent disease, the appearance of stromal keratitis is more common and associated with more significant morbidity.

Primary Ocular Herpes Simplex Virus

Primary ocular herpes is the first exposure of the body to herpes simplex. This first exposure can occur at birth, or more commonly in childhood ususally secondary to HSV Type II, or more commonly in childhood by a HSV Type I infection. These primary ocular herpes infections are described below.

Neonatal Herpes Simplex

Neonatal primary herpes simplex virus occurs in approximately 1 in 10,000 births, with a great majority associated with HSV Type 2. It is acquired by passage through an HSV infected birth canal, especially in those who have had a manipulation completed, such as with a fetal scalp electrode. There may be dermatologic vesicles to help establish the diagnosis. Disseminated HSV can involve the visceral organs or the central nervous system. Despite antiviral therapy, the disease has a mortality rate of 50% in disseminated disease and 10% in patients with central nervous system disease. An increased rate of residual central nervous system damage occurs in the children who survive (23, 432).

The ocular manifestations of neonatal disease are most frequently conjunctivitis with an epithelial keratitis either as a punctate epithelial keratitis or diffuse microdendrites. Stromal keratitis is rare and suggests prolonged intrauterine infection (178). Later ocular complications include a necrotizing chorioretinitis, optic neuritis, cataracts, and strabismus (284). Approximately 37% of patients will have visual acuity of 20/200 or less because of various ocular sequela (23).

The diagnosis must be considered in the appropriate clinical setting and with an appropriate venereal disease history in the parents. Diagnostic skin or ocular cytology or culture will reveal the virus from vesicles. Serologic tests are confirmatory. Therapy requires treatment of the local ocular disease with topical antiviral therapy. A pediatric or infectious disease consult needs to assess the presence of systemic disease and the need for intravenous therapy with acyclovir (also see section on Neonatal Conjunctivitis).

Primary Ocular Herpes Simplex Type 1

Primary ocular herpes simplex virus represents the first association of a nonimmune host with the HSV. It usually begins approximately 1 week after exposure to an infected carrier (frequently a parent). Only approximately 1% of primary ocular herpes simplex virus presents as an overt disease. It presents with an intense (occasionally hemorrhagic) blistering, periocular dermatitis or blepharitis, a follicular conjunctivitis, and preauricular lymphadenopathy. The skin eruption tends to remain localized in an immunocompetent host and resolves without specific therapy (39). An epithelial keratitis will develop in approximately 60% of patients with primary ocular herpes simplex virus, usually manifest as a diffuse microepithelial dendritic, or rarely as a geographic, keratitis.

Primary ocular herpes simplex virus must be distinguished from a patient who has previously had primary herpes simplex virus (with no ocular involvement) and is having a recurrence of herpes simplex virus being manifested in the eye for the first time. In this latter group, the disease more frequently has the appearance and behavior of recurrent ocular herpes simplex virus which is discussed below.

The diagnosis of primary ocular herpes simplex virus can be confirmed by viral culture, measurement of circulating antibodies, or by examination of the skin, conjunctiva or corneal scrapings. External ocular scrapings from vesicles are taken with a sterile platinum (Kimura) spatula or the edge of a surgical blade. They are smeared on a slide and can then be evaluated by Giemsa stain, revealing the multinucleated giant epithelial cells with balloon degeneration and a mixed polymorphonuclear and mononuclear reaction. A Papanicolaou stain is better for evaluating the eosinophilic viral inclusion bodies of Lipschutz (Cowdry A inclusions) within the nucleus (232, 234). Fluorescent antibody staining is a rapid and reliable technique to detect herpes antigen in the nucleus or cytoplasm; it requires an ultraviolet microscope and cannot be permanently stored. Immunodiagnostic tests are available as commercial kits for the specific diagnosis of herpes simplex virus. This includes the Herpchek, Virogen, and an enzyme-linked immunoassay (104, 215). A color change or agglutination is used as an endpoint for the detection of HSV antigen. The sensitivity and specificity of these tests vary.

Viral culture is the most definitive test but requires several days and is not readily available. The sensitivity can be increased if the specimen is collected early in the course of the disease, and before the use of antiviral agents (87). Serologic testing is useful although this requires paired samples for confirmation. The appearance of decreased initial titers in the first sample followed by a four-fold rise in the second titer confirms primary infection with HSV (232). In recurrence of herpes simplex virus, there is often no change in the serologic titer.

The therapy of the skin in primary ocular herpes simplex virus is usually not required except for the use of general good hygiene and wet soaks. Topical antiviral ointments to the skin is not of proven benefit. In the presence of eyelid and eyelid margin involvement, it is appropriate to use a topical ophthalmic antiviral for prophylaxis in an attempt to avoid ocular involvement. Studies to establish the efficacy of this prophylaxis are not available. Conjunctival involvement is treated with topical ophthalmic antivirals as is any evidence of corneal epithelial involvement. Choices available include trifluorothymidine (Viroptic) 1% drops nine times a day, vidarabine (Vira-A) 5% ointment five times a day, or idoxuridine .5% ointment five times a day, or Idoxuridine 0.1% drops every one hour. Ophthalmic acyclovir ointment is not available in the United States. The dermatologic preparation of acyclovir should not be used in the eye. A corneal debridement with a sterile cotton-tipped applicator after anesthetic drops followed by full therapy with topical antiviral therapy is another alternative. A shield may be appropriate for young children to avoid manipulation. In the presence of iritis or stromal involvement (rare with primary ocular herpes simplex virus), more intensive therapy with cycloplegics (homatropine, scopolamine) or with corticosteroids may be required.

Recurrent Ocular Herpes Simplex Virus

Once the facial skin or mucous membranes of the mouth and nose are infected with herpes simplex virus, the virus has access to the sensory nerve endings and travels by retrograde axoplasmic flow to the sensory or trigeminal ganglion, to the ciliary ganglion, and to the mesencephalic nucleus of the brain stem or to the sympathetic nerve fibers where it remains in a latent state (236). An initial oral or facial infection with HSV allows access of the virus to the trigeminal ganglion, probably in the maxillary division. There can be cross infectivity between the three divisions of the trigeminal nerve with the virus gaining access through the maxillary division and spreading to the mandibular or ophthalmic division. Recurrences of the virus in the ophthalmic division may occur in an acute ocular infection, in the absence of a prior ocular infection (236). Bilateral ocular disease is rare and more common in atopic individuals. During latency, active transcription of the virus takes place continually so the virus is not really dormant. Individual neurons are infected; with recurrent infection, some of the neurons may reactivate, but not necessarily all that are latently infected.

There is debate about whether the cornea can be the site of latency and serve as a source of virus during reactivation. Although viral DNA has been found in corneas during latency, there are multiple other criteria needed to confirm latency, most important being the presence of latency associated transcripts. The question has not been completely resolved (88, 89, 126, 309).

The mechanisms causing viral reactivation from latency are not well established but probably occur at the cellular level because of immune deficiency or because of chemical messenger systems (239, 309). Emotional and physical stress and immunodeficiency are associated with recurrent HSV and trigger factors in individual patients can include ultraviolet light, fever, cold wind, surgery, trigeminal nerve sectioning for trigeminal neuralgia, and immunosuppressive therapy. Neither passive immunization nor existing circulating antibodies have an influence on the development of recurrent herpes simplex virus disease. Antibody titers do not correlate with recurrence of HSV (270).

The reactivation of HSV may result in different manifestations of disease including surface epithelial disease, stromal disease, or intraocular involvement with uveitis and glaucoma, all depending on the specific neurons reactivated (Table 51–7) The deeper disease pattern of stromal and intraocular herpes simplex virus is more common after multiple recurrences.

Different viral strains provide different forms of ocular disease in laboratory animals. Strains of virus that produce large amounts of glycoprotein on the viral envelope are effective inducers of humoral and cell mediated responses and are more frequently associated with

TABLE 51–7

Classification of Ocular Involvement with Herpes Simplex Virus

Viral disease
Blepharitis
Conjunctivitis
Epithelial disease
Punctate
Stellate
Dendritic
Geographic
Stromal disease
Disciform keratitis (central endotheliitis)
Necrotizing keratitis (interstitial keratitis)
Peripheral endotheliitis (trabeculitis)
Uveitis
Focal iritis
Diffuse iritis
Nonviral disease (metaherpetic)
Erosions
Indolent ulceration
Trophic ulceration
Permanent altered corneal structure
Permanent trabecular damage

severe stromal disease (195). The response to topical steroids may also be determined by the viral genome (196). The individual virus, however, may not have the same effect in both humans and animals. Both viral strains and a local host immune response play a role in determining the clinical outcomes in an individual patient. The epithelial dendritic and geographic epithelial diseases are caused by active viral replication. The development of stromal disease and iritis appears related primarily to an immune reaction to viral byproducts with a possible role of infective viral particles. Viral antigenic material may alter corneal keratocytes and fibroblasts in concert with active viral replication to set the stage for the cascade of humoral and cellular immune responses that occur with HSV infection (209). Mechanical damage to the epithelium and stroma may result in trophic ulceration of the surface or to neurotrophic changes in the corneal substance.

Clinical Manifestations of Ocular Herpes Simplex

Herpes simpex blepharitis presents as focal clusters of vesicles or weeping ulcers can be seen on the eyelids and can occur in either primary or recurrent ocular HSV (Table 51–7). With recurrent disease, the vesicles are usually more closely clustered and run a shorter course of approximately 1 week. Recurrent disease may be limited to the lids (108, 182). Usually recurrent blepharitis is self-limited and requires no therapy. The use of prophylactic topical antiviral drops is reasonable in the presence of eyelid or eyelid margin involvement to prevent corneal infection. There has been no study to indicate the usefulness of systemic acyclovir in preventing recurrent HSV blepharitis. In a parallel study for preventing HSV labialis, oral acyclovir started within several hours of symptoms and continued at five times a day for several days hastened resolution of pain and duration of HSV labialis, although it did not affect the development of new lesions or the maximum size of lesions (382).

Recurrent follicular conjunctivitis secondary to recurrent HSV is a definite clinical entity (11, 54). This may be associated with a watery discharge, with an occasional patient developing dendritic or geographic conjunctival ulcers. Therapy is with full doses of topical antiviral.

Corneal disease from HSV may be caused by infectious virus, or the immune response to the virus or viral particles. Corneal epithelial disease is the most common form and presents as punctate, dendritic, or geographic patterns of infection of the corneal epithelium. Epithelial disease represents active HSV replication in epithelial cells. The dendrites may be single and linear or have multiple linear branches and multiple small dendrites is another pattern of epithelial involvement. Enlargement, spread, and coalescence of the dendritic pattern results in the geographic (ameboid) pattern (Figure 51–17). Rose bengal will stain the swollen infected epithelial cells while fluorescein stains primarily the central ulceration which is devoid of epithelial cells. Under the epithelial lesions, there is frequently a faint stromal infiltrate which probably represents soluble antigen diffusing into the stroma with a corresponding immune response. Corneal sensation is frequently depressed in the area of prior dendrites, probably because of neuronal cell death at the time of recurrence, versus a structural damage to the nerve ending because of the viral infection. The pattern of epithelial involvement is not related to neuronal distribution, so the pattern of viral spread on the surface suggests contiguous cell to cell transmission of the virus (32, 413). Epithelial disease may resolve without significant stromal involvement. Epithelial lesions closer to the limbus appear to be more resistant to therapy for unclear reasons. Patients with immune deficiency (for example, AIDS, organ transplantation, atopic disease) frequently have more persistent and florid manifestations of epithelial herpes simplex virus.

The diagnosis of HSV epithelial disease is based on the specific corneal findings and the appropriate clinical setting. Diagnostic laboratory studies are usually not necessary. The therapy of HSV epithelial disease is best accomplished with a gentle debridement of the involved epithelium followed by topical antiviral therapy with trifluorothymidine, vidarabine, or idoxuridine. Use of debridement removes the infected cells and antigen load, but the antiviral agents are only virustatic. The disease can be self-limited and resolves in many without significant morbidity. The use of debridement and antiviral therapy hastens the healing process.

Herpes simplex virus stromal disease is commonly

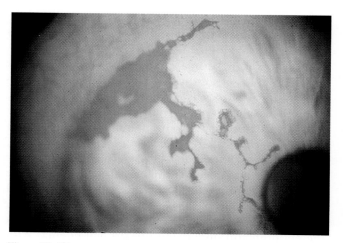

Figure 51–17.
Herpes simplex virus dendrite and geographic keratitis. A 20-year-old immunosuppressed patient with herpes simplex viral epithelial dendritic and geographic keratitis at the corneal limbus with his first known episode of ocular herpes simplex virus.

divided into necrotizing stromal keratitis and disciform stromal keratitis. Both forms are largely immune in nature as a hypersensitivity reaction to the fixed herpes antigen within stromal keratocytes or fibroblasts or within the endothelium (396). The role of active viral infection in the stroma or endothelial cells resulting from reactivation in the trigeminal ganglion or within the corneal stroma remains a topic of debate. Intact viral particles have been detected in the stroma by electron microscopy and grown by tissue cultivation techniques. Herpes simplex virus DNA and latency associated transcripts have been detected in corneal stroma (4, 98, 353, 397, 410).

Although almost all patients with herpes simplex virus stromal disease will have a prior history of herpes simplex viral epithelial disease; an occasional patient may present de novo with stromal keratitis or disciform keratitis. In this setting, there are many other disease processes to consider (437). Laboratory diagnostic tests are only occasionally helpful in sorting out the different entities; a good history and examination are most important.

Necrotizing herpes simplex viral stromal keratitis is characterized by necrotic, cheesy-white stromal infiltrates, immune rings of Wessley (ring stromal infiltrates), limbal vasculitis, and interstitial keratitis. It appears to be mediated in large part by antigen-antibody-complement mechanisms. The stromal response may occur sequential to overlying epithelial disease, or occur independent or isolated from epithelial herpes simplex virus. In some instances, the smoldering stromal reaction incites deep corneal neovascularization. Immune rings can increase the necrotic response leading to corneal thinning. The limbal vasculitis can also produce localized thinning. Mild necrotizing stromal keratitis can resolve on its own over a week or smolder for months with minimal scarring. Persistent or severe stromal inflammation may persist and progress despite pharmacologic attempts to mute the immunologic response.

HSV disciform stromal keratitis shows characteristics of a delayed hypersensitivity reaction to lymphocytes attacking localized areas of the corneal endothelium. There is usually no concurrent epithelial disease. The stimulus that precipitates the immune response is not obvious, perhaps a viral infection of the endothelium, or an antigenic alteration of the endothelial surface or stromal cells may elicit the inflammatory response. The disciform lesions are focal disk-shaped areas of stromal edema without necrosis or neovascularization. Keratic precipitates of lymphocytes and plasma cells are seen on the endothelium underlying the stromal edema. With further endothelial compromise, folds in Descemet's membrane develop. The disease may develop into necrotizing stromal keratitis with the development of necrosis, thinning, neovascularization, and corneal edema.

The histopathologic study of stromal herpes simplex viral keratitis has been reviewed in several studies although the precise pathophysiologic mechanism still remains unknown. In tissue submitted for histopathologic examination (usually because of advanced disease at the time of penetrating keratoplasty) Bowman's membrane is usually absent. There is usually marked epithelial cell loss, thickened basement membranes, and marked infiltration of inflammatory cells, subepithelial fibrous formation, stromal neovascularization, and breaks or reduplications in Descemet's membrane (106, 172). Herpes simplex viral particles have been seen throughout all layers of the cornea in approximately 20% of corneal buttons; herpes simplex virus can be cocultured in up to 60% of corneal buttons (106).

The therapy of stromal herpes simplex viral keratitis can be frustrating. With mild disease, the inflammation may spontaneously resolve without treatment. In more severe or progressive disease, cycloplegia alone may be sufficient. More severe inflammatory reactions require topical corticosteroids. The antiinflammatory effect of corticosteroids prevent and control the abnormal immune response and enzyme release which can lead to permanent corneal scarring. Persistent inflammation promotes continued corneal neovascularization which can reduce the effectiveness of future corneal transplantation (84, 225). The least effective dose of topical corticosteroid to relieve corneal inflammation should be used, followed by a gradual taper. The steroid dose needs to be adjusted up or down depending on the clinical response. These patients cannot tolerate abrupt withdrawal of corticosteroids and frequently need a prolonged, small (homeopathic) dose. A topical antiviral probably has no effect on the stromal keratitis but is used for prophylactic treatment of herpes simplex viral epithelial disease which has a tendency to recur in the presence of topical steroid use. Systemic acyclovir has not proven to be of benefit in patients with stromal keratitis. Corneal transplantation may be required as an emergency in the presence of continued stromal inflammation or corneal perforation. It is preferable, however, to operate when the eye is quiet and has as little inflammation as possible (see role of surgery below).

Metaherpetic keratitis herpes simplex viral indolent ulceration is an epithelial and anterior stromal defect in association with active stromal inflammation. This stromal infiltration causes persistent structural changes in the anterior stroma and the basement membrane with loss of corneal sensation and persistent epithelial and stromal ulceration. Treatment of the inflammatory and stromal condition with topical corticosteroids and antivirals will frequently lead to epithelialization of the corneal surface.

Herpes simplex viral trophic ulceration is a structural epithelial and superficial stromal ulceration in the absence of significant stromal inflammation. It is related to neurotropic damage and scarring which inhibits epithelialization because of marked basement membrane damage. During this period of ulceration, the inflammatory cells attached to this area release lytic enzymes with subsequent stromal melting or perforation. It is important to establish a surface epithelium as quickly as possible. Methods to enhance epithelialization include the removal of toxic agents (e.g., the antiviral), lubrication with nontoxic agents, therapeutic use of soft contact lenses, and the use of a tarsorrhaphy, conjunctival flap, conjunctival transplant, or penetrating keratoplasty. If a corneal perforation occurs, the use of cyanoacrylate tissue adhesive with a bandage contact lens is appropriate.

Herpes simplex virus may involve the anterior chamber resulting in an endothelial infection centrally (endotheliitis) or a peripheral endothelial and trabecular meshwork involvement (trabeculitis). Herpes simplex virus may be isolated from the anterior chamber. This may be associated with corneal edema from endothelial decompensation or with acute glaucoma secondary to obstruction of the trabecular meshwork by inflammatory debris or swelling from inflammatory cells (338, 397, 398, 415). Topical antivirals have not been effective for anterior chamber disease; oral acyclovir is reasonable to try, but, this treatment has not been fully evaluated. Topical corticosteroids are effective in controlling some elements of the inflammatory reaction. Glaucoma medications are necessary to lower the intraocular pressure during this inflammatory reaction and may be required on a permanent basis.

Nongranulomatous anterior uveitis can be caused by herpes simplex virus either isolated or in a recurrent pattern. There may or may not be a prior history of ocular herpes simplex virus. Viral particles have been cultured from the aqueous humor of some of these cases, but there is also an inflammatory component. The iritis may be diffuse or focal. In diffuse iritis, there is widespread infiltration of the iris stroma with lymphocytic cells. In focal iritis, there are areas of swollen hyperemic iris, an irregular pupil, and localized posterior synechia. Cells, flare, and keratic precipitates may be present in both forms. In severe forms, there may be fibrin, hyphema, hypopyon, extensive peripheral anterior synechia, iris edema, and glaucoma (308, 396). Intraocular cultures may be needed to establish this diagnosis in the absence of other or prior signs of herpes simplex virus ocular disease. Therapy is empiric including systemic antivirals, topical corticosteroids, and topical cycloplegics (79, 365).

Ocular Herpes Simplex Virus in Immunosuppressed Patients

Epithelial herpes simplex virus in patients with AIDS tends to be marginal, as opposed to central, and the epithelial ulcers are more resistant to therapy. Recurrences are also more frequent in this population with recurrences of longer duration (276, 364, 459). There appears, however, to be a lower tendency to stromal keratitis probably because of T-lymphocyte suppression. The role of corticosteroids in stromal keratitis in these patients is more suspect.

Patients with atopic dermatitis are particularly susceptible to infection with herpes simplex virus probably because of multiple immune malfunctions. Patients with atopic dermatitis can develop severe local herpetic reaction with secondary bacterial infection and widespread herpetic infection known as Kaposi's varicelliform eruption or eczema herpeticum (234, 256, 417). Bilateral ocular disease is more frequent in patients with atopic disease (140, 436). There is a tendency to delayed epithelial healing and more frequent stromal scarring. Systemic acyclovir should be considered in the treatment program (292).

Role of Surgery in Ocular Herpes Simplex Virus

Penetrating keratoplasty is a viable alternative in patients who fail to respond to medical therapy or who have significant stromal scarring. Improved regimens with topical antiviral, topical corticosteroids, therapeutic contact lenses, and the use of fine nylon sutures have improved the success with penetrating keratoplasty (225). Recurrences of the herpes simplex virus or graft rejection are both common events which need to be monitored closely after surgery. A lateral tarsorrhaphy is recommended in patients with neurotrophic keratitis. Conjunctival flaps or conjunctival transplants are alternatives in patients with prior failed corneal transplants.

■ VARICELLA ZOSTER VIRUS

Epidemiology

The varicella zoster virus causes two distinct but related clinical syndromes in humans, varicella (chickenpox) and herpes zoster (shingles). The VZV is identical morphologically to the herpes simplex virus, differing only in segments of the DNA content. Both are alpha members of the herpes class of viruses. Studies reveal that the identical virus that causes varicella recurs as the virus in herpes zoster. Varicella represents the first encounter by the patient with the VZV and positive seroconversions approach 100% by age 60 in the United States. Local infection of the nasopharynx is followed by a viremia and seeding of the reticuloendothelial cells, skin, viscera, and ganglia. This is a common childhood disease which is usually well tolerated. There can be major complications of primary VZV infection, however, especially in adults which include pneumonia and encephalitis and account for 100 to 200 deaths per year (117). The varicella virus recurs as zoster in approximately 2 to 4% of the population, with the majority being in the older age group (176, 330, 429). The trigeminal nerve is involved in 10 to 50% of the total cases of herpes zoster with a predominance in females and in the seventh to ninth decade (59, 447). The risk of developing herpes zoster is directly related to a depressed immune response (272). Other factors associated with the development of zoster include emotional or physical trauma, systemic disease, and trauma to the involved ganglion (107).

Varicella

Maternal varicella infection during pregnancy, especially during the first or second trimester, may result in congenital varicella syndrome in the child (224). There are cicatricial skin lesions in a dermatomal distribution, hemiparesis, bulbar palsies, developmental delays, and learning difficulties. Ocular findings include chorioretinitis, optic nerve atrophy, congenital cataracts, and Horner's syndrome. There is no therapy for congenital varicella syndrome.

Chickenpox usually occurs in children and has an incubation period of 2 weeks before the onset of fever, malaise, and a mucocutaneous exanthem. The maculopapular rash appears in successive crops. The vesicular lesions can affect the lids or conjunctiva and occasionally the cornea. Varicella keratitis can appear as a superficial punctate keratitis or a branching dendritic lesion (288, 412). A late epithelial keratitis and disciform keratitis have been seen in varicella (100). Rarely, an iritis, interstitial keratitis, or corneal scarring can be seen. Rarely posterior segment and even retinal involvment occurs.

Therapy of ocular complications of varicella are not presently established. The epithelial lesions will resolve on their own, but use of a topical antiviral seems appropriate. Systemic acyclovir given early in the course of varicella disease may shorten the overall course. The disciform keratitis may require topical corticosteroids.

Herpes Zoster Ophthalmicus

Varicella Zoster Virus Latency

During the primary infection with the VZV, the virus gains access to the trigeminal sensory ganglion where it resides in a latent state. The virus is probably actively latent rather than in a truly dormant state (238). Distur-bance of the host-virus relationship, usually by a decrease in cell mediated immunity, results in reactivation of the virus from the ganglion and subsequent necrotic ganglionitis and centripetal movement of the virus to the affected dermatome. The VZV is latent in many ganglia but has a propensity for the trigeminal ganglion, probably because of the extensive facial rash of varicella (251). The ophthalmic division of the trigeminal nerve is affected 20 times more frequently than the maxillary or mandibular divisions. The nasociliary branch of the ophthalmic nerve supplies most of the eye and involvement of this branch with nasal lesions is associated with a increased risk of ocular disease (Hutchinson's sign). Viral reactivation causes significant inflammation of the ganglion (in distinction to herpes simplex virus), and the virus can travel distally down the affected sensory nerve but also proximally to the brain stem or spinal cord (242). The ocular involvement is characterized by elements of viral infection, immune response, host inflammatory response, and vasculitis (161) (Table 51–8). A retinitis may also occur (see Retina section; "ARN").

Clinical Manifestations of Herpes Zoster Ophthalmicus

Multiple crops of clear vesicles develop in the affected dermatome (dermatitis). This may be preceded by a hyperesthesia or deep pain in the dermatome. Occasionally the dermatitis is aborted but ocular signs may still develop (zoster sine herpete) (238). Virus can be cultured from the vesicles for several days until the vesicles become yellow and turbid. Late deep dermal scars occasionally result and may become pigmented.

Conjunctival hyperemia with occasional petechial hemorrhages and a follicular or papillary hypertrophy with preauricular lymphadenopathy are common in herpes zoster ophthalmicus.

A sectoral episcleritis may be either flat or slightly nodular. The scleritis may involve several areas in the perilimbal area. The scleritis may progress onto the cornea. Scleral thinning may result from the scleritis or the scleritis may become prolonged.

There are multiple corneal manifestations of herpes zoster probably resulting from multiple mechanisms of disease. These corneal lesions begin within a few days after the skin rash but may continue for several months after resolution of the rash. Epithelial keratitis is a fine or coarse punctate epithelial keratitis layered on the corneal surface (237).

Unlike the branching dendrite with terminal bulbs of HSV, HZV produces a pseudodendrite which has a coarser, ropy appearance without terminal bulbs. The raised epithelial plaque of the pseudodendrites stain poorly with fluorescein in contrast to the vivid staining of the epithelial ulceration caused by HSV. Zoster virus has been isolated from these lesions and viral antigen

TABLE 51–8
Classification of Ocular Involvement with Herpes Zoster Ophthalmicus

Lids
Blepharitis, lid edema
Cicatricial ectropion
Cicatricial entropion
Ptosis
Upper lid lagophthalmos
Lacrimal
Canalicular scarring
Dacryoadenitis
Conjunctiva
Papillary of follicular conjunctivitis
Vesicular conjunctivitis
Conjunctival edema
Cornea
Punctate epithelial keratitis
Pseudodendritic mucous plaques
Anterior stromal infiltrates (nummular)
Keratouveitis–endotheliitis
Disciform keratitis
Neurotrophic keratopathy
Exposure keratopathy
Seripiginous peripheral ulceration
Interstitial keratitis
Sclerokeratitis
Lipid keratopathy
Band keratopathy
Corneal scars, edema
Sclera
Episcleritis
Scleritis
Uvea
Iridocyclitis
Sectoral iris atrophy
Anterior segment necrosis
Trabeculitis
Secondary glaucoma
Phthisis bulbi
Hypotony
Lens
Secondary cataract
Pupil
Zoster ciliary ganglion involvement
Irregular pupil
Muscle
Extraocular muscle palsies
Orbital apex syndrome
Ptosis
Neurologic
Acute neuralgia
Cranial nerve palsy
Contralateral hemiplegia
Postherpetic neuralgia
Facial palsy
Guillain–Barré syndrome
Segmental cerebral arteritis
Encephalitis
Encephalomyelitis

has been detected by immunofluorescence (412). Anterior stromal infiltrates are frequently seen later, either underlying the epithelial lesions or independent of their location. Delayed pseudodendrites (mucous plaques) appear several months after herpes zoster. They are migratory and transitory and frequently associated with neurotropic keratitis. Keratouveitis with or without endotheliitis is seen in approximately 1/3 of patients with acute or chronic herpes zoster ophthalmicus. Corneal manifestations include keratic precipitates, folds in Descemet's membrane, and focal stromal edema. Endothelial cell loss may result in corneal edema. There may be a viral infection of the endothelium in some instances (261). A severe inflammatory vasculitis and trabeculitis with hypopyon, hyphema, and ischemia may develop resulting in an anterior segment ischemia (237). A necrotizing interstitial keratitis with antigen-antibody-complement mediated inflammation may be seen. This end-stage disease may progress to lipid deposits and fibrovascular scarring of the cornea. Disciform keratitis may occur without keratic precipitates or anterior chamber reaction several months after the initial infection and may evolve into a diffuse interstitial keratitis. Peripheral ulcerative keratitis can occur probably as a result of limbal vasculitis, but may be more likely in patients with collagen vascular disease.

Neurotrophic keratitis is one of the most severe and prolonged consequences of herpes zoster keratitis. It is a result of severe ganglion cell necrosis. Patients may recover but approximately 25% of patients will develop some clinical signs of a neurotrophic keratitis. Early findings include a dull appearance to the corneal surface caused by a mild punctate epithelial keratitis. The tear film becomes unstable and the epithelium develops oval defects with a propensity to melting or corneal thinning. There are multiple factors in the development of neurotrophic keratitis including abnormal epithelial turnover, meibomian gland destruction, decreased blink frequency, reduced wettability of cells, and reduced neurotransmitter substances (237, 248). Exposure keratitis is seen in association with cicatricial retraction of the upper lid or in lagophthalmos of the lower lid. A frozen upper lid with dermal contracture makes lid closure impossible. Additional problems of trichiasis, punctal eversion, and thickening of the lids cause additional insult to the exposed eye.

Uveitis occurs in approximately 50% of patients with ocular complications of herpes zoster ophthalmicus and includes characteristic findings of vascular dilatation of the iris vessels, posterior synechiae, Descemet's folds, sectoral atrophy of the iris, and an irregular pupil. Fluorescein angiography has revealed occluded iris vessels probably from direct viral invasion. Patients may complain of photophobia and pain in the more severe cases. Because of the overall pain of herpes zoster ophthalmicus, patients may not be aware of the onset of this complication.

Glaucoma is most commonly seen in the presence of corneal involvement, although isolated cases are seen associated with peripheral trabeculitis. The trabecular meshwork is swollen and clogged with inflammatory cellular debris. In some instances damage to the pars plicata may balance damage to the trabecular meshwork resulting in hypotony. Palsies of the third, fourth, and sixth cranial nerve are not uncommon with herpes zoster ophthalmicus but usually resolve. The fundus may show involvement with optic neuritis or a vascular occlusive or necrotizing retinitis. Central nervous system complications include a cerebral vasculitis resulting in a transient ischemic attack or a hemiparesis; less commonly a meningitis or meningoencephalitis is seen.

Postherpetic Neuralgia

The acute pain accompanying the dermatologic reaction in herpes zoster ophthalmicus is caused by the inflammatory reaction in the nerve tissue with a predominant lymphocytic response. Sympathetic hyperreactivity may accompany the acute pain. Postherpetic neuralgia is defined in varying ways but best considered the pain which persists after the acute pain has resolved. It persists in approximately 17% of patients with herpes zoster ophthalmicus, and is more common in the elderly and patients with acute pain (447). The pain may be boring, lancinating, or pulsating. It is frequently associated with behavioral disturbances (425).

Herpes Zoster Ophthalmicus in AIDS

The presence of herpes zoster in patients under age 50 has become a marker for consideration of AIDS, especially in high risk groups, such as homosexuals, IV drug abusers, Haitians, or patients with hemophilia A (131, 356). Herpes zoster ophthalmicus in patients with AIDS is more prolonged, associated with an increased risk of severe complications, and an increased risk of recurrences (244).

Medical Therapy of Herpes Zoster Ophthalmicus

Systemic acyclovir is the drug of choice in herpes zoster ophthalmicus. It is most beneficial if given within the first 72 hours and at full dose (800 mg five times a day for 10 days) (238). Acyclovir leads to more prompt resolution of skin rash, earlier cessation of pain, more rapid healing, and reduced duration of viral shedding. There is also a reduction in the incidence of episcleritis, keratitis, and iritis (78). Acyclovir, however, does not eliminate all complications of herpes zoster ophthalmicus, and is only slightly better than placebo for many of the ocular complications. Most studies report no effect on postherpetic neuralgia although further studies with increased doses of acyclovir are in progress.

Effective topical antiviral therapy for herpes zoster ophthalmicus is presently not available in the United States. Studies by McGill suggest a beneficial effect of topical ophthalmic acyclovir, although other studies show no benefit (22, 265). Topical corticosteroids are useful for many of the immune, inflammatory, and vascular responses to the varicella zoster virus; for example, interstitial keratitis, disciform keratitis, keratouveitis, anterior stromal infiltrates, episcleritis, scleritis. They are, however, useless in treating other aspects such as mucous plaques, and dendritic keratitis, and are potentially harmful in neurotrophic keratitis, and exposure keratitis.

The use of systemic corticosteroids in patients with herpes zoster ophthalmicus to reduce the inflammatory components of the disease has a long history in the medical literature (197). Further studies by Esmann question the usefulness of systemic corticosteroids (109). In view of the frequency of immunodeficient disease and the potential for disseminated disease with the use of corticosteroids, and the availability of antiviral agents, it seems prudent to restrict corticosteroids to patients who are immunocompetent. Postherpetic neuralgia has been a frustrating element of herpes zoster ophthalmicus. Multiple modalities are presently suggested. Recurrent stellate ganglion block have been effective in the treatment of both acute neuralgia and postherpetic neuralgia. It is best administered by a pain specialist. Cimetidine (Tagamet), a histamine-2 blocker, has been used in uncontrolled studies. Capsaicin cream deletes substance P from small sensory neurons and is effective in some patients in alleviating postherpetic neuralgia after several weeks of topical application (425). The use of psychotropic medications has been effective in many patients with postherpetic neuralgia. Amitriptyline has been the most effective, but alternatives include imipramine, nortriptyline, or desipramine (283, 426).

Surgical therapy of herpes zoster ophthalmicus. Surgical options are occasionally necessary in the treatment of complications of herpes zoster ophthalmicus. Exposure or neurotrophic keratitis is best treated with a lateral tarsorrhaphy to protect the globe. Cicatricial retraction of the upper lid may require skin grafts. Cryotherapy for trichiasis may be indicated. Plastic lid procedures to correct ectropion or entropion are occasionally necessary. Patients may get punctal and canalicular stenosis as a result of the infection so a dacryocystorhinostomy with Jones tube may be necessary.

Corneal thinning and perforation can be treated with sterile tissue adhesives or, alternatively, corneal thinning can be treated with a conjunctival flap. Penetrating keratoplasty has a limited role in treatment of herpes zoster keratitis because of problems with neurotrophic change and increased risk of poor healing, wound dehiscence, and corneal melt (252). In selected circumstances, a penetrating keratoplasty can be helpful, usually combined with a lateral tarsorrhaphy at the time of surgery (333).

Epstein-Barr Virus

The Epstein-Barr virus is another member of the herpes family which has been associated with nasopharyngeal carcinoma, African Burkitt's lymphoma, and with infectious mononucleosis (271). It has an affinity for B lymphocytes with the capacity to transform them. Epstein-Barr virus in childhood produces a mild clinical disease. In adolescents and adults, the clinical picture of infectious of mononucleosis is more marked with fever, lymphadenopathy, sore throat, hepatitis, pericarditis, polyarthritis, and myositis. Although Epstein-Barr virus does not go into latency, it does persist as a chronic low-grade infection in the lymphocytes.

Ocular manifestations of infectious mononucleosis include a unilateral or bilateral follicular conjunctivitis, nodular episcleritis, iridocyclitis, oculoglandular syndrome, dendritic epithelial keratitis, and a stromal keratitis (2, 259, 433, 448). Neuro-ophthalmic manifestations include optic neuritis, papilloedema, and cranial nerve palsies. Epstein-Barr virus has been cultured or detected by ELISA from conjunctival, corneal or tear film samples of patients with the dendrites. The ocular disease may manifest 1 to 4 weeks after the onset of infectious mononucleosis with symptoms of photophobia, irritation, watering, conjunctival hyperemia, and blurring of vision. The stromal keratitis, and indeed most of the ocular disease, is based on an immune response to the Epstein-Barr virus antigen bearing cells located in the cornea.

The serologic diagnosis of infectious mononucleosis is dependent on the detection of heterophile antibody (Paul Bunnell test). The slide agglutination test using horse erythrocytes (Monospot test), the antibody against EB virus (VCA) capsid antigen, or against EB virus nuclear antigens (EBNA) are highly reliable. Patients with acute infectious mononucleosis will have elevated VCA antibodies but EBNA antibodies develop weeks after the onset of the disease. Both persist for life (74). Culture of the Epstein-Barr virus is a research tool at present.

Therapy of Epstein-Barr virus epithelial keratitis has included topical acyclovir, trifluorothymidine, or corticosteroids with good results (74). This epithelial infection also has a self-limited course. Many of the complications of stromal keratitis will respond to steroids since an immune reaction is the etiology (74).

Cytomegalovirus

Cytomegalovirus is another herpes virus which has a predisposition for lymphocytes. Asymptomatic cytomegalovirus infection is common in immunocompetent patients with 50 to 100% of normal adults having antibody indicative of previous infection (300). In patients with immune deficiency, especially AIDS, cytomegalovirus chorioretinitis is a serious and potentially blinding condition. Anterior segment complications of cytomegalovirus infection are uncommon but include follicular conjunctivitis in a patient with cytomegalovirus infection-mononucleosis-like syndrome (135). Corneal manifestations have not yet been recognized, although the virus is shed in the tears. Transmission of cytomegalovirus has been reported through corneal transplantation (174).

Adenovirus

There are a large number of adenoviruses which have a propensity to cause upper respiratory infections and conjunctivitis with keratitis. They are the most common cause of acute viral infections of the conjunctiva and cornea. Most are self-limited although prolonged infections have been reported (318). There are two major syndromes: pharyngoconjunctival fever and epidemic keratoconjunctivitis. Since they present as a conjunctivitis, they have been discussed under conjunctival disease.

Aids Associated Infection

The etiologic agent of AIDS is a retrovirus (HIV Type 1) which is transmitted by blood, semen, and possibly other body fluids such as saliva and tears. The HIV virus has been recovered from tears, conjunctiva, iris, cornea, vitreous, and retina (67). The virus strikes the immune cells, especially the T-helper lymphocytes with a resultant decrease in lymphokine production, inhibition of antigen response, depressed clonal expansion, and decreased ability to assist B lymphocytes in immunoglobin production. Multiple other abnormalities in the immune response to infection result, making the body subject to multiple opportunistic infections and malignant diseases which are normally held in check by an appropriate immune response.

The most common ocular findings in patients with AIDS are in the posterior segment of the eye and include cotton-wool spots (immune complex infarction), retinal hemorrhages (Roth's spots, ischemic maculopathy, retinal periphlebitis, and papilledema). Opportunistic infections in the posterior segment include herpes simplex virus, varicella zoster virus, cytomegalovirus, pneumocystis, cryptococcus, toxoplasma, candida, and mycobacterium avium-intracellulare (175, 304). Also see Retina section for further discussion.

The anterior segment complications of AIDS are less common than the posterior segment complications but include opportunistic infections with herpes simplex virus, varicella zoster virus, microsporidia and increased frequency of bacterial and fungal infections (sometimes spontaneous). An epithelial keratitis has also been described which may be caused by epithelial invasion by HIV. A diffuse interstitial keratitis, anterior iridocyclitis, and peripheral ulcerative keratitis has been described which may relate to a vascular microinfarctions (320). A nonspecific conjunctivitis is seen which may be transient. Kaposi's sarcoma can affect the eyelids or the conjunctiva. Conjunctival involvement may occur in approximately 10% of patients with AIDS, usually in the lower cul-de-sac. The sarcoma presents as a bright red subconjunctival mass with an associated subconjunctival hemorrhage (102, 103). The HIV virus has been seen in the conjunctiva in association with Kaposi's sarcoma (102, 103). Sarcoma has been treated with cryotherapy, radiotherapy, local excision, and azidothymidine.

Because of the potential to transfer the virus by multiple mechanisms, corneal transplantation donors and corneal transplantation tissue are being carefully screened (145). At present there has been no HIV transmission by a penetrating keratoplasty. High risk donor population screening is still recommended.

The specific treatment of the opportunistic infections associated with AIDS is the same as in other patients with a recognition of the slow response, need for prolonged therapy, and vigilance for unusual complications.

Paramyxovirus

The paramyxoviruses include the RNA virus of measles, mumps, and Newcastle's disease, all of which have been associated with anterior segment infection. The measles virus causes an acute catarrhal conjunctivitis, superficial punctate keratitis, and the presence of Koplik's spots on the conjunctiva or caruncle. The disease is usually self-limited in developing countries. In patients living in undeveloped countries or with nutritional deficiencies, or the presence of severe immunosuppression, measles keratitis can be a blinding disease (101). Malnutrition, vitamin A deficiency, and the application of traditional folk medication all contribute to a severe blinding keratitis in undeveloped countries. In this situation, persistent stromal keratitis can lead to scarring and/or perforation. The diagnosis is made under the appropriate clinical setting and confirmed by a viral cultures or serologic response. There is no specific treatment necessary or required, but in malnourished children, the use of systemic vitamin A and topical antibiotics and lubricating agents is warranted with close monitoring. Measles vaccine is highly effective as a prophylaxis against this disease.

Mumps virus has been associated with a severe dacryoadenitis, a catarrhal conjunctivitis, punctate epithelial keratitis, severe stromal keratitis, iridocyclitis, optic neuritis, episcleritis, and scleritis (399). The majority of cases show spontaneous resolution although optic atrophy may leave residual poor vision. The clinical setting is usually sufficient to make the diagnosis (i.e., enlarged parotid gland) but in atypical cases, the diagnosis can be established by viral culture, immunologic detection of viral antigen, and rising serologic titers of varied antibodies against the mumps virus. There is no specific treatment, but the use of topical corticosteroids may relieve some of the ocular symptoms. The mumps vaccine has been highly effective in preventing this disease in the United States.

The Newcastle disease virus is a rare cause of unilateral follicular conjunctivitis in poultry workers and laboratory technicians. There may be an associated fine epithelial keratitis and subepithelial infiltrates. The disease is self-limited with no evident sequela.

Picornavirus

Picornavirus include the RNA enteroviruses consisting of poliovirus, coxsackie virus and the echovirus. Enterovirus 70 and Coxsachie A24 have been associated with an acute hemorrhagic conjunctivitis which is highly contagious. During epidemics, large populations of patients can be affected with a hyperemic conjunctival chemosis and subconjunctival hemorrhages encircling the corneal limbus. The cornea may be affected with a superficial punctate keratitis. The incubation period and the disease itself is of short duration. There is no specific treatment (30).

Poxvirus

The poxvirus includes the DNA viruses of variola (smallpox), the vaccinia vaccine virus, and the virus of molluscum contagiosum. They have an affinity for the skin and rarely cause conjunctival or corneal involvement. The variola virus is now extinct except for a laboratory sample. The vaccinia virus is now also a laboratory-contained virus which can cause lesions of the lid, conjunctiva, and cornea. Significant corneal scarring can result from an epithelial keratitis and a late onset immune keratitis. Therapy of ophthalmic vaccinia would be with hyperimmune vaccinia immune globulin, topical antiviral therapy (trifluorothymidine), and a topical corticosteroid reserved for the late onset disciform keratitis.

The virus of molluscum contagiosum primarily causes a wartlike growth along the lid margin with an associated serous follicular conjunctivitis and punctate keratitis. Rarely, the molluscum virus can cause growths in the conjunctiva at the limbus. Treatment of lid-margin lesions with surgical removal of the core, provides resolution of the conjunctivitis.

Togavirus

The togavirus include the virus of rubella (German measles) and the arbovirus (yellow fever, dengue, sandfly fever). The congenital rubella syndrome results from a maternal infection with the virus during the first or second trimester of pregnancy. Ocular abnormalities in the congenital rubella syndrome include retinopathy, subretinal neovascularization, cataracts, glaucoma, microcornea, microphthalmia, keratoconus, and corneal scarring (160).

Acquired German measles produces ocular disease in 70% of patients after a short incubation period. A catarrhal or follicular conjunctivitis is common with several patients developing a punctate epithelial keratitis. The disease is self-limited (379).

■ BACTERIAL INFECTIONS OF THE CORNEA (BACTERIAL KERATITIS)

The bacterial infections range from mild disease to destructive diseases leading to permanent loss of vision or loss of the eye. Although bacterial infections of the cornea frequently produce characteristic clinical appearances, accurate diagnosis and successful therapeutic management is best accomplished with rapid identification of the specific organism and appropriate antibiotic therapy.

Epidemiology, Risk Factors, and Pathogenesis of Bacterial Keratitis

The bacterial species causing corneal ulceration vary from geographic regions and vary with the risk factors. Staphylococcal species are the most frequent bacterial organism isolated from corneal ulcers in the northern United States and in Canada. Pseudomonas is the most common organism in the southern United States and is becoming more frequently seen in other areas associated with soft contact lens use. Pneumococcus, a common cause of corneal ulcerations in the past, especially in association with nasolacrimal obstruction, has decreased in frequency. Moraxella is seen in association with malnutrition, alcohol abuse, and compromised corneal conditions. Almost 90% of cases of bacterial keratitis fall into one of four groups identified by Jones (187): the Micrococcaceae (Staphylococcus, Micrococcus), the Streptococcus species, the Pseudomonas species, and the Enterobacteriaceae (Citrobacter, Klebsiella, Serratia, Proteus, Enterobacter). Knowledge of the potential organisms that can cause a bacterial keratitis is an important guide to directing therapy (Table 51–9).

Bacteria must adhere to the epithelial surface before they can initiate an infection. The lids and conjunctiva are colonized by bacteria, but corneal ulcers are relatively infrequent because of the various ocular and systemic immune mechanisms to protect the epithelium. Factors which disturb these natural protective mechanisms include alterations in the lids (entropion, ectropion, seventh nerve palsy), ocular surface disorders (keratitis sicca, pemphigoid, erythema multiforme), corneal disease (bullous keratopathy, neurotrophic keratitis, exposure keratitis), and systemic diseases (alco-holism, diabetes, immune deficiency, nutritional deficiency, and neurologic or psychiatric diseases).

The majority of patients with bacterial corneal ulcers have an additional predisposing risk factor (155) (Table 51–10). Corneal trauma from foreign body or abrasions are prominent risk factors (241). The greatest and increasing risk of bacterial keratitis is the use of contact lenses, especially soft contact lenses, contact lenses worn overnight, and perhaps disposable extended wear contact lenses. Patients with aphakic soft contact lenses have an even higher risk of bacterial keratitis (26, 56, 58, 94, 95, 96, 360, 361, 362, 377). The factors involved in the increased risk with contact lenses are complex, but involve compromised epithelial integrity via hypoxia, osmotic, and mechanical factors, the facilitation of bacterial adherence to the epithelium, and the introduction of an inadequately sterilized lens onto the surface of the eye. Contact lens related keratitis is frequently caused by Pseudomonas, which tends to cause a more severe keratitis. Patients with immunosuppression, especially AIDS, may be at an increased risk for bacterial keratitis, either spontaneously, or in association with various ocular risk factors. They may also follow a more fulminant course (285).

A few bacteria, notably Neisseria, Corynebacterium, Haemophilus, and Listeria can invade an intact epithelium by specialized surface attachments. Most pathogens, however, require a break in the epithelial barrier followed by adherence of the organism to the damaged epithelium and the underlying stroma. After entry into the stroma, there is multiplication, diffusion of toxins and enzymes, and resultant tissue destruction (205). Polymorphonuclear cells respond to the insult but produce their own destructive enzymes adding to the corneal insult. Under appropriate therapy, bacterial multiplication ceases, the necrotic areas slough and are replaced by scar tissue, and a new epithelium is laid down. Bowman's layer does not regenerate, so a permanent fibrotic scar results.

Clinical Features of Bacterial Keratitis

Symptoms of a corneal ulcer vary with the specific organism and the severity of the corneal infection. Symp-

TABLE 51-9
Principal Organisms in Bacterial Keratitis

Gram-positive (aerobic)	**Gram-positive cocci (anaerobic)**
Micrococcus	*Peptococcus*
Staphylococcus aureus	*Peptostreptococcus*
Staphylococcus epidermidis	
Streptococcus	
Steptococcus pneumoniae	
Alpha-, beta-nonhemolytic streptococci	
Gram-positive bacilli (aerobic)	**Gram-positive bacilli (anaerobic)**
Bacillus (B. cereus, B. subtilis)	*Propionibacterium acnes*
Corynebacterium (C. diphtheriae, C. xeroses)	*Actinomyces* (branching filaments)
Listeria monocytogenes	*Clostridium* (rare)
Gram-negative bacilli (aerobic)	**Gram-negative (anaerobic)**
Pseudomonas (especially, *P. aeruginosa*)	*Fusobacterium*
Acinetobacter	*Bacteroides*
Enterobacteriaceae	
Klebsiella	
Serratia	
Proteus	
Citrobacter	
Enterobacter	
Escherichia	
Gram-negative diplococci (aerobic)	**Acid-fast bacilli**
Neisseria	*Mycobacterium*
	Nocardia
Gram-negative diplobacillus (aerobic)	
Moraxella	
Gram-negative coccobacillus (aerobic)	
Haemophilus	

toms usually include decreased vision, photophobia, pain, redness, swelling of the lids and conjunctiva, and discharge. An associated conjunctivitis may be seen in infection with gonococcus, pneumococcus, and haemophilus. Clinical examination will reveal a conjunctival injection, a prominent ciliary flush of perilimbal vessels, a discharge of purulent material, debris in the preocular tear film, a corneal ulceration with variable amount of stromal infiltration, and a variable reaction in the anterior chamber from cells and flare to a hypopyon.

Clinical examination can provide strong evidence to support the diagnosis as well as to suggest a specific organism as the cause. Confirmation of the organism to direct therapy requires isolation of the organism by Gram stain and culture. Ulcers caused by Streptococcus pneumoniae usually follow trauma with a dense white infiltrate beginning at the site of the injury. The anterior chamber reaction is usually brisk with a fibrinous reaction or hypopyon. This bacteria as well as the beta-hemolytic streptococcus have a tendency to progress to corneal perforation. Alpha-hemolytic streptococcus tends to cause an indolent ulceration or crystalline ker-

atopathy. Staphylococcal ulcers tend to occur in compromised corneas with bullous keratopathy or ocular surface disease. There is a dense white infiltration which is fairly localized and distinct. Staphylococcus aureus causes a more severe infiltrate than Staphylococcus epidermidis with a tendency to produce intrastromal abscesses, small satellite lesions, and perforation with prolonged infection.

Pseudomonas (especially P. aeruginosa) tends to cause a rapidly involving infection that can lead to perforation if the organism elaborates destructive enzymes such as protease, lipase, and elastase. This is the most common organism associated with contact lens associated bacterial keratitis. The infection begins as superficial edema and microinfiltration of the epithelium and stroma which then extends peripherally and deeper. The anterior chamber reaction tends to be severe with hypopyon formation. The entire cornea may be involved with a diffuse epithelial graying, a ring ulcer, or melting of the cornea in association with a greenish-yellow discharge. There may be a descemetocele and perforation within days of the initial infection. Other strains of Pseudomonas which do not have these dis-

TABLE 51–10
Risk Factors for Bacterial Keratitis

Trauma
Contact lens wear
Corneal trauma
Extensive skin burns

Abnormal Lid Function
Blepharitis
Entropion, ectropion
Trichiasis

Abnormal Tear Function
Dry eye
Lacrimal duct obstruction

Corneal Diseases
Corneal edema
Exposure keratopathy
Neurotrophic keratopathy
Viral keratitis
Topical steroid or immunosuppressive

Systemic Abnormalities
Alcoholism
AIDS
Erythema multiforme major
Drug addiction
Diabetes
Malnutrition
Age
Systemic immunosuppressive therapy

---

tinctive enzymes and other gram negative rods such as Klebsiella, Serratia, and Proteus have milder, nonspecific features. Moraxella is a gram negative diplobacillus that produces corneal ulcerations most often after trauma in debilitated patients, diabetics, and alcoholics. It tends to be a mild indolent oval ulcer in the inferior portion of the cornea.

Anaerobic and higher order bacteria are rare causes of keratitis usually in association with corneal injuries from soil contamination (316). They may have some specific features to suggest the cause of the organism. The nonspore forming anaerobes of Propionibacterium, Peptococcus, and Peptostreptococcus can occur isolated or in association with other organisms with no distinct patterns. The spore-forming Clostridium may have identifiable bubbles under the epithelium or within the anterior chamber. Listeria may cause a corneal ulcer with a black hypopyon in the anterior chamber. The aerobic Bacillus cereus is associated with a rapidly progressive and devastating corneal infection and ring abscess with intraocular penetration.

Nocardia tends to produce an indolent, infiltrative disease with a cracked-windshield appearance (306, 314). Mycobacterial infection of the cornea tends to be indolent and persistent. Mycobacterium fortuitum tends to cause a roughened surface (cracked windshield) with only moderate corneal infiltrates (411). More recent reports have identified Mycobacterium chelonei and other atypical mycobacterium from chronic indolent keratitis (260, 282).

Laboratory Evaluation of Microbial Keratitis

The definitive diagnosis can be achieved only with the use of corneal scrapings and culture. Although many small ulcerations can be treated with antibiotics in the absence of obtaining a culture, moderate and large ulcers as well as indolent ulcers require a full evaluation to direct therapy. In many instances, it is necessary to distinguish some of the other clinical entities which can mimic bacterial keratitis such as immune infiltrates associated with blepharitis or contact lenses. Smears and cultures should be taken before starting therapy. The yield on cultures is lower if the patient is already taking antibiotics. Cultures appear to be more sensitive than the yield from smears with the Gram stain being positive approximately 50% of the time and cultures being positive 40 to 73% of the time (19, 154, 240, 361). A corneal culture may not be positive despite the presence of a bacterial keratitis. A positive culture is helpful; a negative culture requires consideration of clinical findings. Occasionally a corneal biopsy is indicated in prolonged, indolent, or deep keratitis.

A scheme for evaluating microbial keratitis should be directed at the recovery of the likely responsible organisms with additional studies indicated under selected circumstances (Table 51–11). The following discussion encompasses the workup of a bacterial, fungal, and parasitic keratitis since clinical acumen may not be able to distinguish the differences. A culture of the lids and conjunctiva of both the infected and unaffected eye is taken for comparative purposes. Calcium alginate swabs moistened with trypticase soy broth are swabbed across the conjunctiva and then the lids and streaked on a blood agar plate (Figure 51–18). Topical anesthetic is then applied and corneal scrapings are done with a sterile platinum Kimura spatula or the use of a calcium alginate swab dipped in trypticase soy broth (34). The material is best plated directly on culture media since there are a few organisms and they may be fastidious. Direct visualization with a slit lamp will aid the scraping. The specimen is C-streaked on the blood agar plate with additional scrapings placed on chocolate agar (for Neisseria, Haemophilus specifically) and Sabouraud's agar (for fungus specifically). An anaerobic broth, such as chopped-meat glucose or thioglycolate medium with hemin and vitamin K are alternatives. A brain-heart infusion broth is an ideal fungal media and has the advantage of eluting any antibiotic present. If mycobacteria is suspected, special media are required (e.g., Lowenstein-Jensen). For Acanthamoeba, a prepared nonnutrient agar with E. coli overlay is the best medium to support growth and identification.

Multiple smears are then taken on slides for evaluation by Gram, Giemsa, methenamine silver, acridine orange or calcofluor white (Table 51–12). The Gram stain is best for bacterial detail while the Giemsa stain is ideal for cellular detail and outlines the fungal walls better than the Gram stain. Methenamine silver is the most sensitive for detection of the cell walls of fungi. The acridine orange stain is sensitive for bacteria and amoeba and fungi but requires a fluorescent microscope. Calcafluor white is effective for detecting fungi and amoeba cysts but also requires a fluorescent microscope. An acid fast stain is needed to detect most mycobacteria and nocardioforms (260).

Therapy of Bacterial Keratitis

Therapy should be directed at the bacterial keratitis as well as the predisposing or risk factors (e.g., discontinuing contact lens wear, correcting corneal exposure). The results of the initial Gram stain is helpful in directing therapy, although total reliance on the Gram stain is unwise (29). If done meticulously, the Gram stain can detect the pathogen in 75% of cases caused by a single organism and approximately 37% of cases caused by mixed organisms (188). There is controversy regarding the reliance on Gram stain in the initial management of corneal ulcers. The potential serious consequences of a bacterial keratitis make it wise to consider the results of the Gram stain, but to deliver wide spectrum antibiotic coverage until the culture results are available. Others believe that the specific therapy avoids additional toxicity hazards. Fortunately, topical broad spectrum antibiotics are usually well tolerated in the short term. Most ophthalmologists now use the Gram stain, but begin initial therapy with a broad spectrum combination of fortified aminoglycoside (gentamicin 14 mg/ml) and a fortified cephalosporin (cefazolin 50 mg/ml) (Table 51–13). More recently, ciprofloxacin is an effective broad spectrum antibiotic available commercially (86, 230). Ciprofloxacin is effective against most corneal pathogens including aminoglycoside-resistant pseudomonas, methicillin-resistant staphylococcus, and it is effective against Neisseria. Ciprofloxacin is less effective against streptococci. Fortified cefazolin provides coverage against gram-positive cocci and some gram-negative rods while the aminoglycosides provides coverage of some gram-positive organisms and gram-negative rods including Pseudomonas.

Antibiotic coverage is modified based on culture results and the relative susceptibility data. More specific antibiotics are effective against selected organisms compared with the broad spectrum coverage.

Resistance to the antibiotics determined on the basis of disc sensitivity patterns or even tube dilution are not necessarily accurate since the topical antibiotic is available in increased concentrations. The goal of antimicrobial therapy is to provide an increased level of antibiotic (preferentially bactericidal) within the tolerance of the host tissues. With bacterial keratitis, this can usually be achieved with the frequent installation of fortified topical antibiotics. Fortified antibiotics are prepared by adding the needed amount of parenteral agent to an artificial tear solution or to a commercially available weaker topical solution. Topical antibiotics are generally applied every 30 minutes for the first few days until a response is seen. Subconjunctival antibiotics can

TABLE 51–11
Culture Media for Microbial Keratitis

Medium	Purpose	Incubation temp (°C)
	Routine Media	
Trypticase soy broth	Saturation of swabs	
Blood agar plate	Aerobic and facultative anaerobic bacteria, fungi	35 (10% CO_2)
Chocolate agar plate	Aerobic and facultative anaerobic bacteria, Neisseria and Haemophilus spp.	35 (10% CO_2)
Thioglycolate broth	Aerobic and anaerobic bacteria	35
Brucella agar plate	Anaerobic bacteria	35 (anaerobic system)
Sabouraud dextrose agar	Fungi	25
	Special Media	
Blood agar plate	Fungi, mycobacteria	25
Thayer-Martin medium	Neisseria spp.	35 (10% CO_2)
Lowenstein-Jensen or Middlebrook 7H10 agar slant	Mycobacteria and Nocardia spp.	35
BHI broth with gentamycin	Fungi	25
Nonnutrient agar plate with E. coli overlay	Acanthamoeba spp.	30 and 35

Figure 51–18.
Lid, conjunctival, and corneal culture plates. The pattern of streaking done with a cotton swab for the lids and conjunctiva and a Kimura-spatula for corneal cultures on an agar plate to allow easy identification of organisms and to distinguish contamination on the plate.

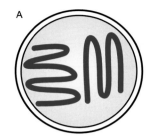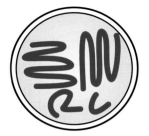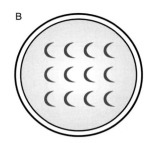

TABLE 51–12
Stains for Microbial Keratitis

Stain	Uses	Comments
Gram stain	Bacteria, yeasts	Gram–positive versus gram–negative bacteria
Giemsa stain	Cytology, fungi, chlamydial inclusions, bacteria (all stain blue)	
Methenamine silver	Fungi	Gelatin–coated slides for modified technique
Acridine orange	Fungi, bacteria, *Acanthamoeba*	Requires fluorescence microscope
Calcofluor white	Fungi, *Acanthamoeba*	Requires fluorescence microscope
PAS (periodic acid–Schiff)	Fungi	
Acid fast (Ziehl-Nielsen)	Mycobacteria, *Nocardia, Actinomyces*	

also achieve therapeutic levels probably by a combination of leakage from the injection site into the tear film and by direct penetration through the sclera or cornea. Subconjunctival antibiotics are added for additional therapeutic enhancement, but have more significant risks and problems with patient tolerance. Systemic therapy is usually even less effective and exposes the patient to potentially greater toxicosis. Systemic antibiotics are indicated if the organism has extended to the limbus (as in Pseudomonas scleritis) or when there is a risk of concurrent septicemia (as with Neisseria infection or with Pseudomonas or Haemophilus in children). Antibiotic impregnated dissolvable collagen shields are an alternative technique for constant bathing of the eye but have a variable dissolution rate from eye to eye resulting in fluctuation in the antibiotic delivered (322).

Adjunctive therapy with cycloplegic agents helps to reduce ciliary spasm and prevent synechiae. Collagenase inhibitors for Pseudomonas keratitis have been the subject of experimental studies but are not clinically useful. Cryotherapy may be indicated for scleral extension of Pseudomonas infection. The most controversial area of adjunctive therapy is the use of topical corticosteroids. Corticosteroids do reduce the polymorphonuclear response and subsequent enzyme release and have been effective in reducing corneal scars. Corticosteroids, however, can enhance bacterial growth and lead to a a recurrence, especially with Pseudomonas. Corticosteroids are much safer to use once the microbial killing is well under way with the appropriate antibiotic. There are different views and approaches to the use of corticosteroids as outlined by some authors (68, 153, 386).

Monitoring the response to therapy allows the ophthalmologist to withdraw the potent medications slowly depending on the response. Occasionally, reevaluation of the clinical situation is necessary with further culture or biopsy or withdrawal of potent antibiotics. With the more aggressive bacteria or with advanced disease, the corneal ulcer may progress to corneal perforation with intraocular or scleral involvement necessitating sterile tissue adhesive (glue) or surgical maneuvers in an attempt to salvage the eye (326).

■ FUNGAL INFECTIONS OF THE CORNEA

Epidemiology, Risk Factors, and Pathogenesis of Fungal Keratitis

Fungal keratitis (keratomycosis) is a rare cause of corneal infection in temperate climates, but is a frequent cause of corneal infections in certain areas of the world such as India and the tropics. The fungi are ubiquitous, both indoors and outdoors, and almost any fungal species is capable of inducing an infection. Fungi are broadly classified as yeasts or molds. Yeasts are unicellu-

TABLE 51–13
Initial Therapy of Bacterial Keratitis*

Gram Stain Cytology	Topical Therapy
Gram-positive cocci	Cefazoline 50 mg/ml (Vancomycin 50 mg/ml for resistant staphylococci)
Gram-negative cocci	Ceftriaxone 50 mg/ml (or Bacitracin 10,000 μ/ml)
Gram-positive rods	Gentamicin 14 mg/ml
Gram-negative rods	Tobramycin 14 mg/ml and Cefazolin 50 mg/ml
Gram-positive filaments	Penicillin 100,000 U/ml
Acid-fast bacilli	Amikacin 10 mg/ml
Two types of bacteria or none	Cefazolin 50 mg/ml and gentamycin 14 mg/ml

* Fluroquinolones may be considered in milder keratitis; intravenous therapy reserved for scleral extension, perforation, or progressing keratitis, or for suspected gonococcal keratitis.

lar fungi characterized by an oval structure called the blastoconidium. Candida is the prototypical yeast and reproduces by budding. In the tissues there is elongation of the buds so that they may appear as hyphae but in truth they are pseudohyphae. Fungi may also invade tissue as a true hyphal form (i.e., molds). The molds are filamentous structures (hyphae) that grow by apical extension and branching. They have a rigid cell wall composed of chitin and an inner layer of sterol-containing cytoplasmic membrane. Fungi reproduce asexually through the formation of various types of spores. The fungi causing fungal keratitis are usually in the sexual phase when they are cultured from the cornea. Primary identification of fungi is not possible from corneal scrapings since identification schemes depend on the appearance of the asexual spore morphology. Under appropriate laboratory conditions, the fungi are induced to undergo sexual reproduction with identification then possible.

The epidemiology of keratomycoses is climate specific. In the southern United States, Fusarium species are the most common cause of keratomycoses. In other areas of the United States, Candida is the most frequent cause of keratomycoses. Worldwide, Aspergillus is the most common cause. Overall, Fusarium and Aspergillus predominate in tropical and subtropical climates whereas Candida and Aspergillus predominate in temperate zones and colder climates. The most common causes of fungal keratitis are listed in Table 51–14.

The molds (filamentous fungi) are most commonly associated with a history of corneal trauma while working with vegetable matter outdoors. Yeast keratitis, on the other hand, is most commonly associated with a compromised or immunocompromised cornea.

The pathogenic mechanisms of fungi include direct physical damage by invasion and growth, chemical damage from fungal toxins and enzymes, and damage from the infiltration of inflammatory cells. The replication of fungi is usually slower than bacteria. Filamentous fungi usually invade and interdigitate between collagen lamel-

lae and lead to disruption of normal collagen fiber arrangement (286). Yeast strain virulence may be associated with the ability to produce hyphae and act as a filamentous fungi (287). Both the yeasts and filamentous fungi inhibit attachment of neutrophils and therefore resist phagocytosis. Infiltration of the corneal stroma with host leukocytes is an important component of the disease which produces ring abscesses and causes release of lysosomal enzymes. Complex mycotoxins and enzymes are released by both filamentous fungi and yeasts (295).

Clinical Features of Funcal Keratitis

Fungal keratitis presents with symptoms of redness, irritation, and photophobia. The onset is usually less ex-

TABLE 51–14
Principal Organisms in the Fungal Keratitis

Moniliaceae (Nonpigmented filamentous fungi)
Fusarium
Aspergillus
Acremonium
Penicillium
Paecilomyces
Dematiaceae (Pigmented filamentous fungi)
Curvilaria
Sphaeropsidales
Melanconiales
Alternaria
Drechslera
Nonseptate Filamentous Fungi (Rare)
Absidia
Mucor
Yeasts
Candida
Geotrichum
Dimorphic Fungi (Rare)
Blastomyces
Cryptococcus

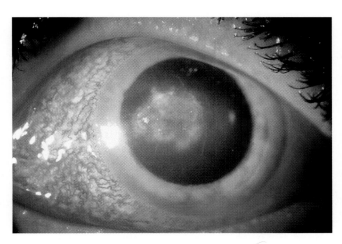

Figure 51–19.
Fungal keratitis. A 20-year-old outdoor laborer who was struck with a branch in his eye one week ago. He was treated with topical antibiotic steroid ointment with worsening of the condition. Culture grew Aspergillus.

plosive than bacterial keratitis, although considerable variation is present. Classic clinical features of filamentous keratitis include a feathery, stromal infiltrate which tends to be dry, gray, and somewhat elevated above the level of the corneal surface (Figure 51–19). There are frequently satellite lesions, hypopyon, and an endothelial plaque. Yeast keratitis tends to be more localized with a small epithelial defect and a much larger discrete and dense white stromal infiltrate. Although distinctive, the features are not enough to forego a careful workup with evaluation for bacteria, fungi, and parasites.

Laboratory Evaluation of Fungal Keratitis

Prompt laboratory evaluation is necessary to confirm the diagnosis. As discussed above under bacterial keratitis, scrapings of the cornea are plated on culture media slides. The media best for fungi is the Sabouraud's

agar plate at room temperature containing gentamicin but without cycloheximide (which inhibits saprophytic fungi). The blood agar plate at room temperature is occasionally successful as is the liquid fungal media such as brain-heart infusion broth. The glass slides are examined with Gram and Giemsa stain, although the more specific and sensitive identification of fungi can be accomplished with the use of the Gomori methenamine silver stain or the calcofluor white stain using a fluorescent microscope.

A corneal biopsy is occasionally necessary in fungal keratitis since the infection frequently is deep in the cornea. A partial thickness trephination with a small trephine (3 to 4 mm) can provide adequate tissue for multiple cultures and slides and histopathologic sections with Periodic acid Schiff or methenamine silver.

The fungal cultures can be positive in either Sabourauds, blood agar, or brain heart infusion or any combination. In fungal keratitis, as opposed to systemic fungal infection, these cultures are frequently available in 48 to 72 hours, although they should be kept for 2 weeks. They are examined with the dissecting microscope to confirm the pattern of growth. A positive smear for fungi is helpful in suggesting the specific type of fungus, but more specific subculturing in media to enhance spores is necessary for confirmatory identification.

Therapy of Fungal Keratitis

Antifungal therapy is significantly hampered by several factors: frequent presence of deep keratitis, poor sensitivity to antifungal, poor solubility and penetrance of antifungals, potential toxicosis of antifungal drugs, and poor correspondence between in vitro and in vivo sensitivity patterns and effectiveness. The major groups of antifungal agents are the polyenes, the imidazoles, the triazoles, and the pyrimidines (Table 51–15). Polyene and imidazoles act on the sterols in the cell wall of fungi.

TABLE 51–15
Antifungal Preparations for Ocular Use

Class	Agents		Mechanism of Action
Polyene	Natamycin	5% suspension	Damage to cell membrane sterol resulting in leakage
	Amphotericin B	0.15% solution	
	Nystatin	—	
Imidazoles	Miconazole	1% solution	Inhibits demethylation preventing formation of cell wall
	Ketoconazole	1% solution 400 mg/day po	
	Clotrimazole	1% cream (vaginal preparation)	
Triazole	Fluconazole	1% solution	Inhibits fungal cytochrome demethylation
		200 mg/day po	
Pyrimidine	5-Fluorocytosine	1% solution	Inhibits RNA synthesis
		150 mg/kg/day po	

The pyrimidines act on fungal RNA and protein synthesis.

The polyenes include natamycin, amphotericin B, and nystatin. Natamycin, as a 5% suspension, is the only FDA-approved antifungal agent for ocular use in the United States. Like all polyenes, it is water insoluble and penetrates ocular tissues poorly. It has a good spectrum against many filamentous fungi, and is most effective against superficial Fusarium infection. Amphotericin B, a large polyene antifungal, is effective and well tolerated at a 0.15% solution prepared from the intravenous preparation and is effective against a broad range of filamentous fungi and candida (184). Previously, higher doses proved to be toxic to the eye. Nystatin is no longer used for fungal keratitis.

Variable results have been achieved with the imidazole and triazole antifungal agents. Several of these agents are available for fungal infection of the skin and vagina in the United States. Clotrimazole is available as a 1% cream for fungal vaginitis and in this formulation has been used for fungal keratitis (122). Miconazole is available as an intravenous preparation in cremophore oil and has a wide spectrum of antifungal activity. It has been used in a variety of keratomycoses (124). Ketoconazole is available as an oral drug for patients with mucocutaneous candidiasis. It has been used topically in combination with other drugs (116, 163). It has also been used in an oral form for fungal keratitis (213).

Fluconazole and Itraconazole are triazole agents. Fluconazole is an oral or intravenous drug available in the United States for systemic treatment for Candida and Cryptococcus infection (296). Topical preparations of a 1% solution in sterile water in combination with oral administration has been effective in selected patients (122). Itraconazole is a triazole which has been effective orally against some fungal keratitis (404).

Flucytosine is a pyrimidine antifungal available as an oral agent and can be mixed into a 1% aqueous solution in the therapy of Candida keratitis (190). Flucytosine needs to be combined with amphotericin because of the frequent emergence of organisms resistant to flucytosine.

Many agents have been tried in fungal keratitis because of poor success with exclusive use of any one regimen. Successful therapy frequently needs to be prolonged for weeks, combination therapy is more frequently effective, and there may be synergism between polyenes and pyrimidines as well as between imidazoles and pyrimidines. Polyenes and imidazoles may have an antagonism. Suggestions for therapy are shown in Table 51–16. Iontophoresis and collagen shields have also been examined as methods to enhance antifungal delivery (366). Therapy for fungal keratitis is generally restricted until a positive smear or culture is obtained. Therapy for filamentous fungi is started with natamycin 5% hourly. If progression is taking place, then further antifungal therapy should be added. For Aspergillus, the addition of miconazole to natamycin is appropriate. For Fusarium, the addition of Amphotericin B is appropriate. For Paecilomyces, miconazole or ketoconazole is appropriate. For yeast keratitis (Candida albicans) the use of Amphotericin B combined with Flucytosine and/or miconazole is appropriate.

Stabilization of the keratitis can take several days and then the antifungal therapy can be gradually weaned over weeks. Despite medical therapy, 10 to 20% of fungal keratitis may progress because of overwhelming disease or poor response to therapy, resulting in corneal perforation. Surgical management of fungal keratitis with therapeutic keratoplasty should be considered in cases of an increasing hypopyon, peripheral corneal involvement, and impending or frank perforation. Conjunctival flaps seem to have a limited role in the treatment of fungal keratitis because of the deep-seated infection.

TABLE 51–16
Therapy of Fungal Keratitis

Organism		Agent
Filamentous Fungi	Topical	Natamycin
	Alternatives:	Amphotericin B, miconazole
	Systemic	Ketoconazole or miconazole
Yeast	Topical	Amphotericin B
	Alternatives:	Flucytosine, miconazole, clotrimazole
	Systemic	Flucytosine or fluconazole

■ PARASITIC INFECTION OF THE CORNEA

Parasitic ocular infections are increasing in frequency from different sources. The more common parasitic infections associated with the cornea include those caused by protozoa (Acanthamoeba, Microsporidia, Leishmania) and by nematodes (Onchocerca, Loa loa). There are other parasites which rarely involve the cornea (302, 435).

Protozoa

Protozoa are unicellular organisms which exist in nature in at least two distinct morphologic phases (mobile trophozoites and cysts). Protozoa species involved in significant corneal infection include Acanthamoeba, Microsporidia, and Leishmania.

Acanthamoeba

Acanthamoeba are small free-living protozoa present in diverse environmental sources as well as found in the throat, gut, and feces of the normal human. They rarely can cause a meningoencephalitis. They have both trophozoites and cysts with the latter occurring under adverse growth conditions in vivo. They have become a frequent cause of corneal infection since the mid-1980s with contaminated water and contact lenses being significant risk factors. Acanthamoeba can adhere to contact lenses and has been found in contact lens cases and nonsterile fluids used by patients. Homemade saline, tap water, and saliva are frequent sources of acanthamoeba and trauma can also be an initiating factor (228, 385).

Symptoms of acanthamoeba keratitis include foreign body sensation, photophobia, and rather severe pain which is out of proportion to clinical findings. Rare cases have been bilateral. Signs of early infection include a granular epithelium with punctate or dendritic figures. After adherence to glycolipids on the corneal epithelium, cytolytic enzymes facilitate transepithelial invasion and other enzymes contribute to stromal damage (435). Patchy stromal infiltrates can coalesce to form an annular pattern. A ring infiltrate and perineural infiltrates are characteristic. Later subepithelial infiltrates and satellite opacities may occur as an immune reaction. Dense stromal suppuration can lead to ulceration and stromal abscess with iritis and hypopyon. Corneal neovascularization may occur. Descemetocele formation and perforation occur rarely.

Corneal scrapings are used for direct examination in smears and for culture. For deeper infections, a corneal biopsy is necessary for both histopathologic examination and microbiologic testing. Material can also be obtained from contact lenses or contact lens cases. The organisms can be seen on a saline wet mount under a cover slip with mobile trophozoites or cysts seen with Nomarski optics. The Gram stain, Giemsa stain, acridine orange, and lactophenol cotton blue stains can reveal both the trophozoites and the cysts (85). Calcofluor white can identify cysts (257). Histopathologic section from corneal biopsies or from sheets of epithelial cells can be used to show organisms using either Periodic acid Schiff, trichrome, or methenamine silver stain. Electron microscopy shows the trophozoites with thorny pseudopodia and double-walled cysts with a wrinkled exocyst and a stellate endocyst. In corneal transplant specimens, the cysts are frequently aligned along Descemet's membrane.

Material for culture can be transported in Page's amaeba saline, but preferably inoculated directly onto a nonnutrient agar seeded with an overlay of gram-negative rods. Acanthamoeba are rarely isolated from other standard media. Culture plates are examined with a dissecting microscope after 24 to 48 hours to show the trails of motile trophozoites on the agar surface. Species classification include cyst morphology and some chemical profiles. The most common corneal isolates have been A. castellani, A. culbertsoni, and A. polyphagia. Sensitivity testing is not reliably established.

Treatment with epithelial debridement early in the disease may remove the infective load and may be curative (24). It can occasionally also help to alleviate some of the severe pain in some of these patients. Medical therapy uses multiple antimicrobial agents for a prolonged duration (227, 416). Diamidines such as propamidine 0.1% solution or dibromopropamidine ointment are used frequently and are occasionally successful. There are many medical failures. Diamidines is not available in the United States but is a nonprescription drug in England. The aminoglycosides, neomycin and paromomycin, have some antiamoebic activity. Neomycin is available as part of the commercially available Neosporin eye drops; Imidazole compounds such as miconazole and clotrimazole are used in 1 to 2% suspension; oral therapy with ketoconazole or fluconazole may be added (180). The polymeric biguanides are available as a swimming pool supplement at 20% concentration; a diluted concentration of 0.02% is useful for acanthamoeba keratitis (229) although there is a risk of ocular surface toxicosis. Chlorhexidine is being evaluated (207). The main problem with therapy is that the drugs are not effective against the cysts; multiple agents are being evaluated for their additive effectiveness (207).

A nonsteroidal antiinflammatory drug such as Sulindac (Clinoril) may help pain and suppress inflammation. Rarely narcotics are needed. The role of steroids remains controversial. They can interfere with replication of trophozoites and cysts and prolong the disease process. They can, however, decrease anterior segment inflammation and are difficult to withdraw once started. Corneal transplantation is best deferred until medical therapy has suppressed the inflammation. It may be required for progressive destructive keratitis with perforation or for persistent nonresponsive infection (111). Cryotherapy can be used along with penetrating keratoplasty. Recurrent Acanthamoeba keratitis can occur; glaucoma and cataract are common complications (111).

The mainstay of treatment is preventive. Since 85% of cases are associated with contact lens use, the education of contact lens patients and the use of appropriate heat or chemical sterilization will lower the risk of Acanthamoeba keratitis.

Microsporidia

Microsporidia are obligate intracellular protozoal parasites which cause two forms of corneal infection; stromal keratitis associated with trauma and superficial keratoconjunctivitis associated with immunosuppression (332). There have been only approximately 20 cases reported in the literature. The onset of the disease has been associated with exposure to livestock, fowl, and household plants. Horizontal transmission can occur in animals via a fecal, urinary or intranasal route. Vertical (congenital) transmission has been shown in animals, although not yet shown in humans. Microsporidia are endemic in the tropics. Serological studies to define the incidence and prevalence are problematic.

Microsporidia are small oval spores. Five species from the phylum Microspora have been associated with human disease (332). The species of genera Nosema, Microsporum, and Encephalitozoon have been associated with ocular infections in humans: Nosema corneum, Nosema ocularum, Microsporidium ceylonensis and Microsporidium africanum, and Encephalitozoon hellem.

Infection with microsporidia results from ingestion or inhalation of organisms which then infect the gastrointestinal or respiratory tract. The ocular infection with encephalitozoon may arise from systemic infections since individuals with ocular infections often shed microsporidia in the urine. The presenting systemic symptoms of encephalitozoon infection include respiratory, urinary, central nervous system, and gastrointestinal symptoms. The slit lamp findings in encephalitozoon infection consists of fine or coarse punctate epithelial opacities, marked conjunctival injection, and superficial corneal infiltration. Infection with nosema and microsporidia may arise from direct contact with a contaminated source or trauma. In microsporidia, the patients are not immunosuppressed. Patients complain of foreign body sensation, photophobia, blurred vision, redness and dryness. The infection involves the stroma with a picture of interstitial keratitis. Without therapy, granulomatous inflammation can lead to necrotic thinning and perforation.

The clinician should suspect AIDS in patients with encephalitozoon infection. Corneal scrapings in either situation may reveal large gram-positive ovoid organisms within conjunctival epithelial cells. The Gram stain of the cornea will also reveal the spores. Other techniques include Weber's chromotrope-based cytology and a fluorescein technique. The most exquisite and confirmatory tests are with electron microscopy. Isolation of the organisms is problematic and requires tissue culture methods. The medical therapy of Microsporidium infection of the cornea has not been extensively investigated. Fumagillin, an antibiotic from Aspergillus fumigatus, at 10 mg/ml has been used to treat encephalitozoon. Itraconazole, propamidine, and a benzimidazole (e.g., Thiobendazole) may have a place in the treatment of microsporidia. For stromal involvement, penetrating keratoplasty with cryotherapy has been used successfully (97).

Leishmania

Leishmaniasis is caused by a protozoa with an animal reservoir and an insect vector. It is endemic in Asia, Africa, South America, and the Mediterranean basin (223). In humans, it occurs in two forms: the cutaneous and visceral. American cutaneous leishmaniasis starts with a papule at the inoculation site that enlarges into a nodule. Mucous membrane later becomes involved, especially around the mouth, nose, pharynx, larynx, and trachea. Eyelid lesions are occasionally present. Keratitis occurs with cutaneous leishmaniasis usually as an ulcerative keratitis or as a phlyctenular-like lesion leading to an interstitial keratitis. Symptoms include pain, hyperemia, photophobia, tearing, and decreased vision. The interstitial keratitis is probably caused by direct invasion of the organism into the host cornea.

Visceral leishmaniasis has an incubation period of several months followed by constitutional symptoms of fever, weight loss, hepatosplenomegaly, leukopenia, jaundice, hair loss, and peripheral edema (kala-azar). Retinal hemorrhages are seen but rarely a keratitis. Limbal episcleral nodules may lead to opacification and neovascularization of the peripheral cornea.

In cutaneous leishmaniasis, the diagnosis is made from a biopsy of the skin ulcer. In visceral leishmaniasis, the organism can be obtained from bone marrow biopsy or lymph node biopsy. The lesions of cutaneous leishmaniasis often resolve without treatment. Pentavalent antimonial agents are useful for large lesions. Topical pentavalent antimony has been used to treat the keratitis. The treatment of visceral leishmaniasis included pentavalent antimony. Splenectomy may be required. The eye findings may respond to this systemic treatment.

Nematodes

Filaria are helminths belonging to the class Nematoda. The filaria have similar life cycles and are transmitted only by blood sucking mosquitos or flies. Onchocerca volvulus and Loa loa can cause ocular manifestations.

Onchocerca

Onchocerciasis is caused by Onchocerca volvulus which is transmitted to humans by the bite of a female black fly. It occurs in Africa, Central and South America, and the Arabian peninsula. Worldwide, almost 500,000 people are blinded from this disease (312). The disease can present as a dermatitis, subcutaneous nodule, and sclerosing lymphadenitis. Ocular findings range from live or dead microfilaria in the stroma without inflammation to a severe inflammation causing an opaque cornea. With death of the microfilaria, a subepithelial infiltrate develops, causing a punctate keratitis. Later, stromal edema occurs with lymphocytes and eosinophils. A form of sclerosing interstitial keratitis is most common in the west African form of this disease, which leads to total corneal scarring and blindness. The diagnosis is confirmed by skin-snip analysis which reveals the microfilaria. Slit lamp examination can reveal live microfilaria in the corneal stroma and anterior chamber. Serologic tests are complicated by cross reactivity with other parasites. Treatment with ivermectin is presently recommended.

Loa Loa

Loa loa is transmitted by the bite of mango flies with human and possibly monkeys as the only definitive hosts. Clinical manifestations are characterized by migration of adult worms under the skin tissue and the conjunctiva of the eye. Other ocular manifestations include migration of the worm into vitreous and anterior chamber as well as retinopathy and uveitis. Laboratory evaluation will reveal microfilaria in the peripheral blood and occasionally in the urine, sputum, and central nervous system. Conjunctival worms can be removed by excision. Systemic therapy with diethylcarbamazine is indicated after the conjunctival worm has been removed; a dying nematode can cause a reactive keratoconjunctivitis.

■ INTERSTITIAL KERATITIS

Interstitial keratitis is a nonulcerative, nonsuppurative inflammation of the corneal stroma. It was originally used to refer to the inflammatory and postinflammatory changes of congenital syphilis but has been broadened over the years to encompass a spectrum of corneal stromal inflammations owing to a variety of causes (Table 51–17). Interstitial keratitis can be caused by a variety of microorganisms which can gain access to the cornea through a exogenous source (for example, contact lens), through endogenous spread from systemic disease by the limbus (onchocerciasis), or by extension from the sclera or iris. The viral causes of interstitial keratitis (herpes simplex virus, varicella zoster virus, Epstein-Barr virus, mumps, measles, variola, vaccinia) have been discussed under viral corneal infections. The parasitic causes of interstitial keratitis (Acanthamoeba, Microsporidia, Leishmania, Onchocerca) have been discussed under parasitic corneal infections. Bacterial causes of interstitial keratitis include Mycobacterium tuberculosis, Mycobacterium leprae, Treponema pallidum, Borrelia burgdorferi, and the multiple causes of infectious crystalline keratopathy. Cogan's syndrome is also presented here although not truly a bacterial cause of interstitial keratitis.

Cogan Syndrome

Cogan's syndrome is a multisystem inflammatory vascular disease characterized by interstitial keratitis and sudden onset of audiovestibular dysfunction (214). It is a rare disorder with no racial, geographic, or gender predilection. The majority of patients are between ages 20 and 40. Systemic vascular involvement varies from 50 to 75%, especially aortic insufficiency.

The etiology is unclear but most likely an immune mediated systemic inflammatory condition. By definition, patients have a negative serologic test for syphilis. Frequent abnormalities include an elevated sedimentation rate, leukocytosis, neutrophilia, increased circulating B and T lymphocytes, anemia, elevated cryoglobulin levels, decreased serum complement levels, and vari-

TABLE 51–17
Principal Causes of Interstitial Keratitis

Viral Disease
Herpes simplex
Varicella zoster virus
Epstein-Barr virus
Rubeola
Mumps
Variola
Vaccinia
Rubella
Bacterial Disease
Mycobacterium tuberculosis
Mycobacterium leprae
Treponemum pallidum
Borrelia burgdorferi
Infectious crystalline keratopathy (multiple causes)
Parasitic Disease
Acanthamoeba
Microsporidia
Leishmaniasis
Onchocerciasis
Trypanosomiasis
Unknown
Cogan syndrome

able abnormalities of serum immunoglobins. Serum antibodies directed against antigen in the cornea and inner ear have been detected (72). A small and medium vessel vasculitis is seen in several tissues (419).

The audiovestibular and ocular symptoms usually occur within 6 months of each other. Patients have sudden unilateral or bilateral ocular irritation, tearing, redness, and photophobia. The most common corneal findings are small (less than 1 mm) faint, peripheral, anterior stromal corneal infiltrates which may be evanescent (77). Rarely does it progress to the patchy, deep, granular corneal infiltrates described by Cogan since steroids alter the course. The audiovestibular dysfunction is manifested with abrupt onset of nausea, vomiting, tinnitus, unsteadiness, vertigo, and hearing impairment. The ear involvement begins unilateral but spreads to bilateral. The hearing loss is progressive over 1 to 3 months with profound loss in half the patients (untreated).

General constitutional symptoms include fatigue, headache, fever, weight loss, rash, arthralgias, myalgias, neck pain, and abdominal discomfort. Cardiac involvement with aortic insufficiency is common. Lymphadenopathy, hepatomegaly, and splenomegaly are present. Neurologic symptoms include cranial neuropathies, meningismus, encephalitis, all of which are rare. Respiratory symptoms include chest discomfort and pleuritis. Prompt recognition is important; there may be an acute phase lasting for months and then a continued phase for years.

There is an atypical Cogan's syndrome which is characterized by ocular inflammatory manifestations other than interstitial keratitis and includes conjunctivitis, episcleritis, scleritis, uveitis, choroiditis, papillitis, proptosis, and retinal vasculitis. The systemic constitutional symptoms are more common in atypical Cogan syndrome.

The ophthalmologist has to have an increased suspicion for the disease to make the diagnosis. Recognizing the audiovestibular symptoms is the key. There are no specific laboratory tests but rather a constellation of clinical and laboratory findings. Untreated, patients have a profound hearing loss whereas early treatment with oral corticosteroids will preserve hearing in most patients. An increased dose is begun initially and tapered slowly. It presumably alters the inflammation in the cochlea. Oral diuretics may also help the hydrops. Immunosuppressive agents such as cytoxan, cyclosporin, azathioprine, and methotrexate have been useful in some patients (9). Some patients may require an aortic valve replacement. The interstitial keratitis, as well as the other ocular inflammatory signs, respond to topical corticosteroids quickly (328). Rarely does the disease now progress to advanced stromal scarring.

Mycobacterium Tuberculosis

Tuberculosis is caused most commonly by Mycobacterium tuberculosis, and less commonly by Mycobacterium bovis and Mycobacterium africanum (162, 275). These organisms are acid fast because mycolic acids in the cell wall form a complex with basic dyes. Infection most commonly occurs by airborne lung infection, but organisms can enter by the conjunctiva, gastrointestinal tract, genitourinary tract, or the skin. Lymph nodes spread and then hematogenous spread occurs with a primary infection. Reactivation from a dormant site results in a secondary infection. The interstitial keratitis of tuberculosis is uncommon and is most likely an immune reaction to tuberculoprotein rather than direct invasion of the cornea. Cellular infiltration of the anterior and deep stroma occur, which is usually unilateral and sectorial, and peripheral. Haze and vascularization occur later. Inflammatory reaction may last for weeks with scarring resulting. Corneal opacification, thinning, and astigmatism frequently result. Other features which may be present include a uveitis, phlyctenular keratoconjunctivitis, scleritis, episcleritis, choroiditis, and retinal vasculitis.

A corneal biopsy cannot reveal diagnostic information since it is an immune response. Tuberculosis needs to be confirmed by evaluation of the organism elsewhere by the Ziehl-Neelsen stains, Löwenstein-Jensen medium for culture, chest radiograph, and skin testing. The systemic disease needs to be treated with multiple antituberculosis drugs. The interstitial keratitis should be treated with topical corticosteroids and cycloplegics varied according to the severity of the keratitis (162).

Mycobacterium Leprae

Leprosy is a chronic mycobacterial infection of the skin and peripheral nerves caused by Mycobacterium leprae. This obligate intracellular parasite has an unusual affinity for monocytes, tissue macrophages, and Schwann cells (275, 366, 368). Leprosy is more common in tropical countries, especially Brazil, Nigeria, India, and Indonesia. The bacillus multiplies slowly over years after entry through the respiratory system. There are different forms, perhaps dependent on the host immune state. The lepromatous form has extensive skin and nerve involvement with a large number of organisms. This form is associated with a disorder of the cell-mediated immunity to Mycobacterium leprae. The tuberculoid form shows few bacilli on biopsy, has a strong cellular reaction, and has more neural involvement than skin involvement. Borderline cases may fall between these forms (336). Interstitial keratitis is most common in the lepromatous form since the bacteria seem to prefer cooler body tissues, such as the peripheral nerves and the anterior segment of the eye. Organisms have been detected in the cornea, so the process may represent either an infectious process, an immune process, or both. It is frequently bilateral, beginning at the upper corneal quadrant and progressing to the center and deep cornea. Vascularization occurs later. The tuberculoid form is associated with nerve damage and exposure keratitis from lagophthalmos with or without corneal hypesthesia. The corneal nerves may become thickened and nodular from direct nerve involvement.

The diagnosis is made from acid fast bacilli seen on skin biopsies. The histologic involvement of the peripheral nerve is pathognomonic. Serodiagnosis for a surface antigen is specific and sensitive in lepromatous disease but not tuberculoid disease. The bacillus cannot be cultured but can be propagated in various animals. The Mycobacterium leprae can be identified from conjunctival smears and corneal biopsy.

Multidrug therapy is indicated. Patients with tuberculoid form require two drugs (dapsone and rifampin) for 6 months and patients with the lepromatous form require three drugs (dapsone, rifampin, and clofazimine) for two years or longer. Topical corticosteroids and cycloplegics are used for the interstitial keratitis and uveitis. The response to therapy is monitored by a skin biopsy. Corneal protection because of exposure keratitis or neurotrophic keratitis is recommended with either medical or surgical therapy. BCG vaccination provides some protection and has been successful in decreasing the incidence of this disease.

Treponemum Pallidum

Syphilis is transmitted by genital, oral, or anorectal sex. There has been an increase recently especially in the inner cities, associated with prostitution and drug use. There has been a marked increase in congenital syphilis in New York City, and an anticipated increase in syphilitic interstitial keratitis may occur in the future. Interstitial keratitis from syphilis is usually associated with congenital infection (255, 331) with approximately 10% resulting from an acquired infection. The Treponema pallidum spirochete can penetrate intact mucous membranes and abraded skin. After a 3 week incubation, primary skin lesions occur (chancre) which are filled with spirochetes. Lesions can also occur on the mouth, eyelid, or conjunctiva. Secondary syphilis develops several weeks later with a generalized maculopapular rash and systemic symptoms. Anterior uveitis may be prominent. Thirty percent of patients will progress to tertiary syphilis which results in skin gumma, cardiovascular disease, or neurosyphilis. Argyll Robertson pupils, optic atrophy, and posterior uveitis are seen in neurosyphilis.

Congenital syphilis is transmitted from the mother through the placenta usually in the second or third trimester. The earliest sign of congenital syphilis occurs within days of birth and includes a generalized rash, rhinitis, jaundice, anorexia, and pseudoparalysis. Chorioretinitis may be evident in the first few months. Late congenital syphilis begins approximately 2 years of age and may also involve the central nervous system. Deformities of the teeth are common (Hutchinson's teeth). Interstitial keratitis is a late finding in congenital syphilis with most cases occurring between age 5 and 18, occurring more commonly in females. Most cases are bilateral with the second eye becoming involved within 1 year. The first sign of interstitial keratitis is conjunctival hyperemia and epiphora with pain and photophobia. Iritis and keratic precipitates are seen in small localized areas. Corneal stromal infiltration later leads to stromal haze and epithelial edema. The peripheral cornea shows the most reaction and is the site of neovascularization with occasional dense accumulation of vessels (salmon patch). Scarring, thinning, and ghost vessels occur as the vessels recede. Rarely, corneal calcification or multilaminated bands of Descemet's membrane at the posterior corneal surface may occur. Recurrent bouts of inflammation can occur. There may be an associated iris atrophy, chorioretinal scars, and optic atrophy. When seen as adults, these patients show corneal ghost vessels, thinning, and diffuse stromal opacification. Patients can usually remember a history of eye inflammation as a child. The interstitial keratitis is thought to arise from a hypersensitivity reaction to treponemal antigens deposited in the corneal stroma and not from an active corneal infection. Interstitial keratitis in acquired syphilis is usually unilateral and occurs months to years after the initial infection. It tends to be milder and more sectoral.

The dark field microscope can be used to identify spirochetes in tissue fluid. The VDRL (Venereal Disease Research Laboratory) test and the RPR (Rapid plasma reagin) test detect nonspecific antibodies to cardiolipin. More specific and sensitive tests are the FTA-ABS (fluorescent treponemal antibody absorption test), and the MHA-TP (microhemagglutination-treponema pallidum assay) but are more expensive. The VDRL decreases over time and is negative after penicillin therapy. The FTA-ABS and MHA-TP remain positive over a long time. A child with acute interstitial keratitis as well as adults with quiescent findings of interstitial keratitis should have an FTA-ABS and cerebrospinal fluid VDRL to confirm or rule out neurosyphilis.

Therapy of the interstitial keratitis consists of topical corticosteroids and cycloplegics. Infants with congenital syphilis should be treated with neurosyphilis doses as should adults with acquired syphilis. There is no evidence that antisyphilitic treatment affects the interstitial keratitis. Patients with interstitial keratitis may require contact lenses or penetrating keratoplasty for rehabilitation.

Borrelia

Lyme disease is an arthropod related disease originally described in patients from Connecticut and now recognized in the United States and Europe. It is a multisystem disorder which follows an expanding red rash resulting from the bite of Ixodes tick with inoculation of the spirochete Borrelia burgdorferi. Although reported in almost all states, the majority of cases have been in the northeast, north central, and the Pacific northwest of the United States. Humans are not normally involved in the life cycle of this spirochete, but ecologic changes have increased the deer population with subsequent increased the tick population. Transmission to humans occurs when the tick bites the human rather than the deer.

There is a wide variety of clinical manifestations with stages defined and variable patterns of exacerbation and spontaneous remission (Table 51–18). Stage 1 is a localized skin rash of erythema migrans. Stage 2 follows months later with varied systemic symptoms including a migratory arthritis, neurologic disease (cranial neuropathy, meningitis), and cardiac arrhythmias. Stage 3 begins months later with prolonged chronic arthritis and long-term neurologic syndromes. Ophthalmic manifestations can occur during each of the three

TABLE 51–18
Stages of Lyme Disease

Stage 1	Systemic Findings	Erythema migrans
		Constitutional symptoms
		Regional lymphadenopathy
Stage 2	Systemic Findings	Skin annular lesions, urticaria, evanescent lesions
		Joint migratory arthralgias
		Regional lymph nodes
		Heart nodal block, pericarditis
		Respiratory symptoms
		Hematuria
		Constitutional symptoms
	Neurologic Findings	Meningitis
		Bell's palsy
		Cranial neuritis
		Encephalitis, myelitis
		Cerebellar ataxia
	Eye Findings	Conjunctivitis
		Iritis, choroiditis, panuveitis
		Retinal hemorrhage
Stage 3	Systemic Findings	Acrodermatitis chronica atrophicans
		Prolonged arthritis
		Fatigue
	Neurologic Findings	Chronic encephalomyelitis, ataxic gait, mental disorder
	Eye Findings	Keratitis

stages. A mild conjunctivitis with photophobia can be seen in stage 1 (461). Neuro-ophthalmic manifestations are common in stage 2 with the seventh nerve palsy, other cranial nerve palsies, optic neuritis, and papilledema. Stage 3 has the most severe ocular inflammatory manifestations. Anterior segment manifestations include episcleritis, symblepharon, keratitis, and iritis. Posterior segment manifestations include vitreitis, choroiditis, panuveitis, endophthalmitis, retinal vasculitis and exudative retinal detachment (1,462).

Lyme keratitis is a rare interstitial keratitis with a nonsuppurative pattern affecting only the corneal stroma. It may be associated with a mild keratitis or keratic precipitates. In some patients, a bilateral keratitis with patchy, nebular, or indistinct hazy stromal infiltrates just below Bowman's membrane or just above Descemet's membrane may be seen (31). There may be late vascularization of the cornea. Lyme keratitis is an immune response as are most stage 3 manifestations. The early diagnosis of Lyme disease is made from the typical skin rash which can reveal the organism on culture (36). In stage 2, Borrelia burgdorferi has been cultured from the cerebrospinal fluid, joint fluid, and heart biopsy. In stage 3, cultures are negative since it is an immune response. Antibody testing with ELISA is the most common antibody test for Lyme disease. The skin rash must be present for at least 2 weeks for the test to be positive. There is a higher frequency of false positives because of cross reactivity with other antigens (other spirochetes). The immunoblotting test against a variety of Borrelia antigen is more specific.

The treatment is with a variety of beta lactam antibiotics or tetracycline for stage 1 or stage 2 disease. Treatment of Lyme keratitis is with topical corticosteroids which can result in corneal clearing. Avoidance of the forest, protection of the skin, and removal of ticks are helpful, preventative measures. A Lyme vaccine is being tested (113).

Infectious Crystalline Keratopathy

Infectious crystalline keratopathy is a microbial infection of the cornea characterized by crystal-like stromal opacities. It could be considered under the category of microbial keratitis, but the needlelike or fernlike lesions with insidious development and no accompanying inflammation are more consistent with interstitial keratitis (147). The cornea is remarkably free of inflammatory response, but organisms have been found in confluent in pockets between collagen lamellae.

Streptococcus viridans has been the most common pathogen recovered in culture from these patients although other pathogens including Peptostreptococcus, Enterococcus, Haemophilus, Mycobacterium fortuitum, staphylococcal species, Candida, and others have been cultured. Prominent risk factors include prior corneal surgery, trauma, epithelial edema, contact lens wear, and the use of topical corticosteroids. The organisms gain access through an epithelial break, replicate, and spread along the plane of dissected collagen lamellae, but do not elicit an inflammatory response because of steroid use. The production of a biofilm material by certain bacteria may limit the immune reaction and the bacterial exopolysaccharide production may cause the visible arborizing pattern (177).

The diagnosis is made by slit lamp findings of hardedged crystalline opacities in the setting of prior corneal surgery and steroid use. The epithelium is intact so corneal scraping is usually not sufficient to obtain material for examination. Corneal biopsy may be necessary with appropriate stain and culture to detect bacteria (including anaerobes), fungi, and mycobacteria. Nutritionally variant streptococci require media with added pyridoxal hydrochloride (301). Electron microscopy may be necessary to detect the ultrastructural features. Therapy is variably successful because of the deep stromal sequestration of the organisms. Vancomycin is effective against most streptococcal species. Other organisms require specific therapy. In general, the corticosteroids should be tapered to allow the antibiotics to have their full effect. Some infections do not respond to antibiotic therapy and patients may require lamellar or penetrating keratoplasty.

■ SURFACE DISEASES OF THE ANTERIOR SEGMENT

The stratified squamous nonkeratinizing epithelium of the cornea and the surface features of the adjacent conjunctiva are a remarkable structure which serve as a protective barrier for the surface of the eye. This layer has complex functions with epithelial cell-cell and cell-substrate interaction, extracellular macromolecule production, and cytoskeletal characteristics to provide a smooth, wet, apical surface that is the major refracting surface of the eye (143). This unique function is best shown when there is loss of function of the specialized barrier by epithelial disadhesions, inadequate healing of surface wounds from insults, and corneal opacification. Diseases to be considered in this section include recurrent corneal erosion, neurotrophic keratitis, Thygeson superficial punctate keritopothy, exposure keratitis, persistent epithelial defects, complications of contact lens wear, toxic reactions to drugs, and drug and metal depositions. Multiple other diseases affect the corneal surface in a secondary fashion (e.g., keratitis sicca, rosacea, erythema multiforme, ocular pemphigoid). These latter diseases have been discussed under conjunctival diseases.

Recurrent Corneal Erosion

The corneal epithelium has specialized attachment complexes anchoring it to Bowman's layer in the stroma (200). This complex is composed of hemidesmosomes of the basal epithelial cell plasma membrane and the extracellular collagenous basement membrane with anchoring fibrils. Any disease, dystrophy, degeneration, or trauma which affects this basement membrane predisposes to poor epithelial adhesion and recurrent erosion. Further inflammation, nerve damage, stromal inflammation, or tear dysfunction states exacerbate this adhesion deficit and can create a vicious cycle of persistent epithelial defects and continuous inflammation.

A partial listing of disorders affecting the epithelium and basement membrane and leading to recurrent or persistent defects of the epithelium as shown in Table 51–19. Most of these have been discussed in other sections. A distinct clinical entity of recurrent corneal erosion syndrome is characterized by abrupt and recurrent attacks of ocular pain and tearing, frequently occurring during sleep or upon awakening without any obvious precipitating cause. There is usually a prior history of corneal abrasion from a fingernail scratch or a tree branch (sometimes in the remote past) (449). Clinical

TABLE 51–19
Disorders Predisposing to Epithelial Erosions

Corneal Epithelial and Basement Membrane Dystrophies
  Epithelial basement membrane disease (anterior membrane dystrophy)
  Meesmann dystrophy
  Reis–Bückler dystrophy
  Lattice corneal dystrophy
Acquired Disease Affecting the Epithelium or Basement Membrane
  Diabetes mellitus
  Neurotrophic (fifth nerve) disease
  Neuroparalytic (seventh nerve) disease
  Exposure keratopathy or trichiasis from lid abnormalities
  1° or 2° keratoconjunctivitis sicca
  Postinfectious corneal damage (herpes simplex, herpes zoster, bacterial, fungal, parasitic)
  Contact lens keratopathy
  Toxic, drug, or allergic keratopathy
  Immune keratopathy (collagen vascular disease, erythema multiforme, pemphigoid)
Trauma
  Chemical, thermal, or radiation injury
  Mechanical abrasion

signs of the recurrent erosion syndrome can vary from a clinically normal examination to a superficial punctate keratitis, to areas of devitalized disadhesive epithelium, or to frank epithelial defects. This all depends on the severity of the erosion and the time the patient is seen after the onset of symptoms. Fluorescein staining of the epithelium and the use of slit lamp retroillumination will sometimes highlight the specific area of the cornea and help reveal an underlying anterior membrane dystrophy. Examination of the other eye may reveal subtle signs of an anterior membrane dystrophy. Defective basement membrane and deficient hemidesmosomal attachment (or production) of the epithelium to the basement membrane and Bowman's layer have been shown in traumatic recurrent erosion.

Recurrent corneal erosion syndrome (as well as other causes of recurrent erosion) usually responds to conservative medical measures including continuous patching for 24 to 72 hours, followed by frequent ocular lubricants during the day, ophthalmic ointments (either hypertonic or tear supplements), and closure of the lid with paper tape at bedtime. This three-fold approach (tears during the day, ointment at bedtime, and taping at night) is continued for 1 month, at which time one of the three can be discontinued. After a further month, another one can be dropped, and after a further month, treatment can be discontinued. If recurrences occur, the regimen is reinstituted. If this conservative treatment is not sufficient, a therapeutic soft contact lens is appropriate on a continuous wear basis with the use of unpreserved artificial tears and a daily antibiotic to help avoid corneal infection. A cycloplegic is frequently helpful the first several days to reduce the risk of tight contact lens syndrome. A topical corticosteroid may reduce the inflammatory component in rare indications. Close followup is necessary because of the risk of infection, toxicosis to medication, loss or tightness of the lens, and the failure to respond appropriately. If the epithelium is loose, a localized debridement with a cellulose sponge can provide a better base for healing.

If patients fail to respond to the medical or bandage contact lens therapy, an alternative is an anterior stromal puncture technique. This involves 15 to 25 micropunctures in the anterior stroma with a hypodermic needle to incite a focal microadhesive scar (spot welding) of the epithelium to the stroma (266). This technique requires that you be able to identify the area of recurrent corneal erosion (sometimes not evident) and it can cause bothersome corneal scars if done in the visual axis. The YAG laser can also perform these micropunctures. When the anterior membrane corneal dystrophy (or other extensive aberrant epithelial basement membrane) is the cause of the erosion, a superficial epithelial keratectomy may be better indicated (60). The epithelium and subepithelial debris is scraped with a disposable blade; a jeweler's forceps may help strip abnormal membranes from the surface. The size of the debridement varies according to the evident slit lamp abnormalities. Patching, or a soft contact lens, is required over several days. Excimer laser phototherapeutic keratectomy has emerged as a treatment option for these dystrophic variants. A surface cautery or diathermy may also be applied but can cause significant corneal scarring so is reserved for eyes with poor visual potential in selected cases. It has also been useful for chronic epithelial edema in patients unsuitable for penetrating keratoplasty.

Thygeson's Superficial Punctate Keratitis

Thygeson's superficial punctate keratitis is a chronic, recurrent, bilateral epithelial keratitis of unknown etiology predominantly affecting individuals 20 to 30 years of age. Patients present with multiple discrete clusters of coarse, punctate, raised epithelial opacities which may stain with fluorescein in the acute period. These opacities may have an associated faint subepithelial haze or infiltrate. The eye appears otherwise quiet with no conjunctival inflammation or anterior chamber reaction. Patients experience symptoms of pain, foreign body sensation, photophobia, and tearing.

Spontaneous recurrences may occur for several years, and in some, the condition may disappear completely. An autoimmune etiology has been postulated associated with HLA DR3. Although it shares characteristics with viral infection, no causative virus has been definitively identified.

Treatment is mainly symptomatic with artificial tears or lubricants. Therapeutic soft contact lenses may provide relief. Decreased doses of topical corticosteroids have been reported to affect rapid resolution of the keratitis. Topical antivirals have not been effective (144a).

Neurotrophic Keratopathy

Whenever corneal sensation is decreased, epithelial dysfunction occurs probably because of some trophic influence on the epithelium, perhaps a chemical release from the sensory nerve endings. With sensory deprivation, cell metabolism is reduced, permeability is increased, mitotic rate decreases, and certain intracellular chemicals are decreased (142). This can lead to poor corneal luster, epithelial defects, and finally vascularization and corneal opacification. Noninfectious stromal ulceration and corneal infections can ensue. There are multiple causes of decreased corneal sensation which can all cause the clinical picture of neurotrophic keratitis (Table 51–20). Patients with congenital forms or longstanding keratrophic changes can adapt well to the condition (Figure 51–20). Patients with acute neurotrophic keratitis can decompensate quickly.

TABLE 51–20
Causes of Neurotrophic Keratopathy

> Congenital Disease
> > Familial dysautonomia
> > Isolated congenital trigeminal anesthesia
> Fifth Nerve Damage
> > Tumors
> > Aneurysm
> > Surgery
> Systemic Disease
> > Diabetes mellitus
> Corneal Disease
> > Herpes simplex keratitis
> > Herpes zoster keratitis
> > Cornea incisions
> > Contact lens wear
> > Any chronic corneal disease
> Toxic
> > Topical anesthetic abuse
> > Timolol
> > Chemical burns

Early signs of neurotrophic damage are corneal haze and conjunctival injection. Later focal loss of epithelial cells and decreased corneal luster is seen. In more severe sensory loss, broad epithelial defects are seen in the interpalpebral area, especially in the inferior paracentral cornea. The defects may have raised, rolled, gray epithelial edges. A sterile hypopyon can occur and with severe disease it may progress to thinning and ulceration, or alternatively, heal with vascularization and scarring. These patients may be relatively asymptomatic since corneal sensation is decreased.

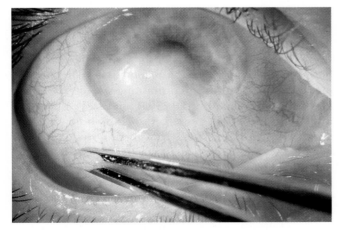

Figure 51–20.
Congenital anesthesia of the cornea. A teenager with congenital absence of fifth nerve function demonstrating severe changes of neurotrophic keratopathy. The patient did not feel the forceps moving the conjunctiva of the eye.

Medical therapy includes methods to promote epithelial healing although there is no specific treatment to reverse the sensory damage. Lubricants, especially nonpreserved, are recommended along with early consideration for lateral and complete tarsorrhaphy, which can be remarkably effective and preserve the globe. Bandage contact lenses are an alternative, but not if the neurotrophic damage is judged to be permanent; it complicates the management of these patients.

Exposure Keratopathy

Exposure keratopathy can result from any prolonged exposure of the corneal surface associated with corneal desiccation. Abnormalities of lid position and function as well as orbital proptosis are the most common causes (Table 51–21). Clinical findings include a punctate epithelial keratopathy that usually involves the inferior third of the cornea or greater. The punctate lesions can coalesce to large epithelial defects with resultant ulceration, melting, and perforation. Patients have more symptoms than neurotrophic keratopathy and complain of foreign body sensation, photophobia, and tearing. Therapy is with artificial tears and ophthalmic lubricating ointments. If the exposure is temporary, taping of the lids can be helpful. Rarely a bandage contact lens is helpful. In most situations, the structural abnormalities in the lid or orbit need surgical correction (35). With temporary exposure keratopathy, a lateral tarsorrhaphy is still sometimes most expedient in resolving the situation.

Persistent Corneal Epithelial Defects

Persistent epithelial defects are associated with a large and heterogenous group of ocular and systemic diseases (Table 51–22). The more common causes are related to

TABLE 51–21
Causes of Exposure Keratopathy

> Abnormal Lid Position or Function
> > Ectropion
> > Post blepharoplasty (upper or lower lids)
> > Chronic skin disorders with shrinkage
> > Lagophthalmos
> > > Seventh nerve palsy
> > > Supranuclear seventh nerve palsy
> > > Nocturnal
> > > Coma
> > > Psychiatric disorder
> > Trauma
> Proptosis
> > Thyroid dysfunction
> > Orbital tumor

TABLE 51–22
Causes of Persistent Epithelial Defects

Abnormal Lid Function
   Lagophthalmos
   Ectropion
   Entropion
   Trichiasis
   Cicatricial lid disease
Corneal Disease
   Corneal damage from infection
   Severe keratoconjunctivitis sicca
   Neurotrophic keratopathy
   Associated with severe conjunctival disease
      Pemphigoid
      Erythema multiforme
      Atopic disease
      Rosacea
      Vernal
   Chemical burns
   Recurrent erosion syndrome
Postsurgical
   Diabetes mellitus
   Anterior segment necrosis
Systemic Disease
   Nutritional disease (vitamin A deficient)
   Collagen vascular disease
   Graft-versus-host disease
Toxic Medicamentosa
   Topical anesthetics
   Topical antimicrobials
   Preservatives

herpetic corneal disease, delayed postsurgical healing, chemical burns, recurrent erosion, dry eye syndrome, anterior segment necrosis, long-term infections, and neuroparalytic disease. This condition is usually seen in more severely damaged corneas. There are varying degrees of symptoms depending on the corneal sensation. On clinical examination, there is a central epithelial defect with rolled, raised edges of piled up epithelium which may be edematous or loosely adherent to the stroma. If the epithelial defect persists, the cornea is prone to infection. The corneal stroma is also at risk of melting from the action of enzymes secreted by the damaged corneal epithelial cells, from stromal keratocytes, or from the inflammatory cells. Alternatively, vascularization may promote corneal scarring.

The therapy requires a recognition of the inciting cause. Structural, inflammatory, infectious, and systemic diseases need to be adequately treated. The promotion of corneal healing takes several approaches, varied according to the precise etiology and response to therapy. Lubricants are appropriate, avoiding those with preservatives. Biologic agents to promote epithelial wound healing and adhesion, such as fibronectin (133)

and epidermal growth factor (363) remain investigational. Pressure patching, bandage contact lens, correction of the lid position are all appropriate. Topical and systemic ascorbate (319) and topical citrate may be helpful in selected severe sterile chemical or thermal burns. Vitamin A analogs can reverse severe keratinization associated with advanced keratoconjunctivitis sicca, erythema multiforme, pemphigoid, and radiation keratitis in selected circumstances (380). Topical corticosteroids may reduce inflammation in selected situations, but generally should be avoided (321). Medroxyprogesterone may be effective in association with the treatment of chemical burns. Immunosuppressive drugs may be useful in the systemic diseases associated with epithelial defects such as Wegener's granulomatosis, Behçet disease, pemphigoid, and other autoimmune diseases (164). Although collagenase has been identified in progressive stromal ulceration, the clinical use of collagenase inhibitors such as EDTA, acetylcysteine, as well as other agents, have been disappointing clinically. Systemic tetracycline may have an anticollagenase effect (313).

Surgical options frequently need to be considered in patients with persistent epithelial defects. Punctal occlusion can be beneficial in some patients with either temporary or a permanent technique. The lateral tarsorrhaphy should be considered early and aggressively designed; it can be opened in portions as desired. Tissue adhesives may prevent stromal ulceration from proceeding to perforation (119). In severe chemical burns, a glued-on hard contact lens can protect the deepithelialized corneal surface until resurfacing can occur from the conjunctivally derived epithelial cells (201, 202). Removal of the limbal conjunctiva has been helpful in postsurgical marginal ulcers and ulcers associated with collagen vascular disease (442). Conjunctival autograft transplantation of the ocular surface epithelium, especially of limbal tissue, has been an effective means of restoring surface integrity to patients with chemical and thermal injuries as well as contact lens keratopathy (442). The transplantation of this "stem cell" in the limbus from the opposite eye has been effective in promoting reepithelialization and promoting stability of the ocular surface epithelium (204,409). In cases of bilateral injury, the use of allogenic keratoepithelioplasty from donor corneal limbal lenticles can promote epithelial healing. A conjunctival flap is especially useful in elderly debilitated patients in whom a quick resolution is desirable. It should not be used in cases of active bacterial, fungal, or parasitic infection, but may be useful in viral keratopathy. Lamellar keratoplasty may be used for tectonic stabilization of the globe in preparation for further rehabilitation with a later penetrating keratoplasty. A keratoprosthesis is used for badly scarred eyes with no hope for a penetrating keratoplasty.

Anterior Segement Complications of Contact Lenses

Contact lenses induce a wide spectrum of changes in the appearance and function of the conjunctiva and cornea. The corneal changes can be caused by multiple pathophysiologic mechanisms including hypoxic, hypercapnic, allergic, toxic, mechanical, and osmotic factors (56) (Table 51–23). These complications are not in a continuum. Selected patients can have none, some, or several of the complications which cannot be predicted in advance. Unfortunately, the majority of contact lens patients are in a mobile population, at an age of medical naivete, and can have lenses refilled by mail order companies without significant medical monitoring. Most of these complications are reversible, especially if detected early. Several of the complications lead to blindness or significant morbidity in the name of cosmetic contact lens wear. Selected complications will be discussed.

Microbial Keratitis

Corneal ulcers are the most serious complications associated with contact lens wear. They are especially frequent with soft contact lenses, lenses worn as extended wear, and perhaps disposable lenses. The corneal ulcer originates with a traumatic insult by a contaminated lens to a cornea already compromised by hypoxia. The most important organisms causing contact lens-related corneal ulcers are Pseudomonas aeruginosa and Acanthamoeba. The symptoms, clinical findings, and treatment have been discussed previously.

Sterile Corneal Infiltrates

Sterile corneal infiltrates related to contact lens wear are predominantly in the periphery and associated with tight contact lens fitting, extended wear contact lenses, and allergic or toxic reactions (28, 38, 56). Several mechanisms may cause this clinical finding including delayed hypersensitivity reaction to chemical disinfectants and their preservatives (Thimerosal), immunologic reaction to lens material, hypersensitivity reaction to bacteria or toxins, and anoxia or mechanical irritation. Increased risk is found in patients with poor lens hygiene and extended contact lens wear. The lens should be discontinued. Occasionally, topical corticosteroids are required.

Contact Lens Induced Superior Limbic Keratoconjunctivitis

Patients with contact lens induced superior limbic keratoconjunctivitis have symptoms of bilateral ocular irritation and conjunctival hyperemia after months or years

TABLE 51–23
Corneal Pathophysiology with Contact Lens Wear

Hypoxia and hypercapnia
  Epithelial metabolic rate reduction
    Mitotic rate decrease
      Epithelial thinning
      Oxygen flux reduction
      Epithelial microcysts
      Increased epithelial fragility
    Compromised junctional integrity
      Diminished electrical potential
      Superficial punctate keratitis
      Epithelial abrasion
      Microbial keratitis
    Epithelial glycogen depletion
  Stromal lactate accumulation
    Stromal edema
      Corneal thickening
      Corneal distortion
      Increased light backscattering
      Stromal striae
      Posterior stromal folds
    Stromal acidosis
      Endothelial edema
      Endothelial polymegethism
  Other hypoxic or hypercapnic effects
    Corneal hypoesthesia
    Vascularization
      Superficial vascularization
      Deep stromal vascularization
      Intracorneal hemorrhage
      Instrastromal opacity
    Stromal thinning
Allergy and Toxicosis
  Immobile lens syndrome
    Limbal vessel hyperemia
    Peripheral corneal infiltrates
    Keratic precipitates
  Thimerosal hypersensitivity
    Epithelial infiltrates
    Contact lens–induced superior limbic keratoconjunctivitis
  Solution toxicosis
    Punctate staining
    Epithelial pseudodendrites
Mechanical Effects
  Direct contact
    Lens edge imprint and corneal distortion
    Epithelial wrinkling
    Corneal wrinkling
  Material trapped under the lens
    Air bubble dimpling
    Foreign body tracks
Osmotic Effects
  Epithelial erosions
    Three- and nine-o'clock fluorescein staining
    Coarse punctate erosions
  Epithelial edema (visual disturbance)

From Bruce AS, Brennan NA. Corneal pathophysiology with contact lens wear. Surv Ophthalmol 35:25–58, 1990.

of successful contact lens wear (370). Findings include a punctate staining around the superior limbus and an extension of dysplastic epithelium toward the central cornea. There may be anterior stromal infiltrates and a vascular pannus. A severe keratopathy may cause a permanent stromal opacification. Conjunctival findings include hyperemia, limbal follicles, and a mild tarsal papillary reaction (38). There is slow improvement after contact lens withdrawal. It is probably a severe form of Thimerosal hypersensitivity. Occasionally, the ocular surface is so damaged that limbal conjunctival transplantation is required (183).

Nummular Keratitis

Nummular keratitis is a sterile inflammatory reaction to components of the lens and/or the lens solution. Macroscopically visible multiple coin-shaped lesions are found at various depths of the corneal stroma, usually centrally. It responds to topical steroids but may take months to clear.

Corneal Abrasions

Corneal abrasions are caused by the mechanical injury of the lens itself or the maneuvers in inserting and removing the lens. Occasionally, a foreign body will get trapped under the lens. Other chemical or hypoxic factors contribute to the epithelial disruption. Although the standard therapy has been to patch the eye after a topical antibiotic, there is an increased risk of Pseudomonas ulcer, perhaps because of a subclinical initial infection. The present suggested therapy is to treat with topical antibiotics without patching and close monitoring.

Superficial Punctate Keratitis

Superficial punctate keratitis manifests with multiple small corneal elevated epithelial lesions. It is related to the lens, lens solution, as well as to mechanical effects. It is best treated by discontinuing contact lens use. Changing disinfection solutions, the lens type, or the lens fit may be helpful. There may be concomitant local eyelid disease or a dry eye.

Corneal Neovascularization

Corneal neovascularization is common in patients with long term soft contact lens wear. A mild degree (less than 2 mm) of superficial pannus can be followed; if the pannus is greater than 2 mm, the contact lens should be discontinued (Figure 51–21). Chronic hypoxia and/or a tight lens is often the cause. Occasionally, a deep stromal neovascularization can occur which may persist and become associated with lipid deposition or occasionally

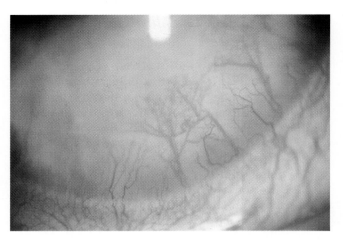

Figure 51–21.
Corneal neovascularization secondary to a soft contact lens. Deep corneal neovascularization in a patient with Fuchs' corneal dystrophy wearing an extended wear soft contact lens to help reduce the irritation from epithelial bulla.

deep interstromal hemorrhages (48). Deep corneal vascularization is an indication to permanently discontinue contact lens wear if at all possible. Topical corticosteroids do not aid in regression of deep vascularization.

Epithelial Microcysts

Epithelial microcysts are seen most frequently with extended wear lenses and are caused by a sustained depression of corneal epithelial metabolism. These translucent irregular-shaped dots are scattered across the cornea. They decrease over months once contact lenses are discontinued (56).

Three and Nine O'Clock Staining

Three and nine o'clock staining occurs in patients with a rigid contact lens with characteristic fluorescein staining within the nasal and temporal margin of the cornea adjacent to the area of lens coverage. If allowed to persist, stromal ulceration, pseudopterygium, and limbal inflammation will develop (56). It is probably similar to a dellen with a breakdown in the tear film adjacent to the lens edge. A lens of smaller diameter and thinner edge design should be fitted.

Contact Lens Overwear Syndrome

Contact lens overwear syndrome can have different manifestations. Some form of corneal swelling is associated with almost all contact lenses within 30 minutes of insertion in most patients. As the eye adapts to contact lens wear, the degree of corneal edema decreases over time. In patients with hard contact lenses it occurs as a central epithelial edema (Sattler's veil) after many hours of contact lens wears. The epithelial edema can progress to an acute epithelial necrosis. Corneal edema associated with soft contact lenses may be more difficult to detect clinically, although a diffuse stromal haze may occur early and corneal striae or folds in the posterior cornea may occur in more advanced cases. The contact lens needs to be discontinued and a new lens needs to be refitted.

Tight Lens Syndrome

The tight lens syndrome, also called the "acute red eye" and the "toxic lens syndrome" is a syndrome generally seen in patients wearing soft contact lenses on an extended basis. An immobile lens may be caused by debris trapped under the lens causing an inflammatory response. There is generally marked limbal vessel hyperemia, peripheral corneal infiltrates, and keratic precipitates in severe cases. The debris is characteristically trapped for 18 to 24 hours and patients are frequently awakened at night with pain, photophobia, and lacrimation. It is seen frequently in therapeutic bandage contact lens use and may be blunted by the prophylactic use of topical cycloplegics.

Toxic Reactions

A toxic reaction to contact lens wear solutions can have multiple manifestations including conjunctival injection, epithelial staining, punctate epithelial keratopathy, erosions, and microcysts. It is frequently accompanied by itching.

Corneal Endothelial Dysfunction

Corneal endothelial dysfunction has been associated with all forms of contact lenses, although less with rigid gas permeable contact lenses. Edema of the corneal endothelial cells is a transient phenomena seen during the initial period of wear and usually resolves. It is probably related to a decrease in the pH at the endothelium. Contact lens wear causes increased polymegathism (variation in cell size), pleomorphism (variation in cell shape) as a result of chronic hypoxia and an acidic stromal pH. These changes may be transient in many but may be irreversible in some and can be associated with irreversible stromal edema in rare patients. The long term significance for the majority of contact lens wearers is unknown (56), although it may imply a stress factor on the cornea predicting possible increased risk of corneal decompensation after future intraocular surgery.

Toxic and Allergic Reactions to Topical Ophthalmic Medications

Toxic reactions are a result of direct chemical irritation of the tissue by drug or preservative. Allergy requires sensitization and the induction of ocular inflammation by the patient's immune system (438, 439, 440). Toxic reactions are far more common and frequently affect both the cornea and the conjunctiva (Table 51–24).

Toxic Papillary Keratoconjunctivitis

Toxic papillary keratoconjunctivitis is the most common of adverse reactions to topical ophthalmic medications. It usually takes at least 2 weeks to develop and is demonstrated by punctate staining on the inferior nasal conjunctiva and cornea (where the drug concentration is the heaviest). It can also produce nonhealing epithelial defects. The conjunctiva is usually hyperemic, with a nonspecific papillary conjunctivitis and scant discharge. The major drug causes are the aminoglycosides, antiviral agents, and benzalkonium chloride. Patients with other ocular surface diseases, especially dry eye, are more prone to this reaction. Withdrawal of the medication and use of nonpreserved artificial tears is recommended. Rarely, a bandage contact lens is necessary.

TABLE 51–24
Causes of Ophthalmic Toxic and Allergic Reactions

Toxic Reaction
Toxic papillary keratoconjunctivitis
Aminoglycoside antibiotics
Antiviral agents
Anesthetic agents
Preservatives
Fortified topical antibiotics
Toxic pseudopemphigoid
Antiglaucoma medications
Toxic follicular conjunctivitis
Antiviral agents
Antiglaucoma agents
Cycloplegic agents
Anesthetic toxic keratoconjunctivitis
Any frequent use of topical anesthetic agents
Allergic Reaction
Allergic contact dermatoconjunctivitis
Aminoglycoside antibiotics
Antiviral agents
Cycloplegic agents
Preservatives
Anaphylactoid blepharoconjunctivitis
Antimicrobial agents
Anesthetic agents

Modified from 438,439,440.

Toxic Pseudopemphigoid

Toxic pseudopemphigoid is a result of prolonged and severe toxic reaction which leads to keratinization and foreshortening of the conjunctiva to give a picture resembling pemphigoid. It has been reported most commonly with glaucoma medications (pilocarpine, epinephrine, timolol, demecarium, echothiophate) and antiviral medications (367). It can occasionally spread onto the cornea with a corneal pannus (pseudotrachoma). Once the offending agent is removed, further progression of the disease does not generally occur. Conjunctival biopsy may be positive for immunoreactants just as true cases of pemphigoid.

Toxic Follicular Conjunctivitis

Toxic follicular conjunctivitis is characterized by a follicular reaction of the bulbar and palpebral conjunctiva as well as in the cul-de-sac. It is a proliferation of subepithelial conjunctival lymphocytes although no true lymphoid follicles. The conjunctiva is usually mildly hyperemic. It is seen most commonly with glaucoma drugs (dipivalyl, epinephrine, pilocarpine, carbachol), antiviral agents, and cycloplegic agents (atropine, homatropine). With prolonged use, these drugs can cause the toxic pseudopemphigoid picture. This toxic follicular response probably results from the ability of certain drugs to act as nonantigenic mitogens (e.g., like pokeweed) to induce mitosis and lymphoblastic transformations. Drug withdrawal is best. Substitution of a fresh product is also helpful.

Anesthetic Toxic Keratoconjunctivitis

Anesthetic toxic keratoconjunctivitis secondary to the abuse of topical anesthetics causes an especially severe form of toxic papillary conjunctivitis. Because of an extensive damage to epithelial microvilli, desmosomes, and cellular physiology, there are elements of tear film dysfunction, as well as neurotrophic and inflammatory keratitis. The clinical manifestations include severe pain, lid swelling, hyperemia, discharge, punctate staining, epithelial defects, inflammatory stromal infiltrates, corneal neovascularization, and anterior chamber reaction. There is usually no large stromal ulceration. This reaction develops days to weeks after the abuse begins and is self perpetuated since the patient continues to take the anesthetic more frequently to try to relieve symptoms. The treatment is to withdraw the anesthetic (once discovered!) and encourage epithelialization with patching, soft contact lenses, and cycloplegia. Patients frequently have underlying psychiatric problems.

Allergic Contact Dermatoconjunctivitis

Allergic contact dermatoconjunctivitis occurs after sensitization of T-lymphocytes in the regional lymph node and represents a Type IV delayed hypersensitivity reaction. The topical medication acts as a hapten and combines with tissue proteins to form complete antigen that sensitizes regional lymphocytes. The lymphocytes return to the eye and produce inflammation by releasing various lymphokines. The reaction may take weeks or years to develop depending on the capacity of the drug to act as a sensitizer. The reaction, however, can occur in 48 hours if the patient has previously been sensitized to the drug. Enhanced susceptibility occurs in patients with inflammatory skin conditions (enhanced penetration of the hapten) and in patients who were previously exposed to a similar drug (cross sensitization). Atopic patients are more predisposed to this reaction. Itching is the prominent symptom with eosinophils in the conjunctiva approximately 25% of the time as a result of lymphocyte-induced eosinophilic chemotactic factor. There is an eczematoid blepharitis and conjunctival hyperemia with a papillary reaction and rarely marginal infiltration and ulceration. Preservatives (thimerosal, EDTA, chlorhexidine), aminoglycosides, antiviral agents, and cycloplegics (atropine, homatropine) are the most common offenders. Treatment is withdrawal of the agent, cool compresses, and topical dermatologic corticosteroids.

True Anaphylactoid Blepharoconjunctivitis

True anaphylactoid blepharoconjunctivitis is rare. It is induced by previously formed immunoglobin E humoral antibody in patients previously sensitized. It can occur upon reexposure within seconds or minutes and is manifested by urticaria or angioedema of the eyelids and chemosis with itching of the conjunctiva. Systemic anaphylactoid reactions are rare. Anaphylactoid con-

TABLE 51–25
Selected Drug and Metal Deposition in the Cornea

Epithelial Deposition
Phenothiazines
Aminoquinolines
Tamoxifen
Amiodarone
Indomethacin
Naproxen
Suramin
Stromal Deposition
Gold
Silver
Copper
Indomethacin
Phenothiazines
Retinoids
Iron

junctivitis is seen most frequently with topical antibiotics (sulfacetamide, bacitracin, penicillin) and anesthetic agents (proparacaine, tetracaine, benoxinate). If recognized, the immediate application of a topical corticosteroid and vasoconstrictor along with cool compresses and oral antihistamine will usually alleviate the reaction.

Drug and Metal Depositions

A wide variety of systemic medications can affect the conjunctiva and cornea causing specific deposits. They need to be distinguished and recognized, although they usually have no effect on vision (14). These are divided into those which cause epithelial deposition and those which result in stromal deposition. The drugs which can cause an epithelial deposition are shown in Table 51–25. The corneal deposits are seen as yellowish, white, or brown deposits in the epithelium usually centrally with the appearance of an epithelial vortex (Figure 51–22). They do not interfere with vision and in themselves are not a reason to discontinue needed therapy. Similar deposits are seen with the different drugs, perhaps all related to "cationic amphiphlia," the formation of polar intracellular lipids which cannot be metabolized by lysosomal phospholipases.

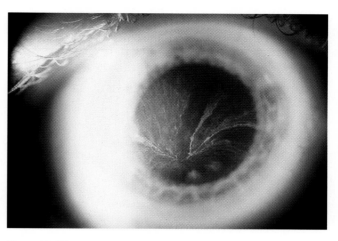

Figure 51–22.
Amiodarone corneal deposits. Deposits in the epithelium with golden brown changes associated with amiodarone. It has a distinct epithelial vortex pattern.

Stromal deposits of metal are seen in association with gold, mercury, copper, silver and iron. They have characteristic clinical appearances at different levels of the cornea either related to deposition from drug or disease (14, 18).

■ PERIPHERAL CORNEAL INFLAMMATORY DISEASE

The peripheral cornea has unique anatomic and physiologic characteristics which allow it to be the target of various local and systemic infections, and local and systemic immune responses (326, 337, 358) (Table 51–26). The blood vessels and lymphatics of the conjunctival allow immunoglobins and complement to reach the corneal periphery. The limbus is the prominent site of Langerhans cells with the capacity of marked immune response. A reservoir of inflammatory cells in the corneal periphery allow a brisk response to inflammatory or infectious particles and cause collagenolytic and proteolytic enzyme release which can result in either infiltration, ulceration, or vascularization. All this sets the stage for a large number of diseases unique to the corneal periphery. Many of these have been discussed in previous sections. A few selected ones will be detailed. A suggested evaluation of patients with these often complex disease presentations is presented elsewhere (123, 337, 354).

Marginal Catarrhal Keratitis

Marginal catarrhal keratitis is seen most frequently in middle-aged patients with blepharoconjunctivitis (73). It begins with one or more peripheral white stromal in-

filtrates parallel to the limbus and usually separated from the limbus by a clear zone. There may be conjunctival hyperemia and chemosis. It can lead to epithelial and stromal ulceration and occasionally heal by vascularization. This may resolve on its own over weeks; it tends to be recurrent. The disease is a hypersensitivity reaction to staphylococci or its toxins, although other organisms have also been implicated (278, 281). The deposition of immune complexes activates the classical complement pathway elaborating multiple enzymes. Therapy is with topical corticosteroids and reduction of antigen load by treatment of the blepharoconjunctivitis. Occasionally, oral tetracycline is indicated.

Corneal Phlyctenulosis (also discussed in Conjunctiva, Chapter 50)

A phlyctenule is an immune response to some prior sensitized antigen (278, 281). In the past, it was associated with a tuberculin antigen but it is now more commonly associated with Staphylococcus aureus. It is usually bilateral and affects the conjunctiva and/or peripheral cornea. The typical phlyctenule is pinkish-white with a limbal nodule, either solitary or multiple. These elevated nodules later ulcerate and resolve; in the cornea,

TABLE 51–26
Causes of Peripheral Corneal Inflammatory Diseases

Local Infections
  Bacteria
  Viruses
  Chlamydia
  Fungi
  Parasites
Systemic Infections
  Bacteria
    Neisseria gonorrheae
    Treponema pallidum
    Mycobacteria tuberculosis
  Viruses
    Varicella zoster virus
  Parasites
    Leishmania
Local Immune Disease
  Marginal "catarrhal" keratitis
  Phlyctenulosis
  Vernal keratoconjunctivitis
  Immune corneal rings
  Mooren ulcer
  Superior limbic keratoconjunctivitis
Systemic Immune Disease
  Vasculitides
    Rheumatoid arthritis
    Juvenile rheumatoid arthritis
    Systemic lupus erythematosis
    Relapsing polychondritis
    Sjögren syndrome
    Wegener granulomatosis
    Polyarteritis nodosa
    Progressive systemic sclerosis
  Dermatologic conditions
    Rosacea
    Psoriasis
    Ichthyosis
  Inflammatory bowel disease
    Crohn's disease
    Ulcerative colitis
  Blood dyscrasia
    Leukemia

this causes a scar, but in the conjunctiva this resolves without scarring. The lesion occasionally wanders to different areas of the limbus. Symptoms depend on location. Corneal involvement is associated with extreme photophobia. Histopathologic tissues show an accumulation of lymphocytes.

In endemic tuberculosis areas, patients should be evaluated for active tuberculosis. The most common cause, staphylococcal blepharoconjunctivitis, is treated with topical corticosteroids, lid hygiene, and occasionally the use of systemic tetracycline (460).

Mooren Ulcer

Mooren ulcer is a rare, chronic and progressive idiopathic ulceration of the peripheral corneal stroma and epithelium without scleral involvement. It begins in the clear cornea at the limbus, and progresses centrally, circumferentially, and posteriorly through the cornea (Figure 51–23). It leaves a thin and vascularized cornea. The edge of the ulcer is undermined with white blood cell infiltration into the advancing edge. There is significant pain and low grade iritis as the destructive process progresses slowly with eventual destruction of the cornea over several months. There appear to be two clinical types of Mooren ulcer (450). The limited form is usually unilateral, in older patients, and of equal sex distribution. It has moderate progression and pain. The second form is seen typically in young, Nigerian, black males; it is usually bilateral, rapidly progressive, with central ulceration and perforation likely. Mooren ulcer may represent a Type III immune complex deposition hypersensitive reaction with immunoglobin and complement found in the peripheral cornea. The neutrophil granules release proteases and collagenase; the peripheral limbus is rich in plasma cells producing immunoglobin. Circulating autoantibodies to cornea, and circulating immune complexes have been reported (37, 358). Mooren ulcer is a diagnosis of exclusion and other causes of peripheral ulcerative keratitis need to be considered, especially potentially lethal systemic vascular disorders.

The initial treatment is with wide conjunctival resection to the bare sclera in the area adjacent, followed by resection of the overhanging lip of the ulcerating cornea. Additionally, the application of a tissue adhesive, a bandage soft contact lens, and the use of a topical

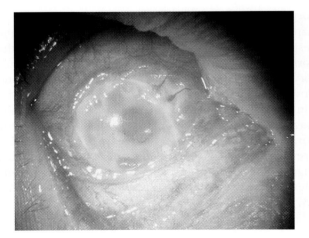

Figure 51–23.
Mooren ulcer. *A severe, painful, progressive idiopathic unilateral deep corneal ulcer in a 70-year-old man. No evident cause after extensive workup. Multiple therapeutic regimens were attempted.*

corticosteroid is recommended. Alternatively, medical treatment regimens include frequent topical corticosteroids, systemic tetracycline, and topical medroxyprogesterone. The surgical approach or medical approach may be curative in the limited unilateral Mooren ulcer. With the bilateral disease, the destructive process resumes when the resected conjunctiva reaches the limbus again. Bilateral progressive Mooren ulcer almost always requires systemic cytotoxic chemotherapy with methotrexate, azathioprine, cyclophosphamide, or cyclosporin (124). Penetrating keratoplasty for visual rehabilitation should only be attempted when the disease is quiescent. Generally, a lamellar tectonic graft is done before definitive central penetrating keratoplasty.

Peripheral Corneal Disease Associated with Systemic Disease

Peripheral corneal ulcers occasionally develop in patients who have systemic vasculitides such as rheumatoid arthritis, Wegener's granulomatosis, systemic lupus erythematosus, polyarteritis nodosa, or an inflammatory bowel disease such as Crohn's disease or ulcerative colitis (123) (Figure 51–24). These ulcers are usually unilateral and limited to one sector of the peripheral cornea although they can be bilateral and extensive. They begin within 2 mm of the limbus and are accompanied by varying degrees of basal occlusion of the adjacent limbal vascular networks. They can progress rapidly even to perforation. There may be an inflammatory infiltrate or a quiescent melt without evident in-

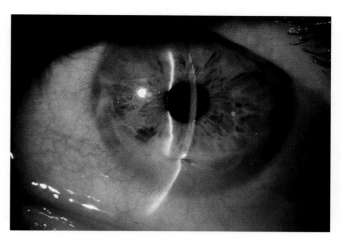

Figure 51–24.
Peripheral ulcerative keratitis secondary to rheumatoid arthritis. A quiet painless melt in the peripheral cornea in a patient with rheumatoid arthritis. The patient responded to a conjunctival resection and supportive therapy.

flammation. If there is infiltration, it may respond to topical corticosteroids. In the absence of an infiltrate, steroids should not be used. The ulcerations may be encouraged to heal with lubricants, patching, and soft contact lenses. Topical collagenase inhibitors or systemic tetracycline have a variable effect. Excision of the adjacent limbal conjunctiva eliminates the source of cells, enzymes, and toxins and may result in healing. Some cases require systemic immunosuppression such as cyclosporin or cyclophosphamide. A lamellar tectonic graft may be indicated.

■ REFERENCES

1. Aaberg, TM: The expanding ophthalmologic spectrum of Lyme disease. Am J Ophthalmol, 1989: 107:77
2. Aaberg, T, O'Brien, W: Expanding ophthalmologic recognition of Epstein-Barr virus infections. Am J Ophthalmol, 1987: 104:420.
3. Abbott, RL, Fine, BS, Webster, RG Jr, et al: Specular microscopic and histologic observations in non-guttate corneal endothelial degeneration. Ophthalmology, 1981: 88:788–800.
4. Abghari, S, Stulting, R: Recovery of herpes simplex virus from ocular tissues of latently infected mice. Invest Ophthalmol Vis Sci, 1988: 29:239.
5. Akiya, S, Brown, SI: The ultrastructure of Reis-Bücklers dystrophy. Am J Ophthalmol, 1971: 72:549.
6. Akiya, SK, Furukawa, H, Sakamoto, H, et al: Histopathologic and immunohistochemical findings in gelatinous drop-like corneal dystrophy. Ophthalmic Res, 1990: 22:371–376.
7. Akova, YA, Kirkness, CM, McCartney, AC, et al: Recurrent macular corneal dystrophy following penetrating keratoplasty. Eye, 1990: 4:698–705.
8. Alfonso, E, Arrellanes, L, Borychoff, SA, et al: Idiopathic

bilateral lipid keratopathy. Br J Ophthalmol, 1988: 72:338–343.
9. Allen, NB, Cox, CC, Cobo, M, et al: Use of immunosuppressive agents in the treatment of severe ocular and vascular manifestations of Cogan's syndrome. Am J Med, 1990: 88:296
10. American Academy of Ophthalmology: Ophthalmic procedures assessment. Corneal endothelial photography. Ophthalmology, 1991: 98:1464–1468.
11. Ameye C, Maudgal P, Missotten L: Primary ocular HSV infections in adults. In Maudgal P, Missotten L (eds): Herpetic Eye Diseases. Dordrecht, The Netherlands, Dr W Junk 1985: 133.
12. Andrews JS: The lipids of arcus senilis. Arch Ophthalmol, 1962: 68:264.
13. Anstice, J: Astigmatism—its components and their changes with age. Am J Optom, 1971: 48:1001.
14. Arffa, RC, Eve, FR: Systemic associations of corneal deposits. Int Ophthalmol Clin, 1991: 31:89–110.
15. Arffa, RC: Grayson's Diseases of the Cornea. Mosby Year Book, St. Louis: 1991: 333–363.

16. Arffa, RC: Grayson's Diseases of the Cornea. Mosby Year Book, St. Louis: 1991: 87–94.

17. Arffa, RC: Grayson's Diseases of the Cornea. Mosby Year Book, St. Louis: 1991: 47–55.

18. Arffa RC: Grayson's Diseases of the Cornea. 3rd ed. St Louis, Mosby Year Book, 1991, chapter 27.

19. Asbell, P, Stenson, S: Ulcerative keratitis. Survey of 30 years' laboratory experience. Arch Ophthalmol, 1982: 100:77.

20. Austin, P, Bron, SI: Inflammatory Terrien's marginal corneal disease. Am J Ophthalmol, 1981: 92:189.

21. Austin, P, Jakobiec, HA, Iwamoto, T: Elastodysplasia and elastodystrophy as pathologic bases of ocular pterygium and pingueculum. Ophthalmology, 1983: 90:96.

22. Aylward, GW, Claoue, CMP, Marsh, RJ: Influence of systemic acyclovir on the complications of herpes zoster ophthalmicus. Eye, 1994: 8:70–74.

23. Azazi, M, Gunilla, M, Forsgren, M: Late ophthalmologic manifestations of neonatal herpes simplex virus infection. Am J Ophthalmol, 1990: 109:1.

24. Bacon, AS, Dart, JKG, Ficker, LA, et al: Acanthamoeba keratitis, the value of early diagnosis. Ophthalmology, 1993: 100:1238–1243.

25. Bahn, CF, Falls, HF, Varley, GA: Classification of corneal endothelial disorders based on neural crest origin. Ophthalmology, 1984: 91:558.

26. Bailey, CS: A review of relative risks associated with four types of contact lenses. Cornea, 1990: 9(suppl):S59-S61

27. Barraquer-Somers, E, Chan, CC, Green, WR: Corneal epithelial iron deposition. Ophthalmol, 1983: 90:729.

28. Bates, AK, Morris, RJ, Stapleton, F, et al: "Sterile" corneal infiltrates in contact lens wearers. Eye, 1989: 3:803–810.

29. Baum, JL: Initial therapy of suspected microbial corneal ulcers: I. Broad antibiotic therapy based on prevalence of organism. Surv Ophthalmol, 1979: 24:97.

30. Baum, J: Hemorrhagic conjunctivitis: A new type of epidemic viral keratoconjunctivitis. Surv Ophthalmol, 1973: 17:489.

31. Baum, J, Barza, M, Weinstein, P, et al: Bilateral keratitis as a manifestation of Lyme disease. Am J Ophthalmol, 1988: 105:75.

32. Baum, J: Morphogenesis of the dendritic figure in herpes simplex keratitis: A negative study. Am J Ophthalmol, 1970: 70:722.

33. Bell, D, Holman, R, Pavan-Langston, D: Herpes simplex keratitis: Epidemiologic aspect. Ann Ophthalmol, 1982: 14:421.

34. Benson, WH, Lanier JD: Comparison of techniques for culturing corneal ulcers. Ophthalmol, 1992: 99:800.

35. Berg JC, Kozarsky A. Exposure Keratopathy. In Abbott RL (ed). Surgical Intervention in Corneal and External Diseases. Orlando: Grune & Straaton Inc. 1987: Chapter 3.

36. Berger, BW, Johnson, RC, Kodner, C, et al: Cultivation of Borrelia burgdorferi from erythema migrans lesions and perilesional skin. J Clin Microbiol, 1992: 30:359.

37. Berkowitz, PJ, Arentsen, JJ, Felberg, NT, Laibson, PR: Presence of circulating immune complexes in patients with peripheral corneal disease. Arch Ophthalmol, 1983: 101:242.

38. Bernauer, W, Dart, JKG: Aseptic keratitis associated with

contact lenses. Ophthalmol Clinic North Am, 1994: 7:661–667.

39. Binder, P: Review of treatment of ocular herpes simplex infections in the neonate and immunocompromised host. Cornea, 1985: 3:178.

40. Boruchoff, SA, Kuwabara, T: Electron microscopy of posterior polymorphous degeneration. Am J Ophthalmol, 1971: 72:879.

41. Boruchoff, SA, Weiner, MJ, Albert, DM: Recurrence of posterior polymorphous corneal dystrophy after penetrating keratoplasty. Am J Ophthalmol, 1990: 109:323.

42. Bourne, WM, Johnson, H, Campbell, J: The ultrastructure of Descemet's membrane. Arch Ophthalmol, 1982: 100:1952.

43. Bourne, WM: Soft contact lens wear decreases epithelial microcysts in Meesmann's corneal dystrophy. Trans Am Ophthalmol Soc, 1986: 84:170.

44. Bourne, WM: Partial corneal involvement in the iridocorneal endothelial syndrome. Ophthalmol, 1982: 94:774.

45. Bowen, RA, Hassard, DTR, Wong, VG, et al: Lattice dystrophy of the cornea as a variety of amyloidosis. Am J Ophthalmol, 1970: 70:822.

46. Boysen, G, et al: Familial amyloidosis with cranial neuropathy and corneal lattice dystrophy. J Neurol, 1979: 42:1020.

47. Bramsen, T, Ehlers, N, Baggesen, KH: Central cloudy corneal dystrophy of Francois. Acta Ophthalmol (Copenh), 1976: 54:221.

48. Braude, L, Sugar, J: Circinate pattern interstitial keratopathy in daily wear soft contact lens wearers. Arch Ophthalmol, 1985: 103:1662–1665.

49. Broderick, JD. Pigmentation of the cornea. Ann Ophthalmol, 1979: 11:855.

50. Bron, AJ. The corneal dystrophies. Curr Opin Ophthalmol, 1990: 1:333.

51. Bron, AJ, Tripathi, RC: Cystic disorders of the corneal epithelium: I. Clinical aspects. Br J Ophthalmol, 1973: 57:361.

52. Brooks, AMV, Grant, G, Gillies, WE: Differentiation of posterior polymorphous dystrophy from other posterior corneal opacities by specular microscopy. Ophthalmology, 1989: 96:1639.

53. Brown, AC, Rao, GN, Aquavella, JV: Peripheral corneal grafts in Terrien's marginal degeneration. Ophthalmic Surg, 1983: 14:931.

54. Brown, D, Nesburn, A, Pavan-Langston, D, et al: Recurrent herpes simplex conjunctivitis. Arch Ophthalmol, 1968: 79:733.

55. Brownstein, S, Fine, BS, Sherman, ME, Zimmerman, LE: Granular dystrophy of the cornea: Light and electron microscopic confirmation of recurrence in a graft. Am J Ophthalmol, 1974: 77:701.

56. Bruce, AS, Brennan, NA: Corneal pathophysiology with contact lens wear. Surv Ophthalmol, 1990: 35:25–58.

57. Bücklers, M: Uber eine weitere familiare Hornhautdystrophic (Reis). Klin Monatsbl Augenheilkd, 1949: 114:386.

58. Buehler, PA, Schein, OD, Stamler, JF, et al: The increased risk of ulcerative keratitis among disposable soft contact lens users. Arch Ophthalmol, 1992: 110:1555–1558.

59. Burgoon, C Jr, Burgoon, J, Baldridge, G: The natural history of herpes zoster. JAMA, 1957: 164:265.

60. Buxton, JN, Fox, ML: Superficial epithelial keratectomy in the treatment of epithelial basement membrane dystrophy: A preliminary report. Arch Ophthalmol, 1983: 101:392.

61. Buxton, JN, Constad, WH: Superficial epithelial keratectomy in the treatment of epithelial basement membrane dystrophy. Cornea, 1987: 6:292.

62. Buxton, JN, Lash, RS: Results of penetrating keratoplasty in the iridocorneal endothelial dystrophy. Am J Ophthalmol, 1984: 98:297.

63. Calandra, A, Chwa, M, Kenney, MC. Characterization of stroma from Fuchs' endothelial dystrophy corneas. Cornea, 1989: 8:90.

64. Caldwell, DR: Postoperative recurrence of Reis-Bücklers dystrophy. Am J Ophthalmol, 1978: 35:567.

65. Cameron, JA, Al-Rajhi, AA, Badr, IA: Corneal ectasias in vernal keratoconjunctivitis. Ophthalmology, 1989: 96:1915.

66. Campbell, DG, Shields, MB, Smith, TR: The corneal endothelium and the spectrum of essential iris atrophy. Am J Ophthalmol, 1978: 86:317.

67. Cantrill, H, Kenry, K, Jackson, B, et al: Recovery of human immunodeficiency virus from ocular tissues in patients with acquired immune deficiency syndrome. Ophthalmol, 1988: 95:1458.

68. Carmichael, TR, Gelfand, Y, Welsh, NH: Topical steroids in the treatment of central and paracentral corneal ulcers. Br J Ophthalmol, 1990: 74:528.

69. Cavanagh, HD, Petroll, WM, Alizadeh, H, et al: Clinical and diagnostic use of in vivo confocal microscopy in patients with corneal disease. Ophthalmology, 1993: 100:1444–1454.

70. Cavara, V: Keratoglobus and keratoconus: a contribution to nosological interpretation of keratoglobus. Br J Ophthalmol, 1950: 34:621.

71. Chandler, PA: Atrophy of the stroma of the iris: endothelial dystrophy, corneal edema, and glaucoma. Am J Ophthalmol, 1956: 41:607.

72. Char, DH, Cogan, DG, Sullivand WR: Immunologic study of nonsyphilitic interstitial keratitis with vestibuloauditory symptoms. Am J Ophthalmol, 1975: 80:491.

73. Chignell, AH, Easty, DL, Chesterton, JR, et al: Marginal ulceration of the cornea. Br J Ophthalmol, 1970: 54:433–440.

74. Chodosh, J: Epstein-Barr virus stromal keratitis. Ophthalmol Clin North Am, 1994: 7:549–556.

75. Cibis, GW, Tripathi, RC: The differential diagnosis of Descemet's tears and posterior polymorphous dystrophy bands. Ophthalmol, 1982: 89:614.

76. Cibis, GW, Krachmer, JA, Phelps, CD, Weingeist, TA: The clinical spectrum of posterior polymorphous dystrophy. Arch Ophthalmol, 1977: 95:1529.

77. Cobo, LM, Haynes, BF: Early corneal findings in Cogan's syndrome. Ophthalmol, 1984: 91:903.

78. Cobo, L, Foulks, G, Liesegang, T, et al: Oral acyclovir in the treatment of acute herpes zoster ophthalmicus. Ophthalmology, 1986: 93:763.

79. Cobo, M: Discussion (Oral acyclovir in the management of herpes simplex infection). Ophthalmology, 1988: 95:429.

80. Cogan, DG: Microcystic dystrophy of the corneal epithelium. Trans Am Ophthalmol Soc, 1964: 62:213.

81. Cogan, DG, Kuwabara, T: Arcus senilis, its pathology and histochemistry. Arch Ophthalmol, 1959: 61:553.

82. Cogan, DG, Reese, AB: A syndrome of iris nodules, ectopic Descemet's membrane, and unilateral glaucoma. Arch Ophthalmol, 1975: 93:963.

83. Cohen, AS, Wegelius, O. Classification of amyloid. Arthritis Rheum, 1980: 23:644.

84. Cohen, E, Laibson, P, Arentsen, J: Corneal transplantation for herpes simplex keratitis. Am J Ophthalmol, 1983: 95:645.

85. Cohen, EJ, Buchanan, HW, Laughrea, PA, et al: Diagnosis and management of Acanthamoeba keratitis. Am J Ophthalmol, 1985: 100:389–395.

86. Cokingtin, CD, Hyndiuk, RA: Insights from experimental data on ciprofloxacin in the treatment of bacterial keratitis and ocular infections. Am J Ophthalmol, 1991: 112:25S.

87. Coleman, V, Thygeson, P, Dawson, C, et al: Isolation of virus from herpetic keratitis: Influence of idoxuridine on isolation rate. Arch Ophthalmol, 1969: 81:22.

88. Cook, SD, Hill, JH: Herpes simplex virus: Molecular biology and the possibility of corneal latency. Surv Ophthalmol, 1991: 36:140

89. Cook, SC: Herpes simplex virus in the eye. Br J Ophthalmol, 1992: 76:365

90. Copeman, PW: Eczema and keratoconus. Br Med J, 1965: 5468:977.

91. Crawford, GJ, Stulting, RD, Cavanagh, HD, Waring, GO III: Penetrating keratoplasty in the management of iridocorneal endothelial syndrome. Cornea, 1989: 8:34.

92. Cross, HE, Maumenee, AE, Cantolino, SJ: Inheritance of Fuchs' endothelial dystrophy. Arch Ophthalmol, 1971: 85:268.

93. Curran, RE, Kenyon, KR, Green, WR: Pre-Descemet's membrane corneal dystrophy. Am J Ophthalmol, 1974: 77:711.

94. Dart, JKG: Disease and risks associated with contact lenses. Br J Ophthalmol, 1993: 77:49–53

95. Dart, JKG: Predisposing factors in microbial keratitis: the significance of contact lens wear. Br J Ophthalmol, 1988: 72:926–930.

96. Dart, JKG, Stapleton, F, Minassian, D: Contact lenses and other risk factors in microbial keratitis. Lancet, 1991: 338:650–653.

97. Davis, RM, Font, RL, Keisler, MS, et al: Corneal microsporidiosis: A case report including ultrastructural observations. Ophthalmol, 1990: 97:953–957.

98. Dawson, C, Togni, B, Moore, T, Jr: Structural changes in chronic herpetic keratitis: Studied by light and electron microscopy. Arch Ophthalmol, 1968: 79:740.

99. Deepak, E, Thonar, EJ-MA, Srinivasan, M, et al: Macular cornea dystrophy of the cornea. A systemic disorder of keratin sulfate metabolism. Ophthalmology, 1990: 97:1194.

100. deFreitas, D, Kelly, L, Pavan-Langston, D, et al: Late-onset varicella-zoster dendritic keratitis. Cornea, 1992: 11:471.

101. Dekkers, NWHM, Teskes, M: Measles keratitis. Ophthalmol Clin North Am, 1994: 7:567–576.

102. Dugel, P, Gill, P, Frangieh, G, et al: Particles resembling retrovirus in conjunctival Kaposi's sarcoma. Am J Ophthalmol, 1990: 110:86.

103. Dugel, P, Gill, P, Frangieh, G, et al: Ocular adnexal Kaposi's sarcoma in acquired immunodeficiency syndrome. Am J Ophthalmol, 1990: 110:500.

104. Dunkel, E, Pavan-Langston, D, Fitzpatrick, K, et al: Rapid detection of herpes simplex virus antigen in human ocular infections. Curr Eye Res, 1988: 7:661.

105. Eagle, RC, Font, RL, Yanoff, M, Fine, BS: Proliferative endotheliopathy with iris abnormalities: the iridocorneal endothelial syndrome. Arch Ophthalmol, 1979: 97:2104–2111.

106. Easty, D, Shimeld, C, Claoue, C, et al: Herpes simplex virus isolation in chronic stromal keratitis: Human and laboratory studies. Curr Eye Res, 1987: 6:69.

107. Edgerton, A: Herpes zoster ophthalmicus: Report of cases and review of literature. Arch Ophthalmol, 1945: 34:40,114.

108. Egerer, U-D, Stary, A: Erosive-ulcerative herpes simplex blepharitis. Arch Ophthalmol, 1980: 98:1760.

109. Esmann, V, Geil, J, Kroon, S, et al: Prednisolone does not prevent post-herpetic neuralgia. Lancet, 1987: 2:126.

110. Fernandez-Sasso, D, Acosta, JEP, Malbran, E: Punctiform and polychromatic pre-Descemet's dominant corneal dystrophy. Br J Ophthalmol, 1979: 63:336.

111. Ficker, LA, Kirkness, C, Wright, P: Prognosis for keratoplasty in Acanthamoeba keratitis. Ophthalmology, 1993: 100:105–110.

112. Fienstra, RPG, Tseng, SCG: Comparison of fluorescein and rose bengal staining. Ophthalmol, 1992: 99:605–617.

113. Fikrig, E, Barthold, SW, Kantor, FS, et al: Long-term protection of mice from Lyme disease by vaccination with OspA. Infec Immun, 1992: 60:773.

114. Fine, BS, Yanoff, M, Pitts, E, Slaughter, FD: Meesman's epithelial dystrophy of the cornea. Am J Ophthalmol, 1977: 83:633.

115. Fishman, RS, Sunderman, FW: Band keratopathy in gout. Arch Ophthalmol, 1966: 75:367.

116. Fitzsimons, R, Peters, AL: Miconazole and ketoconazole as a satisfactory first line treatment for keratomycosis. Am J Ophthalmol, 1986: 101:605–608.

117. Fleisher, G, Henry, W, McSorley, H, et al: Life-threatening complications of varicella. Am J Dis Child, 1981: 135:896.

118. Fogle, JA, Kenyon, KR, Stark, WJ, Green, WR: Defective epithelial adhesion in anterior corneal dystrophies. Am J Ophthalmol, 1975: 79:925.

119. Fogle, JA, Kenyon, KR, Foster, CS: Tissue adhesive arrests stromal melting in the human cornea. Am J Ophthalmol, 1980: 89:795.

120. Forsius, E, Eriksson, AW, Karna, J, et al: Granular corneal dystrophy with late manifestation. Acta Ophthalmol (Copenh), 1983: 61:514–528.

121. Foster, CS: Systemic immunosuppressive therapy for progressive bilateral Mooren's ulcer. Ophthalmology, 1985: 92:1436.

122. Foster CS: Fungal keratitis. In: Albert DM, Jakobiec FA (eds): Principles and Practice of Ophthalmology. Philadelphia: W.B. Saunders 1994, Volume 1 Chapter 8.

123. Foster CS: Immunologic disorders of the conjunctiva, cornea, and sclera. In Principles and Practice of Ophthalmology Clinical Practice, Albert DM, Jakobiec FA (eds): Vol 1, Chapter 10. Philadelphia, WB Saunders Company, 1994; 190.

124. Foster, CS: Miconazole therapy for keratomycosis. Am J Ophthalmol, 1981: 91:622–629.

125. Franceschetti, AT: La cornea verticillata (Gruber) et ses relations avec la maladie de Fabry. Ophthalmologica, 1968: 156:232.

126. Fraser, NW, Spivack, JG, Wroblewska, Z, et al: A review of the molecular mechanism of HSV-1 latency. Curr Eye Res, 1990: 9:1.

127. Fraunfelder, FT, Hanna, C: Spheroidal degeneration of cornea and conjunctiva: III. Incidences, classification and etiology. Am J Ophthalmol, 1973: 76:41.

128. Fraunfelder, FT, Hanna, C, Parker JM: Spheroid degeneration of the cornea and conjunctiva. I. Clinical course and characteristics. Am J Ophthalmol, 1972: 74:821.

129. Freedman, A: Climatic droplet keratopathy. Arch Ophthalmol, 1973: 89:193.

130. Friedlaender, MH, Cavanagh, HD, Sullivan, WR, et al: Bilateral central lipid infiltrates of the cornea. Am J Ophthalmol, 1977: 84:781.

131. Friedman-Kein, A, Lafleur, F, Gendler, E, et al: Herpes zoster: A possible early clinical sign for development of acquired immunodeficiency syndrome in high-risk individuals. J Am Acad Dermatol, 1986: 14:1023.

132. Fuchs, E: Dystrophia epithelialis corneal. Graefes Arch Clin Exp Ophthalmol, 1910: 76:478.

133. Fujikawa, LS, Foster, CS, Harris, TJ, et al: Fibronectin in healing rabbit corneal wounds. Lab Invest, 1981: 45:120.

134. Funderburgh, JL, Panjwani, N, Conrad, GW, Baum, J: Altered keratin sulfate epitopes in keratoconus. Invest Ophthalmol Vis Sci, 1989: 30:2278–2281.

135. Garau, J, Kabins, S, DeNassquo, S, et al: Spontaneous cytomegalovirus mononucleosis with conjunctivitis. Arch Intern Med, 1977: 137:1631.

136. Garner, A: Histochemistry of macular dystrophy. Invest Ophthalmol, 1969: 8:475.

137. Garner, AL: Histochemistry of corneal granular dystrophy. Br J Ophthalmol, 1969: 53:799.

138. Garner, A, Fraunfelder, FT, Barras, TC, Hinzpeter, EN: Spheroidal degeneration of cornea and conjunctiva. Br J Ophthalmol, 60: 473–478.

139. Garner, A: Amyloidosis of the cornea. Br J Ophthalmol 1969: 53:73.

140. Garrity, J, Liesegang, T: Ocular complications of atopic dermatitis. Can J Ophthalmol, 1984: 19:21.

141. Gass, JD: The iron lines of the superficial cornea. Arch Ophthalmol, 1964: 71:348.

142. Gilbard, JP, Rossi, SR: Tear film and ocular surface changes in a rabbit model of neurotrophic keratitis. Ophthalmol, 1990: 97:308–312.

143. Gipson IK, Sugrue SP: Cell biology of the corneal epithelium. In Principles and Practice of Ophthalmology, Albert DM, Jakobiec FA eds., W B Saunders Co Philadelphia, 1994, Chapter 1.

144. Gjone, E, Bergaust, B: Corneal opacity in familial plasma cholesterol ester deficiency. Acta Ophthalmol (Copenh), 1969: 47:222.

144a. Goldberg DB, Schanzlin DJ, Brown SI: Management of

Thygeson's superficial punctate keratitis. Am J Ophthalmol 1980: 98:22–24.

145. Goode, S, Hertzmark, E, Steinert, R, et al: Adequacy of the ELISA test for screening corneal transplant donors. Am J Ophthalmol, 1988: 106:463.

146. Gorevic, PD, Rodrigues, MM, Krachmer, JH, et al: Lack of evidence for AA reactivity in amyloid deposits of lattice corneal dystrophy and corneal amyloid degeneration. Am J Ophthalmol, 1984: 98:216.

147. Gorovoy, MS, Stern, GA, Hood, CI, et al: Intrastromal noninflammatory bacterial colonization of a corneal graft. Arch Ophthalmol, 1983: 101:1749

148. Grayson, M: The nature of hereditary deep polymorphous dystrophy of the cornea: its association with iris and anterior chamber dysgenesis. Trans Am Ophthalmol Soc, 1974: 72:516.

149. Grayson, M, Wilbrandt, H. Dystrophy of the anterior limiting membrane of the cornea. Am J Ophthalmol, 1966: 61:345.

150. Greenfield, G, et al: Blue sclera and keratoconus: key features of a distinct heritable disorder of connective tissue. Clin Genet, 1973: 4:8.

151. Greiner JV, Kenyon KR: Corneal aging. In: Principles and Practice of Ophthalmology. Albert, DM, Jakobiec FA (eds): Philadelphia: W. B. Saunders Co., 1994: V 1, Chapter 3.

152. Griffith, DG, Fine, BS: Light and electron microscopic observations in a superficial corneal dystrophy: Probable early Reis-Bücklers type. Am J Ophthalmol, 1967: 63:1659.

153. Gritz, DC, Lee, TY, Kwitko, S, McDonnell, PJ: Topical anti-inflammatory agents in an animal model of microbial keratitis. Arch Ophthalmol, 1990: 108:1001.

154. Groden LR, Rodnite J, Brinser JH, Genvert GI: Acridine orange and Gram stains in infectious keratitis. Cornea, 1990: 9:122–124.

155. Gudmundsson, OG, Ormerod, LD, Kenyon, KR, et al: Factors influencing predilection and outcome in bacterial keratitis. Cornea, 1989: 8:115.

156. Haddad, R, Font, RL, Fine, BS: Unusual superficial variant of granular dystrophy of the cornea. Am J Ophthalmol, 1977: 83:213.

157. Hall, P: Reis-Bucklers' dystrophy. Arch Ophthalmol, 1974: 91:170.

158. Hanna, C, Fraunfelder, FT: Spheroid degeneration of the cornea and conjunctiva. II. Pathology. Am J Ophthalmol, 1972: 74:829.

159. Hansen, TE. Posterior polymorphous corneal dystrophy. Acta Ophthalmol (Copenh), 1983: 61:454.

160. Hara, J, Fujimoto, F, Ishibashi, T, et al: Ocular manifestations of the 1976 rubella epidemic in Japan. Am J Ophthalmol, 1979: 87:642.

161. Hedges, T, III, Albert, D: Progression of the ocular abnormalities of herpes zoster: Histopathologic observations of nine cases. Ophthalmology, 1982: 89:165.

162. Helm, CJ, Holland, GN: Ocular Tuberculosis. Surv Ophthalmol, 1993: 38:229.

163. Hemady, RK, Foster, CS: Intraocular penetration of ketoconazole in rabbits. Cornea 1992: 11:329–333.

164. Hemady, R, Tauber, J, Foster, CS: Immunosuppressive drugs in immune and inflammatory ocular disease. Surv Ophthalmol 1991: 35:369.

165. Hida, T, Proia, AD, Kigasawa, K, et al: Histopathologic and immunochemical features of lattice corneal dystrophy type III. Am J Ophthalmol 1987: 104:241.

166. Hirsch, MJ: Changes in astigmatism after the age of forty. Am J Optom, 1959: 36:395.

167. Hirst, LW, Quigley, HA, Stark, WJ, Shields, MB: Specular microscopy of iridocorneal endothelial syndrome. Am J Ophthalmol 1980: 89:11–21.

168. Hirst, L, Waring, GO: Clinical specular microscopy of posterior polymorphous endothelial dystrophy. Am J Ophthalmol, 1983: 95:143.

169. Hoffer, KJ, Kraff, MC: Normal endothelial cell count range. Ophthalmol, 1980: 87:861.

170. Hogan, MJ, Wood, I: Reis-Bücklers corneal dystrophy. Trans Ophthalmol Soc UK, 1971: 91:41.

171. Hogan, MJ, Wood, I, Fine, M: Fuchs' endothelial dystrophy of the cornea. Am J Ophthalmol, 1974: 78:363.

172. Hogan, M: Corneal transplantation in the treatment of herpetic disease of the cornea. Am J Ophthalmol, 1957: 43:147.

173. Holbach, LM, Font, RL, Shivitz, IA, Jones, DB: Bilateral keloidlike myofibroblastic proliferations of the cornea in children. Ophthalmol, 1990: 97:1198.

174. Holland, E, Bennett, S, Brannian, R, et al: The risk of cytomegalovirus transmission by penetrating keratoplasty. Am J Ophthalmol, 1988: 105:347.

175. Holland, G: Ocular manifestations of the acquired immune deficiency syndrome. Int Ophthalmol Clin, 1985: 25:179.

176. Hope-Simpson, R: The nature of herpes zoster: A long-term study and a new hypothesis. Proc Roy Soc Med, 1965: 58:9.

177. Hunts, JH, Matoba, AY, Osato, MS, et al: Infections crystalline keratopathy. Arch Ophthalmol, 1993: 111:528.

178. Hutchison, D, Smith, R, Haughton, D: Congenital herpetic keratitis. Arch Ophthalmol, 1975: 93:70.

179. Isakow, I, Romen, M: Ultrastructure of Groenouw II type corneal dystrophy. Metab Pediatr Ophthalmol, 1981: 5:27.

180. Ishibashi, Y, et al: Oral itraconazole and topical miconazole with debridement for Acanthamoeba keratitis. Am J Ophthalmol, 1990: 109:121.

181. Iwamoto, T, Devoe, AG: Electron microscopical study of the Fleisher ring. Arch Ophthalmol, 1976: 94:1579.

182. Jakobiec, F, Srinivasan, D, Gamboa, E: Recurrent herpetic angular blepharitis in an adult. Am J Ophthalmol, 1979: 88:744.

183. Jenkins, C, Tuft, S, Liu, C, et al: Limbal transplantation in the management of chronic contact-lens-associated epitheliopathy. Eye, 1993: 7:629–633.

184. Johns, KJ, O'Day, DM: Pharmacologic management of keratomycoses. Surv Ophthalmol, 1988: 33:178–188.

185. Johnson, BL, Brown, SI: Posterior polymorphous dystrophy: A light and electron microscopic study. Br J Ophthalmol, 1978: 62:89.

186. Johnson, GJ, Overall, M: Histology of spheroidal degeneration of the cornea in Labrador. Br J Ophthalmol, 1978: 62:53.

187. Jones DB: Strategy for the initial management of suspected microbial keratitis. In New Orleans Academy of Ophthalmology, Symposium on Medical and Surgical Diseases of the Cornea. St Louis: CV Mosby, 1980: 86.

188. Jones, DB: Initial therapy of suspected microbial corneal ulcers. II. Specific antibody therapy based on corneal scrapings. Surv Ophthalmol, 1979: 24:97.

189. Jones, ST, Zimmerman, LE: Histopathologic differentiation of granular, macular, and lattice dystrophies of the cornea. Am J Ophthalmol, 1961: 51:394.

190. Jones, ER: Principles in the management of ocular mycosis. Am J Ophthalmol, 1975: 79:719–751.

191. Jones, ST, Stauffer, LK: Reis-Bücklers corneal dystrophy: A clinicopathologic study. Trans Am Acad Ophthalmol Otolaryngol, 1970: 74:417.

192. Judisch, GF, Maumenee, IH: Clinical differentiation of recessive congenital hereditary endothelial dystrophy and dominant hereditary endothelial dystrophy. Am J Ophthalmol, 1978: 85:606.

193. Katsev, DA, Kinkaid, MC, Fouraker, BD, et al: Recurrent corneal erosion: Pathology of corneal puncture. Cornea, 1991: 10:418–423.

194. Kaufman, HE, Thomas, IB: Vitreous opacities diagnostic of familial primary amyloidosis. N Engl J Med, 1959: 261–1267.

195. Kaufman, H, Centifanto-Fitzgerald, Y, Varnell, E: Herpes simplex keratitis. Ophthalmology, 1983: 90:700.

196. Kaufman, H, Varnell, E, Centifanto, Y, et al: Effect of the herpes simplex virus genome on the response of infection to corticosteroids. Am J Ophthalmol, 1985: 100:114.

197. Keczkes, K, Basheer, A: Do corticosteroids prevent postherpetic neuralgia? Br J Dermatol, 1980: 101:551.

198. Kennedy, RE, Roca, PD, Platt, DS: Further observations on atypical band keratopathy in glaucoma patients. Trans Am Ophthalmol Soc, 1975: 72:107.

199. Kenyon, KR, Maumenee, AE: Further studies of congenital hereditary corneal dystrophy of the cornea. Am J Ophthalmol, 1973: 76:419.

200. Kenyon KR, Starck T, Wagoner MD: Corneal epithelial defects and noninfectious ulcerations. In Principles and Practice of Ophthalmology Clinical Practice, Albert DM, Jakobiec FA (eds), Philadelphia: WB Saunders Company, 1994: Vol 1, chapter 11.

201. Kenyon, KR, Wagoner, MD, Hettinger, ME: Conjunctival autograft transplantation for advanced and recurrent pterygium. Ophthalmol, 1985: 92:1461.

202. Kenyon, KR, Berman, M, Rose, J, et al: Prevention of stromal ulceration in the alkali-burned rabbit cornea by glued-on contact lens. Evidence for the role of polymorphonuclear leukocytes in collagen degradation. Invest Ophthalmol Vis Sci, 1979: 18:570.

203. Kenyon, KR, Van Horn, DL, Edelhauser, HF: Endothelial degeneration and posterior collagenous proliferation in aphakic bullous keratopathy. Am J Ophthalmol, 1978: 85:329.

204. Kenyon, KR, Tseng, SCG: Limbal autograft transplantation for ocular surface disorders. Ophthalmology, 1989: 96:709.

205. Kenyon, KR. Inflammatory mechanisms in corneal ulceration. Trans Am Ophthalmol Soc, 1985: 83:610–663.

206. Kirk, JG, Rabb, M, Hattenhauer, J, et al: Primary familial amyloidosis of the cornea. Trans Am Acad Ophthalmol Otolaryngol, 1973: 77:411.

207. Kirkness, CM, Hay, J, Seal, DV, Aitken, D: Acanthamoeba keratitis. Ophthalmol Clin North Am, 1994: 7:605–616.

208. Kirkness, CM, McCartney, A, Rice, NS, et al: Congenital hereditary corneal oedema of Maumenee: its clinical features, management, and pathology. Br J Ophthalmol, 1987: 71:130–144.

209. Klein, R: Pathogenic mechanisms of recurrent herpes simplex virus infections. Arch Virol, 1976: 51:1.

210. Klintworth, GK: Lattice corneal dystrophy: An inherited variety of amyloidosis restricted to the cornea. Am J Pathol, 1967: 50:371.

211. Klintworth, GK, Reed, J, Stainer, GA, Binder, PS. Recurrence of macular corneal dystrophy within grafts. Am J Ophthalmol, 1983: 95:60–72.

212. Klintworth, GK, Smith, CF: Macular corneal dystrophy: Studies of sulfated glycosaminoglycans in corneal explant and confluent stromal cell cultures. Am J Pathol, 1977: 89:167.

213. Komadina, TG, Wilkes, TDI, Shock, JP, et al: Treatment of Aspergillus rheumagutus keratitis in rabbits with oral and topical ketoconazole. Am J Ophthalmol, 1985: 99:476–479.

214. Kowal, VO, Laibson, PR: Keratitis due to Cogan's Syndrome. Ophthalmol Clin North Am, 1994: 7(4): 649–656.

215. Kowalski, R, Gordon, YJ: Evaluation of immunologic tests for the detection of ocular herpes simplex virus. Ophthalmology, 1989: 96:1583.

216. Krachmer, JH, Dubord, PJ, Rodrigues, MM, Mannis, MJ: Corneal posterior crocodile shagreen and polymorphic amyloid degeneration. Arch Ophthalmol, 1983: 101:54.

217. Krachmer, JH: Posterior polymorphous corneal dystrophy: a disease characterized by epithelial-like endothelial cells which influence management and prognosis. Trans Am Ophthalmol Soc, 1985: 83:413.

218. Krachmer, JH, Purcell, JJ Jr, Young, CW, Bucher, KD: Corneal endothelial dystrophy. A study of 64 families. Arch Ophthalmol, 1978: 96:2036–2039.

219. Lafferty, W, Coombs, R, Benedetti, J, et al: Recurrences after oral and genital herpes simplex viral infection. N Engl J Med, 1987: 316:1444.

220. Laibson, PR: Microcystic corneal dystrophy. Trans Am Ophthalmol Soc, 1977: 74:488.

221. Laibson, PR, Krachmer, JH. Familial occurrence of dot, map, fingerprint dystrophy of the cornea. Invest Ophthalmol, 1975: 14:397.

222. Laing, RA, Sandstrom, MM, Berrospi, AR, Leibowitz, HM: Changes in the corneal endothelium as a function of age. Exp Eye Res, 1976: 22:587.

223. Lam, S: Keratitis caused by Leishmaniasis or trypanosomiasis. Ophthalmol Clin North Am, 1994: 7:635–639.

224. Lambert, S, Taylor, D, Kriss, A, et al: Ocular manifestations of the congenital varicella syndrome. Arch Ophthalmol, 1989: 107:52.

225. Langston, R, Pavan-Langston, D, Dohlman, C: Penetrating keratoplasty for herpetic keratitis: Prognostic and therapeutic determinants. Trans Am Acad Ophthalmol Otolaryngol, 1975: 79:577.

226. Lanier, JD, Fine, M, Togni, B: Lattice corneal dystrophy. Arch Ophthalmol, 1976: 94:921.

227. Larkin, DFP: Acanthamoeba keratitis. Int Ophthalmol Clin, 1991: 31:163.

228. Larkin, DF, Kilvington, S, Easty, DL: Contamination of contact lens storage cases by Acanthamoeba and bacteria. Br J Ophthalmol, 1990: 74:133.

229. Larkin, DFP, Kilvington, S, Dart, JKG: Treatment of Acanthamoeba keratitis with polyhexamethylene biguanide. Ophthalmology, 1992: 99:185.

230. Leibowitz, HM: Clinical evaluation of ciprofloxacin 0.3% ophthalmic solution in the treatment of bacterial conjunctivitis. Am J Ophthalmol, 1991: 112:34S.

231. Lemp, MA, Ralph, RA: Rapid development of band keratopathy in dry eyes. Am J Ophthalmol, 1977: 83:657.

232. Lennette, E, VanAllen, A: Laboratory diagnosis of herpetic infections of the eye. Am J Ophthalmol, 1957: 43:118.

233. Levenson, JE, Chandler, JW, Kaufman, HE: Affected asymptomatic relatives in congenital hereditary endothelial dystrophy. Am J Ophthalmol, 1973: 76:976.

234. Leyden, J, Baker, B: Localized herpes simplex infections in atopic dermatitis. Arch Dermatol, 1979: 115:311.

235. Liesegang, T, Melton, J III, Daly, P, et al: Epidemiology of ocular herpes simplex: Incidence in Rochester, Minnesota, 1950 through 1982. Arch Ophthalmol, 1989: 107:1155.

236. Liesegang, TJ: Biology and molecular aspects of herpes simplex and varicella-zoster virus infections. Ophthalmology, 1992: 99:781.

237. Liesegang, T: Corneal complications from herpes zoster ophthalmicus. Ophthalmol, 1985: 92:316.

238. Liesegang, TJ: Diagnosis and therapy of herpes zoster ophthalmicus. Ophthalmol, 1991: 98:1216–1229.

239. Liesegang, T: Ocular herpes simplex infection: Pathogenesis and current therapy. Mayo Clin Proc, 1988: 63:1092.

240. Liesegang, TJ, Forster, RK: Spectrum of microbial keratitis in South Florida. Am J Ophthalmol, 1980: 90:38–47.

241. Limberg, MB: A review of bacterial keratitis and bacterial conjunctivitis. Am J Ophthalmol, 1991: 112:2S.

242. Linnemann, C Jr, Alvira, M: Pathogenesis of varicella-zoster angiitis in the CNS. Arch Neurol, 1980: 37:239.

243. Lisch, W, Weidle, EG, Lisch, C, et al: Schnyder's dystrophy: Progression and metabolism, Ophthalmic & Paediatr Genet, 1986: 7:45–56.

244. Litoff, D, Catalano, R: Herpes zoster optic neuritis in human immunodeficiency virus infection. Arch Ophthalmol, 1990: 108:782.

245. Lohse, E, Stock, EL, Jones, JC, et al: Reis-Bücklers corneal dystrophy: Immunofluorescent and electron microscopic studies. Cornea, 1989: 8:200.

246. Lorenzetti, DW, Uotila, MH, Parikh, N, Kaufman, HE: Central cornea guttata: incidence in the general population. Am J Ophthalmol, 1967: 64:1155–1158.

247. Luxenburg, M: Hereditary crystalline dystrophy of the cornea. Am J Ophthalmol, 1967: 63:507.

248. Mackie, I: Role of the corneal nerves in destructive disease of the cornea. Trans Ophthalmol Soc UK, 1978: 98:343.

249. Macsai, MS, Varley, GA, Krachmer, JH: Development of keratoconus after contact lens wear. Arch Ophthalmol, 1990: 108:534.

250. Maguire, LJ, Bourne, WM: Corneal topography of early keratoconus. Am J Ophthalmol, 1989: 108:107.

251. Mahalingam, R, Wellish, M, Wolfe, W, et al: Latent varicella-zoster viral DNA in human trigeminal and thoracic ganglia. N Engl J Med, 1990: 323:627.

252. Makensen, G, Sundmacher, R, Witschel, D: Late wound complications after circular keratotomy for zoster keratitis. Cornea, 1984: 3:95.

253. Malbran, ES, Meijide, RF, Croxatto, JO. Atypical corneal dystrophy with stromal amyloid deposits. Cornea, 1988: 7:210.

254. Mannis, MJ, Krachmer, JH, Rodrigues, MM, Pardos, GJ: Polymorphic amyloid degeneration of the cornea. A clinical and histopathologic study. Arch Ophthalmol, 1981: 99:1217.

255. Margo, CE, Hemed, LM: Ocular syphilis. Surv Ophthalmol, 1992: 37:203–220.

256. Margolis, T, Ostler, B: Treatment of ocular disease in eczema herpeticum. Am J Ophthalmol, 1990: 110:274.

257. Marines, HM, Osato, MS, Font, RL: The value of calcofluor white in the diagnosis of mycotic and Acanthamoeba infections of the eye and ocular adnexa. Ophthalmol, 1987: 94:23.

258. Mashima, Y, Hida, T, Akiya, S, Uemura, Y: Specular microscopy of posterior polymorphous endothelial dystrophy. Ophthalmic Pediatr Genet, 1986: 7:101–107.

259. Matoba, A, Wilhelmus, K, Jones, D: Epstein-Barr viral stromal keratitis. Ophthalmology, 1986: 93:746.

260. Matoba, A: Mycobacterium chelonae keratitis. Am J Ophthalmol, 1987: 103:595.

261. Maudgal, P, Missotten, L, DeClercq, E, et al: Varicella-zoster virus in the human corneal endothelium: A case report. Bull Soc Belge Ophthalmol, 1980: 190:71.

262. Maury, CPJ, Teppo, AM, Kariniemi, AL, et al: Amyloid fibril protein in familial amyloidosis with cranial neuropathy and corneal lattice dystrophy (FAP type IV) is related to transthyretin. Am J Pathol, 1988: 89:359.

263. McCartney, MD, Wood, TO, McLaughlin, BJ: Moderate Fuchs' endothelial dystrophy ATPase pumpsite density. Invest Ophthalmol Vis Sci, 1989: 30:1560.

264. McDonald, MB, Kaufman, HE, Durrie, DS, et al: Epikeratophakia for keratoconus. The nationwide study. Arch Ophthalmol, 1986: 104:1294.

265. McGill, JI: Topical acyclovir in herpes zoster ocular involvement. Br J Ophthalmol, 1981: 65:542–545.

266. McLean, EN, MacRae, SM, Rich, LF: Recurrent erosion. Treatment by anterior stromal puncture. Ophthalmol, 1986: 93:784.

267. McPherson, SD Jr, Kiffney, GT Jr, Freed, CC: Corneal amyloidosis. Am J Ophthalmol, 1966: 62:1025–1033.

268. Meisler, DM, Fine, M: Recurrence of the clinical signs of lattice corneal dystrophy (type I) in corneal transplants. Am J Ophthalmol, 1984: 97:210.

269. Meretoja, J: Comparative histopathological and clinical findings in eyes with lattice corneal dystrophy of the two different types. Ophthalmologica, 1972: 165:15.

270. Meyers, R: Immunology of herpes simplex virus infection. Int Ophthalmol Clin, 1975: 15:37.

271. Miller G: Epstein-Barr virus; Biology, pathogenesis, and medical aspects. In Fields BN, Knite DM, et al (eds): Virology, ed 2. New York: Raven Press, 1990: 1921.

272. Miller, A: Selective decline in cellular immune response to varicella-zoster in the elderly. Neurology, 1980: 30:582.

273. Millidot, M: The influence of age on the sensitivity of the cornea. Invest Ophthalmol, 1977: 16:240.

274. Millidot, M, Owens, H: The influence of age on the fragility of the cornea. Acta Ophthalmol, 1984: 62:819.

275. Mills, RAD: Tuberculosis and leprosy. Ophthalmol Clin North Am, 1994: 7:583–589.

276. Mines, J, Kaplan, H: Acquired immune deficiency syndrome (AIDS): The disease and its ocular manifestations. Int Ophthalmol Clin, 1986: 26:73.

277. Moller, HU: Interfamilial variability and intrafamilial similarities of granular corneal dystrophy Graenow type I with respect to biomicroscopical appearance and symptomatology. Acta Ophthalmol (Copenh), 1989: 67:669.

278. Mondino, BJ, Kowalski, HV, Peters, J, et al: Rabbit model of phlyctenulosis and catarrhal infiltrates. Arch Ophthalmol, 1981: 99:891–895.

279. Mondino, BJ, Raj, CV, Skinner, M et al: Protein AA and lattice corneal dystrophy. Am J Ophthalmol, 1980: 89:377–380.

280. Mondino, BJ, Rabb, MF, Sugar, J et al: Primary familial amyloidosis of the cornea. Am J Ophthalmol, 1981: 92:732.

281. Mondino, BJ, Kowalski, RP: Phlyctenulae and catarrhal infiltrates. Arch Ophthalmol, 1982: 100:1968–1971.

282. Moore, MB, Newton, C, Kaufman, HE: Chronic keratitis caused by Mycobacterium gordonae. Am J Ophthalmol, 1986: 102:516.

283. Murphy, T: Post-herpetic neuralgia. JAMA, 1989: 262:3478.

284. Nahmias, A, Visintine, A, Caldwell, D, et al: Eye infections with herpes simplex viruses in neonates. Surv Ophthalmol, 1976: 21:100.

285. Nanda, M, Pflugfelder, SC, Holland, S: Fulminant pseudomonal keratitis and scleritis in human immunodeficiency virus-infected patients. Arch Ophthalmol, 1991: 109:503.

286. Naumann, G, Green, WR, Zimmerman, LE: Mycotic keratitis: A histopathologic study of 73 cases. Am J Ophthalmol, 1967: 64:668.

287. Nelson, RD, Shibata, N, Podzorski, RP, Herron, MJ: Candida mannan: Chemistry, suppression of cell-mediated immunity, and possible mechanisms of action. Clin Microbiol Rev, 1991: 4:1.

288. Nesburn, A, Borit, A, Pentelei-Molnar, J, et al: Varicella dendritic keratitis. Invest Ophthalmol, 1974: 13:764.

289. Neubauer, L, Lund, O-E, Leibowitz, HM: Specular microscopic appearance of the corneal endothelium in iridocorneal endothelial syndrome. Arch Ophthalmol, 1983: 101:916.

290. Nevins RC, Jr, Davis, WH Jr, Elliott, JH: Coat's white ring of the cornea: Unsettled metal fettle. [correspondence] Arch Ophthalmol, 1968: 80:145.

291. Nicholson, DH, Green, WR, Cross, HE, et al: A clinical and histopathological study of Francois-Neetens speckled corneal dystrophy. Am J Ophthalmol, 1977: 83:554.

292. Nimura, M, Nishikawa, T: Treatment of eczema herpeticum with oral acyclovir. Am J Med, 1988: 85:49.

293. Norn, MS: Spheroid degeneration, pinguecula, and pterygium among Arabs in the Red Sea territory, Jordan. Acta Ophthalmol (Copenh), 1982: 60:949.

294. O'Connor, GR: Calcific band keratopathy. Trans Am Ophthalmol Soc, 1972: 70:58.

295. O'Day DM, Burd EM: Fungal keratitis and conjunctivitis: In: Smolin T, Thoft RA (eds): The Cornea. Boston: Little, Brown, & Co. 1994: 229–239.

296. O'Day, DM: Orally administered antifungal therapy for experimental keratomycosis. Trans Am Ophthalmol Soc, 1990: 88:685.

297. O'Grady, RB, Kirk, HQ. Corneal keloids. Am J Ophthalmol, 1972: 73:206.

298. Olsen, T, Ehlers, N, Favini, E. Long-term results of corneal grafting in Fuchs' endothelial dystrophy. Acta Ophthalmol (Copenh), 1984: 62:445.

299. Olson, RJ, Kaufman, H: Recurrence of Reis-Bücklers corneal dystrophy in a graft. Am J Ophthalmol, 1978: 85:349.

300. Onorato, I, Morens, D, Martone, W, et al: Epidemiology of cytomegalovirus infections. Recommendation for prevention and control. Rev Infect Dis, 1985: 7:479

301. Ormerod, LD, Ruoff, KL, Meisler, DM, et al: Infectious crystalline keratopathy: Role of nutritionally variant streptococci and other bacterial factors. Ophthalmol, 1991: 98:159.

302. Osato, MS: Parasitic keratitis and conjunctivitis. Parasitology. In: Smolin T, Thoft RA (eds): The Cornea Third Edition. Boston: Little, Brown & Co., 1994: 253–262.

303. Ostler, HB: Diseases of the external eye and adnexa. Baltimore: Williams and Wilkins. 1993, 143–145.

304. Palestine, A, Rodrigues, M, Macher, A, et al: Ophthalmic involvement in acquired immune deficiency syndrome. Ophthalmology, 1984: 91:1092.

305. Panjwani, N, Drysdale, J, Clark, B, et al: Protein-related abnormalities in keratoconus. Invest Ophthalmol Vis Sci, 1989: 30:2481–2487.

306. Parsons, MR, Holland, EJ, Agapitos, PJ: Nocardia asteroides keratitis associated with extended wear soft contact lenses. Can J Ophthalmol, 1989: 24:120.

307. Patel, A, Kenyon, KR, Hirst, LW, et al: Clinicopathologic features of Chandler's syndrome. Surv Ophthalmol, 1983: 27:327.

308. Pavan-Langston, D, Brockhurst, R: Herpes simplex panuveitis: A clinical report. Arch Ophthalmol, 1969: 81:783.

309. Pavan-Langston, D, Rong, B, Dunkel, E: Extraneuronal herpetic latency: Animal and human corneal studies. Acta Ophthalmol Suppl (Copenh), 1989: 192:135.

310. Pavan-Langston D: In Principles and Practice of Ophthalmology Clinical Practice: Viral Disease of the Cornea and External Eye, Albert DM, Jakobiec TA (eds), Philadelphia, W B Saunders Company, 1994: Vol 1, Chapter 6.

311. Pearce, WG, Tripathi, RC, Morgan, G: Congenital endothelial corneal dystrophy: clinical, pathological and genetic study. Br J Ophthalmol, 1969: 53:477.

312. Pearlman, E, Lass, JH: Keratitis due to onchocerciasis. Ophthalmol Clin North Am, 1994: 7:641–648.

313. Perry, HD, Kenyon, KR, Lamberts, DW, et al: Systemic tetracycline hydrochloride as adjunctive therapy in the treatment of persistent epithelial defects. Ophthalmol, 1986: 93:1320–1322.

314. Perry, HD, Nauheim, JS, Donnenfeld, ED: Nocardia asteroides keratitis presenting as a persistent epithelial defect. Cornea, 1989: 8:41.

315. Perry, HD, Fine, BS, Caldwell, DR. Reis-Bucklers' dystrophy. Arch Ophthalmol, 1979: 97:664.

316. Perry, LD, Brinser, JH, Kolodner, H: Anaerobic corneal ulcers. Ophthalmology, 1982: 89:636.

317. Perry, HD, Buxton, JN, Fine, BS: Round and oval cones in keratoconus. Ophthalmology, 1980: 87:905.

318. Pettit, T, Holland, G: Chronic keratoconjunctivitis associated with ocular adenovirus infection. Am J Ophthalmol, 1979: 88:748.

319. Pfister, RR, Paterson, CA: Ascorbic acid in the treatment of alkali burns of the eye. Ophthalmology, 1980: 87:1050.

320. Pflugfelder, S, Saulson, R, Ullman, S: Peripheral corneal ulceration in a patient with AIDS-related complex. Am J Ophthalmol, 1987: 104:542.

321. Philips, K, Arffa, R, Cintron, C: Effects of prednisolone and medroxyprogesterone on corneal wound healing, ulceration, and neovascularization. Arch Ophthalmol, 1983: 101:640.

322. Phinney, RB, Schwartz, SD, Lee, DA, Mondino, BJ: Collagen-shield delivery of gentamicin and vancomycin. Arch Ophthalmol, 1988: 106:1599.

323. Pitts, JF, Jay, JL: The association of Fuchs' corneal endothelial dystrophy with axial hypermetropia, shallow anterior chamber, and angle closure glaucoma. Br J Ophthalmol, 1990: 74:601.

324. Plotkin, J, Reynaud, A, Okumoto, M: Cytologic study of herpetic keratitis. Arch Ophthalmol, 1971: 85:597.

325. Polack, FM: Contributions of electron microscopy to the study of corneal pathology. Surv Ophthalmol, 1976: 20:375.

326. Portney, SL, Insler, MS, Kaufman, HE: Surgical management of corneal ulceration and perforation. Surv Ophthalmol, 1989: 34:47–58.

327. Purcell, JJ Jr, Krachmer, JH, Weingeist, TA: Fleck corneal dystrophy. Arch Ophthalmol, 1977: 95:440.

328. Rabinovitch, J, Donnenfeld, ED, Laibson, PR: Management of Cogan's syndrome. Am J Ophthalmol, 1986: 101:494.

329. Rabinowitz, YS: Corneal topography in family members of patients with keratoconus using computer assisted corneal topography analysis. Invest Ophthalmol Vis Sci 1989;30(suppl):188.

330. Ragozzino, M, Melton, M, Kurland, L, et al: Population-based study of herpes zoster and its sequelae. Medicine, 1982: 61:310.

331. Raryman, MB, Whitcup, SM: Syphilitic keratitis. Ophthalmol Clin North Am, 1994: 7:591–595.

332. Rastrelli, PD, Didier, E, Yee, RW: Microsporidial keratitis. Ophthalmol Clin North Am, 1994: 7:617–633.

333. Reed, J, Joyner, S, Knauer, W III: Penetrating keratoplasty for herpes zoster keratopathy. Am J Ophthalmol, 1989: 107:257.

334. Reis, W: Familiare, fleckige Hornhautentartung. Dtsch Med Wochenschr, 1917: 43:575.

335. Rice, NSC, Ashton, N, Jay, B, Blach, RK: Reis-Bücklers dystrophy. A clinicopathologic study. Br J Ophthalmol, 1968: 52:577.

336. Ridley D, Jopling, W: Classification of leprosy according to immunity. A five group system. Int J Lepr, 1966: 58:319.

337. Robin, JB, Schanzlin, DJ, Verity, SM, et al: Peripheral corneal disorders. Surv Ophthalmol, 1986: 31(1):1–36.

338. Robin, J, Stergner, J, Kaufman, H: Progressive herpetic corneal endotheliitis. Am J Ophthalmol, 1985: 100:336.

339. Robin, AL, Green, WR, Lapsa, TP, et al: Recurrence of macular corneal dystrophy after lamellar keratoplasty. Am J Ophthalmol, 1977: 84:457–461.

340. Rodrigues, MM, Phelps, CD, Krachmer, JH et al: Glaucoma due to endothelialization of the anterior chamber angle: a comparison of posterior polymorphous dystrophy of the cornea and Chandler's syndrome. Arch Ophthalmol, 1980: 98:688–696.

341. Rodrigues, MM, McGavic, JS: Recurrent corneal granular dystrophy: A clinicopathologic study. Trans Am Ophthalmol Soc, 1975: 73:306.

342. Rodrigues, MM, Streeten, BW, Spaeth, GL: Chandler's syndrome as a variant of essential iris atrophy. Arch Ophthalmol, 1978: 96:643.

343. Rodrigues, MM, Waring, GO, Laibson, PR, Weinreb, S: Endothelial alterations in congenital corneal dystrophy. Am J Ophthalmol, 1975: 80:678–689.

344. Rodrigues, MM, Newsome, DA, Krachmer, JH, Sun, TT: Posterior polymorphous dystrophy of the cornea. Exp Eye Res, 1981: 33:535–544.

345. Rodrigues, MM, Krachmer, JH: Recent advances in corneal stromal dystrophies. Cornea, 1988: 7:19.

346. Rodrigues, MM: Lack of evidence for AA reactivity in amyloid deposits of lattice corneal dystrophy and corneal amyloid degeneration. Invest Ophthalmol Vis Sci, 1984: 25(suppl):6.

347. Rodrigues, MM, Sun, TT, Krachmer, J, Newsome, D: Epithelialization of the corneal endothelium in posterior polymorphous dystrophy. Invest Ophthalmol Vis Sci, 1980: 19:832–835.

348. Rodrigues, MM, Gaster, RN, Pratt, MV. Unusual superficial confluent form of granular corneal dystrophy. Ophthalmol, 1983: 90:1507.

349. Rodrigues, MM, Kruth, HS, Krachmer, JH et al. Cholesterol localization in ultrathin frozen sections in Schnyder's corneal crystalline dystrophy. Am J Ophthalmol, 1990: 110:513–517.

350. Rodrigues, MM, Fine, BS, Laibson, PR, Zimmerman, LE: Disorders of the corneal epithelium. A clinicopathologic study of dot, geographic, and fingerprint patterns. Arch Ophthalmol, 1974: 92:475.

351. Rodrigues, MM, Jester, JV, Richards, R, et al. Essential iris atrophy. A clinical, immunohistologic, and electron microscopy study in an enucleated eye. Ophthalmology, 1988: 95:69–78.

352. Rodrigues, MM, Kruth, HS, Krachmer, JH, Willis, R. Unesterified cholesterol in Schnyder's corneal crystalline dystrophy. Am J Ophthalmol, 1987: 104:157.

353. Sabbaga, E, Pavan-Langston, D, Bean, K, et al: Detection of HSV nucleic acid in the cornea during acute and latent ocular disease. Exp Eye Res, 1988: 47:545.

354. Sainz de la Maza, M, Foster, CS: The diagnosis and treatment of peripheral ulcerative keratitis. Seminars in Ophthalmology 1991: 6(3):133–141.

355. Sajjadi, SH, Javadi, MA: Superficial juvenile granular dystrophy. Ophthalmol 1992: 99:95.

356. Sandor, E, Millman, A, Croxson, S, et al: Herpes zoster

ophthalmicus in patients at risk for the acquired immune deficiency syndrome (AIDS). Am J Ophthalmol, 1986: 101:153.

357. Savino, DF, Fine, BS, Alldredge, OC: Primary lipidic degeneration of the cornea. Cornea, 1986: 5:191.

358. Schaap, OL, Feltkamp, TEW, Breebaart, AC: Circulating antibodies to corneal tissue in a patient suffering from Mooren's ulcer. Clin Exp Immunol, 1969: 5:365–370.

359. Scheie, HG, Yanoff, M: Iris nevus (Cogan-Reese) syndrome: a cause of unilateral glaucoma. Arch Ophthalmol, 1975: 93:963.

360. Schein, OD, Buehler, PO, Stamler, JF, et al: The impact of overnight wear on the risk of contact lens—associated ulcerative keratitis. Arch Ophthalmol, 1994: 112:186–190.

361. Schein, OD, Glynn, RJ, Poggio, EL, et al: The Microbial Keratitis Study Group. The relative risk of ulcerative keratitis among users of daily-wear and extended-wear soft contact lenses. A case-control study. N Engl J Med, 1989: 321: 773–778.

362. Schein, OD, Poggio, EC: Ulcerative keratitis in contact lens wearers. Cornea, 1990: 9(Suppl 1):S55-S58.

363. Schultz, GS, Davis, JB, Eiferman, RA: Growth factors and corneal epithelium. Cornea, 1988: 7:96.

364. Schuman, J, Orellana, J, Friedman, A, et al: Acquired immune deficiency syndrome (AIDS). Surv Ophthalmol, 1987: 31:384.

365. Schwab, I: Oral acyclovir in the management of herpes simplex ocular infections. Ophthalmology, 1988: 95:423.

366. Schwab, IR: Ocular leprosy. Infect Dis Clin North Am, 1992: 6:953–61.

367. Schwab, IR, Linberg, JV, Gioia, VM, et al: Foreshortening of the inferior conjunctival fornix associated with chronic glaucoma medications. Ophthalmology, 1992: 99:197–202.

368. Schwab, IR, Nassar, E, Malaty, R, et al: Leprosy in a trachomatous population. Arch Ophthalmol, 1984: 102:240–4.

369. Schwartz, SD, et al: Collagen shield delivery of amphotericin B. Am J Ophthalmol, 1990: 109:701.

370. Sendele, D, Kenyon, K, Mobilia, E, et al: Superior limbic keratoconjunctivitis in contact lens wearers. Ophthalmol, 1983: 90:616–622.

371. Severin, M, Kirchhof, B: Recurrent Salzmann's corneal degeneration. Graefes Arch Clin Exp Ophthalmol, 1990: 228:101.

372. Sheilds, MB, Campbell, DG, Simmons, RJ: The essential iris atrophies. Am J Ophthalmol, 1978: 85:749.

373. Shields, MB, Campbell, DG, Simmons, RJ, Hutchinson, BT: Iris nodules in essential iris atrophy. Arch Ophthalmol, 1976: 94:406–410.

374. Shields, MB, Hurst, LW, Quigley, HA, Stark, WJ: Endothelial specular microscopy of iridocorneal endothelial syndrome. [Abstract] Invest Ophthalmol Visual Sci, 1979: 18(Suppl):40.

375. Shields, MB: Progressive essential iris atrophy, Chandler's syndrome, and the iris nevus (Cogan-Reese) syndrome: A spectrum of disease. Surv Ophthalmol, 1979: 24:3.

376. Shuster, J, Kaufman, H, Nesburn, A: Statistical analysis of the rate of recurrence of herpes virus ocular epithelial disease. Am J Ophthalmol, 1981: 91:328.

377. Smith, RE, MacRae, SM: Contact lenses—convenience and complications. N Engl J Med, 1989: 321(12): 824–826.

378. Smolin G: Corneal dystrophies and degenerations. In: The Cornea. Third edition. Smolin, G, Thoft, RA (eds): Boston: Little, Brown & Co, 1994: 499–533.

379. Smolin, G: Report of a case of rubella keratitis. Am J Ophthalmol, 1972: 74:436.

380. Soong, HK, Martin, NF, Wagoner, MD, et al: Topical retinoid therapy for squamous metaplasia of various ocular surface disorders. A multicenter, placebo-controlled double-masked study. Ophthalmology, 1989: 95:1442.

381. Spencer, WH, Fisher, JJ: The association of keratoconus with atopic dermatitis. Am J Ophthalmol, 1959: 47:332.

382. Spruance, S, Stewart, J, Rowe, N, et al: Treatment of recurrent herpes simplex labialis with oral acyclovir. J Infect Dis, 1990: 161:185.

383. Starck, T, Kenyon, KR, Hanninen, LA, et al: Clinical and histopathological studies of two families with lattice corneal dystrophy and familial systemic amyloidosis (Meretoja syndrome). Ophthalmology, 1991: 98:1197.

384. Starck, T, Hersh, PS, Kenyon, KR: Corneal dysgenesis, dystrophies, and degenerations. In Principles and Practice of Ophthalmology. Albert DM, Jakobiec FA (eds). Philadelphia: W. B. Saunders Co, 1994: V1, Chapter 3.

385. Stehr-Green, JK, Bailey, TM, Visvesvara, GS: The epidemiology of Acanthamoeba keratitis in the United States. Am J Ophthalmol, 1989: 107:331.

386. Stern, GA, Buttross, M: Use of corticosteroids in combination with antimicrobial drugs in the treatment of infectious corneal disease. Ophthalmol 1991: 98:847.

387. Stock, EL, Feder, RS, O'Grady, RB et al: Lattice corneal dystrophy type III A. Arch Ophthalmol 1991: 109:354–358.

388. Stocker, FW, Irsh, A: Fate of successful corneal graft in Fuchs' endothelial dystrophy. Am J Ophthalmol, 1969: 68:820.

389. Stocker, FW, Holt, LB: Rare form of hereditary epithelial dystrophy: Genetic, clinical, and pathologic study. Arch Ophthalmol, 1955: 53:536.

390. Stone, DL, Kenyon, KR, Stark, WJ: Ultrastructure of keratoconus with healed hydrops. Am J Ophthalmol, 1976: 82:450.

391. Strachan, IM: Central cloudy corneal dystrophy of Francois: five cases in the same family. Br J Ophthalmol, 1969: 53:192.

392. Streeten, BW, Falls, HF: Hereditary fleck dystrophy of the cornea. Am J Ophthalmol, 1961: 51:275.

393. Stulting, RD, Sumers, KD, Cavanagh, HD, et al: Penetrating keratoplasty in children. Ophthalmology, 1984: 91:1222–1230.

394. Sturrock, GD, Sherrard, ES, Rice, NSC: Specular microscopy of the corneal endothelium. Br J Ophthalmol, 1978: 62:809.

395. Sugar, HS, Kobernick, S: The white limbus girdle of Vogt. Am J Ophthalmol, 1960: 50:101.

396. Sundmacher R: A clinico-virologic classification of herpetic anterior segment disease with special reference to intraocular herpes. In Sundmacher R (ed): Herpetic Eye Disease. Munich: J F Bergmann 1981: 203.

397. Sundmacher, R, Neumann-Haefelin, D: Herpes simplex

virus isolation from the aqueous of patients suffering from focal iritis, endotheliitis, and prolonged disciform keratitis with glaucoma. Klin Monatsbl Augenheilkd, 1979: 175:448.

398. Sutcliffe, E, Baum, J: Acute idiopathic corneal endotheliitis. Ophthalmology 1984: 91:1161.

399. Sutphin, JR: Mumps keratitis. Ophthalmol Clin North Am, 1994: 7:557–566.

400. Suveges, I, Levai, G, Alberth, B: Pathology of Terrien's disease: Histochemical and electron microscopic study. Am J Ophthalmol, 1972: 74:1191.

401. Taylor, HR. Aetiology of climatic droplet keratopathy and pterygium. Br J Ophthalmol, 1980: 64:154.

402. Taylor, HR, West, SK, Rosenthal, FS et al: Corneal changes associated with chronic UV irradiation. Arch Ophthalmol, 1989: 107:1481–1484.

403. Thiel, HJ, Behnke, H. Eine bisher unbekannte subepitheliale hereditare Hornhautdystrophie. Klin Monatsbl Augenheilkd, 1967: 150:862.

404. Thomas, PA, Abraham, BJ, Kalavathy, CM, Rajasekaran, J: Oral itraconazole therapy for mycotic keratitis. Mycoses, 1988: 31:271–279.

405. Thonar, E, Meyer, RF, Dennis, RF, et al. Absence of normal keratin sulfate in the blood of patients with macular corneal dystrophy. Am J Ophthalmol, 1986: 102:561–569.

406. Tour, RI: Astigmatism. Int Ophthalmol Clin, 1965: 5:369.

407. Tremblay, M, Dube, I: Meesmann's corneal dystrophy: ultrastructural features. Can J Ophthalmol, 1982: 17:24.

408. Tripathi, RC, Garner, A: Corneal granular dystrophy: A light and electron microscopical study of its recurrence in a graft. Br J Ophthalmol, 1970: 54:361.

409. Tsai, RJ-F, Sun, T-T, Tseng, SCG: Comparison of limbal and conjunctival autograft transplantation in corneal surface reconstruction in rabbits. Ophthalmology, 1990: 97:446.

410. Tullo, A, Easty, D, Shimeld, C, et al: Isolation of herpes simplex virus from corneal discs of patients with chronic stromal keratitis. Trans Ophthalmol Soc UK, 1985: 104:159.

411. Turner, L, Stinson, I: Mycobacteria fortuitum: As a cause of corneal ulcer. Am J Ophthalmol, 1965: 60:329.

412. Uchida, Y, Kaneko, M, Hayashi, K: Varicella dendritic keratitis. Am J Ophthalmol, 1980: 89:259.

413. Van Horne, D, Edelhauser, H, Schultz, R: Experimental herpes simplex keratitis: Early alterations of corneal epithelium and stroma. Arch Ophthalmol, 1970: 84:67.

414. Vannas, A, Hogan, MJ, Wood I: Salzmann's nodular degeneration of the cornea. Am J Ophthalmol, 1975: 79:211.

415. Vannas, A, Ahonen, R: Herpetic endothelial keratitis. Acta Ophthalmol, 1981: 59:296.

416. Varga, JH, Wolf, TC, Jensen, HG, et al: Combined treatment of Acanthamoeba keratitis with propamidine, neomycin, and polyhexamethylene biguanide. Am J Ophthalmol, 1993: 115:466–470.

417. Vestey, J, Howie, S, Norval, M, et al: Immune responses to herpes simplex virus in patients with facial herpes simplex and those with eczema herpeticum. Br J Dermatol, 1988: 118:775.

418. Vihlen, FS, Wilson G: The relation between eyelid tension, corneal tonicity, and age. Invest Ophthalmol Vis Sci, 1983: 24:1367.

419. Vollerstsen, RS: Vasculitis and Cogan's syndrome. Rheum Dis Clin North Am 1990: 16:433.

420. Wakefield, D, Robinson, LP: Cyclosporin therapy in Mooren's ulcer. Br J Ophthalmol: 1987: 71:415–417.

421. Waring, GO, Rodrigues, MM: Patterns of pathologic response in the cornea. Surv Ophthalmol, 1987: 31:262–266.

422. Waring, GO, Rodrigues, MM, Laibson, PR: Corneal dystrophies. I. Dystrophies of the epithelium. Bowman's layer, and stroma, Surv Ophthalmol, 1978: 23:71.

423. Waring, GO, Bourne, WM, Edelhauser, HG, Kenyon, KR: The corneal endothelium. Normal and pathologic structure and function. Ophthalmology, 1982: 89:531.

424. Waring, GO, Rodrigues, MM, Laibson, PR: Anterior chamber cleavage syndrome: A stepladder classification. Surv Ophthalmol, 1975: 20:3–27.

425. Watson, P, Ross, D, Soltani, K, et al: Therapeutic advances in the management of post-herpetic neuralgia. Geriatr Med Today, 1988: 7:20.

426. Watson, C, Evans, R, Reed, K, et al: Amitriptyline vs placebo in post-herpetic neuralgia. Neurology, 1982: 32:671.

427. Weale, RA: The aging eye. London, HK Lewis, 1963.

428. Weber, FL, Babel, J: Gelatinous drop-like dystrophy: A form of primary corneal amyloidosis. Arch Ophthalmol, 1980: 98:144.

429. Weller T: Varicella and herpes zoster: Changing concepts of the natural history, control, and importance of a not-so-benign virus. N Engl J Med, 1983: 309:1362,1434.

430. Werblin, TP, Hirst LW, Stark WJ, Maumenee IH. Prevalence of map-dot-fingerprint changes in the cornea. Br J Ophthalmol, 1981: 65:401–409.

431. Wheeler, GE, Eiferman, RA: Immunohistochemical identifications of the AA protein in lattice dystrophy. Exp Eye Res, 1983: 36:181.

432. Whitley, R, Nahmias, A, Visintine, A, et al: The natural history of herpes simplex virus infection of mother and newborn. Pediatrics, 1980: 4:489.

433. Wilhelmus, K: Ocular involvement in infectious mononucleosis. Am J Ophthalmol, 1981: 91:117.

434. Wilhelmus, K, Coster, D. Donovan, H, et al: Prognostic indicators of herpetic keratitis: Analysis of a five-year observation period after corneal ulceration. Arch Ophthalmol, 1981: 91:1578.

435. Wilhelmus KR: Parasitic keratitis and conjunctivitis. Clinical Disease. In: Smolin T, Thoft RA (eds) The Cornea, Third Edition. Boston: Little, Brown & Co., 1994: 262–275.

436. Wilhelmus, K, Falcon, M, Jones, B: Bilateral herpetic keratitis. Br J Ophthalmol, 1981: 65:385.

437. Wilhelmus, KR, Liesegang, TJ (eds): Interstitial keratitis. Ophthalmol Clin North Am, 1994: 7:1–669.

438. Wilson, FM II: Adverse external ocular effect of topical ophthalmic therapy: an epidemiologic, laboratory, and clinical study. Trans Am Ophthalmol Soc, 1983: 81:854.

439. Wilson FM II: Toxic and allergic reactions to topical ophthalmic medications. In Arffa RC (ed) Grayson's Diseases of the Cornea. 3rd edition. St. Louis, Mosby Year Book 1991, Chapter 28.

440. Wilson, FM II: Adverse external ocular effects of topical ophthalmic medications. Surv Ophthalmol, 1979: 24:57.

441. Wilson FM II: Congenital anomalies of the cornea and conjunctiva. In: Smolin, G, Thoft, RA. The Cornea. 3rd ed. Boston: Little, Brown & Co, 1994: 535–553.

442. Wilson, FM, Grayson, M, Ellis, FD: Treatment of peripheral corneal ulcers by limbal conjunctivectomy. Br J Ophthalmol, 1976:60:713.

443. Wilson, SE, Bourne, WM: Fuchs' dystrophy. Cornea, 1988: 7:2.

444. Wilson, SE, Klyce, SD: Advances in the analysis of corneal topography. Surv Ophthalmol, 1991: 35:269–277.

445. Wittebol-Post, D, Van Schooneveld, MJ, Pels, E. The corneal dystrophy of Waardenburg and Jonkers. Ophthalmic Paediatr Genet, 1989: 10:249.

446. Wittebol-Post, D, Van der Want, JJ, Van Bijsterveld, OP. Granular dystrophy of the cornea. Is the keratocyte the primary source after all? Ophthalmol, 1987: 195:169.

447. Womack, L, Liesegang, T: Complications of herpes zoster ophthalmicus. Arch Ophthalmology, 1983: 101:42.

448. Wong, K, D'Amico, D, Hedges, T III, et al: Ocular involvement associated with chronic Epstein-Barr virus disease. Arch Ophthalmol, 1987: 105:788.

449. Wood, TO: Recurrent erosion. Trans Am Ophthalmol Soc, 1984: 82:850–898.

450. Wood, TO, Kaufman, HE: Mooren's ulcer. Am J Ophthalmol, 1971: 71:417.

451. Wood, TO, Fleming, JC, Dotson, RS, Cotten, MS: Treatment of Reis-Bücklers' corneal dystrophy by removal of subepithelial fibrous tissue. Am J Ophthalmol 1978: 85:360.

452. Wood, TO, Walker, GG: Treatment of band keratopathy. Am J Ophthalmol, 1975: 80:553.

453. Wood, TO: Salzmann's nodular degeneration. Cornea, 1990: 9:17.

454. Wood TO, Griffith, ME. Surgery for corneal epithelial basement membrane dystrophy. Ophthalmic Surg, 1988: 19:20.

455. Yamaguchi, TR, Polack, FM, Rowsey, JJ: Honeycomb-shaped corneal dystrophy: a variation of Reis-Buckler's dystrophy. Cornea, 1982: 1:71.

456. Yamaguchi, T, Polack, FM, Valenti, J: Electron microscopic study of recurrent Reis-Bücklers corneal dystrophy. Am J Ophthalmol, 1980: 90:95.

457. Yang, CJ, Sundor, Raj N, Thonar, EJ, Klintworth, GK. Immunohistochemical evidence of heterogeneity in macular corneal dystrophy. Am J Ophthalmol, 1988: 106:65–71.

458. Yanoff, M: Iridocorneal endothelial syndrome: Unification of a disease spectrum. Surv Ophthalmol, 1979: 24:1.

459. Young, T, Robin, J, Holland, G, et al: Herpes simplex keratitis in patients with acquired immune deficiency syndrome. Ophthalmol, 1989: 96:1476.

460. Zaidman, GW, Brown, SI: Orally administered tetracycline for phlyctenular keratoconjunctivitis. Am J Ophthalmol, 1981: 92:173–182.

461. Zaidman, GW, Wormser, GP: Lyme keratitis. Ophthalmol Clin North Am, 1994: 7:597–603.

462. Zaidman, GW: The ocular manifestations of Lyme disease. Int Ophthalmol Clin, 1993: 33:9.

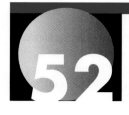

52 Corneal And Refractive Surgery

Procedures for Corneal Disease

Thomas J. Liesegang

The corneal diseases presented previously may require a surgical repair if medical therapy is not completely effective. This section is not written as an atlas of surgery but will include most of the commonly done surgical procedures with an assessment of the indications, contraindications, complications, and success rate. There are many other complex features which encompass surgical procedures, such as the decisions for surgery, preoperative preparation, the medical clearance, the preparation and administration of anesthesia, the setup of the operating room, the selection of instruments and sutures, and most importantly, the postoperative care. These cannot be presented in any detailed fashion.

◼ PENETRATING KERATOPLASTY

Penetrating keratoplasty is a surgical procedure in which the abnormal full thickness cornea is removed from the host and substituted with a full thickness donor corneal tissue. Homografts are tissues from another human, whereas autografts are donor cornea material from the same individual. These autografts may be contralateral (from the other eye) or rotating ipsilateral (rotated from the same eye). Isografts are transplantations between homozygous twins. Zenografts (from different species) are not done. Penetrating keratoplasties are done for different purposes such as optical (vision purposes), tectonic (restoration of altered corneal structure), therapeutic (tissue substitution for refractive corneal disease), and cosmetic (replacement without hope of visual improvement). Many times the penetrating keratoplasty is done for several indications.

There are approximately 40,000 penetrating keratoplasties in the United States each year. The advent of the surgical microscope, advances in microsurgical instrumentation, improved preoperative and postoperative care (especially with corticosteroids and immunosuppressive agents), and eye banking techniques have contributed to an increased success rate for this procedure.

Indications

The diagnostic indications for penetrating keratoplasty have changed over the past 40 years. In the earlier years, it was primarily for herpes scarring, regrafts, and keratoconus. Now in the United States the most common indications are pseudophakic bullous keratopathy, Fuchs' corneal dystrophy, and keratoconus. In both England and Australia, however, the most common indication for penetrating keratoplasty is keratoconus followed by regrafts and bullous keratopathy (15,17). Patients can be grouped according to the diagnostic indications for penetrating keratoplasty and also according to the prognosis for long-term postoperative graft clarity (Table 52–1) (Table 52–2).

There is no strict visual acuity criteria for completing optical penetrating keratoplasty; it is generally indi-

TABLE 52–1
Diagnostic Indications for Penetrating Keratoplasty

Frequent	Pseudophakic bullous keratopathy
Common	Repeat keratoplasty
	Keratoconus
	Corneal dystrophies and degenerations
	Herpes simplex keratopathy
	Corneal scarring from microbial keratitis
	Corneal scarring from trauma
	Interstitial keratitis
Rare (poor prognosis)	Chemical burns
	Herpes zoster keratopathy
	Autoimmune cicatricial disease
	Active microbial keratitis

cated when the corneal disease is causing sufficient social, economic, or visual suffering. Preoperative evaluation of the whole eye is completed to assess the best visual potential, to detect any associated ocular conditions, and to plan the size of the penetrating keratoplasty. In patients with a lens (or cataract) in place, a decision has to be made about whether to remove the

TABLE 52–2
Long–Term Prognosis for Graft Clarity

Excellent	Keratoconus
(>90% prognosis)	Inactive scars
	Early Fuchs' dystrophy
	Granular dystrophy
Very Good Prognosis	Advanced Fuchs' dystrophy
	Pseudophakic bullous keratopathy
	Aphakic bullous keratopathy
	Inactive herpes simplex keratitis
	Interstitial keratitis
	Macular dystrophy
	Iridocorneal endothelial syndrome
Fair Prognosis	Active bacterial keratitis
	Active herpes simplex keratitis
	Active fungal keratitis
	Mild chemical burns
	Moderate dry eye
	Lattice dystrophy
Poor Prognosis	Severe chemical burns
	Radiation burns
	Erythema multiforme major
	Ocular pemphigoid
	Neurotrophic disease
	Multiple graft failures
	Epithelial downgrowth
	Severe dry eye

cataract during a triple procedure (penetrating keratoplasty, removal of the cataract, and placement of an intraocular lens). If a moderate cataract is present, especially if the patient is over age 65, a triple procedure is generally done. Conversely, in a patient with a moderate or severe cataract who has concomitant corneal disease such as Fuchs' corneal dystrophy, the decision to do a triple procedure is usually made on the basis of corneal edema. If there is already epithelial edema, a triple procedure is recommended. Measurement of axial length and corneal keratometry are required to determine the intraocular lens power. Corneal surgeons may be better able to predict the postoperative keratometry based on prior patients having the same technique done. Decisions about how to handle the intraocular lens which is in place, advanced synechia, vitreous in the anterior segment, and glaucoma, are all made in advance of surgery. Ocular surface problems (dry eye, trichiasis, blepharitis) must be recognized before penetrating keratoplasty. Active keratitis and uveitis is best controlled before surgery because of an increased risk of graft failure,

TABLE 52–3
Criteria Contraindicating Donor Cornea Use

Death of Unknown Cause

Unknown Central Nervous System Disease

Certain Infectious Diseases of the Central Nervous System
Creutzfeldt-Jakob disease
Subacute sclerosing panencephalitis
Progressive multifocal leukoencephalopathy
Congenital rubella
Reye syndrome
Infectious encephalitis
Rabies

Systemic Infections
Septicemia
Endocarditis
AIDS
Viral hepatitis

Intrinsic Eye Disease
Ocular malignancies
Scleritis
Conjunctivitis
Uveitis
Retinitis
Choroiditis

Eye Disorders which Preclude a Clear Graft
Keratoconus
Corneal scars
Pterygia
Corneal dystrophies

Prior Intraocular or Anterior Segment Surgery

Active Leukemia or Disseminated Lymphoma

Social, Clinical, or Laboratory Evidence Suggestive of HIV Infection, Syphilis, or Viral Hepatitis

TABLE 52–4
Complications of Penetrating Keratoplasty

Wound leak
Flat chamber or iris incarceration
Glaucoma
Endophthalmitis
Primary endothelial failure
Persistent epithelial defects
Suture related problem
   Excessive tightness
   Excessive looseness
   Suture abscesses
   Toxic suture infiltrates
   Vascularization
Wound dehiscence
Microbial infection
Recurrence of primary disease
Late nonimmune endothelial failure
Corneal astigmatism
Graft rejection

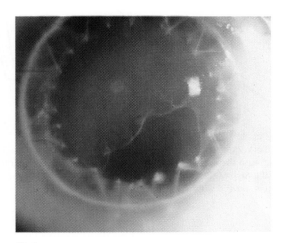

Figure 52–1.
Corneal graft rejection. An endothelial rejection line on the back of a previously clear corneal transplant. This rejection was reversed with frequent topical corticosteroids.

glaucoma, and cystoid macular edema in the postoperative period.

Eye Banking Techniques

Storing enucleated globes in a moist chamber at 4° centigrade usually leads to endothelial deterioration within 3 days. McCarey Kaufman tissue culture media was developed 20 years ago to nurture the endothelial cells in a friendly media which permitted transplantation up to 4 to 5 days later. Other storage media have now extended the viable storage period to as long as 2 weeks. Clinical investigation with storage media containing insulin and epidermal growth factor are investigatory and may prolong the storage time longer. Organ culture (at 37° centigrade) and cryopreservation (at −197° centigrade) have been used for some years but are complicated and expensive.

The criteria for screening donor corneas before distribution continue to undergo periodic reevaluation. Criteria contraindicating donor corneal use include those listed in Table 52–3 (58). The ultimate responsibility for accepting tissue still resides with the operating surgeon. Factors to consider include the slit lamp appearance of the donor tissue, specular microscopy, death to preservation time, storage time before surgery, and the donor age (58).

Surgical Considerations

Decisions are made before surgery about multiple aspects of the procedure. The specific technique varies from surgeon to surgeon and includes the preparation of the donor button (technique of cutting, size of the button), the choice of lid speculum and scleral support ring, the preparation of the recipient eye (size of the button and technique of cutting), the handling of cataracts, intraocular lenses, vitreous, and iris tissue, as well as suture closure techniques (running, continuous, or combined). These are discussed in surgical texts.

Postoperative Complications

The postoperative care of corneal transplant patients is complex with multiple decisions required. Some of the common complications are listed in Table 52–4. There are multiple considerations in handling these problems as outlined in surgical texts (16). Corneal graft rejection remains the highest cause of graft failure. Many episodes of graft rejection can be reversed if detected early. There are three clinical forms of corneal transplant rejection: endothelial rejection, subepithelial rejection, and epithelial rejection. Frequent topical administration of corticosteroids is the mainstay of therapy (Figure 52–1). In severe episodes, the use of periocular or systemic steroids may be additive. Topical cyclosporine has been used prophylactically in high-risk grafts.

■ LAMELLAR KERATOPLASTY

Lamellar keratoplasty involves replacement of the patient's diseased anterior corneal stroma and Bowman's membrane with donor material (Figure 52–2). The host endothelium, Descemet's membrane, and part of the

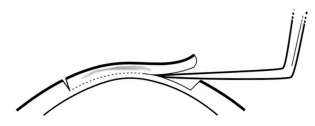

Figure 52–2.
Lamellar keratoplasty. A trephine is used to make a partial thickness incision into the cornea, followed by a Paufique knife to separate the corneal lamellae containing the diseased tissue. The new donor cornea is sutured with nylon sutures.

deep stroma are preserved. The donor lamellar graft is later repopulated with host keratocytes and the recipient epithelium covers the anterior corneal surface. With improvements in the techniques of penetrating keratoplasty, lamellar keratoplasty is rarely done today. It is technically more difficult. The rise in refractive surgery, however, has led to an increase in some forms of lamellar keratoplasty. An onlay lamellar keratoplasty is a technique in which a lamellar lenticule is placed on the corneal surface after removal of the epithelium. It is sutured to the corneal periphery. It is used as a refractive technique and will be described under refractive procedures.

Indications and Contraindications

The lamellar keratoplasty is indicated for optical, tectonic, or therapeutic reasons. An optical lamellar keratoplasty is useful in superficial scars, superficial degenerations and dystrophies (such as Salzmann's nodular degeneration, Reis-Bückler dystrophy). In these circumstances, the lamellar dissection is done to sufficient depth to remove the pathologic tissue and a partial thickness (lamellar) donor cornea of similar thickness is sutured to the dissection bed (6). Lamellar keratoplasty is indicated for tectonic purposes when building up a corneal base is necessary because of a previous stromal melt or perforation. It can be used for keratoconus to flatten the corneal surface. It helps reestablish the integrity of the globe and can be followed, if necessary, by optical penetrating keratoplasty for visual rehabilitation

once the disease is quiescent. A therapeutic lamellar keratoplasty has also been used in the removal of a large pterygium or corneal tumor when there is extensive infiltration of the host cornea.

The advantages of the lamellar keratoplasty over penetrating keratoplasty are primarily the minimal requirements for donor material (since the endothelium does not have to be healthy), the avoidance of entry into the anterior chamber, the shorter wound healing and convalescence, and the reduced incidence of graft rejection. The disadvantages are that it is technically more difficult than penetrating keratoplasty, and there may be opacification and vascularization at the interface which may limit vision. Lamellar keratoplasty is contraindicated in patients with deep stromal or endothelial disease and any active bacterial or fungal keratitis.

Surgical Considerations

A lamellar graft can be taken from a whole donor globe; it is technically more difficult to obtain from a corneoscleral rim. Preground stromal buttons for lamellar grafting may be available. Automated lamellar microkeratomes are available for refractive procedures and aid in the dissection of the recipient and donor dissection. The precision of this instrument has significantly reduced the opacification at the graft host interface. Penetration into the anterior chamber remains the major operative complication and may require conversion to a penetrating keratoplasty. Lamellar grafts can be of any size to fit a specific hole, but they are generally slightly larger. Depending on the area of corneal thinness, the lamellar graft can be placed centrally, peripherally, as an annular graft of the periphery, or as a total corneal lamellar graft.

Postoperative Complications

The major postoperative complication is opacification and vascularization of the interface. This can be reduced with sharper cuts and meticulous surgery. Allograft rejection of the endothelium cannot take place, but epithelial rejection and subepithelial rejection may occur and respond to corticosteroid therapy. Inflammatory necrosis of the graft can occur for unclear reasons.

■ KERATOPROSTHESIS

Indications and Techniques

Eyes with corneal disease not amenable to corneal transplantation may be candidates for the rarely done keratoprosthesis. In the keratoprosthesis, a biocompatible

material of glass, methylmethacrylate, or ceramic is used. Patients who are bilaterally blind from pemphigoid, Stevens-Johnson syndrome, trachoma, chemical burns, and repeated graft failure are reasonable candidates. Patients with severe glaucoma or diabetic

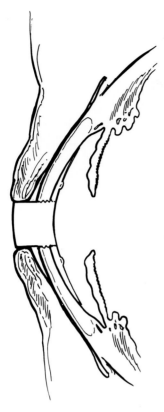

Figure 52–3.
Keratoprosthesis. A keratoprosthesis which is inserted through the skin of the eyelid for added support.

retinopathy are excluded. There are different designs for the keratoprosthesis, but most have a stem supported by a meshwork that is inserted into the corneal stroma. The optical portion can be screwed into the stem, resulting in different dioptric focal lengths (Figure 52–3). The prosthesis is covered with a conjunctival flap at the completion which can later be opened. Alternatively, in patients with poor conjunctiva, the prosthesis is placed through the lids (24). It is labor-intensive but can help a few patients with no other visual alternatives.

This is a rare procedure. Techniques have been described by individual surgeons with variation depending on the type of prosthesis (5, 24, 47).

Complications

The complication most commonly found is intraocular hemorrhage in these diseased and scarred eyes. Severe vitreitis must be distinguished from endophthalmitis. A sterile membrane behind the prosthesis is a frequent occurrence and may need a vitrectomy for removal. Retinal detachment is difficult to detect and repair. Glaucoma is a frequent complication and difficult to monitor. Extrusion from tissue necrosis is the most common complication and requires complex revisions to salvage the eye (48).

Conjunctival and Limbal Surgery for Corneal Disease

There are several surgical procedures done for corneal scarring, vascularization, stromal loss, chemical injury, and surface failure which involve the conjunctival tissue. The epithelial layer of the cornea and conjunctiva are morphologically dissimilar, but the conjunctival epithelium has the capacity to transdifferentiate into corneal epithelium. Corneal reepithelialization takes place from the limbus and many corneal diseases are caused by abnormalities in the limbal, immune, or vascular response. The two surfaces are intimately related with an interplay and exchange. Several effective conjunctival procedures bring to resolution many pesky corneal disorders (66).

■ CONJUNCTIVAL FLAP

Conjunctival flaps have been used for decades in the treatment of recalcitrant corneal ulceration including herpetic ulceration and stromal keratitis, neuroparalytic keratitis, neurotrophic keratitis (Figure 52–4), severe keratitis sicca, severe peripheral marginal ulceration, and ulcerations associated with collagen vascular disease. They are not used for unresponsive bacterial, fungal, or parasitic ulcers. The conjunctiva can be a to-

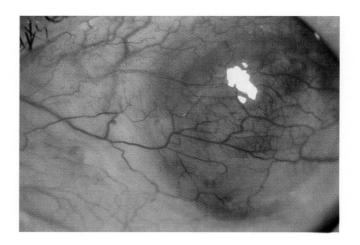

Figure 52–4.
Conjunctival flap. A thin conjunctival flap done for persistent neurotrophic keratitis in a patient with herpes zoster keratitis. The patient is comfortable and pain free.

tal or partial flap. Conjunctival flaps are remarkably effective in controlling pain, infection, and stromal ulcer- ation. Complications include ptosis, conjunctival cyst formation, and retraction of the flap (29).

■ CONJUNCTIVAL RESECTION

Conjunctival resection has been proposed as a procedure to eliminate conjunctival reactive products and immune response. It has been used effectively in peripheral marginal ulceration, especially associated with rheumatoid arthritis (26) and may alleviate the need for systemic immunosuppression. Superior limbic keratoconjunctivitis may be alleviated by multiple techniques, but probably the most definitive is with conjunctival resection. The mechanism of relief is debated.

■ CONJUNCTIVAL TRANSPLANTATION

Conjunctival transplantation may permit resurfacing of damaged cornea from chemical and thermal injury by drawing healthy epithelial cells from the conjunctival surface. In addition to use in chemical and thermal injuries, it has also been useful for recalcitrant epithelial defects associated with herpes simplex, contact lens induced keratopathy, and those associated with corneal surgery, such as penetrating keratoplasty. The flap frequently can achieve a smooth corneal surface helping to improve vision and prevent epithelial breakdown. There are many modifications of this technique. The corneal epithelium of the diseased eye is removed, as well as the conjunctival epithelium for several millimeters from the limbus. Small conjunctival grafts are then taken from the uninjured fellow eye in four quadrants, usually covered by the lids. These grafts are then sutured to the cornea at the limbus (65,68).

■ PTERYGIUM SURGERY

Pterygia appear to be associated with ultraviolet light exposure. They can cause visual loss by growth onto the cornea and production of irregular and regular astigmatism. Some patients report irritation, foreign body sensation, or complain of the cosmetic defect. The pterygium can be removed with a bare sclera technique and then approximation of the remaining conjunctiva. Concurrent radiation or antimetabolites such as mito- mycin have been used (50, 56). Conjunctival autotransplantation has emerged as a popular technique because of the decreased recurrence rate. The free graft of conjunctiva with minimal subepithelial tissue is taken from the superior temporal conjunctiva, slid into the recipient bed, and sutured with interrupted sutures. It has been used for both primary and recurrent pterygia (31, 60).

■ KERATOEPITHELIOPLASTY

Keratoepithelioplasty is a technique to offer ocular surface replacement to patients who have bilateral disease and do not have any donor sites. Healthy corneal epithelium is used to supply cells to treat persistent epithelial defects, as well as the superficial pannus in aniridia. The epithelium is derived from donor eyes by carving four lenticules from the peripheral cornea with

a sharp cataract knife. After the host eye has had the diseased epithelium removed, the lenticules are sutured in place and oriented the same way they were on the donor eye. This epithelium gradually replaces the host epithelium. The indications and techniques for this procedure are still undergoing evaluation (64, 67, 72).

■ KERATOREFRACTIVE SURGERY

The field of refractive surgery has undergone dramatic growth and is now a subspecialty within ophthalmology. There are multiple options to correct refractive errors

of myopia, hyperopia, aphakia, and astigmatism with newer ones developing rapidly. This section will outline some of the techniques of refractive corneal surgery.

TABLE 52–5
Refractive Corneal Surgery Terms

Refractive Keratotomy

Radial keratotomy—partial thickness incisions into the cornea to flatten it and reduce the refractive power. Incisions are radial to the center of the cornea.

Transverse keratotomy—partial thickness incisions into the cornea to flatten a steep corneal meridian. Incisions are straight or arcuate and parallel to the equator of the globe.

Circumferential hexagonal keratotomy—partial thickness incisions in a nonconnected pattern around a 7–mm zone.

Lamellar Keratoplasty

Keratomileusis—removal of anterior disc of corneal tissue which is then carved on its posterior stromal surface to change its radius of curvature and then replaced. The carving can be done with a cryolathe, planar microkeratome, or an excimer laser.

Keratophakia—a human or synthetic lenticule is placed within the corneal stroma (beneath a corneal disc removed by microkeratome) or placed in a lamellar pocket incision. A modification of this is an intracorneal ring in a circular lamellar dissection in the peripheral cornea.

Epikeratoplasty—a lenticule with a power is sewn on the surface of the deepithelialized Bowman's membrane. This lenticule can be human donor cornea or synthetic material.

Plano lamellar keratoplasty—a lenticule with no power is used to diminish myopia and irregular astigmatism of keratoconus. (Also called epikeratoplasty with lenticule of no power.)

Laser Refractive Surgery

Phtorefractive keratectomy—the central removal of a specific profile of Bowman's membrane and anterior stroma to change the anterior curvature of the cornea.

Laser assisted in situ keratomileusis—the removal of a corneal cap or creation of a flap with automated lamellar keratotomy and the ablation of tissue in the stromal bed or the cap to create the desired refractive change.

Intrastromal photorefractive keratectomy—the removal of stromal tissue without disrupting the surfaces of the cornea by creating an intrastromal cavity of photodisruption.

Thermokeratoplasty

Intrastromal thermal coagulation—hot–tipped probe that penetrates deeply into the stroma and shrinks the collagen; when done in the midperiphery it steepens the central cornea.

Laser thermokeratoplasty—a holmium:YAG laser to create focal spots of intrastromal thermal coagulation resulting in flattening the peripheral cornea and steepening the central cornea to treat hyperopia.

Refractive Procedures after Penetrating Keratoplasty

Relaxing keratotomy—arcuate transverse incisions in the donor or in the graft–host junction to decrease astigmatism.

Crescentic wedge resection—a wedge–shaped removal of tissues to decrease astigmatism after penetrating keratoplasty.

Intraocular Lens (not a corneal procedure)

Clear lens extraction—the removal of clear lenses in high myopia with placement of low power or plano intraocular lens to more closely approximate emmetropia.

Phakic intraocular lens—the placement of an intraocular lens into the anterior or posterior chamber of the eye to change the refractive error of myopia with the natural lens left in place.

TABLE 52–6
Options for Various Refractive Errors

	1–8 Diopters	8–20 Diopters	>20 Diopters
Myopia	Radial keratotomy	Keratomileusis	Keratomileusis
	Photorefractive keratectomy	ALK	ALK
	Intrastromal ring	LASIK	LASIK
		Intrastromal implants	Epikeratoplasty
		Intraocular lens	Intraocular lens
	Low to Moderate		**High Hyperopia/Aphakia**
Hyperopia	Hexagonal keratotomy		Epikeratoplasty
	Thermokeratoplasty		Keratophakia
	Holmium		Intracorneal inlay
	Photorefractive keratectomy		Intraocular lens
	Hyperoptic keratomileusis		
Astigmatism	Transverse keratotomy, arcuate keratotomy		
	Ruiz procedure		
	Postkeratoplasty relaxing incisions with or without compression sutures		
	Wedge resection		
	Photorefractive keratectomy		

Some terms are used in jargon which make communication within the field somewhat difficult. (Table 52–5).

Most of the optical focusing power of the eye (probably 75%) resides in the cornea. Although the cornea as a whole is an aspherical surface, the central cornea is nearly spherical with two axes of differing spherical power (astigmatism). Three optical zones are present: a central spherical zone, a midperipheral aspheric zone, and a limbal flatter zone. Through the use of retinoscopy, refraction, keratometry, photokeratoscopy, computer-assisted corneal topographic analysis, contrast sensitivity, and pachymetry measurements, the preoperative corneal state is determined to assess the appropriate surgical procedure. Multiple procedures have been developed and evolved because earlier ones have not been sufficiently predictive or reliable (Table 52–6).

The selection of the appropriate patient is important in refractive surgery. In many instances, these patients have good visual acuity with glasses or contact lenses. Realistic expectations and a reasonable comprehension of potential risks and benefits is a prerequisite. The patients usually cannot go back to their preoperative state and many can no longer wear contact lenses. Refractive surgery will also not eliminate presbyopia, and in some instances, will enhance its onset. Refractive surgery is major surgery with all of the serious, as well as minor complications including corneal perforation. Patients with some specific ocular conditions (e.g., ocular surface diseases) should be excluded, or at least controlled before surgery. The major risk of the procedures are overcorrection and undercorrection. Fluctuation in central curvature can cause cyclical daily fluctuations in vision. Patients may regress over time (lose the effect of the procedure) or progress over time (get a further undesirable correction). Irregular corneal astigmatism may cause glare and halos around lights, especially with the pupil dilated. Contact lenses frequently cannot be fit after a refractive corneal procedure because of altered surfaces.

■ INCISIONAL TECHNIQUES

Radial Keratotomy

Radial keratotomy is currently the most common procedure for myopia less than 8 diopters. Radial keratotomy consists of deep, equally spaced, radially oriented, incisions in the paracentral and peripheral cornea with a diamond blade set at approximately 95% depth of the cornea. The corneal incisions sever collagen fibrils in the stroma; the intraocular pressure produces a wound gape that increases the radius of curvature in the central cornea, decreasing the refractive power by flattening the central optical zone and thereby, decreasing the myopia. There have been several large studies documenting the effectiveness of the procedure in reducing myopia (7, 23, 52, 54, 59, 75, 76). A summary of these studies indicates that the predictability of the desired outcome is best with decreased degrees of myopia (1). Most important, the procedure is not precisely predictable in any one patient. Complications that decrease best-corrected visual acuity occur in less than 3%. Long

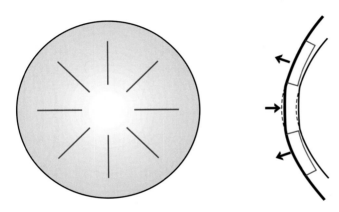

Figure 52–5.
Radial keratotomy. A schematic drawing of an eight-incision radial keratotomy showing the flattening effects on the central cornea.

TABLE 52–7
Complications of Radial Keratotomy

Loss of best corrected visual acuity
Overcorrections
Undercorrections
Diurnal fluctuation of visual acuity
Mild glare, halos
Poor contact lens fit/Contact lens intolerance
Disabling glare
Irregular astigmatism/Induced astigmatism
Corneal perforation
Corneal neovascularization
Microbial keratitis
Endothelial damage
Cataract
Endophthalmitis
Traumatic globe rupture (dimished corneal strength)
Regression of effect
Progression of effect
Stromal melting

term stability is a problem in that 15 to 31% of patients may have a shift towards hyperopia (farsightedness) over 1 to 5 years.

Two principal techniques for performing radial keratotomy have evolved: the American style, in which incisions are made from the center optical zone to the periphery, and the Russian style in which incisions are made from the limbus to the desired optical zone. Debate continues around nomograms developed to determine centering techniques, clear zone diameter, the number of incisions, depth of incision, the style of the blade, and specific cutting maneuvers based on factors of degree of myopia, patient age, keratometry readings, intraocular pressure, and sex (Figure 52–5) (Figure 52–6).

The major complications of radial keratometry are listed in Table 52–7 (8). Radial keratotomy continues to evolve with marked improvements in techniques and in-

strumentation. The incisions can be more reliable with newer techniques and multifaceted thinner gemstone knives with better footplates. Although not embraced by all ophthalmologists, the procedure has a definite position in refractive surgery.

Hexagonal Keratotomy

Hexagonal keratotomy is a form of refractive surgery used to treat hyperopia (20, 28). Six nonintersecting corneal incisions in the midperiphery of the cornea are completed around the central corneal apex, forming a hexagonal pattern (Figure 52–7). This produces steepening of the central cornea. This procedure has been as-

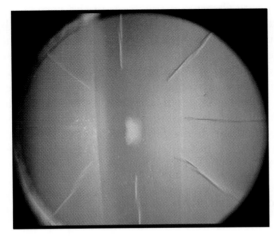

Figure 52–6.
Radial keratotomy. A patient with an eight-incision radial keratotomy.

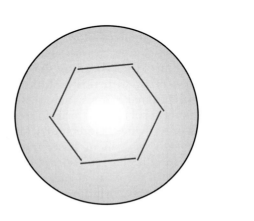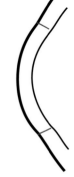

Figure 52–7.
Hexagonal keratotomy. A schematic drawing of the six incisions in a hexagonal keratotomy which permits a steepening of the central cornea and to treat hyperopia.

sociated with an increased incidence of complications including glare, photophobia, polyopia, fluctuations in visions, overcorrections, irregular astigmatism, corneal edema, corneal perforations, bacterial keratitis, cataract, and endophthalmitis (11). Anterior displacement of the cornea and wound healing abnormalities are common. Currently, this procedure appears to be unpredictable with an increased complication rate. It has been largely abandoned.

Astigmatic Keratotomy

Corneal astigmatism can be reduced by incisional techniques on the cornea. Transverse incisions at 95% depth in either a linear or arcuate pattern create an incision which is concentric to the visual axis and parallel to the equator. The incisions, generally only 3 mm in length, are usually done in pairs at 5 to 7 mm from the center of the cornea. This causes flattening of the central cornea in that axis and steepening in the cornea 90° away, thus producing cylindrical (astigmatic) changes without affecting the spherical equivalent of refraction. Arcuate cuts, by virtue of the uniform distance of the optical center throughout their length, have a much greater effect than transverse cuts of the same length and optical zone (2, 25, 35, 41, 69, 70).

Decreasing the distance to the central visual axis, increasing the length or depth of the incision, and using multiple incisions all increase the cylindrical change. Astigmatic keratotomy can be done alone or in combi-

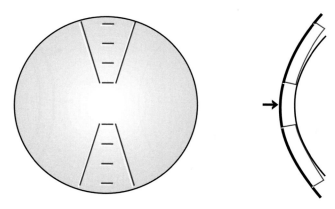

Figure 52–8.
Astigmatic keratotomy. A trapezoidal keratotomy with two semiradial incisions and four transverse incisions that flatten the corneal curvature and decrease its refractive power.

nation with radial keratotomy. There are numerous tables and nomograms for the procedure. Currently it is less predictable in an individual eye than radial keratotomy alone.

The trapezoidal keratotomy, popularized by Ruiz, consists of two pairs of semiradial incisions, coupled with pairs of equally spaced transverse incisions centered on the steep axis of the cornea (51) (Figure 52–8) This procedure can reduce large amounts of astigmatism but is unpredictable. It can be used for astigmatism after penetrating keratoplasty (19, 34, 40).

■ LASER CORNEAL SURGERY

Pulsed laser, especially the argon fluoride (193 nanometers) excimer laser can create accurate and precise excisions of corneal tissue to an exact length or depth, with minimal disruption of the remaining tissue. This minimal disruption and smooth edges allow more uniform stromal wound healing compared with incisional keratotomy. Computers control the procedure so there is less chance of surgeon error with this technique. Lasers are being developed to make linear incisions, to make surface area ablations in specific patterns to treat myopia or hyperopia (laser refractive keratectomy), and to remove surface pathologic assessment (laser therapeutic keratectomy). The specific characteristics of laser light that allow it to be useful for corneal surgery are monochromaticity, directionality, brightness, coherence, and mode structure. Laser light is created by an active medium of gas (e.g., argon fluoride), a solid (e.g., neodymium yttrium aluminum-garnet (YAG)), or a liquid (e.g., a dye laser). An energy source or pump is needed to excite the atoms and an optical resonator allows the emitting beam to amplify and create a more powerful beam. Laser light can then be emitted either continuously or in pulses. A laser is selected with the appropriate absorption spectrum of the cornea to allow ablation to take place. Absorption of laser light by the cornea produces three molecular events: photothermal (breaking chemical bonds and producing protein denaturization), photodisruption (electrons torn from their atoms with a plasma collection), and photochemical. Numerous types of lasers are under investigation for corneal surgery, including the excimer laser, carbon dioxide laser, hydrogen fluoride laser, erbium: YAG laser, pulsed holmium: YAG laser, and the dye laser (77).

Excimer Laser for Myopia

"Excimer" is derived from two words (excited and dimer). A dimer consists of a two-molecule structure (in this situation, argon and fluoride). An increased voltage electrical discharge induces dimers to form an unstable bond, which produces a photon of ultraviolet energy upon release. These photons of ultraviolet energy are guided through an aperture and a series of lenses and mirrors that optimize excimer laser homogeneity before striking the cornea. The photon energy is increased, enabling layer-by-layer tissue removal with minimal adjacent tissue damage. Various excimer wave lengths have been evaluated, with the 193 nanometer having the best performance. The etching of the cornea with this laser is precise and shows absence of thermal injury and preservation of normal morphology. The cornea does mount a controlled and moderate wound healing response with new collagen formation and epithelial hyperplasia in the bed of the ablation. Haze in the ablation zone is presumably related to this new collagen deposition.

The most active clinical research with the excimer has been with photorefractive keratectomy for spherical myopia (Figure 52–9). This is more accurately termed laser anterior myopic keratomileusis. Large area ablation for myopia creates a flattening of the central cornea relative to its original curvature, with progressively less flattening toward the periphery of the optical zone. The size of the ablation is determined by a diaphragm, a rotating wheel, the use of sweeping slits, or with an ablatable mask. The depth of the ablation is highly dependent on the size of the optical zone. Earlier experience in the United States indicates less stability and predictability for myopia exceeding 5 to 6 diopters. With lower degrees of myopia, the procedure has been fairly reliable. Human myopic corrections are usually made hyperopic initially, and then predictably regress towards emmetropia over several months. They become stable in 2 to 4 months with approximately 90% achieving 20/40 visual acuity or better. With corrections exceeding 6 diopters, there is eventually undercorrection because of regression which is variable and not predictable. Pharmacologic modulation of the corneal response to myopic photorefractive keratectomy has been controlled with steroids and other nonsteroidal agents.

There have been two primary clinical problems with photorefractive keratectomy for myopia: subepithelial haze and regression. Subepithelial haze in the visual access can limit visual acuity, reduce contrast sensitivity, and cause glare. The regression of the corneal refractive power occurs as remodeling takes place in the wound. FDA-approved studies are underway for both correction of myopia and for the smoothing of irregular corneal surfaces (phototherapeutic keratectomy). Phototherapeutic keratectomy for anterior corneal stromal diseases that compromise the visual axis have been successful in some patients (61). The initial results for myopic photorefractive keratectomy are also promising (12, 14, 53). Regular astigmatism can also be treated with an ablatable toric mask or a scanning laser slit beam.

In comparison with radial keratotomy, most series of photorefractive keratectomy for myopia have 70 to 80% success rate with an uncorrected acuity of 20/40 or better (slightly worse than radial keratotomy) and 85% of eyes are within one diopter of emmetropia (slightly better than radial keratotomy). The predictability is good and reoperations are less common. Postoperative pain takes longer to resolve with photorefractive keratectomy. Improved pain control with Voltaren has improved this postoperative complication. Visual recovery is much slower with photorefractive keratectomy. The long-term stability of the refractive errors may be better with photorefractive keratectomy and there is less diurnal fluctuation in vision. While central stromal scarring is a concern with photorefractive keratectomy, traumatic wound rupture is more of a concern with radial keratotomy. Glare and decreased contrast sensitivity are seen after both procedures. More postoperative care is required with photorefractive keratectomy, relating primarily to modulation of wound healing with topical corticosteroids or nonsteroidal antiinflammatory agents. Overall, there are fewer postoperative complications with photorefractive keratectomy. The cost of photorefractive keratectomy is much higher but the procedure

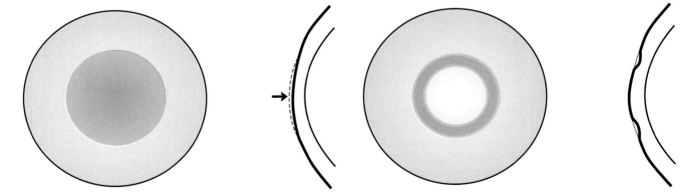

Figure 52–9.
Excimer laser for myopia. The shaving of the anterior central corneal surface with the excimer laser to treat myopia.

Figure 52–10.
Excimer laser for hyperopia. The shaving of the peripheral cornea to make the central cornea relatively steeper to treat hyperopia.

is computerized and inherently less risky than radial keratotomy. The debate will continue.

Excimer Laser for Hyperopia

The principles of hyperopic correction require steepening the anterior cornea (Figure 52–10). This is achieved by a furrow-like ring zone in the corneal periphery. For the sculpturing of this ring zone, a larger ablation zone is required than in myopic photorefractive keratectomy. The excimer has been used to create the annular deepening of the peripheral cornea without ablation of the central cornea (30). Accurate centration of the ablation area is critical and the source of most complications. Slow rehabilitation is another drawback to this procedure. The technique is feasible, although not as successful or predictable as myopic photorefractive keratectomy (22).

Holmium-YAG Laser for Hyperopia

The holmium-YAG laser thermokeratoplasty accomplishes steepening of the central cornea through coagulative shrinkage of the stromal collagen in the paracentral cornea (21) (Figure 52–11). Thermokeratoplasty is a concept used for years in the treatment of keratoconus, but with unstable and/or transient effects (4). Radial thermokeratoplasty for hyperopia was introduced by Fyodorov with a retractable cautery probe used to penetrate the cornea up to 90% depth (44). The holmium-YAG laser is a flashlight pumped solid-state laser with a pulse precisely focused into the core of a fiberoptic handpiece, producing coagulation spots in the cornea. Eight spots of irradiation are placed around the circumference of each of two circles centered on the optical axis. The radius of the inner diameter varies to achieve the desired final correction. The amount of treatment is based on empiric studies (42). Although the Holmium-YAG laser thermokeratoplasty can achieve a hyperopic correction, the long-term stability has not been judged (3).

Excimer Laser for Presbyopia

Observations that radial keratotomy may help some presbyopic patients have both good uncorrected distance and near acuity, it is evident that the corneal power can have multifocal lens effects. A defined multifocal surface is potentially possible by a bifocal sculpturing of the human cornea. Different patterns have been tried on the cornea. Procedures to treat both myopia and presbyopia with a multifocal photorefractive keratectomy with the excimer have been reasonably safe and effective, provided that patients have pseudoaccommodation (the ability to receive and process different images on the retina simultaneously). Patients who do not have pseudoaccommodation are likely to have visual distortion or monocular diplopia (3).

Excimer laser for combined hyperopia and presbyopia correction, or for presbyopia correction alone, has also been attempted by varying the ablation zones to create a steepening of the inferior cornea followed by a further ablation area in the inferior cornea for the presbyopic correction. The side effects of all these presbyopic corrections have been the presence of ghost images and double contours. With decentration, there is a resulting loss of best-corrected visual acuity.

Intrastromal Photorefractive Keratectomy

The neodymium-yttrium lithium fluoride (Nd:YLF) is a new laser instrument that can remove tissue within the corneal stroma. Since Bowman's membrane can be left minimally injured, the cornea can maintain its clarity over the long-term (27); since the epithelium remains intact, this procedure is relatively painless. This laser can be used to create iridotomies and sclerostomies, ablate vitreous floaters, remove epiretinal membranes, and open posterior capsules. The YLF laser creates a microplasma, or electron-stripped medium, when the collagen lamellae are ablated. Patterns of ablation which can be used include a line, curved, rectangle, spot, hole, ring, or spiral. The correction of hyperopia using intrastromal photorefractive keratectomy involves the use of a ring pattern applied to the peripheral cornea; this causes flattening peripherally and steepening centrally. Myopic intrastromal photorefractive keratectomy involves the use of a spiral pattern centrally, resulting in central corneal flattening (27). Good results have been obtained in the cat model; FDA clinical trials are underway in the United States.

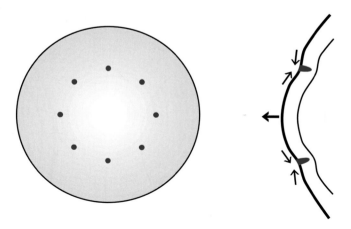

Figure 52–11.
Holmium YAG for hyperopia. A heat shrinkage is done in a peripheral intrastromal pattern to cause central steepening of the cornea.

■ LAMELLAR REFRACTIVE SURGERY

Lamellar refractive surgery corrects myopia and hyperopia by altering the anterior curvature of the cornea. In myopia, there is flattening at the tear film-air interface by removing stroma from the central corneal stroma, leaving the epithelium and Bowman's membrane intact. In hyperopia, there is steepening of this interface by removing stroma from the peripheral cornea.

The first lamellar refractive work was done by Barraquer for correction of hyperopia (keratophakia) (9, 63). This procedure changes the anterior surface of the cornea by placing an insert of synthetic material between layers of the corneal stroma. In the original procedure of keratophakia, a microkeratome made a cut to remove tissue and then a precut lenticule, calculated to correct the hyperopia, was inserted and covered by the first layer. The lenticule could be human tissue or other inserts.

The classic myopic keratomileusis was developed by Barraquer (10, 62). A corneal disc was removed using a complex suction microkeratome, reshaped on a cryolathe aided by a computer program, and then resutured onto the patient's eye. This was a time-consuming and complex procedure which was not effective for the average keratorefractive surgeon (57). The Barraquer-Krumeich-Swinger keratomileusis technique used two microkeratome cuts but was also technically difficult.

Keratomileusis in situ involved cutting a single lamellar disc of tissue as a cap, or a hinged flap (Figure 52–12). The suction ring allows fixation as the microkeratome (automated guillotine knife) glides to dissect an anterior stromal cap or hinged flap. A second cut on the bed thins out the central cornea (49). The cap or hinged flap is then draped back on the resected bed, causing a final alteration in the anterior curvature of the

cornea. This technique has become more accurate and consistent with the development of automated geared microkeratomes that control the speed of the pass across the cornea so a consistent cut is possible. The keratome cut from this automated lamellar machine is smooth and precise. Improvements in the suction ring to hold the cornea add to the ease of this complex procedure. The cap or flap does not need to be sutured

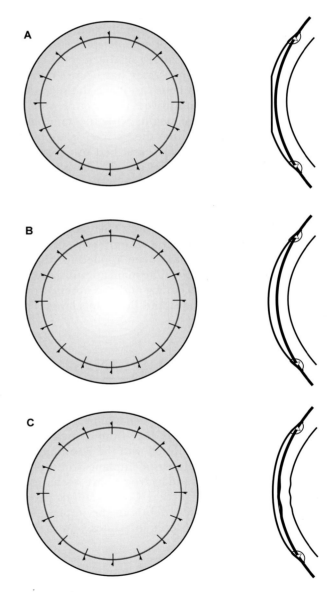

Figure 52–13.
Epikeratoplasty. A. Epikeratoplasty for myopia with an onlay lamellar graft to create a central flattening of the cornea. B. Epikeratoplasty for hyperopia with an onlay lamellar graft used to create a central steepening of the cornea. C. Epikeratoplasty for keratoconus with an onlay plano lamellar graft used to create a smooth surface and reduce the myopia.

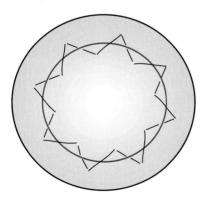

Figure 52–12.
Keratomileusis. Keratomileusis for myopia with excision of a lamellar disc, carving the disc to create the flattening centrally, and resuturing the disc back on the cornea.

back in place. The accuracy of this automated lamellar keratoplasty (ALK) depends completely on the thickness of the resected disc. The automated keratome has improved the technical complexity of the procedure, improved recovery times, and enhanced the accuracy of the procedure. It has the advantage of a wide spectrum of correction up to 25 diopters of myopia. Major complications of the procedure include irregular astigmatism and loss of the caps.

Photorefractive In Situ Keratomileusis

Although the in situ keratomileusis (or ALK) has improved the predictability and capability of increased myopic corrections, it is still not completely accurate, primarily because of the accuracy of the second critical refractive cut. The excimer laser has been combined with the in situ keratomileusis to make the second refractive cut and has improved the accuracy of the surgery. The procedure begins with the same automated lamellar cut and then the excimer is applied to the exposed interlamellar stromal bed to accomplish the refractive cut. The excimer can also make ablations in the cap, but the preferred site is now the stromal bed. The flap of the cornea is then laid back in position. The technique has been called LASIK (laser assisted in situ keratomileusis) or "flap and zap." This technique has been successful in rabbits and a large series of human eyes (45,18). LASIK has also been applied for the correction of astigmatism (57). The main advantages of the LASIK technique are accuracy and the absence of effects on the epithelial layer and Bowman's layer. Thus,

healing is not the major variable it is with surface ablation. The cornea is not weakened. The technique can be used to correct hyperopia or myopia. The advantages of photorefractive in situ keratomileusis compared with ALK must be weighed against the cost and availability of the laser equipment.

Epikeratoplasty

Epikeratoplasty, or superficial corneal lens, is an onlay lamellar graft of predetermined parameters, lathe cut and sutured to the top of a denuded Bowman's membrane (Figure 52–13). The graft is sutured in a 7.0 to 7.5 mm circumferential ridge. Epikeratoplasty has been used in correction of myopia, hyperopia, and aphakia in both adults and children. Epikeratoplasty plano lenticules are used to correct the irregular astigmatism and myopia of keratoconus and provide a smooth anterior corneal contour. In theory, it is a reversible procedure, and in practice, it is relatively straightforward to perform. Care must be taken to obtain a symmetric keratotomy, good optical centering, a clear graft interface, and a firm attachment of the edge of the graft (30, 39, 43).

Varying degrees of success are reported with epikeratoplasty. It does not appear to give predictable refractive outcomes to the same degree as other keratorefractive procedures. There is prolonged visual recovery and, in some instances, poor healing. A synthetic material for the lenticule may give more accurate and predictable results (74).

■ INTRACORNEAL IMPLANTS

Inserts have been placed within corneal pockets to alter the refractive power, by either changing the anterior curvature or the refractive index of the cornea. This is similar to what is accomplished with the Barraquer keratophakia technique. Alloplastic implants with polysulfone, plexiglass, silastic, and hydrogel have been used in myopic and aphakic correction. Complications have included scarring, refractive debris in the implant, subluxation of the implant, sterile infiltrates, and vascularization (33).

A synthetic intracorneal ring can also alter the anterior corneal surface without direct surgical intervention to the central visual axis. A small, optically transparent polymethylmethacrylate intrastromal ring is inserted through a single incision into a 360° intrastromal channel at approximately 60% depth, with the aid of a circular channeling blade. The refractive effect may be reversible after explantation of the device (46).

■ CATARACT SURGERY AS REFRACTIVE SURGERY

Cataract surgery has the ability to correct preexisting refractive errors by using proper intraocular lens calculations, performing astigmatically neutral cataract

surgery, or adjusting preoperative astigmatism based on wound construction or astigmatic keratotomy incisions. Cataract surgery, then, is being increasingly judged as a refractive surgical procedure. The current evolving techniques of refractive surgery can be applied to cataract surgery to alleviate astigmatic and spherical refractive errors.

Clear lens extraction, with or without an intraocular lens, is being used as a method of reducing increased myopic refractive errors. These patients are prone to retinal detachment and this intraocular procedure may increase the risk. Intraocular lenses have also been placed in phakic eyes, either in the anterior chamber, or in the posterior chamber to correct increased myopic errors. These procedures give large optical zones with fairly predictable, reproducible, and stable visual acuities. It is a reversible procedure, although it requires another intraocular procedure. It has all the disadvantages of an intraocular procedure and is a major procedure in a highly myopic eye. The accuracy of the intraocular lens calculation is tenable with increased myopia.

■ REFRACTIVE PROCEDURES FOR PENETRATING KERATOPLASTY

Increased and irregular astigmatism can result from donor and recipient corneal pathologic process, trephination technique, donor-recipient wound disparity, irregular suture placement, unequal suture tension, and irregular wound healing. There are operative measures and techniques to improve on astigmatism but it is still a significant problem after otherwise successful penetrating keratoplasty (55).

After surgery, the astigmatism can be evaluated and monitored with keratometry and computer-assisted corneal topography to suggest the adjustment of the running suture or the removal of individual interrupted sutures to help steepen the flatter areas of the graft or to flatten the steeper areas of the graft (13, 73).

Once all sutures are removed, there are some alternative methods of reducing increased graft astigmatism. Relaxing incisions flatten the steeper meridian and steepen the flatter meridian an equal amount (Figure 52–14). This can be done on both sides of the corneal graft host interface in the axis of the steepest meridian, usually extending for approximately 60 to 90° on each side. If relaxing incisions alone are not sufficient, nylon compression sutures are placed on each side of the graft host interface 90° away from the relaxing incisions (32, 38). With higher degrees of astigmatism, a .5 to 2 mm crescentic wedge resection (Figure 52–15) is done in the axis of the flattest meridian for 60° in the donor-host interface and in the wound suture tightly with nylon suture to overcorrect the astigmatism. Selective suture removal is done in the postoperative period (72).

Astigmatic keratotomies, similar to those described in virgin eyes, can also be used within the corneal donor tissue margin to correct astigmatism after penetrating keratoplasty (36, 37).

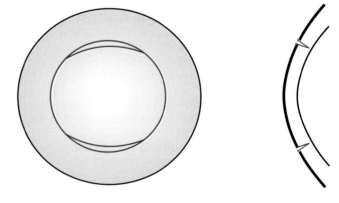

Figure 52–14.
Relaxing incision. Arcuate relaxing incisions at the interface of the host donor graft after penetrating keratoplasty to flatten the steeper axis and to reduce the astigmatism.

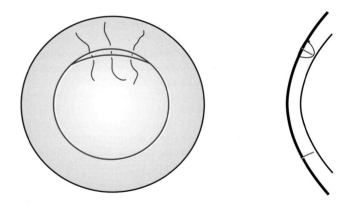

Figure 52–15.
Wedge resection. A crescentic wedge resection in the area of the flattest meridian of astigmatism to reduce the astigmatism by creating a central steepening of the cornea in the same axis.

■ REFERENCES

1. American Academy of Ophthalmology: Radial keratotomy for myopia. Ophthalmic Procedures Assessment. Ophthalmology, 1993: 10:1103–1115.

2. Agapjitos P, Lindstrom R, Williams P, et al: Analysis of astigmatic keratotomy. J Cataract Refract Surg 1989;15:13–18.

3. Anschutz T. Laser Correction of Hyperopia and Presbyopia, Int'l Ophthalmol Clin 1994;34:107–137.

4. Aquavella J, Smith R, Schaw E. Alterations in corneal morphology following thermokeratoplasty. Arch Ophthalmol 1976;94:2082–2085.

5. Aquavella JV: Keratoprosthesis. In: Smolin G, Thoft RA (eds): Cornea. Boston: Little, Brown and Company, 1994;665.

6. Arentsen JJ: Lamellar grafting. In Brightbill FS (ed): Corneal Surgery: Theory, Technique, and Tissue. St Louis, CV Mosby 1992, pp 360–368.

7. Arrowsmith PN, Marks RG: Visual, refractive, and keratometric results of radial keratotomy. Five-year follow-up. Arch Ophthalmol 1989;107:506–511.

8. Assil KK, Parks, RA: Sidestepping the complications of incisional keratotomy, Sem Ophthalmol 1994;9:67–75.

9. Barraquer JI. Modification of refraction by means of intracorneal inclusions. Int Ophthalmol Clin 1966;6:53–78.

10. Barraquer JI. Keratomileusis for myopia and aphakia. Ophthalmology 1981:88:701–708.

11. Basuk WL, Zisman M, Waring III GO, et al: Complications of hexagonal keratotomy. Am J Ophthalmol 1994; 117:37–49

12. Binder PS: Excimer laser photoablation. Clinical results and treatment complications in 1992. Arch Ophthalmol 1992;110:1221–1222.

13. Binder PS: Selective suture removal can reduce postkeratoplasty astigmatism, Ophthalmology 1985;92: 1412–1416.

14. Binder PS: Radial keratotomy and excimer laser photorefractive keratectomy for the correction of myopia. J Refr Corn Surg 1994; 10:443–464.

15. Brady SE, Rapuano DJ, Arentsen JJ, et al: Clinical indication for and procedures associated with penetrating keratoplasty 1983–1988, Am J Ophthalmol 1989;108: 118–122.

16. Brightbill ES: Corneal Surgery: Theory, Technique, and Tissue. St Louis, CV Mosby, 1992.

17. Brooks AM, Weiner JM: Indications for penetrating keratoplasty: a clinicopathological review of 511 corneal specimens, Aust NZ J Ophthalmol 1987;15(4):277.

18. Buratto L, Ferrari M, Rama P. Excimer laser intrastromal keratomileusis. Am J Ophthalmol 1992;113:291–295.

19. Buzard K, Haight D, Troutman R: Ruiz procedure for post-keratoplasty astigmatism. J Refract Surg 1987;3:40.

20. Casebeer JC, Phillips SG: Hexagonal keratotomy. A historical review and assessment of 46 cases. Ophthalmol Clin North Am 1992;5:727.

21. Cavanaugh TB, Durrie DS: Holmium Yag Laser Thermokeratoplasty: Synopsis of Clinical Experience, Sem Ophthalmol 1994;9:110–116.

22. Dausch J, Klein R, Schroder E. Excimer laser photorefractive keratectomy for hyperopia. Refract Corneal Surg 1993;9:2028.

23. Deitz, MR, Sanders DR, Raanan MG: A consecutive series (1982–1985) of radial keratotomies performed with the diamond blade. Am J Ophthalmol 1987;103:417–422.

24. Dohlman CH: Keratoprostheses. In Principles and Practice of Ophthalmology Clinical Practice, Albert DM, Jakobiec FA (eds), Philadelphia, WB Saunders, 1994, Vol 1, Chapter 19.

25. Duffey R, Jain V, Tchah H, et al: Paired arcuate keratotomy. Arch Ophthalmol 1988;106:1130–1135.

26. Feder RS, Krachmer JH. Conjunctival resection for the treatment of the rheumatoid corneal ulceration. Ophthalmology 1984;91:111.

27. Gimbel HV, Beldavs RA. Intrastromal photorefractive keratectomy with the Nd: YLF Laser, Int'l Ophthalmol Clin, 1994;34:139–145.

28. Grady FJ: Hexagonal keratotomy for corneal steepening. Ophthalmic Surg 1988:19:622–623.

29. Gundersen, T. Conjunctival flaps in the treatment of corneal disease with reference to a new technique of application. Arch Ophthalmol 1958;60:880.

30. Kaufman HE, Werblin TP: Epikeratophakia for the treatment of keratoconus, Am J Ophthalmol 1982;93:342.

31. Kenyon KR, Wagoner MD, Hettinger ME: Conjunctival autograft transplantation for advanced and recurrent pterygium. Ophthalmology 1985;92:1461.

32. Krachmer JH, Fenzl RE: Surgical correction of high post-keratoplasty astigmatism, Arch Ophthalmol 1980;98: 1400–1402.

33. Lane SS, McCarey BE, Lindstrom RL. Alloplastic corneal lenses. In: Schwab IR, ed. Refractive keratoplasty. New York: Churchhill Livingstone, 1987:95–124.

34. Lavery G, Lindstrom R: Clinical results of trapezoidal astigmatic keratotomy. J Refract Surg 1985;1:70.

35. Lindquist T, Rubenstein J, Rice S, et al: Trapezoidal astigmatic keratotomy: Quantification in human cadaver eyes. Arch Ophthalmol 1986;104:1534–1539.

36. Lindstrom RL: Surgical correction of refractive errors after penetrating keratoplasty, Int Ophthalmol Clin 1994;34:35–53.

37. Lindstrom RL: The surgical correction of astigmatism: a clinician's perspective. Refract Corneal Surg 1990;6: 441–454.

38. Lustbader JM, Lemp MA: The effect of relaxing incisions with multiple compression sutures on post-keratoplasty astigmatism, Ophthalmic Surg 1990;21:416–419.

39. McDonald MB: Epikeratophakia: the surgical correction aphakia, Ophthalmology 1983;90:668.

40. Merck M. Williams P, Lindstrom R: Trapezoidal keratotomy: A vector analysis. Ophthalmology 1986;93:719.

41. Merlin U: Curved keratotomy procedure for congenital astigmatism. J Refract Surg 1987;3:92–97.

42. Moreira H, Campos M, Sawusch MR, et al. Holmium laser thermokeratoplasty. Ophthalmology 1993;100:752–761.

43. Morgan KS et al: Epikeratophakia in children, Ophthalmology 1984;91:780.

44. Neumann AC, Fyodorov S, Sanders DR. Radial thermokeratoplasty for the correction of hyperopia. Refract Corneal Surg 1990;6:404.

45. Pallikaris IG, Papatzanaki ME, Stathi EZ, et al. Laser in situ keratomileusis. Lasers Surg Med 1990;10:463–468.

46. Parks RA, Assil KK, Schanzlin, DJ: Intracorneal implants, Sem Ophthalmol 1994;9:125–129.

47. Polack FM, Keratoprosthesis. In: Brightbill FS (ed): Corneal Surgery. St Louis: CV Mosby, 1993; Chapter 33.

48. Rao GN, Blatt HL, Aquavella JV: Results of keratoprosthesis. Am J Ophthalmol 1979;88:190.

49. Rozakis GW, Slade SG. Refractive lamellar keratoplasty. Thorofare, NJ: Slack, Inc., 1994.

50. Rubinfeld RS, Pfister RR, Stein RM, et al. Serious complications of topical mitomycin-C after pterygium surgery. Ophthalmology 1992;99:1645–1646.

51. Ruiz LA: The astigmatic keratotomies (Ruiz procedure). In Boyd B (ed): Highlights of Ophthalmology, vol. 2 Refractive Surgery with the Masters. Coral Gables, FL 1987, pp 162–193.

52. Salz JJ, Salz JM, Salz M, et al: Ten years experience with a conservative approach to radial keratotomy. Refract Corneal Surg 1991;7:12–22.

53. Salz J, Maguen E, Newburn A, et al. A two-year experience with excimer laser photorefractive keratectomy for myopia. Ophthalmology 1993;100:873–882.

54. Salz JJ: Radial keratotomy: a different point of view (letter). J Cat Refr Surg 1987;13:374–580.

55. Serdarevic ON: Refractive corneal transplantation: control of astigmatism and ametropia during penetrating keratoplasty, Int Ophthalmol Clin. 1994;34:13–33.

56. Singh G, Wilson MR, Foster CS. Long-term follow-up study of mitomycin eye drops as adjunctive treatment of pterygia and its comparison with conjunctival autograft. Cornea 1990;9:331.

57. Slade SG, Updegraff SA. Advances in lamellar refractive surgery. Int Ophthalmol Clin 1994;34:147–182.

58. Soong HK: Penetrating keratoplasty. In Focal Points: Clinical Modules for Ophthalmologists, vol X, module 6. San Francisco, American Academy of Ophthalmology, 1992.

59. Spigelman AV, Williams PA, Lindstrom RL: Further studies of four incision radial keratotomy. Refract Corneal Surg 1989;5:292–295.

60. Starck T, Kenyon KR, Serrano F: Conjunctival autograft for primary and recurrent pterygia: Surgical techniques and problem management. Cornea 1991;10:196.

61. Stark WJ. Gilbert ML, Goodman GL, et al: Phototherapeutic keratectomy preliminary report. Invest Ophthalmol Vis Sci 31(Suppl) 1990;243.

62. Swinger CA, Barker BA. Prospective evaluation of myopic keratomileusis. Ophthalmology 1984;91:785–792.

63. Taylor D, Stern A, Romanchuk K. Keratophakia: clinical evaluation. Ophthalmology 1981;88:1141–1150.

64. Thoft RA, Sugar J. Epithelial graft reaction in keratoepithelioplasty. Cornea 1993;12:363.

65. Thoft RA. Indications for conjunctival transplantation. Ophthalmology 1982;89:335.

66. Thoft RA. Conjunctival and limbal surgery for corneal diseases. In: Smolin G, Thoft RA (eds): Cornea. Boston: Little, Brown & Co., 1994; Chapter 25.

67. Thoft RA: Keratoepithelioplasty. Am J Ophthalmol 1984;97:1.

68. Thoft RA, Friend J: The X, Y, Z hypothesis of corneal epithelial maintenance. Invest Ophthalmol Vis Sci 1983;24:1008.

69. Thornton S. Inverse arcuate incisions, a new approach to the correction of astigmatism. Refract Corneal Surg 1994;10:27–30

70. Thornton S. Astigmatic keratotomy: a review of basic concepts with case reports. J Cataract Refract Surg 1990;16:430–435.

71. Troutman RC: Corneal wedge resections and relaxing incisions for postkeratoplasty astigmatism. Int Ophthalmol Clin 1983:23–161.

72. Turgeon PW, Nauheim RC, Roat MI, et al. Indication for keratoepithelioplasty. Arch Ophthalmol 1990;108:233.

73. Van Meter WS, Gussler JR, Soloman KW, Wood TO: Postkeratoplasty astigmatism control. Single continuous suture adjustment versus selective interrupted suture removal, Ophthalmology 1991;98:177–183.

74. Verity SM, Schanzlin DJ: Onlay lamellar refractive keratoplasty, Sem Ophthalmol 1994;9:130–138.

75. Waring GO III, Lynn MJ, Nizam A, et al: Results of the Prospective Evaluation of Radial Keratotomy (PERK) Study five years after surgery. Ophthalmol 1991;98:1164–1176.

76. Waring GO III: Radial keratotomy for myopia. In Focal Points: Clinical Modules for Ophthalmologists, vol X, Module 5. San Francisco, American Academy of Ophthalmol 1992.

77. Waring GO III: Development of a system of excimer laser corneal surgery. Trans Am Ophthalmol Soc 1989;87:854–983.

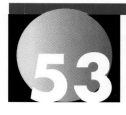

Lens and Cataract

Thomas A. Deutsch

■ BASIC SCIENCE OF THE LENS

The lens is one of the most unusual organs in the body; it matures "inside out," never discarding any of the tissue. As we shall see, it is this pattern of growth that results both in its clarity as well as its opacities.

The crystalline lens is an asymmetrical oblate spheroid with the anterior surface flatter than the posterior surface (5). The capsule of the lens is a true basement membrane, the thickest basement membrane in the body. It is secreted by epithelial cells, the most active of which are at the equator. It is the transformation of these cells into fibers that become the "guts" of the lens.

The lens is subdivided into the nucleus, the cortex, and the capsule for surgical purposes. However, the true anatomy of the lens results from a series of growth periods from fetal development through adulthood. This tissue actually consists of former cortical fibers that have been compressed over time into the nuclear portions which are seen at the slit lamp.

The epithelial cells at the equator elongate and transform into fiber cells. These grow anteriorly and posteriorly to create the fiber mass that we clinically call cortex. This is accomplished through terminal differentiation, that is, amplification and modification of specific proteins (the lens crystallins), as well as cell-to-cell interactions that allow these cells to adapt their structure for the function of producing and maintaining a clear lens. Unfortunately, the proteins and cell walls eventually fail, and this results in cataract.

As the lens grows, the fibers are laid down in a more and more complex arrangement. In the early stages, three seams or "sutures" develop both anteriorly and posteriorly where the fiber ends meet. Over time, 6, then 9, and then 12 sets of sutures are formed (Figure 53–1). Errors in the development of an individual suture line result in an area of cortical cataract which appears as a loop, a wedge, or a spoke.

The concentric growth shells, which are made from the fibers, overlay older shells; therefore, every lens fiber within every shell which is formed during life, is pushed deeper and deeper into the lens substance, and yet must be fed from outside of the lens (Figure 53–2). It is no wonder that even minor insults result in changes in these fiber relationships, the forerunner of cataractous opacities.

Cataract Types

In the normal lens, the intricate pattern formed by the radial cell columns of fiber cells, the growth shells which they make up, and the "sutures," are the result of the ends of these fibers lining up in a stereotypical way (6). This complex structure results in the transparency of the lens.

Unfortunately, as previously noted, small changes in the cell-to-cell interactions result, ultimately, in opacification. The three most common kinds of cataractous opacifications that are noted clinically are nuclear sclerosis, posterior subcapsular cataract (PSC), and cortical cataracts.

Nuclear Sclerosis

Over the course of a person's life, the growth shells are packed tighter and tighter together. The lens, however, increases both in width and thickness, as the older fibers are compressed centrally. In addition, metabolic

779

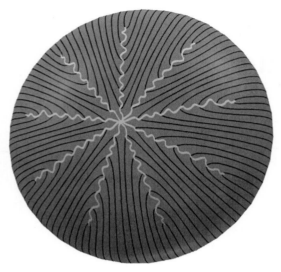

Figure 53–1.
Computer-generated drawing depicting the anterior cortex at the nine suture stage. The close arrangement of the fibers results in the clarity of the lens, but some diffraction of light is at the sutural interfaces. (Courtesy of Jerome R. Kuszak, PhD)

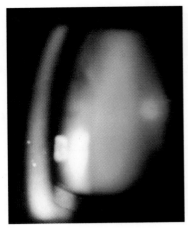

Figure 53–3.
Slit lamp appearance of a dense nuclear sclerotic cataract. Note the deep yellow-brown color to the central nucleus. Note also that the cortex anterior to the nucleus is clear in this pure nuclear cataract.

changes within the cells lead to color changes, most commonly yellow and brown, which further attenuate the passage of light through the lens (Figure 53–3). The result of these changes is clinical nuclear sclerosis. Nuclear sclerosis results in a reduction in the amount of light that reaches the retina, but also increases the refractive power of the lens. The result is increased myopia early on without a reduction in the patient's best corrected visual acuity until later. This increasing myopia negates presbyopia and is what many patients refer to as "second sight."

Posterior Subcapsular Cataract

As fiber cells migrate posteriorly, they may become dysplastic and enlarged. Histologically, they adopt the appearance of fat "bladder" or "Wedl" cells. These dysplastic fiber cells tend to congregate in nests, surrounded by normal fiber cells. The clinical appearance at the slit lamp is a posterior subcapsular cataract (Figure 53–4). PSC-repetitive cataracts may be clinically asymptomatic, but more commonly, they result in glare from diffraction and scatter of light rays as they pass through the posterior part of the lens. Since the posterior capsule is close to the nodal point of the eye, central PSC cataracts often result in distortion or blurring of vision, particularly for reading, even when they are small.

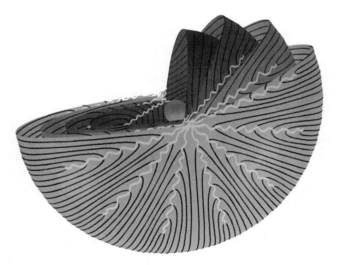

Figure 53–2.
Cutaway of the lens at the twelve suture stage. Note that the fibers do not go from pole to pole, but end at the sutures, making a twist at the terminal. (Courtesy of Jerome R. Kuszak, PhD)

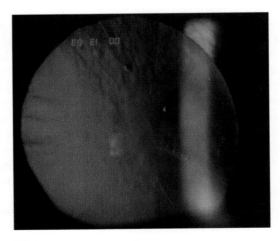

Figure 53–4.
Retroillumination view of a posterior subcapsular cataract. The grainy appearance to the central lens is characteristic.

Cortical Cataract

The development of each fiber cell, its relationship to its neighbors, and the ultimate formation of the concentric growth shells is a tempermental process. However, since the process proceeds at a snail's pace, unless there is a break in the capsule, injuries to the fiber cell mass in the teenage years will not result in clinical opacity until middle age. Such opacities are cortical cataracts which may be either anterior or posterior, depending on the location of the first injured fiber cell (Figure 53–5) (Figure 53–6). As the fiber cells insert into sutures, an injured fiber cell may be slightly crooked. Since it is the template for the insertion of every fiber cell that comes after it, the sutural architecture will be permanently disturbed. Because of this manner of growth, the opacities usually are peripheral in the lens. Therefore, they are not seen nor are they clinically significant unless the pupil is widely dilated, or until a sufficient build up of abnormal suture insertions has encroached into the center of the pupil; that is where these opacities can disturb the transmission of light through the lens and disrupt vision.

Classification Systems

The classification of cataracts is difficult because of the many issues that are involved in describing them. The most common classifications use the age of onset, the location of the opacity, and the extent (4).

In terms of age of onset, cataracts can be broken down into congenital, developmental, and adult. Congenital cataracts are present at or around the time of birth and are discussed in the pediatric section of this book. Developmental cataracts, also discussed in the pediatric section, do not become manifest until after the "critical period" for the development of the densest amblyopia. Therefore, the visual potential for an eye with a

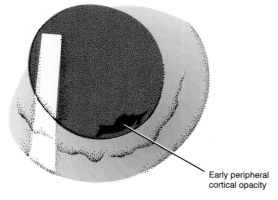

Early peripheral cortical opacity

Figure 53–5.
Retroillumination view of a cortical cataract. The dark smudge-like opacity could not be seen before dilation and is not visually significant.

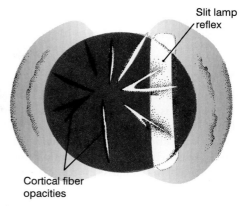

Slit lamp reflex

Cortical fiber opacities

Figure 53–6.
Retroillumination view of another cortical cataract which consists of spokes of cortical fiber opacities. This patient in her mid-forties had a febrile illness as a teenager which may have resulted in a chain of events leading to this cataract.

developmental cataract is usually good. Adult cataracts are the majority of those treated by ophthalmologists. It is acceptable to use this term for any cataracts that develop after the age of 20.

A classification based on the "kind" of cataract, including its location and extent, is usually the most useful for describing cataracts. One begins by noting the predominant location (nuclear, cortical, subcapsular), and then describes the location. For instance, one might have "a posterior subcapsular cataract which is central, with mild nuclear sclerosis and some peripheral cortical spokes." Such a description accurately portrays the cataract to any other practitioner who understands this classification.

Lately, mostly for the purpose of research, some classification schemes have been proposed. The most commonly used in the United States is the Lens Opacities Classification System (LOCS). This system, which has gone through several iterations, takes into account both the color and the density (opalescence) of the nucleus, the extent of cortical opacities, and the extent of PSC opacities. For the purposes of research, this is a powerful classification which seems to correlate well with the clinical manifestations of cataract. The Wilmer classification is similar to LOCS, but it puts much more emphasis on the kind, location, and extent of the cortical opacities. However, these are too cumbersome for routine clinical use.

Etiologies of Cataract in Adults

Aging is, of course, the most common reason adults develop cataracts. This relates to factors that have already been described. First, there is progressive packing of the developing fiber mass and its growth shells. As the packing progresses, the nucleus becomes denser and denser and hence, less transparent. Second, as has been described, small errors in the formation or insertion of any individual fiber cell becomes magnified, since that mistake is copied over and over again. This results in focal, and eventually, diffuse cortical opacities.

Metabolic

Metabolic abnormalities can cause cataracts in adults as well (1). The lens is continuously bathed in nutrients, mostly from the aqueous humor. If the aqueous becomes spiked with chemicals that are harmful, the delicate balance is disturbed and opacification may result. A common and well-known cause of metabolic lens opacity is Wilson's disease, with the deposition of copper in the capsule, sometimes referred to as a "sunflower cataract." Recall that copper is also deposited in Descemet's membrane (Figure 53–7), and that both the lens capsule and Descemet's membrane are basement membranes.

Sugar cataracts, particularly from diabetes, develop because increased glucose levels in the anterior chamber result in an accumulation of sugar in the lens. The glucose is transformed by the enzyme aldose reductase into sorbitol. Sorbitol is unable to cross back through the capsule and into the anterior chamber, and thus, remains in the lens creating an osmotic gradient. Subsequent hydration of the fibers results in swelling of the lens, and, more importantly, separation of the lens fiber cells. Contrary to conventional wisdom, acute elevations in systemic glucose levels, and the attendant changes in the lens, are usually associated with acute hyperopia as the lens loses its refractive power to some extent. These changes often take approximately 6 weeks to resolve, during which time many patients need to have a temporary pair of new glasses. For unknown reasons, some patients do become more myopic during acute hyperglycemia, resulting in a need for a temporary distance correction. Chronically, these changes result in damage to the elongating fiber cells. The most common type of cataract that results is a PSC, in which this damage has

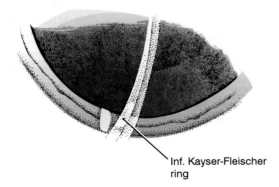

Figure 53–7.
A Kayser-Fleischer ring in Wilson's disease. The grainy yellow changes represent copper deposited in Descemet's membrane.

caused the development of the fat Wedl cells previously described.

Galactosemia is another cause of sugar cataract. There are two types: galactokinase deficiency which does not have systemic manifestations, and galactose-l-phosphate uridyl transferase deficiency which is life-threatening. Both result in "oil droplet" cataracts in infancy.

Pseudoexfoliation of the lens capsule is a mysterious condition that results in deposition of material in the trabecular meshwork, on the anterior lens capsule, and other anterior segment structures. This material is associated with open-angle glaucoma. It is unilateral in approximately one-third of cases. In addition to glaucoma, some patients with pseudoexfoliation develop nuclear sclerotic cataracts sooner than in the fellow eye. The condition is characterized by a peeled appearance to the anterior lens capsule which occurs in a ring or bull's eye pattern, seen when the pupil is dilated. The evidence is that both the capsule and zonules are weaker in these eyes, possibly resulting in a greater rate of complications in cataract surgery. The exact source of the material is unknown, but it is interesting that conjunctival biopsies in these patients show the presence of this material, indicating that it is not purely an intraocular problem.

Trauma

Trauma is an important cause of cataracts in adults. The concussive force of blunt trauma may cause disruption of the fiber architecture and eventual cataract formation. More commonly, a perforation of the lens capsule results in immediate overhydration of the fiber mass with loss of the normal relationships and, therefore, loss of transparency. In addition, liquification of the cortex may result, leading to profound and permanent local or diffuse changes in the cortical structure. In either case, cataract formation often progresses rapidly.

Trauma may also cause dislocation of the lens. Since the lens is held in place by zonules that may be easily broken, even relatively innocent blunt trauma can result in movement of the lens out of its normal position. In many cases, the lens remains clear and no clinical sequelae occur. However, should the lens opacify or become completely dislocated out of the pupil, intervention may be necessary to restore good visual acuity.

Inflammation

Prolonged inflammation is a common cause of cataract in adults. Uveitis can result in posterior subcapsular changes that are referred to as a "complicated cataract." In addition, the treatment of uveitis may also be a cause of cataract.

Toxic Cataracts

Drugs may result in a toxic type of cataract. Systemic drugs such as corticosteroids not uncommonly result in PSC cataracts. However, the effect is somewhat idiosyncratic; some patients who are on steroids for many, many years never develop any PSC changes, while others who are on systemic corticosteroids for only a few months will begin to show cataractous changes. When patients have chronic uveitis and have been treated with systemic steroids, it may be difficult to differentiate between the etiology of the cataract as being inflammatory or toxic.

Long-term use of topical corticosteroids has also been implicated as a cause of cataract, but this has never been proven and the phenomenon may have been observed only because most patients treated with long-term corticosteroid drops also have prolonged intraocular inflammation.

Topical miotic drops such as pilocarpine and, more commonly, the anticholinesterase inhibitors cause cataract with extended usage. Because the stronger anticholinesterases often cause cataract, they are only rarely used in phakic patients.

Ultraviolet exposure and, to some extent, smoking have also been implicated as toxic causes of cataract. In both cases, long-term exposure may be related to the development of nuclear lens opacities, but the association is not strong enough to dictate clinical recommendations.

Systemic Diseases

Some systemic diseases are associated with lens changes. Diabetes and Wilson's disease have already been discussed. Myotonic dystrophy is associated with lens opacities in 90% of cases. These tend to be small, colorful opacities scattered throughout the cortex, and usually are not clinically significant.

Cataract Decision-making

Indications

Every patient is different, each with individual goals, needs, and concerns about vision. Obviously, it is necessary to consider lifestyle, the vision in the other eye, support at home, and many other factors when making a decision to proceed with cataract surgery. In addition, the relationship between risks and benefits, the risk/benefit ratio, should be evaluated in every case. Although these measures are qualitative, one usually prefers to do cataract surgery in a case where the potential benefit is much greater than the known risks. In all cases, a patient should proceed with cataract surgery only if the current level of visual functioning is insuffi-

cient for everyday needs, and it can be reasonably expected that the visual acuity will be improved sufficiently to meet those needs if cataract surgery is successful (2).

In some cases there are medical indications for cataract surgery, beyond the patient's visual needs. An example would be in the situation of an eye with diabetic retinopathy, in which the retina cannot be visualized well enough for adequate examination or treatment may require surgery to facilitate management.

Preoperative Evaluation

Every patient should have a complete ophthalmological examination by the operating surgeon before discussing and scheduling cataract surgery. The goal of this examination is to convince the surgeon, and ultimately the patient, that there is sufficient cataract present to explain the level of visual acuity. By far, refraction is the best test that is available to the ophthalmologist. This should be followed by pupillary testing to ensure that there is no afferent pupillary defect, and a thorough examination of the macula for any abnormalities. In some cases, visual field testing and/or fluorescein angiography will be necessary to show that the preoperative reduction of visual acuity is secondary to the cataract.

Assessment of Macular Function

When the macula can be seen and examined, it is usually possible to determine the potential for visual acuity after surgery. When media opacities obscure the macula, prognostication becomes more difficult. In these cases, there are tricks that can be used to develop a sense about whether there is normal macular function.

The good, old-fashioned approach is to determine whether the patient can perceive colored lights. This can most easily be accomplished by placing a bright flashlight into different colored eye drop bottle caps. Red, yellow, blue, and green are readily available to the ophthalmologist. Patients who can perceive and differentiate between colors are likely to have a relatively normal set of cones in the foveal area suggesting good potential acuity.

A red Maddox rod is sometimes useful for detecting macular abnormalities, since the line that is created by the lens cylinders will appear broken or distorted by a macular lesion.

Finally, the entoptic phenomenon can be elicited by gently moving a bright penlight over closed eyelids. The perceptive patient will see the leaflike pattern of macular vessels. A large lesion in the macula may be perceived as a blank spot within those vessels.

Recently, the Watzke-Allen sign has been popularized as a test for macular holes. A narrow vertical slit beam is directed onto the retina and the patient is asked to look at the line. If the line is perceived as being broken, this is sensitive for the presence of a macular hole. Patients with macular scars may note disruption of the central part of the line.

Over the past decade, more macular function tests have become popular. The laser interferometer uses a bright laser light to create an interference fringe pattern on the retina. The fringes can then be varied in frequency, and the patient asked to what frequency level the fringes can be detected. The Potential Acuity Meter (PAM) is a device which uses a bright light to project a miniature eye chart onto the macula. Both of these tests have drawbacks, however. The laser interferometer and PAM may give a falsely optimistic prediction of acuity because only small patches of intact photoreceptors are necessary to see the pattern or letters. Conversely, when the cataract is so dense that the macula cannot be examined, the PAM will often give a falsely pessimistic prediction. Therefore, again, when the macula can be examined the results of that examination are the best predictor of macular function.

Glare testing has become popular in the past few years as a way of simulating the glare produced by headlights in patients with cataracts, particularly those with PSC and cortical opacities. While shining a bright light during performance of Snellen acuity testing may exacerbate the perceived visual deficit, there is no clear evidence that the glare test reflects real world situations. Indeed, a far more accurate approach to the evaluation of glare is the patient's own history.

When the retina cannot be visualized at all, an ultrasound examination must be done to rule out the presence of a tumor or a retinal detachment.

Surgical Choices

Anesthesia

Until approximately 100 years ago, anesthesia for cataract surgery consisted of a rag placed between the patient's teeth with several assistants to hold the patient's arms and head still during the procedure. Things have progressed somewhat since then.

General anesthesia is sometimes used for cataract surgery, particularly when the patient is disoriented, retarded, or young. However, it is rarely necessary with modern techniques of sedation.

In most cases, adequate sedation with mild agents are more than adequate to relieve anxiety, induce amnesia for the period of the anesthetic injection, and induce unconsciousness for the immediate moment of the injection.

Retrobulbar anesthesia has been used for many decades and is the gold standard for efficacy of regional ocular anesthesia. While techniques vary, the most reliable is to insert a blunted needle approximately one-third of the way from the lateral orbital rim through the inferior orbital septum near the inferior orbital rim. Once through the septum, the needle is directed towards the apex of the orbit until the tip is in the muscle cone. Entrance into the muscle cone is noted because passage through the inferior intermuscular septum results in temporary inferoduction of the globe followed by an immediate recentration fixation. Three to 5 ml of anesthetic may then be injected into this space. The result is immediate anesthesia and akinesia of the eye. The duration is dependent on the type of anesthetic.

One must be cautious when giving a retrobulbar injection of local anesthetic. An injection directly into a rectus muscle can cause necrosis of the muscle, scar and secondary contracture (3, 7). The inferior rectus muscle is most commonly involved with this complication. Initially the inferior rectus muscle will show paresis and there will be an ipsilateral hyperdeviation. Over the next several weeks the muscle contracts and the small hypertropia will change to an ipsilateral hypodeviation. The incidence of this complication has been reduced by the use of peribulbar injections (see below) and retrobulbar injections keeping the needle away from the inferior rectus muscle.

A facial block may be given at the same time. This can be directed behind the ear lobe near the stylomastoid foramen to block the entire excursion of the seventh nerve (Nadbath), anterior to the tragus to block only the superior portion of the seventh nerve (O'Brien), or around the lateral, superior, and inferior lids to block only the periocular portion of the nerve (Van Lint). While one of these is usually used, the necessity in modern cataract surgery is uncertain.

The peribulbar block has become popular lately. This block is given either through the conjunctiva or the lower lid with a short needle directed into the inferior orbit. It is thought that there is less chance of perforation of the globe and certainly no chance of perforation of the optic nerve. However, this block is more uncertain and requires more anesthetic volume and time to become effective. Many authors are now advocating "mini blocks" in which the conjunctiva is opened with a scissors and a blunt cannula is used to instill anesthetic into the sub-Tenon's space.

The newest approach to anesthesia for cataract surgery is the use of only topical anesthetic. This is particularly popular for clear corneal phacoemulsification in which no manipulation of the conjunctiva or sclera is necessary. It appears as though topical anesthetic, either tetracaine or 4% lidocaine is effective in producing anesthesia of the cornea and intraocular structures. No akinesia results, but using two-handed phacoemulsification techniques and continuous communication with the patient, the eye position can be stabilized sufficiently to complete the surgery.

Surgical Approaches

Until approximately 1980, most cataract surgery was done using an intracapsular technique in which the entire lens including the capsule was removed. For a variety of reasons, this has been almost completely abandoned in the United States.

Extracapsular cataract extraction (ECCE) refers to the removal of the clinical nucleus with cortical cleanup using either manual or automated vacuuming techniques. The posterior and equatorial capsule is left intact as an envelope, the "bag" into which a posterior chamber intraocular lens can be inserted. If the posterior capsule and zonules are intact, this lens will ordinarily remain in place throughout the patient's life without any complications.

To gain access to the nucleus and cortex, an opening must be created in the anterior lens capsule. This capsulotomy is classically made by perforating the capsule multiple times in a circular fashion like a can opener. Alternatively, a continuous circular tear capsulorhexis gives the advantage of being a tough annulus that resists tearing peripherally to the zonules.

Phacoemulsification is increasing in popularity. In this technique the clinical nucleus is emulsified in situ by ultrasound created by a vibrating needle. The cortex is then removed with an automated irrigation/aspiration unit leaving the posterior capsule intact. The advantage of phacoemulsification is that the nucleus does not have to be removed in one piece, thus negating the necessity for a 10 mm wound. The size of the wound is dictated only by the size of the intraocular lens which will be placed in the eye. Current intraocular lenses can be placed through openings which range from 3.5 mm to 7 mm. Phacoemulsification has the potential for faster rehabilitation of the patient's visual acuity. However, the learning curve is long for development of the necessary skills, and when intraoperative complications occur they tend to be more serious than in ECCE.

Many surgeons are now moving from the traditional superior incision site to a temporal approach. The advantage of the temporal approach is that the surgeon needn't wrestle with the eyebrow in a deep set eye, and hence the instruments may be placed into the eye more easily. In addition, it is easy to make a clear corneal entry temporally which eliminates most of the dissection of the conjunctiva, the potential for bleeding, and may be helpful in controlling astigmatism. Because the optic nerve is not blocked, many patients who have clear corneal cataract surgery with topical anesthesia will have instant rehabilitation of vision. The clinical significance of this approach is important in some instances, but is not appropriate for every patient.

Prevention of Endophthalmitis

Endophthalmitis is a devastating complication of intraocular surgery. Some approaches for the prevention of endophthalmitis have been proposed. Most surgeons give an injection of an antibiotic in the periocular region either before or after surgery. There has never been any evidence to indicate that this prevents endophthalmitis, but it is standard therapy in many areas.

The use of topical antibiotics both before surgery and after surgery reduces the ocular surface flora. Again, there is no evidence that this reduces the chance of endophthalmitis, but since the vast majority of postoperative endophthalmitis is caused by organisms which are resident in the patient's own tear film, this approach makes a certain amount of sense. Some surgeons place a drop of diluted povidone (Betadine) in the cul-de-sac before surgery, as this has been shown to reduce the bacterial colony counts recovered from the conjunctiva.

Lately, cataract surgeons have begun adding antibiotics to the infusion solution during surgery. If this is done in a sterile manner, and if the person adding the antibiotics is able to do so safely and accurately, this is potentially the best way of cleansing the anterior chamber during and at the conclusion of cataract surgery. In addition, the newer approach of giving no anesthetic injections also means that the surgeon may also wish to avoid antibiotic injection. Such an approach adds further justification for placement of antibiotics in the infusion solution. However, there remains no proof that this actually results in a lower incidence of endophthalmitis.

Intraocular Lenses

The classic manner of correcting aphakia was the use of spectacle lenses. However, the correction of a monocular aphake with a spectacle lens creates too much aniseikonia (image size disparity) to be tolerated. In addition, bilateral aphakes have some difficulties with the ring scotomas and other distortions associated with aphakic lenses.

Contact lenses can be used effectively and are still useful in children and in some traumatic situations. However, there are fewer and fewer indications for the use of aphakic contact lenses.

Since 1980 almost all cataract surgeons have adopted the use of intraocular lenses for the correction of aphakia. The most commonly used are made of polymethylmethacralate (PMMA) or silicone. The PMMA lenses come as unifocal or multifocal lenses, although the multifocal lenses never achieved FDA approval and will probably never be marketed in the United States. The majority of patients who have cataract surgery have been wearing bifocal glasses for many years, and readily accept an overcorrection for near, distance, or both. In addition, the surgeon can opt for "monovision" in which one eye is left slightly nearsighted and one eye is corrected for distance allowing the patient to do almost all tasks without any glasses.

The advent of flexible lenses which may be folded and therefore placed through small incisions has hastened the changeover to phacoemulsification surgery. Many surgeons prefer the short rehabilitation time and have become so proficient at phacoemulsification that the rate of complications is nearing that for extracapsular cataract extraction.

The correct power of intraocular lens selected depends on the refractive power of the cornea as measured with a keratometer, and the length of the eye measured with ultrasound. There are formulas for using these numbers to calculate the intraocular lens power. In addition, some formulas factor in the anterior chamber depth or the distance from the corneal endothelium to the implant, and this measurement must be made by ultrasound at the time of axial length determination.

Cataract Combined with Glaucoma

Since both cataract and glaucoma are conditions of the aging eye, it is not unusual to face the combined problem of the need for better glaucoma control in a patient requiring cataract surgery. There are three basic approaches. First, one can do the cataract surgery and then return when the eye is quiet and perform a glaucoma procedure; however, glaucoma surgery in previously operated eyes has a decreased success rate. Second, one can do the filtration surgery and then remove the cataract when the eye has recovered. The difficulties are that the patient may require improved vision soon, yet have to wait for visual rehabilitation through cataract surgery, and that there is at least a 50% chance of losing pressure control after cataract surgery in an eye with a functioning filter. Finally, one can combine cataract and glaucoma surgery at one sitting. The difficulty is that the success rate of the glaucoma portion of the surgery is less than that in primary surgery.

There is no single correct answer to this issue, but some rules of thumb are useful. If the pressure is well controlled on limited medication, there seems little benefit to subjecting an eye to the extra surgery of a combined procedure. In this case, simple cataract extraction is warranted. If the pressure is out of control, but the cataract is minimal, it seems prudent to perform glaucoma surgery alone, and deal with the cataract when it become significant. However, if the extent of the two conditions is roughly equal, or if the patient is unlikely to be able to withstand two separate procedures, then combined surgery seems the best alternative.

Suture Techniques

The classic technique for closing cataract wounds consists of interrupted 10–0 nylon sutures. This remains an excellent way to close the eye and allows the surgeon to selectively remove sutures to control postoperative astigmatism. However, many surgeons have found that various combinations of running or figure of eight sutures result in little or no postoperative astigmatism. Where there is no astigmatism there is no need to cut sutures, and consequently there is faster visual rehabilitation.

Small incisions may be closed either with interrupted sutures, a figure of eight technique, or a horizontal closure. A horizontal suture is somewhat more difficult to place, but in some surgeons' hands results in less astigmatism.

Finally, by making a small, shelved or tunnel incision, many surgeons have found that they can construct wounds which require no sutures and only leak when the intraocular pressure becomes either increased or decreased. Since the wound tends to seal over the first several days, suturing in many cases may be unnecessary.

The prudent surgeon will develop techniques for dealing with the particular goals which are set for each patient and will construct the wound and suture it as necessary for each individual case.

Postoperative Follow-up

The goals of postoperative follow-up include early diagnosis of complications, management of postoperative medications, and refraction for the purpose of prescribing spectacles. In most cases cataract patients are examined on the day after surgery to be certain that there is no wound dehiscence, intraocular hemorrhage, intraocular lens dislocation, or other untoward event. Subsequent examinations ordinarily occur 3 to 7 days later and several weeks after surgery to dispense glasses if they are necessary.

Obviously, patients who develop complications will need to be seen more often. The frequency will be determined by the seriousness of the situation.

Complications of Cataract Surgery
Intraoperative Complications

The most common intraoperative complications revolve around tears or ruptures of the posterior capsule.

In some cases the posterior capsule tears without vitreous loss. In most of these eyes the remainder of the operation can continue and an intraocular lens placed as usual into the capsular bag. When vitreous actually enters the anterior chamber and surges towards the wound, it is necessary to remove the prolapsing vitreous. This is most efficiently and safely done using an automated vitrectomy instrument, although small prolapses can be reflected back into the eye with a cyclodialysis spatula and then a viscoelastic can be used to force it back through the rent in the posterior capsule.

Because the goal of vitrectomy is to reduce the level of anterior vitreous to below the posterior capsule, it is important to avoid hydrating the vitreous with excessive irrigation. For this reason, many surgeons avoid any irrigation, or use a second port for irrigation and only minimal vacuum to minimize the amount of fluid which enters the eye during the vitrectomy. In addition, it is useful to avoid excessive vacuum as this tends to pull more vitreous from the posterior part of the globe and into the anterior chamber. Once the vitreous has been reduced to below the level of the posterior capsule, a viscoelastic should be placed over the tear to prevent further prolapse and a careful inspection of the wound made to ensure that no vitreous strands continue into the wound.

When a large tear in the posterior capsule occurs during phacoemulsification there is danger that the nucleus can drop into the vitreous cavity. The best way to avoid this is through careful phacoemulsification, but if a hole does develop and the nucleus appears to be ready to fall, the wound should be enlarged and the entire nucleus expressed from the eye as an extracapsular procedure. Under no circumstances should an attempt be made to irrigate the nucleus into the anterior segment, nor should phacoemulsification be done in the vitreous. This creates traction on the vitreous which further places traction on the peripheral retina and can easily lead to retinal detachment.

If, after the nucleus, vitreous, and cortex have been removed, there is insufficient capsular support for a sulcus-fixated posterior chamber lens, an anterior chamber lens can be placed in the eye. Alternatively, several suturing techniques have been developed to facilitate sewing a posterior chamber lens into the ciliary sulcus. This places the lens in the normal location, and removes it from the vicinity of the cornea and chamber angle. Theoretically, there is less chance of late glaucoma and corneal decompensation.

In some cases an intraocular lens may be placed into the eye, and it is subsequently found that the capsular support is insufficient to keep the intraocular lens from falling into the vitreous. If this is suspected, it may be prudent to loop a suture around one of the haptics so that the lens may be retrieved if it begins to fall before placement of the lens. Should a lens completely dislocate into the vitreous where it cannot be retrieved through the anterior segment, the eye should be closed and a posterior segment surgeon enlisted to do a vitrectomy so that manipulation of the lens does not place traction on the vitreous and retina.

Suprachoroidal hemorrhage can occur rarely in eyes during cataract surgery and can result in prolapse of blood, anterior segment structures, and retina. When this happens, it is referred to as an "expulsive hemorrhage". Risk factors for expulsive hemorrhage include old age, arteriosclerosis, glaucoma, increased myopia, and prolonged hypotony. In addition, patients with increased blood pressure during the procedure may be at an increased risk.

The signs of expulsive hemorrhage include sudden vitreous loss, sudden collapse of the anterior chamber with inability to deepen even with viscoelastics, iris prolapse, bright red blood in the anterior chamber, and a rock hard eye by palpation. In addition, any loss of part or all of the red reflex should be regarded with alarm.

If an expulsive hemorrhage appears to be occurring, the surgeon should place a finger on the eye and press with great force to raise the intraocular pressure. This may tamponade the bleeding arteries and expulsion may be aborted. The eye should be closed as tightly and rapidly as possible, and in most cases an intraocular lens should not be placed in the eye at that time. If the eye can be successfully closed without prolapse of retina, the intraocular contents may be able to be repositioned after several days by a retinal vitreous surgeon.

Common Postoperative Side Effects

Many times the surgeon and patient are disappointed by the surgical results. In some cases, side effects have occurred which happen so commonly that they cannot be referred to as complications.

Posterior Capsular Opacification

After cataract surgery, epithelial cells at the equator of the lens continue to transform into fiber cells and begin migrating towards the posterior capsule. However, without normal cell-to-cell interactions and sutures to insert upon, they amass along the posterior capsule as an opacity.

Posterior capsular opacification occurs in approximately 50% of patients by 2 years after cataract surgery and results in increasing glare and reduced vision (Figure 53–8). The timing of a posterior capsulotomy is dependent on the patient's needs, just as was the initial decision for cataract surgery. There is no convincing evidence that an early posterior capsulotomy results in cystoid macular edema or retinal detachment, but there is no need to be hasty. Two to four percent of patients will develop retinal detachment after YAG laser poste-

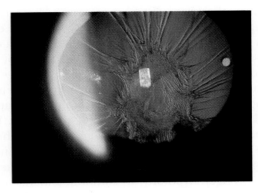

Figure 53–8.
Retroillumination view of the posterior capsular opacification in an aphakic eye.

rior capsulotomy, a rate approximately the same as after cataract surgery. Therefore, patients should be advised of this possibility, and the risk/benefit ratio should be judged before laser surgery.

The patient and surgeon should be clear on what the goals of treatment are, and it is important for the surgeon to attempt to rule out any other cause of decreased vision before the capsulotomy. There is no advantage to a large capsulotomy unless the patient needs to have extensive peripheral retinal examinations. Therefore, a capsulotomy which is only slightly larger than the size of the pupil in a darkened room should be sufficient.

Astigmatism is, of course, a common side effect of cataract surgery. Patients with astigmatism in the axis of the incision can have the astigmatism reduced by selective suture lysis. If a large amount of astigmatism appears against the axis of the incision, or if all of the sutures have already been removed, astigmatic keratotomy may be useful. Most studies have shown suture removal after cataract surgery hastens the return to the baseline astigmatism of the patient before surgery. While many surgeons attempt to manipulate astigmatism by clever placement of the wound or sutures, in most cases patients revert to their original astigmatic axis and power.

Cystoid macular edema occurs in 10 to 20% of eyes of nondiabetic patients after cataract surgery. The incidence may be highest in eyes that have vitreous loss, or vitreous or iris incarceration in the wound. However, it is clinically significant in only approximately 5%. In the majority of cases, the visual acuity falls 8 to 12 weeks after the procedure. If left untreated, the vast majority of patients will return to their best potential visual acuity within approximately 2 months. Therefore, the majority of patients who develop clinically important cystoid

macular edema will have returned to their best potential visual acuity by 4 months after surgery.

Cystoid macular edema can be diagnosed clinically with a contact lens or indirect biomicroscopy lens at the slit lamp. Swelling, particularly in a cystlike or petal-like arrangement is characteristic. If further documentation is necessary, a fluorescein angiogram will show leakage in the macula, often with the characteristic petaloid appearance of cystoid macular edema.

The majority of patients with cystoid macular edema will recover spontaneously within approximately 2 months. However, there is some evidence that this response may be hastened, or that refractory cases might be treated with nonsteroidal antiinflammatory eye drops. Further studies are necessary to show the efficacy of these medications.

Cataract surgeons have been aware for some time that diabetic retinopathy may worsen after cataract surgery. Patients with minimal nonproliferative diabetic retinopathy may develop severe intractable macular edema in the months after cataract surgery that is poorly responsive to therapy. In addition, patients with preproliferative retinopathy may develop neovascularization of the retina or iris after cataract removal. For this reason, cataract surgeons should be cautious before recommending surgery to patients with diabetic retinopathy. Diabetics must be informed that the risk of visual loss after cataract surgery is greater than in the nondiabetic population.

Pseudophakic corneal edema occurs after cataract surgery, because of traumatic loss of endothelial cells. Patients with preexisting Fuchs' Endothelial Dystrophy are at an increased risk, but eyes which have had complicated or prolonged surgical procedures, or have had anterior chamber or iris fixated lenses are also prone to corneal edema. In many cases, the edema progresses to the point of significant visual loss, and penetrating keratoplasty is indicated to rehabilitate the vision. If the intraocular lens is considered to have been at fault, it will usually be exchanged for a new lens of more modern design with less tendency to cause edema.

Strabismus after cataract surgery is an uncommon, though important, side effect. Reported causes include a bridle suture placement through the superior rectus muscle, direct myotoxic effect of local anesthetics to the inferior rectus muscle, preexisting amblyopia or strabismus. One of the more common causes of vertical strabismus is the myotoxic effect of a local anesthetic injection into the inferior rectus muscle (3) (see retrobulbar infection above). Preexisting strabismus which presents after cataract surgery can include decompensated congenital fourth nerve paresis, and phorias which decompensate because of changes in postoperative refraction. Monocular diplopia can occur secondary to decentration of the intraocular lens, posterior capsule opacification or induced irregular astigmatism.

Unexpected Complications

Dislocation of the intraocular lens can occur either early or late. In most cases the lens slips off center. When the lens subluxes inferiorly, it is referred to as a "sunset syndrome." These case can often be repaired from an anterior approach, with fixation of the loops of the lens to the sclera. Occasionally, the lens can become completely dislocated into the vitreous cavity. In this case a pars plana vitrectomy must be done to mobilize the lens and reposit it in the proper anatomic location (Figure 53–9).

Retinal detachment occurs in 2 to 4% of eyes after cataract extraction. It is reported that highly myopic eyes (those with axial lengths greater than 25 mm) are at increased risk of retinal detachment. All patients should have a thorough peripheral retinal examination before contemplation of cataract surgery. Those who are highly myopic may benefit from prophylactic closure of otherwise benign retinal holes. After cataract surgery, every patient should have a thorough dilated fundus exam within 3 months to rule out the new development of retinal holes or tears. Because the rate of retinal detachment in patients who have had cataract extraction is higher than in the general population, it is prudent to closely observe and sometimes close holes which otherwise would not be treated in phakic patients.

Endophthalmitis occurs in approximately 1 in 750 cataract operations. Approximately three-fourths of all cases stem from the external ocular flora of the patient.

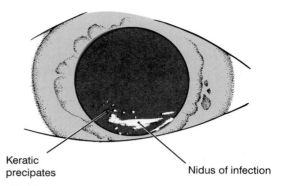

Figure 53–10.
Propionibacterium acnes endophthalmitis. Note the KPs which can be seen on the corneal endothelium, and also the chalky white opacity inferiorly. This opacity is the nidus of infection, caught between the anterior and posterior leaflets of the lens capsule.

Keratic precipates

Nidus of infection

Despite this, there is no clear evidence that reduction of that flora has any effect on the rate of development of endophthalmitis. The rate of recovery of organisms from the anterior chamber at the conclusion of surgery appears to be greater in extracapsular cataract extraction than in phacoemulsification surgery. However, there has not been a reduction in the incidence of endophthalmitis with the increasing popularity of phacoemulsification. It remains to be seen whether the rate of recovery of organisms has any relationship to the development of endophthalmitis.

Most cases of endophthalmitis present as increasing pain, redness, and decreased vision 2 to 7 days after surgery. Some patients will have increasing inflammation over the first 48 hours, while others will not have any signs for 2 to 4 weeks. The variability of presentation appears to be a result of several factors, including the virulence of the organism and the regimen of corticosteroids.

There is an increasing incidence of decreased virulence endophthalmitis caused by anaerobic bacteria, primarily propionibacterium acnes. In many cases endophthalmitis does not present for 6 to 12 months and is characterized only by inflammation, keratitic precipitates, and a white, chalky placque within the capsular bag (Figure 53–10).

The presentation of endophthalmitis can be variable, with increasing inflammation, corneal edema, and a dense anterior chamber reaction. The development of an hypopyon is characteristic and can never be ignored. The hallmark of endophthalmitis is a lessening of the red reflex when observed either at the slit lamp or with an indirect ophthalmoscope. Therefore, it behooves the surgeon responsible for follow-up to continuously monitor and document the quality of the red reflex throughout the postoperative period.

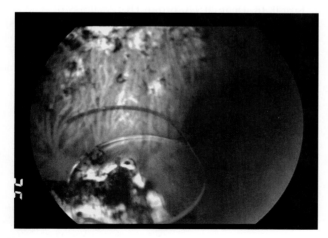

Figure 53–9.
A dislocated intraocular lens lying on the retina. The lens dislocated two years after surgery. This eye previously had undergone scleral buckling surgery for a retinal detachment.

Endophthalmitis is both a clinical and laboratory diagnosis. With good culture technique, approximately 75% of cases of true bacterial endophthalmitis should be culture positive from the vitreous. The rate of bacterial recovery from the aqueous is less than from the vitrous. Those who are culture negative are often treated as though they were culture positive, but the surgeon never is really sure whether a bacterial endophthalmitis was present. When cultures are positive, bacteria are more likely to grow from the vitreous than the aqueous, possibly because of the more rapid turnover of the aqueous humor. There is also evidence that the external ocular flora correlates well with the causative organism, and therefore culturing the conjunctiva at the time of diagnosis and before the use of intraocular antibiotics may be helpful. The most common organism in acute postoperative endophthalmitis, by far, is coagulase negative staph.

It is not entirely clear what is the best treatment for bacterial endophthalmitis. At the present time, most vitreoretinal surgeons recommend either injection of intraocular antibiotics or vitrectomy with intraocular antibiotic lavage. Data to support one or the other of these treatments is pending. It is also unclear whether subconjunctival or systemic antibiotics are useful. In addition, the use of intraocular steroids as well as systemic steroids is controversial.

Delayed nonexpulsive suprachoroidal hemorrhage occurs in some cases, usually in susceptible individuals with multiple risk factors as noted above. Prolonged hypotony during surgery, or postoperative hypotony may be contributing factors.

Patients ordinarily present with decreased vision on the first postoperative day, there is a diminished red reflex, and examination of the fundus reveals hemorrhagic choroidal detachments. Because this suprachoroidal blood usually does not clot, vitreoretinal surgeons often will wait several days before draining the choroidal hemorrhages and using intraocular gas to reform the posterior segment.

Since cataract surgery is ordinarily done on older patients, all of the ocular diseases which are characteristic of the elderly may reduce the postoperative visual result. Glaucoma, ischemic optic neuropathy, and macular degeneration are all potential causes of postoperative reduction in visual acuity, and may disappoint an otherwise excellent surgical result.

■ REFERENCES

1. Berger BB: The lens, cataract, and its management. In: Peyman GA, Sanders DR, Goldberg MF (eds): Principles and Practice of Ophthalmology. Philadelphia: WB Saunders, 1980: 489–632.
2. Cataract Management Guideline Panel: Cataract in adults: management of functional impairment. Rockville, Md: US Dept HHS, Agency for Health Care Policy and Research, 1993.
3. Hamed LF, Mancuso, A. Inferior rectus muscle contracture syndrome after retrobulbar anesthesia. Ophthalmology. October 1991, 98:10 p.1506–1512.
4. Khu PM, Chylack LT: Subjective classification and objective quantification of human cataract. In: Albert DM, Jakobiec FA (eds): Principles and Practice of Ophthalmology, Clinical Sciences. Philadelphia: WB Saunders, 1994: 591–602.
5. Kuszak JR, Brown HG: Embryology and anatomy of the lens. In: Albert DM, Jakobiec FA (eds): Principles and Practice of Ophthalmology, Basic Sciences. Philadelphia: WB Saunders, 1994: 82–96.
6. Kuszak JR, Deutsch TA, Brown HG: Anatomy of aged and senile cataractous lenses. In: Albert DM, Jakobiec FA (eds): Principles and Practice of Ophthalmology, Clinical Sciences. Philadelphia: WB Saunders, 1994: 564–575.
7. Lewen RM, Eifrit DE. Scleral buckling of failed pneumatic retinopexy. Arch Ophthalmol 106:18–19, Jan 1988.

X Retina

Section Editor: Eugene de Juan Jr.

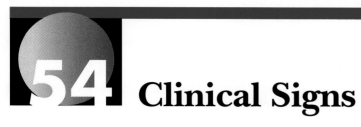

54 Clinical Signs

Eugene de Juan Jr., Stuart W. Noorily,
William P. Townsend-Pico, Kenneth C. Chern

The retina and choroid can react to injury or damage in only a limited number of ways. Below are clinical signs that are commonly found. Each sign may be found in a number of different conditions.

■ RETINAL FINDINGS

The retina is normally transparent allowing the choroid and RPE to be visible. With injury, the retina may become opaque, obscuring the retinal vessels and underlying details.

A. Cotton-wool spots. These are localized, fluffy, white areas of nerve fiber layer edema usually caused by focal ischemia and resultant swelling of the axons of the ganglion cells. Cotton-wool spots may be found in many vascular diseases (hypertension [Figure 60–13], diabetes, sickle cell disease, central retinal vein occlusion), collagen-vascular diseases (SLE), and infectious processes (HIV retinopathy) (Figure 38–3).

B. Retinal edema. Thickening and slight opacification of the retinal layers from edema may be found in association with leakage of fluid in diabetes (Figure 60–5), retinal artery occlusion (Figure 60–8), and cystoid macular edema (Figure 59–6).

C. Myelinated nerve fiber layer. Myelination appears as white, wispy opacities following the radiating pattern of the nerve fiber layer often originating from the optic disc. Myelination is usually non-progressive and a normal variant.

D. Epiretinal membrane (macular pucker). Proliferation of cells on the retinal surface can cause surface wrinkling and distortion. Ophthalmoscopically, this may appear as a thin, glistening cellophane membrane with straightening of retinal vessels (Figure 59–7). Epiretinal membranes may result following retinal tears, vitreous hemorrhage, or ocular surgery.

E. Lipid. Intraretinal lipid has a bright yellow appearance and represents a localized breakdown of the blood brain barrier. It is an important sign of vascular leakage in diabetic retinopathy (Figure 60–4) and age related macular degeneration (Figure 59–1).

F. Pigment. Pigment in the retina usually arises as a result of a disturbance of the pigment epithelium. It is a non-specific sign of isolation; however, there are characteristic pigment changes in diseases such as retinitis pigmentosa (Figure 57–4), and pattern dystrophies.

■ HEMORRHAGES

Localization of hemorrhages is critical in determining the etiology and dictating the treatment.

A. Vitreous hemorrhage. With an acute vitreous hemorrhage, red blood cells are visible moving freely behind the posterior lens capsule. Blood may obscure the view of the optic disc and retinal details. With time, vitreous blood will settle inferiorly and appear as grey-white globular vitreous opacities. Causes of vitreous hemorrhage include retinal breaks, proliferative diabetic retinopathy, trauma, Valsalva retinopathy, and any cause of nevascularization (See table on vitreous hemorrhage).

B. Preretinal hemorrhage. Preretinal blood collects between the retina and the posterior vitreous face often producing a red, boat-shaped hemorrhage obscuring the retina below. This may be found with trauma, Valsalva retinopathy, shaken baby syndrome, and macroaneurysms.

C. Flame-shaped hemorrhage. Blood in the nerve fiber layer will follow the radiating pattern of the axons. Central retinal vein occlusion (Figure 60–6), hyper-

tensive retinopathy, and diabetes may have these hemorrhages.

D. Dot and blot hemorrhage. Hemorrhage in the outer plexiform layer of the retina will track vertically and produce round or oval hemorrhages. These are associated with diabetes mellitus (Figure 60–1), venous stasis, and hypertension.

E. Subretinal hemorrhage. Collections of blood underneath the retina appear as darker, sharply circumscribed areas with the overlying vasculature visible. Subretinal hemorrhage may indicate a choroidal neovascular membrane (Figure 59–3), macroaneurysm, or trauma.

F. White-centered hemorrhage. Hemorrhages with white centers (Roth spots) can be seen with leukemia, diabetes, and septic emboli.

■ VASCULAR CHANGES

A. Tortuous. Retinal vessels normally follow a gentle arc from the optic nerve. Increased curvature and sinuosity of the vessels may be found with vein occlusions (Figure 60–6), Wyburn-Mason syndrome, and ocular ischemia.

B. Attenuated. Thinning of the retinal arterioles and veins can be associated with hypertension, retinal artery occlusion, and retinitis pigmentosa (Figure 57–4).

C. Sheathed. Whitish perivascular cuffing, known as sheathing, is a sign of inflammation. Periphlebitis and periarteritis can be seen in a number of inflam-

matory conditions: sarcoidosis (Figure 36–2), Behcet's disease, tuberculosis, and syphilis.

D. Neovascularization. The growth of new vessels from the optic disc or retina is neovascularization. This usually indicates focal or general ischemia as in proliferative diabetic retinopathy (Figure 60–4), branch retinal vein occlusion, and sickle cell disease (Figure 60–12A) (See table on neovascularization of the retina).

E. Ghost. Ghost vessels are the sclerosed remnants of the vasculature occurring with branch retinal vein occlusions sickle cell (Figure 60–12), and sarcoid.

■ EMBOLI

A. Calcific. Dull, white emboli of calcium are most frequently from a calcified cardiac valve.

B. Platelet-fibrin. Dull, white, elongated emboli originate from a carotid plaque or the heart.

C. Cholesterol. Bright, yellow birefringent emboli,

lodged at the bifurcation of an arteriole, are frequently from the carotid (Figure 60–9).

D. Talc or cornstarch. Multiple white or yellow particles often lodged in the parafoveal capillaries associated with intravenous drug abuse.

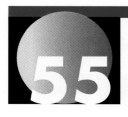

55 Retinal Imaging

Eugene de Juan Jr., Stuart W. Noorily,
William P. Townsend-Pico, Kenneth C. Chern

■ ULTRASONOGRAPHY

Ophthalmic ultrasound is an important tool in the evaluation of ocular and orbital disorders. Diagnostic ophthalmic ultrasound usually uses frequencies in the range of 8 to 10 MHz. This allows excellent resolution of the ocular structures. A new, high frequency (50–100 MHz) B-scan method called ultrasound biomicroscopy is available for high resolution evaluation of the anterior segment.

Ultrasonography is especially useful in the evaluation of the posterior segment in cases with media opacification. Other important indications include the evaluation of intraocular tumors, the determination of the configuration and extent of retinal detachments, the evaluation of serous and hemorrhagic choroidal detachments, the evaluation of eyes after trauma, and endophthalmitis. Ultrasonography is also commonly used for the measurement of axial lengths for intraocular lens calculations.

Ophthalmic ultrasonography uses both A- and B-scan instruments. A-scanning is a one-dimensional acoustic study in which the echoes are displayed as vertical spikes and the height of the spikes indicates the amplitude of the echoes (Figure 55–1). It permits the evaluation of a lesion's internal constitution and size.

B-scan ultrasonography is a two-dimensional study with both horizontal and vertical dimensions. It is useful in the topographic evaluation of intraocular structures and lesions (Figure 55–2) (Figure 55–3).

Quantitative echography evaluates the lesions reflectivity, internal structure, and sound attenuation. Reflectivity is determined by the A-scan spike height, whereas the internal structure is evaluated for regularity and homogeneity. A lesion's mobility and vascularity can also be studied on A/B scanning.

■ FLUORESCEIN ANGIOGRAPHY

Fluorescein angiography (1) is an invaluable tool in the evaluation of diseases of the retinal and choroid. Sodium fluorescein is a molecule which is 70 to 80% protein bound and which has an absorption and emission spectra of 465 to 490 nm and 530 nm, respectively. The fundus camera emits a white light which passes through a blue filter and thus, emerges as a blue light. This blue light then enters the eye and excites the sodium fluorescein molecule to a higher energy level which causes the fluorescein molecule to emit light in the green section of the light spectrum at 530 nm. While

both blue and yellow-green light emerge from the eye, a yellow-green filter blocks the blue light and allows only yellow-green light to be recorded on high-resolution black and white film.

The procedure of fluorescein angiography itself involves an initial, preinjection, red-free photograph followed by the injection of 5 ml of 10% sodium fluorescein (3 ml of 20% fluorescein can also be used) into the antecubital vein. The photographs are then taken in a rapid-fire sequence seconds after the injection. Late images are captured 5 to 15 minutes later.

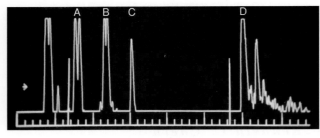

Figure 55–1.
Immersion A-scan ultrasound of a normal eye. The spikes occur at interfaces between changes in tissue density. The immersion scan allows visualization of the cornea (A, 2 spikes), anterior lens capsule (B), posterior lens capsule (C), and retina/choroid/sclera complex (D).

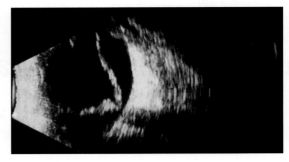

Figure 55–3.
B-scan ultrasound of a rhegmatogenous retinal detachment. The retina can be seen attached at the optic nerve and anteriorly at the ora.

Fluorescein dye is a compound unrelated to radiographic dye and patients allergic to radiologic contrast materials may tolerate fluorescein angiography without difficulty. The risks and side effects associated with fluorescein angiography include yellow coloring of the skin and urine, nausea and vomiting, pain if extravasation occurs, and allergic reactions ranging from itching to hives to bronchospasm and anaphylaxis. Serious allergic reactions (anaphylactic shock, myocardial infraction, seizures, etc.) occur in less than 1% of all cases. Fluorescein angiography should be avoided in pregnant women.

The fluorescein molecule will normally enter through the ophthalmic artery passing through the short posterior ciliary arteries into the choroidal circulation and through the central retinal artery into the retinal circulation. Normal arm-to-eye circulation time is approximately 10 to 15 seconds. Several stages are noted during fluorescein angiography: the choroidal phase (10 to 15 seconds after the injection), arterial phase (15 seconds after injection) (Figure 55–4A), arteriovenous phase (20 to 25 seconds after injection) (Figure 55–4B), late venous phase, and the recirculation

phase (Figure 55–4C). Cilioretinal arteries will fill during the choroidal phase.

Fluorescein leakage is restricted by the inner and outer blood-retinal barriers which are comprised of the retinal capillary endothelial and retinal pigment epithelial tight junctions, respectively. Fluorescein will, however, normally leak through the permeable choriocapillaris.

The fovea will usually appear darker and more hypofluorescent than the rest of the retina due to three factors: blockage by xanthophyll pigment, blockage by taller retinal pigment epithelial cells with a greater amount of melanin than the extramacular RPE cells, and the avascularity of the foveal avascular zone.

When interpreting a fluorescein angiogram, a distinction must initially be made whether the lesion is hypofluorescent or hyperfluorescent. Hypofluorescence may be the result of blocking defects secondary to pigment (xanthophyll, melanin), blood, exudates, or lipofuscin, hypoperfusion of the choroidal or retinal circulation, and retinochoroidal tissue loss (choroideremia, gyrate atrophy, myopic degeneration, Bietti's crystalline dystrophy). Hyperfluorescence can be seen as a result of window defects, leakage, staining of tissues, and pooling. Window defects are the result of retinal pigment epithelial loss or atrophy and show early hyperfluorescence which fades slowly as the angiogram progresses. The size and margins of hyperfluorescent window remain constant throughout the study. Leakage is manifested as an increase in the intensity of the fluorescence with blurring and increase in size of the margins of the hyperfluorescent lesion. Leakage can be seen in a great variety of lesions including retinal neovascularization, choroidal neovascularization, retinal vascular diseases, idiopathic central serous chorioretinopathy, retinal or choroidal neoplasms, and optic neuropathies. Staining represents the accumulation of fluorescein into a tissue and usually displays constant margins of hyperfluorescence throughout the study. Pooling is the accumulation of fluorescein dye within an anatomic space, usually subretinal or sub-RPE.

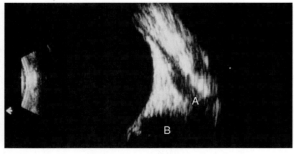

Figure 55–2.
B-scan ultrasonography of a normal eye provides a two-dimensional longitudinal cross section of the structures in the eye. The retina cannot be separated from the choroid or sclera in a normal eye. The medial rectus muscle (A) and the optic nerve (B).

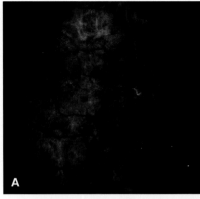

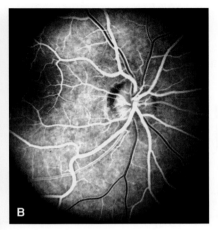

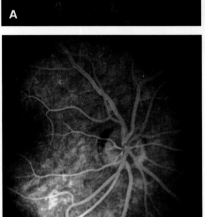

Figure 55–4.
Fluorescein angiogram of anormal
patient. Early phase (A): the choroid has
already started filling in a patchy pattern
and dye is visible in the arteries. Arteriovenous (laminar venous) phase (B): the
veins can be identified by the parallel
column of dye within. Late phase (C): the
dye has left the vessels with slight staining
of the vessel walls and optic disc.
Leakage, pooling, and staining are best
evaluated in the late phases.

■ INDOCYANINE GREEN ANGIOGRAPHY

Indocyanine green dye (ICG) angiography is another useful modality to study the choroidal vasculature.
ICG dye is injected intravenously where it is highly protein bound and remains predominantly in the retinal
and choroidal vasculature. ICG absorbs infrared light at
805 nm and emits at 835 nm. Special infrared film and
cameras are needed to observe this fluorescence.

Abnormalities of choroidal circulation, especially
subretinal choroidal neovascular membranes, may be
better delineated by ICG than by conventional fluorescein angiography since the infrared wavelengths are
transmitted better through blood, exudates, and
melanin.

■ ELECTRORETINOGRAM

The retina converts light energy into electrical energy
transmitted by neurons to the brain. These electrical im-
pulses can be detected as changes in electric potential
of the eye. An electroretinogram (ERG) is the recording
of the changes in potential of the retina stimulated under different conditions. This is measured using special
contact lens electrodes and displayed as a waveform on
an oscilloscope.

The ERG is best for evaluating retinal function as a
whole. The depolarization of photoreceptors generates
the a-wave. The subsequent b-wave is a result of the interneurons and bipolar cells. The implicit time is the delay from the stimulus to the trough of the a-wave or the
peak of the b-wave.

The cone or rod systems can be specifically evaluated by altering the testing conditions. Light adaptation
bleaches the rods and only the cone response is detected (photopic ERG). The use of a dim white or blue
flash below the cone threshold in a dark-adapted eye
isolates the rods producing a scotopic ERG (Figure
55–5). A flickering light stimulus can also be used to
evaluate the cone system. Rods can respond to slow
flicker rates (usually less than 10 Hz). The cones can cycle at higher rates up to approximately 70 Hz.

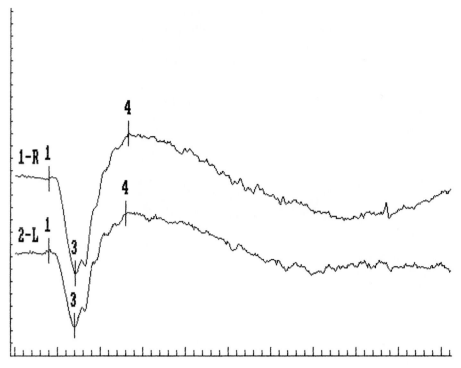

Figure 55–5.
Normal scoptopic ERG. In the dark-adapted state (scotopic), the light flash stimulates both rods and cones. Since rods greatly outnumber cones, the waveform is predominantly a result of stimulation of the rods. The negative a-wave corresponds to photoreceptor depolarization. The positive b-wave results from interneuron and bipolar cell depolarization.

Because the ERG measures the mass response of the retina, focal retinal processes may not be recordable. Abnormal ERGs may be found in photoreceptor degeneration (retinitis pigmentosa), retinal ischemia (CRVO), and toxicity (siderosis). The ERG can be helpful in the diagnosis of hereditary retinal disorders since ERG changes may be present before ophthalmoscopic findings are evident.

■ ELECTRO-OCULOGRAM (EOG)

The retinal pigment epithelium and photoreceptors generate a steady transretinal voltage that results in a 10 mv positive potential at the cornea and a negative potential at the retina. This positive potential at the cornea can be used to measure eye movements. Skin electrodes placed at the medial canthus and the lateral canthus record electrical potential changes as the eye rotates medially and laterally. The change in electrical potential correlates with the change in eye position and can be plotted to measure eye movement velocities.

The EOG can also be used to measure retinal function thought to be based on the integrity of the retinal pigment epithelium. In the dark, the EOG potential is small (dark trough); however, under photopic condition, the potential is large (light peak). The EOG is calculated by dividing the light peak potential by the dark trough potential. A normal ratio is 2 : 1 and values less than 1.5 are almost always abnormal. The EOG light : dark ratio will be abnormal in retinal degenerations that involve large areas of the retinal pigment epithelium. In cases of severe photoreceptor degeneration, there will also be secondary retinal pigment epithelial degeneration; therefore, late stages of retinitis pigmentosa will have an abnormal EOG. Retinal degeneration associated with an abnormal EOG and a normal ERG include butterfly dystrophy, pattern dystrophy of Marmour and Byers, and most notably Best's disease (vitellaform dystrophy).

■ VISUAL EVOKED POTENTIAL

The visual evoked potential (VEP) is a specialized averaged electroencephalogram (EEG). Scalp electrodes over the occipital cortex measures the integrity of the entire visual system. Abnormalities on VEP are nonlocalizable and can occur at any point from the retina to the occipital lobe.

VEP, which, by virtue of recording from the more superficially represented macular cortical neurons, may be most helpful in estimating visual acuities in nonverbal patients (infants or individuals with mental retardation), and cases of malingering.

■ REFERENCE

1. Berkow JW, Orth DH, Kelley JS: Fluorescein Angiography. Ophthalmology monograph 5. San Francisco: American Academy of Ophthalmology, 1991.

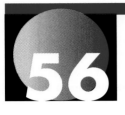

56 Development Disorders

Eugene de Juan Jr., Stuart W. Noorily,
William P. Townsend-Pico, Kenneth C. Chern

■ PERSISTENT HYPERPLASTIC PRIMARY VITREOUS

Persistent hyperplastic primary vitreous (6,11) (PHPV) is a descriptive classification for a sporadic, usually unilateral disorder characterized by abnormal regression of the tunica vasculosa lentis (hyaloid artery, vasa hyaloidea propria, and anterior ciliary vessels) and primary vitreous. Ninety percent of cases are unilateral. No gestational risk factors are noted. Systemic associations are absent.

Cases typically come to medical attention in the neonatal period when leukocoria, microphthalmos, or strabismus may be noted. Nystagmus is present in bilateral cases. Anterior and posterior variants of disease are recognized, with the purely posterior variant of disease representing only 10 to 20% of cases. Delayed presentation is not uncommon for the posterior variant.

Anterior PHPV is characterized by a pinkish-white retrolental plaque of variable size, centered just nasal to the visual axis. Vessels may radiate from its center. Abnormally long ciliary processes extend toward or into the fibrovascular plaque. Large radial blood vessels are seen on the iris. The globe invariably exhibits some degree of microphthalmia. At birth the lens is clear, but progressively becomes cataractous. With age, the posterior capsule of the lens may dehisce with secondary lenticular swelling and cataractous changes and subsequent anterior chamber shallowing with resultant glaucoma or corneal decompensation. The appearance of buphthalmos or uveitis may confuse the diagnosis in its later stages. Contraction of retrolental tissue can result in vitreous hemorrhage, typically several months after birth. Early in the disease, the retina is attached with a well-formed fovea, despite the frequent involvement of retinal tissue in the peripheral aspect of the retrolental fibrovascular mass. In later stages of disease, however, fibrosis and hemorrhage may lead to total retinal detachment.

Posterior PHPV (9) does not directly involve anterior structures, although microcornea and an immature filtration angle are often present. Ciliary processes are normal and the lens is clear. The disorder is characterized by white intravitreal membranes originating from the optic nerve head and extending radially out to the periphery. The retina is pulled up into discrete radial folds beneath the membranes. The macula is typically directly or indirectly involved. Vessels are often visible along the crest of folds and appear to represent persistent remnants of the vasa hyaloidea propria.

Experimental studies implicate overdevelopment and subsequent incomplete regression of the tunica vasculosa lentis in the pathogenesis of PHPV. Formation of retinal folds in the posterior variant of disease may be explained by persistent adhesion of a portion of the "proto"-retina to the primary vitreous as it regresses anteriorly toward its retrolental location during development. Retinal elements encompassed by the fold never achieve contact with the underlying pigment epithelium during development and thus, may fail to undergo normal cellular differentiation. This results in histopathologic evidence of retinal dysplasia.

The disorder must be differentiated from other causes of leukocoria including retinoblastoma, congenital cataract, retinopathy of prematurity, familial exudative vitreoretinopathy, shaken baby syndrome, Coat's disease, toxocariasis, and syndromes of retinal detachment associated with systemic disease (trisomy 13, Meckel syndrome, Warburg syndrome, Norrie's disease, and incontinentia pigmenti). See also Pediatrics, Retina Chapter 22, Table 22–4). Differentiation from retinoblastoma is of critical importance. Both disorders may show calcification on computed tomography (CT). The presence of microphthalmia can be helpful given its rarity in retinoblastoma except in phthisical eyes. The differentiation of findings of PHPV from those of solid or cystic tumors seen in retinoblastoma, is usually straightforward by means of ophthalmoscopy and ultrasonography; however, differentiation of advanced cases with vitreous hemorrhage can be difficult. CT of the

brain may be useful in excluding neurologic abnormalities which should be absent in PHPV.

Without treatment, severely affected eyes invariable progress to phthisis bulbi. The implementation of modern vitreoretinal techniques, together with amblyopia therapy has dramatically improved the prognosis for patients with these eyes. The majority of infants with anterior PHPV are able to achieve 20/30 to 20/200 vision when surgery is undertaken within the first months of life (7). Unfortunately, the visual results of surgery have been uniformly poor for posterior PHPV with macular involvement (see also Pediatrics Retina, Chapter 22, Figure 22–6).

■ NORRIE'S DISEASE

Norrie's disease is a rare, bilateral X-linked recessive syndrome of ocular dysgenesis associated with progressive auditory and mental impairment. Only males are affected. Females are silent carriers. Unaffected males do not pass the genetic defect to their offspring (13).

Typically, bilateral blindness is observed at birth. Rarely, an infant may retain some vision into its early teens. Ocular findings include retinal folds or detachment, persistent hyperplastic primary vitreous, vitreous hemorrhage, iris atrophy, and corneal opacities (5). The lens is clear. The globe is of normal size. Progressive cataract and microphthalmos subsequently ensue in the first years of life, secondary to phthisis bulbi.

The pathogenesis of disease appears to involve developmental abnormality of the inner layer of the optic cup during the fifth through seventh weeks of gestation (2). Primary failure of neurosensory differentiation with subsequent lack of induction of the secondary vitreous has been suggested. Molecular studies have localized the Norrie's disease gene to an area near the DXS7 locus in the proximal short arm of the X chromosome (13). Other studies have identified deletions near this gene locus in some affected patients. Further study is

required to precisely identify the gene or genes involved.

Histopathologic examination of biopsies of detached retinas in neonates show retinal immaturity with lack of differentiation of the normal layered neurosensory architecture. Retinal rosettes may be seen (1).

Systemic findings include mental retardation (60%) and impaired hearing (30%). Mental development in preschool years may be no different from visually impaired controls, but then follows a steady decline in the teens. Other infants may maintain superior mental ability, enabling them to proceed to the college level. Sensorineural hearing deficits, when present, typically do not appear until the second through fifth decades of life. Lifespan is normal.

Females within the lineage of an affected male are at risk of having an affected son or carrier daughter. Dramatic advances in recent years now allows determination of carrier status in selected females. Surgical intervention for retinal detachment in infants with the disease has not been successful. Moreover, the visual prognosis of such intervention is tenuous, given evidence for widespread retinal immaturity.

■ INCONTINENTIA PIGMENTI

Incontinentia pigmenti (2,3) (Block-Sulzberger syndrome) is a rare, bilateral, asymmetric disorder of pigmentary skin abnormalities with associated ocular, central nervous system, and dental abnormalities. Inheritance is sporadic (45%) or X-linked dominant with gestational lethality in males (55%).

Erythema with linear bullae and vesicles appear on the torso and extremities within the first 2 weeks of life. A transient peripheral blood eosinophilia may occur. Demonstration of intraepithelial eosinophils upon biopsy of skin lesions establishes the diagnosis. Lesions

are replaced by hypertrophic warts which disappear in several months leaving small papules, particularly on the feet. In the fourth month of life a bizarre pattern of chocolate brown splashes of pigment with jagged margins appears on the torso and extremities. The pigmentation fades with time and may disappear completely by adulthood.

Ocular involvement occurs in 30% of cases (10). Findings include peripheral fibrovascular proliferation with traction retinal detachment, strabismus, nystagmus, peripheral vascular abnormalities (capillary nonperfusion, microaneurysms, arteriovenous shunts, and neovascularization), pigmentary changes of the RPE and conjunctiva, macroaneurysms, foveal hypoplasia, congenital cataract, corneal opacities, and vitreous hemorrhage. The onset of ocular disease is always within the first year of life. Progression of ocular disease after the first year of life is unusual.

Histopathologic examination of pigmented skin lesions shows a decrease in basal epithelial melanin with an increase in melanin in the upper dermis. The term "incontinentia pigmenti" was originated by Bloch to conceptualize his observations that pigmented cells of the epithelium become "incontinent" of melanin, permitting it to drop into the upper dermis.

Molecular studies have localized the incontinentia pigmenti gene to the q28 region of the X chromosome. Sporadic cases, though clinically indistinguishable, appear to be related to a separate genetic defect involving translocations about the p11 region of the X chromosome. The pathogenesis of ocular disease is unclear. Theories include both a retinovascular and a pigment epithelial basis for disease. Others have suggested an inflammatory response to an abnormal gene product.

The differential diagnosis includes retinopathy of prematurity, familial exudative vitreoretinopathy, posterior PHPV, and Norrie's disease. In older individuals, peripheral retinal findings may be confused with those of sickle cell disease, systemic lupus erythematosus, and sarcoidosis.

Systemic associations involve other ectodermal components including teeth, hair, nails, and the central nervous system. Missing or pegged teeth are manifest in 65% of cases. Alopecia is seen in 38% of cases. Flattened or spoon shaped nails occur in 7% of cases. Neurologic findings include spastic or paralytic motor disorders, convulsive disorders or mental retardation in 30% of cases. The majority of patients exhibit normal or increased intelligence.

Except for its ocular and CNS associations, the clinical course is benign. Cryotherapy or photocoagulation to areas of peripheral nonperfusion, if present, has been suggested in order to avert progression to traction retinal detachment. Genetic counseling should integrate the knowledge that women with incontinentia pigmenti have a 25% spontaneous miscarriage rate and will transmit the disease to 50% of their female offspring, and that healthy offspring, regardless of gender, cannot transmit the disease.

■ FAMILIAL EXUDATIVE VITREORETINOPATHY

Familial exudative vitreoretinopathy (4,8,12) (FEVR) is a bilateral, autosomal-dominant, slowly progressive disorder of peripheral retinal vascular development, often associated with retinal traction. The patients have no history of prematurity or of oxygen supplementation. Systemic findings are absent. Phenotypic expression is highly variable among family members. Fluorescein angiography is often required to document peripheral retinovascular abnormalities in asymptomatic individuals.

The disease is characterized by abrupt termination of the temporal retinal vasculature with scalloped borders. Fluorescein angiography shows formation of a vascular-avascular border occurring a variable distance from the ora serrata. The vasculature just posterior to this zone appears dilated and straightened. Vessels end abruptly in arteriovenous anastomoses which may leak fluorescein dye, and from which neovascularization may develop. Unlike other disorders affecting the peripheral vasculature, vitreous hemorrhage is rare. Just anterior to the avascular border, a fibrovascular mass may develop with prominent, large caliber arterial and venous feeders associated with marked retinal exudation. The mass may encompass the ciliary body and peripheral lens capsule. Dragging of the macula, disc, and retinal vessels often occurs. Retinal folds and traction or rhegmatogenous retinal detachment develops in 10 to 20% of patients.

The fundamental abnormality in FEVR is unclear. Despite the similar appearance of the peripheral retinovascular findings to ROP, the two disorders follow a different time course and natural history. A notable difference is the tendency of ROP to either progress to cicatricial stages or to abort and vascularize the periphery. In contrast, the avascular zone in FEVR remains a permanent feature throughout life. Persistence of the avascular zone continues to stimulate peripheral neovascularization after the neonatal period, a finding never seen in ROP.

Retinal folds seen in FEVR are distinguished from those of posterior PHPV by the absence of their association with remnants of the hyaloid vascular system and the lack of histopathologic evidence for retinal dysplasia.

The majority of patients with FEVR suffer no visual impairment. Those which do, manifest their disease at an early age. Retinal folds presenting in infancy or childhood may progress rapidly, slowly, or remain stable. Despite unpredictability of its initial course, eventual stability is the rule. Visual loss after the second or third decade of life is rare and usually relates to the development of rhegmatogenous retinal detachment. The benefit of prophylactic ablation of avascular areas of peripheral retina is unclear, given the typically stable course of disease.

Despite the name, the retinal detachments are usually tractional and not exudative (8). The appearance of subretinal lipid at the posterior edge of the tractional retinal detraction is a sign of chronicity in the detachment and will resorb if the detachment is repaired. The prognosis for successful reattachment is poor (8). Rhegmatogenous retinal detachments may also be seen.

■ REFERENCES

1. Apple DJ, Fishman GA: Ocular histopathology of Norrie's disease. Am J Opthalmol 1974; 78:196–203.
2. Carney RG Jr. Incontinentia pigmenti: a world statistical analysis. Arch Dermatol 1976;112:535–542.
3. Catalano RA. Incontinentia pigmenti. Am J Ophthalmol 1990;110:696–700.
4. Criswick VG, Schepens Cl. Familial exudative vitreoretinopathy. Am J Ophthalmol 1969;68:578–594.
5. Enyedi LB, de Juan E, Gaitan A. Ultrastructural study of Norrie's disease. Am J Ophthalmol 1991;111:439–445.
6. Haddad R, Font RL. Persistent hyperplastic primary vitreous: a clinicopathologic study of 62 cases and review of the literature. Surv Ophthalmol 1978; 23: 123–134.
7. Karr DJ, Scott WE. Visual acuity results following treatment of persistent hyperplastic primary vitreous. Arch Ophthalmol 1986;104:662–667.
8. Ober RR, Bird AC. Autosomal dominant exudative vitreoretinopathy. Br J Ophthalmol 1980; 64:112–120.
9. Pruett RC, Schepens CL. Posterior hyperplastic primary vitreous. Am J Ophthalmol 1970; 69: 535–543.
10. Rosenfeld SI, Smith ME. Ocular findings in incontinentia pigmenti. Ophthalmology 1985; 93:543–546.
11. Stark WJ, Lindsey PS. Persistent hyperplastic primary vitreous. Ophthalmology 1983;90:452–457.
12. van Nouhuys CE. Signs, complications, and platelet aggregation in familial exudative vitreoretinopathy. Am J Ophthalmol 1991; 111:34–41.
13. Warburg M, Friedrich U. Norrie's disease: delineation of carriers among daughters of obligate carriers by linkage analysis. Trans Ophthalmol Soc UK 1986; 105: 88–93.

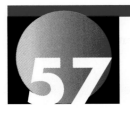

57 Hereditary Disorders In Children And Young Adults

*Eugene de Juan Jr., Stuart W. Noorily,
William P. Townsend-Pico, Kenneth C. Chern*

■ STARGARDT'S DISEASE—FUNDUS FLAVIMACULATUS

Stargardt's disease (11) is the most common hereditary macular dystrophy. Recent molecular genetic studies indicate that the disease may be heterogenous (similar to RP). Stargardt's and fundus flavimaculatus represent a varying spectrum of the same disease. Inheritance is typically autosomal recessive though, rarely, it may be autosomal dominant. Both sexes are equally affected. The disorder is bilaterally symmetric.

Stargardt's disease presents in adolescence with complaints of slowly progressive decreased central vision, often associated with mild impairment of color vision. Later, nyctalopia may develop.

Initially, the only ophthalmoscopic finding may be a mottled appearance of the macula. Over time, this progresses to the classic "beaten bronze" appearance. Later in the disorder, geographic atrophy may be present. Small, drusenoid, yellow pisciform (fishtail) flecks are present in one-half of cases, predominantly in the posterior pole (Figure 57–1). Occasionally, flecks may extend out to the equator.

Fluorescein angiography is particularly helpful in two regards. It distinguishes the flecks from those of drusen by the absence of hyperfluorescense related to window defect or late staining. Typically, there is a striking lack of correspondence of lesions seen ophthalmoscopically to their angiographic appearance. In over four-fifths of cases, fluorescein angiography is characterized by obscurance of choroidal fluorescence, otherwise referred to as the "dark choroid" effect.

Electroretinographic findings are typically normal, although subnormal values of the EOG may be present as an artifact of poor central acuity (17).

Histopathologic studies suggest the accumulation of an acid mucopolysaccharide (lipofuscin) in retinal pigment epithelial cells, thereby explaining the dark choroid effect (8).

The differential diagnosis includes dominant cone dystrophy, dominant drusen, retinitis punctata albescens, and fundus albipunctatus.

The prognosis for maintaining good central acuity in either eye is uniformly poor with the majority of patients dropping to the 20/200 level, usually by the third decade of life. No treatment exists.

■ BEST'S DISEASE

Best's disease (15) is an autosomal dominant, bilateral macular dystrophy widely known for its vitelliform or "egg yolk" macular lesion but actually encompasses a wide spectrum of disease with variable penetrance. It is

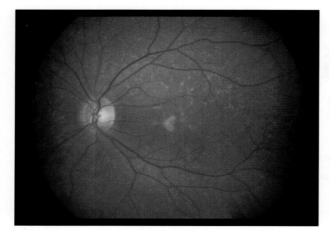

Figure 57–1.
Fundus flavimaculatus in a 42-year-old patient with 20/100 vision. Color photograph showing multiple yellow flecks at the level of the RPE, visible throughout the posterior pole.

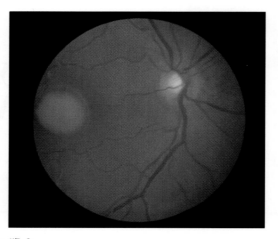

Figure 57–2.
The vitelliform macular lesion of Best's disease is an accumulation of lipofuscin within the RPE. At a later stage, the "egg yolk" may be partially resorbed, producing a scrambled egg appearance.

the second most common macular dystrophy. Onset is from early childhood to the mid-teens, although late onset may occur.

Symptoms include diminished central vision and metamorphopsia, though typically less marked than suggested by the ophthalmoscopic appearance. The classic egg yolk macular lesion at the level of the RPE is usually associated with good vision (Figure 57–2). Over time, the pigment epithelial lesion breaks through into the subretinal space and partial resorption of the lesion

produces a "pseudohypopyon" appearance. Further absorption of the lesion creates a "scrambled egg" appearance which ultimately resolves to leave an area of geographic atrophy. The process may be complicated by development of a choroidal neovascular membrane, with subsequent disciform scarring.

Fluorescein angiography shows blockage of choroidal fluorescence by the yellowish material and window defect hyperfluorescence in areas of atrophic change. The diagnosis is confirmed by marked reduc-

TABLE 57–1
The Hereditary White Dot Syndrome

	Retinitis Punctata Albescens	Fundus Albipunctatus	Alport's Disease	Kandori's Flecked Retina	Basal Laminar Drusen	Hypovitaminosis A	Pseudoxanthoma Elasticum
History	Progressive visual field loss and nyctalopia	Autosomal recessive form of CSNB, acuity and visual field normal, nonprogressive	Deafness, nephropathy, hematuria	Nyctalopia	Metamorphopsia, middle-aged	Malnutrition, nyctalopia	'Plucked' chicken skin, elastic fiber abnormalities, gastrointestinal hemorrhage
ERG	Reduced amplitude, delay in implicit time	Regeneration of scotopic ERG after full dark adaptation	Normal	Normal a-wave, reduced photopic and scotopic b-wave	Normal	Reduced scotopic a- and b-waves	Normal
Ocular manifestations	Multiple, 50–100 micron, hypopigmented dots at level RPE, arteriolar attenuation, bonespicule pigmentary changes	Multiple hypopigmented dots level RPE, CSNB	Anterior lenticonus, superficial paramacular and midperipheral hypopigmented flecks	Equatorial yellowish irregular flecks deep to retina	Multiple, hypopigmented 50–100 micron spots level RPE, pseudovitelliform macular detachment, reactive RPE hyperplasia	Xerophthalmia, Bitot's spots, keratomalacia, peripheral yellow-white dots deep to the retina	Angioid streaks, multiple, yellow lesions at mid-periphery, reticular pigmentary dystrophy, crystalline bodies, optic nerve head drusen

tion in the light-dark adapted ratio of the electro-oculogram in the presence of a normal electroretinogram. This test may be particularly useful in detecting otherwise silent carriers of the disease.

Histopathologic studies suggest the abnormal accumulation of lipofuscin granules within the retinal pigment epithelium, reminiscent of findings in Stargardt's disease (9).

The differential diagnosis includes a similar appearing disease in older individuals, often associated with multifocal lesions and good visual acuity. These patients do not have a family history of disease and do not exhibit an abnormality of the electro-oculogram.

Although there is no treatment, the prognosis for vision is good. The majority of affected individuals maintain acuity in the 20/40 to 20/100 range.

■ X-LINKED RETINOSCHISIS

X-linked recessive retinoschisis (5) is a bilateral, congenital disorder consisting of foveal and peripheral retinal splitting (schisis) at the level of the nerve fiber layer (Figure 57–3). It is almost exclusively a disorder of males. Although structural abnormalities are thought to be present at birth, symptoms of decreased vision, strabismus, or vitreous hemorrhage typically develop in childhood.

Foveal schisis is pathognomonic of the disease and consists of spokelike cystoid spaces that do not accumulate fluorescein on angiography. Fine folds of the internal limiting membrane may be seen radiating from the fovea in the area overlying the microcysts. One-half of patients have peripheral schisis, typically involving the inferotemporal quadrant. Ophthalmoscopic detection of a shallow area of peripheral schisis may be difficult. Scleral depression and a search for absolute scotomas on visual field testing can be helpful. Large inner breaks are common. Vitreous veils, representing free floating portions of inner retina may be observed.

The propensity for vitreous hemorrhage is explained by histopathologic evidence of splitting within the blood vessel rich nerve fiber layer. This contrasts with the infrequency of vitreous hemorrhage in acquired retinoschisis, in which splitting occurs at the level of the outer plexiform layer. Primary involvement of the inner retina also supports the characteristic finding of diminished b-wave amplitudes on the electroretinogram.

In advanced cases, differentiation from X-linked retinitis pigmentosa may be difficult. Pigment clumping can develop in areas of retinoschisis. Rarely, the electroretinogram may be extinguished. In these cases, preservation of the a-wave in light of an extinguished b-wave is particularly supportive of a diagnosis of retinoschisis.

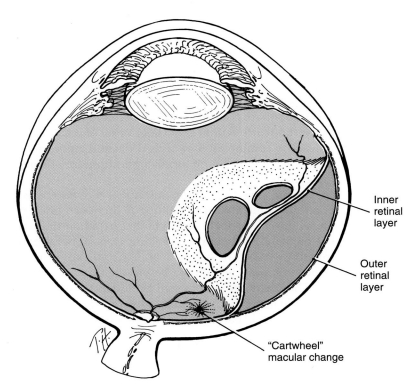

Inner retinal layer

Outer retinal layer

"Cartwheel" macular change

Figure 57–3.
Drawing—X-linked retinoschisis. The splitting occurs at the nerve fiber layer.

Vision often remains in the 20/70 range. In most cases, the peripheral schisis is not progressive. Laser photocoagulation (3) or cryopexy is reserved for bridging vessels causing vitreous hemorrhage or outer layer breaks in conjunction with inner layer breaks. Vitreous hemorrhages are managed conservatively whenever possible, unless the risk of amblyopia is great. Rarely, tractional or rhegmatogenous retinal detachment occurs beneath the area of schisis. When extensive, scleral buckling or vitreous surgery may be indicated. No reliable means exist to identify female carriers.

■ RETINITIS PIGMENTOSA

Retinitis pigmentosa (19) (RP) is the name given to a group of heritable disorders of progressive retinal degeneration characterized by bilateral nyctalopia constricted visual fields and abnormality of the electroretinogram. Disease may be confined to the eye or associated with systemic abnormalities. The incidence of disease is estimated at 1 in 4000. Inheritance in the United States is roughly 20% autosomal dominant, 20% autosomal recessive, 8% X-linked recessive, and 50% with only one affected family member. Both onset and clinical course appear to be related to mode of inheritance. Patients with autosomal recessive and X-linked recessive cases tend to have a childhood or adolescent onset and a severe course. Autosomal dominant cases tend to have a later onset and a slower, milder course.

RP represents a varied group of diseases whose common thread is the abnormal production of at least one protein in photoreceptor outer segments critical to light transduction (7). Molecular studies in one family with autosomal dominant RP have shown a point mutation in the rhodopsin gene on chromosome 3, resulting in the substitution of the amino acid proline for histidine at a highly conserved site in the rhodopsin protein in rod outer segments with theorized effects on the molecule's three-dimensional configuration and its interaction with vitamin A. Subsequently, other pedigrees have been found with different mutations in the rhodopsin or peripherin gene.

Early symptoms include difficulty with dark adaptation and midperipheral visual field loss. As the disease progresses, visual field loss advances, typically leaving a small central field of vision until eventually even central vision is affected. Central acuity may also be affected earlier in the course of disease either by cystoid macular edema, macular atrophy, or development of a posterior subcapsular cataract.

Ophthalmoscopic findings include bone spicule hyperpigmentary changes in the midperiphery, arteriolar attenuation, waxy pallor of the optic nerve, pigmented vitreous cells, and macular epiretinal membranes (Figure 57–4). Early in the disease, ophthalmoscopic signs may be minimal or absent. Some cases of RP may never develop the classic pigmentary abnormalities, despite an extinguished electroretinogram, arteriolar attenuation, and disc pallor. This variant, so-called retinitis pigmentosa sine pigmento, appears to be associated with a more pronounced cone dysfunction than typical RP. Sector RP, or pigmentary involvement of the inferior quadrant of the fundus is associated with absent or slow progression. Female carriers of X-linked recessive RP may show a golden reflex in the posterior pole. This finding is present in only one-half of obligate carriers, whereas the electroretinogram is abnormal in over 90%.

Electroretinography in affected individuals shows diminished or extinguished a-wave and b-wave responses, particularly in the dark adapted state, with a delay in b-wave implicit time. Quantitative diminishment of the ERG over time provides information regarding the course of progression, as will comparison of serial visual fields. Fluorescein angiography can rarely be helpful in detecting subtle peripheral pigmentary abnormalities. Cystoid macular edema accompanying RP characteristically does not accumulate fluorescein dye.

Retinitis pigmentosa may be associated with a wide variety of systemic associations. A few of these are of particular importance for either their treatment or counseling implications.

Usher's syndrome describes the association of autosomal recessive RP and congenital deafness in as many as 5% of patients. Type I Usher's syndrome consists of profound neurosensory deafness and absent vestibular function, whereas type II has less profound deafness, intact vestibular function, and a later onset of visual symptoms. The combination of both visual and auditory deprivation has devastating social implications for affected individuals.

Refsum's syndrome is an autosomal recessive defect in fatty acid metabolism, resulting in increased levels of phytanic acid throughout the body (including the retinal pigment epithelium), resulting in peripheral neuropathy, cerebellar ataxia, deafness, and the onset of atypical retinitis pigmentosa before the third decade of life. The diagnosis is confirmed by elevated levels of phytanic acid in serum. Implementation of a diet decreased in phytanic acid early in life may slow progression of disease.

Bassen-Kornsweig disease or abetalipoproteinemia is a rare autosomal recessive disorder of intestinal fat

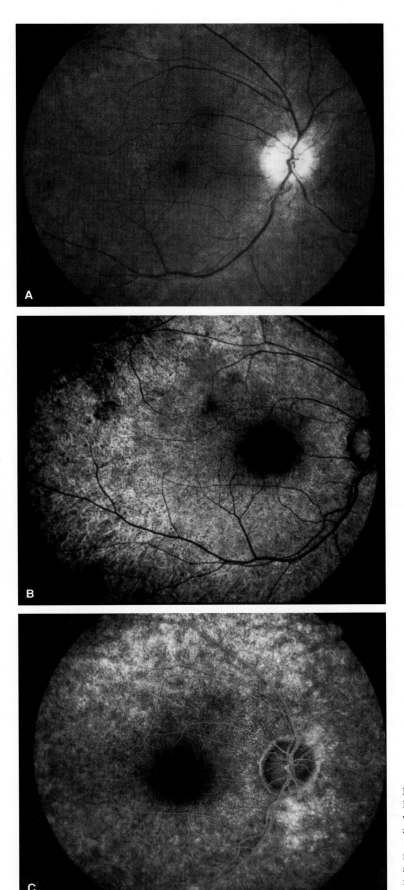

Figure 57–4.
Retinitis pigmentosa in a 17-year-old female with 20/20 vision, constricted visual fields, and extinguished scotopic and photopic electroretinography. Red-free photograph (A) showed marked arterial attenuation and diminished fundus reflexes for the patient's age. Fluorescein angiography shows window defect from a mottled pattern of retinal pigment epithelial atrophy in the early (B) and late (C) phases.

malabsorption resulting in decreased serum levels of cholesterol, triglycerides, and the fat-soluble vitamins A, E, and K. Diagnosis is confirmed by serum lipoprotein electrophoresis. Patients present with steatorrhea, acanthocytosis, ataxia, and childhood onset RP. Supplementation with vitamin A may have some visual benefit in this ultimately fatal disease.

Lawrence-Moon-Biedl-Bardet syndrome is a disorder of mental retardation, obesity, hypogenitalism, polydactyly, and spastic paraplegia associated with retinitis pigmentosa in approximately 90% of patients.

The differential diagnosis of retinitis pigmentosa includes syphilis, cancer-associated retinopathy, congenital stationary night blindness, and vitamin A deficiency.

Treatment is directed toward decreased vision aids, genetic counseling, and cataract surgery when appropriate. Preliminary evidence supports the utility of acetazolamide in the treatment of RP-related cystoid macular edema (6). Other studies suggest that vitamin A supplementation may slow deterioration of the electroretinogram over time (1). The functional visual benefit of such supplementation in patients with typical RP is not yet known.

■ PROGRESSIVE CONE DYSTROPHY

Cone dystrophy (13) is a rare, typically autosomal dominant disorder of progressive cone dysfunction heralded by diminished central vision and color vision in the first through third decades of life. Additional symptoms include photophobia, dark-to-light adaptation difficulty, and a history of better vision at night. Color vision may be affected out of proportion to the visual loss. Visual field examination may show central scotomas with preservation of the peripheral visual field.

Ophthalmoscopy is characterized by central macular pigment epithelial atrophy, although early cases may appear normal. In some cases only a faint granular appearance may be present in the macula, while in others a bull's eye maculopathy or profound geographic atrophy is evident (Figure 57–5). Additional findings include arteriolar attenuation, temporal pallor of the optic nerve head, and peripheral, sectoral granular or bone spicule pigmentary changes.

The differential diagnosis includes Stargardt's disease, retinitis pigmentosa, chloroquine toxicosis, North Carolina macular dystrophy, (20) and central areolar choroidal dystrophy. The history can be helpful in distinguishing among these possibilities. Presence of the dark choroid effect on fluorescein angiography suggests Stargardt's disease. Early constriction of the peripheral visual field suggests retinitis pigmentosa.

The course of disease is variable, even among members of the same family. Vision often declines to the

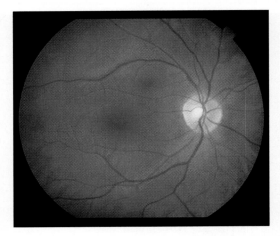

Figure 57–5.
Cone dystrophy in a 19-year-old female with progressive nyctalopia and 20/60 visual acuity. Note the mild pigmentary mottling of the subfoveal RPE, loss of the foveal reflex, and mild attenuation of arterioles concerning the patient's age. Color vision was only 1 of 14 plates. Electroretinography showed markedly diminished photopic and flicker responses with only minimally reduced scotopic responses.

20/200 level by the end of the third decade. No treatment is known. Tinted glasses may help reduce photophobic symptoms.

■ ACHROMATOPSIA (ROD MONOCHROMATISM)

Achromatopsia (rod monochromatism) is at the extreme end of the cone dystrophies. It is an autosomal recessive, stationary disorder associated with reduced vision, nystagmus, photophobia, and absent color vision since birth. Although initially the fundus may be normal or show minimal pigmentary changes, there may be a progression to a pigmentary retinopathy, reminiscent of retinitis pigmentosa. The ERG findings are characteristic and show an absent photopic (cone) flicker response with a reduced photopic single-flash response and a normal scotopic response. Window defect hyperfluores-cence on fluorescein angiography may highlight the bull's-eye maculopathy.

■ CENTRAL AREOLAR CHOROIDAL DYSTROPHY

Central areolar choroidal dystrophy (18) (CACD) is an autosomal dominant progressive disorder which usually presents at ages 30 to 40 and is associated with a wide range of presenting visual acuities ranging from 20/30 to 20/200. It is a bilateral, symmetric disorder not associated with peripheral white spots or drusen. CACD presents initially with mild macular retinal pigment epithelial mottling which slowly progresses to a well-circumscribed round or oval-shaped area of atro-phy of the RPE and choriocapillaris. Fluorescein angiography reveals early well-circumscribed hyperfluorescence with easy visualization of the large choroidal vessels and mild late leakage from the remaining choriocapillaris at the margins of the lesion. The ERG and EOG are usually normal. The differential diagnosis includes the cone dystrophies, Best's disease, Stargardt's, North Carolina macular dystrophy, and atrophic ARMD.

■ ADULT-ONSET FOVEOMACULAR DYSTROPHY

Adult-onset foveomacular dystrophy (10) is an autosomal dominant disorder which usually presents between age 40 to 50 with mild decreased vision and/or metamorphopsia. Ocular findings include bilateral, minimally elevated, symmetric, subfoveal, round or oval-shaped yellowish lesions with a central hyperpigmented spot. These lesions are typically one-third to 1 disc diameter in size and have a characteristic fluorescein angiographic finding of a ring of hyperfluorescence surrounding a central hypofluorescent spot. The ERG is usually normal and the EOG may be slightly subnormal. The visual prognosis of AOFMD is reasonably good with preservation of reading vision in at least one eye in most cases. Best's disease, in contrast, commonly presents earlier, has larger vitelliform lesions, and has a markedly abnormal EOG.

■ PATTERN DYSTROPHIES

The pattern dystrophies (4,22) are most likely a phenotypic spectrum of an inherited autosomal dominant retinal pigment epitheliopathy which usually presents in midlife, associated with mild-to-moderate visual changes, and manifest with bilateral, symmetric geometric retinal pigment epithelial changes. Many different titles have been placed on this entity including butterfly-shaped pigment dystrophy, reticular dystrophy of the pigment epithelium, macroreticular dystrophy of the pigment epithelium, and fundus pulverulentus. However, they are likely just a result of variable expressivity of the same gene. The characteristic RPE changes are often highlighted on fluorescein angiography. The ERG is normal and the EOG may be abnormal. Choroidal neovascularization is an occasional complication of this disorder. Systemic associations are few but include pseudoxanthoma elasticum and myotonic dystrophy.

■ CONGENITAL STATIONARY NIGHT BLINDNESS

Congenital stationary night blindness (4) (CSNB) is a rare, bilateral, nonprogressive disorder of hereditary nyctalopia in the absence of diminished vision, color, or visual fields. The disorder may be autosomal dominant, autosomal recessive, or X-linked. Two unique variants of CSNB, Oguchi's disease and fundus albipunctatus, are associated with an abnormal appearing fundus and autosomal recessive inheritance.

Patients typically present in the first decade of life with the isolated complaint of nyctalopia. Initially, cases may be difficult to distinguish from early retinitis pigmentosa, except for the progressive nature of the latter, and information elicited from the family history. A paradoxical pupil may be present. Myopia is common.

Oguchi's disease shows a characteristic golden-yellow sheen which normalizes after prolonged dark adaption (Mizuo phenomenon). Fundus albipunctatus exhibits abundant, discrete 50 micron white dots in the midperiphery, typically sparing the macula. The dots do not hyperfluoresce or block choroidal fluorescence on fluorescein angiography.

Electroretinography shows diminution of the scotopic response in the presence of a normal photopic response. Oscillatory potentials may be lost from both sco- topic and photopic waveforms. Dark adaptation exhibits a normal early cone phase, but absence of the rod phase.

Since visual fields and acuity do not become affected, the overall prognosis is good. No treatment is known. In older individuals, the condition must be distinguished from acquired causes of nyctalopia including cancer-associated retinopathy (12).

■ CHOROIDEREMIA

Choroideremia (14) is an X-linked recessive, bilateral disorder characterized by progressive degeneration of the choriocapillaris and its overlying retinal pigment epithelium. Typically, only males are affected. Obligate female carriers often show patchy mottling of the pigment epithelium with mild peripheral pigment clumps but are without visual symptoms in most cases.

The onset of disease is in the first decade of life. The symptoms and course are similar to retinitis pigmentosa. Nyctalopia and midperipheral visual field loss occur early in the disease. Central vision is unaffected until later in the course of disease.

Molecular studies have shown deletions in a gene contained with the Xq21 band of the X chromosome. The product of this gene is expressed in the retina, as well as the choroid and pigment epithelium. Its role in the pathogenesis of disease is still unclear.

Ophthalmoscopy shows diffuse loss of the choriocapillaris and overlying retinal pigment epithelium, be- ginning in the midperiphery then spreading both anteriorly and posteriorly. Bone spicules are characteristically absent. Often, the macula is spared until late in the disease. Loss of the pigment epithelium and choriocapillaris allows the underlying, large choroidal vessels to be easily visualized.

Electroretinography resembles the findings in retinitis pigmentosa with reductions in a-wave and b-wave amplitudes and prolonged b-wave implicit time. Fluorescein angiography is particularly helpful in illustrating prominent, nonleaking, large choroidal vessels in the absence of the typical "choroidal flush" normally provided by an intact choriocapillaris.

The differential diagnosis includes retinitis pigmentosa, gyrate atrophy, increased myopia, and ocular albinism. These conditions can be easily differentiated on the basis of their inheritance pattern and the results of fluorescein angiography. No treatment is known.

■ GYRATE ATROPHY

Gyrate atrophy (21,23) is a rare, autosomal recessive, bilateral disorder characterized by progressive, well-demarcated, scalloped atrophy of the pigment epithelium and choriocapillaris. The symptoms and clinical course of disease are similar to those of retinitis pigmentosa and choroideremia.

The onset of disease is typically in the first two decades of life with symptoms of nyctalopia and diminished midperipheral visual field. Central visual acuity is relatively spared until late in disease. Ophthalmoscopy shows scalloped areas of pigment and choriocapillaris loss in the midperiphery with a characteristic border of surrounding hyperpigmentation. Atrophic areas ultimately coalesce with corresponding worsening of the visual field. Central vision becomes affected in the fifth decade with expansion of lesions into the macula, or the development of posterior subcapsular cataracts or cystoid macular edema.

All patients show a deficiency of the enzyme ornithine aminotransferase, resulting in tenfold to twenty- fold elevations of normal plasma ornithine levels (2). The gene for the enzyme has been localized to chromosome 10. Multiple point mutations in the ornithine aminotransferase gene have been identified in gyrate atrophy patients. The extraocular effects of hyperornithinemia appear to be minimal; however, alternations in hair and muscle fibers have been documented. Carriers may be diagnosed by identifying decreased levels of ornithine aminotransferase in skin fibroblasts.

Electroretinography shows reduced or extinguished responses. Fluorescein angiography is useful to confirm focal areas choriocapillaris loss.

Associated systemic findings related to elevated levels of ornithine include borderline decreased intellectual function, electroencephalographic abnormalities, mild myopathy affecting type-2 fibers, and fine scalp hair.

Treatment is directed at reducing serum ornithine levels. This may be accomplished in one of two ways. Daily supplementation with 300 to 500 mg of pyridoxine (vitamin B_6) improves ornithine aminotransferase activity in some patients, with a resultant 30 to 50% fall in serum ornithine levels. Unfortunately, most patients are not vitamin B_6 responsive. All patients, however, are responsive to dietary modification, since, in the absence of functioning ornithine aminotransferase, arginine becomes the major source of ornithine, by way of the urea cycle. Implementation of a decreased arginine diet has been shown to be successful in significantly reducing serum ornithine levels, with preliminary evidence suggesting a beneficial effect on the development and progression of ocular disease.

■ REFERENCES

1. Berson EL, Rosner B, Sandberg MA, et al: A randomized trial of vitamin A and vitamin E supplementation for retinitis pigmentosa. Arch Ophthalmol 1993; 111: 761–772.
2. Berson EL, Schmidt SY, Shih VE: Ocular and biochemical abnormalities in gyrate atrophy of the choroid and retina. Ophthalmology 1978; 84: 1018–1027.
3. Brockhurst RJ: Photocoagulation in congenital retinoschisis. Arch Ophthalmol 1970; 84: 158–165.
4. Carr RE: Congenital stationary night blindness. Trans Am Ophthalmol Soc 1974; 72: 448–487.
5. Condon GP, Brownstein S, Wang NS: Congenital hereditary (juvenile X-linked) retinoschisis: histopathologic and ultrastructural findings in three eyes. Arch Ophthalmol 1986; 104: 576–583.
6. Cox SN, Hay E, Bird AC: Treatment of chronic macular edema with acetazolamide. Arch Ophthalmol 1988; 106: 1190–1195.
7. Dryja TP, McGee TL, Hahn LB: Mutations within the rhodopsin gene in patients with autosomal dominant retinitis pigmentosa, N Engl J Med 1990; 323: 1302–1307.
8. Eagle RC, Lucier AC, Bernardin o VB, Yanoff M: Retinal pigment epithelial abnormali ties in fundus flavimacu latus: a light and electron microscopic study. Ophthalmology 1980; 87: 1189–1200.
9. Frangieh GT, Green WR, Fine SL: Histopathologic study of Best's macular dystrophy. Arch Ophthalmol 1982; 100: 1115–1121.
10. Gass, JDM: A clinicopathologic study of a peculiar foveomacular dystrophy. Trans Am Ophthalmol Soc 1974; 72: 139–156.
11. Hadden OB, Gass JDM: Fundus flavimaculatus and Stargardt's disease. Am J Ophthalmol 1976; 82: 527–539.
12. Keltner JL, Thirkill CE, Tyler NK: Management and monitoring of cancer-associated retinopathy. Arch Ophthalmol 1992; 110: 48–53.
13. Krill AE, Deutman AF: Dominant macular degenerations: the cone dystrophies. Am J Ophthalmol 1972; 73: 352–369.
14. McCulloch C: Choroideremia: a clinical and pathologic review. Trans Am Ophthalmol Soc 1969; 67: 142–195.
15. Maloney WF, Robertson DM, Duboff SM: Hereditary vitelliform macular degeneration. Arch Ophthalmol 1977; 95: 979–983.
16. Marmor MF, Byers B: Pattern dystrophy of the pigment epithelium. Am J Ophthalmol 1977; 84: 32–44.
17. Moloney JBM, Mooney DJ, O'Connor MA: Retinal function in Stargardt's disease and fundus flavimaculatus. Am J Ophthalmol 1983; 96: 57–65.
18. Noble KG: Central areolar choroidal dystrophy. Am J Ophthalmol 1977; 84: 310–318.
19. Pagon RA: Retinitis pigmentosa. Surv Ophthalmol 1988; 33: 137–177 .
20. Small KW, Killian J, McLean WC: North Carolina's dominant progressive foveal dystrophy: How progressive is it? Br J Ophthalmol 1991; 75: 401–406.
21. Takki KK, Milton RC: The natural history of gyrate atrophy of the choroid and retina. Ophthalmology 1981; 88: 292–301.
22. Watzke RC, Folk JC, Lang RM: Pattern dystrophy of the retinal pigment epithelium. Ophthalmology 1982; 89: 1400–1406.
23. Wilson DJ, Weleber RG, Green WR: Gyrate atrophy of the choroid and retina: a clinicopathologic correlation. Am J Ophthalmol 1991; 111: 24–35.

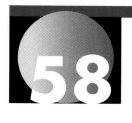

58 Hereditary Vitreoretinal Degenerations

Eugene de Juan Jr., Stuart W. Noorily,
William P. Townsend-Pico, Kenneth C. Chern

The hereditary vitreoretinal degenerations encompass a continuum of related disorders. The key features distinguishing the different entities is outlined in Table 58–1.

■ GOLDMANN-FAVRE SYNDROME

Goldmann-Favre (2) is an autosomal recessive, bilateral, vitreo-tapeto-retinal degeneration which affects both sexes equally and usually presents in the first decade of life with night blindness. Characteristic clinical findings include progressive cataracts, an optically-empty vitreous with bands, macular and peripheral retinoschisis, peripheral retinal pigmentary degeneration, waxy pallor of the optic nerve head, and attenuation of the retinal vessels. Perimetry may show an absolute scotoma corresponding to the peripheral retinoschisis. Fluorescein angiography is normal without evidence of macular leakage. The ERG, particularly scotopic, is significantly abnormal as is the EOG. X-linked retinoschisis can be distinguished by the lack of peripheral pigmentary changes, nyctalopia, recessive inheritance, and the abnormal EOG seen in Goldmann-Favre and not in X-linked retinoschisis. Prophylactic treatment of retinal tears in these patients is recommended since the retinal detachments often seen with this disorder are difficult to treat and are frequently associated with proliferative vitreoretinopathy.

■ WAGNER'S DISEASE

Wagner's disease (3) is an autosomal dominant disorder which consists of myopia, glaucoma, cataracts (usually cortical and PSC), an optically-empty vitreous, preretinal membranes, retinal perivascular pigmentary changes, and lattice-like retinal degeneration. Patients with Wagner's disease, by definition, have no systemic associated disorders. Progressive loss of vision may be seen owing to a panretinal degeneration. Wagner's is not associated with a higher risk of retinal detachments. The ERG may become progressively reduced as the patient ages. The EOG is characteristically normal.

Jansen's disease is a related disorder with clinical characteristics indistinguishable from Wagner's disease. Retinal detachments are, however, very commonly associated with this disorder and may be bilateral.

TABLE 58–1
The Hereditary Vitreoretinal Degenerations

	Wagner's disease	Jansen's disease	Stickler's disease	Congenital, X-linked retinoschisis	Goldmann-Favre
Inheritance	Autosomal dominant	Autosomal dominant	Autosomal dominant	X-linked	Autosomal dominant
Ocular features	Myopia, glaucoma, cataracts, vitreous and preretinal membranes, lattice-like retinal degeneration	Same as Wagner's	Same as Wagner's	Stellate maculopathy, peripheral retinoschisis, recurrent vitreous hemorrhage	Cataract, empty vitreous, stellate, maculopathy, peripheral retinoschisis, waxy pallor of optic nerve head, attenuation retinal vessels, peripheral pigmentary changes
Risk of retinal detachment	–	+	+	Low-risk	Low-risk
Systemic manifestations	None	None	Facial abnormalities, cleft palate, Pierre-Robin sequence, hearing loss, skeletal, joint abnormalities	None	None
ERG	Reduced	Reduced	Reduced	Normal a-wave, reduced b-wave	Reduced
EOG	Normal	Normal	Normal	Normal	Abnormal

■ STICKLER'S SYNDROME (HEREDITARY PROGRESSIVE ARTHRO-OPHTHALMOPATHY)

Stickler's syndrome (1) is a progressive autosomal disorder with complete penetrance but marked variability in expression. An association with abnormal production of type 2 collagen has been associated. Ocular features are essentially the same as Wagner's and Jansen's disease and include myopia, cataracts, strabismus, an optically-empty vitreous with transvitreal and epiretinal bands, lattice-like retinal degeneration, an increased risk (75%) of multiple retinal breaks, and retinal detachment (42% bilateral) (Figure 58–1). Systemic manifestations are key in making this diagnosis and include facial abnormalities (maxillary and mandibular hypoplasia), cleft palate, neurosensory hearing loss, the Pierre-Robin sequence, and skeletal abnormalities including joint hyperextensibility, a marfanoid habitus with arachnodactyly, and bony dysplasias.

■ THE HEREDITARY WHITE DOT SYNDROMES

The differential diagnosis of the hereditary white dot syndromes includes retinitis punctata albescens, fundus albipunctatus, Alport's disease, Kandori's flecked retina, pseudoxanthoma elasticum with peau d'orange lesions, basal laminar drusen, and hypovitaminosis A. All of these entities may present with multiple, punctate, yellow-white lesions at the level of the retina and/or retinal pigment epithelium. They may be differentiated by several historical, funduscopic, and electroretinographic findings (Table 58–1).

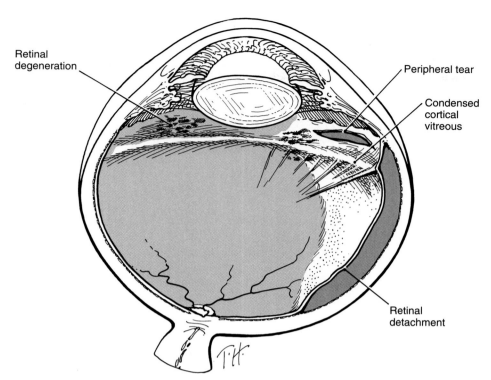

Figure 58–1.
Stickler's syndrome.

■ REFERENCES

1. Blair NP, Albert DM, Lieberfarb RM, Hirose T: Hereditary progressive arthrophthalmopathy of Stickler. Am J Ophthalmol 1979; 88: 876–888.

2. Fishman GA, Jampol LM, Goldberg MF: Diagnostic features of the Favre-Goldmann syndrome. Br J Ophthalmol 1976; 60: 345–353.

3. Hirose T, Lee KY, Schepens CL: Wagner's hereditary vitreoretinal degeneration and retinal detachment. Arch Ophthalmol 1973; 89: 176–185.

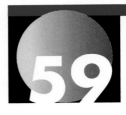

59 Acquired Macular Disorders

Eugene de Juan Jr., Stuart W. Noorily,
William P. Townsend-Pico, Kenneth C. Chern

■ THE CRYSTALLINE RETINOPATHIES

Intraretinal crystals may be the result of a variety of etiologies including hereditary, retinovascular, and toxic. The differential diagnosis includes cystinosis, primary hyperoxaluria, Bietti's crystalline dystrophy, idiopathic juxtafoveal telangiectasis type 2, diabetic macular edema, talc retinopathy, canthazanthine toxicosis, tamoxifen toxicosis, and methoxyflurane toxicosis.

■ RETINAL TOXICOSIS OF SYSTEMIC MEDICATIONS

Several medications have important ocular toxic side effects of which every clinician should be aware. These medications include chloroquine (Aralen), hydroxychloroquine (Plaquenil), thioridazine (Mellaril), chlorpromazine (Thorazine), tamoxifen (Nolvadex), nicotinic acid (niacin), canthazanthine, methoxyflurane, methanol, and clofazimine.

Chloroquine and hydroxychloroquine were first used for the prophylaxis and treatment of malaria and now are more commonly used in the treatment of the connective tissue diseases (55). Both produce identical retinopathies which may progress from a mild macular pigmentary abnormality to the classic bull's-eye maculopathy which consists of a central, foveal area of hyperpigmentation surrounded by hypopigmentation (Figure 59–1A). These findings may be better visualized on fluorescein angiography. Cornea verticillata may also be seen (see Cornea section). Toxicosis from chloroquine or hydroxychloroquine usually does not occur with daily doses of 250 mg or less (cumulative dose 100 gm) and 400 mg per day, respectively. Follow-up examinations with testing of visual acuity, central visual field with a red Amsler grid, and EOG should be done approximately every 6 months. Once toxicosis is noted, progression may be seen even after discontinuation of the drug.

Thioridazine toxicosis may present with a history of decreased vision and/or nyctalopia (57,59). Fundus findings may range from mild granularity of the retinal pigment epithelium, posterior to the equator, to a patchy, nummular, atrophic retinal pigment epitheliopathy with associated atrophy of the RPE and choriocapillaris. This retinopathy usually develops with the long-term use of thioridazine with a dosage greater than 800 mg per day. The retinopathy may progress even upon discontinuation of the drug. The differential diagnosis of these retinal findings include choroideremia and Bietti's Crystalline Retinopathy.

Chlorpromazine toxicosis is usually limited to the anterior segment with a characteristic pigmentary deposition in the corneal endothelium and the lens capsule. Rare posterior segment manifestations include a pigmentary retinopathy with RPE atrophy and reversible pigmentary clumping.

Tamoxifen (20 to 30 mg/day) (9), canthazanthine (3) (total dose greater than 37 g/day), and methoxyflurane have all been associated with a crystalline retinopathy.

The use of nicotinic acid for the lowering of serum cholesterol has been associated with a cystoid maculopathy which clinically appears similar to cystoid mac-

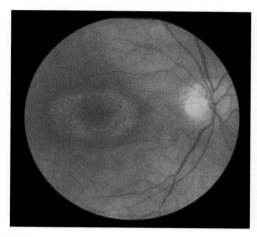

Figure 59–1A.
Bull's-eye macular lesion in a 28-year-old patient who had received a cumulative dose of almost 700 g chloroquine over 6 years. The pigmentary changes in the macular remain, even after discontinuation of the drug.

ular edema but on fluorescein angiography shows no leakage (6). This retinopathy is usually associated with a dose greater than 1.5 grams per day and is reversible upon discontinuation of the drug.

Methanol toxicosis is associated systemically with a metabolic acidosis and mental status changes, which may even progress to coma and death. Early ocular manifestations include bilateral optic disc edema with occasional concomitant retinal edema, with subsequent progression to optic atrophy.

Clofazimine is used in the treatment of leprosy and Mycobacterium avium-intracellulare in patients with AIDS. Doses greater than 200 mg per day have been reported to cause bilateral bull's-eye maculopathies with normal central and color vision and reduction in the ERG b-wave amplitudes.

■ AGE-RELATED MACULAR DEGENERATION

Age-related macular degeneration (2, 3, 22) (AMD) is the most common cause of legal blindness in adults. The underlying abnormality of AMD is the development of involutional changes at the level of Bruch's membrane and the retinal pigment epithelium (RPE). The hallmark lesion of such changes is the druse (plural, drusen). Clinically, drusen appear as small, yellow-white deposits at the level of the RPE. Drusen may be categorized as hard drusen, soft drusen, or basal laminar drusen.

Hard drusen have well-defined borders and are typically 50 microns or smaller in size. Histopathologically, hard drusen represent focal accumulation of hyaline material in the inner and outer collagenous zones of Bruch's membrane. Intervening areas of Bruch's membrane appear normal. The accumulation of hyaline material is thought to result from the extrusion of debris from RPE cells. The presence of hard drusen is not associated with neovascular complications of AMD.

Soft drusen are poorly demarcated lesions greater than 63 microns in diameter (Figure 59–1B and C). Histopathologically, soft drusen represent diffuse thickening of the inner aspect of Bruch's membrane with overlying RPE hypopigmentation. Focal detachments of the inner aspect of Bruch's membrane may occur. The presence of soft drusen is indicative of global thickening of inner Bruch's membrane throughout the macula. Soft drusen are associated with an increased prevalence of neovascular complications of AMD.

Basal laminar drusen are small, round, uniform, translucent, innumerable lesions 25 to 75 microns in size. Histopathologically, they represent diffuse thickening of the inner aspect of Bruch's membrane with

overlying, nodular sub-RPE excrescences. Basal laminar drusen are infrequently associated with neovascular complications of AMD. They may, however, be associated with the development of peculiar exudative detachments of the RPE which mimic Best's disease. Such RPE detachments pool fluorescein dye in the mid frames of the angiogram and must be differentiated from true choroidal neovascularization.

Visual loss in AMD may result from nongeographic or geographic atrophy ("dry" AMD) or neovascular complications of AMD ("wet" AMD). Nongeographic atrophy refers to stippled areas of RPE hyperpigmentation and hypopigmentation corresponding to atrophy of the RPE overlying a diffusely thickened inner aspect of Bruch's membrane. Geographic atrophy refers to a pattern of well-demarcated RPE atrophy with associated choriocapillaris and photoreceptor atrophy (Figure 59–2). Areas of RPE atrophy may often develop from coalescence of areas of soft drusen, with diffuse thickening of Bruch's membrane replaced by fibrous tissue. Geographic atrophy typically spreads in a horseshoe pattern with the central fovea spared until late in the disease. Large areas of atrophy may be associated with a diminished risk of choroidal neovascularization.

Although affecting only 10% of patients with AMD, neovascular complications of AMD account for the overwhelming majority of cases of severe visual loss. Risk factors include increasing age, soft drusen, nongeographic atrophy, family history, hyperopia, and pigment epithelial detachments. The incidence of the fellow eye involvement in neovascular AMD is 12% per year.

The pathogenesis of choroidal neovascularization in AMD appears to be related to the development of cracks

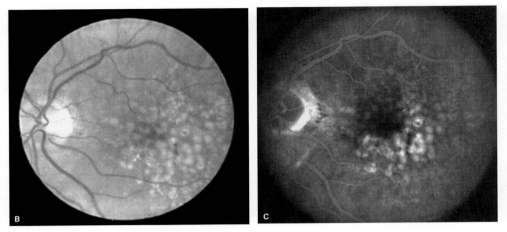

Figure 59–1. *(continued)*
Age-related macular degeneration in a 74-year-old patient. Multiple and confluent soft drusen are present in the macula (B). On fluorescein angiography (C), the soft drusen stain in the late frames without leakage of dye. This patient should be monitored closely since soft drusen are associated with formation of choroidal neovascular membranes.

in an abnormally thickened Bruch's membrane. Ingrowth of new vessels from the choriocapillaris into the sub-RPE and subretinal space is associated with mechanical and cellular damage of the outer retina. Gass has recently proposed a classification of choroidal neovascular membranes into two types: type 1 is a subretinal pigment epithelium CNVM, while type 2 is located under the neurosensory retina. Ultimately, the neovascularization undergoes a process of fibrous involution with formation of a disciform scar.

Symptoms of choroidal neovascularization in AMD include metamorphopsia, paracentral scotomas or diminished central vision. Ophthalmoscopic findings include subretinal fluid, blood, or exudate; RPE detachment, cystic retinal changes, or the presence of grayish-green subretinal neovascular membrane. Type 2 neovascular membranes, which are located anterior to the RPE, are frequently surrounded by a pigmented ring.

An understanding of the fluorescein angiographic features of choroidal neovascularization is critical to the management of the disease. Choroidal neovascularization can be categorized either as well-defined or occult. Classic choroidal neovascularization describes well-demarcated areas of hyperfluorescence discernible in the early phase of the angiogram. Progressive pooling of dye in the subretinal space is seen in the late frames of the angiogram often blurring the boundaries of the lesion. Occult choroidal neovascularization consists of either fibrovascular pigment epithelial detachment (PED) or late leakage of undeterminable source. Fibrovascular PED is an area of irregular elevation of the RPE (appreciated in the stereo views of the angiogram) associated with a characteristic pattern of stippled hyperfluorescence in the late frames of the angiogram. Late leakage of undetermined source denotes fluorescence leakage at the level of the RPE in the late phase of the angiogram which does not correlate with any well-defined areas of hyperfluorescence in the early phase of the angiogram.

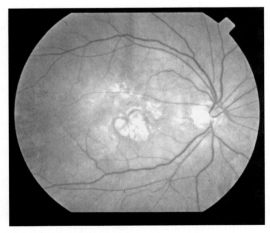

Figure 59–2.
Age-related macular degeneration with geographic atrophy in an elderly patient. In the macula is an area of RPE atrophy with the underlying choroidal vasculature visible. Photorecepter degeneration in this region results in decreased acuity to 20/200.

Additional components of choroidal neovascular membranes as delineated by fluorescein angiography include elevated blocked fluorescence, flat blocked fluorescence, serous PED, blood, and disciform scar. Elevated blocked fluorescence is thought to represent hypertrophic, opacified pigment epithelial cells overlying fibrovascular tissue. Flat blocked fluorescence represents hypertrophic pigment epithelial cells in the absence of underlying fibrovascular proliferation. Serous PED describes a smooth, circular elevation of the pigment epithelium associated with uniform pooling of dye and well-defined borders in the early phase of the angiogram.

Our present understanding of neovascular AMD suggests that classic choroidal neovascularization is the lesion component most strongly associated with rapid visual deterioration and that treatment must encompass all neovascular and fibrovascular components of the lesion. At present, treatment is only indicated when classic neovascularization has boundaries that are well demarcated. The Macular Photocoagulation Study (24, 28, 32, 36, 55) has shown the benefit of focal laser photocoagulation in various clinical scenarios.

In eyes with extrafoveal choroidal neovascularization (>=200 microns from the foveal center), argon laser photocoagulation diminished the incidence of severe visual loss, (≥6 lines) at 5 years from 64% to 46%. Recurrent neovascularization developed in one-half of laser-treated eyes, usually in the first year after treatment. Recurrent neovascularization was invariably associated with the development of severe visual loss (Figure 59–3).

In eyes with juxtafoveal choroidal neovascularization (1 to 199 microns from the foveal center), krypton laser photocoagulation diminished the incidence of severe visual loss from 45% to 31% at 1 year, although the difference between untreated and treated groups was less marked at 5 years. The benefit of treatment was di-

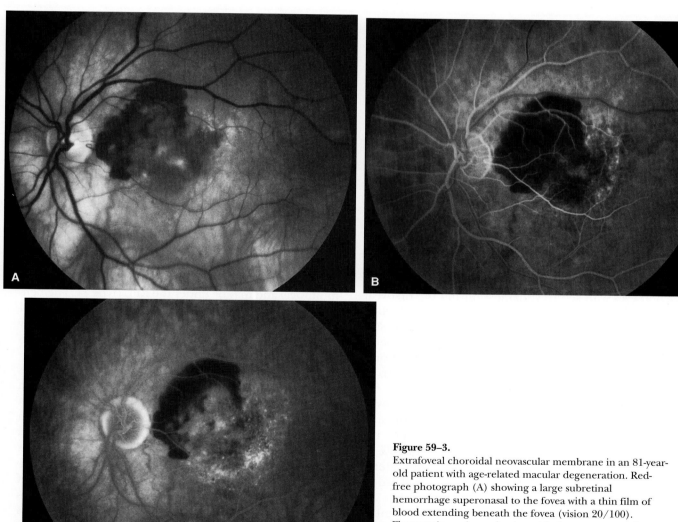

Figure 59–3.
Extrafoveal choroidal neovascular membrane in an 81-year-old patient with age-related macular degeneration. Red-free photograph (A) showing a large subretinal hemorrhage superonasal to the fovea with a thin film of blood extending beneath the fovea (vision 20/100). Fluorescein angiography shows blockage corresponding to subretinal hemorrhage in the early phase (B) with leakage superonasal to the fovea in the late phase (C). Prominent staining of drusen and window defects are present elsewhere. One year later, red-free photograph *(continued)*

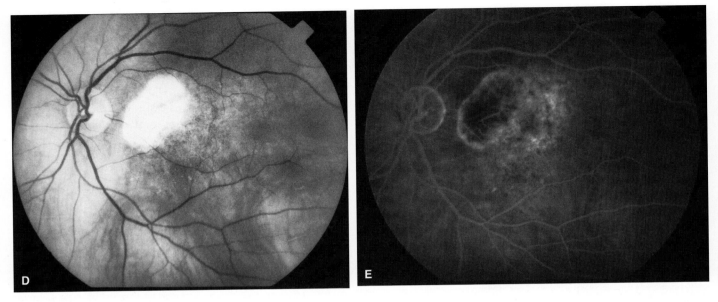

Figure 59–3. *(continued)*
(D) illustrates the laser scar and later phases of the angiogram (E) show blockage corresponding to a 2 disc area extrafoveal laser lesion nasal to the fovea with prominent staining of drusen in the foveal area, but no sign of recurrence (vision 20/60).

minished in patients diagnosed with hypertension. As in the extrafoveal study, recurrences occurred in one-half of the laser-treated eyes, though in 32% of laser-treated eyes such events were thought to represent persistent neovascularization instead of true recurrences owing to their development shortly after the initial treatment.

In eyes with subfoveal choroidal neovascularization of less than 3.5 disc areas, krypton or argon laser photocoagulation reduced the incidence of severe visual loss at 2 and 3 years, from 38% to 21% and 42% to 28%, respectively. Of note was the higher proportion of laser-treated eyes with severe visual loss during the first year of follow-up because of the immediate visual reduction associated with foveal ablation. Subgroup analysis suggests that smaller lesions may exhibit a treatment benefit sooner than larger lesions. Again, approximately one-half of laser-treated eyes developed recurrent neovascularization (Figure 59–4).

In eyes with recurrent subfoveal choroidal neovascularization of less than 6 disc areas total lesion size, krypton or argon laser photocoagulation reduced the incidence of severe visual loss at 2 years from 28% to 9%. Treatment benefit was not observed until after 6 months, because of an average immediate visual reduction of 3 lines associated with foveal ablation.

The role of surgical excision in the management of choroidal neovascular membranes is unclear. Vitreoretinal surgery with excision of the CNVM is a viable and technically feasible alternative for patients with well-defined, large subfoveal neovascular membranes (16,

50). This procedure involves completing a pars plana vitrectomy with stripping of the posterior hyaloid (if still attached), making a small access retinotomy with a 36 G sharp spatula, and grasping and excising the CNVM with horizontal subretinal forceps. Preliminary results of small, nonrandomized studies have suggested a benefit of this procedure in patients with POHS, inflammatory and idiopathic CNVMs. All of these neovascular membranes are usually located under the neurosensory retina (type 2) and unifocal in origin, as opposed to the neovascular membranes in ARMD, which are usually multifocal and may be under the RPE (type 1). The benefit of vitreoretinal surgery with excision of the CNVM in patients with ARMD is unanswered and is currently under study in the Submacular Surgery Study, a multicenter, randomized clinical trial.

The hypothesized role of oxidative stress on the RPE in the pathogenesis of AMD has stimulated interest in the medical treatment of the early stages of AMD with antioxidants including zinc, beta carotene, and vitamin E. Zinc interacts with proteins to protect sulfhydryl groups from oxidative damage. Beta carotene reduces light toxicosis in experimental models. Clinical evidence suggests that patients with higher serum levels of beta carotene may have a lower risk of neovascular complications of ARMD. Vitamin E deficiency exacerbates light toxicosis in experimental models. Nonetheless, to date, no evidence conclusively supports or refutes the benefit of dietary supplementation with antioxidants.

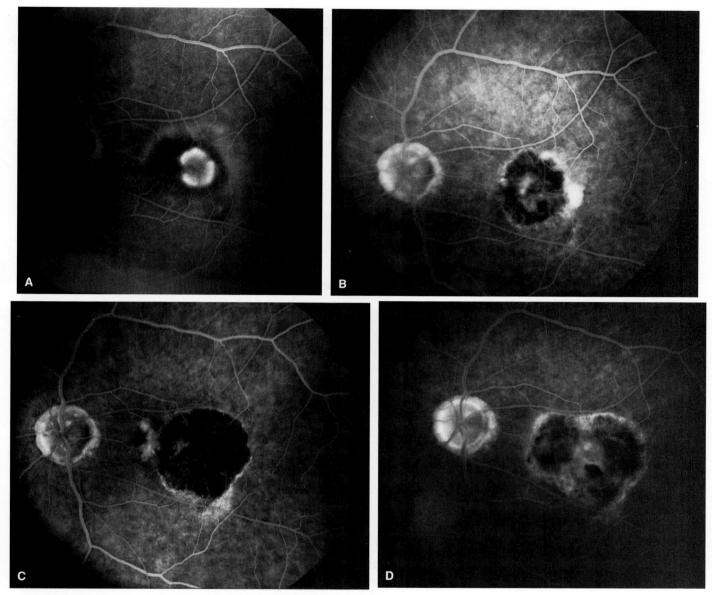

Figure 59–4.
Subfoveal choroidal neovascular membrane in a 74-year-old patient with age-related macular degeneration. Fluorescein angiograms before laser photocoagulation (A) (vision 20/200), temporal recurrence 3 months after treatment (B) nasal recurrence 16 months after treatment (C) and stable laser scar without recurrence 20 months after treatment (D) (vision 2/200).

■ IDIOPATHIC CENTRAL SEROUS CHOROIDOPATHY

Idiopathic central serous choroidopathy (ICSC) is a fairly common disorder characterized by the development of a small, shallow, neurosensory detachment in the central macula. Affected patients are 20 to 50 years old. Males are 10 times more likely to be affected than females. The disorder is uncommon in blacks. Although bilaterality is common, typically, both eyes are not simultaneously affected.

Presenting symptoms include mildly decreased vision associated with micropsia, metamorphopsia, mild color deficits, paracentral scotomas, and difficulties with stereopsis (12). Some patients may be correctable to 20/20 with the addition of plus sphere (hyperopic shift).

Ophthalmoscopy shows loss of the foveal reflex associated with a round, well-demarcated, shallow, serous elevation of the neurosensory retina, typically of approximately 3 disc areas (Fig. 59–5). Beneath the detachment one or more 200 to 300 micron yellow-gray focal detachments of the RPE may be observed. Dotlike subretinal precipitates may be present. Less commonly, the subretinal fluid may be turbid. Atrophic subretinal tracts may be seen as well.

Fluorescein angiography shows one or more focal

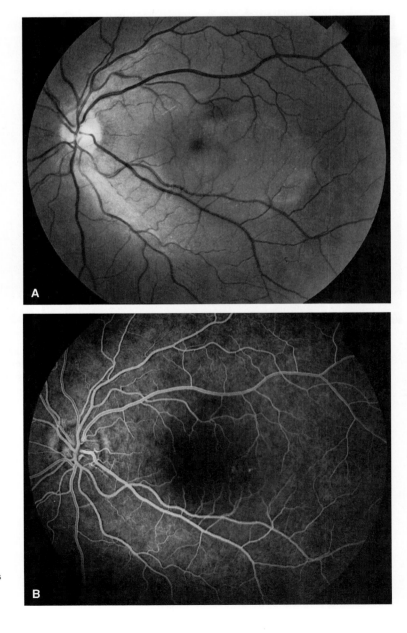

Figure 59–5.
Idiopathic central serous choroidopathy in a 34-year-old male. Red-free photograph (A) shows a well-demarcated oval area of subretinal fluid with small white subretinal precipitates. Fluorescein angiography shows late development of pinpoint hyperfluorescence which diffuses like a flume of smoke to gradually pool within the area of neuruosensory detachment (B through E). *(continued)*

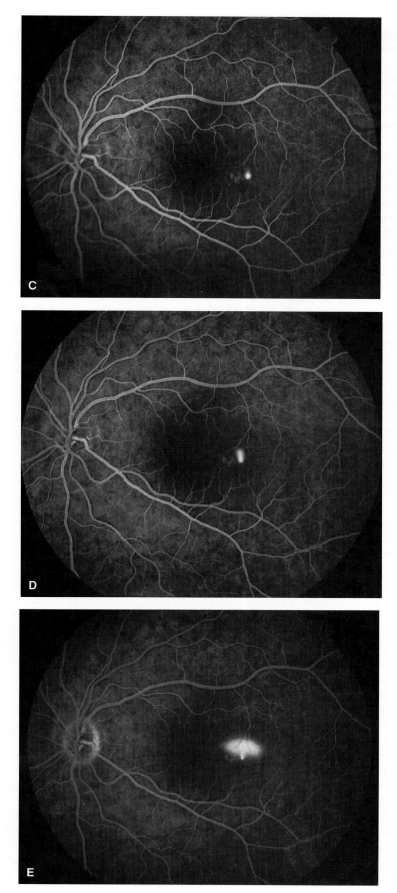

Figure 59–5. *(continued)*

spots of hyperfluorescence at the level of the pigment epithelium in the arteriovenous phase of the angiogram which gradually leak and irregularly pool in the space defined by the neurosensory detachment (Figure 59–5). In less than 10% of cases a "smokestack pattern" of leakage is observed in which a plume of fluorescein dye first heads superiorly from the leakage site before fanning out to occupy the subretinal detachment. Theoretically, this phenomenon is the result of an osmotic density gradient formed by the gravitational pull on the proteinaceous component of the subretinal fluid inferiorly. A leakage site should be definable in every case. A solitary leakage site is seen in nearly three-quarters of cases. If a leakage site is not observed it is often helpful to look for tracts of atrophic RPE with whose help one may occasionally identify an extramacular leakage site. More typically, leakage sites occur within the area of neurosensory detachment.

The etiology and pathophysiology of ICSC is controversial. Focal disruptions of the RPE, as in a photocoagulation burn, do not typically produce serous retinal detachment since the net oncotic and hydrostatic forces still favor flow in a retinochoroidal direction. For this reason some have suggested a reversal of the active transport function of RPE at the leak site with consequent active pumping of ions and water into the subretinal space by these cells. Still others have implicated a more global dysfunction of the surrounding pigment epithelium since one would expect the normally vigorous pumping function of these cells to compensate for the additional fluid load. One final proposed pathophysiologic theory is that ICSC may be the result of an abnormality in the choroidal circulation with choriocapillaris hyperpermeability.

An intriguing association is the predominance of type A behavioral characteristics in affected patients (54). Moreover, patients will often concede that their ocular disease coincided with a period of particular stress. Pregnancy, organ transplantation, and the use of corticosteroids have also been reported to induce or in association with ICSC. The ability of repeated intravenous epinephrine injections in monkeys to induce an experimental model of ICSC has given credibility to the stress theories of disease and may implicate responsiveness of the choriocapillaries to stress hormones in the ultimate pathobiology of this disease.

In the majority of patients the disease is self-limited with resolution of the serous detachment occurring in 2 to 6 months (21, 30). However, despite the return of vision to 20/20 to 20/25 in most cases, permanent deficits in color vision and contrast sensitivity often remain. Prospective randomized trials (42) of focal laser treatment directed at the site of leakage have shown that while treatment is successful in shortening the course of disease, it has no long-term visual benefit, does not decrease the rate of recurrence, which may be seen in 40 to 50% of the patients, and does not diminish the risk of development of chronic disease. The side effect of laser treatment in ICSC is the small but present risk of iatrogenic choroidal neovascularization. Currently, indications for laser rely upon the immediate visual needs of the patient.

■ CYSTOID MACULAR EDEMA

Cystoid macula edema (CME) is a common ocular abnormality resulting from a diverse group of etiologies. Strictly defined, these etiologies share an ability to perturb the integrity of the blood-retinal barrier of the perifoveal capillaries and the optic nerve head such that leakage of fluorescein dye can be observed by angiography with accumulation of fluid as microcysts in the outer plexiform layer. Causes include postcataract or laser capsulotomy (Irvine-Gass syndrome), diabetic macular edema, uveitis, branch or central vein occlusion, topical epinephrine use, severe hypertension, radiation retinopathy, perifoveal telangiectasia, and retinitis pigmentosa. Syndromes which exhibit cystic spaces in the fovea, but do not exhibit pooling of fluorescein dye on angiography, should be separated from our discussion as they likely represent an altogether separate pathobiological category. These include juvenile retinoschisis, nicotinic acid maculopathy, and some cases of retinitis pigmentosa.

The Irvine-Gass syndrome is the most common cause of poor visual outcome after uncomplicated cataract surgery (25, 26). Angiographic evidence of CME is present in one-half of intracapsular surgeries and one-fifth of extracapsular surgeries, occurring 4 to 12 weeks after the operation. The vast majority of these cases resolve spontaneously without treatment with only 1% percent of patients progressing to chronic disease. Causes include vitreous incarceration to the cataract wound, vitreous adhesion to the iris, mechanical irritation of the iris by the intraocular lens, vitreoretinal traction, or nonspecific postoperative inflammation. Rupture of the posterior capsule and anterior hyaloid face either at the time of surgery or by subsequent laser capsulotomy may contribute to the pathogenesis of disease by facilitating diffusion of inflammatory mediators from the anterior segment back to the retina. Presently, prostaglandins have been singled out as the most likely inflammatory mediators involved given their propensity to increase capillary permeability and the detection of increased anterior chamber levels of prostaglandin in patients with CME. The diminished incidence of CME after placement of an ultraviolet-blocking intraocular lens compared with an uncoated lens suggests that the ability of ultraviolet light to stimulate the release of free radicals at the level of the retina may also contribute to this disease.

Symptoms consist of blurred central vision with significantly delayed reading speeds. Ophthalmoscopy shows loss of the foveal light reflex with a translucent appearance. Occasionally, a yellowish appearance to the fovea is seen. A few perifoveal dot hemorrhages may be present. Rarely, one may be aware of a small amount of disc edema. Contact lens biomicroscopy is the preferred method of examination since this allows the stereopsis and magnification required to visualize the individual cystic compartments. Rarely, cystic spaces coalesce and advance to produce a lamellar hole but more commonly this may represent a failure to be aware of the thin anterior wall of a large, intact cyst.

Fluorescein angiography (Figure 59–6) shows multiple focal areas of hyperfluorescence at the level of the retina in the perifoveal area during the arteriovenous phase which increases in fluorescence and pools dye in a flower petal ("petaloid") pattern in the recirculation phase of the study. Typically late fluorescein staining of the disc is also present (Figure 59–6c).

Histopathologic studies show the presence of extracellular cystic spaces containing proteinaceous material in the inner nuclear and outer plexiform layers. Subsequent photoreceptor cell loss is well described.

Given the spontaneous resolution of most cases of postoperative CME, evaluation of the efficacy of various treatments is difficult. In lieu of evidence showing clear benefit to any one therapy, one should seek to identify the specific etiology of CME in a given patient, and then begin with the least toxic therapeutic alternatives. Cases in which vitreous incarceration, iridic irritation, or vitreomacular traction can be identified, and CME which is not responsive to topical antiinflammatory agents, should undergo pars plana vitrectomy to correct the anatomic alterations (14). Occasionally, YAG laser lysis of a strand of incarcerated vitreous may be successful. Cases in which no anatomic etiology can be found may benefit from therapeutic trials of topical nonsteroidal antiinflammatory agents, topical steroids, oral acetazolamide, (7) posterior subtenons steroid injection, or pars plana vitrectomy.

■ MACULAR EPIRETINAL MEMBRANE

Epiretinal membranes (45, 48) (ERMs), also known as macular puckers, cellophane membranes, or preretinal macular fibrosis, represent cellular proliferation and collagen deposition on the retinal surface. Autopsy studies have shown that approximately 2% of the normal population have ERMs, although the vast majority of ERMs do not impair vision. In addition to the idiopathic development of ERMs, some conditions appear to stimulate ERM growth including vitreous hemorrhage, retinal tears, cryopexy, photocoagulation, trauma, proliferate vitreoretinopathy, diabetic retinopathy, papillitis and uveitis. ERMs are commonly encountered after retinal detachment repair where they complicate 4 to 8% of cases.

Clinical symptoms depend on membrane location and thickness, as well as the degree of retinal distortion. Thin membranes with no distortion are frequently completely asymptomatic. In more advanced cases, symptoms include diminished central vision and metamorphopsia.

Early membranes are seen best as a cellophane-like reflection on the retinal surface. Often red-free photographs or green illumination with the direct ophthalmoscope is helpful. With more progressive disease, retinal striae, distortion of the perifoveal vessels, and focal tractional detachment may be seen (Figure 59–7). Membranes which complicate proliferative vitreoretinopathy tend to be the thickest and most opaque. Idiopathic ERMs tend to be thinner. Macular edema may be present. Pseudoholes are often present in idiopathic membranes. These often occur over the fovea, perhaps relating to attachments of the posterior cortical vitreous fibers in the perifoveal regions. Macular cysts and holes are known to be associated with macular ERMs and in certain cases thought to be involved in their development. Previous teachings emphasized the requirement of a posterior vitreous detachment (PVD) to allow cellular access to the epiretinal space for membranes to grow. While approximately three-quarters of ERMs are associated with a PVD, ERMs may clearly develop in the absence of a PVD as is frequently encountered with ERMs associated with macular cysts and holes (See Section IV). In these instances the ERM appears to represent cellular infiltration of the remaining attached posterior cortical vitreous. As such these membranes can be seen to insert at the optic nerve head as does cortical vitreous.

Fluorescein angiography can be helpful both in

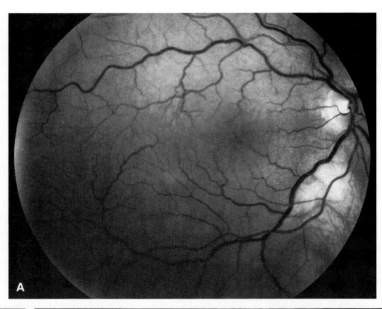

Figure 59–6.
Pseudophakic cystoid macular edema seen 5
weeks after uncomplicated cataract surgery in
a healthy 67-year-old patient. Note the
absence of the foveal depression in the red-
free photograph (A). The arteriovenous phase
of the angiogram (B) shows pinpoint areas of
hyperfluorescence surrounding the fovea, and
intense pooling of fluorescein dye within
cystic foveal spaces (the so-called petaloid or
flowerlike pattern). Characteristic staining of
the optic disc is seen in the late phase (C).

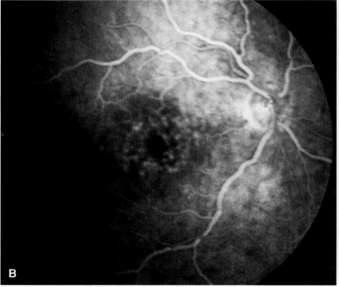

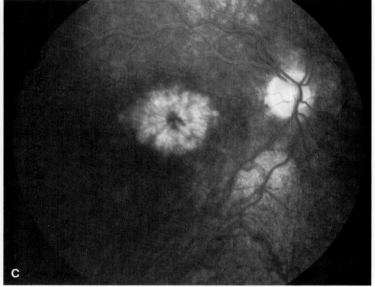

highlighting the degree of mechanical distortion of the
retinal vasculature and in evaluating the presence of
retinovascular leakage associated with the membrane.
When present, this usually appears as a poorly-defined
area of late leakage with no defined origin. The absence
of leakage on angiography portends a better visual prognosis after surgery.

Histopathologic characterization of the cells responsible for epiretinal membrane development has been a
longstanding area of interest and debate. Although earlier studies showed the presence of fibroblasts, extracellular collagen deposition, and pigment clumps, im-
munocytochemical and electron microscopic studies
have now shown that the cellular component of epiretinal membranes actually represent cells of both retinal
glial and pigment epithelial origin. Glial cell types tend
to predominate idiopathic membranes, whereas pigmented epithelial cells tend to predominate retinal detachment associated membranes. Although the origin
of the pigmented epithelial cells is thought to be a result
of dispersion and migration of RPE through the retinal
breaks, such cell types are also present in idiopathic
membranes in which no retinal breaks can be identified. This suggests that both glial and epithelial cell

types within epiretinal membranes gain access to the retinal surface by migration though the retina or ciliary body, or are derived by transformation of other cell types such as vitreous hyalocytes.

The treatment of visually significant ERMs requires surgical excision by pars plana vitrectomy with membrane peeling (25). Recurrence of membranes after surgical excision is uncommon except in the case of children, diabetic retinopathy, proliferative vitreoretinopathy and peripheral vasculopathies including retinopathy of prematurity (9).

Retinal reattachment rates and visual results have improved significantly with the development and the use of newer, more refined vitreoretinal techniques and instrumentation, panoramic viewing systems, and the perfluorocarbon liquids (PFCL) (6). The PFCLs are heavier than water liquids with an increased specific gravity (1.76 to 1.92), decreased viscosity, and increased vapor pressures which are excellent for flattening the retina without the need for posterior drainage retinotomies. The PFCLs can also be used to stabilize the retina if anterior membrane dissection and/or relaxing retinotomies are needed. These liquids are also helpful in the evaluation of any residual traction from preretinal or subretinal membranes.

The perfluorocarbon liquids are also an invaluable tool in the surgical management of giant retinal tears, dislocated lens fragments and IOLs, combined tractional/rhegmatogenous retinal detachments, and traumatic retinal detachments.

■ PRESUMED OCULAR HISTOPLASMOSIS SYNDROME
(see Uveitis, Chapter 34)

Histoplasmosis (46, 51) is a typically self-limited minimally symptomatic, respiratory and systemic fungal infection often occurring in childhood in certain endemic areas including the Ohio and Mississippi river valleys and western Maryland. Humans appear to be infected by inhalation of aerosolized spores from soil contamination with the excrement of birds and chickens. Epidemiologic evidence supports an etiologic relationship of this infection with the later development of a characteristic syndrome of multifocal, atrophic chorioretinal lesions, peripapillary atrophy, and macular choroidal neovascularization.

Histoplasmosis capsulatum is a dimorphic fungus occurring in a filamentous form in soil and as an intracellular yeast form in humans. After pulmonary infection, the organism undergoes hematogenous spread to multiple organs including the choroid. Experimental studies suggest that hematogenous spread to the choroid is quickly followed by focal granuloma formation which destroys the organism and often leaves behind an area of focal choroidal atrophy. These findings explain both the occurrence of characteristic chorioretinal scars in 2 to 3% of individuals in endemic areas, as well as the inability to conclusively identify the presence of fungi later in the disease when ocular symptoms occur.

Patients are not aware of ocular symptoms unless the disease is complicated by choroidal neovascularization. The average age of presentation is the fourth or fifth decade of life. Usual complaints include blurred vision and metamorphopsia. Ophthalmoscopic findings include subretinal hemorrhage, fluid, or exudates within the macula. A grayish-green area of subretinal neovascularization may be identifiable (Figure 59–8). Sharply-defined, "punched out," depigmented 400 to 750 micron diameter lesions are present in the midperiphery and posterior pole. A variable amount of pigment clumping may be present in the center of the lesion. Peripapillary choroidal atrophy and hyperpigmentation is typically present. Vitreous cells are absent.

Fluorescein angiography is essential to identify and characterize choroidal neovascularization in symptomatic patients. In the vast majority of cases, neovascularization arises from an atrophic macular lesion. In other cases it may arise from peripapillary neovascularization.

Histoplasmin antigen skin testing will reliably identify the majority of those patients with endemic exposure. Skin testing is no longer done, however, since such exposure information is also obtainable from the history and because of the risk of reactivation of an immune response to ocular lesions in response to skin testing. Assays for circulating antibody levels against histoplasmosis are present in only one-third of patients, presumably related to the distant nature of the exposure. An increase prevalence of HLA-B7 and HLA-DR2 antigens have been noted in patients with neovascular complications of POHS.

The Macular Photocoagulation Study (31,33,37) has shown laser photocoagulation to be of benefit in treating certain extrafoveal and juxtafoveal choroidal neovascular membranes complicating POHS. Five-year results from the extrafoveal study ≥200 microns from the foveal center) show that treatment is associated with a 68% versus 43% chance of maintaining 20/40 vision and a 6% versus 22% risk of losing six or more lines of

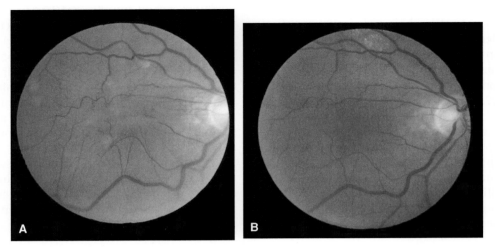

Figure 59–7.
Epiretinal membrane in a 70-year-old. Proliferation of cells on the surface of the retina prodcues the glistening sheen visible (A). Contraction of the fibrous component of the membrane causes distortion of the parafoveal vessels. After vitrectomy with membrane peeling (B), the configuration of the retinal vasculature is restored.

Snellen acuity. Recurrences after treatment occurred in 26% of cases with 80% of recurrences occurring with the first year. Three year results from the juxtafoveal study (1–199 microns from the foveal center) show that treatment versus no treatment is associated with a 50% versus 41% chance of maintaining <=20/40 vision and a 5% versus 25% risk of losing six or more lines of Snellen acuity.

Unlike age-related macular degeneration, no studies are available which support photocoagulation of subfoveal choroidal neovascular membranes in POHS. The lower incidence of severe visual loss in POHS, as well as the documented occurrence of spontaneous membrane involution in some (14%) patients, largely precludes any visual benefit from foveal ablation. This group of patients may benefit from surgical excision of the subfoveal membrane; however, the long-term benefit of such intervention awaits further study. Treatment of choroidal neovascularization with steroids is of unproven benefit. A 1 in 5 risk is present for the developing choroidal neovascularization in the fellow eye within 10 years. Patients with atrophic chorioretinal lesions present in the macula of the fellow eye appear to be at highest risk.

■ MACULAR HOLE

The thinness and avascularity of the foveal region predisposes it to the development of full-thickness dehiscence known as a macular hole (18, 19, 28). This condition usually occurs idiopathically in women in their sixth through eighth decades; however, it may also occur after trauma, solar injury, lightning injury, scleral buckling, or in staphylomatous eyes. Symptoms include metamorphopsia and diminished acuity. Often the visual deterioration is gradual rather than abrupt.

Full-thickness macular holes appear ophthalmoscopically as a reddish, round foveal lesion 500 to 750 microns in diameter (13). A cuff of neurosensory detachment surrounding the hole is usually present. Cystic retinal change and epiretinal membrane formation are often observed. Yellow deposits are invariably present at the base of the hole and probably represent lipofuscin-laden macrophages or nodular proliferations of the retinal pigment epithelium. When a thin slit beam is projected across the hole, patients will describe a break in the beam (positive Watzke sign). When presented with a small point of light, patients will often reliably fixate upon it, typically at the inferior or superior edge of the hole.

Attempts to better understand the pathobiology of macular hole formation has led to the clinical staging of macular hole lesions (Table 59–1). Stage 1 describes loss of the foveal depression associated with a yellow foveal spot or ring, perhaps because of increased visibility of xanthophyll pigment. With progressive thinning of the fovea the lesion may obtain a reddish appearance. At this stage patients will not report a Watzke sign. Fluorescein angiography appears normal or may show faint hyperfluorescence. Stage 2 describes the early development of an eccentric full thickness dehiscence. The rate of progression of stage 1 to stage 2 lesions is unclear; however, perhaps as many as one-third undergo sponta-

TABLE 59–1
Stages of Idiopathic Macular Holes

Stage I	Premacular hole, impending hole
IA	Foveal yellow spot
IB	Foveal yellow ring
	Loss of foveal depression
	Negative Watzke's sign
	Visual acuity 20/25 to 20/70
Stage II	Eccentric full-thickness macular hole
Stage III	Full-thickness macular hole
	Cuff of subretinal fluid
	Yellow deposits at base of hole
	Operculum anterior to fovea
	Positive Watzke's sign
	Visual acuity 20/70 to 20/400
Stage IV	Full-thickness macular hole with posterior vitreous detachment
	Positive Watzke's sign

neous resolution. Stage 3 represents a round full-thickness macular hole, characteristically with yellow deposits at its base and a cuff of neurosensory detachment (Figure 59–9). A complete posterior vitreous detachment is lacking, although a partial vitreous detachment may be present over the fovea. When this occurs one can usually see a small operculum from the macular hole suspended just anterior to the fovea. Development of a complete posterior vitreous detachment with a Weiss ring defines stage 4. The vast majority of patients with full thickness macular holes do not have complete posterior vitreous detachments. In contrast, most do have a prominent posterior vitreous syneretic cavity.

While this may be confused with a PVD, no Weiss ring is present.

The pathophysiology of macular hole formation is now thought to be explained by tangential traction across the retinal surface induced by the posterior cortical vitreous with involvement of fluid movement within the posterior vitreous syneresis cavity. The rationale for this theory rests upon the protective effect of PVD development on future hole development and the lack of evidence for foveal elevation anterior to the surface of the surrounding retina in stages 1 and 2 as would be expected if anteroposterior traction were the culprit.

The development of full-thickness macular holes from macular cysts should probably be considered as an altogether separate pathobiologic category. Such cysts are often associated with anteroposterior vitreoretinal traction. Fluorescein angiography shows distortion of the perifoveal capillaries but is otherwise normal. Faint foveal hyperfluorescence may be seen but petaloid edema is absent. In these patients, macular hole formation can be associated with progression to a complete posterior vitreous detachment.

The differential diagnosis of macular holes includes pseudoholes in epiretinal membranes, thin-walled cystoid macular edema, and macular cysts.

The treatment of macular holes is unclear. Preliminary results of vitreous surgery with peeling of the posterior cortical vitreous and gas tamponade for full thickness holes are encouraging (29). The use of tissue adhesives such as autologous serum, and plasma/thrombin may be a valuable adjunct in their surgical treatment. Surgical intervention may be reasonable for the 20 to 30% of patients in whom bilateral disease develops.

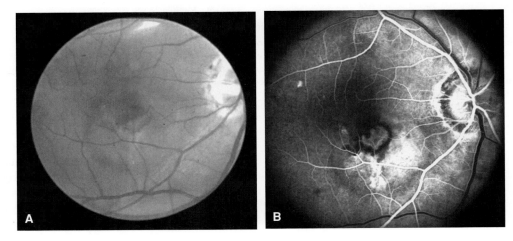

Figure 59–8.
Presumed ocular histoplasmosis syndrome in a middle-aged patient. A gray-green subfoveal lesion with adjacent subretinal hemorrhage (A) can be better delineated on angiography (B) as a choroidal neovascular membrane. Other stigmata of POHS include peripapillary atrophy and punched-out chorioretinal scars.

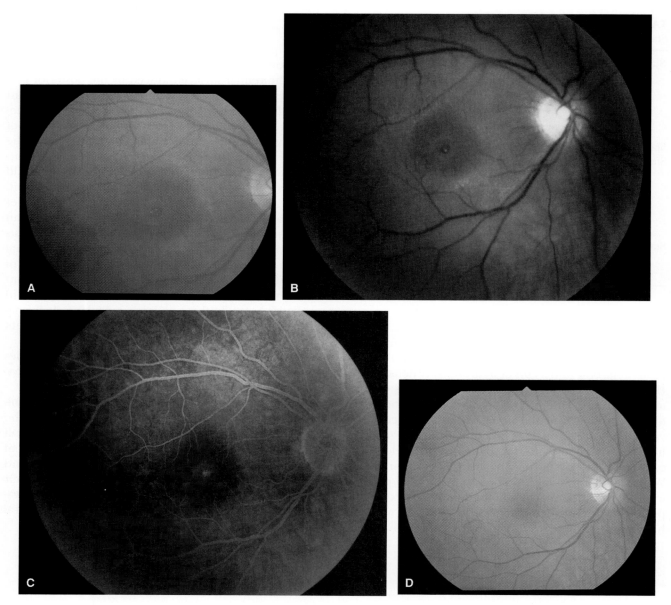

Figure 59–9.
Stage 3 macular hole in a 45-year-old female. Color photograph (A) shows a 400 micron full-thickness hole, small cuff of subretinal fluid and yellow precipitates on the retinal pigment epithelium within the hole (vision 20/80). Red-free photograph (B) shows a reflective sheen corresponding to an intact shell of posterior hyaloid vitreous on the macular surface. Fluorescein angiography (C) highlights abnormal transmission of choroidal fluorescence within the fovea because of absence of overlying xanthophyll pigment. After surgical repair (D), the hole is no longer apparent (vision 20/30).

■ ANGIOID STREAKS

Angioid streaks (5) are red-brown, spoke-like lesions with irregular contours which emanate from the peripapillary region in a radial fashion. They derive their name from their misleading resemblance to blood vessels. Angioid streaks represent cracklike dehiscences in Bruch's membrane with secondary calcification. Additional findings include an "orange-peel" (peau d'orange) appearance of the retinal pigment epithelium in the midperipheral region as well as optic disc drusen.

Patients are typically asymptomatic unless they experience central visual loss related to choroidal neovascularization. The incidence of choroidal neovascularization is increased, occurring in over half of the patients. Minor trauma may be associated with subretinal hemorrhages which are likely related to the increased susceptibility of the eyes to choroidal rupture.

Systemic associations are found in over half of patients with angioid streaks (Table 59–2). Pseudoxanthoma elasticum (PXE) is the most commonly found association. PXE is a rare autosomal recessive or dominant connective tissue disorder affecting elastic tissues of the skin, heart and gastrointestinal systems. Patients with PXE have redundant, "plucked chicken" skin, often apparent on the neck or axilla. Skin biopsy shows pathognomonic elastic tissue staining with associated calcification. Myocardial infarction and gastrointestinal bleeding may occur. Patients with PXE have an 85% incidence of angioid streaks. Other conditions associated with angioid streaks include Paget's disease, sickle cell disease (most commonly the SS form), and rarely, the Ehlers-Danlos syndrome, an uncommon dis-

TABLE 59–2
Differential Diagnosis of Angioid Streaks

Diagnosis	Key Clinical Features
Pseudoxanthoma	redundant, "plucked chicken" skin
	hypertension
	weak peripheral pulses
	gastrointestinal bleeding
Ehlers-Danlos syndrome	blue sclera
	joint hyperextensibility
	fragile, elastic skin
	excessive bruising
Paget's disease	extraskeletal calcification
	bony erosion and abnormal formation
	osteoarthritis
	hearing loss, vertigo, tinnitus
	slurred speech, difficulty swallowing
Sickle cell disease	hemoglobin SS (most frequently)
	anemia
Idiopathic	vaso-occlusive crises

order of skin elasticity, joint flexibility, blue sclera, and retinal detachment.

The differential diagnosis of angioid streaks includes choroidal rupture and lacquer cracks in myopes.

Laser treatment of extrafoveal choroidal neovascularization associated with angioid streaks appears to be successful; however recurrences are unusually frequent (20) (Figure 59–10). Safety glasses and abstinence from contact sports should be considered.

■ MYOPIC DEGENERATION

Myopia is a common ocular abnormality; however, pathologic changes occur in only a small fraction. Myopic degeneration encompasses a spectrum of changes associated with increased axial length and enlargement of the globe. Manifestations include posterior staphyloma and increased incidence of retinal breaks. Staphyloma occur secondary to scleral thinning and ectasia. Myopic fundi may appear less pigmented because of

thinning and atrophy of the retina. Breaks in Bruch's membrane, known as lacquer cracks, may be found in pathologic myopia. Subretinal hemorrhages and the subsequent chorioretinal scarring at these sites are called Fuchs spots. Subretinal choroidal neovascularization may occur secondarily at sites of lacquer cracks (Figure 59–11).

■ ACUTE POSTERIOR MULTIFOCAL PLACOID PIGMENT EPITHELIOPATHY (see uveitus chapter, Chapter 35)

Acute posterior multifocal placoid pigment epitheliopathy (15, 44) (APMPPE) is a rare, self-limited, inflammatory disease of otherwise young, healthy adults. One or both eyes may be affected. Patients present with

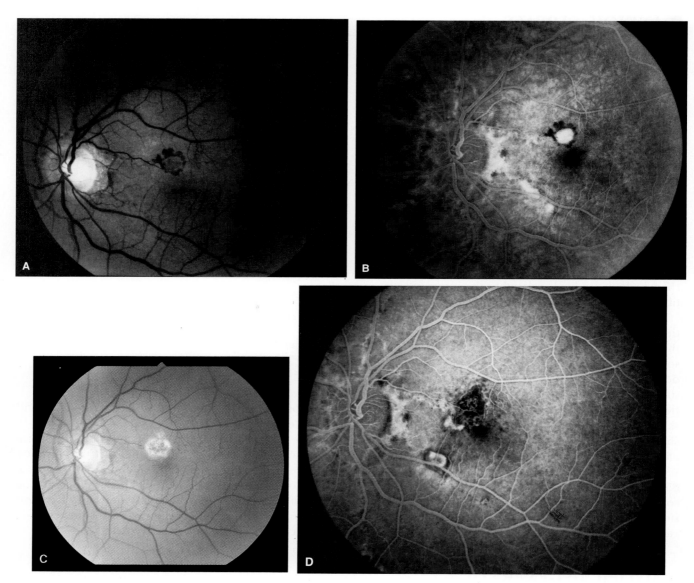

Figure 59–10.
Angioid streaks with a choroidal neovascular membrane in a 44-year-old female. Red-free photograph (A) shows an extrafoveal choroidal neovascular membrane surrounded by a halo of subretinal hemorrhage. The midphase angiogram (B) illustrates window defect along angioid streaks, as well as hyperfluorescence from a choroidal neovascular membrane arising from an angioid streak, just superior to the fovea. Color photograph (C) shows the area of laser photocoagulation. Six months later, the fluorescein angiogram (D) shows two areas of choroidal neovascularization.

a history of abrupt central or paracentral visual loss, often after a flulike illness. Central vision may drop profoundly, occasionally to the count fingers level.

Ophthalmoscopy shows patchy, creamy yellow lesions with soft borders at the level of the retinal pigment epithelium in the posterior pole and macula. Individual lesions may be 750 to 2000 microns in size but often become confluent. Over the subsequent 1 to 2 weeks, the lesions fade, leaving behind granular pigment epithelial changes.

Fluorescein angiography shows blockage of choroidal fluorescence by the lesions in the arterial phase of the angiogram with late staining of the edges of the lesions.

Associated findings include uveitis, serous retinal detachment, cerebral vasculitis, cerebrospinal fluid pleocytosis, headache, dysacousia, and tinnitus.

The differential diagnosis includes serpiginous choroiditis and Vogt-Koyangi-Harada disease. These diseases are distinguished by their somewhat different clinical appearance and their different clinical course.

Debate has ensued regarding whether APMPPE represents a disorder of the retinal pigment epithelium or choroidal vasculature. Angiographic evidence lends support to either theory as the blockage of lesions early in the angiogram might be explained by swollen opaque pigment epithelial cells or by focal hypoperfusion of discrete lobules of the choriocapillaris. Current opinion favors a pigment epithelial origin of the disorder.

The natural history of APMPPE is one of spontaneous improvement over several weeks in the majority of patients. Eighty percent of patients regain 20/40 or better acuity. Recurrences are unusually rare. The disease is not associated with later development of choroidal neovascularization.

Typically, no treatment is indicated. The use of oral corticosteroids for particularly severe cases of APMPPE is of unproven benefit.

■ MULTIPLE EVANESCENT WHITE DOT SYNDROME (see Uveitis, Chapter 36)

Multiple evanescent white dot syndrome (MEWDS) described by Jampol et al (10) predominantly affects young women often with a history of a previous viral infection. Patients present with sudden, unilateral decrease in vision.

Fundoscopy shows many discrete 50 to 100 micron dots at the level of the RPE or outer retina in the posterior pole. The dots may appear and disappear over several days. There may be a mild vitritis (see Tables 2–1, 4–3).

No treatment is available. Recovery of vision over several months is the general rule. Recurrences may occur in 10%.

■ LEBER'S IDIOPATHIC STELLATE NEURORETINITIS

Leber's idiopathic stellate neuroretinitis (11) (LISN) is a rare, predominantly unilateral, self-limited, benign condition usually affecting patient in their 20s and 30s. A viral etiology has been postulated since many patients have a flulike prodrome. Cat-scratch disease and leptospirosis have also been reported in association with LISN.

Patient present with an acute decrease in vision and an afferent pupillary defect. Optic disc edema occurs early with exudation of subretinal fluid. Formation of a macular star follows a week later (Figure 59–10a). Mild anterior and vitreous inflammation may be present.

Leakage on fluorescein angiography occurs from the optic nerve capillaries and not from the parafoveal capillaries.

Visual acuity returns to normal in the majority of patients as the exudative fluid resorbs over 6 to 8 weeks. The macular star resolves more slowly. Retinal pigment epithelial atrophy and optic disc pallor are uncommon sequelae.

Differential diagnosis includes anterior ischemic optic neuropathy, systemic hypertension, syphilis, and papillophlebitis.

■ MULTIFOCAL CHOROIDITIS WITH PANUVEITIS (see Uveitis, Chapter 36)

In the mid-1980s, a clinical picture was described which resembled the presumed ocular histoplasmosis syndrome but differed from it in several important respects. Like POHS, the syndrome was characterized by

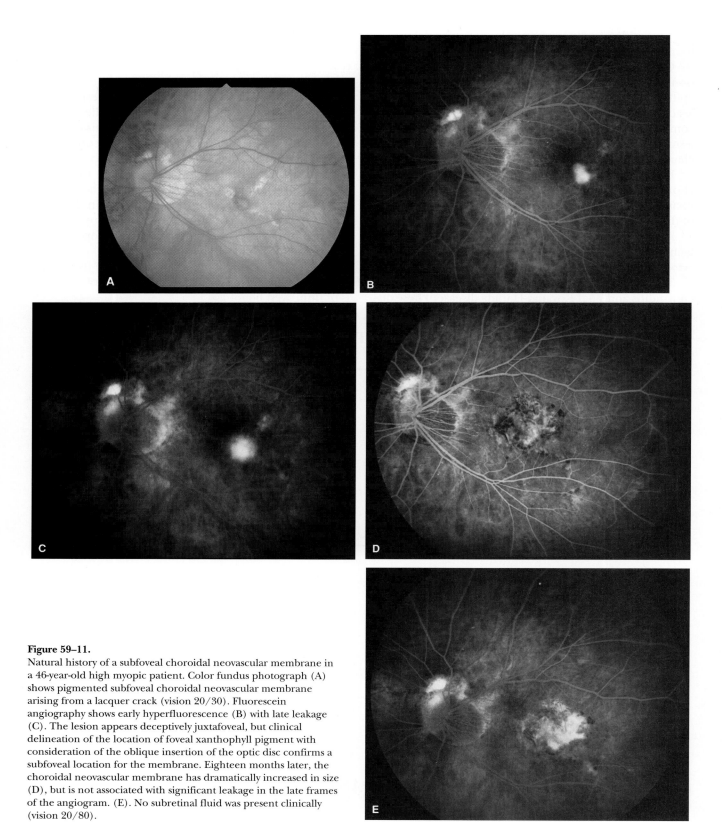

Figure 59–11.
Natural history of a subfoveal choroidal neovascular membrane in
a 46-year-old high myopic patient. Color fundus photograph (A)
shows pigmented subfoveal choroidal neovascular membrane
arising from a lacquer crack (vision 20/30). Fluorescein
angiography shows early hyperfluorescence (B) with late leakage
(C). The lesion appears deceptively juxtafoveal, but clinical
delineation of the location of foveal xanthophyll pigment with
consideration of the oblique insertion of the optic disc confirms a
subfoveal location for the membrane. Eighteen months later, the
choroidal neovascular membrane has dramatically increased in size
(D), but is not associated with significant leakage in the late frames
of the angiogram. (E). No subretinal fluid was present clinically
(vision 20/80).

TABLE 59–3
White Dot Syndromes

	Multiple Evanescent White Dot Syndrome	Acute Posterior Multifocal Placoid Pigment Epitheliopathy	Punctate Inner Choroidopathy	Birdshot Chorioretinopathy
Demographics	Female:Male 4:1 15–45 years old	male=female 15–40 years old	Female ≫ male 15–40 years old myopic	male=female young, white adults, + HLA–A29
Etiology	unknown, ? viral	unknown, ? recent viral illness	unknown	unknown, ? autoimmune
Symptoms	photopsias visual loss	loss of central vision	blurred vision, photopsias, scotomas	Painless, bilateral blurred vision and floaters
Clinical Features	unilateral 100–200 μ white dots at level of RPE, granular appearance of macula with orange specks, optic nerve hyperemia, venous sheathing mild vitreous cell	bilateral, asymmetric, large yellow-white placoid lesions at level of RPE concentrated in posterior pole, associated with vitritis, anterior uveitis, perivasculitis	bilateral small discrete yellow lesions at level of RPE and inner choroid, concentrated in the posterior pole	bilateral, symmetric, multiple small creamy lesions at level of RPE localized nasally and radiating toward the equator, minimal to mild vitritis, papillitis
IVFA Findings	early hyperfluorescence with late staining of dots	block early, stains late	early leakage with late staining	spots not very remarkable on IVFA, leakage from disc
Treatment	None	None	None	Cyclosporine A
Complications			CNVM	CNVM, ERM, NV
Other		May be recurrent	No recurrences	Chronic disease with exacerbations and remissions

	Diffuse Unilateral Subacute Neuroretinitis	Ophthalmomyiasis	Acute Retinal Pigment Epitheliitis	Presumed Ocular Histoplasmosis Syndrome	Multifocal choroiditis and panuveitis
Demographics	Young, male:female 1.5:1		Young, male=female	Middle age, Ohio/Mississippi valley, HLA-B7	Young, female:male 3:1
Etiology	motile, nematode, racoon ascarid	Rodent bot fly maggot	? viral etiology	Histoplasmosis capsulatum	Unknown, ? association with EBV
Symptoms	Unilateral, slow decrease in vision, often loss of peripheral vision first	Unilateral decrease in vision	Unilateral sudden decrease in vision	Asymptomatic, unless recurrence of infection; metamorphopsia with formation of CNVM	Acute loss of vision, metamorphopsia when CNVM present
Clinical Features	Mild vitritis and papillitis, multiple clusters of white dots along track of nematode Late—massive RPE disruption, optic atrophy	Mild inflammation of anterior chamber and vitreous, subretinal RPE tracks, maggot in vitreous	Clusters of small hyperpigmented lesions in macula with surrounding RPE edema	Atrophic punched-out chorioretinal scars, peripapillary crescent, disciform macular scar. No vitritis	Bilateral, multifocal white chorioretinal lesions, anterior uveitis and vitritis
IVFA Findings			Small hypofluorescent dots with halo, no CME	CNVM, staining of punched-out lesions	
Treatment	Photocoagulation of the worm	Surgical resection phtocoagulation, steroids	None	laser photocoagulation or surgical excision	Steroids
Complications		severe inflammatory response to death of worm			CNVM
Other			Recurrent	Recurrence possible, involvement of fellow eye	

	Serpiginous choroiditis	Vogt-Koyanagi-Harada Syndrome	Sympathetic ophthalmia
Demographics	Middle age, male=female	Young, male=female, pigmented races (oriental, hispanic, black)	Men>Women
Etiology	unknown	? autoimmunity to melanin	Penetrating ocular trauma, intraocular surgery
Symptoms	bilateral, progressive, recurrent decrease in vision	decreased vision, photophobia	photophobia, pain, decreased accomodation
Clinical Features	peripapillary, ill-defined yellow-grey lesion with inflammation along edges, mild vitritis, RPE and choriocapillaris atrophy late	Severe anterior and posterior uveitis, exudative retinal detachments, pigment scarring Poliosis, alopecia, vitiligo, dysacousis	diffuse granulomatous panuveitis, Dalen-Fuchs nodules, vitritis, perivasculitis
IVFA Findings	hyperfluorescence of edge of lesion, active lesions block early and stain late		leakage from optic nerve, multiple choroidal spots
Treatment	None effective	Corticosteroids, other immunosuppressives	Enucleate blind, inciting eye; Prednisone or other immunosuppression
Complications Other	CNVM, multiple recurrences		

multifocal chorioretinal scars and a propensity for the development of choroidal neovascularization (49,42). Unlike POHS, however, the syndrome was associated with vitritis, anterior uveitis, and occurrence in patients without exposure to regions endemic for the histoplasmosis organism.

Compared with POHS, patients tended to be younger with an overwhelming predilection for females. Most patients tend to become symptomatic in their thirties. Myopia is common. Presenting complaints include photopsias, floaters, and paracentral scotomas in contrast to patients with POHS who invariably present for symptoms related to the development of choroidal neovascularization. Often, an antecedent flulike illness is reported. Bilateral involvement is typical.

Ophthalmoscopic examination shows 100 to 300 micron size punched-out chorioretinal lesions scattered in the posterior pole and midperiphery. These lesions tend to be smaller than typical POHS lesions. A prominent vitritis and anterior uveitis may be present. Choroidal neovascularization is common. Some patients may have a particularly severe course associated with the development of profound subretinal fibrosis in the macula and surrounding the optic nerve.

Punctate inner choroidopathy may represent a subgroup of patients with multifocal choroiditis (47). This syndrome, which characteristically lacks vitreous cells, consists of the bilateral development of small, yellow chorioretinal lesions confined to the macula which heal leaving punched-out chorioretinal lesions. Spontaneously resolving serous macular detachments may occur. Choroidal neovascularization develops in 40% of eyes. Subretinal fibrosis may similarly occur.

The association of multifocal choroiditis with Epstein-Barr virus infection has been reported but remains unsubstantiated (40). Whether this potential association represents an etiologic relationship or an epiphenomenon caused by more widespread alterations in the immune system is unclear. Histopathologic examination of a chorioretinal biopsy from a patient with subretinal fibrosis showed the presence of B lymphocytes and plasma cells without the detection of viral particles.

The typical course of multifocal choroiditis is poor. While the panuveitis and choroiditis may respond to systemic steroids, recurrences are common. Treatment of choroidal neovascularization with laser photocoagulation is often unsuccessful in preserving central vision.

■ VOGT-KOYANAGI-HARADA SYNDROME (See Uveitus, Chapter 36)

The Vogt-Koyanagi-Harada (VKH) (41, 47). syndrome is a systemic immunologic disorder characterized by the association of a bilateral panuveitis with meningeal and cutaneous findings. In 1906, Vogt described the association of bilateral uveitis with premature graying and balding hair. In 1926, Harada published five cases of bilateral posterior uveitis associated with exudative retinal detachment and cerebrospinal fluid pleocytosis in the Japanese literature. Koyanagi's 1929 description of bilateral uveitis with headache, fever, vitiligo, dysacousia, balding, and premature graying suggested that these reports likely represented the same disorder and eventually to the acceptance of the disorder as the VKH syndrome.

The incidence of VKH is estimated to represent roughly 4% of the uveitis cases in the midwestern United States and 8% of uveitis cases in Japan. The onset of disease is usually in the third decade of life. The disorder has a predilection for darkly pigmented races, particularly Asians, Hispanics, and American Indians. Sixty percent of patients are female. Ocular involvement is invariably bilateral; however, the fellow eye may present weeks or even years later. Patients typically present with complaints of abrupt decreased vision.

Ocular involvement often begins primarily as a posterior uveitis progressing quickly to a panuveitis. Mutton-fat keratic precipitates may be present on the

corneal endothelium. Posterior synechia are common. Hyperemia or edema of the optic nerve heads is invariably present. Exudative macular detachments occur in 75% of patients. The subretinal fluid can be seen to shift with changes in positioning. Focal retinal pigment epithelial detachments commonly occur in the posterior pole. Nodular yellow choroidal lesions may be seen in the retinal periphery, particularly inferiorly, reminiscent of Dalen-Fuchs nodules seen in sympathetic ophthalmia. Evidence of old, inactive disease may be afforded by a "leopard skin" pigment epithelial change in areas of previous longstanding exudative retinal detachment or more widespread pigment epithelial atrophy giving a "sunset glow" appearance.

Fluorescein angiography shows pinpoint or focal areas of hyperfluorescence at the level of the RPE in the arterial phase which coalesce and pool fluorescein dye within the neurosensory detachment. Ultrasonography shows choroidal thickening.

Neurologic findings are present in 60% of cases. Meningeal signs are characterized by stiff neck, headache, nausea, and vomiting. Transient deafness and tinnitus may occur. Personality changes include psychosis and suicidal ideation. Spinal tap can show cerebrospinal fluid pleocytosis, increased intracranial pressure, and increased cerebrospinal fluid protein.

Cutaneous findings are often delayed for 3 to 6 weeks after the onset of disease. They include premature balding (alopecia) in 50%, premature greying of body hair (poliosis) in 50%, and patchy depigmentation of skin with hyperpigmented borders (vitiligo) in 50%.

Histopathologic study of globes shows localized choroidal granulomas with a predominant plasma cell infiltrate. This differs from the pathologic study of sympathetic ophthalmia by the scarcity of epithelioid cells, lack of diffuse choroidal thickening, and involvement of the choriocapillaris in cases of VKH.

The etiology of VKH is unknown. Attempts to show an infectious cause have been unsuccessful. Limited studies have shown a cell-mediated response from T cells obtained from patients with VKH against melanin-containing cells in culture. Increased prevalence of the HLA-BW54 and HLA-DR4 antigens have been noted in Japan. Current opinion supports an autoimmune pathogenesis for this disorder (4).

The differential diagnosis includes posterior scleritis, metastatic carcinoma, idiopathic central serous choroidopathy, uveal effusion syndrome, sympathetic ophthalmia, leukemia, and benign lymphoid hyperplasia of the choroid.

Treatment with 80 to 100 mg of oral prednisone often elicits a prompt clinical response, first evidenced by resolution of the exudative detachment and normalization of the angiographic changes. Initiation of treatment with intravenous pulse corticosteroids may occasionally be indicated. Cycloplegics and topical steroids should be administered if an anterior uveitis is present. Refractory cases may benefit from the use of immunosuppressive agents including cyclosporine. Long-term treatment is usually required to prevent relapse.

■ POSTERIOR SCLERITIS (see also Ocular Inflammation Chapter 39)

The sclera is an avascular collection of collagen and elastic tissue which derives its nutrition from the underlying choroid and overlying episclera. The episclera, or Tenon's capsule is the vascular coat of the sclera which facilitates an inflammatory response in disease states. The episclera is comprised of both a deep layer with vessels and a superficial layer with radially oriented vessels.

Posterior scleritis (1,43) is a relatively uncommon inflammatory disorder of the sclera posterior to the ora serrata. While posterior scleritis may occasionally represent a posterior extension of anterior scleritis, particularly in patients with rheumatoid arthritis or relapsing polychondritis, it commonly presents as an isolated disorder. Women are more commonly affected than men. Twenty to 30% of cases are bilateral. The average patient with posterior scleritis presents in the third or fourth decade of life; however, both childhood and elderly patients are reported.

Symptoms include decreased vision and pain. Pain is often proportional to the extent of anterior involvement. Complaints of photophobia are not uncommon. Diffuse posterior scleral thickening without exudative detachment may produce a hyperopic shift in refraction.

Ocular findings include exudative retinal detachment, choroidal folds, and optic disc edema. The subretinal fluid associated with exudative detachment in this disease tends to be cloudy. Cells are typically present in the vitreous. Focal elevation of an intact choroid and RPE by thickened sclera may give the appearance of an orange mass lesion. Overlying choroidal inflammation may occur. Involvement of the extraocular muscles may produce limitations of ocular movements, proptosis, and eyelid edema. Unlike thyroid myopathy, which primarily involves the posterior belly of the extraocular muscles, posterior scleritis tends to first involve the tendinous insertion of the muscle onto sclera. Scleritis may induce overlying anterior ciliochoroidal detachment. This produces anterior rotation of the iris-lens diaphragm with shallowing of the anterior chamber and the threat of angle closure glaucoma.

Ultrasonography is particularly helpful in demonstrating the scleral thickening pathognomonic of the disease. Scleral thickening can be realized as a widened echolucent space between the choroid and Tenon's capsule on B-scan echography. Extension of scleral thickening to the peripapillary region produces the so-called "T-sign" as the echolucent area defined by the posterior displacement of Tenon's capsule and its insertion on the echolucent optic nerve shadow is highlighted. In cases of exudative retinal detachment, fluorescein angiography shows pinpoint areas of hyperfluorescence at the level of the choroid which coalesce to pool fluorescein dye in the area defined by the detachment. The pattern is identical to that seen in the Vogt-Koyanagi-Harada syndrome. Fluorescein angiography may also highlight the presence of choroidal folds whose peaks and valleys display alternating lines of hyperflouorescence and normo-fluorescence, respectively.

Unlike anterior scleritis, the likelihood of uncovering systemic association in posterior scleritis is decreased. Nonetheless, the implications of identifying an associated systemic disorder warrant limited medical workup. They should seek to exclude the diagnosis of rheumatoid arthritis, relapsing polychondritis, Wegener's granulomatosis, inflammatory bowel disease, and syphilis.

The differential diagnosis includes the Vogt-

Koyanagi-Harada syndrome, choroidal tumors including malignant melanoma and metastatic carcinoma, uveal effusion syndrome, benign reactive lymphoid hyperplasia, and hypotony.

Treatment with systemic corticosteroids is usually effective in controlling the disease. Severely affected or bilaterally visually impaired patients may benefit from initiation of treatment with pulse intravenous corticosteroids. Oral nonsteroidal antiinflammatory agents such as indomethacin may also be effective. Refractory patients, particularly those associated with rheumatoid arthritis may require the use of immunosuppressive agents such as cyclophosphamide to control their ocular disease.

■ SERPIGINOUS CHOROIDITIS (See Chapter 34)

Serpiginous choroiditis (23, 39, 53) is a rare, long-term, alternating bilateral disorder of the retinal pigment epithelium and choriocapillaris often associated with profound visual loss. The onset of disease is in the fourth through seventh decades of life. Men are affected more commonly than women. There is no racial predilection.

Presenting symptoms include paracentral scotomas or diminished central vision. Scotomas precisely correspond to the observed ophthalmoscopic lesions. As lesions often begin in the peripapillary region, patients may remain asymptomatic until macular extension of the lesions occurs. Although the disorder is bilateral, only one eye is affected at a time. A family history of disease is absent.

Active disease on ophthalmoscopy shows irregular, edematous, whitish-gray lesions at the level of the RPE and choroid in the peripapillary and macular region. Typically, the lesions are contiguous with evidence of an active edematous portion of the lesion adjacent to areas of punched out, scalloped scars. The propensity for successive recurrences to occur, in pseudopodal fashion, at the border of inactive scarring explains the use of the term "serpiginous" to describe the disease. Active lesions evolve into areas of RPE and choroidal atrophy with variable amounts of hyperpigmentation over weeks to months. Cells are present in the vitreous in one-third of cases. Occasionally a mild anterior uveitis can occur. Retinal periphlebitis or branch venous occlusive disease occasionally occur. Choroidal neovascularization may complicate the disease in 25% of cases. Systemic associations are typically absent.

Fluorescein angiography shows hypofluorescence of active lesion early in the angiogram with evidence of late staining beginning at the lesion borders and spreading centrally. This angiographic pattern has been alternatively suggested to represent either blockage of choroidal fluorescence by swollen, opaque pigment epithelial cells or by ischemia of the choriocapillaris (Figure 59–13).

Histopathologic studies show atrophy of the choriocapillaris, retinal pigment epithelium, and photoreceptors in areas of the lesion. Lymphocytic infiltration of the choroid is present.

The etiology of disease is unknown. An autoimmune mechanism is suspected. An increased prevalence of the HLA-B7 antigen has been reported in Finland where the antigen was present in roughly half of patients with serpiginous choroidopathy compared with one-quarter of the population at large.

The differential diagnosis chiefly includes acute posterior multifocal placoid pigment epitheliopathy (APMPPE). In APMPPE, however, acute lesions resolve in only 1 to 2 weeks, simultaneous bilateral involvement is common, lesions are rounder and more scattered, atrophic scarring is milder, visual prognosis is excellent, and recurrences are uncommon.

Treatment of serpiginous choroidopathy with systemic or periocular steroid is of unproven benefit but believed by many to speed the resolution of active disease (24). Attempts to prevent recurrences by treatment with systemic immunosuppressive agents such a cyclophosphamide or cyclosporine may be a reasonable approach in patients with bilateral foveal-threatening disease.

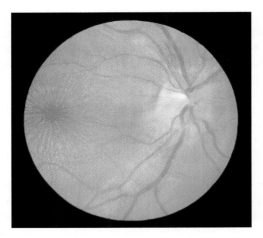

Figure 59–12.
Leber's idiopathic stellate neuroretinitis in a 12-year-old girl. Visual acuity measured 5/200. Precipitation of lipid from fluid leaking from the optic nerve results in the yellow, radial pattern of exudates in the macular star. Four months later, after resolution of the exudation, her vision returned to 20/20.

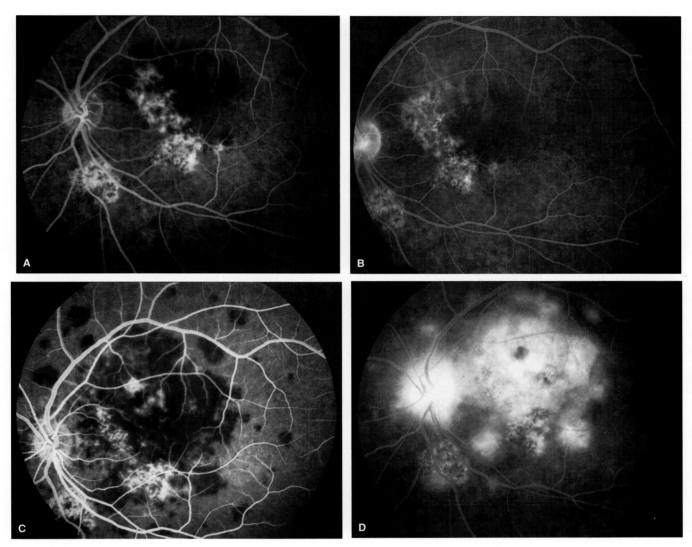

Figure 59–13.
Serpiginous choroidopathy in a 46-year-old female who presented with abrupt onset of diminished central vision. A similar episode had occurred 4 years previously in the same eye. Fluorescein angiography shows window defect, corresponding to the existing retinal pigment epithelial atrophy, with an area inferonasal to the fovea at the edge of this atrophy which blocks in the early (A) and stains in the late (B) phases of the study. Vision improved and inflammation subsided on oral corticosteroids. Fifteen months later, an extensive recurrence ensued, illustrated by blockage of area of RPE and choroidal inflammation in the early phases of the study (C) with leakage in the late (D).

■ DIFFUSE UNILATERAL SUBACUTE NEURORETINITIS (See Chapter 34)

Diffuse unilateral subacute neuroretinitis (17), a term coined by Gass and Scelfo, is an inflammatory entity characterized by extensive, unilateral destruction of the retinal pigment epithelium. Patients have subacute loss of vision first affecting the periphery. A mild vitritis or papillitis may be present. Loss of the b-wave on ERG may help to confirm the diagnosis. Late in the disease, optic atrophy and massive RPE disruption with an afferent pupillary defect is present.

Nematode larvae have been observed to migrate under the retina in areas of active inflammation leaving subretinal tracts.

Laser photocoagulation of the worm is effective in treating this condition. In some patients, the worm spontaneously disappears and the retinal damage stabilizes.

■ REFERENCES

1. Benson WE: Posterior scleritis. Surv Ophthalmol 1988; 32: 297–316.

2. Bressler SB, Bressler NM, Alexander J. Green WR: Clinicopathologic correlation of occult choroidal neovascularization in age related macular degeneration. Invest Ophthalmol Vis Sci 1991; 32: 689.

3. Bressler SB, Maguire MG, Bressler NM, Fine SL: The Macular Photocoagulation Study Group: Relationship of drusen and abnormalities of the retinalpigment epithelium to the prognosis of neovasculamaculardegeneration. Arch Ophthalmol 1990; 108:1444–1447.

4. Chan CC, Palestine AG, Nussenblatt RB: Anti-retinal autoantibodies in Vogt-Koyanagi-Harada syndrome, Behcet's disease, and sympathetic ophthalmia. Ophthalmology 1985; 92: 1025–1028.

5. Clarkson JG, Altman RD: Angioid streaks. Surv Ophthalmol 1982; 26: 235–246.

6. Coll GE, Chang S, Sun J, Wieland MR, Berrocal M: Perfluorocarbon liquid in the management of retinal detachment with proliferative vitreoretinopathy. Ophthalmology 1995; 102: 630–639.

7. Cox SN, Hay E. Bird AC: Treatment of chronic macular edema with acetazolamide. Arch Ophthalmol 1988; 106: 1190–1195.

8. deBustros S. Thompson JT, Michels RG: Vitrectomy for idiopathic epiretinal membranes causing macular pucker. Br J Ophthalmo l 1988; 72: 692–695.

9. de Juan E. Lambert HM, Machemer R: Recurrent proliferations in macular pucker, diabetic retinopathy and retrolental fibroplasialike disease after vitrectomy. Graefe's Arch Clin Ophthalmol 1985; 223: 174–183.

10. Dreyer RF, Gass JDM: Multifocal choroiditis and panuveitis: A syndrome that mimics ocular histoplasmosis. Arch Ophthalmol 1984, 102: 1776- 1787.

11. Dreyer RF, Hopen G, Gass JDM, Smith JL: Leber's idiopathic stellate neuroretinitis. Arch Ophthalmol 1984; 102: 1140–1145.

12. Folk JC, Thompson HS, Han DP, Brown CK: Visual function abnormalities in central serous choroidopathy. Arch Ophthalmol 1984; 102: 1299–1302.

13. Frangieh GT, Green WR, Engel HM: A histopathologic study of macular cysts and holes. Retina 1981; 1: 311–336.

14. Fung WE: Vitrectomy for chronic aphakic cystoid macular edema. Results of a national, collaborative, prospective, randomized investigation. Ophthalmology 1985; 92: 1102–1111.

15. Gass JDM: Acute posterior multifocal placoid pigment epitheliopathy. Arch Ophthalmol 1968; 80: 177–185.

16. Gass JDM: Biomicroscopic and histopathologic considerations regarding the feasibility of surgical excision of subfoveal neovascular membranes. Am J Ophthalmol 1994; 118: 285–298.

17. Gass JDM, Gilbert WR Jr, Guerry RK, et al: Diffuse unilateral subacute neuroretinitis. Ophthalmology 1978; 85: 512–545.

18. Gass JDM: Idiopathic senile macular holes: Its early stages and pathogenesis. Arch Ophthalmol 1988; 106: 629–639.

19. Gass JDM, Joondeph BC: Observations concerning patients with suspected impending macular holes. Am J Ophthalmol 1990; 109: 638–646.

20. Gelisken O, Hendrikse F, Dutman AF: A long-term follow-up study of laser coagulation of neovascular membranes in angioid streaks. Am J Ophthalmol 1998; 105: 299–303.

21. Gilbert CM, Owens SL, Smith PD, Fine SL: Long-term follow-up of central serous chorioretinopathy. Br J Ophthalmol 1984; 68: 815–820.

22. Green WR, McDonnell PH, Yeo JH: Pathologic features of senile macular degeneration. Ophthalmology 1985; 92: 615–627.

23. Hardy RA, Schatz H: Macular geographic helicoid choroidopathy. Arch Ophthalmol 1987; 105: 1237–1242.

24. Hooper PL, Kaplan HJ: Triple agent immunosuppression in serpiginous choroiditis. Ophthalmology 1990; 98: 944–951.

25. Jaffe NS, Clayman HM, Jaffe MS: Cystoid macular edema after intracapsular and extracapsular cataract extraction with and without an intraocular lens. Ophthalmology 1982; 89: 25–29.

26. Jampol LM: Cystoid macular edema after cataract surgery. Arch Ophthalmol 1988; 106: 894–895.

27. Jampol LM, Sieving PA, Pugh D, et al: Multiple evanescent white dot syndrome. I. Clinical findings. Arch Ophthalmol 1984; 102: 671–674.

28. Johnson RN, Gass JDM: Idiopathic macular holes: Observations, stages of hole formation, and implications for surgical intervention. Ophthalmology 1988; 95: 917–924.

29. Kelly NE, Wendel RT: Vitreous surgery for idiopathic macular holes: Results of a pilot study. Arch Ophthalmol 1991; 109: 654–659.

30. Levine R, Brucker AJ, Robinson F: Long-term follow-up of idiopathic central serous chorioretinopathy by fluorescein angiography. Ophthalmology 1989; 96: 854–859.

31. Macular Photocoagulation Study Group: Argon laser photocoagulation for neovascular maculopathy—three year results. Arch Ophthalmol 1986; 104: 694–701.

32. Macular Photocoagulation Study Group: Argon laser photocoagulation for neovascular maculopathy after five years. Results from randomized clinical trials. Arch Ophthalmol 1991; 109: 1109–1114.

33. Macular Photocoagulation Study Group: Krypton laser photocoagulation for neovascular lesions of ocular histoplasmosis. Arch Ophthalmol 1987; 105: 1499–1507.

34. Macular Photocoagulation Study Group: Krypton laser photocoagulation for neovascular lesions of age-related macular degeneration. Results of a randomized clinical trail. Arch Ophthalmol 1990; 108: 816–824.

35. Macular Photocoagulation Study Group: Laser photocoagulation of subfoveal neovascular lesions in age-related macular degeneration. Results of a randomized clinical trial. Arch Ophthalmol 1991; 109: 1219–1231.

36. Macular Photocoagulation Study Group: Laser photocoagulation of subfoveal recurrent neovascular lesions in age-related macular degeneration. Results of a randomized clinical trial. Arch Ophthalmol 1991; 109: 1232–1241.

37. Macular Photocoagulation Study Group: Persistent and recurrent neovascularization after krypton laser photocoagulation for neovascular lesions of ocular histoplasmosis. Arch Ophthalmol 1989; 107: 344–352.

38. Macular Photocoagulation Study Group: Subfoveal neovascular lesions in age-related macular degeneration: Guidelines for evaluation and treatment in the Macular Photocoagulation Study. Arch Ophthalmol 1991; 109: 1242–1257.

39. Mansour AM, Jampol LM, Packo KH: Macular serpiginous choroiditis. Retina 1988; 8: 125–131.

40. Morgan CM, Schatz H: Recurrent multifocal choroiditis. Ophthalmology 1984, 93: 1138–1147.

41. Perry HD, Font RL: Clinical and histopathologic observations in severe Vogt-Koyanagi-Harada syndrome. Am J Ophthalmol 1977; 83: 242–254.

42. Robertson DM: Argon laser photocoagulation treatment in central serous chorioretinopathy. Ophthalmology 1986; 93: 972–974.

43. Rosenbaum JT, Robertson JE: Recognition of posterior scleritis and its treatment with indomethacin. Retina 1993; 13: 17–21.

44. Ryan SJ, Maumenee AE: Acute posterior multifocal placoid pigment epitheliopathy. Am J Ophthalmol 1972; 74: 1066–1074.

45. Smiddy, WE, MaGuire AM, Green WR: Idiopathic epiretinal membranes. Ophthalmology 1989; 96: 811–821.

46. Smith RE, Dunn S, Jester JV: Natural history of experimental histoplasmic choroiditis in the primate II: Histopathological features. Invest Ophthalmol Vis Sci 1984; 25: 810–819.

47. Snyder DA, Tessler HH: Vogt-Koyanagi-Harada syndrome. Am J Ophthalmol 1980: 89:69–75 .

48. Trese MT, Chandler DB, Machemer R: Macular Pucker: prognostic criteria. Graefe's Arch Clin Exp Ophthalmol 1983; 221: 16–26.

49. Tiedeman JS: Epstein-Barr viral antibodies in multifocal choroiditis and panuveitis. Am J Ophthalmol 1987, 103: 659–663.

50. Thomas MA, Dickinson JD, Melberg NS, et al: Visual results after surgical removal of subfoveal choroidal neovascular membranes. Ophthalmology 1994; 101: 1384–1396.

51. Watzke RC, Claussen RW: The long-term course of multifocal choroiditis (presumed ocular histoplasmosis). Am J Ophthalmol 1981; 91: 750–760.

52. Watzke RC, Packer AJ, Folk JC: Punctate inner choroidopathy. Am J Ophthalmol 1984, 98: 572–584.

53. Weiss H, Annesley WH, Shields JA: The clinical course of serpiginous choroidopathy. Am J Ophthalmol 1987; 87: 133–142.

54. Yanuzzi LA: Type A behavior and central serous chorioretinopathy. Trans Am Ophthalmol Soc 1986; 84: 799–845.

55. Bernstein HN: Chloroquine ocular toxicity. Surv Ophthalmol 1967; 12: 415–447 .

56. Daiker B, Scheidt K, Adnet JJ, et al: Canthaxanthine retinopathy. An investigation by light and electron microscopy and physiochemical analysis. Graefes Arch Clin Exp Ophthalmol 1987; 225: 189–197.

57. Davidorf FH: Thioridazine pigmentary retinopathy. Arch Ophthalmol 1973; 90: 251–255.

58. Gass JDM: Nicotinic acid maculopathy. Am J Ophthalmol 1973; 76: 500–510.

59. Kozy D, Doft BH, Lipkowitz J: Nummular thioridazine retinopathy. Retina 1984; 4: 253–256.

60. McKeown CA, Swartz M, Blom J, et al: Tamoxifen retinopathy. Br J Ophthalmol 1981; 65: 177–179.

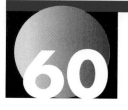

60 Retinovascular Diseases

Eugene de Juan Jr., Stuart W. Noorily,
William P. Townsend-Pico, Kenneth C. Chern

■ DIABETIC RETINOPATHY

Diabetes mellitus is the most common serious metabolic disease in humans. Twelve million Americans have diabetes mellitus. Ten to fifteen percent of these patients have juvenile-onset, insulin-dependent, type I diabetes, whereas the remainder have non-insulin-dependent, type II diabetes which is usually diagnosed after the age of 40. Type I diabetes results from autoimmune destruction of the insulin-producing beta cells of the pancreatic islets of Langerhans. A family history is usually lacking. Type II diabetes has no known cause although it usually occurs in middle-aged, overweight individuals with a strong family history. The multisystem effects of diabetes are related to microvascular consequences of chronic hyperglycemia: basement membrane thickening, endothelial pericyte loss, and increased platelet aggregation.

Diabetic retinopathy is the leading cause of blindness in working age Americans. Some degree of retinopathy is present in 50% of diabetics who have had their disease for 7 years. This figure increases to 90% in those with diabetes for over 20 years. Proliferative retinopathy develops in one-quarter of patients with diabetes of over 25 years duration and affects an esitmated 700,000 Americans. Diabetic macular edema affects an estimated 500,000 Americans.

The retinovascular consequences of diabetes essentially consist of microvascular leakage and capillary nonperfusion. Microvascular leakage follows the impairment of the structural integrity of retinal capillaries heralded by the development of microaneurysms. Microaneurysms may either become thrombosed or may leak serum components into the surrounding retina. Retinal edema, lipid exudates and dot-blot intraretinal hemorrhages are the result of such breakdown of the blood-retinal barrier (Figure 60–1). Capillary nonperfusion, on the other hand, results in the formation of arteriovenous shunts known as intraretinal microvascular abnormalities (IRMA) (Figure 60–2). Elaboration of vascular endothelial growth factor from hypoxic retina in areas of capillary nonperfusion results in the development of extraretinal neovascularization. These new vessels may arise from the optic disc (NVD) or elsewhere in the retinal periphery (NVE) (Figure 60–3). Such neovascularization and its associated fibrous component may spontaneously involute or be complicated by vitreous hemorrhage or traction retinal detachment. Neovascularization may be easily seen on fluorescein angiogram by the profuse leakage of dye from these new vessels since they lack the tight endothelial junctions of the retinal vasculature. Impaired axoplasmic flow in areas of retinal hypoxia result in cotton wool spots.

Until the late stages of its development, diabetic retinopathy remains largely asymptomatic. For this reason, uniform classification and careful screening of diabetics is required in order to identify those patients who would benefit from timely treatment. Diabetic retinopathy is classified into two main groups: nonproliferative and proliferative based on the presence of neovascularization. Macular edema may be associated with either group. Areas suspicious for neovascularization may be confirmed by their marked leakage of fluorescein dye by angiography.

Nonproliferative diabetic retinopathy (NPDR) can be further divided into mild NPDR, moderate NPDR, and severe NPDR in an effort to predict which eyes are at higher risk of developing proliferative retinopathy.

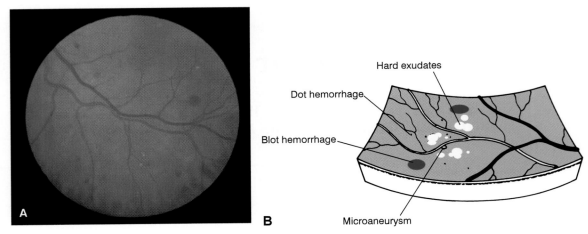

Figure 60–1.
Among the earliest microvascular changes in diabetes is the formation of microaneurysms, and dot and blot hemorrhanges (A & B). Microaneurysms may leak fluid and may sometimes be identified at the center of a ring of exudates.

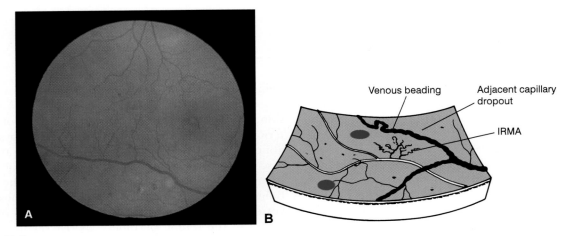

Figure 60–2.
In areas of capillary dropout, intraretinal microvascular abnormalities (IRMA) form representing dilated telangiectactic capillaries (A & B). Unlike extraretinal neovascularization, IRMA do not leak on fluorescein angiography.

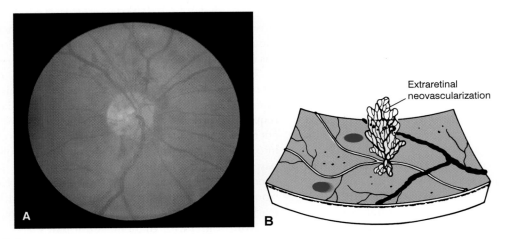

Figure 60–3.
Extraretinal neovascularization may form at the optic disc (A) or elsewhere in the retina (B). These new vessels extend from the retina into the vitreous. Extraretinal neovascularization is associated with vitreous hemorrhage and production of fibrovascular traction.

Mild NPDR describes eyes with scattered hemorrhages and microaneurysms. Moderate NPDR contains hemorrhages and microaneurysms and mild degrees of soft exudates, venous beading, and IRMA. Severe NPDR is defined by the presence of venous beading in 2 or more quadrants, IRMA in one or more quadrants, or microaneurysm and dot hemorrhages in all 4 quadrants. The importance of these distinctions is that 52% of severe NPDR, versus 27% and 5% of moderate or mild NPDR, respectively, progress to proliferative diabetic retinopathy within 1 year. The Early Treatment Diabetic Retinopathy Study (11) (ETDRS) evaluated the benefit of early panretinal photocoagulation (PRP) in patients with mild-to-severe NPDR. While early PRP, compared with deferral of treatment, was associated with a small reduction in the rates of severe visual loss to the 5/200 level or worse over 5 years, the incidence of such loss was decreased in both the treatment and deferral groups (2.6% and 3.7%, respectively).

Proliferative diabetic retinopathy (PDR) can be divided into nonhigh risk PDR and high risk PDR, in order to identify those eyes at greater risk of severe visual loss and, therefore, most likely to benefit from panretinal photocoagulation. PRP may be successful by ablating areas of ischemic retina, reducing the production of growth factors responsible for neovascularization. High risk PDR (Figure 60–4) is defined by the presence of three or more of the following characteristics: new vessels, new vessels on or within one disc diameter of the optic nerve, severe new vessels (as defined by one-third disc area neovascularization at the optic nerve or one-half disc area neovascularization elsewhere), and preretinal or vitreous hemorrhage (Table 60–1). The Diabetic Retinopathy Study (1) (DRS) evaluated the

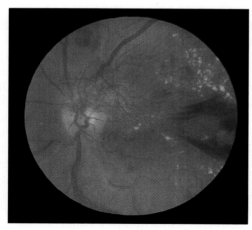

Figure 60–4.
Proliferative diabetic retinopathy. In this color photograph, several high-risk characteristics are apparent: severe neovascularization of the disc and preretinal hemorrhage. Immediate panretinal photocoagulation is indicated to induce regression of the new vessels.

TABLE 60–1
High-Risk Characteristics for Proliferative Diabetic Retinopathy

Presence of three or more of the following characteristics indicates high-risk PDR which requires panretinal photocoagulation without delay.
- any neovascularization
- neovascularization on or within 1 disc diameter of the optic disc (NVD)
- NVD greater than one third to one half disc area
- neovascularization of the retina (NVE) greater than one half disc area
- vitreous or preretinal hemorrhage

benefit of panretinal photocoagulation in eyes with PDR (see Chapter 63 on retinal surgery). Treated eyes with high risk PDR were half as likely to sustain severe visual loss to the 5/200 level or worse at 4 years (20% versus 44%). All eyes with PDR should undergo detailed examination of the iris and angle for signs of growth of new vessels (rubeosis) in order to avert the devastating development of neovascular glaucoma in severely ischemic eyes or those with extensive retinal detachment.

The presence of diabetic macular edema is a clinical determination made by the stereoscopic observation of retinal thickening by contact lens fundus examination or stereophotography. Clinically significant macular edema (CSME) is defined by the presence of retinal thickening within 500 microns of the foveal center, hard exudates within 500 microns of the foveal center associated with retinal thickening, or retinal thickening of one disc area or greater located partially within one disc diameter of the foveal center (Figure 60–5), (Table 60–2). The ETDRS (3) evaluated the benefit of focal or grid laser photocoagulation for the treatment of macular edema (see chapter on retinal surgery). At 3 years, treated eyes with CSME were half as likely to sustain moderate visual loss (doubling of the visual angle) as untreated eyes (12% versus 24%). In eyes with CSME and foveal thickening, treatment tripled the chance of moderate visual gain compared with untreated eyes (17% versus 5%). Panretinal photocoagulation was

TABLE 60–2
Clinically Significant Macular Edema

ETDRS Definition:
1. Thickening of the retina 0–500 μm from the center of the macula
2. Hard exudates located 0–500 μm from the center of the macula with associated thickening of the adjacent retina
3. Retinal thickening, 1 disc area or larger, any part of which is within 1 disc diameter from the center of the macula

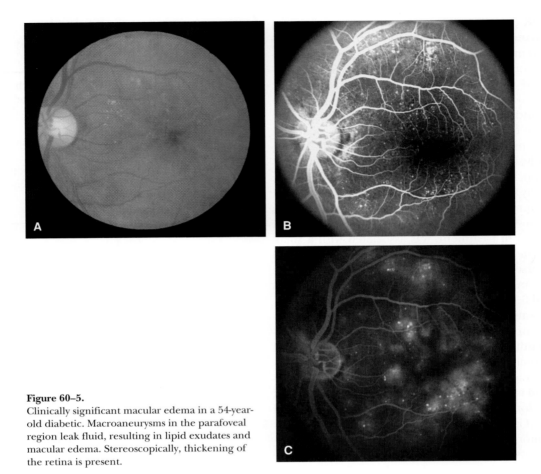

Figure 60–5.
Clinically significant macular edema in a 54-year-old diabetic. Macroaneurysms in the parafoveal region leak fluid, resulting in lipid exudates and macular edema. Stereoscopically, thickening of the retina is present.

found to exacerbate diabetic macular edema. Moreover, focal laser treatment benefit is delayed until after the placement of panretinal photocoagulation. As such, efforts should be made to treat diabetic macular edema before the institution of panretinal photocoagulation, if at all possible.

Fluorescein angiography is useful in identifying sites of focal leakage from microaneurysms, as well as diffuse areas of leakage and cystoid macular edema. Areas of diffuse leakage may benefit from treatment with a grid pattern of laser in those areas. Extensive diffuse edema and cystoid macula edema are less likely to respond to treatment.

The EDTRS also prospectively evaluated the effect of daily aspirin in diabetics. Aspirin did not slow the progression of retinopathy, nor did it increase the risk of vitreous hemorrhage. Aspirin was associated with a decreased risk of cardiovascular disease.

Despite treatment with panretinal photocoagulation, a small portion of eyes still progress to nonclearing vitreous hemorrhage or traction retinal detachment. Vitreous surgery may be indicated when these complications occur. The Diabetic Retinopathy Vitrectomy Study (9, 10) (DRVS) examined the timing and benefit

of vitrectomy in eyes with advanced proliferative diabetic retinopathy. At 2 years, early vitrectomy for vitreous hemorrhage compared with deferral, was associated with a threefold increased likelihood of achieving 20/40 or better visual acuity (36% versus 12%). This benefit was only present in type I diabetics and no difference in the ability to prevent severe visual loss was observed (28% versus 26%) for type II diabetics. Four-year results of early vitrectomy for eyes with severe PDR characterized by extensive neovascularization with fibrovascular proliferation, showed an improved likelihood of achieving 20/40 or better visual acuity compared with the deferral group (44% versus 28%); but again no benefit in the prevention of severe visual loss was observed. In another arm of the study, the expected stability of extrafoveal traction retinal detachments without persistent neovascularization was confirmed, with only 14% of these eyes progressing to severe visual loss over 2 years.

Current indications for vitreoretinal surgery for complications of diabetic retinopathy include macular tractional retinal detachment, nonclearing vitreous hemorrhage, combined tractional/rhegmatogenous retinal detachments, severe progressive fibrovascular proliferation, neovascular glaucoma with vitreous hemorrhage, dense premacular hemorrhages, continuous macular edema with a thickened posterior hyaloid, and anterior hyaloidal fibrovascular proliferation.

Cataract extraction in patients with diabetic retinopathy may contribute to progression of retinopathy, worsening of diabetic macular edema, and an increased likelihood of neovascular glaucoma. Whenever possible, treatment of preexisting macular edema, PDR, or severe NPDR should be undertaken before cataract removal.

The Diabetes Control and Complications Trial (7) (DCCT) was a multicenter, randomized study which showed that intensive therapy with tight control of blood sugars, as compared with conventional therapy, in patients with type I IDDM delayed the onset and slowed the progression of diabetic retinopathy, nephropathy, and neuropathy; however, intensive therapy was associated with a higher incidence of severe hypoglycemia.

■ CENTRAL RETINAL VEIN OCCLUSION

Central retinal vein occlusion (CRVO) is a common retinovascular disorder characterized by impaired venous outflow. A spectrum of overlapping or independent clinical presentations may occur including nonischemic CRVO, ischemic CRVO, hemiretinal vein occlusion, papillophlebitis, venous stasis retinopathy, and combined central venous and arterial occlusion (19).

Nonischemic (perfused) CRVO is characterized by dilation and tortuosity of the retinal venules with mild-to-moderate dot-blot and flame-shaped intraretinal hemorrhages in all quadrants (Figure 60–6). This variant represents roughly one-half of all CRVOs. Optic nerve and macular edema may be present. Cotton wool spots are absent or minimal. Venous pulsations are absent. Patients usually present in the fifth or sixth decades of life with complaints of acute or insidious painless loss of central vision. Fluorescein angiography shows prolongation of the arteriovenous transit time, patchy retinovascular leakage and late staining of the optic nerve, and occasionally, retinal venules. Blockage of choroidal fluorescence by intraretinal hemorrhages is present. Capillary nonperfusion is absent or minimal.

Over a period of time, opticociliary collaterals develop at the optic nerve. Unlike neovascularization, these vessels do not have a lacy, branching appearance and do not leak fluorescein dye. Intraretinal hemorrhages clear slowly over time. The visual prognosis is varied. If the initial visual acuity corresponds with maintained fovea vision (e.g., better than 20/200), then the majority of patients will recover at least 20/60 vision. Iris or retinal neovascularization occurs in less than 3% of nonischemic CRVO.

Ischemic (nonperfused) CRVO appears as a much more dramatic clinical picture with more extensive intraretinal hemorrhages and more profound visual loss, often to the count finger or hand motion level. Cotton wool spots are usually present. As in nonischemic CRVO, disc edema, macula edema, and opticociliary collaterals may occur. Unlike the nonischemic CRVO, however, ischemic CRVO is characterized by the presence of severe capillary nonperfusion on fluorescein an-

giography, and the frequent presence of an afferent pupillary defect. Electroretinography shows reduction in the b/a wave ratio consistent with functional impairment of the inner retina with relative preservation of the choroidally nourished outer retina. Two-thirds of ischemic CRVOs will develop iris neovascularization. Untreated, the majority of such patients will progress to the devastating complication of neovascular glaucoma, often within 3 months of the occlusion. Retinal neovascularization may occur as well but is quite uncommon. The visual prognosis is poor.

Hemi-vein occlusion represents the occurrence of a CRVO in an eye in which the central retinal vein has branched in the retrolaminar portion of the nerve. Hemi-vein occlusions may be either ischemic or nonischemic. Their clinical course behaves more like a CRVO than a branch vein occlusion. Ischemic hemi-vein occlusions are associated with a 30 to 40% incidence of retinal neovascularization and 10% incidence of iris neovascularization.

Venous stasis retinopathy is not a form of central venous occlusion. Although its appearance of dot-blot hemorrhages scattered throughout the mid-periphery of all four quadrants is reminiscent of venous occlusive disease, a number of features are unique. These include lack of tortuosity of the retinal veins, absence of disc edema, and prolongation of the injection time to arterial onset of the fluorescein angiogram. As its name implies, the disorder is one in which flow through the venous system is indeed impaired, however, not because of outflow obstruction, but because of inadequate arterial perfusion. This may be clinically shown by observing premature closure of the central retinal artery perfusion pressure with ophthalmodynamometry. The etiology of impaired arterial perfusion is carotid artery stenosis. Such patients should undergo carotid imaging and flow studies.

Papillophlebitis describes the occurrence of dilated, tortuous veins, optic nerve edema, and scattered dot-blot hemorrhages in healthy, young adults without associated systemic disease. A mild cellular reaction may be present in the vitreous. Most patients undergo sponta-

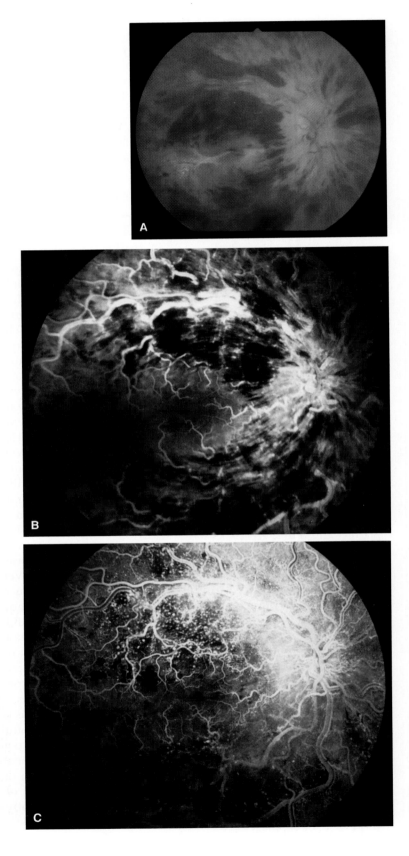

Figure 60–6.
Perfused central retinal vein occlusion. Color photograph (A) shows extensive flame-shaped nerve fiber layer hemorrhages, dilated and tortuous veins, and disc edema. Fluorescein angiography (B) shows blockage corresponding to intraretinal hemorrhage, but no evidence of capillary nonperfusion. Five months later, angiogram (C) illustrates clearing of intraretinal hemorrhages and areas of focal telangiectasis within the capillary bed with preservation of good acuity.

neous recovery over several weeks with an excellent visual prognosis. Aside from its occurrence and improved prognosis in young patients there is nothing to distinguish these patients from nonischemic CRVO. Speculation that the disorder may represent an inflammatory condition of the optic nerve or central retinal artery remains unproven.

Combined central venous and arterial occlusion is an unusual finding which may result from traumatic retrobulbar injection or infiltrative or compressive optic nerve processes.

Histopathologic studies suggest that the etiology of CRVO is thrombus formation in the central retinal vein at, or posterior to, the level of the lamina cribrosa (18). Narrowing of the central retinal vein as it passes through the lamina cribrosa may induce turbulent flow and subsequent thrombus formation.

Sixty percent of patients with CRVO have hypertension and 40% have primary open-angle glaucoma. Other commonly coexistent diseases in patients with CRVO include diabetes and cardiovascular disease (13). Nonetheless, these associations have not been clearly established as risk factors for disease development. On the other hand, CRVO, particularly when bilateral, may herald the presence of an underlying hyperviscosity state or collagen vascular disease. Both polycythemia vera and Waldenstrom's macroglobulinemia may produce hyperviscosity syndromes associated with CRVO. The association of CRVO with systemic lupus erythematosus is well established. CRVO with severe vaso-occlusion and rapid development of neovascularization may suggest the presence of antiphospholipid antibody associated disease.

The use of corticosteroid, anticoagulant, or thrombolytic therapy for the treatment of CRVO remains unproven. Present treatment consists of searching for and treating associated systemic diseases, as well as managing the complications of CRVO: retinal neovascularization, neovascular glaucoma, and macular edema. Panretinal photocoagulation is effective in averting neovascular glaucoma in eyes with ischemic CRVO if instituted before closure of the filtration angle by neovascular proliferation. Determination of the optimum timing of panretinal photocoagulation in ischemic CRVO, as well as the benefit of grid laser photocoagulation for macular edema in nonischemic CRVO, is currently under evaluation in the Central Vein Occlusion Study.

■ BRANCH RETINAL VEIN OCCLUSION

Branch retinal vein occlusion (BRVO) is the second most common retinovascular disorder after diabetic retinopathy. BRVO results from thrombotic occlusion of the vein at the site of arteriovenous crossing, where the artery and vein share a common sheath. Such crossing sites may be altered by hypertension-induced arteriosclerosis with subsequent impingement on the vein. Nonetheless, the exact pathogenesis of venous obstruction is unclear. The disorder usually presents in the fifth or sixth decade of life. Hypertension is present in one-half to two-thirds of cases (22).

Patients seek treatment for symptoms of diminished central vision or visual scotomas above or below fixation. The onset of symptoms is typically acute. Initial visual acuity is often in the 20/40 to 20/200 range.

Ophthalmoscopy shows a wedge-shaped area of intraretinal flame and dot-blot hemorrhage, dilated retinal veins, retinal edema, exudates and cotton wool spots. The apex of the lesion points to the site of venous occlusion (Figure 60–7). Typically, the site of occlusion is found within one to two disc diameters from the optic nerve. The supertemporal vein is involved in two-thirds of cases. The fovea may be involved secondary to edema, hemorrhage, or capillary nonperfusion.

Histopathologic study shows an intact or recanalized thrombus present at the site of occlusion (14).

Fluorescein angiography displays prolongation of the arteriovenous transit time through the involved circulatory branches. Retinovascular leakage is seen in the involved areas. Cystoid macular edema may be present. A variable amount of capillary nonperfusion may occur. One-half of BRVOs show greater than five disk areas of capillary nonperfusion. Early in the course of the disor-

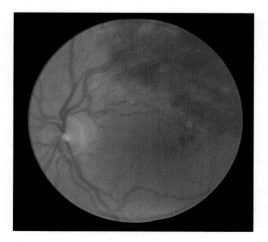

Figure 60–7.
Branch retinal vein occlusion in a 52-year-old patient. The superotemporal arcade, as in this patient, is most frequently affected. Edema and hemorrhages appear in a sectoral pattern with the apex pointing to the site of obstruction. Visual acuity was 20/200, limited by macular edema.

der, before the intraretinal hemorrhages have cleared, angiography is of limited value secondary to blockage of choroidal and retinal fluorescence by blood. Later in the course of the disease, angiography may be particularly useful in assessing the amount of capillary nonperfusion and in distinguishing neovascularization from collateral vessels which will not leak fluorescein.

The differential diagnosis of a branch retinal vein occlusion includes hemicentral vein occlusion, Coat's disease, macular hemorrhage, disciform age-related macular degeneration, and CMV retinitis.

The recovery phase involves the formation of collateral vascular channels across the horizontal raphe. Intraretinal hemorrhages usually resorb over the subsequent 4 to 6 months. Occasionally, intraretinal hemorrhages may spread into the subretinal space or vitreous cavity. Visual recovery depends on the extent of foveal involvement in the edematous, hemorrhageous, and ischemic processes. Recovery may be complicated by the development of retinal neovascularization, by persistence of macular edema, or rarely, by rhegmatogenous retinal detachment.

The Branch Vein Occlusion Study (23,31) (BVOS) observed that 31% of BRVOs with more than 5 disc areas of capillary nonperfusion on fluorescein angiography will develop retinal neovascularization. Moreover, of those which develop neovascularization, 61% will progress to visually significant vitreous hemorrhage—the BVOS randomized nonperfused BRVOs both before and after the development of neovascularization. The study found that treatment of nonperfused patients before the development of neovascularization, lowered the incidence of neovascularization from 22% to 12%, with an estimated 13% versus 7% progressing to vitreous hemorrhage. Given the limited benefit of this treatment effect, the study concluded that peripheral scatter laser in the affected retinal sector should be deferred until the development of neovascularization, when treatment was shown to significantly lower the incidence of visually significant vitreous hemorrhage from 61% to 29%.

The BVOS also studied the benefit of macular grid laser photocoagulation on nonclearing macular edema, involving the fovea of at least 3 month's duration associated with impairment of visual acuity to at least the 20/40 level. At 3 years, treated eyes were more likely to gain 2 or more lines of vision (65% versus 37%), and less likely to deteriorate to 20/200 or worse acuity (12% versus 23%). The mechanism by which grid laser works is unclear, but may include autoregulation of retinal vessels, retinal thinning secondary to cellular destruction with improved access to choroidal blood flow, and stimulation of increased pigment epithelium pumping.

■ RETINAL ARTERIAL OBSTRUCTION

Central, branch, cilioretinal, and ophthalmic arterial obstruction constitute a spectrum of related vaso-occlusive disorders which may result from embolic, thrombotic, vasculitic, hypoperfusive, or compressive processes (1). Each is characterized by the acute onset of painless visual loss. Given the thromboembolic etiology of the majority of arterial occlusions, most patients experience symptoms in the sixth or seventh decade of life. Systemic hypertension is present in the majority of these patients. Ten percent of arterial obstructions occur in children and young adults. The etiology of arterial obstruction in young patients is different, since it is often associated with migraine, coagulation disorders, hemoglobinopathies, or prepapillary arterial loops (4). The prognosis of arterial obstructions appears to depend most on which portion of the circulation is involved, with less regard to age or etiology.

In cases of central retinal or ophthalmic artery occlusion, an afferent pupillary defect develops immediately. No light perception is typically encountered with ophthalmic artery occlusion. Visual acuity in central retinal artery occlusion drops to the hand motion or light perception level, since the peripheral retina may receive adequate oxygen from the choroidal circulation to function. Central retinal artery obstruction in eyes in which the fovea is supplied by a cilioretinal artery, may have preservation of central vision. Conversely, isolated occlusion of the cilioretinal artery may occur. Branch arterial occlusions almost always affect the temporal circulation (27). Visual acuity is often diminished to the 20/50 to 20/100 level, although 80% will eventually improve to 20/40 or better.

Since the inner two-thirds of the retina is supplied by the retinal circulation, retinal arterial obstruction results in inner retinal opacification and edema within hours of the event (2). Opacification is thought to be related to impaired axoplasmic flow. Opacification is most dramatic in areas where nerve fibers and ganglion cells are the most concentrated, namely, the posterior pole. When the fovea is involved, a cherry red spot may occur as a result of the absence of opacified ganglion cells in this area, which allows the intact underlying choroidal circulation to be seen (Figure 60–8). Varying degrees of arteriolar narrowing is observed, owing to diminishment of the blood column. Often, flow is so sufficiently slowed that individual clumps of blood cells may be observed to move along the arteriole, representing so-called "boxcar" formation. When the etiology of the oc-

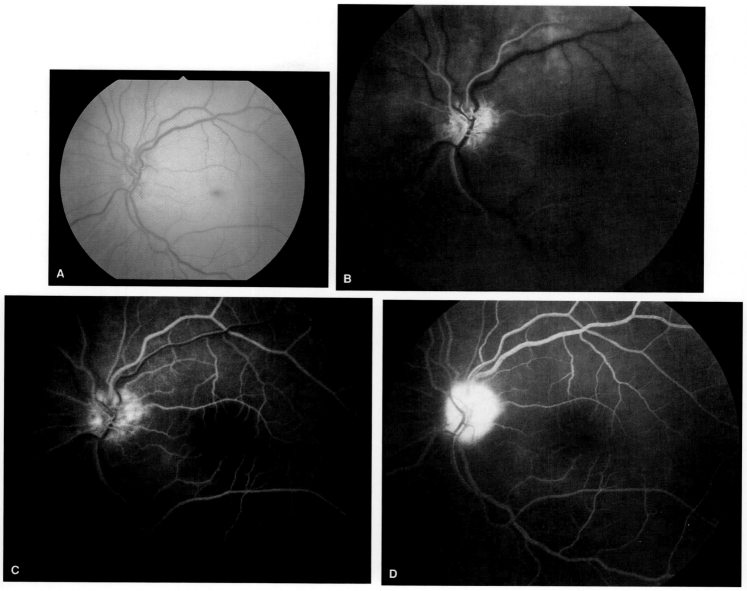

Figure 60–8.
Central retinal artery occlusion in a 71-year-old female with cardiac valvular disease. Color photograph (A) shows opacification of the nerve fiber layer, producing a cherry red spot in the fovea. Fluorescein angiography (B through D) illustrates normal filling of the choroidal circulation, delayed filling of the retinal arterial tree, and prolongation of the arteriovenous transit time.

clusion is thromboembolic, emboli may be seen at arterial branching sites or at the optic nerve head.

Over a period of weeks, inner retinal opacification subsides. Recanalization of the artery may occur with reestablishment of arterial circulation, though capillary circulation usually remains impaired. Such changes occur too late to impact functional recovery. Arterial-arterial shunts between normal and affected areas may occasionally develop after branch arterial obstruction and are pathognomonic of previous obstruction. While retinal neovascularization is rare, iris neovascularization occurs in 10 to 15% of central retinal artery occlusions.

Fluorescein angiography shows delayed arterial filling and prolongation of the arteriovenous transit time (Figure 60–6) (IVFA). Rarely, a precapillary arterial loop may represent the etiology of a branch artery obstruction. Ophthalmic artery occlusion differs from that of central, branch, or cilioretinal occlusion in that choroidal fluorescence is impaired, as well.

Histopathologic study of the acute phase of occlusion shows inner retinal edema and pyknotic inner retinal layer nuclei. Months later, inner nuclear and ganglion cell loss is observed.

The most common etiology of arterial obstruction is embolic disease. Carotid artery stenosis is present in 75% of adults with retinal artery obstruction. Emboli derived from atheromatous plaques in stenotic carotid arteries may lodge near the lamina cribrosa, in branch retinal arteries, or rarely, in the ophthalmic artery. Emboli from the carotid arteries may be composed of cholesterol (Hollenhorst plaques), fibrinoplatelet aggregates, or calcium deposits. The most important of these are the calcific emboli which appear as single, white, nonrefractile, angular deposits which give the illusion of being of larger diameter than the vessel they occupy. Cholesterol emboli are large, elongated, matted gray-white deposits along vessel walls (Figure 60–9). They are often associated with transient visual loss.

Less commonly, though particularly in younger patients, emboli may be derived from cardiac vegetations associated with mitral valve prolapse, rheumatic heart disease, arrhythmia, congenital heart defects, and left atrial myxoma. Rarer causes of embolic arterial obstruction include Purtcher's retinopathy, which is believed to result from activation of complement C5a in patients with severe trauma or acute pancreatitis.

Bilateral arterial vaso-occlusion may have associated systemic collagen vascular diseases, including systemic lupus erythematosus, polyarteritis nodosa, Wegener's granulomatosis, and giant cell arteritis. Also paranasal steroid injections of eyelid. A syndrome of bilateral arterial obliterative vaso-occlusion, often associated with early neovascularization, has been reported in patients with collagen vascular disease, some of whom test positive for antiphospholipid antibodies or the lupus anticoagulant.

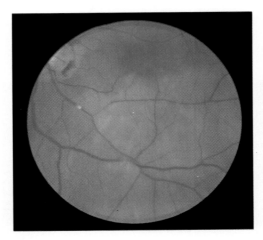

Figure 60–9.
Branch retinal artery occlusion in a 72-year-old patient with carotid atherosclerosis. Note the sectoral retinal edema, distal to the site of obstruction by the bright yellow, refractile Hollenhorst plaque.

Giant cell arteritis is an important etiology of central retinal artery occlusion in the elderly. Although it occurs in only 2% of cases, the propensity for undiagnosed cases to affect the fellow eye makes the detection of affected patients critical. Invariably, some complaints of systemic collagen vascular disease can be elicited from the history including long-term malaise, proximal myalgia, headache, jaw claudication, scalp tenderness, and temporal artery tenderness. Elevation of the erythrocyte sedimentation rate increases suspicion of the diagnosis. Diagnosis is made by biopsy of one or both temporal arteries. Since long-term oral steroid therapy is the treatment of choice, pathologic confirmation of disease is preferable before committing the patient to the potential side effects of continuous steroid use. Once the diagnosis is suspected, steroids should be instituted immediately since pathologic assessment changes on biopsy will still be present if completed within 2 weeks. Pathologic examination findings include inflammatory cellular infiltration of the media and adventitia with fragmentation of the internal elastic lamina.

Compressive events such as retrobulbar injection, traumatic optic nerve sheath hemorrhage, or coexistent central retinal vein occlusion, may also result in central retinal artery occlusion. Arterial obstructions may be the result of local retinitis from CMV, toxoplasmosis, herpes zoster, or syphilis. Lastly, a syndrome of idiopathic bilateral, recurrent, multiple branch retinal artery occlusion associated with tinnitus, hearing loss, and vertigo, in otherwise healthy individuals, has been described.

Hypoperfusion as a result of carotid artery stenosis may result in dot-blot hemorrhages in the retinal midperiphery, producing so-called venous stasis retinopathy. Impaired arterial perfusion with subsequent pool-

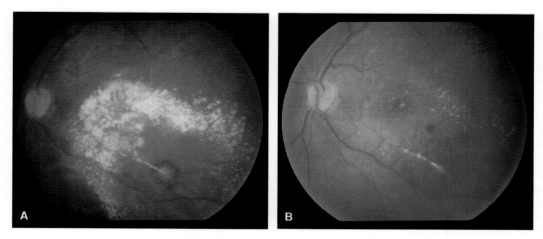

Figure 60–10.
Acquired retinal arterial macroaneurysm with marked lipid exudation into the fovea (A). One year after laser photocoagulation along the edges of the macroaneurysm, no sign of persistent exudation is seen (B).

ing of blood in the venous circulation causes the clinical picture. More advanced stenosis of the carotid artery may result in severe ophthalmic artery hypoperfusion, producing the ocular ischemic syndrome. The syndrome consists of retinal venous dilation without tortuosity, dot-blot mid-peripheral hemorrhages, lowered intraocular pressure, cataract, iris and retinal neovascularization, mild uveitis, and corneal clouding. Symptoms of profound visual loss typically develop insidiously, often associated with episodes of transient visual loss. Decreased ocular perfusion may be shown by premature closure of the central retinal artery with slight digital pressure, or by ophthalmodynamometry.

The treatment of arterial obstruction is disappointing. Experimental models suggest irreversible cell in-jury occurs after 90 minutes of deprived perfusion (20). Anterior chamber paracentesis or ocular massage has been advocated in order to increase the relative arterial pressure head and dislodge the embolus, but is of unproven benefit. Breathing 5% CO_2 and 95% oxygen in order to dilate retinal arteries and improve oxygen is of limited use. Currently, treatment should be largely directed at elucidating the underlying etiology of the obstruction. The medical workup must be tailored to the individual patient from an extensive list of possible studies, including carotid ultrasonography and Dopplers, cardiac echography, erythrocyte sedimentation rate, temporal artery biopsy, hemoglobin electrophoresis, coagulation tests, antinuclear antibody assay, and anticardiolipin antibody assay.

■ RETINAL ARTERIAL MACROANEURYSMS

Retinal arterial macroaneurysms (19A, 20A, 24) are acquired round or fusiform dilatations of the arterial tree. Patients present in the sixth or seventh decade of life. Women outnumber men 3:1. Seventy-five percent of cases are associated with systemic hypertension. Bilaterality is present in 10% of cases.

Leakage of serum components or hemorrhage causes patients to seek medical attention. Occasionally, symptoms may be precipitated by acute rises in retinal arterial perfusion pressure, as with Valsalva maneuvers.

Ophthalmoscopy may show retinal exudates, subinternal limiting membrane hemorrhage, intraretinal hemorrhage, subretinal hemorrhage, vitreous hemorrhage, cystoid macular edema, or serous macular detachment (Figure 60–10). The presence of both preretinal and subretinal hemorrhage should raise the suspicion of arterial microaneurysm. The macroaneurysm is noted most commonly along supertemporal branch points or arteriovenous crossings. Emboli may be present distal to the aneurysm. Occasionally, the macroaneurysm may not be initially identified because it is obscured by hemorrhage or is present outside the macula. Multiple macroaneurysms occur in 20% of cases. Secondary branch vein occlusion may complicate the clinical picture. Epiretinal membranes may develop.

Fluorescein angiography may show filling of the aneurysm in the early arterial phase with leakage or staining in the late phase of the study. Overlying hemorrhage may obscure the aneurysm. Distal arterial flow may be impaired or normal. Aneurysms which have spontaneously thrombosed may show relatively normal transit of dye.

Histopathologic examination demonstrates a break in the arterial wall with thrombus formation in the surrounding aneurysmal dilation.

Thrombosis and closure of the aneurysm often eventually occur spontaneously. Eyes with visual loss related to hemorrhage from a ruptured macroaneurysm associated with retinal exudation, may develop chronic macular edema accompanied by continued leakage and a poorer visual prognosis.

The differential diagnosis includes branch vein occlusion, diabetic retinopathy, radiation retinopathy, Coats' disease, Von Hippel's retinal capillary angioma, uveitis with retinal arteritis, and choroidal neovascularization.

Focal argon or yellow laser is applied to the peripheral margin of the aneurysm (20). Direct treatment of the aneurysm may induce branch arterial occlusion or hemorrhage. No clear indications for laser treatment have yet been established. Treatment of active, visually threatening aneurysms, particularly when associated with foveal threatening exudation, is reasonable. Patients with asymptomatic lesions do not require treatment.

■ COATS' DISEASE

Coats' disease (6, 29A) is a nonheritable, unilateral, congenital vasculopathy characterized by the presence of telangiectatic and aneurysmal retinal vessels. The majority of cases present before age 10. Males outnumber females 3:1. Eighty percent of cases are unilateral. No systemic associations are present.

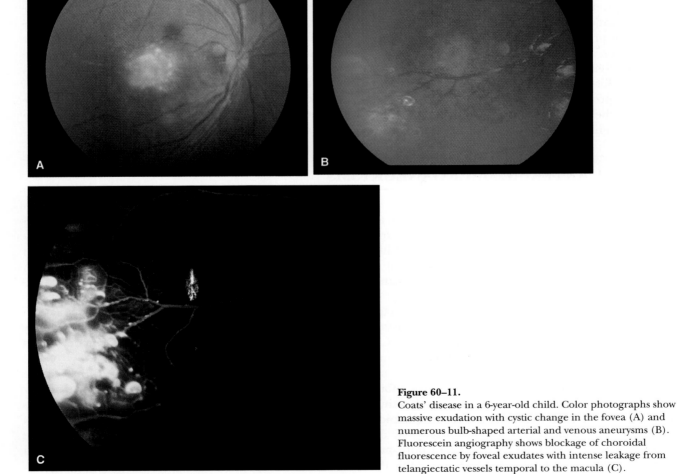

Figure 60–11.
Coats' disease in a 6-year-old child. Color photographs show massive exudation with cystic change in the fovea (A) and numerous bulb-shaped arterial and venous aneurysms (B). Fluorescein angiography shows blockage of choroidal fluorescence by foveal exudates with intense leakage from telangiectatic vessels temporal to the macula (C).

In his initial classification, Coats separated the disorder into three groups. Type I included eyes with massive subretinal exudation and mononuclear infiltration of the choroid (Figure 60–11). Often, in a young child, these eyes present as leukocoria with exudative retinal detachment, which must be differentiated from retinoblastoma. Type II represents a less severe picture of retinal telangiectasis which may be associated with lipid exudation. These eyes essentially represent Leber's miliary retinal aneurysms, although, strictly defined, Leber's description did not include lipid exudation. Type III includes eyes with lipid exudation surrounding a retinal capillary angioma. These eyes essentially represent Von Hippel's angiomatosis retinae or acquired retinal capillary hemangiomas.

Most cases come to medical attention for leukocoria or strabismus in childhood. Milder cases may go unrecognized until adulthood. Vascular abnormalities are probably present at birth. The ophthalmoscopic appearance is variable. A localized yellow exudative retinal elevation is often present. Retinal hemorrhages may be associated. In more severe cases, extensive exudative retinal detachment may occur. Telangiectatic and tortuous retinal vessels may be observed or may be obscured by massive exudation and hemorrhage. Vascular sheathing or signs of inflammation are absent.

Fluorescein angiography (Figure 60–11 IVFA) may show typical "light bulb" aneurysmal dilations of arterioles and venules with associated capillary nonperfusion. The anomalous vessels leak fluorescein dye.

Histopathologic features include loss of endothelial integrity and thickening of capillary walls.

The differential diagnosis includes retinoblastoma, familial exudative vitreoretinopathy, retinopathy of prematurity, incontinentia pigmentosa, Toxocara canis, branch retinal vein occlusion, and parafoveal telangiectasia. [See also Pediatrics chapter, Table 22–4].

Given the progressive nature of the disorder, together with the increasing difficulty of controlling advanced lesions, early intervention is advisable (26). Treatment consists of laser photocoagulation, triple freeze-thaw cryopexy, or retinal reattachment surgery as indicated. Ablative treatment results in resolution of the vascular anomalies and exudate in half of cases, although the presence of retinal detachment often imparts a poor prognosis. Multiple treatment sessions are often required to obliterate the abnormal vessels.

■ PARAFOVEAL TELANGIECTASIA

Parafoveal telangiectasia (5, 15, 16) describes a rare group of disorders characterized by ectasia of juxtafoveal capillaries, primarily in the temporal macula, and usually associated with retinovascular leakage. Unlike Coats' disease, adults, not children, are affected. The disorder may be bilateral, and either sex may be involved. Only capillaries which border the foveal avascular zone are involved. The pathogenesis of disease is unknown. No family history is present.

Unilateral Congenital Parafoveal Telangiectasia (Group 1A) occurs in men in their 40s. Edema and exudates are present, temporal to the fovea. Patients complain of mild blurring of vision to the 20/25 to 20/40 level. Fluorescein angiography shows capillary telangiectasia at the temporal border of the fovea, associated with the early leakage of dye. The disorder most likely represents a mild presentation of Coats' disease. The disorder does not necessarily progress. Spontaneous improvement may occur. The benefit of laser photocoagulation of the telangiectatic capillaries is unclear.

Unilateral Idiopathic Parafoveal Telangiectasis (Group 1B) occurs in middle-aged men. The area of temporal telangiectasis is small and may not be associated with much leakage. Visual acuity is typically 20/25 of better. Photocoagulation is not indicated.

Bilateral Acquired Parafoveal Telangiectasia (Group 2) occurs in either sex in the fifth or sixth decade of life.

A visual acuity of 20/30 to 20/60 is present. Telangiectatic capillaries are seen at the temporal foveal border but may extend along the nasal border, as well. Retinovascular leakage occurs, but without liquid exudates. White intraretinal dots may be observed. Some patients may develop a yellow, pseudovitelliform lesion in the fovea. Fluorescein angiography shows leakage from the telangiectatic capillaries. Right-angled venules may be seen to drain the telangiectatic capillaries. Intraretinal pigment migration may develop around these right angle venules. Visual decline typically occurs gradually over many years but may drop rapidly should the process be complicated by choroidal neovascularization. The disorder is usually not amenable to laser photocoagulation. A significant number of Group 2 patients will have diabetes or an abnormal glucose tolerance test. Histopathologic study of a Group-2 eye showed capillary basement membrane abnormalities, similar to those of diabetes. The significance of these observations to the pathogenesis of disease is unclear.

Bilateral Perifoveal Telangiectasis with Capillary Occlusion (Group 3) represents an even rarer condition characterized by obliteration and telangiectasia of the perifoveal capillary network in the fifth decade. No leakage of fluorescein dye is present. Optic disc pallor and hyperactive deep tendon reflexes may be present.

The differential diagnosis of parafoveal telangiectasis includes diabetic macular edema, Coat's disease, collateral vessel development following BRVO, radiation retinopathy, sickle cell retinopathy and age-related macular degeneration.

■ SICKLE CELL RETINOPATHY

The sickling hemoglobinopathies are the result of diminished red blood cell deformability under conditions of hypoxia and acidosis, as a result of genetic errors in hemoglobin structure. Normal hemoglobin or hemoglobin A is a protein composed of two alpha and two beta chains. Substitution of the amino acid valine for glutamic acid at the sixth position of the beta chain results in hemoglobin S. A similar substitution of lysine for glutamic acid produces hemoglobin C. Failure of production of one of the alpha or beta chains results in thalessemia. Combination of these various hemoglobin molecules in individuals results in sickle cell trait (AS), sickle cell anemia of SS disease (SS), SC disease (SC), or S-thal disease.

Sickling hemoglobinopathies are essentially a disease of black individuals. Sickle trait occurs in 8% of

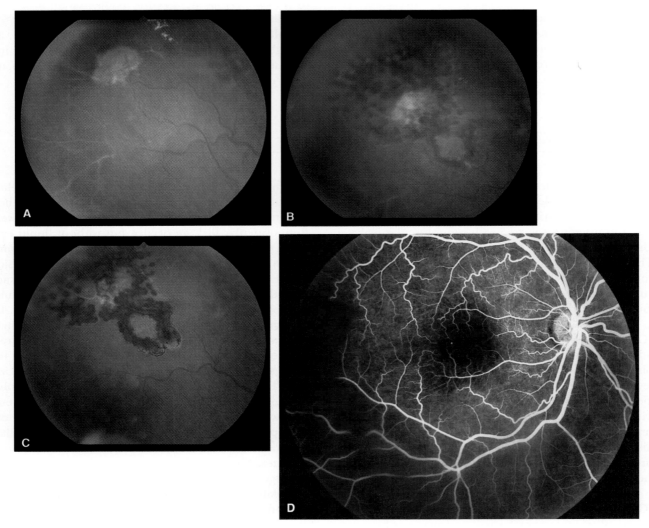

Figure 60–12.
Sickle cell retinopathy. Peripheral neovascularization (A) with involution after laser phtocoagulation at 1 month (B) and 1 year (C). Fluorescein angiography in a 33-year-old black male with SC disease shows a normal macula (D), abrupt termination of the peripheral retinal vasculature, arteriovenous anastomoses, leakage from an area of neovascularization, and blockage corresponding to peripheral preretinal hemorrhage (E & F).

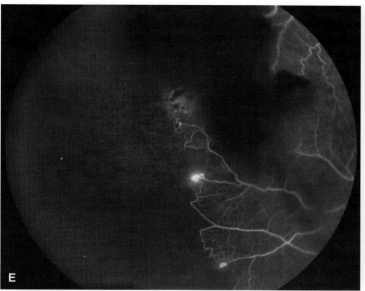

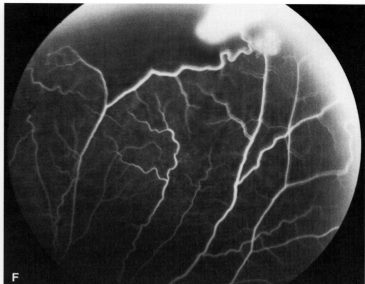

Figure 60–12. *(continued)*

American blacks; S-thal disease in 0.5%; SS disease in 0.4%; and SC disease in 0.2%. While SS disease is most likely to produce severe systemic manifestations including anemia and ischemic crisis, SC and S-thal disease are usually responsible for the development of retinovascular disease.

Abnormalities may be grouped into nonproliferative and proliferative categories. Nonproliferative findings include abruptly terminating, "comma-shaped" conjunctival or optic nerve head vessels, perifoveal arteriolar occlusion, mid-peripheral salmon patch hemorrhages or iridescent spots, and mid-peripheral black sunbursts. Salmon patch hemorrhages represent preretinal or internal lining membrane hemorrhages which occur near an occluded arteriole. Over 1 to 2 months these hemorrhages resorb, leaving iridescent spots of hemosiderin within a small schisis cavity. Black sunbursts represent retinal pigment epithelial hyperplasia in response to subretinal extension of the hemorrhage.

Proliferative sickle retinopathy (17) is largely confined to the retinal periphery. It can be divided into five stages, which chart the pathogenesis of disease.

(a) Stage 1 is characterized by peripheral arteriolar occlusion.

(b) Stage 2 shows peripheral arteriovenous anastomoses at the border of posteriorly perfused and anteriorly nonperfused retina. At this stage, fluorescein angiography does not show any leakage of dye.

(c) Stage 3 is characterized by the development of neovascularization from the network of anastomoses. Often, neovascular tufts are served by a single feeding arteriole and draining venules. Typically, they develop a frond-like, "sea-fan" appearance akin to

the similarly shaped marine invertebrate. Fluorescein angiography shows leakage of dye from these tufts. Neovascularization appears to develop as a response to local factors since distant neovascularization in the posterior pole, or at the optic nerve, does not occur. Autoinfarction of neovascular tufts with spontaneous regression of disease often accompanies this stage of the disorder.

(d) Some patients, however progress to stage 4 with the occurrence of vitreous hemorrhage, secondary to vitreous traction on the neovascular tufts.

(e) Stage 5 represents the development of rhegmatogenous retinal detachment, secondary to progressive vitreous traction at sites of neovascularization and accompanying fibrous proliferation.

The differential diagnosis includes sarcoidosis, pars planitis, systemic vasculitis, diabetes mellitus, hyperviscosity syndromes, retinopathy of prematurity, Eales' disease, familial exudative vitreoretinopathy, incontinentia pigmenti, Norrie's disease, longstanding detachments, and talc retinopathy.

Treatment is indicated for active peripheral neovascularization, nonclearing vitreous hemorrhage, or retinal detachment. Peripheral nonperfusion in the absence of active neovascularization does not warrant treatment. Involution of peripheral neovascularization may be induced by 360° panretinal photocoagulation applied to the nonperfused areas of the anterior retina (25) (Figure 60–12). Direct photocoagulation of the feeder arteriole of sea fans has also been used. However, this method of treatment may be associated with a higher rate of complications, including hemorrhage and retinal tear formation (21). Scleral buckling surgery may be complicated by anterior segment ischemia (28). The use of general anesthesia may aggravate ocular and systemic hemodynamics, particularly if mild acidosis develops. Whenever possible, encircling buckles should be avoided and anesthesia techniques which minimize acidosis and maximize oxygenation, should be sought. Preoperative plasmapheresis is occasionally a useful adjunct.

■ HYPERTENSIVE RETINOPATHY

Acute or chronic elevations of systemic blood pressure lead to characteristic ophthalmoscopic alterations (32, 33). Chronic hypertension usually does not produce any visual symptoms or dysfunction. Ocular findings are minimal. Ophthalmoscopy shows generalized and focal arterial narrowing through autoregulation, in response to elevated perfusion pressure. Narrowing is best appreciated in relative arterial-to-vein diameters, the so-called A/V ratio. A normal value is approximately 2/3 Over time, arterial walls lose their luster, assuming first a copper color, and finally a silver wire appearance. Depression of underlying veins a crossing sites by thickening arterial walls typically occurs, referred to as A-V nicking (Figure 60–13).

Acute, severe (malignant) hypertension produces visual symptoms. Affected patients may complain of transient obscuration of diminished central vision. Systemic complaints may include headache, nausea and vomiting, alterations in mental status, and convulsions. Ophthalmoscopic findings include prominent cotton wool spots, nerve fiber layer hemorrhages, and lipid exudation in the posterior pole (Figure 60–14). Both eyes are involved, typically symmetrically. Disc edema may be present. Rarely, hypertensive choroidopathy with secondary exudative retinal detachments can occur. Focal areas of choroidal and choriocapillaris infarction with secondary fibrinoid necrosis of the retinal pigment epithelium may occur. This RPE necrosis and pigment clumping represents the so-called Elsching's spots.

Fluorescein angiographic findings in acute, severe hypertensive retinopathy include capillary nonperfusion, microaneurysm formation, telangiectasis, and retinovascular leakage. Fluorescein angiographic findings of hypertensive choroidopathy will characteristically show early, multiple punctate areas of hyperfluorescence, which leak later in the study.

Histopathologic examination shows thickening and fibroblastic infiltration of the intima. Fibrinoid necrosis of precapillary arterioles occurs. Swollen nerve fibers with accumulation of organelles (cytoid bodies) are noted in the area corresponding to cotton wool spots as a result of ischemic interruption of axoplasmic flow (3).

The differential diagnosis includes systemic lupus erythematosus, polyarteritis nodosa, toxemia of pregnancy, diabetic retinopathy, and neuroretinitis.

Hypertension may also be associated with central

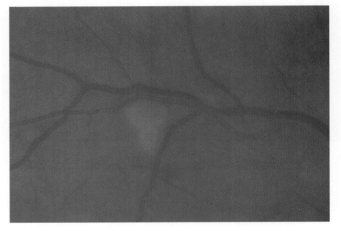

Figure 60–13.
Arteriovenous nicking seen in severe hypertension. The artery and vein share a common sheath at sites of crossing. The atherosclerotic artery compresses the vein, producing this picture.

retinal vein occlusion, branch retinal occlusion, retinal macroaneurysms, and ischemic optic neuropathy.

Treatment consists of gradual normalization of blood pressure. Patients with acute, severe hypertension mandate emergent medical evaluation and often require hospitalization.

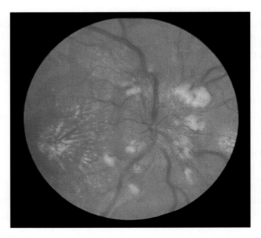

Figure 60–14.
Malignant hypertension with blood pressure of 220/140 in a 52-year old patient. Bilateral disc edema, multiple cotton wool spots, and lipid deposition in the formation of a macular star are indicative of severely uncontrolled blood pressure. This patient needs immediate evaluation and treatment for hypertension.

■ FROSTED BRANCH ANGIITIS

Frosted branch angiitis (FBA) is a striking condition with bilateral sheathing of all of the retinal vessels, like the branches of a tree. Young, healthy patients present with profound visual loss often worse than 20/200. Anterior chamber and vitreous inflammation is also present.

FBA can be effectively treated with systemic steroids with recovery of normal vision in most cases.

The etiology is not known. Other conditions producing phlebitis, such as sarcoidosis, Eales' disease, tuberculosis, syphilis, and multiple sclerosis, should be excluded.

■ REFERENCES

1. Appen RE, Ray SH, Cogan DG: Central retinal artery occlusion. Am J Ophthalmol 1975; 79: 374–381.
2. Arruga J, Sanders M: Ophthalmoscopic findings in 70 patients with evidence of retinal embolism. Ophthalmology 1982; 89: 1336–1347.
3. Ashton N, Harry J: The pathology of cotton-wool spots and cytoid bodies in hypertensive retinopathy and other diseases. Trans Ophthalmol Soc UK 1963; 83: 91.
4. Brown GC, Magargal LE, Shields JA, et al: Retinal arterial obstruction in children and young adults. Ophthalmology 1981; 88: 18–25.
5. Chew EY, Murphy RP, Newsome DA, Fine SL: Parafoveal telangiectasis and diabetic retinopathy. Arch Ophthalmol 1986; 104: 71–75.
6. Coats G: Forms of retinal disease with massive exudation. Roy Lond Ophthalmol Hosp Rep 1908; 18: 440–525.
7. The Diabetes Control and Complications Trial Research Group: The Effective Intensive Treatment of Diabetes on Development and Progression of Long-term Complications and Insulin-dependent Diabetes Mellitus. New Engl J Med 1993, 329: 977–986.
8. Diabetic Retinopathy Study Research Group: Four risk factors for severe visual loss in diabeticretinopathy. The third report from the DRS. Arch Ophthalmol 1979; 97: 654–655.
9. Diabetic Retinopathy Vitrectomy Study Research Group: Early vitrectomy for severe proliferative diabetic retinopathy in eyes with useful vision: Clinical application of results of a randomized trial—Diabetic Retinopathy Vitrectomy Study Report 5. Ophthalmology 1988; 95: 1321–1334.
10. Diabetic Retinopathy Vitrectomy Study Research Group: Early vitrectomy for severe vitreous hemorrhage in diabetic retinopathy. Four years results of a randomized trial-Diabetic Retinopathy Vitrectomy Study Report 5. Arch Ophthalmol 1990; 108: 958–964.
11. Early Treatment Diabetic Retinopathy Study Group: Early photocoagulation for diabetic retinopathy. Early Treatment Diabetic Study report number 9. Ophthalmology 1991; 98: 766.
12. Early Treatment Diabetic Retinopathy Study Group: Photocoagulation for diabetic macular edema. Early Treatment Diabetic Study report number 1. Arch Ophthalmol 1985; 103: 1796–1806.
13. Elman MJ, Kaur Bhatt A, Quinlan PM: The risk of systemic vascular disease and mortality in patients with central retinal vein occlusion. Ophthalmology 1990; 97: 1543–1548.
14. Frangieh GT, Green WR, Barraquer-Somers E, Finkelstein D: Histopathologic study of nine branch retinal vein occlusions. Arch Ophthalmol 1982; 100: 1132–40.
15. Gass JDM, Blodi BA: Idiopathic juxtafoveolar retinal telangiectasis: update of classification and follow-up study. Ophthalmology 1993; 100: 1536–1546.
16. Gass JD, Oyakawa RT: Idiopathic juxtafoveal retinal telangiectasis. Arch Ophthalmol 1982; 100: 769–780.
17. Goldberg MF: Classification and pathogenesis of proliferative sickle retinopathy. Am J Ophthalmol 1971; 71: 649–65.
18. Green WR, Chan CC, Hutchins GM, et al: Central retinal vein occlusions: A prospective histopathologic study of 29 eyes in 28 cases. Trans Am Ophthalmol Soc 1981, 79: 371–422.
19. Hayreh SS: Classification of central retinal vein obstruction. Ophthalmology 1993; 90: 458–474.
19A. Palestine AG, Robertson DM, Goldstein BG: Macroaneurysms of the retinal arteries. Am J Ophthalmol 1982; 93: 164–71.
20. Hayreh SS, Kolder HF, Neingeist TA: Central retinal artery occlusion and retinal tolerance time. Ophthalmology 1982; 89: 1336–1347.
20A. Abdel-Khalek MN, Richardson J: Retinal microaneurysm: natural history and guidelines for treatment. Br J Ophthalmol 1986; 70: 2–11.
21. Jacobson MS, Gagliano DA, Cohen SB: A randomized clinical trial of feeder vessel photocoagulation of sickle cell retinopathy. A long-term follow-up. Ophthalmology 1991; 98–581.
22. Johnston RL, Brucker AJ, Steinmann W: Risk factors of branch retinal vein occlusion. Arch Ophthalmol 1985; 103: 1831–2.
23. Depression of underlying veins a crossing sites by thickening arterial walls typically occurs, referred to as A-V nicking (Figure 60–13).
24. Rabb MF, Gagliano DA, Teske MP: Retinal arterial macroaneurysms. Surv Ophthalmol 1988; 33: 73–96.
25. Rednam KR, Jampol LM, Goldberg MF: Scatter retinal photocoagulation for proliferative sickle cell retinopathy. Am J Ophthalmol 1982; 93: 594–9.
26. Ridley JE, Shields JA, Brown GL: Coats' disease: evaluation of management. Ophthalmology 1982; 89: 1381–1387.

27. Ros MA, Magargal LE, Uram M: Branch retinal artery occlusion: a review of 201 eyes. Ann Ophthalmol 1989; 3: 103–107.

28. Ryan SJ, Goldberg MF: Anterior segment ischemia following scleral buckling in sickle cell hemoglobinopathy. Am J Ophthalmol 1971; 72: 35–50.

29A. Tarkkanen A, Laatikainen L: Coats' disease: clinical, angiographic, histopathological findings and clinical management. Br J Ophthalmol 1983; 67: 766–76.

29. Magargal LE, Brown GA, Augsburger JJ: Efficacy of panretinal photocoagulation in preventing neovascular glaucoma following ischemic central retinal vein obstruction. Ophthalmology 1982; 89: 780–4.

30. The Branch Vein Occlusion Study Group: Argon laser photocoagulation for macular edema in branch vein occlusion. Am J Ophthalmol 1984; 98:271–282.

31. The Branch Vein Occlusion Study Group: Argon laser scatter photocoagulation for prevention of neovascularization and vitreous hemorrhage in branch vein occlusion. Arch Ophthalmol 1986; 104: 34–41.

32. Tso MOM, Abrams GW, Jampol LM: Hypertensive retinopathy, choroidopathy, and optic neuropathy: a clinical and pathophysiological approach to classification. In: Singerman LJ and Jampol LM (eds): Retinal and Choroidal Manifestations of Systemic Disease. Baltimore: Williams & Wilkins, 1991.

33. Walsh JB: Hypertensive retinopathy: description, classification, and prognosis. Ophthalmology 1982; 89: 1127–31.

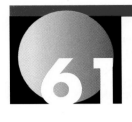

Peripheral Vitreoretinal Disorders

*Eugene de Juan Jr., Stuart W. Noorily,
William P. Townsend-Pico, Kenneth C. Chern*

■POSTERIOR VITREOUS DETACHMENT

The vitreous is a matrix of collagen fibers interspersed with molecules of negatively-charged hyaluronic acid. The outer surface of the vitreous gel, the cortical vitreous, is firmly attached to the retinal surface and pars plana in a 4 to 6 mm area straddling the ora serrata known as the vitreous base. Less firm attachment is present at the optic disc, over the macula, and along the larger retinal vessels. Depletion of the hyaluronic acid concentration in vitreous as a result of aging, vitreous hemorrhage, vitreous inflammation, or laser capsulotomy, induces aggregation of collagen fibers with collapse (syneresis) of the vitreous gel (Figure 61–1A). Separation of the cortical vitreous gel from the macula and optic disk constitutes a posterior vitreous detachment (PVD) (7) (Figure 61–1B).

PVDs occur in 27% of persons between 60 and 69 years of age, and 63% of persons over age 70. The majority of PVDs are asymptomatic. Symptomatic patients may report the onset of floaters or of photopsia ("flashing lights") exacerbated by ocular movement. Floaters are caused by clumps of vitreous collagen, or secondary to hemorrhage from avulsed blood vessels. Photopsia results from retinal stimulation secondary to vitreoretinal traction. Often a well-defined central translucent floater is noted corresponding to the condensed cortical vitreous which separated from the optic disc. Referred to as the Weiss ring, this structure is the only nonsurgical clinical sign pathognomonic of a PVD.

The significance of a PVD is the potential of retina tears (16) (Figure 61–1C). Retinal tears develop in 10 to 15% of patients with a symptomatic PVD. The presence of red blood cells in the vitreous is an important diagnostic clue, since 70% of such eyes will harbor a retinal tear, compared with 2 to 4% without hemorrhage. Clumps of retinal pigment epithelial cells, in the vitreous, so-called "tobacco dust," are pathognomonic of a retinal break or detachment.

All patients with symptoms of PVD should undergo careful indirect ophthalmoscopy with scleral depression to search for retinal breaks. If none are found, patients should be educated as to the symptoms of retinal breaks and detachment. An additional examination with scleral depression should be done in 4 weeks since 6 weeks appears to be the period of highest risk for the onset of retinal detachment after PVD.

■ ASTEROID HYALOSIS

This degenerative process is a common, primarily unilateral (75%) condition seen in elderly patients and rarely associated with any significant decrease in vision. Its incidence is 1/200 patients. Ocular examination shows multiple yellow-white opacities in the vitreous which, on histopathologic study, are found to consist of calcium soaps (Figure 61–2). The differential diagnosis includes synchysis scintillans and amyloidosis.

Figure 61–1.
A. Liquifaction and syneresis of the vitreous gel. B. Remnants of glial tissue after the separation of the vitreous from the optic nerve can be seen ophthalmoscopically as a Weiss ring.

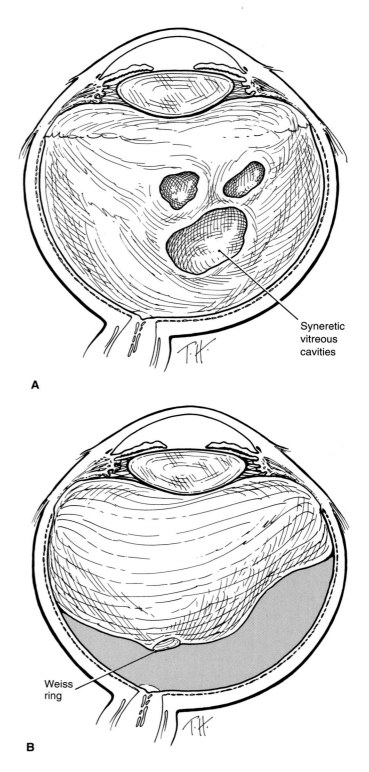

Syneretic
vitreous
cavities

A

Weiss
ring

B

■ SYNCHYSIS SCINTILLANS

Synchysis scintillans consists of an accumulation of yellow, refractile cholesterol crystals in the anterior chamber, vitreous cavity, and occasionally, in the subretinal space after a vitreous hemorrhage, ocular trauma, or chronic uveitis. The crystals may settle inferiorly since many of these patients have liquified vitreous and a posterior vitreous separation.

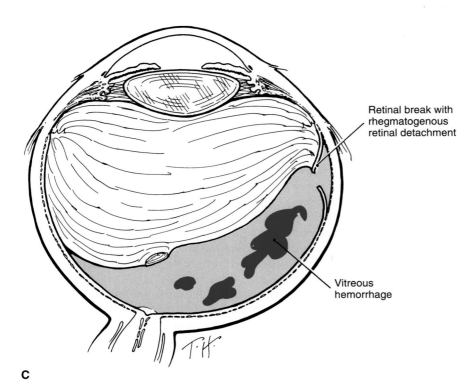

Retinal break with rhegmatogenous retinal detachment

Vitreous hemorrhage

C

Figure 61–1. *(continued)* C. Traction at the vitreous base during vitreous separation may create a retinal break allowing liquified vitreous to flow under the retina creating a rhegmatogenous retinal detachment. Tearing of vessels can result in vitreous hemorrhage in these instances.

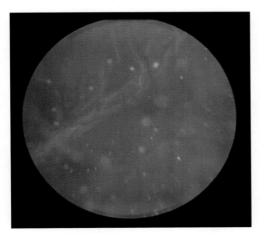

Figure 61–2.
Asteroid hyalosis. Precipitation of calcium soaps in the vitreous produces these white opacities suspended in the vitreous gel. These usually do not affect visual acuity. A rhegmatogenous retinal detachment is also visible.

■ VITREORETINAL AMYLOIDOSIS

Vitreous opacification may be the presenting sign of heredofamilial amyloidosis, an autosomal dominant disorder associated with abnormal accumulation of prealbumin-associated amyloid in the vitreous cavity. The source of the protein is thought to be the retinal vasculature and possibly, the ciliary body. Vitreoretinal amyloidosis is usually bilateral and presents with a sheetlike opacification of the vitreous, with a significant reduction in visual acuity. Although pars plana vitrectomy is usually effective in clearing the vitreous and improving the visual acuity, recurrence of the amyloidosis is common and is believed to originate from the retrolenticular vitreous in phakic patients. Uveitis with vitritis and large cell lymphoma should be included among the differential diagnosis.

■ LATTICE AND OTHER PERIPHERAL RETINAL DEGENERATIONS

Peripheral retinal degenerations encompass a broad range of peripheral retinal changes that include thinning and atrophy of the retina, as well as areas of increased vitreoretinal adhesions (Figure 61–3). An understanding of these degenerations is critical to differentiate those lesions which benefit from prophylactic treatment of retinal detachment. The distinguishing feature between innocuous and high-risk peripheral retinal lesions is the presence of focal vitreoretinal traction.

Lesions without vitreous traction, and thereby, considered benign, include cobblestone or pavingstone degeneration, cystoid degeneration, and white with or without pressure. Cobblestone or pavingstone degeneration consists of areas of outer retinal thinning associated with loss of the RPE and choriocapillaris. They occur in one-fifth of the population and are usually located inferiorly. Hyperpigmentation occurs at the borders of the lesions. Cystoid degeneration represents the development of cystic spaces in the outer plexiform layer. Clinically, these appear as small vesicles associated with mild retinal opacification. Cystoid degeneration is the precursor of retinoschisis. White with or without pressure consists of circumferential bands of retinal whitening. The explanation of this phenomenon is unclear, but may result from the normal attachment of collagen fibrils to retinal Mueller cells.

Lesions associated with vitreous traction and, therefore, predisposed to retinal detachment, include retina flap tears, lattice degeneration, snail track degeneration, zonular traction tufts, and cystic retinal tufts. Retinal flap tears (horseshoe tear) occur as the vitreous pulls anteriorly during formation of a vitreous separation (Figure 61–4). Continued traction on the anterior flap

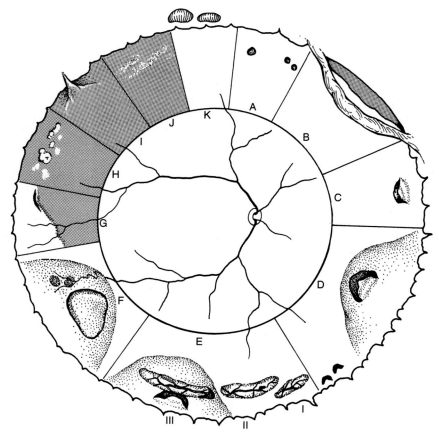

Figure 61–3.
Peripheral retinal changes. A. atrophic hole, B. avulsed vitreous base, C. horseshoe tear, D. horseshoe tear with rhegmatogenous and rhegmat retinal detachment, E. I. Lattice degeneration; II. Lattice with atrophic holes; III. Lattice with horseshoe tear at anterior border of lesion, F. retinoschisis with inner layer breaks, G. white without pressure, H. cobblestone degeneration, I. meridional fold, J. snailtrack degeneration, K. pars plana cysts.

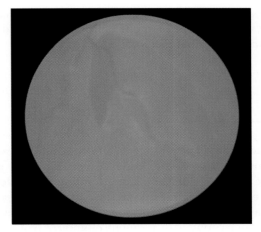

Figure 61–4.
Horseshoe retinal tear with bridging vessel. Retinal traction during a posterior vitreous detachment caused a tear in the retina. A bridging vessel can be seen spanning the break. Shearing of these vessels can lead to vitreous hemorrhage. Liquified vitreous can enter through the break causing a rhegmatogenous retinal detachment.

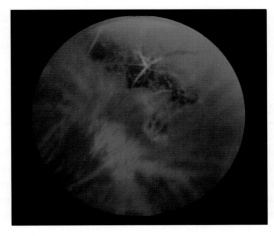

Figure 61–5.
Lattice degeneration. Lattice appears in the peripheral retina as areas of RPE atrophy and pigment clumping with the typical sclerosed vessels traversing the lesion. Vitreous adhesions along the edges of lattice may predispose to formation of retinal breaks.

of the tear allows liquified vitreous access to the potential space between the RPE and photoreceptors, thereby creating a retinal detachment. Flap tears tend to develop at sites of strong vitreoretinal adhesion, such as the posterior border of the vitreous base, the posterior border of lattice degeneration, or at cystic retinal tufts. Operculation of a flap tear typically signals resolution of vitreous traction and decreased risk of retinal detachment; however, care must be taken to ensure that no residual vitreous attachment to the borders of the retinal break remains.

Lattice degeneration occurs in 7 to 8% of the population and in 30% of patients with retinal detachment. The disorder is bilateral in 45% of cases. Lattice degeneration is characterized by circumferential bands of retinal thinning associated with vitreoretinal adhesion at its borders and an overlying pocket of syneretic vitreous. A "lattice" of fine, white, hyalinized blood vessels may be seen within the lesion, although their presence is not required (Figures 61–4 and 61–5). Atrophic holes are often present and may be surrounded by a cuff of subretinal fluid. Eyes with lattice have an increased risk of developing flap tears both associated and independent of lattice patches, particularly at the time of posterior vitreous detachment (2). Nonetheless, the risk of developing retinal detachment in the overall population of patients with lattice degeneration is less than 1%. Risk factors for retinal detachment in patients with lattice include retinal flap tears, increased myopia, and a history of retinal detachment in the fellow eye.

Snail track degeneration consists of circumferential lines of frosty, fine white dots, typically in myopic eyes. While flap tears do not occur, large round, atrophic retinal holes may develop and are associated with an in-

creased risk of retinal detachment. Unlike lattice degeneration, such eyes do not appear to be predisposed to retinal breaks outside the areas of degeneration.

Cystic retinal tufts are congenital, small, granular elevations of retinal tissue located posterior to the vitreous base. Typically, they are bilateral and symmetric. Pigment clumping may or may not be present at the base of the lesion. Vitreous strands strongly attach to these lesions and may cause the development of a retinal break during formation of a PVD. Although cystic retinal tufts are thought to account for 10% of primary retinal detachments, they may be present in as much as 5% of the population. The risk of development of retinal detachment from a cystic retinal tuft is approximately 0.3%.

The decision of when to prophylactically treat lesions predisposing to retinal detachment must balance the likelihood of retina detachment against the success rate and side effects of treatment. Since in most cases, the incidence of retinal detachment is decreased, treatment should be reserved only for those patients at the highest risk of detachment (6). As such, consideration must be given to symptoms, a history of retinal detachment in the fellow eye, the extent of myopia, the state of the vitreous, and a family history of retinal detachment. Symptoms of light flashes are perhaps the most important risk factor, since they are indicators of vitreous traction. The presence of a longstanding PVD dramatically diminishes the risk of detachment. Patients who have sustained a giant retinal tear in one eye should undergo peripheral 360° photocoagulation to the retina, just posterior to the vitreous base, given the risk of bilaterality in 75% of patients.

Treatment of appropriate cases may be done with

cryopexy or laser. Care should be taken to adequately treat retina anterior to the lesion, since this is the area onto which vitreous traction will extend. Cryopexy in the bed of the tear should be avoided since this may disperse viable retinal pigment epithelial cells and contribute to epiretinal membrane formation.

■ RETINAL DETACHMENT

Accumulation of fluid in the potential space between the retinal pigment epithelium (RPE) and the photoreceptors defines a retinal detachment (1). In a rhegmatogenous retinal detachment, liquified vitreous gains access to the subretinal space through a retinal break (Figure 61–6). Rhegmatogenous retinal detachments are the most common variant of detachment with an estimated incidence of 1 in 10,000 persons. Both retinal traction and areas of retinal atrophy are predisposed to the formation of breaks. Retinal breaks characteristically develop during detachment of the posterior vitreous. Eyes at increased risk include myopes, aphakes or pseudophakes, and traumatized eyes.

Symptoms of a rhegmatogenous retinal detachment result from vitreous traction on the retinal break and the spread of subretinal fluid. Symptoms related to traction include photopsias ("flashing lights") and floaters, secondary to vitreous hemorrhage. The spread of subretinal fluid distorts the retinal surface and separates it from its metabolic relationship with the pigment epithelium. This results in a blurred or dark peripheral scotoma often described by the patient as a "curtain." Rhegmatogenously detached retina usually assumes a bullous contour as continued fluid movement through the retinal break attempts to overwhelm normal forces of RPE-photoreceptor attachment. Clumps of pigment epithelial cells of "tobacco dust" can often be seen in the anterior vitreous, having been liberated through the retinal break. Intraocular pressure is typically diminished secondary to increased access of intraocular fluid to trans-RPE uveoscleral outflow passing through the retinal breaks. Localization of retinal breaks invariably dictates the configuration of the detachment (10) (Figure 61–6). Superior detachments result from breaks within one and one-half clock hours of the highest meridian of detachment. If a superior detachment crosses the 12:00 meridian, the primary retinal break will be found between 11:00 and 1:00. The highest border of an inferior detachment dictates which inferior quadrant will harbor the retinal break. The exception to this rule is the presence of a peripheral gutter of subretinal fluid, allowing an inferior detachment which results from a superior break.

Histologically, a detached retina will develop inner nuclear layer edema within a few days. Edema causes folds in the outer retina which can be observed clinically as a corrugated appearance. White dots may be seen on the outer surface of the retina, corresponding to metaplastic RPE histologically. Longstanding retina detachment results in full thickness retinal atrophy, and retinal cysts and peripheral neovascularization may develop. RPE hypertrophy with pigment clumping typically develops at the border of attached retina resulting in a demarcation line.

Rhegmatogenous retinal detachments must be differentiated from traction and exudative retinal detachments. Traction retinal detachment results from mechanical separation of the retina from the underlying RPE because of pulling from fibrous or fibrovascular epiretinal or subretinal proliferations. The clinical appearance of such detachments is characterized by fixed, immobile retinal folds. Unlike rhegmatogenous detachments, the retinal contour is concave and detachment does not extend to the ora serrata. Typically, the detachments result from proliferative diabetic retinopathy or proliferative vitreoretinopathy (PVR) (see PVR section). Traction retinal detachments may additionally be complicated by retinal breaks, resulting in a combined traction-rhegmatogenous retinal detachment.

Exudative retinal detachment results from disturbances of vitreochoroid fluid flow as a result of abnormality of the retinal pigment epithelium or sclera. Exudative detachments are characterized by shifting fluid, which results from gravity dependent movement of the protein-rich subretinal fluid. Also unlike rhegmatogenous detachments, the retinal contour appears smooth, rather than corrugated (Figure 61–7). Occasionally, the retina may become highly elevated, appearing at the posterior lens surface. Longstanding exudative retinal detachments result in characteristic "leopard spot" RPE changes. Causes of exudative retinal detachments include Vogt-Koyangi-Harada syndrome, posterior scleritis, metastatic carcinoma, central serous choroidopathy, serous retinal detachments associated with optic pits, and uveal effusion syndrome.

Other entities in the differential diagnosis of retina detachment include retinoschisis, choroidal detachment, choroidal melanoma, Coat's disease, and retinoblastoma.

Treatment of rhegmatogenous retinal detachment consists of localizing all the retinal breaks, inducing a chorioretinal seal around the retinal breaks with laser

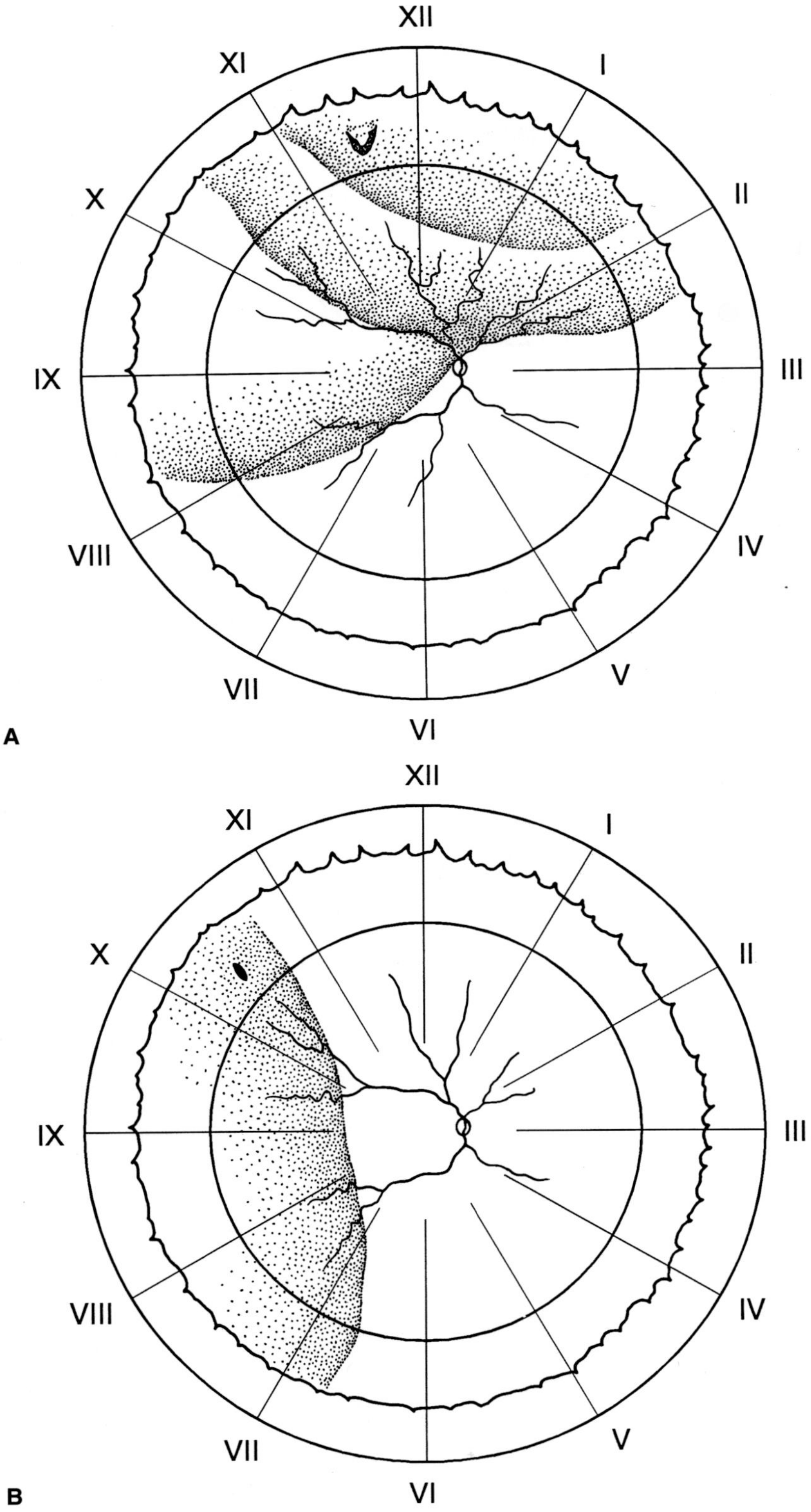

Figure 61–6.
Configuration of rhegmatogenous retinal detachment and localization of breaks. A and B. Superior detachment with retinal break within one and a half clock hours of the highest meridian of detachment.

Figure 61–6. *(continued)* C. The break for an inferior detachment may be located at the meridian of the higher border of the detachment. D. An inferior break can produce equal elevation nasally and temporally.

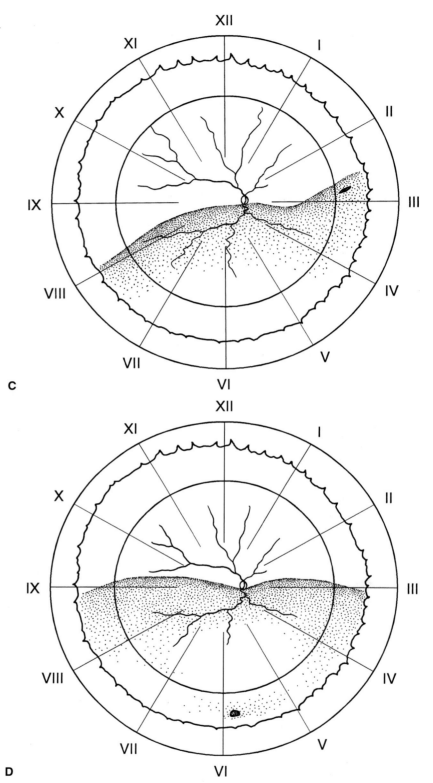

C

D

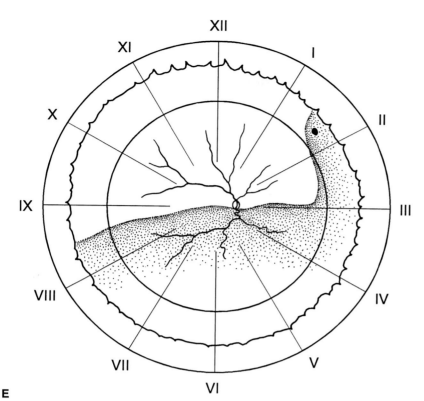

E

Figure 61–6. *(continued)* E. A peripheral gutter of subretinal fluid from an inferior detachment may track superiorly to the retinal break.

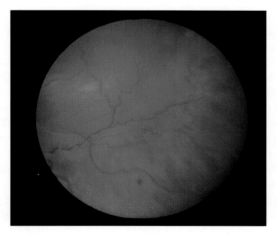

Figure 61–7.
Exudative RD.

or cryopexy (9), relieving vitreous traction, and placing the retina and pigment epithelium in proximity to one another by means of scleral indentation, intravitreal gas tamponade, and/or drainage of subretinal fluid. Choices of surgery include a scleral buckling procedure, pneumatic retinopexy (17), or temporary episcleral balloon procedure (11). In instances of dense vitreous hemorrhage, giant retinal tears, or very posterior breaks, pars plana vitrectomy may be indicated as a primary procedure. Present surgical techniques afford an excellent prognosis for the treatment of rhegmatogenous retinal detachment, with retinal reattachment able to be achieved in 90 to 95% of cases. Failures usually result from the development of proliferative vitreoretinopathy.

■ RETINAL DIALYSIS

Full-thickness separation of the retina at the ora serrata is called a retinal dialysis (see also retinoschisis). Blunt trauma to the eye in the anteroposterior direction causes expansion and contraction of the vitreous gel producing traction at the points of attachment to the retina, especially at the ora serrata, resulting in a dialysis. Traumatic dialyses most commonly occur in the superonasal quadrant. Idiopathic dialyses, in contrast, are more commonly found in the inferotemporal quadrant. Such dialyses occur bilaterally in young patients often with a strong family history of dialyses.

Retinal dialyses can often be closed by application of cryotherapy to the base of the dialysis followed by scleral buckling.

■ GIANT RETINAL TEARS

Giant retinal tears are essentially large horseshoe tears that encompass over 90° of retina. These occur from extensive circumferentially traction at the posterior border of the vitreous base. The posterior edge of giant retinal tears is not attached to the vitreous base and commonly rolls over itself (Figure 61–8).

Repair of giant retinal tears may require scleral buckling or vitrectomy, which combined with the use of perfluorocarbon liquids or silicone oil helps unroll the curled retina. Repair may be complicated by proliferative vitreoretinopathy.

■ PROLIFERATIVE VITREORETINOPATHY

Proliferative vitreoretinopathy (12) (PVR) is a dramatic disorder in which contractile cellular membranes grow on both surfaces of the retina after rhegmatogenous retinal detachment. PVR is the primary cause of failure of retinal reattachment surgery. Risk factors for the development of PVR include failure to achieve initial retinal reattachment after scleral buckling surgery, giant retinal tears, choroidal detachment, and vitreous hemorrhage (5). PVR membranes are composed of cells of retinal pigment epithelium (RPE), glial and macrophage origin. The cellular events important in the evolution of PVR include dispersion, chemotaxis, proliferation, and contraction.

Dispersed pigmented cells, clinically evident as "tobacco dust" are present in the vitreous of most eyes after retinal detachment. Cryopexy has been shown to enhance the dispersion of viable RPE (4).

The importance of chemotaxis in the evolution of PVR is unclear. Nonetheless, in-vitro studies have shown a chemotactic response of RPE to serum, fibronectin, platelet derived growth factor (PDGF), macrophage conditioned culture media, interleukin-1, normal vitreous, and vitreous aspirates from eyes with PVR. Glial cells are less responsive to chemotactants but do respond to PDGF. The origin of chemotactants in the vitreous cavity is unclear; however hemorrhage and breakdown of the blood-ocular barrier have been suggested as the source of such factors.

Cellular proliferation is paramount to the development of vitreoretinal membranes. Proliferation of RPE has been shown in response to PDGF, vitreous, subretinal fluid, and other humoral factors. Glial proliferation is stimulated by vitreous hemorrhage and breakdown of the blood-ocular barrier. Cell-cell interaction may be an equally important stimulus for proliferation as suggested by RPE-glial co-culture experiments.

Metaplastic, proliferating RPE can assume fibroblastic characteristics in PVR membranes (8). Such cells are motile, moving by extension of lamellipodia. Within the vitreous cavity, such extension and retraction of lamellipodia results in "reeling-in" of vitreous collagen fibrils with subsequent contraction of the gel. This process enables quite dramatic vitreous contraction despite relatively hypocellular appearing membranes. Cell-mediated gel contraction requires the presence of fibronectin, a protein which mediates cell-cell and cell-collagen adhesion. Fibronectin levels are increased after cryopexy of breakdown of the blood-ocular barrier. Characteristically, the contractile phase of the evolution of PVR occurs 6 to 8 weeks after retinal reattachment surgery.

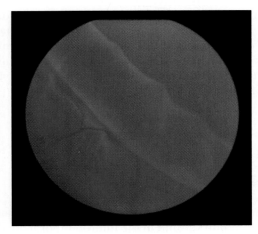

Figure 61–8.
Giant retinal tear in a 35-year-old man hit in the eye with a racquetball. Vitreous traction on the extensive vitreous adhesion to the anterior border creates a large circumferential giant tear. The posterior edge has no vitreous attachments and curls over itself. This rolled retina makes closure of giant retinal tears more difficult.

TABLE 61–1
Types of Grade C PVR (Fig. 61–9)

Type 1: Focal posterior contraction
Type 2: Diffuse posterior contraction
Type 3: Subretinal membranes and proliferation
Type 4: Circumferential contraction along vitreous base with radial retinal folds
Type 5: Anterior retinal displacement with trough

PVR may be systemically classified (13). Grade A represents RPE clumps in the vitreous and on the retinal surface in the setting of vitreous flare. Grade B denotes transparent surface wrinkling and rolled edges of tears. Grade C specifically describes five configurations, all with full-thickness retinal folds, with regard to extent of folds (in clock hours) and its anterior or posterior position to the equator (Figure 61–9).

Proliferative vitreoretinopathy occurs in approximately 7% of patients after initial retinal detachment surgery. Risk factors for PVR include previous retinal surgery, excessive cryotherapy, retinal breaks larger

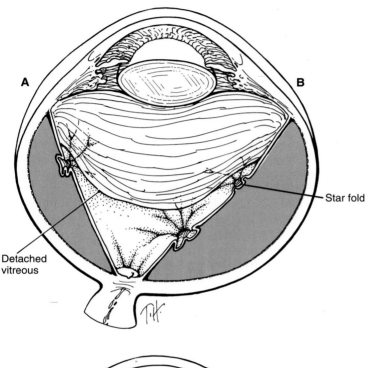

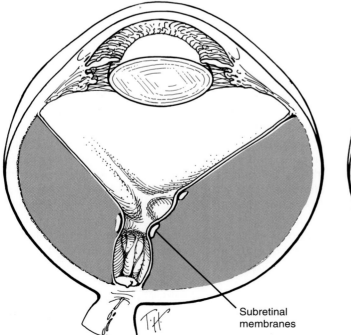

Figure 61–9.

Types of Grade C proliferative vitreoretinopathy. A. Type 1. Radial folds from a focal area of traction create a star fold. B. Type 2. Diffuse posterior contraction producing multiple radial folds posteriorly. C. Type 3. Subretinal membranes encircle the posterior retina in a funnel over the disc. D. Type 4. Circumferential contraction along vitreous base with radial folds posteriorly.

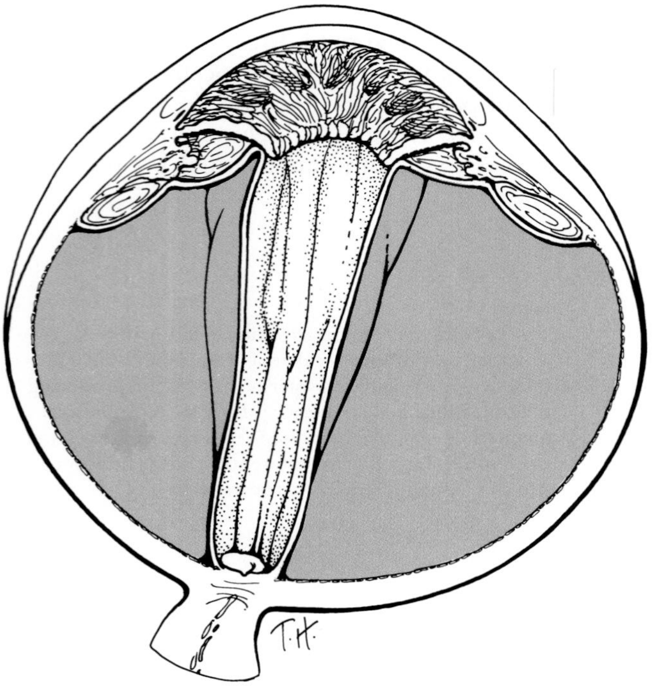

E

Figure 61–9. *(continued)* E. Type 5. Severe contraction of membranes encircling anterior and posterior retina. Traction of ciliary body may produce hypotony.

than 3 disc diameters, and preoperative vitreous hemorrhage and choroidal detachment.

Vitreoretinal surgery for PVR is successful initially in 70 to 80% of cases. The most common cause of anatomic failure and redetachment is anterior PVR.

Twenty-two percent of eyes with primary PVR will have an anterior component as opposed to 86% of eyes with recurrent PVR. Final retinal reattachment rates for recurrent PVR range from 63 to 96% with three-fourths of patients achieving a final visual acuity better than 5/200. Fourteen to 37% of these patients will end up with final visual acuities of 20/100 or better.

Subretinal membranes are present in half of all cases with PVR. However, they are noted to prevent retinal reattachment in only one-third of cases. Long-term reattachment can be achieved in 65% of these cases. Unfortunately, a visual acuity of greater than or equal to 5/200 is achieved in less than one-quarter of these difficult cases.

The primary treatment of early PVR is still the use of scleral buckling or revision scleral buckling surgery. Detached retina often accentuates the appearance of contractile membranes which might otherwise remain stable if all retinal breaks are identified and closed and the retina attached. For eyes which fail scleral buckling surgery, vitreous surgery combined with intraocular gas of silicone oil tamponade has improved the anatomic success rate of such eyes to 80% or 90%, although often more than one operative procedure may be required. The Silicone Study (14) investigated the selection of intraocular tamponade in eyes with PVR in a randomized, prospective, clinical trial. While the study suggested that both C_3F_8 gas and silicone oil are superior to SF_6 gas for intraocular tamponade, C_3F_8 gas and silicone oil appear to be equivalent to one another with regard to anatomic results, visual results, and the prevalence of complications.

■ ACQUIRED RETINOSCHISIS

Acquired retinoschisis (3) represents the degenerative splitting of neurosensory retina at the level of the outer plexiform layer (see X-linked retinoschisis in Section 2). Acquired retinoschisis is present in about 5% of the population, representing the extreme of the clinical spectrum of coalesced peripheral cystoid degeneration. The majority of patients experience bilateral movement. Seventy percent of patients are hyperopic.

Patients are characteristically asymptomatic. The asymptomatic nature of the disorder helps to differentiate it from retina detachment. Nonetheless, photopsias or symptomatic scotomas may develop in the setting of coexistent retinal detachment or macular extension of schisis.

Acquired retinoschisis appears as a smooth, fixed, dome-shaped, translucent, peripheral retinal elevation in contrast to the corrugated mobile, opaque appearance of retinal detachment (18). Typically, the temporal quadrants are affected. Retinal blood vessels are always contained in the elevated, inner layer of schisis.

Blood vessels may be sheathed or occluded. Snowflake-like dots may be son on the undersurface of the inner layer, representing Muller cell remnants. The outer layer has an irregular surface exhibiting a pockmarked appearance and white with pressure on scleral depression. In contrast to retinal detachment, vitreous cells are absent. In contrast to congenital retinoschisis, in which splitting occurs at the level of the blood vessel rich nerve fiber layer, vitreous hemorrhage is a rare occurrence.

Inner wall breaks are a common occurrence in retinoschisis. Unless associated with an outer wall break, these holes are not of consequence and need not be treated. Outer wall breaks occur in one-quarter of cases. By themselves, or in conjunction with inner wall breaks, outer wall breaks may be associated with retinal detachment. Retinal detachment in such cases, so-called schisis-detachment, consists of an underlying outer wall detachment beneath a schisis cavity. Patients may or may not be symptomatic. Continued accumulation of subphotoreceptor fluid may progress to generalized retinal detachment. In such cases, outer wall breaks may be difficult to identify and treat. The presence of retinal pigment epithelial demarcation lines is always a sign of associated retinal detachment since the pigment epithelium is not distributed in isolated retinoschisis.

Since splitting occurs at the level of the outer plexiform layer, continuity between the photoreceptors and the outer nuclear layer is destroyed. This is manifest by the presence of absolute scotomas on visual field testing. As such, visual field testing may provide a useful measure of progression of the disorder.

The overwhelming majority of patients with acquired retinoschisis do not sustain visual impairment. In a study of 218 patients with retinoschisis followed for an average of 9 years, visual loss related to retinoschisis did not occur in any eye. Nonetheless, uncommonly, individuals are at risk for visual loss either from schisis detachment or rarely, from posterior extension of retinoschisis. Treatment consists of identifying and treating outer wall breaks with photocoagulation or cryopexy. Since areas already affected by retinoschisis exhibit irreparable disruption of photoreceptor-nuclear connections, flattening areas of retinoschisis does not result in return of visual function as does retinal detachment. In select cases, scleral buckling techniques may be useful in treating more extensive configurations of schisis detachment (15).

■ REFERENCES

1. Foos RY: Posterior vitreous detachment. Trans Am Acad Ophthalmol Otolaryngol 1972; 76: 460.
2. Tasman WS: Posterior vitreous detachment and peripheral retinal breaks. Trans Am Acad Ophthalmol Otolaryngol 1968; 72: 217.
3. Davis MD: Natural history of retinal breaks without detachment. Arch Ophthalmol 1974; 92:183–194.
4. Byer NE: Long-term natural history of lattice degeneration of the retina. Ophthalmology 1989; 96: 1396–1401.
5. Lincoff H, Gieser R: Finding the retinal hole. Arch Ophthalmol 1971; 85: 565–569.
6. Gonin J: The treatment of detached retina by sealing the retinal tears. Arch Ophthalmol 1930; 4: 621–625.
7. Tornambe PE, Hilton GF: The Retinal Detachment Study Group: Pneumatic retinopexy: a multicenter randomized controlled clinical trial comparing pneumatic retinopexy with scleral buckling. Ophthalmology 1988; 96: 772–784.
8. Lincoff H, Kreissig I, Farber M: Results of 100 aphakic detachments treated with a temporary balloon buckle: a case against routine encircling operations. Br J Ophthalmol 1985; 69: 798–804.
9. Benson WE: Retinal Detachment: Diagnosis and Management. Hagerstown: Harper and Row, 1980.
10. Machemer R: Pathogenesis and classification of massive preretinal proliferation. Br J Ophthalmol 1978;62: 737–747.
11. Cowley M, Conway BP, Campochiaro PA: Clinical risk factors for proliferative vitreoretinopathy. Arch Ophthalmol 1989; 107: 1147–51.
12. Campochiaro PA, Kaden IH, Vidaurri-Leal J, Glaser BM: Cryotherapy enhances intravitreal dispersion of viable retinal pigment epithelial cells. Arch Ophthalmol 1985; 103: 434–436.
13. Silicone Study Group: Vitrectomy with silicone oil or perfluoropropane gas in eyes with severe proliferative vitreoretinopathy: results of a randomized clinical trial. Silicone Study Report No. 2. Arch Ophthalmol 1992; 110: 770–779.
14. Machemer R, Aaberg TM, Freeman MH: An updated classification of retinal detachment with proliferative retinopathy. Am J Ophthalmol 1991; 112: 159–165.
15. Glaser BM, Cardin A, Biscoe B: Proliferative vitreoretinopathy. The mechanism of development of vitreoretinal traction. Ophthalmology 1987; 94: 327–332.
16. Byer NE: Long-term natural history of senile retinoschisis with implications for management. Ophthalmology 1986; 93: 1127–1137.
17. Zimmerman LE, Spencer WH: The pathologic anatomy of retinoschisis. Arch Ophthalmol 1960; 63: 10–19.
18. Sned SR, Blodi CF, Folk JC, et al: Pars plana vitrectomy in the management of retinal detachments associated with degenerative retinoschisis. Ophthalmology 1990; 97: 470–474.

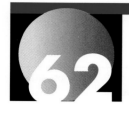

62 Choroidal and Retinal Tumors

Eugene de Juan Jr., Stuart W. Noorily,
William P. Townsend-Pico, Kenneth C. Chern

■ METASTATIC TUMORS

Patients with underlying systemic malignancy may experience metastasis of tumor cells to the eye (9, 14). The rich vascular supply of the posterior choroid makes it the most likely site for ocular metastasis. Metastatic lesions to the choroid are more common than primary ocular malignancies, including choroidal melanoma. While most patients with metastatic tumors of the choroid have already been diagnosed with cancer. Others have not. Metastases most commonly arise from carcinomas of the breast or lung.

Presenting symptoms include metamorphopsia, diminished central vision, visual field defects, and photopsia. Pain is typically absent. Serous retinal detachment represents the most frequent clinical representation. Beneath the retinal detachment, the tumor can be visualized as a creamy-yellow irregular elevation of the choroid. In contrast to primary choroidal melanoma, metastases commonly exhibit multifocal involvement, bilaterality, and lateral growth with an irregular surface. Nonetheless, differentiation on purely ophthalmoscopic grounds is often impossible. Fluorescein angiography shows early leakage of dye from the surface of the choroidal mass in a nonspecific pattern, common to choroidal masses of numerous etiologies. Ultrasonography is particularly helpful since metastatic choroidal tumors characteristically show a pattern of moderate to increased reflectivity, often with intralesional variability, in contrast to decreased, uniform reflectivity seen with standardized A scan sonography of choroidal melanomas (Table 62–1).

The systemic prognosis of patients with metastatic tumors of the choroid is poor. Median survival is 8.5 months. Palliative treatment of choroidal metastases with external beam radiation can improve vision and control tumor growth.

■ CHOROIDAL MALIGNANT MELANOMA

Choroidal malignant melanoma is the most common primary malignancy of the eye. White individuals are preferentially affected. A hereditable tendency for the disorder is typically absent. The incidence of disease is approximately 7 per million whites per year.

Most patients remain symptomatic unless the tumor involves the central macula by means of direct extension, surrounding retinal detachment, or cystoid macular edema. Large, anterior tumors may induce lenticular astigmatism, cataract, or glaucoma. The typical lesion is an elevated, brown, oval, dome-shaped choroidal mass. Not infrequently, tumors may be amelanotic (Figure 62–1). The presence of orange, lipofuscin pigment at the level of the RPE is characteristic of choroidal melanoma. Mushroom-shaped eruption of the tumor through Bruch's membrane is also highly characteristic of melanoma (Figure 62–2A).

Differentiation of choroidal melanoma from benign nevi is most reliably based upon the height of the lesion, significant growth in height, and the presence of orange

TABLE 62–1
The Differential Diagnosis of Choroidal Tumors on Standardized Echography

	Choroidal Melanoma	Choroidal Hemangioma	Choroidal Metastases	Choroidal Nevus	Disciform Scar
Reflectivity	Low to medium	High	Medium to high	High	Initially low later high
Internal Structure	Regular	Regular	Irregular	Minimal height	Regular to irregular
Vascularity	+	+/−	−	−	+/−
Shape	Mushroom or collar-button	Mild to moderate elevation	Flat to elevated, lobulated	Flat to minimally elevated	Elevated

lipofuscin pigment on the tumor surface. Lesions greater than 2.5 mm in height are unlikely to represent nevi, whereas atypical lesions less than 2 mm in height should probably be considered suspicious nevi, rather than melanomas. Approximately 10% of suspicious nevi of 1 to 2 mm in height progress to melanoma. The presence of subretinal fluid or drusen is not a reliable differentiating sign since they can be associated with both nevi and melanoma.

The differential diagnosis of choroidal melanomas include choroidal nevi, congenital hypertrophy of the RPE, choroidal metastasis, choroidal hemangioma, age-related extramacular degeneration with choroidal neo-vascularization, posterior scleritis, Vogt-Koyangi-Harada disease, choroidal osteoma, and combined hamartoma of the retina and RPE (13).

The fluorescein angiographic appearance of choroidal melanomas is highly variable and not particularly useful in differentiating nevi from melanomas. The classic appearance of intrinsic tumor circulation or multiple pinpoint leaks on the surface of the tumor, while supportive of the diagnosis of melanoma, may occasionally be observed in benign nevi.

Ultrasonography is far and away the most important diagnostic modality in the evaluation of suspected choroidal melanoma. Standardized A-scan ultrasonography can reliably differentiate the low-medium internal tumor reflectivity of melanomas (Figure 62–2B) from medium-to-high internal tumor reflectivity of metastatic tumors, and the high internal reflectivity of choroidal hemangiomas. In contrast to hemorrhagic choroidal detachments, intrinsic vascular pulsations are often demonstrable with A-scan ultrasonography. Ultrasonography also provides an objective measurement of interval changes in tumor height and size.

Evaluation of a patient in whom a diagnosis of choroidal melanoma has been made should address the possibility of systemic metastasis. The most common site of metastasis is the liver, followed by the lung. A systemic diagnostic workup should include a physical examination, serum liver enzyme levels, and a chest radiograph. Abdominal CT scanning is not as sensitive as serum liver

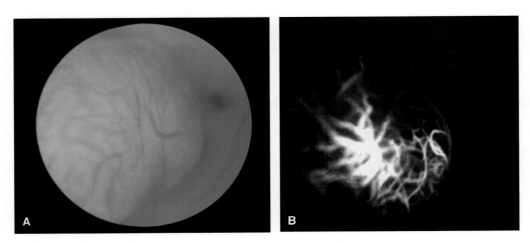

Figure 62–1.
Large amelanotic choroidal melanoma. (A) Angiogram. (B) Early filling of the tumor vessels with the choroidal circulation. This eye was subsequently enucleated.

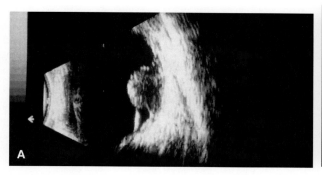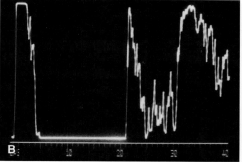

Figure 62–2.
Malignant melanoma. The melanoma assumes a mushroom shape configuration on B-scan ultrasound (A) as it breaks through Bruch's membrane. A retinal detachment is also visible adjacent to the tumor. A-scan ultrasonography demonstrates the steep attenuation and low to medium reflectivity typical of melanomas.

enzymes in detecting metastases. The prognosis of patients who develop metastatic disease is dismal, with most surviving less than 1 year.

Treatment options for choroidal melanomas include observation, episcleral radioactive plaque therapy, enucleation (19), local tumor resection (10), external proton beam irradiation, and photocoagulation. The selection of treatment modality depends on the size and location of the tumor, as well as the life expectancy and preference of the patient. Each of the treatment options is associated with its own profile of local side effects. Moreover, the relative benefit of treatment options on systemic survival is unclear. The preconception that enucleation should minimize the risk of systemic tumor spread has been contested by those who believe that enucleation may promote metastatic activity. The mechanism by which enucleation could promote metastatic activity is unclear but may include ceasation of immunologic suppression of preexistent microscopic metastases.

■ CHOROIDAL HEMANGIOMA

Choroidal hemangiomas (2) are benign tumors which appear as localized or diffuse red-orange lesions with distinct margins. Choroidal hemangiomas are typically located within or near the macula, where they may produce symptoms related to the development of subretinal fluid, cystoid macular edema, or degenerative changes of the overlying pigment epithelium. Involvement is typically unilateral.

Fluorescein angiography shows a characteristic pattern of hyperfluorescence of vascular channels in the tumor in the earliest frames of the angiogram, followed by diffuse leakage of dye as the study progresses.

Ultrasonography shows a classic appearance of increased internal reflectivity with A-scan techniques. Choroidal hemangiomas are usually less than 3 mm in height.

Diffuse hemangiomas produce relatively flat, widespread choroidal thickening, imparting a reddish appearance to the entire fundus which may be overlooked, unless compared with the fellow eye. Diffuse choroidal hemangiomas are associated with the Sturge-Weber syndrome (see also Pediatric Syndromes, chapter 23). The Sturge-Weber syndrome is a sporadic unilateral developmental disorder associated with cutaneous, ocular, and central nervous system (CNS) findings. Cutaneous findings are characterized by nevus flammeus (port wine stain), a congenital dermal capillary hemangioma which involves the first and second division of the trigeminal nerve. The side of the lesion typically dictates the side of ocular involvement. In addition to diffuse choroidal hemangiomas, ocular involvement includes glaucoma in 30% of patients. The mechanism of glaucoma may involve elevated episcleral venous pressure or anomalous development of the filtration angle. CNS involvement is characterized by meningeal hemangiomas. These may be associated with seizures or mental retardation.

Histopathologically, choroidal hemangiomas are composed of large choroidal vessels which blend with the normal surrounding choroidal vasculature at the borders of the tumor (18).

Laser treatment of choroidal hemangiomas is indicated when the tumor is associated with the development of subretinal fluid which threatens the macula (11). Treatment consists of moderately intense grid photocoagulation over the tumor with the aim of diminishing serous leakage from the tumor, rather than obliterating it entirely.

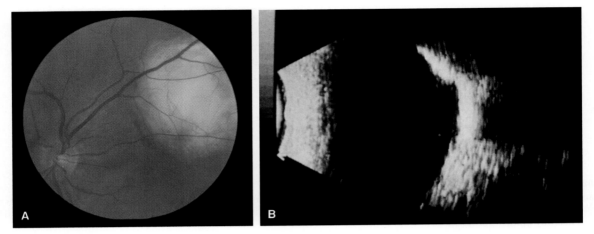

Figure 62–3.
Choroidal osteoma in a 35-year-old woman with 20/40 visual acuity. This bright, white, slightly elevated choroidal mass is an ectopic rest of cancellous bone (A). On B-scan ultrasonography (B), the dense osteoma is present with retrolesional shadowing.

■ CHOROIDAL OSTEOMA

Choroidal osteomas (15) are rare, benign, yellow-white choristomatous tumors with well-defined borders which preferentially involve the peripapillary region in adolescents or young adults. Females are more commonly affected. Symptoms include metamorphopsias or scotomas associated with the development of subretinal fluid. Twenty percent of cases are bilateral.

Ophthalmoscopically, the tumors appear as white, mildly raised lesions with overlying hypopigmentation of the RPE. Fine vessels may be seen on the tumor surface (Figure 62–3A). Fluorescein angiography shows mottled hyperfluorescence of the lesion with staining in the late frames of the study. Fine vessels on the tumor surface do not exhibit early hyperfluorescence. Choroidal neovascularization frequently complicates the disorder. Ultrasonography shows a highly reflective surface spike with retrolesional shadowing (Figure 62–3B). CT scanning dramatically illustrates the calcium-dense lesions.

Histopathologically, tumors are composed of cancellous bone located between the choriocapillaris and outer choroid.

The etiology of choroidal osteomas is unknown. Low-grade choroidal inflammation has been suggested as a causative factor (16). Typically, no systemic associations are identified. The differential diagnosis includes metastatic or dystrophic choroidal ossification, idiopathic sclerochoroidal calcification, choroidal metastases, amelanotic choroidal melanoma, choroidal granulomas, and choroiditis.

The visual prognosis is variable. The tumors tend to enlarge slowly over time. Since they represent benign growths, they do not have the potential to metastasize. Laser treatment is reserved for choroidal neovascular complications of the disease.

■ RETINAL CAPILLARY HEMANGIOMA

Retinal capillary hemangiomas (3,6) are red, vascular tumors which arise from the inner retina and extend above the retinal surface. Tumors may be solitary or multiple. The disorder may be acquired or inherited in an autosomal dominant fashion as part of Von Hippel's disease. Twenty percent of patients with the hereditary form of this disorder will develop cerebellar hemangioblastomas (Von Hippel-Lindau syndrome).

Retinal capillary hemangiomas are rarely detected

before the third decade of life. Presenting symptoms relate to the development of vitreous hemorrhage, foveal extension of retinal edema, or exudative retinal detachment. Fluorescein angiography shows rapid filling of the tumor in the arterial phase of the angiogram, associated with leakage of dye in the mid and late phases of the study.

In the hereditable form of the disorder, these tumors may be multifocal, are bilateral in approximately

50% of cases, and are usually accompanied by a prominently dilated and tortuous arterial feeder and draining venule. Tumors are usually located in the mid-peripheral but may occasionally involve the posterior pole. Systemic association include cerebellar hemangioblastoma (the Lindau tumor), renal cell carcinoma, pheochromocytoma, and epididymal, pancreatic, or renal cysts.

Acquired tumors are typically solitary, unilateral, and without systemic associations. These lesions involve the retinal periphery and are not associated with prominent feeder vessels. By definition, systemic associations are absent.

Because the natural history of the hereditary tumors is continued growth, early ablation of the tumors with laser or triple freeze cryotherapy is indicated (1). Treatment should be done over several sessions in a gentle fashion, since overaggressive laser photocoagulation may result in an exudative retinal detachment. Medical evaluation should include a thorough physical examination, computer tomography (CT) or magnetic resonance imaging (MRI) scan of the brain, and an abdominal imaging study.

■ COMBINED HAMARTOMA OF THE RETINA AND RPE (CHRRPE)

Combined hamartoma of the retinal and RPE (4,12) (CHRRPE) is a rare, partly pigmented, slightly elevated, ill-defined, peripapillary or macular lesion. Retinal vessels included within the lesion are both distorted by an associated epiretinal membrane, and inherently tortuous and anomalous. Affected patients range in age from 10 months to 66 years. Symptoms typically consist of metamorphopsia or diminished vision related to fovea traction from epiretinal membranes. Vitreous hemorrhage occurs infrequently. CHRRPE has been associated with neurofibromatosis II. However, a hereditary pattern is usually absent.

Fluorescein angiography shows early filling of dilated, large caliber, anomalous retinal vessels associated with leakage of dye in the mid and late phases of the study. Choroidal neovascularization may occasionally complicate the disorder.

Histopathologically, lesions consist of retinal disorganization, RPE hyperplasia, toxocara canis, Coat's disease, and exaggerated epiretinal membranes.

The visual prognosis is variable. While the majority of cases do not progress, visual deterioration occurs in one-quarter of eyes. When visual deterioration is the result of distant foveal effects of an epiretinal membrane, vitreous surgery with membrane peeling may occasionally be beneficial (8).

■ INTRAOCULAR LYMPHOMA (see Uveitis, Chapter 37)

Primary intraocular lymphoma (5, 7, 17) is a rare disorder which presents the development of primary ocular-CNS non-Hodgkin's lymphoma. Previously, multiple names have been used to refer to the disorder including large cell lymphoma and reticulum cell sarcoma. Affected patients are usually in the sixth or seventh decade of life. Ocular involvement precedes the appearance of CNS lymphoma in most cases. Although 80% of patients have bilateral involvement, unilateral involvement may be present initially.

Ocular signs and symptoms mimic those of posterior uveitis. Presenting complaints include floaters and diminished central vision. Vision may be impaired as a result of vitreous opacities, cystoid macular edema, or exudative retinal detachment. Additional findings include creamy, focal, solid pigment epithelial detachments from sub-RPE collection of tumor cells, atrophic, hypopigmented lesions of the RPE, anterior uveitis, retinal vasculitis, necrotizing retinitis, and disc edema. Fluorescein angiography of RPE lesions may show early staining of tumor cell collections or window defects in areas of atrophy.

Histopathologic examination of cells obtained by vitreous biopsy show relatively large cells with nuclear-cytoplasmic disproportion, nuclear membrane abnormalities, and one or more nucleoli. Immunocytologic studies suggest the tumor cells are of B-cell origin.

The early diagnosis of intraocular lymphoma necessitates an increased degree of suspicion and a willingness to proceed with diagnostic vitrectomy in cases of vitritis associated with characteristic sub-RPE accumulations or in cases of idiopathic vitritis unresponsive to treatment. The diagnostic sensitivity of vitreous biopsy is improved by discontinuing steroid therapy before vitrectomy. Patients in whom diagnostic vitrectomy is suggestive of large cell lymphoma, should undergo MRI of the brain and cytologic examination of cerebrospinal fluid.

The differential diagnosis includes birdshot choroidopathy, sarcoidosis, multifocal choroiditis, pars planitis, pneumocystitis choroiditis, fungal endophthalmitis, syphilis, tuberculosis, and Whipple's disease.

The systemic prognosis of primary intraocular lymphoma is dismal. Despite treatment with CNS radiation, the mean survival time after diagnosis is less than 2 years. The tendency for ocular involvement to precede CNS involvement by 2 years and the historical tendency for definitive vitreous diagnosis, coupled with improved chemotherapeutic treatments, will lead to improved survival of these patients in the future.

■ REFERENCES

1. Mewis L, Young SE: Breast carcinoma metastatic to the choroid: Analysis of 67 patients. Ophthalmology 1982; 89: 147–151.

2. Stephens RF, Shields JA: Diagnosis and management of cancer metastatic to the uvea: A study of 70 cases. Ophthalmology 1979; 86: 1336–1349.

3. Zimmerman LE, McLean IW: An evaluation of enucleation in the management of uveal melanomas. Am J Ophthalmol 1979; 87: 741–760.

4. Peyman GA, Juarez CP, Diamond JG, Raichand M: Ten years experience with eye wall resection for uveal malignant melanomas. Ophthalmology 1984; 91: 1720–1724.

5. Shields JA, Augsburger JJ, Brown GC, Stephens RF: The differential diagnosis of posterior uveal melanoma. Ophthalmology 1980; 87: 518–522.

6. Augsburger JJ, Shields JA, Moffat KP: Circumscribed choroidal hemangiomas: long-term visual prognosis. Retina 1981; 1: 56.

7. Sanborn BE, Augsburger JJ, Shields JA: Treatment of circumscribed choroidal hemangiomas. Ophthalmology 1982; 89: 1374–1380.

8. Witschel H, Font RL: Hemangioma of the choroid: A clinicopathologic study of 71 cases and review of the literature. Surv Ophthalmol 1976; 20: 415–431.

9. Teich SA, Walsh JB: Choroidal osteoma. Ophthalmology 1981; 88: 696–698.

10. Trimble SN, Schatz H: Choroidal osteoma after intraocular inflammation. Am J Ophthalmol 1983; 96: 759–764.

11. Hardwig T, Robertson DM: von Hippel-Lindau disease: A familial, often lethal, multisystem phakomatosis. Ophthalmology 1984; 91: 263–270.

12. Annesley WH, Leonard BC, Shields JA, Tasman WS: Fifteen year review of treated and untreated cases of retinal angiomatosis. Trans Am Acad Ophthalmol Otolaryngol 1977; 83: 446–453.

13. Campochiaro PA, Conway BP: Hemangiomalike masses of the retina. Arch Ophthalmol 1988; 106: 1409–1413.

14. Schachat AP, Shields JA, Fine SL: Combined hamartomas of the retina and retinal pigment epithelium. Ophthalmology 1984; 91: 1609–1615.

15. Flood TP, Orth DH, Aaberg TM, Marcus DF: Macular hamartomas of the retinal pigment epithelium and retina. Retina 1983; 3: 164–170.

16. McDonald HR, Abrams GW, Burke JM, Neuwirth J: Clinicopathologic results of vitreous surgery for epiretinal membranes in patients with combined retinal and retinal pigment epithelial hamartomas. Am J Ophthalmol 1985; 100: 806–813.

17. Freeman LN, Schachat AP, Knox DL: Clinical features, laboratory investigations, and survival in ocular reticulum cell sarcoma. Ophthalmology 1987; 94: 1631–1639.

18. Whitcup SM, de Smet MD, Rubin BI: Intraocular lymphoma: Clinical and histopathologic diagnosis. Ophthalmology 1993; 100: 1399–1406.

19. Lang GK, Surer JL, Green WR: Ocular reticulum cell sarcoma: Clinicopathologic correlation of a case with multifocal lesions. Retina 1985; 5: 79–86.

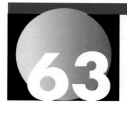

63 Retinal Surgery

Eugene de Juan Jr., Stuart W. Noorily,
William P. Townsend-Pico, Kenneth C. Chern

Retinal surgery encompasses a wide variety of procedures and techniques. The particular instruments and methods are as numerous as there are surgeons. In this section, the basic premises behind the major procedures will be outlined. Combinations and modifications of these procedures are common, as indicated by the particular case.

■ PHOTOCOAGULATION

Laser photocoagulation has emerged as an important element of retinal surgery. Current lasers used for retinal surgery include the argon green (614 nm), argon blue-green (488 and 514 nm), krypton red (647 nm), tunable dye, diode and xenon arc lasers. Laser energy is absorbed predominantly by tissues containing pitment (melanin, xanthophyll, or hemoglobin) producing thermal effects on adjacent structures. The wavelength of the krypton red laser is better able to penetrate nuclear sclerotic cataracts and vitreous hemorrhage and, therefore, requires less energy than the argon laser to achieve the same degree of photocoagulation. Argon blue-green and xenon arc lasers are less frequently used today.

Laser parameters may be modified depending on the goal of photocoagulation (see Table 63–1). At decreased energy levels (lower power settings, longer duration, larger spot size), the laser has a coagulative effct on small vessels. Focal laser photocoagulation is used in diabetes to stop leakage of microaneurysms. The laser spot is placed directly over the macroaneurysm to achieve a slight whitening and closure of the aneurysm. When applied as a grid over an edematous area of retina, the laser may reduce microvascular leakage. At higher energy levels, laser ablation of tissue is possible. Panretinal photocoagulation is thought to be effective by destroying retinal tissue, reducing the amount of ischemic tissue in the eye. Confluent laser spots may be used over a neovascular membrane to obliterate the abnormal vessels. Laser-induced chorioretinal adhesions are useful for the treatment of retinal tears or breaks. A triple row of overlapping laser burns is usually created around a tear. It is critical to ensure adequate laser burns at the anterior extent of a horseshoe tear since vitreal traction will extend tears in this direction.

Complications of laser photocoagulation include inadvertent laser burns (especially disastrous in the macula), burns on other ocular tissues, retinal breaks, and exudative retinal detachment from exuberant panretinal photocoagulation.

■ RETINAL DETACHMENT SURGERY

Several techniques are available to repair retinal detachments. The particular procedure chosen depends on the type of retinal detachment, location and number of breaks, and presence of tractional forces. The basic principles are the same: 1) creation of chorioretinal adhesions to close the breaks (usually with cryotherapy or

883

TABLE 63–1
Laser Parameters

	Spot Size	Duration	Power	Endpoint
Focal	50–100 μm	0.1 s	50–100 mW	Light blanching of microaneurysm
Grid	50–200 μm	0.1 s	50–250 mW	Light to moderate retinal whitening
PRP	250–500 μm	0.2–0.5 s	100–1000 mW	Moderate retinal burn
Wall-off	250–500 μm	0.1–0.5 s	100–1000 mW	Moderate retinal burn

Laser power should be started at the lowest possible level and titrated upward to the desired effect.

photocoagulation), 2) reapproximation of the retina to the RPE, and 3) relief of tractional forces. All three of these must be satisfied in order to achieve successful anatomic reattachment of the retina.

■ PNEUMATIC RETINOPEXY

Pneumatic retinopexy (2) can be used successfully in selected cases. Cryotherapy or laser photocoagulation is used to create an area of adhesion at the site of the break. Intraocular air or longer lasting gas (C_3F_8, C_2F_6, SF_6) is injected into the vitreous cavity and the patient is positioned so that the gas bubble tamponades the site of the retinal break. Resorption of the subretinal fluid occurs via the RPE pump, thus flattening the detachment.

This procedure has been used for breaks less than one clock hour in size and located in the upper two-thirds of the fundus without significant PVR. The reattachment rate after the primary pneumatic retinopexy compares favorably with scleral buckling (73% versus 82%) (7). Patients failing pneumatic retinopexy may successfully undergo subsequent scleral buckling with good results. Complications include subretinal gas, new break formation, and macular detachment.

■ SCLERAL BUCKLE

Scleral buckles are commonly employed for rhegmatogenous retinal detachments. An encircling silicone band around the eye provides relief of the intravitreal tractional forces by indentation of the sclera, as well as reapposition of the retina and choroid. Radial elements or sleeves can be added to provide localized support for breaks posterior to the band. Laser photocoagulation or cryotherapy, again, is used to create chorioretinal adhesions. Drainage of subretinal fluid by means of a sclerotomy may help to flatten bullous elevations.

Complications include creation of new retinal tears or breaks, retinal folds, retinal perforation, and retinal vascular occlusion. Hemorrhage, retinal incarceration, and vitreous loss may complicate drainage of subretinal fluid. Postoperative anterior segment ischemia may result if the band is too tight.

Prognosis (visual and anatomic) is dependent on many factors, among which is whether the macula was detached preoperatively (5). In general, visual potential declines the longer the macula is detached. Giant retinal tears, the presence of proliferative vitreoretinopathy, and preoperative choroidal detachment are associated with less successful reattachment of the retina.

■ VITRECTOMY

Pars plana vitrectomy is able to achieve all three elements critical to the reattachment of the retina. Vitrectomy, with scleral depression, allows relief of transvitreal traction at sites of adhesion such as lattice or chorioretinal scars. Tangential retinal traction can be released with membrane peeling, incision of fibrous membranes, or retinotomy (4). Endophotocoagulation allows creation of chorioretinal adhesions. Intraocular gas, silicone oil (1), and perfluorocarbon liquids may be useful in expressing subretinal fluid through a break and placing the retina in proximity to the RPE.

Techniques for the removal of the vitreous gel have

evolved greatly over the last decade. Current techniques are based on a three-port pars plana approach. An infusion canula occupies one port and maintains the intraocular pressure via an infusion of balanced salt solution or air. The two other ports allow bimanual surgery with specialized instruments. Fiber optic light pipes provide illumination within the eye. Automated vitreous cutters allow removal of the vitreous gel with minimal traction on the retina. Intraocular forceps, scissors, and picks have been developed to peel epiretinal membranes, lyse fibrovascular bands, and manipulate intraocular foreign bodies. A view of the posterior pole through the binocular operating microscope is possible with a variety of contact lenses.

There are many indications for vitrectomy. A diagnostic vitrectomy may be used to obtain specimens for culture from a case of endophthalmitis. Vitrectomy may be used to remove media opacities such as vitreous hemorrhage, amyloid, or inflammatory debris. Neovascularization of the iris with vitreous hemorrhage may require vitrectomy to allow retinal photocoagulation and perhaps debulk angiogenic factors. Vitrectomy with stripping of the posterior hyaloid may relieve tangential traction in macular holes.

■ CHOROIDAL EFFUSION AND HEMORRHAGE

Choroidal effusions are collections of blood or serum in the choroidal or suprachoroidal space as a result of shearing damage to choroidal vessels or branches of the posterior ciliary arteries, secondary to hypotony. Effusions and hemorrhages most commonly result after anterior segment surgery and glaucoma filtering operations (especially with setons or mitomycin C), and especially when there is wound leakage and hypotony. Effusions may also form after scleral buckling surgery associated with hypotony, and draining of large amounts of subretinal fluid, or compression of the vortex veins by the encircling element.

Choroidal effusions range in severity from small localized effusions to large, bullous elevations that bow inward and almost touch (kissing choroidals) (Figure 63–1). Serous effusions can be distinguished from hemorrhagic choroidals by transillumination.

Effusions and hemorrhages will usually resolve slowly after restoration of intraocular pressure and closure of any leaking tracts. Drainage of choroidals may be indicated if the choroidals continue to enlarge to form kissing choroidals, to threaten the macula, or to shallow the anterior chamber. Sclerotomies over the pars plana in the affected quadrants allows drainage of the fluid. A trial of oral steroids may slow or halt enlarging choroidals.

■ EXPULSIVE HEMORRHAGE

Suprachoroidal expulsive hemorrhage is one of the most feared complications of intraocular surgery. It usually presents rapidly with forward movement of the lens-iris diaphragm, dulling of the red reflex viewed through the pupil, and subsequent expulsion of intraocular contents. Immediate closure of the corneoscleral incision is imperative to restore intraocular pressure and tamponade the bleeding. Sclerotomies over the quadrants of hemorrhage may allow external drainage of blood.

Expulsive hemorrhages are rare with an incidence

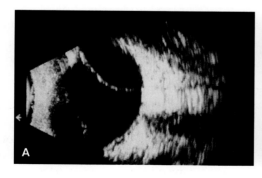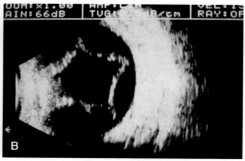

Figure 63–1.
Choroidal effusions as seen in a patient with postoperative hypotony. Longitudinal B-scan ultrasound view (A) of the choroidals. Note the bullous elevation and attachment of the uvea at the posterior ciliary arteries (and not the optic nerve). Transverse view (B) shows choroidal effusions in all four quadrants.

estimated at 0.19% for all cases. Risk factors include glaucoma, increased axial length, atherosclerosis, and elevated intraoperative pulse rate (6).

Prevention is critical. Normalization of intraocular pressure reduces the sudden decompression of the eye. Preplacement of safety sutures may allow more rapid closure of the wound. Scleral support using Flieringa rings may help to lessen distortion of the globe. Intraoperative regulation of the pulse may be helpful in high-risk patients.

■ REFERENCES

1. Cox MS, Trese MT, Murphy PL: Silicone oil for advanced proliferative vitreoretinopathy. Ophthalmology 1986; 93: 646–650.

2. Hilton GF, Grizzard WS: Pneumatic retinopexy: a two-step outpatient operation without conjunctival incision. Ophthalmology 1986; 93: 626–641.

3. Michels RG: Scleral buckling methods for rhegmatogenous retinal detachment. Retina 1986; 6: 1–49.

4. Pesin SR, Olk RJ, Grand MG, et al: Vitrectomy for premacular fibroplasia: prognostic factors, long-term follow-up and time course of visual improvement. Ophthalmology 1991; 98: 1109–1114.

5. Schwartz PL, Pruett RC: Factors influencing retinal redetachment after removal of buckling elements. Arch Ophthalmol 1977; 95: 804–807.

6. Speaker MD, Guerriero PM, Met JA, et al: A case-control study of risk factors for intraoperative suprachoroidal expulsive hemorrhage. Ophthalmology 1991; 98: 202–210.

7. Tornambe PE, Hilton GF, Brinton DA, et al: Pneumatic retinopexy: a two-year follow-up study of the multicenter clinical trial comparing pneumatic retinopexy with scleral buckling. Ophthalmology 1991; 98: 1115–1123.

XI Ocular Trauma

Section Editor: Kenneth W. Wright

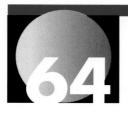

64 Ocular Trauma

Kenneth W. Wright

■ GENERAL APPROACH

As in all aspects of medicine, history is important, and it is especially important when evaluating ocular trauma. Clarify exactly what, when, and how the trauma occurred. Document the timetable of events, and if there was an antecedent ocular disease. Other important history includes coexisting systemic disease, allergy, and previous tetanus prophylaxis. Ocular trauma is often associated with head trauma. Loss of consciousness, amnesia, or headache should prompt further neurological workup and neuro-imaging.

The first goal of the ocular examination is to determine the overall extent of the trauma, and to rule out a ruptured globe. If a ruptured globe is identified or suspected, then the rest of the examination should be limited and done carefully in order to avoid further extrusion of intraocular contents. If the globe is ruptured, obtain a visual acuity, assess pupillary responses (check consensual response and APD), place a shield over the eye for protection, obtain a CT scan to rule out foreign body, and schedule emergency surgery. If the patient does not have a ruptured globe, a complete ocular examination should be done, including a dilated fundus examination.

A CT scan of the head and orbits is indicated in patients who sustain a penetrating injury to the eye or orbit, to rule out the presence of an intraocular or orbital foreign body. It is preferable over an MRI because the magnetic field associated with MRI can move a metallic intraocular foreign body, resulting in further ocular trauma. Blunt orbital trauma may also call for a CT scan to diagnose orbital fractures, since plain radiograph films will miss approximately 50% of floor fractures. Ocular ultrasound should not be used to examine the posterior pole if there is a possibility the globe is ruptured. Pressure from the ultrasound probe can cause extrusion of intraocular contents (see Chapter 26 for discussion of periorbital and orbital injuries).

■ CHILD ABUSE (BATTERED CHILD SYNDROME)

Unfortunately, child abuse or the battered child syndrome is a significant cause of pediatric ocular trauma. Warning signs of child abuse include an injury that is not consistent with the alleged accident, multiple admissions at different hospitals for trauma, delay in presentation to the physician, multiple fractures and soft tissue injuries at different stages of healing, and skin burns which may be secondary to a cigarette (2,4,6,16).

If child abuse is suspected, the workup should consist of a complete pediatric examination, with genital examination, and long bone radiographs looking for fractures. Neuro-imaging should be considered if there are central nervous system signs such as lethargy. A complete ocular examination including a dilated fundus examination is critical to the evaluation of a child with possible battered child syndrome. Retinal hemorrhages in

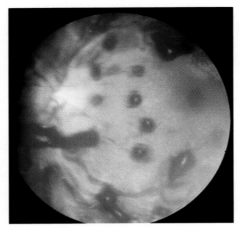

Figure 64–1.
Fundus photograph of a battered infant. Just inferior to the optic disc is a preretinal boat-shaped hemorrhage. Note the presence of multiple preretinal hemorrhages with white light reflexes off the dome of the hemorrhage giving the appearance of Roth spots. These are not true Roth spots which are localized hemorrhages with a central white spot which represent an accumulation of white blood cells or an area of ischemia (cotton wool spot). Roth spots are usually associated with subacute bacterial endocarditis, leukemia, or anemia.

infants are highly suggestive of battered child syndrome, and include; dot and blot hemorrhages, preretinal (boat-shaped) hemorrhages, and vitreous hemorrhages (2,6,10,13) (Figure 64–1). Other retinal findings are chorioretinal scars, optic atrophy, retinoschisis, and cotton wool spots (2,4,5). Infants who present with lethargy, subdural hematomas or subdural effusions, and/or retinal hemorrhages of unknown etiology, should be evaluated for child abuse. Birth trauma, leukemia, increased intracranial pressure, malignant hypertension, bacterial endocarditis, idiopathic thrombocytopoenia, and rarely cardiopulmonary resuscitation are other causes for pediatric retinal hemorrhages (8). It should be emphasized that it is the physician's responsibility to report all suspected battered children to social services or the police department immediately. Most states have laws which require physicians and health professionals to report all suspected battered children. Battered child syndrome is almost always a recurrent problem. If not identified early, children continue to be abused causing physical and psychological devastation, which too often ultimately results in death.

■ PERFORATING TRAUMA

There are two general catagories of ocular trauma: penetrating and perforating. A perforating injury passes all the way through a structure, whereas a penetrating wound passes into a structure. An ice pick injury through the cornea, stopping in the center of the lens, for example, is a perforating injury to the cornea, and a penetrating injury of the lens.

Perforating Injures of the Globe/Ruptured Globe

A ruptured globe is defined as a perforating injury of the cornea and/or sclera, so the integrity of the eye is violated. This can be the result of blunt trauma, a sharp object, or a missile. Signs of a ruptured globe include chemosis, pigment under the conjunctiva, deep anterior chamber (posterior rupture), shallow anterior chamber (anterior rupture), peaked pupil, vitreous hemorrhage, and decreased intraocular pressure. The areas of the eye wall which are most susceptible to rupture are the sclera, posterior to the rectus muscle insertions, the corneoscleral limbus, and areas of previous surgical incisions (previous cataract surgery, corneal graft, and radial keratotomy incisions). Blunt trauma will often produce wounds that extend from the corneoscleral limbus posteriorlly behind a rectus muscle insertion, because the sclera is thinnest directly behind the rectus muscles measuring only 0.3 millimeters.

When exploring for a ruptured globe, it is important to look behind the rectus muscles for an occult rupture.

Perforating injuries can be divided into anterior segment trauma (injuries to the cornea, anterior chamber, iris and lens), and posterior segment trauma (injuries involving the sclera, retina and vitreous). Posterior segment trauma carries a much higher risk of postoperative retinal detachment and has a poorer prognosis than anterior segment trauma, especially if a vitreous hemorrhage is present (1). The poor prognosis of posterior perforating injuries is secondary to cellular proliferation and retinal fibrosis which can lead to retinal detachment (1,12).

Repair of Corneal and Limbal Lacerations

A corneal laceration is usually associated with a shallow anterior chamber, iris prolapse, and a peaked pupil. The first step is to reposit the prolapsed iris and reform the anterior chamber with viscoelastic substance or air. Once the anterior chamber is formed, then the corneal laceration is closed with 10–0 nylon suture, burying the knots within the cornea. A cyclodialysis spatula may be used to sweep the iris from the wound. If the lens capsule is ruptured, and there is an obvious cataract, one may remove the cataract primarily at the time the corneal laceration is sutured, with or without IOL insertion. A staged approach, closing the wound, then performing cataract surgery at a later date, may be a better alternative if the injury is severe.

Limbal (corneoscleral) lacerations are repaired in a similar manner to corneal lacerations except the first suture is placed at the limbus to align and anchor the limbal anatomy (usually a 9–0 or 8–0 nylon) (Figure 64–2). Once the limbus is repaired, then the cornea and sclera can be sutured. If the corneoscleral laceration involves the lens and anterior vitreous, a lensectomy and anterior vitrectomy is usually necessary to reconstruct the anterior chamber and remove the vitreous from the wound. First, close the corneoscleral laceration and establish a watertight seal. Next, use vitrectomy instrumentation through a limbal approach to remove the lens material and vitreous.

Repair of Posterior Scleral Laceration

If a posterior rupture is suspected, the first step is to do a 360° peritomy, explore the quadrants between the muscles, and inspect behind the rectus muscle insertions. Once a rupture is identified, reposit uveal prolapse with a cyclodialysis spatula, and close the scleral wound with interrupted sutures (usually 8–0 silk). Complete a full exploration of the entire globe after repairing a scleral laceration, since more than one laceration may be present. In cases of severe and/or multiple lacerations, try to close the sclera as best as possible to avoid a primary enucleation. In some cases of severe

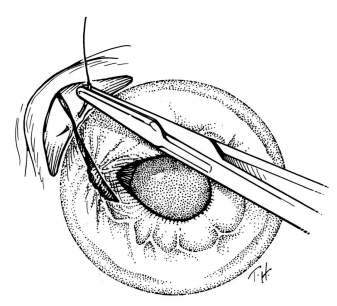

Figure 64–2.
Drawing of a corneoscleral laceration. First align the cut edges at the limbus and secure with a limbal suture. Then close the corneal laceration, and lastly explore and repair the scleral laceration. (From Color Atlas of Ophthalmic Surgery, KW Wright Editor in Chief, Chapter 15 Page 222, LP Chong, and WE Smiddy, JP Lippincott Co. Philadelphia PA, 1995).

trauma the globe can not be repaired, and a primary enucleation is indicated.

Scleral and Corneal Wound Healing

Because the sclera, and especially the cornea, are essentially avascular, wound healing is slow, requiring 6 months to a year. The anterior aspect of the corneal wound heals in a similar manner to skin, with the epithelium being a major contributor, while the posterior wound may heal by endothelial cell fibrous metaplasia. Histologically, healing occurs as fibrous tissue fills the corneal or scleral wound with the fibrous tissue oriented perpendicular to the stromal lamellae.

Postoperative Management of a Ruptured Globe

The incidence of posttraumatic endophthalmitis after a ruptured globe is approximately 10%. Therefore, postoperative antibiotics are indicated. After closure of a ruptured globe give subconjunctival injections of antibiotics. Coricosteroids are given (gentamicin 20 mg, vancomycin 20 mg or cefazolin 100 mg, and dexamethasone 2 mg), as well as broad spectrum IV antibiotics, which should be continued for at least 3 days ciprofloxacin and an aminoglycoside (gentamicin or tobramycin). Clindamycin should be considered if there is a possibility of a bacillus cereus contamination (15).

Secondary surgery: Posterior Vitrectomy and Enucleation

If the rupture is posterior, a retina consultation should be obtained. Lacerations that involve the retina and are associated with a vitreous hemorrhage usually require a posterior vitrectomy to reduce the possibility of cellular proliferation, intraocular fibrosis, and retinal detachment (1,12). The timing of the vitrectomy is controversial. Some advocate early surgery within the first week, while others wait for 7 to 10 days. Early surgery has the advantage of preventing irreversible retinal damage, but delaying 10 to 14 days allows for less inflammation, less hemorrhage, and posterior vitreous separation that facilitates vitrectomy surgery.

A severely traumatized globe with uveal prolapse and documented no light perception (NLP) postoperatively has no visual function, yet there is a small but significant risk of developing sympathetic ophthalmia and losing vision in the good eye. Because of the risk of sympathetic ophthalmia, consider performing a secondary enucleation if the eye remains NLP after the primary repair. Enucleation should be done within 2 weeks after the trauma to prevent sympathetic ophthalmia.

Phthisis Bulbi: A blind eye, shrunken, and hypotonous eye is termed phthisis bulbi. This end stage eye is often painful and can be treated with enucleation, or in the case of post endophthalmitis or end stage glaucoma, retrobulbar alcohol.

Intraocular Foreign Bodies

The management of intraocular foreign bodies starts with careful documentation as to the nature and position of the foreign body. Taking a detailed history will help identify if the foreign body is magnetic, vegetable, or organic material, and whether it is radio-opaque. In cases where the foreign body is secondary to hammering or high speed machinery, the foreign body is usually metallic, even if the hammering or cutting was on rock or concrete. Forged steel can crack under stress, sending a small piece of the steel flying at increased velocity. A CT scan is critical for determining the nature and location of the foreign body. Plain radiographs do not localize radio-opaque foreign bodies well and results can be deceiving.

Retained intraocular foreign bodies cause various degrees of inflammation, depending on its composition. Sterile nontoxic foreign bodies such as stone, glass, and plastic are especially well tolerated. Zinc and aluminum are also fairly well tolerated and cause minimal inflammation. Any large foreign body, however, has the risk of inciting an infection and producing fibrovascular proliferation (15). Copper and vegetable material can cause severe inflamation. As a general rule, all acute foreign bodies should be removed to prevent endophthalmitis.

Copper and copper alloys (containing more than 85% copper) can produce a severe inflammatory reaction which presents like endophthalmitis. Alloys containing less than 85% copper will produce a chronic condition termed chalcosis. Copper has an infinity for accumulating in basement membranes. Signs of chalcosis include deposits around Descemet's membrane (Kayser-Fleischer ring), green discoloration of the iris, a sunflower cataract, and retinal degeneration. Early removal of a copper foreign body is indicated to prevent permanent ocular damage.

Siderosis is ocular disease caused by iron toxicosis. Over time, the iron breaks down and ferric ions disseminate throughout the eye. Cell membrane damage and enzyme inactivation occurs. Signs of siderosis include deep corneal stromal staining (rust colored), decreased iris pigmentation (heterochromia), pupillary mydriasis with poor reactivity, lenticular deposits, and retinal changes. If the foreign body is in the posterior chamber, especially if it is in contact with the retina, retinal siderosis can be severe and the foreign body must be removed. The retinal photoreceptors and retinal pigment epithelial cells are sensitive to ferric ions and will undergo progressive degeneration. Findings associated with retinal siderosis include night blindness, constricted visual field, and late central visual loss. Early electroretinogram (ERG) changes include a large a wave and normal b wave. As the siderosis progresses, the b wave amplitude diminishes, eventually becoming extinguished. Serial ERGs are useful for following small retained intraocular foreign bodies. Small anterior metallic foreign bodies may be cautiously observed.

Vegetable (organic) foreign bodies cause a severe inflammatory response. More importantly, vegetable materials are contaminated and carry pathogens such as Bacillus cereus and fungi (15). Bacillus endophthalmitis is commonly associated with vegetable or soil intraocular foreign bodies, and has a rapid onset, and carries poor visual prognosis.

Nonperforating Anterior Segment Trauma

Corneal abrasion

Corneal abrasions occur when the corneal epithelium is removed. Corneal abrasions heal by the sliding of existing epithelium to fill in the areas of abraded epithelium. After careful slit lamp examination to rule out corneal foreign body or infiltrate, antibiotic ointment and a pressure patch are placed on the eye. In most cases, a corneal abrasion will heal after 24 to 48 hours of patching. Remember to rule out herpes keratitis as a cause of unilateral corneal abrasion.

Corneal Hydrops

Traumatic corneal hydrops is localized corneal edema caused by blunt trauma that produces breaks in Descemet's membrane. Birth trauma with the forceps being placed on the infant's eye can cause corneal hydrops. Traumatic forceps breaks tend to be vertically aligned, in contrast to Haab's striae of congenital glaucoma which are usually horizontal.

Subconjunctival Hemorrhage

A subconjunctival hemorrhage may be related to trauma, but in most cases it occurs spontaneously of unknown etiology. Rarely a subconjunctival hemorrhage is associated with a systemic disease such as systemic hypertension, a bleeding diathesis, or diabetes mellitus. In the vast majority of cases no systemic evaluation is necessary, but a systemic evaluation is indicated if the hemorrhages are recurrent. There is no treatment for subconjunctival hemorrhages except to reassure the patient, since the hemorrhage will resolve spontaneously by approximately 2 weeks.

Hyphema

A hyphema is simply blood in the anterior chamber (Figure 64–3). Hyphemas are most frequently caused by

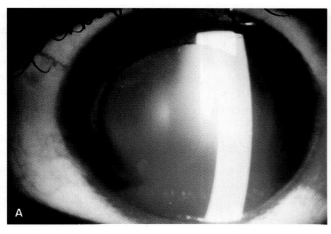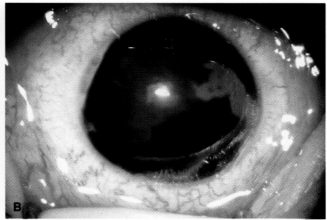

Figure 64–3.
(A) Photograph of a small hyphema which is layered inferiorly, plus some diffuse blood. A small hyphema is a hyphema that occupies less than or equal to one third of the anterior chamber. (B) Total hyphema secondary to blunt trauma. The anterior chamber is full of clot and takes on a black or "eight ball" appearance. This patient required surgical evacuation of the clot.

ocular trauma; however, nontraumatic causes include iris neovascularization (associated with diabetes, intraocular tumors, or retinal vascular occlusive disease), iris tumors such as juvenile xanthogranuloma, or anterior spill over from a vitreous hemorrhage. The mechanism of bleeding associated with blunt trauma is thought to be external compression, and secondary expansion of the angle with tearing of the iris root. This results in rupture of the vascular arcade of the iris, the recurrent choroidal arteries, and possibly ciliary body veins. A hyphema indicates severe ocular trauma, and concurrent injuries to the retina or other ocular tissues can occur.

The two most important complications of a hyphema include increased intraocular pressure and corneal blood staining. Increased intraocular pressure can occur from red blood cells, red blood cell remnants (ghost cells), or sickled erythrocytes blocking the trabecular meshwork outflow, or from pupillary block glaucoma, secondary to a large central blood clot that occludes the pupil. Damage to the trabecular meshwork associated with angle recession can cause glaucoma that presents acutely, or late, months or even years after the trauma.

Corneal blood staining occurs as hemoglobin and hemosiderin from the hyphema infiltrate through the endothelial cells into the posterior aspect of the corneal stroma (Figure 64–4). Corneal blood staining is usually associated with large hyphemas and increased intraocular pressure; however, corneal blood staining has been reported in patients with normal intraocular pressure. Often corneal blood staining will be seen in the area where a blood clot is in direct contact with the corneal epithelium. In children, it is important to avoid the complication of corneal blood staining, since this can produce a severely blurred retinal image and amblyopia.

Another important complication of hyphema is optic neuropathy associated with sickle cell hemoglobinopathies. Patients with SC, SS or S-thal are predisposed to optic neuropathy even with slightly elevated intraocular pressures (greater than 25mm Hg) (3). The intraocular pressure must be monitored closely and kept under 25mm Hg in patients with sickle cell hemoglobinopathies. A sickle cell prep should be part of the workup of patients at risk for having a sickle cell hemoglobinopathy.

Medical Management of Traumatic Hyphemas. Controversy persists as to the medical management of traumatic hyphemas. The classic treatment is hospitalization with bed rest for at least 5 days. Hyphemas resolve as blood is absorbed via the iris and trabecular meshwork. Hyphema clots contract at approximately 3 to 5

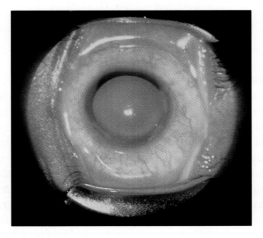

Figure 64–4.
Photograph of corneal blood staining several weeks after removal of an eight ball hyphema. Note the yellowish-amber appearance of the cornea.

days posttrauma. Therefore, the greatest incidence of rebleeds occur at this time. An alternative to hospitalization is treatment with bed rest at home. This outpatient treatment has been shown to be safe; however, it should be used in patients who are reliable and can return to the office for daily checkups (18). In general, small hyphemas have a good prognosis (hyphemas less than one-third of the anterior chamber), and these patients can be safely followed as outpatients. Hyphemas larger than one-third, however, have an increased risk of developing rebleeds. These patients with large hyphemas may benefit from hospitalization and bed rest. Some authorities advocate no medical treatment, not even topical drops, while others suggest long-acting cycloplegic agents in order to minimize ciliary spasm and topical corticosteroids to reduce inflammation (17, 18).

The use of systemic antifibrinolytic agents such as aminocaproic acid is also controversial (9, 11). These agents may decrease the incidence of rebleeding. Unfortunately, adverse effects such as nausea, emesis, hypotension, and prolonged absorption of the clot can occur. Those who advocate the use of fibrinolytic agents restrict their use to small hyphemas less than one-third of the anterior chamber. These agents are contraindicated in patients who are pregnant, have renal failure, blood dyscrasia, coagulopathies, and thrombotic disease. Previous reports have stated that fibrinolytic agents reduce the rebleed rate in patients with small hyphemas from 33% to 4% (11). Others, however, have shown that the rebleed rate of small hyphemas is approximately 10 to 15% and others could not document significant improvement in the rebleed rate when patients were treated with aminocaproic agents (9).

If the hyphema is causing increased intraocular pressure, the pressure may be lowered with topical or oral glaucoma medications. Methazolamide is preferred over acetazolamide in patients with sickle cell disease, because methazolamide slightly raises the intracameral pH, while acetazolamide lowers the pH, thus, predisposing to sickling.

Surgical Management of Hyphemas. In most cases, hyphemas can be managed medically, and the hyphema will resolve within 3 to 5 days after trauma. Indications for surgery include increased intraocular pressure, unresolved clot, and corneal blood staining. The timing of the surgery is somewhat arbitrary and each case must be individualized. Surgery should be considered in the following situations: total hyphema with IOP greater than 25mm Hg for 6 days, large hyphema IOP greater than 50mm Hg for 2 days, sickle cell disease or trait with IOP greater than 25mm Hg for 1 day, or intermittent IOP greater than 30mm Hg. The surgical procedure should depend on the type of hyphema. The hyphema clot can be surgically removed with automated vitrectomy instrumentation using an anterior approach. Alternatively, small hyphemas associated with sickle cell can be evacuated by simple irrigation wash out. Finally, some have advocated a trabeculectomy and removal of the clot with forceps. The author prefers the closed vitrectomy instrumentation for clot evacuation.

Traumatic Iritis

Blunt, nonperforating ocular trauma can result in an acute iritis. Symptoms include tearing photophobia and eye pain. The intraocular pressure is variable since it can be increased or decreased. Treatment is topical cycloplegics, usually with a topical coricosteroid. The iritis typically lasts for 1 to 2 weeks.

Angle Recession

Angle recession occurs when blunt trauma pushes the lens-iris diaphragm posteriorly, thus, tearing the iris root between the longitudinal and circular ciliary muscles. If the angle recession is more than 50% of the circumference of the angle, then the patient is at risk for developing posttraumatic glaucoma. Glaucoma can occur months or even years after the trauma, so these patients must be followed closely long-term. Angle recession can only be diagnosed by the use of gonioscopy.

Cyclodialysis Cleft

A cyclodialysis cleft is a separation of the iris root and ciliary body from the scleral spur, so aqueous percolates through the angle between the sclera and ciliary body. Local ciliary body detachment reduces ciliary body aqueous production, causing hypotony. Persistent hypotony after blunt trauma is an indication of a possible cyclodialysis cleft. Cyclodialysis clefts are treated by laser or cryotherapy over the area of the cleft, approximately 2 mm posterior to the limbus. Recalcitrant clefts may be sutured closed.

Traumatic Cataracts

Traumatic cataracts can occur after blunt or penetrating injuries to the anterior segment. A blunt injury can cause a cataract, which occurs several weeks or even months after the injury. If there is a large rupture of the lens capsule, the lens will usually need to be removed. Rarely will a small anterior capsule tear heal with a local opacity, and the lens can be preserved.

Traumatic Subluxation of the Lens

See Pediatric Lens, chapter 21.

Retinal Trauma

Commotio Retinae (Berlin's Edema)

This is a retinal contusion as a result of pressure waves emanating from anterior trauma. Commotio retinae appears grayish-white and can involve the macula or peripheral retina. There may be associated retinal hemorrhages or a choriodal rupture. Macular commotio retinae will reduce central vision, but vision usually improves as the edema resolves, unless there is a macular hole or retinal pigment epithelial disruption of the fovea. Animal studies have shown the cause of commotio retinae is probably a disruption of photoreceptor outer segments, not true extracellular edema. Fluorescein angiograms of humans show early blockage in areas of white retina, and no alteration of retinal vascular permeability.

Choroidal Rupture

Choroidal rupture can occur associated with blunt anterior trauma. These ruptures represent crescent-shaped curvilinear lines which usually transect the macula. They are deep and gray in appearance. Hemorrhages may be associated with an acute choroidal rupture. Choroidal ruptures represent a break in Bruch's membrane. Subretinal neovascular membranes may develop months or years after a traumatic choroidal rupture occurs.

Chorioretinitis Sclopetaria

If the retinal and choroid are both damaged by severe injury, usually an increased velocity projectile or object, the resultant diffuse necrosis and tissue disruption is termed chorioretinitis sclopetaria. This can occur after blunt injury, from a missile glancing off the scleral wall, or a penetrating injury. This is the most severe form of a choroidal retinal contusion.

Whiplash Retinopathy

Whiplash retinopathy is caused by a sudden acceleration/deceleration head injury. There is an acute shift of the vitreous, thus, causing traction on the macula and fovea. Ocular examination may show a small pit in the central foveal area with or without a small overlying vitreo retinal wisp of tissue. The visual prognosis is good with visual acuity usually 20/50 or better.

Traumatic Retinal Breaks

Retinal breaks can occur from direct retinal perforation, vitreous traction, or retinal contusion (see Commotio Retinae previously). Blunt injury can cause retinal breaks indirectly in the area of trauma, most often located at the equator, in the inferior temporal quadrant (area most exposed). One of the most common retinal breaks associated with blunt trauma is a retinal dialysis. This is a circumferential linear break at the vitreous base. As traumatic shock waves pass through the vitreous, tears occur along the vitreous base where there are strong retino-vitreal attachments. Since dialyses are located in the periphery, visualization almost always requires scleral depression. The dialysis may be small, only a few clock hours, or may extend beyond 90. Other retinal tears associated with trauma include horseshoe tears, operculated tears, and macular holes (see following). Retinal detachment after trauma usually occurs late, with most appearing between 1 month and 2 years after trauma.

Macular Hole

A macular hole may occur after blunt trauma associated with commotio retinae, whiplash retinopathy, or subfoveal hemorrhage. A full-thickness hole results in loss of central vision (VA= 20/100 to 20/200).

Purtscher's Retinopathy

Purtscher's retinopathy occurs secondary to mechanical injury elsewhere in the body, such as multiple fractures with fat embolism, or severe chest compression. Purtscher's retinopathy is associated with soft exudates throughout the posterior pole which are often concentrated around the optic disc. Nerve fiber layer hemorrhages are a consistent finding, often with preretinal hemorrhages. Purtscher's retinopathy may be caused by microembolism such as fat or blood aggregate, which cause ischemia and hemorrhage, or from increased venous pressure secondary to chest compression. The treatment of Purtscher's retinopathy is conservative observation since the retinal lesions disappear within a few weeks to months after the injury.

Terson's Retinopathy

This is a hemorrhagic retinopathy caused by an intracranial subarachnoid hemorrhage with increased intracranial pressure. Blood dissects anteriorly through the lamina cribrosa into the eye. Nerve fiber layer and preretinal hemorrhages are typically seen emanating from the optic nerve.

Optic Nerve Injury

Traumatic optic neuropathy is acute optic nerve injury that occurs after blunt head trauma, usually after a frontal blow. Decreased vision is associated with an afferent pupillary defect and a relatively normal fundus appearance. The head trauma is usually severe, associated with loss of consciousness or amnesia. Most authorities recommend a course of high dose corticosteroids (14). If a short course of corticosteroids does not improve vision, then optic nerve decompression may be considered in selective cases (7). Patients who have no light perception have a poor prognosis for visual recovery, regardless of treatment. Injury to the chiasm can occur after frontal head trauma, resulting in a bitemporal visual field defect. This is an unusual complication of severe closed head trauma, often associated with diabetes insipidus and a skull fracture.

Optic nerve avulsion is caused by severe blunt anterior trauma which produces a pressure wave that pushes the optic disc posteriorly behind the lamina cribosa. Visual acuity is usually no light perception. On fundus examination the optic disc appears to be absent.

Chemical Burns

Acid or alkaline solutions that come into direct contact with the surface of the eye can cause severe damage. A chemical burn is one of the true ophthalmic emergencies and deserves immediate irrigation and lavage in the field before the patient arrives at the emergency room. Once in the emergency room, lavage should be continued using at least 3 liters of normal saline. Litmus paper can be used to check the pH of the conjunctival fornix.

Alkaline solutions are especially damaging because the base will denature proteins and lyse cell membranes. This enhances the alkaline penetration into the eye, furthering the damage. Surface damage includes removal of the corneal epithelium and obliteration of conjunctival blood vessels. The prognosis is proportional to the clock hours of avascular conjunctiva and sclera whitening. If more than 50% of the limbus is blanched, the prognosis is poor. After the acute burn, damage and corneal breakdown continues. Collagenase is released from regenerating tissue which produces even more destruction. Over time, symblepharon and cicatricial entropion may occur. In severe cases, the cornea undergoes progressive degeneration and melt, leading to eventual perforation. The treatment for late alkaline burns includes a conformer to prevent symblepharon and preserve the conjunctival fornix, anticollagenases such as mucomist, artificial tears of dry eye, and topical antibiotics to prevent infection.

Acid solutions can also cause severe damage. However, because the acid tends to precipitate proteins, the area and depth of necrosis is more limited than with alkaline burns. The treatment is generally the same as alkaline burns.

Radiation Injury

Radiation therapy of ocular tumors (e.g., retinoblastoma and choroidal melanoma), and orbital tumors (e.g., rhabdomyosarcoma and lymphoma) can cause ocular injury. Radiation cataracts can form with a single fraction dose as decreased as 200 rads, but they are usually not progressive and are not visually significant. Doses over 800 rads can cause a progressive cataract which develops over 2 to 3 years. Injury to the lacrimal gland usually occurs with doses over 5000 rads, resulting in a dry eye syndrome within a year after radiation therapy. Radiation retinopathy is caused by retinal vascular ischemia, initiated by damage to retinal capillary endothelial cells. Radiation retinopathy develops 2 to 3 years after increased dose radiation therapy (usually over 5000 rads). The majority of patients receiving over 8000 rads will develop retinopathy. The retinopathy begins with areas of cotton wool spots which are the first sign of radiation retinopathy, representing early retinal ischemia. As the retinal ischemia progresses, large areas of capillary nonperfusion develop. Next, microaneurysms and telangiectatic neovascularization occur. Late changes include iris rubeosis, glaucoma, hyphema, and vitreous hemorrhage. The retinal appearance is similar to diabetic retinopathy. Radiation optic neuropathy is uncommon but can occur with doses over 6000 rads.

■ REFERENCES

1. Cleary PE, Ryan SJ: Vitrectomy in penetrating eye injury: results of a controlled trial of vitrectomy in an experimental posterior penetrating eye injury in the rhesus monkey. Arch Ophthalmol 1981;99:287.
2. Friendly DS: Ocular manifestations of physical child abuse. Trans Am Acad Ophthalmol Otolaryngol 1971;75:318–332.
3. Goldberg MF: Sickled erythrocytes, hyphema, and secondary glaucoma: I. The diagnosis and treatment of sickled erythrocytes in human hyphemas. Ophthal Surg 1979;10:17.
4. Greenwald MJ, Weiss A, Oesterle CS, Friendly DS: Traumatic retinoschisis in battered babies. Ophthalmology 1986;93:618–625.
5. Harcourt B, Hopkins D: Permanent chorio-retinal lesions in childhood of suspected traumatic origin, Trans Ophthalmol Soc UK 1973;93:199–205.
6. Harley RD: Ocular manifestations of child abuse. J Pediatr Ophthalmol Strabismus 1980;17:5–13.
7. Joseph MP, et al: Extracrainial optic nerve decompression for traumatic optic neuropathy. Arch Ophthalmol, 108: 1091- 1093, 1990.

8. Kanter RK: Retinal hemorrhage after cardiopulmonary resuscitation or child abuse. J Pediatr, 1986;108:430–432.

9. Kraft SP, Christianson MD, Crawford JS, et al: Traumatic hyphema in children—treatment with epsilon-aminocaproic acid. Ophthalmology 1987;94:1232.

10. Lambert SR, Johnson TE, Hoyt CS: Optic nerve sheath and retinal hemorrhages associated with the shaken baby syndrome. Arch Ophthalmol 1986;104:1509–1512.

11. McGetric JJ, Goldberg MF, Frenkel M, Fiscella RG: Aminocaproic acid decreases secondary hemorrhage after traumatic hyphema. Arch Ophthalmol 1983;101:1031.

12. Michels RG: Vitrectomy methods in penetrating ocular trauma. Ophthalmology 1980;87:629.

13. Ober RR: Hemorrhagic retinopathy in infancy: a clinicopathologic report. J Pediatr Ophthalmol Strabismus 1980, 17:17–20.

14. Spoor TC, et al Treatment of traumatic optic neuropathy with corticosteroids. Am J Ophthalmol, 110: 665–669, 1990.

15. Thompson JT, et al: Infectious endophthalmitis after penetrating injuries with retained intraocular foreign bodies. Ophthalmol. 100: 1468–1474, 1993.

16. Tongue AC: The ophthalmologist's role in diagnosing child abuse. Ophthalmology 1991;98:1009–1010.

17. Usitalo RJ, Ranta-Kemppainen L, Tarkkanen A: Management of traumatic hyphema in children: An analysis of 340 cases. Arch Ophthalmol 1988;106:1207–1209.

18. Wright KW, Sunalp M, Urrea PT: The ambulatory treatment of small hyphemas. Ann Ophthalmol 1988;20: 143–145.

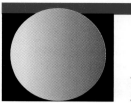

Index

Note: Page numbers in italics indicate figures; Page numbers followed by *t* indicate tables.